# Quinolone Antimicrobial Agents

SECOND EDITION

# Quinolone Antimicrobial Agents

SECOND EDITION

EDITED BY

David C. Hooper and
John S. Wolfson

Infectious Disease Unit, Medical Services,
Massachusetts General Hospital and
Harvard Medical School,
Boston, Massachusetts

American Society for Microbiology
*Washington, D.C.*

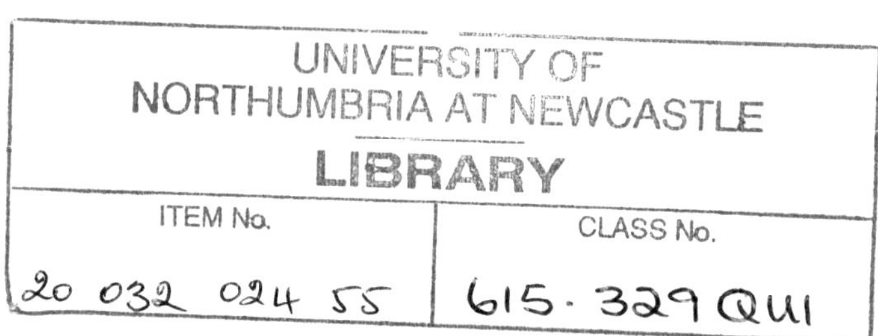



1325 Massachusetts Avenue, N.W.
Washington, DC 20005

**Library of Congress Cataloging-in-Publication Data**

Quinolone antimicrobial agents/edited by David C. Hooper and John S. Wolfson.—2nd ed.
p. cm.
Wolfson's name appears first on the earlier edition.
Includes bibliographical references and index.
ISBN 1-55581-059-4
1. Quinolone antimicrobial agents—Testing. 2. Bacterial diseases—Chemotherapy—Evaluation. I. Hooper, David C. II. Wolfson, John S.
[DNLM: 1. Anti-Infective Agents, Quinolone—pharmacology. 2. Bacterial Infections—drug therapy. 3. Quinolones—pharmacology. QV 250 Q66 1993]
RM666.Q55Q56 1993
616.9'2061—dc20
DNLM/DLC
for Library of Congress 93-10990
CIP


*Printed in the United States of America*

*Cover figure:* Stereoview of the crystal structure of nalidixic acid (reprinted with permission from Shen et al., *Biochemistry* **28:**3886–3894, 1989)

# Contents

# Contributors

*Michael Barza*
Department of Medicine, Division of Geographic Medicine and Infectious Diseases, New England Medical Center Hospital, Tufts University School of Medicine, Boston, MA 02111

*Arnold S. Bayer*
UCLA School of Medicine, Los Angeles, CA 90024, and Division of Infectious Diseases, LAC Harbor-UCLA Medical Center, Torrance, CA 90509

*Steven C. Budsberg*
Department of Small Animal Medicine, College of Veterinary Medicine, University of Georgia, Athens, GA 30602

*Pratik Devasthale*
Department of Medicinal Chemistry, School of Pharmacy, University of Kansas, Lawrence, KS 66045-2506

*George L. Drusano*
Division of Clinical Pharmacology, Department of Medicine, Albany Medical College, Albany, NY 12208

*Herbert L. DuPont*
Center for Infectious Diseases, Medical School and School of Public Health, University of Texas Health Science Center, Houston, TX 77030

*C. T. Eliopoulos*
Department of Medicine, New England Deaconess Hospital, Boston, MA 02215, and Harvard Medical School, Boston, MA 02115

*G. M. Eliopoulos*
Department of Medicine, New England Deaconess Hospital, Boston, MA 02215, and Harvard Medical School, Boston, MA 02115

*Alan Forrest*
The Clinical Pharmacokinetics Laboratory, Millard Fillmore Hospital, and Center for Clinical Pharmacy Research, State University of New York at Buffalo, Buffalo, NY 14209

*Layne O. Gentry*
Infectious Disease Section, St. Luke's Episcopal Hospital, and Baylor College of Medicine, Houston, TX 77030

*Thomas D. Gootz*
Department of Immunology and Infectious Diseases, Central Research Division, Pfizer Inc., Groton, CT 06340

*Jennifer R. Grandis*
Department of Otolaryngology, School of Medicine, University of Pittsburgh, Pittsburgh, PA 15213

*Craig E. Greene*
Department of Small Animal Medicine, College of Veterinary Medicine, University of Georgia, Athens, GA 30602

*David C. Hooper*
Infectious Disease Unit and Medical Services, Massachusetts General Hospital, Harvard Medical School, Boston, MA 02114-2696
*Seiji Hori*
Division of Clinical Pharmacology, Institute of Medical Science, St. Marianna University School of Medicine, Kawasaki 216, Japan
*Nigahus Karabalut*
Division of Infectious Diseases, University of Maryland School of Medicine, Baltimore, MD 21201
*Marc LeBel*
Laboratoire de Pharmacocinétique Clinique, École de Pharmacie, Université Laval, Québec, Québec G1K 7P4, Canada
*Daniel Lew*
Infectious Diseases Division and Clinique Médicale 2, Department of Medicine, University Hospital, CH-1211 Geneva 14, Switzerland
*Lester A. Mitscher*
Department of Medicinal Chemistry, School of Pharmacy, University of Kansas, Lawrence, KS 66045-2506
*Robert C. Moellering, Jr.*
Department of Medicine, New England Deaconess Hospital and Harvard Medical School, Boston, MA 02215
*K. G. Naber*
Urologic Clinic, Elisabeth Hospital, D-8440 Straubing, Germany
*David E. Nix*
The Clinical Pharmacokinetics Laboratory, Millard Fillmore Hospital, and Center for Clinical Pharmacy Research, State University of New York at Buffalo, Buffalo, NY 14209
*S. Ragnar Norrby*
Department of Infectious Diseases, University of Lund, Lund University Hospital, S-22185 Lund, Sweden
*Neil Osheroff*
Department of Biochemistry, Vanderbilt University School of Medicine, Nashville, TN 37232-0146
*Rosanna W. Peeling*
National Laboratory for Sexually Transmitted Diseases, Laboratory Centre for Disease Control, Ottawa, Canada K1A 0L2
*Lance R. Peterson*
Clinical Microbiology Laboratory, Northwestern Memorial Hospital, Northwestern University Medical School, Chicago, IL 60611
*Monique Richer*
Laboratoire de Pharmacocinétique Clinique, École de Pharmacie, Université Laval, Québec, Québec G1K 7P4, Canada
*Allan R. Ronald*
Division of Infectious Diseases, St. Boniface Hospital, Winnipeg, Manitoba R2H 2A6, Canada
*Ethan Rubinstein*
Infectious Disease Unit, Sheba Medical Center, Tel-Hashomer, Israel

*W. Michael Scheld*
Division of Infectious Diseases, Departments of Internal Medicine and Neurosurgery, University of Virginia Health Sciences Center, Charlottesville, VA 22908
*Jerome J. Schentag*
The Clinical Pharmacokinetics Laboratory, Millard Fillmore Hospital, and Center for Clinical Pharmacy Research, State University of New York at Buffalo, Buffalo, NY 14209
*Brian E. Scully*
Infectious Diseases/Epidemiology Division, College of Physicians and Surgeons of Columbia University, New York, NY 10032
*Itamar Shalit*
Tel-Aviv Sourasky Medical Center, Tel-Aviv University, Tel-Aviv, Israel
*Linus L. Shen*
Anti-infective Research Division, Abbott Laboratories, Abbott Park, IL 60064
*Jingoro Shimada*
Division of Clinical Pharmacology, Institute of Medical Science, St. Marianna University School of Medicine, Kawasaki 216, Japan
*Allan R. Tunkel*
Division of Infectious Diseases, Department of Internal Medicine, Medical College of Pennsylvania, Philadelphia, PA 19129
*Francis Waldvogel*
Clinique Médicale 2, Department of Medicine, University Hospital, CH-1211 Geneva 14, Switzerland
*Mark P. Wentland*
Medicinal Chemistry, Sterling Winthrop Pharmaceuticals Research Division, Collegeville, PA 19426-0900
*Drew J. Winston*
Department of Hematology/Oncology, UCLA Medical Center, Los Angeles, CA 90024
*John S. Wolfson* (deceased)
Infectious Disease Unit and Medical Services, Massachusetts General Hospital, Harvard Medical School, Boston, MA 02114-2696
*Michael R. Yeaman*
UCLA School of Medicine, Los Angeles, CA 90024, and Division of Infectious Diseases, LAC Harbor-UCLA Medical Center, Torrance, CA 90509
*Victor L. Yu*
Infectious Disease Section, Veterans Affairs Medical Center, and School of Medicine, University of Pittsburgh, Pittsburgh, PA 15261
*Robin Zavod*
Department of Medicinal Chemistry, School of Pharmacy, University of Kansas, Lawrence, KA 66045-2506

# In Memoriam: John Stone Wolfson, M.D., Ph.D.

15 March 1946–11 October 1991

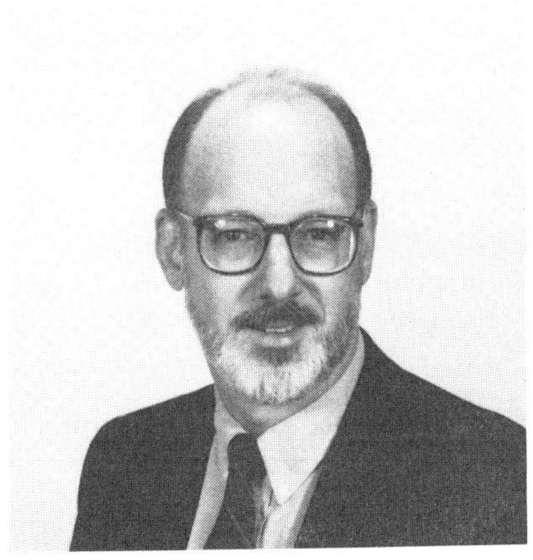

The sudden and untimely death of John Wolfson on 11 October 1991 at age 45 was a great loss to his many friends and colleagues and to the field of antimicrobial action and resistance.

John graduated summa cum laude from Harvard College and then went on to receive his Ph.D. in biology in the laboratory of David Dressler at Harvard University, where he worked defining the modes of replication of bacteriophages $\phi$X174 and T7. He subsequently received his M.D. degree from Johns Hopkins University. After training as a medical house officer at Massachusetts General Hospital, he stayed on at the hospital for a fellowship in infectious diseases and joined the staff of the Infectious Disease Unit and the faculty of Harvard Medical School. It was at this point that his interests turned to DNA gyrase. Morton Swartz, who was then chief of the Infectious Disease Unit, had observed that novobiocin was able to eliminate or "cure" some plasmids that encoded antibiotic resistance. Novobiocin had recently been shown by Martin Gellert, Nicholas Cozzarelli, and their associates to target the newly identified enzyme DNA gyrase. These same groups soon thereafter had also identified this enzyme as the target of nalidixic and oxolinic acids. Thus began John's initial studies of the role of DNA gyrase in plasmid replication and maintenance and his abiding interest in its inhibitors and their mode of action. As the potency and numbers of quinolones grew, his studies began to focus on how quinolones kill bacteria, a question that nearly 2 decades after the discovery of nalidixic acid by the late George Lesher remains only partially answered, and on the ways in which bacteria can circumvent quinolone action.

John was a dedicated scientist and scholar, and his efforts resulted in 76 scientific publications covering a range of topics from bacteriophage replication to inhibition of trypanosome growth to human infectious diseases. Some 40 of his publications dealt with the action of quinolones, resistance to them, or clinical aspects of their use and included editorship of the American Society for Microbiology book *Quinolone Antimicrobial Agents*. His expertise was also recognized in his 7 years of service on the editorial board of *Antimicrobial Agents and Chemotherapy.* In addition to his research activities, John also served as director of the Clinical Parasitology Laboratory and was active as an infectious disease consultant at Massachusetts General Hospital. He was a member of a number of scientific societies and was elected directly to fellowship in the Infectious Diseases Society of America.

Although these credentials are impressive, they tell only part of the story. To know John was to respect and admire him for his uncompromising intellectual honesty and conscientiousness. He was a sensitive and deeply caring man, always courteous and gracious, and with a strong sense of honor.

There was also a lighter, even whimsical, side to John. There were the ties he wore, which at a distance looked conventional enough but upon closer inspection contained tiny figures of Kermit the Frog of Sesame Street fame or multiple interlocked circles, representations of catenated DNA molecules produced by the actions of DNA gyrase. There also was an inscription in the wedding book of a newly married colleague who had worked on DNA gyrase in the lab: having drawn the interlocked circular symbols for male and female, John wrote beneath these symbols "congratulations on your catenation." His office, too, contained some surprises, for example, a small gold towel neatly hung. Although neatness was one of John's hallmarks, this gold towel seemed somehow out of place in his office until one saw the label, "aureus," denoting an organism in which he had a particular interest. On his bookshelf, stemming from his interests in parasitology, stood a large model of an anophelene mosquito, which he referred to as the state bird of Massachusetts.

One particularly memorable aspect of John Wolfson that was evident to me each day and I was sure to many others, even those who met him only briefly, was his love of ideas, of new hypotheses to be tested, of new information and clues to be found in the biomedical literature that he, as no one else, could attack, organize, and devour. There was always delight and excitement whenever it was time to discuss experiments and new ideas, and for John, that was anytime. Ideas are the engine of science, and John Wolfson was a scientist to the core. John made us richer for having known him. He will be dearly missed but never forgotten.

**David C. Hooper**

# In Memoriam: George Y. Lesher, Ph.D.

22 February 1926–17 March 1990

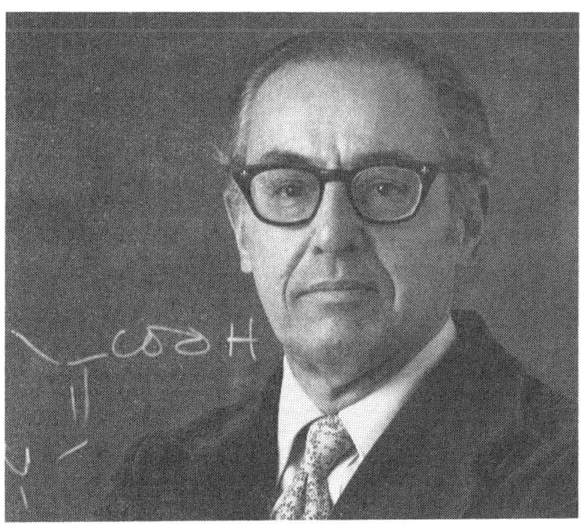

George Y. Lesher pioneered the discovery of the first therapeutically useful quinolone, nalidixic acid; however, his contributions to medicinal chemistry and medicine went far beyond that achievement. It was a great loss to the scientific community when he died at the age of 64 as a result of a tragic canoe accident near Albany, N.Y.

George Lesher was born in Norman, Ill., on 22 February 1926. He earned his B.S. degree in chemistry in 1950 at the University of Illinois. In 1952, following studies at Dartmouth College, where he received his M.S. in organic chemistry, he began his 38-year tenure in the medicinal chemistry department of Sterling-Winthrop Research Institute (now Sterling Winthrop Pharmaceuticals Research Division, Sterling Winthrop Inc.). During his first 4 years at Sterling, he earned his Ph.D. in organic chemistry at Rensselaer Polytechnic Institute (RPI).

In September 1986 at the International Symposium on Quinolone Antibiotics in Chicago, George Lesher gave his account of the discovery of nalidixic acid. As part of a study at Sterling in the late 1950s aimed at the identification of by-products of the synthesis of the important antimalarial drug chloroquine, he and his coworkers isolated and characterized 7-chloro-l-ethyl-1,4-dihydro-4-oxo-3-quinolinecarboxylic acid. This by-product was a regioisomer of the normal intermediate in the process, ethyl 7-chloro-1,4-dihydro-4-oxo-3-quinolinecarboxylate. The by-product exhibited modest in vitro antibacterial properties and served as the lead structure for the design and synthesis of additional analogs. Among those new derivatives was the 1,8-naphthyridine analog nalidixic acid.

While the discovery of nalidixic acid is perhaps his most notable achievement, George Lesher made other significant contributions to quinolone research. He and his coworkers discovered rosoxacin, the first 7-pyridinylquinolone, and, more recently, WIN 57273, an agent possessing exceptional properties against gram-positive bacteria.

It is truly a rare event when a scientist discovers a novel class of therapeutic agents such as the quinolones, yet among George Lesher's achievements is the discovery of another totally new category of therapeutic agents, the bipyridine class of phosphodiesterase inhibitors. Two commercial products used in the treatment of congestive heart failure, amrinone and milrinone, emanated from that research.

George Lesher authored more than 40 scientific publications and held 160 U.S. patents. His contributions to medicinal chemistry, Sterling Winthrop, and RPI are most appropriately memorialized in the recently founded Lesher Lecture Series at RPI.

**Mark P. Wentland**

*Quinolone Antimicrobial Agents, 2nd ed.*
Edited by David C. Hooper and John S. Wolfson


*Chapter 1*

# Introduction

***David C. Hooper***

Information about the quinolone antimicrobial agents has continued to increase at a remarkable rate since the publication of the first edition of *Quinolone Antimicrobial Agents* in 1989. For this reason, an expanded second edition has been organized to bring together in a single volume current information on a larger number of compounds and their expanding clinical applications as well as new information on the limitations to the use of quinolones, including problems with bacterial resistance and new adverse-effect profiles of some quinolones. Like the first edition, this edition is designed for use by clinicians, clinical microbiologists, pharmacologists, pharmacists, basic scientists, and others needing information about these drugs.

The quinolones (also called fluoroquinolones, 4-quinolones, and quinolone carboxylic acids) are analogs of the earlier developed agent nalidixic acid. Nalidixic acid was originally isolated by Lesher and associates (1) from a distillate during chloroquine synthesis and thus was a by-product of antimalarial research (2). Additional older analogs include oxolinic acid, pipemidic acid, and cinoxacin. These older or first-generation analogs are not considered further in this book except for purposes of comparison with the newer agents.

The second generation of quinolones, about which we have the most information, includes norfloxacin, ciprofloxacin, ofloxacin, enoxacin, and pefloxacin. These agents are substantially more potent in vitro and have broader antibacterial spectra than nalidixic acid but maintain the favorable property of being absorbed after oral administration. Additional advantageous pharmacologic properties include relatively long half-lives, which allow twice-daily dosing; excellent distribution into many tissues; and penetration into human cells, resulting in antimicrobial activity against intracellular pathogens. Although differences in spectra of activity exist, this generation of quinolones in general exhibits striking potency against enteric gram-negative bacilli, additional lesser activity against nonenteric gram-negative bacilli and staphylococci, and generally marginal activity against streptococci and anaerobes.

The third generation of quinolones, the most recently developed, has maintained many of the favorable properties of the second generation. Some compounds (e.g., lomefloxacin and fleroxacin) differ from those in the second generation in having sufficiently long half-lives to allow once-daily dosing, and others (e.g., sparfloxacin, tosufloxacin, and PD 127,391) have en-

***David C. Hooper*** • Infectious Disease Unit, Massachusetts General Hospital, 14 Fruit Street, Boston, Massachusetts 02114-2696.

hanced activities against gram-positive cocci and anaerobic bacteria. Also recently recognized have been other quinolone congeners with enhanced potency against mammalian topoisomerase II, the homolog of the bacterial target enzyme DNA gyrase. This finding raises the possibility that some members of the quinolone class will be suitable for use as antitumor agents.

In general, the tolerability of the antibacterial quinolones has been good and comparable to that of other commonly used classes of antimicrobial agents, with many of the second-generation agents having been given to millions of patients. Adverse effects have been seen with some more recently developed compounds, however. These have included the rare, severe hemolytic and nephrotoxic reactions that occurred unexpectedly after the marketing of temafloxacin and the photosensitivity reactions that are being recognized with lomefloxacin and fleroxacin. Thus, the tolerability of each member of the quinolone class must be considered individually.

The second edition of *Quinolone Antimicrobial Agents* is organized similarly to the first edition, with chapters dealing with laboratory aspects, pharmacology, clinical applications, and adverse effects. As dictated by the larger body of data accumulated since the first edition, earlier chapters have been divided into separate topics and new chapters have been added. The single chapter on mechanisms of action and resistance in the first edition has been expanded to separate chapters on mechanisms of action, binding of quinolones to DNA gyrase and DNA, basic and clinical aspects of bacterial quinolone resistance, and interactions of quinolones with eukaryotic topoisomerases. A comprehensive chapter on structure-activity relationships has been added.

The pharmacology section now includes separate chapters on pharmacokinetics in selected patient populations, pharmacodynamics, and drug-drug interactions. In the clinical applications section, uses of quinolones for treatment of prostatitis and urinary tract infections are now dealt with in separate chapters. Chapters on uses of quinolones in head and neck infections (particularly malignant otitis externa), central nervous system infections, and animal infections have also been added. In the section on adverse effects, there are now separate chapters on adverse effects in the central nervous system and the effects of quinolones on the immune system.

With chapter 29, the book concludes as before with an updated overview of the current and future roles of quinolone agents in the therapy of bacterial infections.

I am grateful for all of the considerable efforts of the authors of the individual chapters and for the assistance and patience of the editors at the American Society for Microbiology. Particular thanks are due my wife, Sally, and my daughters, Allison and Brook, who remain my inspiration and who have put up with all too many intrusions on their time. And finally, I shall always remain indebted to my friend, colleague, and coeditor, the late John Wolfson, who always set a standard for excellence and to whom I dedicate this volume.

## REFERENCES

1. **Lesher, G. Y., E. D. Forelich, M. D. Gruet, J. H. Bailey, and R. P. Brundage.** 1962. 1,8-Naphthyridine derivatives. A new class of chemotherapeutic agents. *J. Med. Pharm. Chem.* **5:**1063–1068.
2. **Neu, H. C.** 1987. Ciprofloxacin: an overview and prospective appraisal. *Am. J. Med.* **82**(Suppl. 4A)**:**395–404.

*Quinolone Antimicrobial Agents, 2nd ed.*
Edited by David C. Hooper and John S. Wolfson


*Chapter 2*

# Structure-Activity Relationships

*Lester A. Mitscher, Pratik Devasthale, and Robin Zavod*

The quinolone era is now nearly a quarter of a century old. Following the announcement of nalidixic acid (NAL) in 1967, about 700 analogs were reported before the first comprehensive review of this group was published by Albrecht in 1977 (2). At that time, these antimicrobial agents were comparatively insignificant economically, being used primarily as urinary tract disinfectants. All this changed dramatically following the discovery of norfloxacin (NOR) in 1980 (44). Feverish international activity followed, and at present, more than 10,000 analogs have been described. These descriptions provide a rich lode of data from which to propose structure-activity relationships. While it is natural for chemists to try to discern broad relationships so as to reduce a mass of data to comprehensible proportions, it is appropriate to remind the reader that the analysis of Albrecht, which was eminently reasonable and fully supported by the data available at that time, would have directed researchers away from the preparation of the *N-tert*-butyl and *N*-aryl series, both of which have subsequently become rather important. Furthermore, the preparation of ciprofloxacin (CIP), one of the best of the analogs in clinical use today, would not have taken place. A more recent and updated analysis (50) may have the same fate. Thus, it cannot be overemphasized that the data and analysis in this chapter reflect only what is known and/or believed at this moment. Although this review can serve as a means of assimilating what has been done in the past and as a tentative guide to future developments, it should not be used to prevent investigators from constructing unusual or unprecedented molecules. Indeed, we are approaching the point of diminishing returns, and successful structural novelty is desperately needed in the quinolone field.

The primary emphasis of this chapter is on developments subsequent to the discovery of NOR. The work of the last decade has concentrated almost exclusively on the production of quinolone analogs possessing a fluorine substituent at C-6 and a base-containing substituent at C-7. This work has been very productive, and a large number of clinical candidates and important lead substances has resulted. The work is presented in tabular form, and each table attempts to relate the potency of individual members to that of an important precedent molecule lacking the novel structural feature of the new substances. It is well known among quinolone chemists and biologists that the activities of quinolones are decreased significantly by acidic pHs and the presence of magnesium ions. The quinolones resemble the tetracyclines in this regard. In addition to the

***Lester A. Mitscher, Pratik Devasthale, and Robin Zavod*** • Department of Medicinal Chemistry, University of Kansas, Lawrence, Kansas 66045-2506.

usual variation between laboratories because of the use of different strains and different medium compositions, these factors make it difficult to make precise distinctions in potency when analogs have been prepared and evaluated in different laboratories. Wherever possible, data in the tables are from the same laboratory in order to avoid these difficulties. This means that the potency attributed to a given agent (NOR, for example) may not be the same in different tables. The differences are seldom large but are nonetheless perceptible.

The choice of particular microorganisms to include in the tables is arbitrary by necessity. There is no consensus among quinolone investigators about which microorganisms and strains to use. The choice is often dictated by the data available rather than the data one would like to have. We have chosen to use *Escherichia coli* and *Klebsiella pneumoniae* as representatives of the gram-negative bacilli that are ordinarily responsive to quinolones and *Pseudomonas aeruginosa* to represent the difficult pathogens lying on the fringe of coverage by many quinolones. *Staphylococcus aureus* represents the gram-positive organisms normally responsive to the fluoroquinolones, and since methicillin-resistant strains often are as responsive as methicillin-sensitive strains, the sensitive strains are used. *Streptococcus pneumoniae* represents gram-positive organisms that are on the fringe of coverage by quinolones. Anaerobes are usually nonresponsive. Where data are available, this group of pathogens is represented by *Bacteroides fragilis* or some other *Bacteroides* sp. Data involving gram-negative cocci (*Neisseria gonorrhoeae* and *Neisseria meningitidis*), gram-positive bacilli (*Corynebacterium diphtheriae*), other gram-negative bacilli (*Proteus vulgaris*, *Salmonella* sp., *Shigella* sp., *Haemophilus influenzae*, *Yersinia pestis*, *Vibrio cholerae*, and *Legionella pneumophila*), acid-fast organisms (*Mycobacterium tuberculosis* and *Mycobacterium leprae*), spirochetes (*Treponema pallidum*), and miscellaneous pathogens (*Mycoplasma pneumoniae*, *Rickettsia* sp., and *Chlamydia trachomatis*) would be of great interest. Such data are often available for compounds that have undergone significant preclinical workup but not for molecules of laboratory interest only. Coverage of these interesting microorganisms is too spotty to provide material for the tables.

The consensus target of the quinolones is bacterial DNA gyrase. Where available, these data are also given. The source of the enzyme in such studies is almost always *E. coli*, so the reader must be careful in extrapolating such data to other bacteria. DNA gyrase has been isolated from a number of other microbes, but data using these enzymes are extremely scarce and are usually limited to prominent quinolones that have seen clinical evaluation. While there are some reversals, the rank order with these enzymes is usually similar to that seen with the *E. coli* enzyme (54).

The potency of a quinolone against intact bacteria is a complex function of the ability of the drug to penetrate the cell, bind to DNA gyrase, and inhibit the function of the gyrase. It is of some comfort that those quinolones that are very potent at killing bacteria are invariably excellent at inhibiting DNA gyrase. On the other hand, some agents inhibit the enzyme at low doses but are poor at killing intact bacteria. Thus, there is a penetration barrier of some consequence that must be taken into account when potencies are compared and molecules are designed. Two parameters are available for measuring DNA gyrase activity: inhibition of supercoiling and cleavage of DNA. Actual cleavage is highly likely to be a lethal event, so doses reflecting this parameter are reported in the tables.

It is also important to bear in mind that the data in the tables reflect in vitro potency only. In vivo and clinical data are presented elsewhere in this book. Thus, the generalizations that follow include important factors such as pharmacokinetics, toxicity, species differences, and the like to only a limited extent. Many compounds that are potent in vitro fail to be developed because of factors not reflected in these tables.

## THE QUINOLONE PHARMACOPHORE

The pharmacophore is the minimum structural unit in a drug that possesses recognizable and typical pharmacological activity. This minimum unit by itself is often of low potency and specificity. The function of the other portions of a drug molecule, the auxopharmacophore, is to provide tighter receptor fit, greater selectivity, more-useful pharmacokinetic characteristics (absorption, distribution, metabolism, excretion, etc.), and solubility. In the quinolones, the pharmacophoric unit, consisting of the pyridone ring and its associated carboxyl group or suitable carboxyl surrogate, is illustrated in structure 1 (Fig. 1). The pyridone nitrogen (N-1) cannot be replaced (although the groups attached to it can be varied substantially), C-2 can be varied only in very limited ways, the carboxyl at C-3 can be replaced only by a fused thiazolidone bioisostere, and C-4 variations have been reported hardly at all. All other positions in the quinolone molecules can be varied fairly widely. This is consistent with auxopharmacophoric status. In structure 1, the auxopharmacophore is primarily a fused aromatic ring of some type with appropriate pendent substituents. It has been postulated that the quinolones self-associate cooperatively into a bioactive tetraplex in the DNA gate created by the action of DNA gyrase on substrate DNA following strand cleavage (79). In this view, illustrated in structure 2 (Fig. 1), the upper margin ("northern front") of the quinolone is complementary to the DNA bases exposed and made available for new hydrogen-bonding partners by the action of the enzyme. This represents the pharmacophoric carboxyl group at C-3 and the ketone at C-4. It is likely that certain small substituents at C-5 also contribute to this. Substituents at C-2 must be small so as not to prevent the carboxyl group at C-3 from lining up in the plane of the quinolone ring as needed. This gives C-2 only a potential "spoiler" role on the "eastern front." The lower margin ("southern front") of the molecule is held to be a lipophilic self-association region consisting of N-1 and is pendent greasy substituent and C-8. The basic substituent at C-7 serves to orient the quinolone molecules so that carboxy and protonated amine line up near each other in adjoining quinolone molecules in the vertical

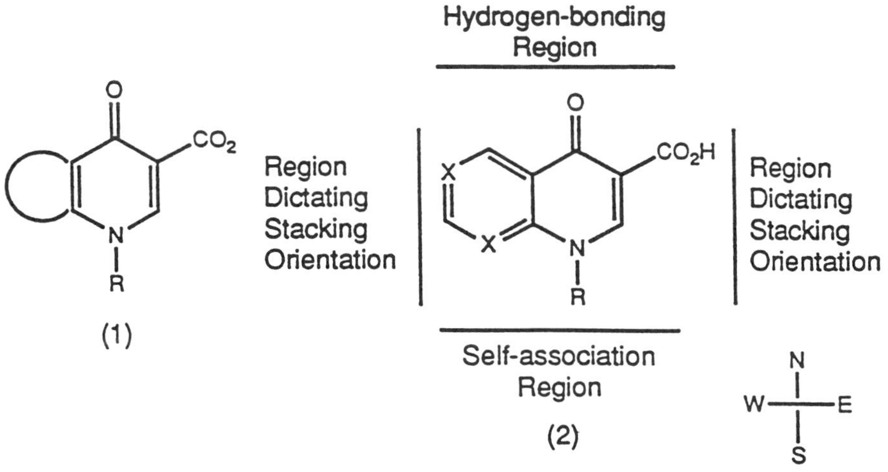

O
$CO_2$
N
R
(1)
Region
Dictating
Stacking
Orientation
Hydrogen-bonding
Region
O
$CO_2H$
X
X
N
R
Region
Dictating
Stacking
Orientation
Self-association
Region
(2)
N
W
E
S

**Figure 1.** Structures 1 and 2.

and horizontal dimensions. The C-7 substituent may also contribute to binding to the enzyme, which is otherwise held in place by its DNA substrate and is not given a role to play in drug binding (in the "western front"). This is in agreement with the observation that quinolones do not bind significantly to DNA gyrase in the absence of DNA. The substituent at C-6 needs to be small so as not to get in the way of either DNA or DNA gyrase. Optical activity, as will be explicated in greater detail later, is expected to exert a more profound influence on potency when attached close to N-1 than when attached close to C-7. This agrees with experience. Perhaps this allows us to modify Pfeiffer's useful rule (72) somewhat by making the seemingly obvious corollary that not only does appropriate optical activity exert a more profound effect on potency when drugs bind tightly to their receptor, as Pfeiffer has enunciated, but also that the effect is more pronounced when the chiral center is closest to one of the essential points of binding.

These rationalizations are in general agreement with what is known about the structure-activity relationships of the quinolones and may assist imaginative scientists in designing new ring systems for exploitation.

Finally, although treating each atom of the quinolone nucleus individually and attempting to define the optimum substituent at each center implies that the centers all contribute independently and that the optimum quinolone ("utopiafloxacin") will emerge by a cut-and-paste assembly of the best individual substituents at each center into a single composite molecule, there is ample and increasing evidence that such is not always the case and that the best collection of substituents needs to be found experimentally by tinkering collectively with all of the variables. Recently, for example, particular attention has been drawn to cooperativity between positions 1 and 5 (21). Consequently, the following tables have been subdivided so that the overall substitution pattern of the rest of the molecule is held constant and the position under particular discussion is the systematically varied feature. For the convenience of the reader, the tables are also numbered to correspond with the numbering of the individual atoms, following quinolone numbering. Where this is not possible, letters are used. To guide the reader to particular entries, specific compounds and their testing results are indicated by listing first the appropriate table and then either the three-letter acronym or the appropriate line number (T1;6, for example, means Table 1, entry 6).

## ABBREVIATIONS

It is often convenient to abbreviate the generic names of quinolones that have received United States Adapted Name status. Three letters are sufficient to differentiate all of the present members of this exclusive club as follows: AMI, amifloxacin; CIN, cinoxacin; CIP, ciprofloxacin; DAN, danofloxacin; DIF, difloxacin; ENO, enoxacin; ENR, enrofloxacin; FLE, fleroxacin; FLU, flumequine; IRL, irloxacin; LOM, lomefloxacin; MIL, miloxacin; NAL, nalidixic acid; NOR, norfloxacin; OFL, ofloxacin; OXO, oxolinic acid; PEF, pefloxacin; PIP, pipemidic acid; PIR, piromidic acid; ROS, rosoxacin; RUF, rufloxacin; SAR, sarafloxacin; SPA, sparfloxacin; TEM, temafloxacin; TOS, tosufloxacin.

In the tables, organism names are abbreviated as follows: Bf, *B. fragilis*; Ec, *E. coli*; EcH, *E. coli* H560; Ef, *Enterococcus faecalis*; Kp, *K. pneumoniae*; Mm, *Morganella morganii*; Pa, *P. aeruginosa*; Pac, *Propionibacterium acnes*; Pv, *P. vulgaris*; Sa, *S. aureus*; Sp, *S. pneumoniae*; Spy, *Streptococcus pyogenes*.

Other abbreviations used in the tables are as follows: Ac, acetyl; DiF, difluoride; Et, ethyl; $IC_{50}$, 50% inhibitory concentration; Me, methyl; Ph, phenyl.

## QUINOLONES OF THE CLASSICAL ERA

Table a compares the antimicrobial potencies of the more prominent quinolones of the classical era (from NAL to NOR) (23). NAL is the only 1,8-naphthyridine example. This very abbreviated spectrum shows that NAL is active mainly against gram-negative cocci and that the MICs are weak. This relegates the drug to treatment of infections in which significant concentrations can be reached and susceptible microorganisms congregate. In practice, this means largely community-acquired urinary tract infections. Gram-positive organisms, anaerobes, and difficult pathogens, such as *P. aeruginosa,* are not susceptible to NAL. Examination of the effect of NAL on the enzyme purified from *E. coli* provides a ready rationale for these various findings, as NAL is not very potent compared with NOR (set by definition to equal 1).

PIR and PIP represent the pyrimidopyridones. Compared with NAL, PIR shows enhanced activity against gram-positive organisms but loses some potency

**Table a.** Comparison of in vitro biological activities of classical quinolones with those of NOR and PEF[a]

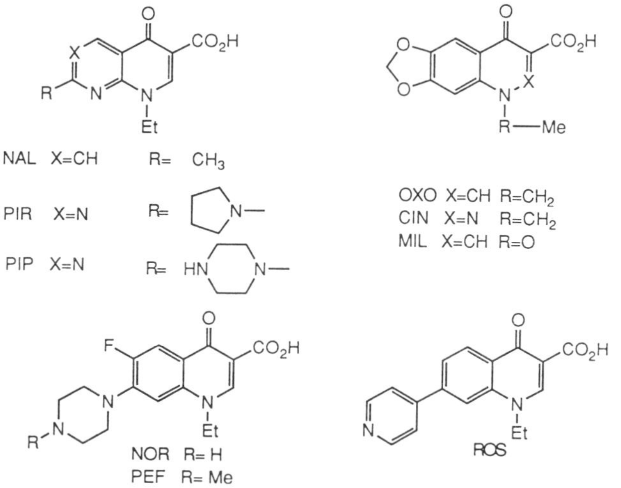

NAL X=CH R= $CH_3$
PIR X=N R= (pyrrolidin-1-yl)
PIP X=N R= (piperazin-1-yl)

OXO X=CH R=$CH_2$
CIN X=N R=$CH_2$
MIL X=CH R=O

NOR R= H
PEF R= Me

ROS

| Drug | MIC (μg/ml) for: EcV | EcH | Pa I.18 | Sa H.228 | Sp sv-1 | Kp MGH-2 | DNA gyrase (μg/ml)[b] Cleavage | $IC_{50}$ |
|---|---|---|---|---|---|---|---|---|
| NAL | 6.3 | 6.3 | >100 | >100 | >100 | 6.3 | 50 | >100 |
| PIR | 25 | 50 | >100 | 12.5 | >100 | 25 | 38 | >100 |
| PIP | 1.6 | 3.1 | 6.3 | 50 | >100 | 6.3 | 50 | >100 |
| OXO | 0.2 | 0.2 | 6.3 | 1.6 | 100 | 0.2 | 10 | 25 |
| CIN | 3.1 | 50 | >100 | >100 | >100 | 1.6 | 43 | >100 |
| MIL | 0.4 | 0.4 | 12.5 | 6.3 | 100 | 0.2 | 10 | 50 |
| ROS | 0.2 | 0.2 | 6.3 | 0.4 | 12.5 | 0.4 | 2.5 | >10 |
| NOR | 0.025 | 0.1 | 0.2 | 0.8 | 1.6 | 0.05 | 1 | 5.5 |
| PEF | 0.025 | 0.1 | 0.4 | 0.2 | 0.8 | 0.05 | 1 | 5.5 |

[a]Data are from reference 23.
[b]The DNA gyrase was from *E. coli* H560.

against gram-negative organisms. It is more effective in promoting DNA cleavage by *E. coli*'s DNA gyrase, suggesting that at least some of the lesser whole-cell potency of PIR is due to a penetration barrier. PIP shows enhanced anti-gram-negative-organism activity but is still unimpressive against gram-positive organisms. There is some suggestion from these data that the piperazinyl moiety at C-7 conveys useful properties. Present theory suggests that the distal nitrogen plays an important role in orienting self-assembled quinolone tetraplexes so that acid is near amine in both vertical and horizontal planes, as illustrated schematically in structure 3 (Fig. 2). Whereas the pyrimidine ring-proximal nitrogen is spatially closer, it is not expected to be very basic, as it is deactivated by the electron-withdrawing carbonyl group at C-4.

OXO, CIN, and MIL represent a group of analogs related to each other through the principle of bioisosterism. OXO is the most potent of this group. Comparing this agent with NAL, one may tentatively conclude that for in vitro potency, when there is no orienting basic substituent in the ring annelated to the pyridone pharmacophore, a benzene ring is superior to either a pyridine or a pyrimidine ring. This conclusion is flawed because no complete set of analogs with identical substitution patterns on the peripheries of all of these rings is available for comparison.

Interestingly, as far as one can glean from the open literature and the nature of the chemistry involved, optimum placement of the methylenedioxy moiety of OXO was fortuitous. Following a more in-depth study requiring, in part, some new chemistry, it was found that the two possible alternative positional isomers of OXO were dramatically less active (51).

## VARIATIONS AT N-1

The original quinolones had nitrogen-bearing a substituents at position 1. This appears to have been a fortunate circumstance. Subsequent work has shown that an oxygen (39) or a carbon (38) cannot substitute for N-1.

Hard-won experience with the first 800 quinolone analogs led to the belief that a small, lipophilic, aliphatic substituent attached to N-1 led to the best activity (2). Ultimately, following the discovery of the outstanding activity profile conveyed by the combination of 6-fluoro-7-piperazinyl substitution (which fits the classic structure-activity rules), it was discovered in several laboratories that other N-1 substituents could be used with excellent results. This finding is an excellent argument against being too rational or too scholarly too soon in a new drug series.

Table 1a compares the in vitro MICs of a

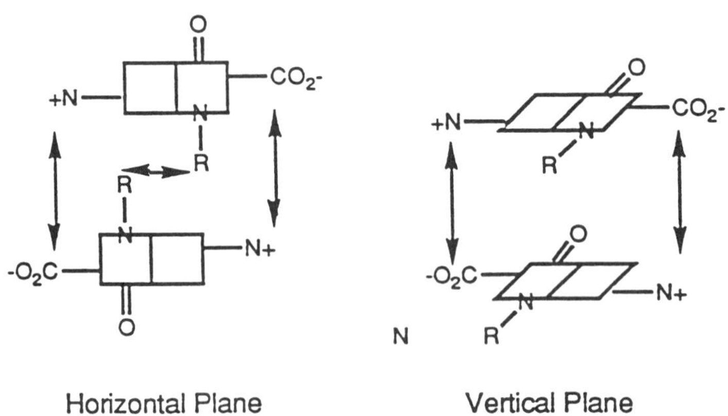


**Figure 2.** Structure 3.

**Table 1a.** Comparison of in vitro MIC for C-6-fluorinated quinolones with nonpolar aliphatic substituents at N-1

| Drug | R | MIC ($\mu$g/ml) for: | | | | Reference(s) |
|---|---|---|---|---|---|---|
| | | Ec | Pa | Sa | Kp | |
| | H | i[a] | i | i | i | |
| | $CH_3$ | 0.39 | 1.56 | 6.25 | | 44 |
| NOR | $C_2H_5$ | 0.05 | 0.39 | 0.39 | | 44 |
| | $CH{=}CH_2$ | 0.1 | 0.39 | 3.13 | | 44 |
| | $CH_2CH_2F$ | 0.10 | 0.78 | 1.56 | | 44 |
| | $n{-}C_3H_7$ | 0.20 | 3.13 | 1.56 | | 44 |
| | $CH_2CH{=}CH_2$ | 0.20 | 1.56 | 3.13 | | 44 |
| | $CH_2Ph$ | 0.78 | 1.56 | 1.56 | | 44 |
| CIP | $CH(CH_2)_2$ | 0.05 | 0.40 | 3.10 | | 22 |
| | | 0.004 | 0.125 | 0.25 | | 22,85 |
| | $CH(CH_3)_2$ | 0.5 | 1 | 1 | | 8 |
| | $C(CH_3)_3$ | 0.06 | 0.5 | 0.06 | 0.13 | 8 |
| | $CH_2CH(CH_2)_2$ | 0.5 | 4 | 1 | | 8 |
| | $CH(CH_2)_3$ | 0.13 | 1 | 0.5 | 0.13 | 8 |
| | $C(CH_3)_2CH_2F$ | 0.016 | 1 | 0.13–0.16 | 0.006 | 73 |
| | $CCH_3(CH_2F)_2$ | 0.13 | 0.5 | 1–2 | 0.13 | 73 |

[a]i, inactive.

series of NOR analogs substituted at N-1 with a variety of nonpolar aliphatic moieties. For the first entries, it can be seen that small saturated or unsaturated alkyl moieties (T1a;4,7) are indeed good, especially against gram-negative microorganisms (44). Activity optimizes roughly at the ethyl, especially against gram-positive organisms. Later work upset this view. The excellent activity of CIP is somewhat surprising when the Albrecht generalizations are considered, and this agent has had outstanding clinical success (24). In the tabulated examples, there is significant scatter in the potency data. At worst, CIP is equivalent to NOR against gram-negative organisms and is less active against gram-positive organisms. Data from other laboratories indicate that CIP is superior across the board to anything else in this table. It is dramatically more active than its *N*-isopropyl analog (T1a;10) (8). This activity may be associated with the compactness and pseudo-olefinic character of the cyclopropyl ring. CIP has now replaced NOR as the "gold standard" of the modern quinolone era. Moving the cyclopropyl ring away from the N-1 atom by a methylene group (T1a;12) decreases anti-gram-negative-organism activity by 1 order of magnitude but increases the anti-gram-positive-organism activity somewhat. Another analog whose publication raised eyebrows was the *N-tert*-butyl analog (T1a;11) (8). On the basis of all that had gone before, one would have predicted confidently that this compound would be poor. In fact, the anti-gram-negative-organism activities of NOR and CIP are retained and the anti-gram-positive-organism activities are enhanced. The hydrogen atoms of the N-1 substituent in this case can be replaced with satisfactory results by fluorine atoms also (T1a;14,15) (73). Thus, the overall length of a nonpolar aliphatic moiety should still not exceed that of an *N*-ethyl group for optimal results, but in some cases, the circumference of the group can be much greater than previously suspected. Efforts to reduce these conclusions to quantitative equations have been made (24).

Table 1b addresses the following question: are the same results obtained in the 1,8-naphthyridine ring system with analogous substitution? The answer is yes. ENO is analogous structurally and antimicrobially to NOR (8, 23, 44, 49). In this series, ethyl is again approximately optimal among the early entries (49), and again, the *N*-1-cyclopropyl (T1b;14) and *N*-1-*tert*-butyl (T1b;13) analogs are unexpectedly superior (73). A few entries in these references deal with anaerobes. The activities revealed are unimpressive.

Comparatively few N-1 substituents with polar aliphatic groups are available for analysis. This lack reflects earlier experience, which suggested that such groups would be deleterious. Such data as are available involving NOR and ENO analogs (Tables 1c and 1d) agree with this proposition (44, 68, 83, 84). These findings are in agreement with

**Table 1b.** Comparison of in vitro MIC for C-6-fluorinated naphthyridines with nonpolar aliphatic substituents at N-1

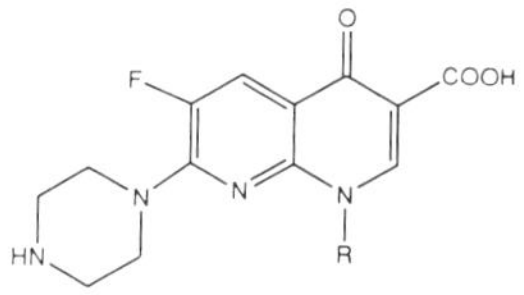

| Drug | R | MIC ($\mu$g/ml) for: | | | | | | Reference(s) |
|---|---|---|---|---|---|---|---|---|
| | | Ec | Pa | Sa | Kp | Sp | Bf | |
| | Me | 0.2 | 6.25 | 6.25 | | | | 49 |
| ENO | Et | 0.05 | 0.39 | 0.39 | | | | 44 |
| ENO | Et | 0.13 | 0.5 | 0.25 | 0.5 | | | 8 |
| ENO | Et | 0.2 | 0.78 | 0.78 | | | | 49 |
| ENO | Et | 0.1 | 0.8 | 3.1 | 0.1 | 3.1 | | 23 |
| | $CH{=}CH_2$ | 0.05 | 0.78 | 1.56 | | | | 49 |
| | $CH_2CH{=}CH_2$ | 0.39 | 3.13 | 3.13 | | | | 49 |
| | $(CH_2)_2CH{=}CH_2$ | 0.39 | 6.25 | 3.13 | | | | 49 |
| | $(CH_2)_2F$ | 0.2 | 0.78 | 0.39 | | | | 49 |
| | $(CH_2)_2Cl$ | 0.1 | 0.78 | 0.39 | | | | 49 |
| | $CHF_2$ | 0.78 | 6.25 | 6.25 | | | | 49 |
| | $CHMe_2$ | 0.25 | 4 | 2 | 1 | | | 8, 73 |
| | $CMe_3$ | 0.015 | 1 | 0.06 | 0.13 | 1 | 8 | 8, 73 |
| | $CH(CH_2)_2$ | 0.06 | 0.06 | 0.25 | 0.06 | | | 8, 73 |
| | $CH(CH_2)_2$ | 0.05 | 0.2 | 0.39 | | | | 49 |
| | $CMe_2CH_2F$ | 0.13 | 1 | 0.25 | 0.25 | 0.5 | 16 | 73 |
| | $CMe(CH_2F)_2$ | 0.13 | 4 | 4 | 0.25 | 16 | 125 | 73 |
| | $C(CH_2F)_3$ | 0.5 | 16 | 8 | 1 | 32 | 125 | 73 |
| | $(CH_2)_2Me$ | 0.2 | 3.13 | 0.78 | | | | 49 |
| | $CHMe_2$ | 0.2 | 6.25 | 3.13 | | | | 49 |
| | $(CH_2)_3Me$ | 0.39 | 25 | 6.25 | | | | 49 |
| | $(CH_2)_4Me$ | 6.25 | $>100$ | 30 | | | | 49 |
| | $(CH_2)_3Cl$ | 0.78 | 6.25 | 6.25 | | | | 49 |
| | $(CH_2)_4Cl$ | 3.13 | 100 | 25 | | | | 49 |

**Table 1c.** Comparison of in vitro MIC for C-6-fluorinated quinolones with polar aliphatic substituents at N-1

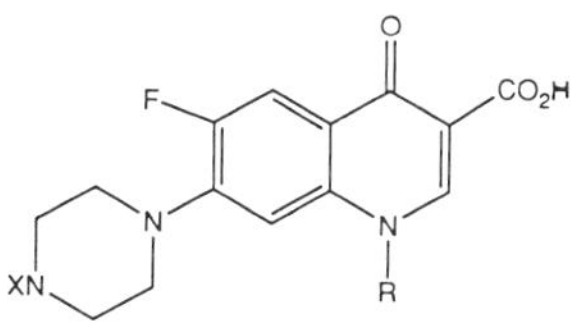

| Drug | R | X | MIC (μg/ml) for: Ec | Pa | Sa | Kp | Reference |
|---|---|---|---|---|---|---|---|
| NOR | $C_2H_5$ | H | 0.05 | 0.39 | 0.39 | 0.5 | 44 |
| | $CH_2CH_2OH$ | H | 0.39 | 3.13 | 1.56 | | 44 |
| | $NHCH_3$ | H | 1.0 | 1.0 | 1.95 | 1.0 | 84 |
| AMI | $NHCH_3$ | Me | 0.25 | 1.0 | 1.0 | 0.25 | 84 |

theory, which requires a hydrophobic interior for suitable self-association (structure 2).

Another group of analogs discovered in recent years to be surprisingly useful is the one with an aromatic ring substituted at N-1. An aromatic ring is bigger in its long dimension and potentially more hydrophobic (depending on the substitution pattern) than an ethyl group. It is, however, capable of pi association not possible with saturated aliphatic groupings. With PEF (N = ethyl group) as comparator, consider SAR, the most potent compound in Table 1e (11). There is a slight falling off in potency against gram-negative organisms but a retention of potency against gram-positive organisms. These differences are smaller in vivo than in vitro. Advantageously, fluorine substitution at C-4′ (T1e;3,4) and particularly at both C-2′ and C-4′ (T1e;7) enhances potency much as it did in the aliphatic examples in Tables 1a and 1b. Larger C-4′ substituents are deleterious (T1e;11). Once again, there are definite limits to the permissible length of the N-1 substituent. Instructive pairs in this regard are C-4′-OH (T1e;10) versus C-4′-*O*-methyl (T1e;11) and C-4′-F (T1e;3) versus C-4′-Cl (T1e;8). There are fewer data available for

**Table 1d.** Comparison of in vitro MIC for C-6-fluorinated naphthyridines with polar aliphatic substituents at N-1

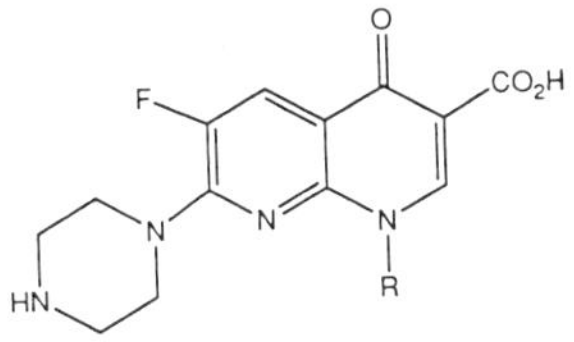

| Drug | R | MIC (μg/ml) for: Ec | Pa | Sa | Kp | Reference |
|---|---|---|---|---|---|---|
| ENO | $C_2H_5$ | 0.1 | 1.56 | 0.78 | | 69 |
| | $CH_2CH_2OH$ | 1.56 | 50 | 6.25 | | 69 |
| | $(CH_2)_3OH$ | 1.56 | 50 | 25 | | 69 |
| | $NHCH_3$ | 0.25–1 | 0.25–16 | 2–8 | 0.25–2 | 83 |

**Table 1e.** Comparison of in vitro MIC for C-6-fluoroquinolones with aromatic substituents at N-1[a]

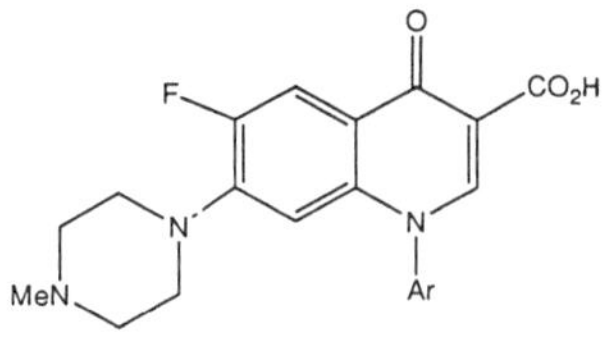

| Drug | Ar | MIC ($\mu$g/ml) for: | | | | |
|---|---|---|---|---|---|---|
| | | Ec | Pa | Sa | Sp | Kp |
| PEF | (Et) | 0.025 | 0.4 | 0.2 | 3.1 | 0.1 |
| | Ph | 0.78 | 6.2 | 0.78 | 3.1 | 0.2 |
| DIF | 4-F-Ph[b] | 0.2 | 1.56 | 0.2 | 1.56 | 0.1 |
| SAR | 4-F-Ph[b] | 0.05 | 0.39 | 0.2 | 0.78 | 0.2 |
| | 3-F-Ph | 6.2 | 50 | 12.5 | 25 | 3.1 |
| | 2-F-Ph | 0.78 | 6.2 | 1.56 | 12.5 | 0.39 |
| | 2,4-DiF-Ph | 0.2 | 1.56 | 0.1 | 0.78 | 0.1 |
| | 4-Cl-Ph | 1.56 | 12.5 | 1.56 | 12.5 | 0.78 |
| | 4-Br-Ph | 6.2 | 50 | 3.1 | 50 | 3.1 |
| | 4-OH-Ph | 0.1 | 0.39 | 0.10 | 0.2 | 0.05 |
| | 4-OMe-Ph | 50 | 200 | 12.5 | 50 | 12.5 |
| | 4-Me-Ph | 1.56 | 12.5 | 1.56 | 12.5 | 0.78 |
| | 2-Me-Ph | 1.56 | 25 | 3.1 | 50 | 1.56 |
| | 2,6-$Me_2$-Ph | >100 | >100 | >100 | >100 | >100 |
| | 3,4-$OCH_2O$-Ph | 0.78 | 6.2 | 0.78 | 12.5 | 0.2 |

[a]Data are from reference 11.
[b]SAR has a *C*-7-piperazinyl moiety instead of the *C*-7-*N*-4-methylpiperazinyl moiety of DIF.

**Table 1f.** Comparison of in vitro MIC for C-6-fluorinated naphthyridines with aromatic substituents at N-1[a]

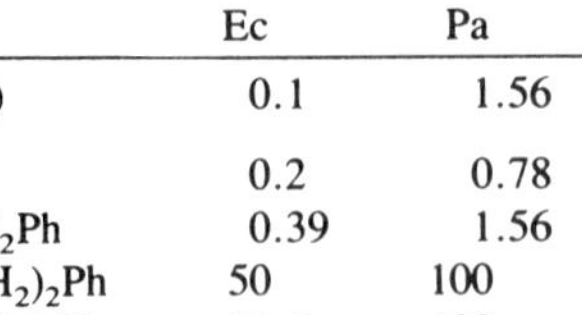

| Drug | Ar | MIC ($\mu$g/ml) for: | | |
|---|---|---|---|---|
| | | Ec | Pa | Sa |
| ENO | (Et) | 0.1 | 1.56 | 0.78 |
| | Ph | 0.2 | 0.78 | 1.56 |
| | $CH_2Ph$ | 0.39 | 1.56 | 3.13 |
| | $(CH_2)_2Ph$ | 50 | 100 | 12.5 |
| | $(CH_2)_3Ph$ | 12.5 | >100 | 1.56 |
| | $(CH_2)_4Ph$ | >100 | >100 | >100 |

[a]Data are from reference 69.

the naphthyridine series as shown in Table 1f (69), but *N*-1-phenyl substitution (T1f;2) produces a potency similar to that of *N*-1-ethyl (ENO). Insertion of methylene spacers progressively decreases potency, with a momentary trend reversal at n = 3 (T1f;5), especially against *S. aureus.*

A small group of ROS-like naphthyridines is available (68). This group has less intrinsic potency than other groups, but the same considerations hold (Table 1g). The naphthyridine analog (T1g;2) is actually slightly superior in vitro to ROS, and replacement of the terminal hydrogen with fluorine (T1g;3) gives equivalent activity. The *N*-cyclopropyl analog (T1g;6) is the most potent substance in the table.

Computer graphic considerations led to the introduction of the C-7-(3′-ethylamino-

**Table 1g.** Effect of varying N-1 substituents of ROS and its 1,8-naphthyridine analogs[a]

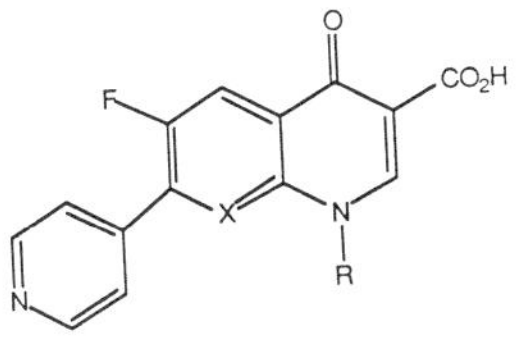

| Drug | X | R | MIC (μg/ml) for: | | |
|---|---|---|---|---|---|
| | | | Ec | Pa | Sa |
| ROS | CH | Et | 0.39 | 3.13 | 0.78 |
| | N | Et | 0.2 | 3.13 | 0.39 |
| | N | $CH_2CH_2F$ | 0.2 | 1.56 | 0.39 |
| | N | $CH_2CH_2OH$ | 1.56 | 50 | 50 |
| | N | $CH{=}CH_2$ | 0.78 | 6.25 | 1.56 |
| | N | $CH(CH_2)_2$ | 0.1 | 0.78 | 0.2 |

[a]Data are from reference 68.

**Table 1h.** MICs of C-6,8-difluorinated quinolones with *C*-7-3′-ethylaminomethyl pyrrolidine moieties and variations in N-1 substituents[a]

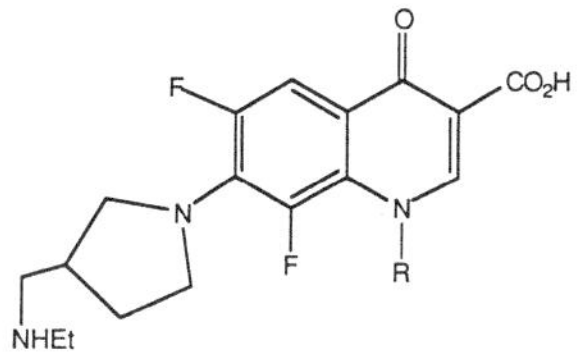

| R | MIC (μg/ml) for: | | | DNA gyrase (μg/ml) | |
|---|---|---|---|---|---|
| | Ec | Pa | Sa | $IC_{50}$ | Cleavage |
| $CH_3$ | 0.4 | 1.6 | 1.6 | 7.5 | 5.0 |
| $C_2H_5$ | 0.1 | 1.6 | 0.1 | 14 | 2.5 |
| $CH{=}CH_2$ | 0.2 | 1.6 | 0.4 | 2.9 | 0.8 |
| $CH_2CH_2F$ | 0.1 | 1.6 | 0.4 | 7.5 | 2.5 |
| $CH_2CF_3$ | 0.8 | 6.3 | 0.4 | 26 | 2.5 |
| $NHCH_3$ | 0.2 | 0.8 | 0.4 | 27 | 2.5 |
| $OCH_3$ | 0.4 | 6.3 | 0.8 | 27 | 2.5 |
| $CH(CH_2)_2$ | 0.05 | 0.4 | 0.05 | 1.4 | 0.25 |
| $CH(CH_3)_2$ | 0.8 | 12.5 | 0.4 | 28 | 5.0 |
| $CH(CH_2)_3$ | 0.2 | 3.1 | 0.1 | 26 | 2.5 |
| $CH(CH_2)_4$ | 3.1 | 12.5 | 0.4 | 28 | 5.0 |
| $CH(CH_2)_5$ | 6.3 | >100 | 6.3 | 30 | 10 |
| Ph | 1.6 | 6.3 | 0.8 | 29 | 7.5 |
| 4-F-Ph | 0.8 | 1.6 | 0.1 | 14 | 2.5 |

[a]Data are from reference 22.

methylpyrrolidines) of Table 1h (22). This moiety roughly overlaps in space with a piperazinyl moiety. Unlike NOR, these compounds contain *C*-8-F atoms. Trends for this series of compounds contain no particular surprises. *N*-Ethyl (T1h;2) is good, and *N*-cyclopropyl (T1h;8,9) is better. All the other analogs are somewhat inferior to these two. One notes with interest the lack of parallelism between the results in intact bacteria and against *E. coli*-derived DNA gyrase. The most potent analogs against bacteria are excellent at inhibiting the enzyme and leading to DNA cleavage, but not all analogs potent against the enzyme are equally potent against the intact bacterium. This disparity is generally attributed to less passage into the cells, although definitive data are lacking.

Thus, contemporary data reaffirm the earlier observation that lipophilic substituents are optimal at N-1, although the Albrecht generalizations are seen in retrospect to have been too restrictive. A wider range of favorable substitutions, including cyclopropyl, *tert*-butyl, and aryl, is now available. These groups exert an activity-enhancing effect in all of the bicyclic ring systems to which they have been attached. The results vary from microorganism to microorganism, but it appears that gram-positive organisms are usually more bulk tolerant than gram-negative organisms. It is also interesting that of the cyclic analogs, the smallest, cyclopropyl, conveys the best potency.

## VARIATIONS AT C-2

Comparatively little work involving C-2 has been done. As Table a shows, bioisosteric replacement of the *C*-2-CH group of oxolinic acid with a nitrogen led to CIN and activity in vitro decreased, even though there was a favorable influence on pharmacokinetics. In Table 2a is another example of this phenomenon. Replacement of the *C*-2-CH of norfloxacin by N (T2a;2) is compatible with activity, but potency is significantly de-

**Table 2a.** MICs of untethered C-2 variants[a]

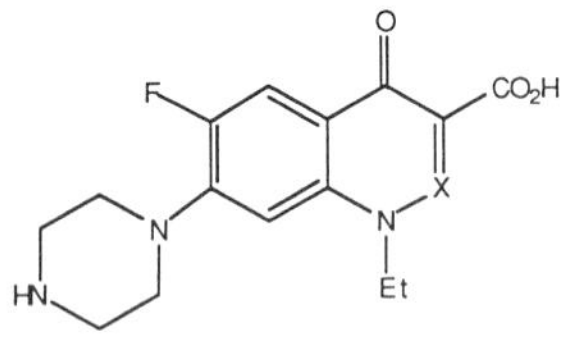

| Drug | X | MIC ($\mu$g/ml) for: | | |
|---|---|---|---|---|
| | | Ec | Pa | Sa |
| NOR | CH | 0.1 | 0.78 | 0.39 |
| | N | 3.13 | 50 | 12.5 |

[a]Data are from reference 48.

creased (48, 57). In the prefluoroquinolone era, single substituent additions to C-2 were shown to be deleterious (50). In more-recent work, similar results have been obtained (data not in tables). Table 2b shows some analogs in which a C-2 aliphatic or aromatic substituent is tethered to N-1. This keeps the substituent more or less in the same plane as the aromatic rings but can interfere with the planarity of the carboxyl substituent at C-3. The potencies of these compounds are compared with those of OFL and free-rotating analogs a, in which the aromatic ring is most probably orthogonal to the bicyclic ring system (10, 13, 45). Compound b and an analogous compound, c, with a sulfur insertion retain significant activity. Use of a smaller oxygen or nitrogen insertion in the c series results in significant loss of potency. Tethering is thus clearly advantageous.

The thiazolidone series tethered between C-2 and C-3 is discussed under Variations at C-3.

## VARIATIONS AT C-3

It was established in the classical era that a carboxyl substituent was superior to esters, phosphonates, and sulfonates (87). A carboxaldehyde moiety turned out to be a prodrug. Excitingly, however, fusing a thiazolidone ring between C-2 and C-3 of quinolones such that the amide linkage, because of its aromatic resonance, can mimic a carboxyl group in acidity results in compounds with outstanding in vitro potencies (Table 3). Compound A is equivalent to CIP (22, 85) when used against *E. coli* but is 1 order of magnitude more active against *P. aeruginosa* and *S.*

**Table 2b.** MICs of tethered C-2 variants

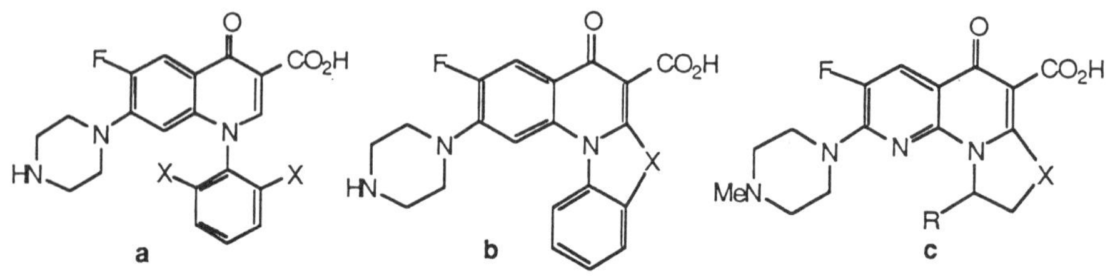

| Drug | X | R | MIC ($\mu$g/ml) for: | | | Reference |
|---|---|---|---|---|---|---|
| | | | Ec | Pa | Sa | |
| OFL | | | 0.2 | 1.56 | 0.39 | 45 |
| a | H | | 0.2 | 1.56 | 0.78 | 10 |
| a | $CH_3$ | | >100 | >100 | >100 | 10 |
| b | S | | 0.2 | 1.56 | 0.39 | 13 |
| c | S | H | 0.2 | 1.56 | 0.39 | 45 |
| c | O | Me | 12.5 | >25 | 12.5 | 45 |
| c | NMe | H | 50 | 100 | 100 | 45 |

**Table 3.** MICs of tethered C-3 variants

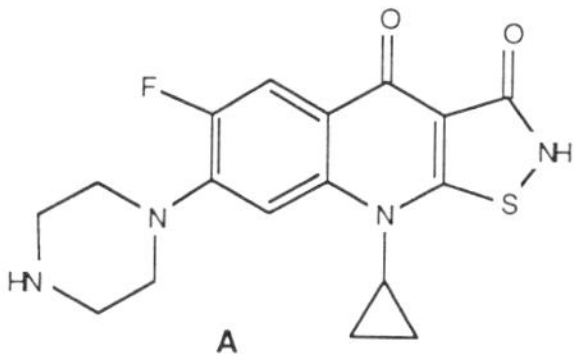

A

| Structure | MIC ($\mu$g/ml) for: | | | DNA gyrase $IC_{50}$ ($\mu$g/ml) | Reference(s) |
|---|---|---|---|---|---|
| | Ec | Pa | Sa | | |
| CIP | 0.004 | 0.125 | 0.25 | 0.3 | 22, 85 |
| A | 0.005 | 0.02 | 0.02 | 0.09 | 12 |

*aureus* (12). The fusion not only activates the NH atom so that it is equivalent in acidity to a weak carboxylic acid but also keeps the moiety in the same plane as the aromatic rings so as to allow effective putative hydrogen bonding to purine and pyrimidine bases.

Almost all of the other work involving C-3 was done in the classical era and gave disappointing results (2). A repetition of some of this work on ring systems of contemporary interest might produce useful substances.

## VARIATIONS AT C-4

There is no Table 4, reflecting the apparent lack of any work involving changes at this center.

## VARIATIONS AT C-5

In the classical era, comparatively little work involved substituent introduction at C-5 aside from the finding that 1,5-naphthyridines (substitution of N for CH at position 5) were relatively uninteresting. Contemporary theory suggests that groups at C-5 must not be big and that they may be advantageous if they can participate actively in putative hydrogen bonding to DNA bases. Recent findings strongly support this idea.

More-recent work is summarized in Table 5a. With CH as standard (T5a;1), primary amine introduction at C-5 (T5a;2) does not change potency against the purified *E. coli* enzyme, but activity in whole microorganisms is improved by 1 order of magnitude over the activities of the other substances listed in the table (23, 33, 56–58). This suggests that one of the contributions of this new moiety is enhanced penetration. Replacement of one of the NH atoms by *N*-methyl (T5a;4) decreases activity both against the enzyme and against microbes, and dimethylation is quite deleterious. Unfortunately, the performance of the C-5 amino analogs in vivo was poorer than the in vitro studies suggested. Use of the small fluorine atom in place of hydrogen (T5a;9) leads to rough equivalency except against pseudomonads, where the F-containing molecule is not as effective. Curiously, use of the larger Cl (T5a;14) and Br (T5a;15) substituents improves activity. Likewise, a methyl group at C-5 (T5a;6) is rather effective. Incorporation of a hydroxyl group (T5a;12), which can participate in hydrogen bonding, is better than incorporation of H, but incorporation of an even larger SH group (T5a;13) leads to poor activity, even though the molecule is quite capable of participating in hydrogen bonding. These findings are hard to rationalize at present.

A rather limited group of analogs with a

**Table 5a.** MICs of C-5 substituents with C-7-piperazinyl moieties

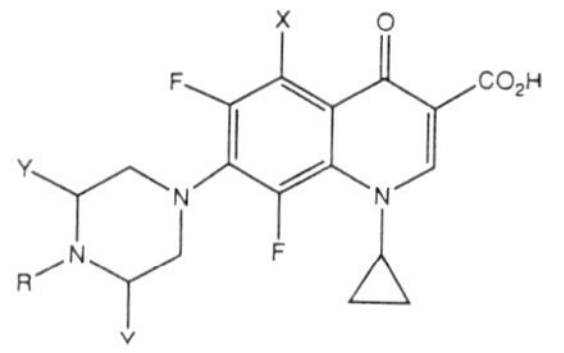

| Drug | R | X | Y | MIC (μg/ml) for: | | | DNA gyrase (μg/ml) | | Reference |
|---|---|---|---|---|---|---|---|---|---|
| | | | | Ec | Pa | Sa | $IC_{50}$ | Cleavage | |
| | H | H | H | 0.1 | 0.2 | 0.4 | 2.8 | 0.5 | 23 |
| | H | $NH_2$ | H | 0.013 | 0.025 | 0.05 | 2.8 | 0.5 | 23 |
| SPA | H | $NH_2$ | Me | 0.0125 | 0.39 | 0.05 | | | 57 |
| | H | $NHCH_3$ | H | 0.1 | 1.6 | 0.8 | 13.8 | 2.5 | 23 |
| | H | NHAc | H | >25 | >25 | >25 | >100 | >100 | 23 |
| | H | $CH_3$ | H | 0.013 | 0.2 | 0.025–0.1 | | 0.3 | 34 |
| | $CH_3$ | $NH_2$ | H | 0.013 | 0.1 | 0.05 | 2.8 | 0.5 | 34 |
| | $CH_3$ | $N(CH_3)_2$ | H | >25 | >25 | >25 | >200 | >200 | 34 |
| | $CH_3$ | F | H | 0.06 | 4 | 0.5 | | | 58 |
| | $CH_3$ | $OCH_3$ | H | 0.2 | 12.5 | 25 | | | 57 |
| | $CH_3$ | $SCH_3$ | H | 0.2 | 12.5 | 3.13 | | | 57 |
| | $CH_3$ | CH | H | 0.05 | 0.78 | 0.2 | | | 57 |
| | $CH_3$ | SH | H | 0.39 | 12.5 | 3.13 | | | 57 |
| | $CH_3$ | Cl | H | 0.025 | 0.78 | 0.2 | | | 57 |
| | $CH_3$ | Br | H | 0.05 | 0.78 | 0.39 | | | 57 |

noncyclic basic substituent at C-7 is illustrated in Table 5b (67). The results are more or less as expected from Table 5a. Compared with a hydrogen at C-5, a primary amino group (T5b;1) enhanced potency. Other groups are somewhat inferior to H.

**Table 5b.** MICs of C-5 substituents with C-7-thioethylamine moieties[a]

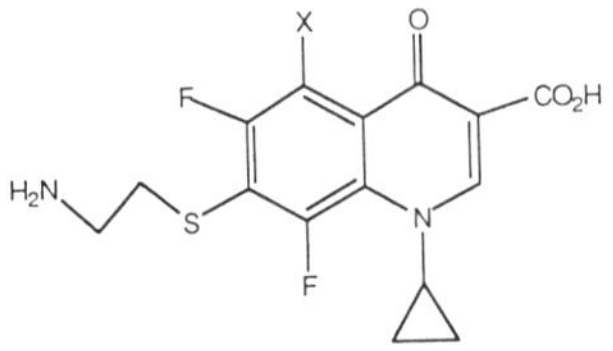

| X | MIC (μg/ml) for: | | |
|---|---|---|---|
| | Ec | Pa | Sa |
| $NH_2$ | 0.025 | 0.1 | 0.05 |
| OH | 1.56 | 6.25 | 1.56 |
| F | 0.78 | 3.13 | 3.13 |

[a]Data are from reference 68.

Curiously, in the pyridopyrimidine series (Table 5c), the very limited data suggest that a 5-amino substituent (T5c;2) is definitely deleterious (23). This reinforces the suggestion that the value of a particular substituent must be determined in each ring system and that it is dangerous to extrapolate too widely, especially from a small sample of analogs.

Table 5d gives a few tricyclic benzothiazine examples and compares them with RUF, a compound recently introduced to the clinic. In conflict with the findings in Table 5a, a C-5 chloro group (T5d;2) is deleterious (9).

## VARIATIONS AT C-6

From Table 6a, the reader will readily perceive the dramatic enhancing and nearly

**Table 5c.** MICs of molecules in the pyridopyrimidine series with C-5 substituents[a]

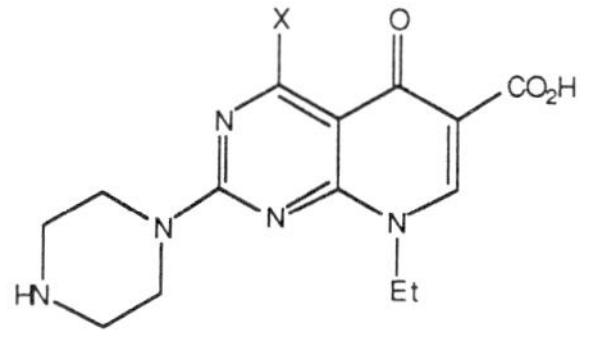

| Drug | X | MIC (μg/ml) for: | | | DNA gyrase (μg/ml) | |
|---|---|---|---|---|---|---|
| | | Ec | Pa | Sa | $IC_{50}$ | Cleavage |
| PIP | H | 1.6 | 6.3 | 50 | >100 | 50 |
| | $NH_2$ | 6.3 | 25 | 50 | | 100 |

[a]Data are from reference 23.

unique contribution of the *C*-6-F moiety (T6a;2) discussed elsewhere (44). A C-6 fluoro substituent is superior to all others tried thus far when C-7 carries a basic substituent. NOR is at least 1 order of magnitude more potent across the board than any of the other analogs in this table. In the naphthyridine series (Table 6b), the fluorine contribution is smaller but still clearly favorable (69). As might be expected by analogy with ROS (Ta;ROS), these compounds do not approximate the potency of ENO, which has a piperazinyl moiety at C-7 usually associated with greater activity (44). With naphthyridines having the more typical *C*-7-piperazinyl moiety (Table 6c), the *C*-6-F (T6c;2) contribution to potency is still significant, and no other substituent contributes so well (23,49). Most interestingly, in the NAL class (Table 6d), incorporation of a *C*-6-F atom (T6d;2) dramatically enhances in vitro potency (23). The effect against intact microorganisms is much more dramatic than that against the en-

**Table 6a.** MICs of molecules in the norfloxacin series with C-6 substituents[a]

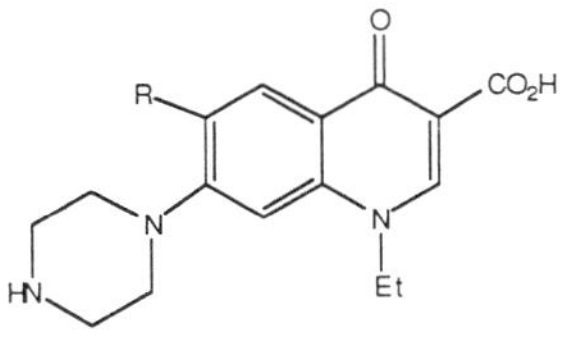

| Drug | R | MIC (μg/ml) for: | | |
|---|---|---|---|---|
| | | Ec | Pa | Sa |
| | H | 0.78 | 3.13 | 12.5 |
| NOR | F | 0.05 | 0.39 | 0.39 |
| | Cl | 0.20 | 3.13 | 1.56 |
| | Br | 0.39 | 12.5 | 3.13 |
| | $CH_3$ | 0.39 | 6.25 | 3.13 |
| | $SCH_3$ | 0.78 | 12.5 | 25 |
| | $COCH_3$ | 100 | >100 | 100 |
| | CN | 0.39 | 6.25 | 12.5 |
| | $NO_2$ | 0.78 | 12.5 | 25 |

[a]Data are from reference 44.

**Table 5d.** MICs for molecules in the benzothiazine series with C-5 substituents[a]

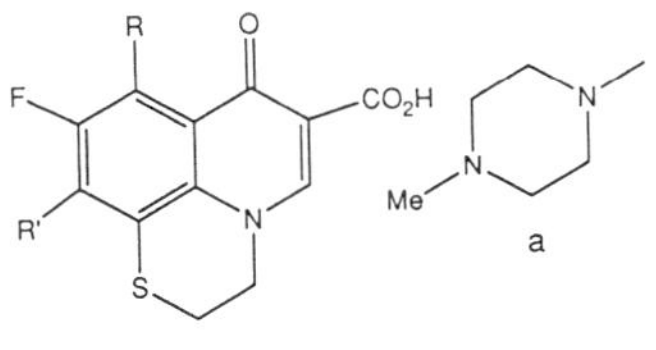

| Drug | R | R′ | MIC (μg/ml) for: | | |
|---|---|---|---|---|---|
| | | | Ec | Pa | Sa |
| | H | H | 0.78 | 50 | 6.25 |
| | Cl | H | >50 | >50 | >50 |
| RUF | H | a | 0.78 | 12.5 | 0.78 |

[a]Data are from reference 9.

**Table 6b.** MICs of molecules in the C-7 4-pyridyl series with C-6 substituents

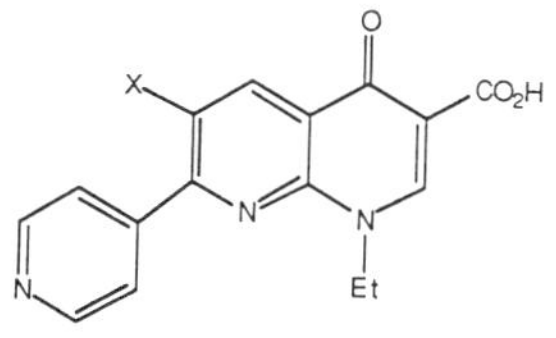

| Drug | X | MIC (μg/ml) for: | | | Reference |
|---|---|---|---|---|---|
| | | Ec | Pa | Sa | |
| | H | 0.78 | 12.5 | 1.56 | 68 |
| | F | 0.2 | 3.13 | 0.39 | 68 |
| ENO[a] | | 0.05 | 0.39 | 0.39 | 44 |

[a]See Table 1c.

**Table 6c.** MICs of molecules in the naphthyridine series with C-6 substituents

| Drug | X | Y | MIC ($\mu$g/ml) for: | | | DNA gyrase ($\mu$g/ml) | | Reference |
|---|---|---|---|---|---|---|---|---|
| | | | Ec | Pa | Sa | $IC_{50}$ | Cleavage | |
| | H | CH | 6.3 | 25 | >50 | | 18 | 23 |
| NOR | F | CH | 0.025 | 0.2 | 0.8 | 1 | 5.5 | 23 |
| | H | N | 6.3 | 12.5 | 50 | | 75 | 23 |
| ENO | F | N | 0.1 | 0.8 | 3.1 | 28 | 5 | 23 |
| | Cl | N | 0.78 | 6.25 | 3.1 | | | 49 |
| | CN | N | 1.56 | 6.25 | 6.25 | | | 49 |
| | $NO_2$ | N | 6.25 | 25 | 6.25 | | | 49 |
| | $NH_2$ | N | 3.13 | 6.25 | >100 | | | 49 |

zyme, suggesting a significant contribution to penetration in addition to the enhancing effect against the enzyme. It is ironic that this substituent change would likely have produced a dramatic result when development began a quarter of a century ago, when the original lead substance had a C-6 chlorine atom. So close and yet so far away!

The effect of the fluoro atom must be at least partly electronic, as F is intermediate in size between H and Cl and the result is outside of each of these.

A concomitant result of the discovery of the dramatic auxopharmacologic effect of a C-6 fluoro is a dramatic decrease in interest in the PIP class, in which a C-6 fluoro substituent is chemically impossible.

**Table 6d.** MICs of molecules in NAL series with C-6 substituents[a]

| Drug | X | MIC ($\mu$g/ml) for: | | | DNA gyrase ($\mu$g/ml) | |
|---|---|---|---|---|---|---|
| | | Ec | Pa | Sa | $IC_{50}$ | Cleavage |
| NAL | H | 6.3 | >100 | >100 | >100 | 50 |
| | F | 0.2 | 12.5 | 1.6 | | 25 |

[a]Data are from reference 23.

## VARIATIONS AT C-7

Position 7 has proven to be the most malleable position in the quinolone series, and a very large amount of information on the influence of structure on activity and systematic changes at that center is available. We have learned that a basic center at C-7 is optimal, although there is some flexibility in the substituent carrying this center, and that there are limits to the size that the substituent may be, although this parameter, too, is somewhat flexible. Seemingly small substituent changes at C-7 can lead to very significant effects on solubility, potency, and pharmacokinetics. In fact, C-7 is one of the best positions in which to make substituent changes for the purpose of adjusting absorption, distribution, metabolism, and excretion problems. Overall, appropriate C-7 substitution is very important for cellular uptake. Optical activity at C-7 is much less influential than at N-1 with regard to potency. The largely aliphatic scaffoldings erected at C-7 present opportunities for metabolism, and aside from the anticipated glucuronidation at C-3, most of the metabolic changes experienced by quinolones take place in the substituents at C-7. Interestingly, a number of the metabolites retain useful activities, and some even exceed the potency of the drug administered. Example m in Table 7a (T7a;22) represents one such active metabolite.

It is somewhat difficult to organize the data associated with C-7 variations into a fully coherent story, as the work has not been done in a systematic fashion. Many of the side-by-side comparisons that an academic wants are not possible, because when various firms investigate the permissible variations in different molecular frameworks, they often do not publish data associated with specific C-7 moieties discussed in the work of others.

Before the discovery of NOR and the subsequent primary focus on various basic groups, a wider variety of C-7 substituents was evaluated. Table 7a shows a comparison of many possible N-1-ethylated entries with NOR and PEF. PEF gives less potent in vitro readings than NOR but is better absorbed. It is convenient, therefore, that demethylation occurs in vivo, thus allowing the best attributes of both drugs to develop progressively in the patient's body. In this grouping, NOR is clearly the best against gram-negative organisms and is bested against gram-positive organisms by only a few entries. As presaged in the classical quinolone era, among the nonbasic (at C-7) analogs, only methyl (T7a;4,5) is much good, and it is at least 1 order of magnitude inferior to NOR both against the enzyme and in intact cells (23, 44). Placing a weakly basic substituent in the molecule by direct attachment of a nitrogen substituent to C-7 through a nucleophilic aromatic displacement reaction (T7a;6,7) improves the situation little against gram-negative organisms but gives improved performance against gram-positive organisms as represented by *S. aureus*. This is particularly true of lipophilic substituents such as piperidinyl (T7a;19). Adding a variety of heteroaromatic ring systems (such as pyrrolyl [T7a;24], 2-furanyl [T7a;34], 3-imidazolyl [T7a;33], and the like) is unfortunately deleterious, even though some of these contain more distal, though feebly basic, amine moieties (16, 23). From a synthetic standpoint, constructing a linkage arm involving sulfur and a more distal amine moiety would be quite convenient. The one entry in Table 7a involving this structure (T7a;8) gave comparatively poor results, even though intact *P. aeruginosa* and, interestingly, the *E. coli*-derived enzyme responded comparatively well to this arrangement (23). This possibility has not been much pursued in the journal literature. When the distal nitrogen substituent is secondary or tertiary, one often gets comparatively good results, and NOR and PEF, of course, represent the best of these in Table 1a. Experience also indicates that groups significantly larger than *N*-methyl at the distal end are poorer in activity, especially against gram-negative organisms, and these are represented by *N*-ethyl (T7a;20) and *N*-benzyl (T7a;21) in Table 7a. These substituents may, however, be removed oxidatively in the body, thus changing the identity and the potency of the drug.

Are these considerations still valid when N-1 carries a cyclopropyl substituent? The data in Table 7b indicate that they basically are. Here CIP is the most prominent member and is the comparator (89). It, of course, carries the same piperazinyl moiety that NOR carries. The *N*-4′-ethyl analog of CIP has been introduced into veterinary practice in Germany under the name enrofloxacin (ENR), but MIC data for this agent are hard to find (26, 32). The principal metabolite of ENR and its methyl homolog is CIP itself.

**Table 7a.** MICs of molecules in the C-6-fluorinated quinolone series with variations at C-7 where N-1 is ethyl

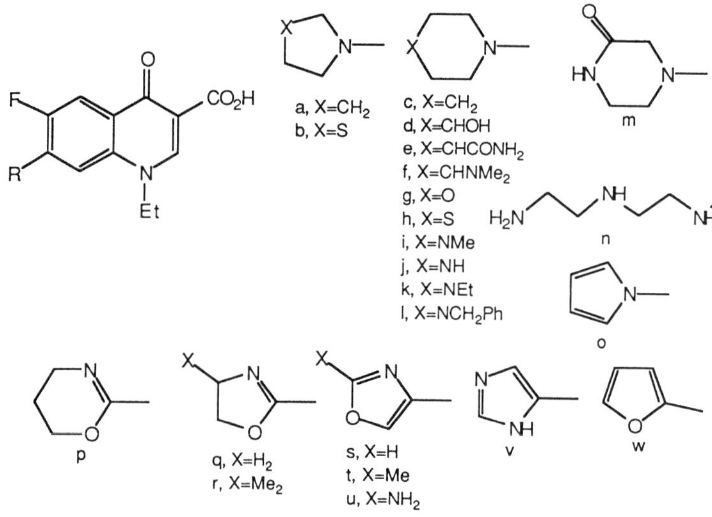

a, X=$CH_2$; b, X=S

c, X=$CH_2$; d, X=CHOH; e, X=$CHCONH_2$; f, X=$CHNMe_2$; g, X=O; h, X=S; i, X=NMe; j, X=NH; k, X=NEt; l, X=$NCH_2Ph$

m; n; o; p

q, X=$H_2$; r, X=$Me_2$

s, X=H; t, X=Me; u, X=$NH_2$

v; w

| Drug | R | MIC (μg/ml) for: Ec | Pa | Sa | Gyrase cleavage (μg/ml) | Reference |
|---|---|---|---|---|---|---|
| | H | 0.8 | >100 | >100 | 50 | 44 |
| | Cl | 1.56 | 100 | 12.5 | | 44 |
| | Cl | 0.8 | 50 | 3.1 | 38 | 23 |
| | Me | 0.39 | 50 | 6.25 | | 44 |
| | Me | 0.2 | 12.5 | 16 | 25 | 23 |
| | $NMe_2$ | 0.39 | 50 | 0.78 | | 44 |
| | NHMe | 3.1 | >100 | 12.5 | 18 | 23 |
| | $S(CH_2)_2NH_2$ | 0.8 | 3.1 | 25 | 5 | 23 |
| | a | 0.39 | 12.5 | 0.2 | | 44 |
| | a | 1.6 | >100 | 0.8 | 5 | 23 |
| | b | 0.2 | 3.1 | 0.2 | 5 | 23 |
| | c | 1.56 | 5.0 | 0.78 | | 44 |
| | d | 0.2 | 12.5 | 0.39 | | 44 |
| | e | 1.56 | 100 | 1.56 | | 44 |
| | f | 0.1 | 3.13 | 0.39 | | 44 |
| | g | 0.2 | 12.5 | 0.78 | | 44 |
| | h | 0.1 | 0.8 | 0.006 | 5 | 23 |
| PEF | i | 0.1 | 1.56 | 0.39 | | 44 |
| NOR | j | 0.025 | 0.2 | 0.8 | 1 | 23 |
| | k | 0.1 | 3.13 | 0.39 | | 44 |
| | l | 0.78 | 50 | 0.39 | | 44 |
| | m | 0.39 | 12.5 | 3.13 | | 44 |
| | n | 6.25 | 50 | >100 | | 44 |
| IRL | o | 1.6 | 12.5 | 0.4 | 2.5 | 23 |
| | $CO_2H$ | >100 | >100 | >100 | | 16 |
| | $CONH(CH_2)_2OH$ | >100 | >100 | >100 | | 16 |
| | p | 50 | >100 | 50 | | 16 |
| | q | 12.5 | >100 | 25 | | 16 |
| | r | >100 | >100 | 25 | | 16 |
| | s | 12.5 | >100 | 6.2 | | 16 |
| | t | 6.2 | 50 | 1.56 | | 16 |
| | u | 50 | >100 | 12.5 | | 16 |
| | v | 25 | >100 | 12.5 | | 16 |
| | w | 12.5 | >100 | 1.56 | | 16 |

**Table 7b.** MICs of molecules in the C-6-fluorinated quinolone series with variations at C-7 where N-1 is cyclopropyl

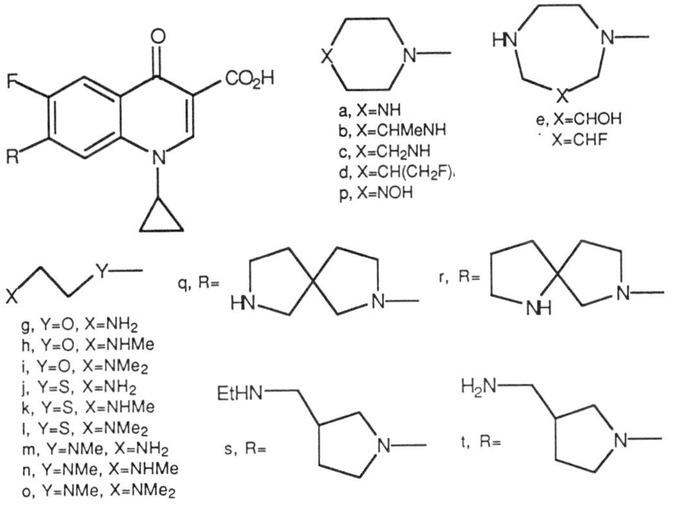

O
$CO_2H$
F
R
N
X
N—
a, X=NH
b, X=CHMeNH
c, X=$CH_2$NH
d, X=CH($CH_2$F)
p, X=NOH
HN
N—
X
e, X=CHOH
X=CHF
Y—
X
g, Y=O, X=$NH_2$
h, Y=O, X=NHMe
i, Y=O, X=$NMe_2$
j, Y=S, X=$NH_2$
k, Y=S, X=NHMe
l, Y=S, X=$NMe_2$
m, Y=NMe, X=$NH_2$
n, Y=NMe, X=NHMe
o, Y=NMe, X=$NMe_2$
q, R=
HN
N—
r, R=
NH
N—
EtHN
s, R=
N—
$H_2N$
t, R=
N—


| Drug | R | MIC (μg/ml) for: Ec | Pa | Sa | Sp | Kp | Reference |
|---|---|---|---|---|---|---|---|
| CIP | a | 0.025 | 0.2 | 0.2 | | 0.012 | 88 |
| | b | 0.015 | 0.25 | 0.12 | | | 92 |
| | c | 0.03 | 1 | 0.25 | | | 92 |
| | d | 0.06 | 2 | 0.12 | | | 92 |
| | e | 0.25 | 2 | 4 | | | 92 |
| | f | 0.03 | 2 | 0.25 | | | 92 |
| | g | 0.2 | 1.56 | 3.13 | | 0.1 | 88 |
| | h | 0.2 | 1.56 | 3.13 | | 0.2 | 88 |
| | i | 0.2 | 3.13 | 1.56 | | 0.1 | 88 |
| | j | 0.1 | 0.39 | 0.78 | | 0.05 | 88 |
| | k | 0.2 | 1.56 | 1.56 | | 0.1 | 88 |
| | l | 0.39 | 6.25 | 3.13 | | 0.1 | 88 |
| | m | 0.78 | 3.13 | 1.56 | | 0.2 | 88 |
| | n | 0.78 | 6.25 | 3.13 | | 0.2 | 88 |
| | o | 0.78 | 25 | 6.25 | | 0.2 | 88 |
| | p | 0.1 | 1.56 | 0.39 | | 0.025 | 81 |
| | q | 0.2 | 1.6 | 0.2 | 0.1 | 0.4 | 19 |
| | r | 0.025 | 0.2 | 0.05 | 0.4 | 0.1 | 19 |
| | s | 0.05 | 0.4 | 0.025 | 0.025 | 0.1 | 19 |
| | t | 0.013 | 0.1 | 0.05 | 0.05 | 0.025 | 19 |

Whereas a number of the entries are equally effective against gram-positive *S. aureus*, only the third entry (T7b;3) (with an expanded ring) (92) and the third-from-last entry (T7b;18) (with a spiroamino moiety) (19) are equivalent when all of the organisms are considered. The latter entry emphasizes the comparative degrees of freedom the chemist has in preparing new structures to evaluate. A number of other bases convey useful activity to this molecule but are not superior to CIP itself. An interesting series (T7b;7–15) addresses a question posed in considering the last table: what connector is best put proximal

**Table 7c.** MICs for molecules in the *C*-6,8-difluoroquinolone series with variants at C-7 where N-1 is cyclopropyl

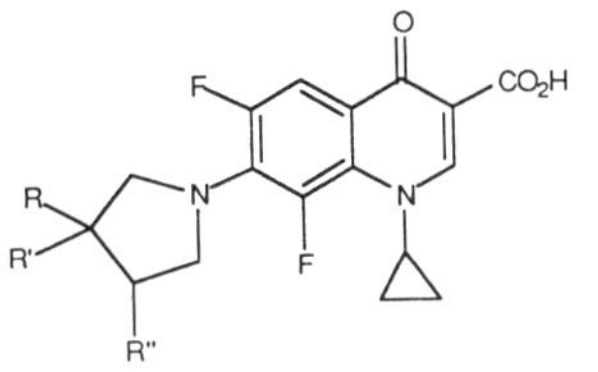

| R | R′ | R″ | MIC (μg/ml) for: Ec | Pa | Sa | Kp | Gyrase cleavage (μg/ml) | References |
|---|---|---|---|---|---|---|---|---|
| $NH_2$ | H | H | 0.013 | 0.1 | 0.05 | 0.025 | 0.1 | 33, 34 |
| $CH_2NH_2$ | H | H | 0.025 | 0.2 | 0.025 | 0.05 | 0.25 | 33, 34 |
| $CH_2NH_2$ | Ph | H | 0.05 | 0.8 | 0.025 | 0.1 | 2.6 | 33, 34 |
| $CH_2NHEt$ | Ph | H | 0.4 | 3.1 | 0.1 | 0.8 | 2.6 | 33, 34 |
| $CH_2NMe_2$ | Ph | H | 0.05 | 0.4 | 0.05 | 0.1 | 2.6 | 33, 34 |
| $NH_2$ | Ph | H | 0.025 | 0.2 | 0.013 | 0.05 | 0.55 | 33, 34 |
| $NH_2$ | H | Ph | 0.1 | 1.6 | 0.05 | 0.2 | 2.7 | 33, 34 |
| $CH_2NH_2$ | H | Ph | 0.1 | 1.6 | 0.013 | 0.1 | 2.6 | 33, 34 |
| $NH_2$ | Me | H | 0.2 | 3.1 | 0.8 | 0.4 | 0.8 | 33, 34 |
| $CH_2NH_2$ | Me | H | 0.5 | 0.4 | 0.013 | 0.1 | 2.6 | 33, 34 |

to the benzene ring? One cannot give a definitive answer from this set of data, but the trend is clearly S > O > N when the chains terminate with identical distal substituents. Unfortunately for extending this concept, only N has sufficient valences to support a heteroaliphatic ring system.

Table 7c includes data for a selection of *N*-1-cyclopropyl analogs related to those in Table 7b but with an additional fluorine substituent at C-8 (33). In this study, the C-7 substituent is a pyrrolidinyl moiety containing an amine substituent at the C-3′ position. The most generally potent of these analogs is that with a C-3′ primary amino group (T7c;1). Relative potency against *S. aureus* differs in this regard. Here, the addition of a phenyl group on the amine-bearing carbon is rather advantageous (T7c;6). Potency against the other organisms is slightly less, however, with this addition. Compared with CIP (data in Table 7b), the best compound in Table 7c (T7c;1) gives better results against gram-negative organisms and *S. aureus*. In terms of directly comparable compounds, entry 2 in Table 7c is analogous to the last entry in Table 7b. They are roughly comparable in potency, and thus a fluorine at C-8 has little effect here.

The data in Table 7d supplement those in Table 7b. Here, a small series demonstrated that an oxygen linker attaching side chain elements to C-7 was intermediate in desirability between N and S. As expected, none of the analogs in Table 7d gives potencies as good as those for CIP. The effect of optical asymmetry at C-7 is minimal in this series (T7d;4,5), which agrees with general experience in the quinolone field. With the exception of *K. pneumoniae*, in which the effect is generally better, this oxygen-linked series is less active (88). It is also interesting that the range of variation in MICs is not very large throughout this whole series, consisting primarily of one tube difference except against *P. aeruginosa*, where a four-tube range is seen.

On the basis of preliminary work in Table 7b and the results illustrated in Table 7d, the sulfur-linked series illustrated in Table 7e

**Table 7d.** MICs of molecules in the *C*-6,8-difluoroquinolone series with variants linked through oxygen at C-7[a]

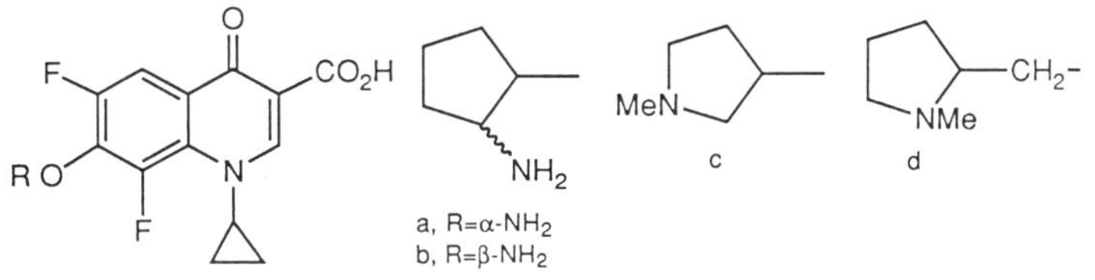

a, R=α-$NH_2$
b, R=β-$NH_2$

| R | MIC (μg/ml) for: | | | |
|---|---|---|---|---|
| | Ec | Pa | Sa | Kp |
| CIP | 0.025 | 0.2 | 0.2 | 0.012 |
| $CH_2CH_2NH_2$ | 0.1 | 0.78 | 1.56 | 0.1 |
| $CH_2CHMeCH_2$ | 0.1 | 0.78 | 1.56 | 0.05 |
| (R) | 0.1 | 0.39 | 1.56 | 0.05 |
| (S) | 0.1 | 0.78 | 1.56 | 0.05 |
| $CH_2CMe_2NH_2$ | 0.2 | 1.56 | 0.78 | 0.05 |
| $CHMeCH_2NH_2$ | 0.2 | 0.78 | 1.56 | 0.1 |
| a | 0.2 | 3.13 | 0.78 | 0.1 |
| b | 0.2 | 1.56 | 1.56 | 0.1 |
| c | 0.2 | 1.56 | 1.56 | 0.1 |
| d | 0.2 | 3.13 | 1.56 | 0.1 |

[a]Data are from reference 89.

would be expected to show a continued increase in potency. SPA (see also Table 7f) is included as comparator; it is more potent than any of the new analogs (67). While there are no directly comparable analogs, the trend is definitely to less potency except against *S. aureus,* where the result is again idiosyncratic. It is generally true with the quinolones that it is often difficult to find a collection of substituents that cause an increase in potency against all of the organisms tested. The directions of responses of gram-negative organisms all too often are opposite those of gram-positive organisms. That is certainly the case in Table 7e.

Table 7f contains a number of *C*-7-piperazinyl-*C*-6,8-difluoroquinolones with an amino group at C-5. SPA is the comparator (57). These data suggest that the piperazinyl group is not in close contact to a space-demanding receptor area, as significant variations in numbers, positions, identities, and stereochemistries of the groups attached to the piperazinyl carbons result in generally satisfactory potency. SPA is one of the better compounds in Table 7f but not against all of the organisms tested. Once again, comparison of absolute stereochemical isomers (T7f;4,5) demonstrates only a twofold difference in potency, i.e., not much different from the general day-to-day variation seen in the test results themselves. One speculates that the inclusion of alkyl groups in the piperazinyl ring is intended primarily to decrease metabolism and/or modulate pharmaceutical properties.

One of the problems seen with some C-8 halogenated derivatives in animal and clinical studies is phototoxicity. This does not seem to be a severe problem, but it is a clear disadvantage in a crowded and highly competitive field. One way to get around this problem is to use a different substituent, such as the C-8 methyl group. Table 7g collects data for a series of these molecules compared with CIP (56). With a comparable C-7 substituent, the C-8 methyl group gives comparable potencies except against *P. aeruginosa,* where

**Table 7e.** MICs of variants in the *C*-6,8-difluoroquinolone series with sulfur at C-7[a]

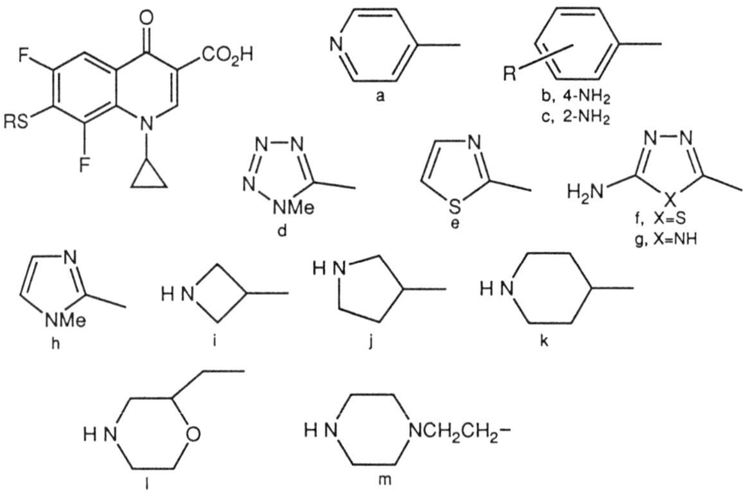

| R | MIC (μg/ml) for: Ec | Pa | Sa |
|---|---|---|---|
| SPA | 0.025 | 0.2 | 0.05 |
| $CH_2CH_2NH_2$ | 0.1 | 0.78 | 0.39 |
| $CH_2CH_2NMe_2$ | 0.39 | 6.25 | 3.13 |
| Me | 0.2 | 1.56 | 0.2 |
| Et | 0.78 | 3.13 | 0.78 |
| $CH_2Ph$ | 3.13 | >100 | 0.78 |
| $CH_2CH_2OH$ | 0.39 | 3.13 | 0.78 |
| a | 3.13 | 12.5 | 0.78 |
| b | 1.56 | 6.25 | 0.2 |
| c | 1.56 | 6.25 | 0.39 |
| d | 6.25 | 100 | 12.5 |
| e | 0.78 | 6.25 | 0.39 |
| f | 12.5 | 100 | 6.25 |
| g | 25 | >100 | 6.25 |
| h | 6.25 | 100 | 6.25 |
| $HO_2CCH(NH_2)CH_2$ | 50 | >100 | 50 |
| i | 0.39 | 0.78 | 0.78 |
| j | 3.13 | 1.56 | 0.78 |
| k | 0.78 | 3.13 | 0.39 |
| l | 0.78 | 3.13 | 0.78 |
| m | 3.13 | 25 | 1.56 |

[a]Data are from reference 67.

some falling off is seen. With *S. aureus,* as is often the case, potency moves in an opposite direction. The usual piperazinyl (T7g;2) and piperidinyl (T7g;8,9) moieties cost potency. When the substituent is changed to a substituted pyrrolidinyl moiety, however, some quite potent analogs are seen (T7g;12–15), especially against gram-positive organisms. These data remind us again that introduction of a given substituent at a given position does not necessarily produce the same potency increment against all organisms. In some cases

**Table 7f.** MICs of molecules related to the 5-amino-6,8-difluoroquinolone SPA with variations at C-7

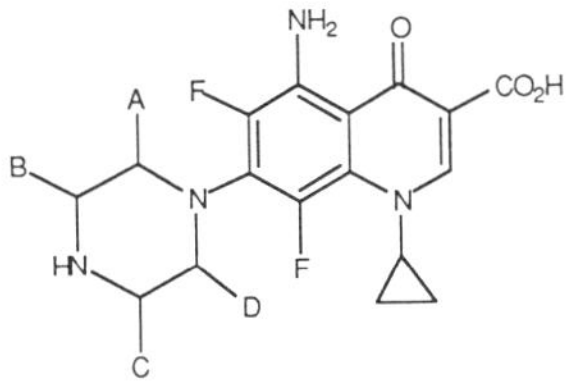

| Drug | A | B | C | D | MIC ($\mu$g/ml) for: | | |
|---|---|---|---|---|---|---|---|
| | | | | | Ec | Pa | Sa |
| | H | H | H | H | 0.0125 | 0.39 | 0.2 |
| | Me | H | H | H | 0.05 | 0.78 | 0.2 |
| | H | Me | H | H | 0.0063 | 0.2 | 0.025 |
| | H | (*S*)-Me | H | H | 0.0063 | 0.1 | 0.025 |
| | H | (*R*)-Me | H | H | 0.0125 | 0.2 | 0.05 |
| | Me | Me | H | H | 0.0125 | 0.78 | 0.025 |
| | H | $Me_2$ | H | H | 0.025 | 0.78 | 0.05 |
| | H | (*R*)-Me | H | (*S*)-Me | 0.39 | 3.13 | 0.78 |
| SPA | H | $\beta$-Me | $\beta$-Me | H | 0.0125 | 0.39 | 0.05 |
| | H | $\alpha$-Me | $\beta$-Me | H | 0.0125 | 0.78 | 0.025 |
| | H | $CH_2OH$ | H | H | 0.025 | 0.2 | 0.05 |
| | H | $CH_2F$ | H | H | 0.0063 | 0.2 | 0.025 |
| | H | $CH_2NMe_2$ | H | H | 0.1 | 1.56 | 0.05 |

[a]Data are from reference 57.

the change is indifferent, in others it is favorable, and in yet others it is unfavorable. Medicinal chemistry is a young science, and precedent carries us only so far. We are often surprised and puzzled when the compounds are actually made and tested.

Attaching a 4′-pyridinyl moiety to C-7 does not ordinarily lead to high in vitro potency (see Ta;ROS and T6b;1–3 for examples). In medicinal chemistry, a sulfur atom is often considered roughly equivalent to an olefinic linkage. Such substitution interchanges that lead to retention of potency are referred to as bioisosterism. Thus, a thiazolyl ring can be considered pharmacologically equivalent to a pyridyl ring or a benzene ring. Table 7h presents a series of analogs in which the orientation of the thiazolyl ring differs. Regardless of whether a basic or nonbasic substituent was appended, none of these analogs had significant antimicrobial potency (90, 91).

In Table 7i, a series of C-7 variants in the *N*-1-*tert*-butyl series is compared with CIP and with the closest analog (structure a) (7). Except against gram-positive *S. aureus,* the *tert*-butyl group gives somewhat less potency. The most difficult organism in Table 7i against which to get good potency is *P. aeruginosa.* None of the analogs comes up to CIP in this regard. On the other hand, compound c (T7i;4) is clearly superior against all the other organisms. In this particular grouping, no data on the two optically active forms of this potentially chiral molecule are given. Judging from experience with other series, the difference will probably not be significant. Given the huge number of analogs with piperazinyl substituents and the resulting congestion of the patent literature, it is interesting that a significant number of bicyclo analogs retain usable activity (T7i;8–11). The variation in potency with antipodes (T7i;10 and 11) is at most fourfold in this series.

**Table 7g.** MICs of molecules in the C-8 methylfluoroquinolone series with variations at C-7[a]

a, X=NH, R=H
b, X=NMe, R=H
c, X=NH, R=Me
d, X=NMe, R=Me
e, X=NCHO, R=Me
f, X=NAc, R=Me
g, X=CO, R=H
h, X=CHOH, R=H
i, X=O, R=H
j, X=O, R=Me

k, R=H, R'=NHMe
l, R=H, R'=$CH_2NH_2$
m, R=Me, R'=$NH_2$
n, R=Me, R'=α-$NH_2$

| R | MIC (μg/ml) for: | | |
|---|---|---|---|
| | Ec | Pa | Sa |
| CIP | 0.024 | 0.2 | 0.2 |
| a | 0.024 | 0.39 | 0.1 |
| b | 0.024 | 0.78 | 0.1 |
| c | 0.024 | 0.39 | 0.1 |
| d | 0.024 | 1.56 | 0.1 |
| e | 0.39 | 6.25 | 0.024 |
| f | 0.78 | 12.5 | 0.05 |
| g | 0.1 | 1.56 | 0.006 |
| h | 0.1 | 1.56 | 0.012 |
| i | 0.1 | 0.78 | 0.012 |
| j | 0.2 | 0.78 | 0.012 |
| k | 0.006 | 0.39 | 0.024 |
| l | 0.012 | 0.39 | 0.006 |
| m | 0.006 | 0.1 | 0.024 |
| n | 0.012 | 0.2 | 0.024 |

[a]Data are from reference 56.

**Table 7h.** MICs of quinolones with benzene bioisosteres at C-7

| R | MIC (μg/ml) for[a]: | | | |
|---|---|---|---|---|
| | Ec | Pa | Sa | Kp |
| H | 6.25 | 50 | 6.25 | 6.25 |
| Me | 50 | >100 | 12.5 | 25 |
| $NH_2$ | 12.5 | 50 | 3.12 | 3.12 |
| $NMe_2$ | >100 | >100 | 6.25 | 25 |
| a | >100 | >100 | 3.12 | >100 |
| Ph | >100 | >100 | 1.6 | >100 |

| R | R′ | MIC (μg/ml) for[b]: | | | |
|---|---|---|---|---|---|
| | | Ec | Pa | Sa | Kp |
| Me | H | 50 | >100 | 6.25 | 25 |
| Me | Me | >100 | >100 | 3.12 | >100 |
| Ph | H | >100 | >100 | 3.12 | >100 |

[a]Data are from reference 90.
[b]Data are from reference 91.

These bicyclic analogs would likely be metabolized in vivo differently from compound a (T7i;2), for example.

Table 7j shows a number of naphthyridine analogs related to the quinolones in Table 7i (7). When similarly substituted analogs in the two series are compared, it is difficult to detect a completely consistent trend between them. In some cases, the quinolone is the more active, and in other cases, the naphthyridine is. The differences are often not large, however. Of all the compounds in the table, the *trans*-3′-amino-4′-methyl analog (T7j;19) stands out as exceptionally potent across the board. It is also superior to the analogs in Table 7i.

One of the more prominent of the *N*-1-aryl analogs is TEM. Its in vitro spectrum is set forth in Table 7k. From this and the other items in the table, it is clear that a *C*-7-piperazinyl (T7k;1) or a 3-aminopyrrolidinyl (T7l;7) group is also superior in the *N*-aryl series. Increasing the steric bulk of the amino group by alkylation decreases activity. In all these series, the piperazinyl or aminopyrrolidinyl substituents consistently produce the most interesting analogs. The data in Table 7l address the question of whether this is also true in the *N*-1-(2′,4′-difluorophenyl) series based on the naphthyridine ring system.

**Table 7i.** MICs of molecules in the *N*-1-*t*-butyl-*C*-6-fluoroquinolone series with variations at C-7[a]

a, R=R'=H
c, R=H, R'=Me
d, R=R'=Me
e, R=H, R'=Ph
f, R=H, R'=$CH_2F$
i, (1R, 4R)
j, (1S, 4S)
k, R=H, R'=$NH_2$
l, R=H, R'=$CH_3$, $NH_2$
m, R=H, R'=$CH_2NH_2$
n, R=H, R'=$CH_2NHEt$

| R | MIC (μg/ml) for: | | | |
|---|---|---|---|---|
| | Ec | Pa | Sa | Kp |
| CIP | 0.03 | 0.13 | 0.13 | 0.03 |
| a | 0.06 | 0.5 | 0.06 | 0.13 |
| b | 0.03 | 0.5 | 0.03 | 0.25 |
| c | 0.008 | 1 | 0.06 | 0.015 |
| d | 0.13 | 4 | 0.25 | 0.5 |
| e | 0.06 | 1 | 0.06 | 0.25 |
| f | 0.25 | 4 | 0.13 | 0.13 |
| g | 0.5 | 4 | 0.13 | 0.13 |
| h | 0.5 | 2 | 0.13 | 0.25 |
| i | 0.5 | 0.5 | 0.5 | 0.13 |
| j | 2 | 1 | 0.25 | 0.5 |
| k | 0.06 | 1 | 0.03 | 0.25 |
| l | 0.5 | 2 | 0.06 | 0.25 |
| m | 0.25 | 0.5 | 0.03 | 0.25 |
| n | 0.25 | 8 | 0.06 | 1 |

[a]Data are from reference 7.

**Table 7j.** MICs of molecules in the *N*-1-*t*-butyl-*C*-6-fluoronaphthyridine series with variations at C-7[a]

a, R=R'=H
c, R=H, R'=Me
d, R=H, R'=Ph
e, R=H, R'=$CH_2F$
i, (1R, 4R)
j, (1S, 4S)
k, R=$NH_2$
l, H=NHMe
m, R=NHEt
n, R=$NMe_2$
o, R=Me,$NH_2$
p, R=$CH_2NH_2$
q, R=$CH_2NHEt$
r, R=Me, R'=$NH_2$
s, R=Me, R'=α-$NH_2$
t, R=Et, R'=$NH_2$
u, R=Et, R'=α-$NH_2$
v, R=F, R'=$NH_2$
w, R=α-F, R'=$NH_2$
x, R=F, R'=$CH_2NH_2$
y, R=α-F, R'=$CH_2NH_2$

| R | MIC (μg/ml) for: | | | |
|---|---|---|---|---|
| | Ec | Pa | Sa | Kp |
| a | 0.015 | 1 | 0.06 | 0.13 |
| b | 0.06 | 1 | 0.06 | 0.06 |
| c | 0.5 | 8 | 0.13 | 2 |
| d | 0.06 | 4 | 0.03 | 0.06 |
| e | 0.13 | 4 | 0.13 | 0.13 |
| f | 0.13 | 4 | 0.06 | 0.13 |
| g | 0.06 | 2 | 0.06 | 0.13 |
| h | 0.13 | 1 | 0.03 | 0.13 |
| i | 0.06 | 0.25 | 0.06 | 0.06 |
| j | 0.13 | 0.5 | 0.13 | 0.13 |
| k | 0.13 | 2 | 0.015 | 0.25 |
| l | 0.06 | 2 | 0.06 | 0.13 |
| m | 0.06 | 4 | 0.06 | 0.06 |
| n | 0.25 | 1 | 0.03 | 0.13 |
| o | 0.06 | 2 | 0.015 | 0.06 |
| p | 0.5 | 1 | 0.03 | 0.25 |
| q | 0.13 | 2 | 0.13 | 0.25 |
| r | 0.25 | 0.5 | 0.015 | 0.03 |
| s | 0.015 | 0.25 | 0.008 | 0.015 |
| t | 0.13 | 1 | 0.015 | 0.13 |
| u | 0.03 | 1 | 0.015 | 0.06 |
| v | 0.25 | 2 | 0.015 | 0.06 |
| w | 0.5 | 2 | 0.003 | 0.5 |
| x | 0.06 | 0.5 | 0.015 | 0.25 |
| y | 0.06 | 0.5 | 0.004 | 0.13 |

[a]Data are from reference 7.

Here, ENO is the comparator (61–65). The 3'-aminopyrrolidyl substituent (T7l;7) gives the best results across the board in vitro, and the best compound, known as TOS, has been examined clinically.

To sum up, then, investigations on variants at the C-7 position carried out over a quarter of a century reinforce the present belief that great latitude is available for successful variation provided that a basic atom is present and that the overall superstructure does not exceed fairly permissive size limits. The attachment of the C-7 substituent is made best through S, less well through O, and most poorly through N. Carbon linkages, presumably because of synthetic inconvenience, have been explored far less. In general, these considerations apply to most of the ring systems and their currently popular subvariants. Simultaneous optimization against gram-positive and gram-negative organisms with a given substituent is not common. The influence of stereochemistry on potency is not pronounced.

**Table 7k.** MICs of molecules in the *C*-6-fluoroquinolone series with variations in the C-7 substituents

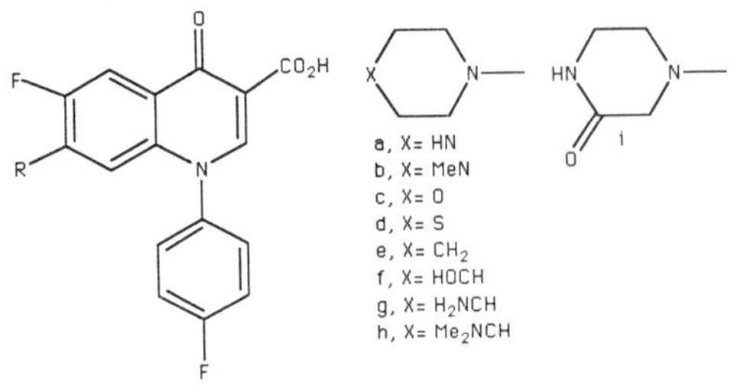
O
$CO_2H$
F
R
N
F
X
N—
HN
N—
O
i
a, X= HN
b, X= MeN
c, X= O
d, X= S
e, X= $CH_2$
f, X= HOCH
g, X= $H_2NCH$
h, X= $Me_2NCH$

| Drug | R | MIC (μg/ml) for[a]: | | |
|---|---|---|---|---|
| | | Ec | Pa | Sa |
| A-56620 | a | 0.05 | 0.39 | 0.20 |
| Difloxacin | b | 0.2 | 1.56 | 0.20 |
| | c | 0.39 | 3.1 | 0.1 |
| | d | 0.78 | 3.1 | 0.05 |
| | e | 1.56 | 6.2 | 0.2 |
| | f | 0.39 | 6.2 | 0.1 |
| | g | 0.02 | 0.2 | 0.05 |
| | h | 0.39 | 25 | 0.39 |
| | i | 0.39 | 6.2 | 0.2 |

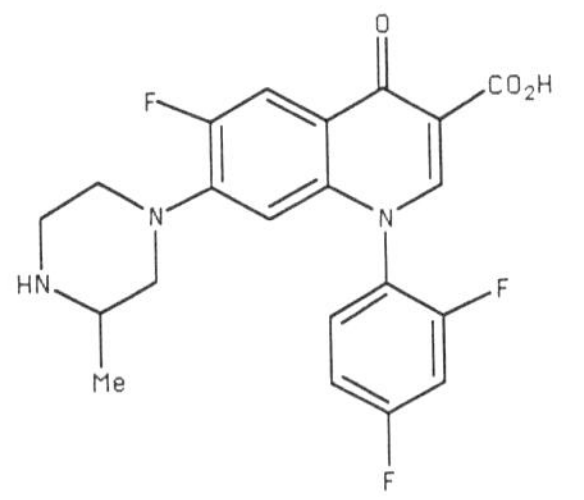
O
$CO_2H$
F
N
N
HN
Me
F
F

| Drug | MIC (μg/ml) for[b]: | | | | |
|---|---|---|---|---|---|
| | Sp | Bf | Ec | Pa | Sa |
| TEM | 1.0 | 1.0 | 0.06 | 1.0 | 0.06 |

[a]Data are from reference 11.
[b]Data are from reference 35.

**Table 7l.** MICs of molecules in the *C*-6-fluoronaphthyridine series with variations in the C-7 substituent where N-1 is 2,4-difluorophenyl[a]

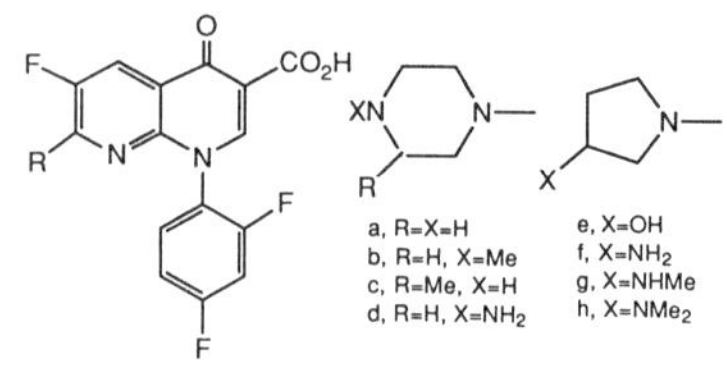
O
$CO_2H$
F
R
N
N
F
F
XN
N—
R
N—
X
a, R=X=H
b, R=H, X=Me
c, R=Me, X=H
d, R=H, X=$NH_2$
e, X=OH
f, X=$NH_2$
g, X=NHMe
h, X=$NMe_2$

| Drug | R | MIC (μg/ml) for: | | |
|---|---|---|---|---|
| | | Ec | Pa | Sa |
| ENO | | 0.05 | 0.78 | 0.78 |
| | a | 0.05 | 0.78 | 0.2 |
| | b | 0.1 | 3.13 | 0.39 |
| | c | 0.05 | 3.13 | 0.39 |
| | d | 0.05 | 0.39 | 0.2 |
| | e | 0.05 | 3.13 | 0.05 |
| TOS | f | 0.05 | 0.2 | 0.05 |
| | g | 0.05 | 1.56 | 0.2 |
| | h | 0.1 | 12.5 | 0.39 |

[a]Data are from reference 62.

## VARIATIONS AT C-8

Table 8a contains a comparison of the most commonly employed structural variants at the C-8 position, with a number of prominent contenders. With this particular substitution pattern, there is little difference in potencies against the indicator organisms between the quinolones, represented by NOR, and the naphthyridines, represented by ENO. When a fluoro atom is attached, represented by CI-934, potency against *E. coli* is roughly maintained, potency against *P. aeruginosa* slips, and activity against *S. aureus* improves (8). Thus, the trends associated with these changes are variable depending on the microorganism. Generally, an 8-aza analog is better absorbed in vivo, providing a complicating feature.

Table 8b continues the comparison of the same structural variations when N-1 contains a cyclopropyl group (8, 24, 85). The result is not the same as with N-1 ethyl. Against *E. coli* DNA gyrase, the order is clearly CH > CF > N, and the same order is seen against intact *E. coli,* as might be expected. Against *S. aureus,* the order is CF > CH = N, whereas against *P. aeruginosa,* the order becomes N > CH > CF. No clear pattern emerges from this small sampling, leading to the conclusion that activity against a given pathogen probably must be optimized in each

**Table 8a.** Comparison of NOR, ENO, CI-934, FLE, and LOM, with variations in C-8 substituents

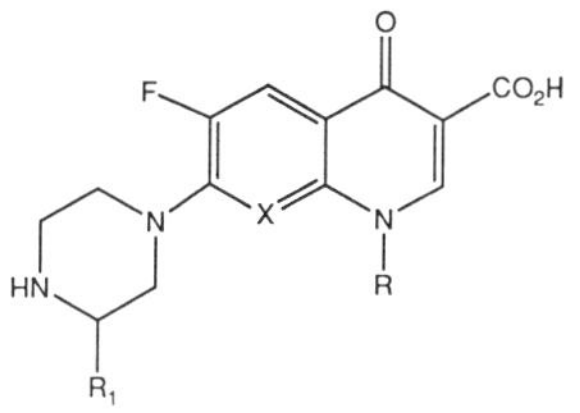

| Drug | X | R | $R_1$ | MIC ($\mu$g/ml) for: Ec | Pa | Kp | Sa | Sp | Bf | Reference |
|---|---|---|---|---|---|---|---|---|---|---|
| NOR | CH | Et | H | 0.13 | 0.5 | | 0.25 | | | 8 |
| | | | | 0.025 | 0.2 | 0.05 | 0.8 | 1.6 | | 23 |
| ENO | N | Et | H | 0.13 | 0.5 | 0.5 | 0.25 | | | 8 |
| CI-934 | CF | Et | H | 0.1 | 1.6 | | 0.05 | | | 8 |
| FLE | CF | $CH_2CH_2F$ | H | 0.05 | 0.39 | 0.1 | 0.1 | 3.13 | 6.25 | 37 |
| | | | | 0.12[a] | 1.0[a] | 0.35[a] | 0.5[a] | 4.0[a] | 8.0[a] | 86 |
| LOM | CF | Et | Me | 0.12[a] | 1.0[a] | 0.25[a] | 1.0[a] | 8.0[a] | 8.0[a] | 86 |

[a]MIC for 50% of isolates.

**Table 8b.** MICs of molecules with variations in C-8 substituents where N-1 is cyclopropyl

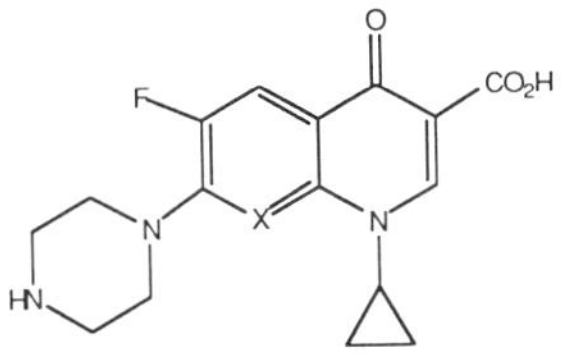

| Drug | X | MIC ($\mu$g/ml) for: Ec | Pa | Sa | Bf | DNA gyrase $IC_{50}$ ($\mu$g/ml) | Reference(s) |
|---|---|---|---|---|---|---|---|
| CIP | CH | 0.004 | 0.125 | 0.25 | 2 | 0.03 | 25 |
| ENO | N | 0.06 | 0.06 | 0.25 | | 5.3 | 8, 24 |
| | CF | 0.03 | 0.25 | 0.13 | | 2.8 | 8, 24 |

ring system specifically and probably in each N-1 substituent subgroup. This is hardly comforting news to quinolone research managers.

In the molecule shown in Table 8c, the N-1 substituent of Table 8b is maintained but the C-7 piperazinyl moiety is changed to 3′-aminopyrrolidyl; a wider range of C-8 substituents is thus available for examination (77). Once again, the rank ordering of N versus CH versus CF gives a different ranking for each organism, but the differences are quite small and may not be meaningful. Within the quinolone series (X = CR), as long as the substituent is comparatively small (chlorine is roughly the size of a methyl group, and fluorine is roughly the size of a hydrogen), there is not much variation in potency. There is a modest tendency to favor the halogens. Against the enzyme, size seems to be more of a factor, as CCl (T8c;3) is disfavored significantly. Since the result is not paralleled with

**Table 8c.** MICs of molecules in the *C*-7-3-aminopyrrolidinyl series with variations in C-8 substituents[a]

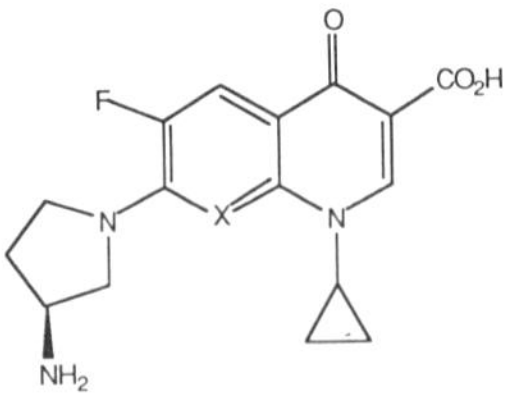

| X | MIC ($\mu$g/ml) for: | | | DNA gyrase cleavage ($\mu$g/ml) |
|---|---|---|---|---|
| | Ec | Pa | Sa | |
| CH | 0.025 | 0.1 | 0.1 | 0.1 |
| CF | 0.013 | 0.1 | 0.05 | 0.1 |
| CCl | 0.013 | 0.05 | 0.05 | 0.5 |
| $CNO_2$ | 0.2 | 1.6 | 0.8 | |
| $CNH_2$ | 0.4 | 1.6 | 3.1 | 18 |
| N | 0.013 | 0.05 | 0.2 | 1.0 |

[a]Data are from reference 77.

**Table 8d.** MICs of molecules in the *C*-7-imidazolyl series with variations in C-8 substituents[a]

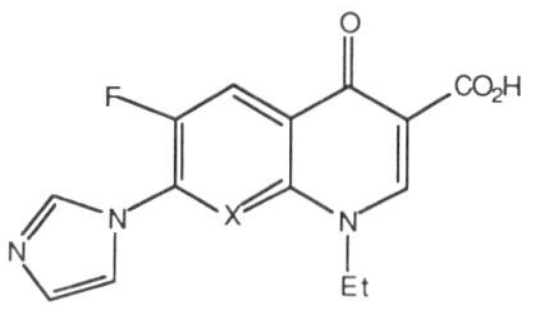

| X | MIC ($\mu$g/ml) for: | | |
|---|---|---|---|
| | Ec | Pa | Sa |
| CH | 1.56 | 12.5 | 6.25 |
| CF | 0.20 | 6.25 | 0.39 |
| $COCH_3$ | 1.56 | 25 | 0.39 |
| $CSCH_3$ | 6.25 | 25 | 3.13 |

[a]Data are from reference 82.

intact *E. coli*, this suggests that there may be facilitated penetration into cells with this substituent. Once the substituent becomes polar or larger, as with nitro (T8c:4) and amino (T8c;5), there is a definite falling off of potency. This parallels the findings for N-1 and may represent operation of the same self-association requirements. When the substances in Tables 8a and 8b with otherwise equivalent substitutions are compared, the results against different microorganisms are variable. The one consistent trend is that activity against *S. aureus* is enhanced by incorporation of a C-7 aminopyrrolidinyl moiety whether C-8 is CH, N, or CF.

Table 8d shows a group of IRL analogs in which CF (T8d;2) at C-8 is preferred across the board (82). The comparative inferiority of CH (T8d;1) against *E. coli* and *S. aureus* is interesting. All other substituents included are inferior except against *S. aureus*, where an *O*-methyl group (roughly the size of an ethyl group) shows good antistaphylococcal activity. The interested reader is reminded that this last is a distant cousin of (surgically altered) OFL (see section below on benzoxazines).

Consider the C-8 methyl substituent again (Table 7g). This substituent is roughly the same size as a chlorine atom, and it has gained in interest lately because of the apparent involvement of C-8 halo substituents in the kind of in vivo phototoxicity that reminds one of the tetracyclines. Table 7g shows that in a case of otherwise identical substitution, CH (T7g;CIP) and *C*-methyl (T7g;2) are roughly equivalent.

In summary, there is some latitude for structural changes at C-8 provided that the groups involved are comparatively small and hydrophobic. The most successful groups to date are F, Cl, and methyl.

## BENZOXAZINES

OFL has been accepted into the clinic in various countries. From the conceptual viewpoint, it can be considered a molecule in which an N-1 ethyl group has been fused with a C-8 methoxy substituent. In other quinolones, N-1-ethyl is, of course, generally favorable, whereas *C*-8-*O*-methyl (T8d;3, for example) was inferior to *C*-8-F (T8d;2) except against *S. aureus*. One might predict a poor result for OFL on the basis of these findings with single substituents. The result, however, is quite favorable. Thus, once

**Table b.** MICs of molecules in the benzoxazine series

a, X=NH
b, X=NMe
e, X=NEt
f, X=N-*n*-Pr
g, X=$CH_2$
h, X=$CHNH_2$
i, X=CHOH

| Drug | Y | R | MIC ($\mu$g/ml) for: | | | Reference |
|---|---|---|---|---|---|---|
| | | | Ec | Pa | Sa | |
| | a | H | <0.05 | 3.13 | 1.56 | 36 |
| OFL | b | $CH_3$ | <0.05 | 1.56 | 0.19 | 36 |
| | b | $CH_3$ | <0.05 | 0.78 | 0.78 | 36 |
| | c | $CH_3$ | <0.05 | 0.39 | <0.05 | 36 |
| | d | $CH_3$ | <0.05 | 6.25 | 0.39 | 36 |
| | b | $-(CH_2CH_2)-$ | 0.125 | 4.0 | 2.0 | 85 |
| | b | $(CH_3)_2$ | 0.5 | 32 | 2.0 | 85 |
| | e | $CH_3$ | <0.05 | 1.56 | 0.39 | 36 |
| | f | $CH_3$ | 0.19 | 6.25 | 0.78 | 36 |
| | g | $CH_3$ | 0.78 | 6.25 | 0.19 | 36 |
| | h | $CH_3$ | 0.19 | 6.25 | 0.39 | 36 |
| | i | $CH_3$ | 0.19 | 6.25 | 0.10 | 36 |
| | $NH_2$ | $CH_3$ | 0.10 | 12.5 | 3.13 | 36 |
| | $N(CH_3)_2$ | $CH_3$ | 0.10 | 6.25 | 0.39 | 36 |

again, fusing substituents produces a better result than is obtained with an independent combination of the individual substituents. The first entry in Table b is equivalent to fusing an 8-*O*-methyl substituent with a methyl at N-1. Prior experience with the classic quinolones suggests that such a change would not be very good, and with the gram-negative organisms in Table b, this is seen to be the case. Against gram-positive *S. aureus,* the OFL *C*-methyl group is definitely helpful (9Tb;2) (36). When the C-7 substituent is changed from a piperazinyl moiety to the equivalent 3′-aminopyrrolidyl (Tb;4), the main consequence is a dramatic enhancement of activity against *S. aureus.* When the less basic imidazolyl group is used (Tb;5), activity falls off somewhat. In general agreement with classical findings, attachment of larger alkyl substituents in place of the methyl leads to significant decreases in in vitro potency across the board (85). When other rings are placed at the carbon equivalent to the quinolone C-7 (Tb;10-12) only potency against *S. aureus* is enhanced (36). As might be surmised, OFL (Tb;2) and its *N*-4′-methyl analog (Tb;3) are the best compromise considering the range of microorganisms represented. Once again, as the size of the substituent becomes excessive or as its basicity decreases substantially, activity generally suffers.

Table c shows a series of OFL analogs in which olefinic linkages are present in the third rings so that no optical isomerism is possible (6, 70, 71). All of these analogs are inferior to their corresponding saturated analogs. When the oxygen linker (Y) is exchanged for a larger sulfur atom, the result is poorer still. Notably, however, when the piperazinyl substituent is exchanged for a

**Table c.** MICs of pyridobenzoxazines and pyridobenzthiazines with variations at C-7

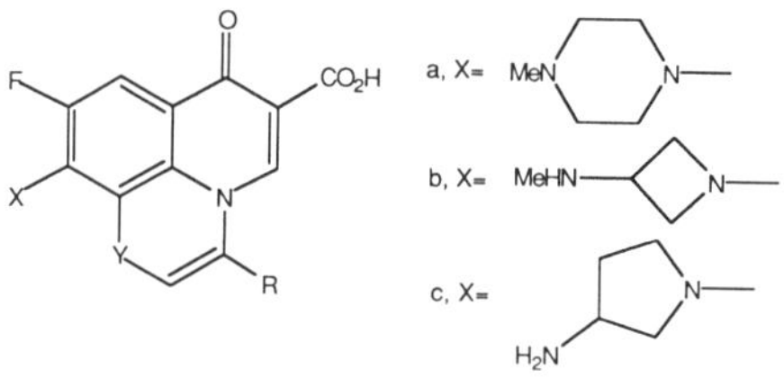

| R | X | Y | MIC ($\mu$g/ml) for: Ec | Pa | Sa | Sp | Reference(s) |
|---|---|---|---|---|---|---|---|
| H | a | O | 0.2 | 6.3 | 1.6 | 25 | 70, 71 |
| H | b | O | 0.2 | 3.1 | 0.8 | 6.3 | 70, 71 |
| Me | a | O | 0.4 | 25 | 6.3 | 12.5 | 70, 71 |
| Me | a | O | 0.39 | 12.5 | 12.5 | | 6 |
| Me | c | O | 0.2 | 3.1 | 0.8 | 6.3 | 70, 71 |
| H | a | S | 50 | >100 | 50 | 50 | 70, 71 |
| H | c | S | 1.6 | 12.5 | 3.1 | 12.5 | 70, 71 |
| H | b | S | 0.05 | 1.6 | 0.2 | 3.1 | 70, 71 |
| Me | b | S | 0.1 | 1.6 | 0.2 | 3.1 | 70, 71 |
| OFL | | | 0.1 | 1.6 | 0.4 | 1.6 | 70, 71 |

3′-methylaminoazetinyl group (Tc;5), greater activity is seen and the result is essentially equivalent to results with OFL itself. This reemphasizes that optimization in a given series of compounds may well not occur with the classical substituents. There is much yet to learn about the quinolones.

Table d shows a series of even more different variants on the OFT system (6, 14, 46, 70, 71). Structure A fuses yet another ring to the nucleus, this one involving sulfur linkage to C-2. Reference to Table 2 reminds us that substituent attachments to structure A are equivalent across the board to OFL. Structure E is essentially 2-methylofloxacin and, in agreement with precedent, is a rather poor molecule. Structures C and D are carried over from Table c for convenience and require no more comment. When the unsaturated linkage of analogs C and D is made exocyclic, as in structure F, activity is enhanced and the analog becomes nearly as potent as OFL. Exchange of the linker from O to S (structure G), however, spoils this improvement except against tolerant *E. coli*.

Table e presents a small additional series of sulfur-linked OFL analogs. These are generally less active in vitro than OFL. Attention is drawn to RUF (9). This analog has recently been introduced into clinics in various countries. When a carbonyl group replaces the hetero atom in the fused third ring, the result (Te;5) is generally inferior (3).

In Table f we see a series of tricyclic derivatives in which the oxygen linker of OFL is replaced by bioisosteric carbon. Historically, the most important of these derivatives is FLU. Although FLU has good in vitro potency against *E. coli* and *S. aureus,* it is not very good against *P. aeruginosa* (30,31). It is interesting that when a piperazinyl moiety is attached to C-7, activity against *P. aeruginosa* is significantly enhanced (Tf;2) (41). The activity-enhancing effect of a C-6 halo group, particularly a fluorine, can be seen by comparing entries 5 through 7 in Table f. Comparing the second and the fifth entries demonstrates again the positive contribution to potency of a branched carbon attached to N-1. Whereas the seventh entry is the most potent against gram-negative organisms, this is not the case against *S. aureus,*

**Table d.** MICs of benzoxazinones

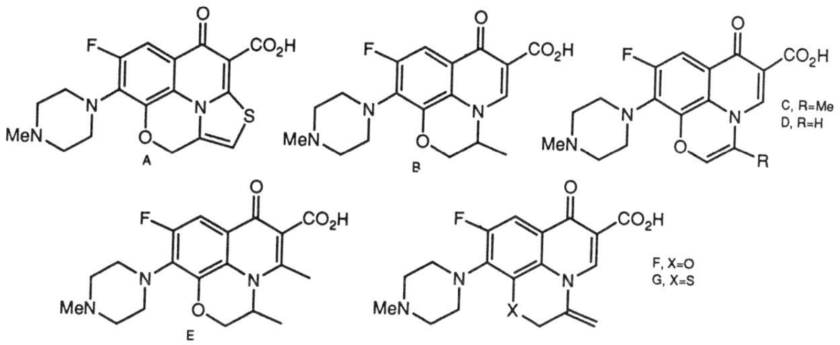

C, R=Me
D, R=H
F, X=O
G, X=S

| Drug | Molecule | MIC (μg/ml) for: Sa | Sp | Ec | Kp | Pa | Bf | Reference |
|---|---|---|---|---|---|---|---|---|
| | A | 0.05–0.39 | 0.39 | 0.013–6.25 | 0.025–0.78 | 0.2–6.25 | 1.56–12.5 | 46 |
| OFL | B | 0.39 | | <0.25 | | 0.25 | | 6 |
| | C | 12.5 | | 0.39 | | 12.5 | | 6 |
| | D | >100 | | 100 | 50 | >100 | | 40 |
| | E | 0.8 | 3.1 | 0.1 | 0.1 | 1.6 | | 71 |
| | F | 0.4 | 1.6 | 0.2 | 0.4 | 3.1 | | 71 |
| | G | 1.6 | 25 | 0.2 | 0.2 | 6.3 | | 70 |

**Table e.** MICs of molecules in the benzothiazine series

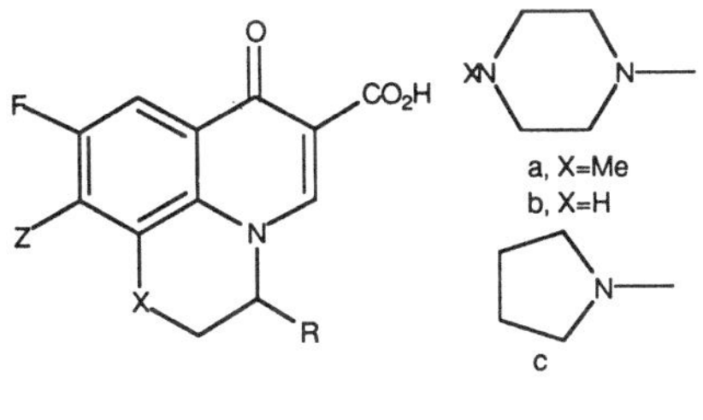

a, X=Me
b, X=H
c

| Drug | R | X | Z | MIC (μg/ml) for: Ec | Pa | Sa | Sp | Bf | Reference |
|---|---|---|---|---|---|---|---|---|---|
| OFL | $CH_3$ | O | a | 0.19 | 1.56 | 0.19 | | | 9 |
| | H | S | c | 1.56 | 3.12 | <0.39 | | | 9 |
| | H | S | b | 0.39 | 12.5 | 0.78 | | | 9 |
| RUF | H | S | a | 0.78 | 12.5 | 0.78 | | | 9 |
| | $CH_3$+ | C=O | a | 0.05–1.56 | 3.13–50 | 0.39–3.13 | 3.13–12.5 | 1.56–25 | 3 |

against which a basic distal nitrogen is not needed. Activity against *P. acnes* in this series likewise follows its own general trend and does not closely parallel that against the other organisms (59).

## OPTICAL ACTIVITY IN THE FLU AND OFL SERIES

The quinolone antiinfective agents are entirely synthetic molecules; thus, they lack in-

**Table f.** MICs of molecules in the FLU series with variations at C-7

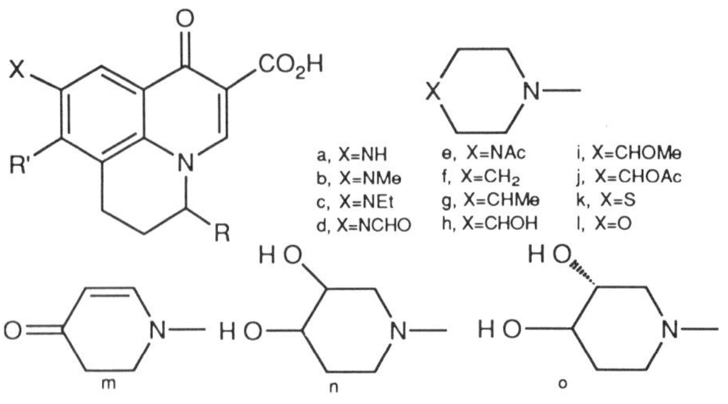

a, X=NH
b, X=NMe
c, X=NEt
d, X=NCHO
e, X=NAc
f, X=$CH_2$
g, X=CHMe
h, X=CHOH
i, X=CHOMe
j, X=CHOAc
k, X=S
l, X=O

| | R | X | R | MIC (μg/ml) for: | | | | Reference |
|---|---|---|---|---|---|---|---|---|
| | | | | Ec | Pa | Sa | Pac | |
| FLU | Me | F | H | 0.2 | 6.2 | 0.05 | | 30 |
| | H | H | a | 3.13 | 6.25 | 12.5 | 12.5 | 41 |
| | H | H | b | 1.56 | 6.25 | 6.25 | 25 | 41 |
| | H | Cl | a | 0.78 | 3.13 | 3.13 | 6.25 | 41 |
| | Me | H | a | 1.56 | 6.25 | 6.25 | 6.25 | 41 |
| | Me | Cl | a | 0.39 | 1.56 | 0.78 | 3.13 | 41 |
| | Me | F | a | 0.2 | 0.78 | 0.39 | 0.76 | 41 |
| | Me | F | b | 0.1 | 1.56 | 0.2 | 0.78 | 41 |
| | Me | F | c | 0.2 | 3.13 | 0.2 | 3.13 | 41 |
| | Me | F | d | 0.39 | 3.13 | 0.05 | 0.2 | 41 |
| | Me | F | e | 0.39 | 3.13 | 0.05 | 0.78 | 41 |
| | Me | F | f | 1.56 | 12.5 | 0.1 | 1.56 | 41 |
| | Me | F | g | 0.78 | 12.5 | 0.2 | 1.56 | 41 |
| | Me | F | h | 0.39 | 3.13 | 0.024 | 0.2 | 41 |
| | Me | F | h | 0.39 | 3.13 | 0.024 | | 59 |
| | Me | F | i | 1.56 | 12.5 | 0.1 | 0.39 | 41 |
| | Me | F | j | 0.39 | 3.13 | 0.1 | 0.78 | 41 |
| | Me | F | k | 0.2 | 3.13 | 0.05 | 0.78 | 41 |
| | Me | F | l | 0.2 | 3.13 | 0.05 | 0.2 | 41 |
| | Me | F | m | 0.78 | 6.25 | 0.2 | | 59 |
| | Me | F | n | 1.56 | 25 | 0.2 | | 59 |
| | Me | F | o | 3.13 | 25 | 0.2 | | 59 |

trinsic optical activity. The targets (DNA and DNA gyrase) are optically active, so it might be expected that such molecules would respond best to compatible chirality, so resolution or chiral synthesis thus appear to be called for.

FLU (30, 31) is a seminal molecule in several senses. It was not only the first fluoroquinolone but also the first quinolone to be resolved and examined as a pair of enantiomers. It was prepared during the classical era but was never developed. More recently, a FLU derivative in which a methyl group is attached to the carbon corresponding to C-7 in the quinolones has been investigated. Methyl FLU racemate (Tg1;1) is equivalent in vitro to FLU (Tf;1) (4, 5, 30, 31, 36, 50, 53, 85). When resolved, the *S*-enantiomer of methyl FLU ranges from a low of four times more active than the *R*-enantiomer against *P. aeruginosa* to a high of 124-fold more active against *S. aureus* (Tg1;2 versus 3). Thus, the

**Table g1.** MICs for optical isomers at N-1 in the FLU series[a]

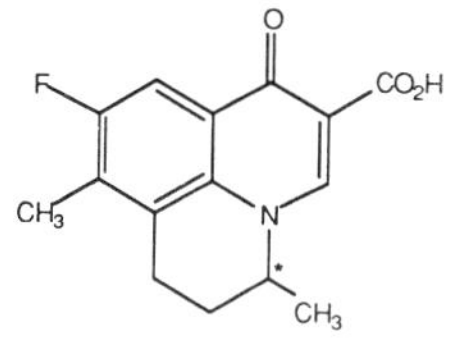

| Enantiomer | MIC (μg/ml) for: | | |
|---|---|---|---|
| | Ec | Pa | Sa |
| *R,S* | 0.2 | 6.2 | 0.05 |
| *R* | 6.2 | 12.5 | 3.1 |
| *S* | 0.1 | 3.1 | 0.025 |

[a]Data are from reference 30.
[b]S-25930.

range of chiral preference is from moderate to profound. With OFL, the same enantiomer is the more active and the range encompassed is from 8- to 250-fold (Table g2). Against the *E. coli* DNA gyrase, this eudismic ratio is 30-fold. This is almost exactly the ratio seen with intact cells, implying that intrinsic activity is more important than penetration with this molecule. The *S*-enantiomer of OFL is advancing toward clinical introduction.

## PYRROLOQUINOLONE SERIES

On a formal basis, the pyrroloquinolones are ring-contracted FLU analogs. In the literature and in Table h, however, the comparator is OFL (42). It is interesting that entry 3 in Table h is within one dilution tube of having the same potency against the indicator organisms. The potencies follow by now relatively anticipated trends, with a basic distal nitrogen of some sort being important for gram-negative organisms and relatively less important for gram-positive organisms. Where there are directly comparable analogs, the pyrroloquinolones are usually equivalent or superior to the FLU analogs against gram-negative organisms but are often inferior against *S. aureus*. The incorporation of an amino group at the position equivalent to the quinolone C-5 (Th;17–21) generally enhances activity.

## NEWER RING SYSTEMS STUDIED RECENTLY

The comparative simplicity and ease of synthetic variation that originally lured researchers into the area of quinolone research have now become a curse. The intense resulting activity has led to a thicket of intertwined patents, and it is difficult to come up with a contribution that would be regarded as truly novel. As a consequence, although it must be regarded as a higher-risk operation than making incremental improvements in established ring systems, reports describing the anti-

**Table g2.** MICs for optical isomers at N-1 in the benzoxazine series[a]

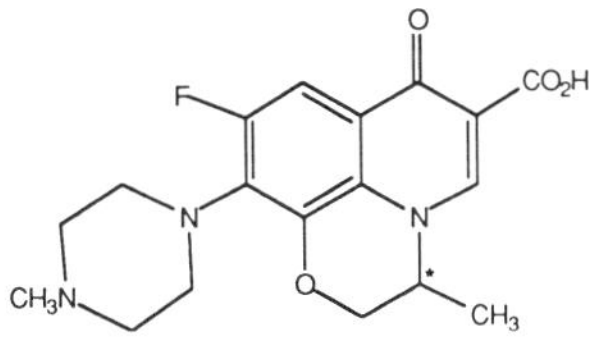

| Enantiomer | MIC (μg/ml) for: | | | DNA gyrase $IC_{50}$ (μg/ml) |
|---|---|---|---|---|
| | Ec | Pa | Sa | |
| *R,S* | 0.5 | 0.78 | 0.39 | |
| *R* | 0.39 | 12.5 | 5.0 | 27 |
| *S* | 0.05 | 0.39 | 0.02 | 0.9 |

[a]Data are from references 5, 36, 53, and 85.

**Table h.** MICs of molecules in the pyrroloquinolone series with variations at C-7[a]

a, X=NH
b, X=NMe
c, X=NEt
d, X=NCHO
e, X=$CH_2$
f, X=CHOH
g, X=O
h, X=S
i, X=$CH_2$NH
j, R=H
k, R=OH
l, R=H
m, R=Me
n, R=H
o, R=Me

| X | R | MIC (μg/ml) for: Ec | Pa | Sa |
|---|---|---|---|---|
| OFL | | 0.1 | 1.56 | 0.2 |
| H | a | 0.1 | 0.78 | 1.56 |
| H | b | 0.05 | 1.56 | 0.39 |
| H | c | 0.1 | 3.13 | 0.2 |
| H | d | 0.39 | 6.25 | 0.78 |
| H | e | 0.2 | 1.56 | 0.05 |
| H | f | 0.39 | 3.13 | 0.2 |
| H | g | 0.2 | 1.56 | 0.1 |
| H | h | 0.2 | 1.56 | 0.1 |
| H | i | 0.39 | 3.13 | 3.13 |
| H | j | 0.78 | 3.13 | 0.2 |
| H | k | 0.39 | 3.13 | 0.39 |
| H | l | 0.78 | 25 | 0.39 |
| H | m | 12.5 | 100 | 1.56 |
| H | n | 0.39 | 6.25 | 0.2 |
| H | o | 0.78 | 6.25 | 0.2 |
| $NH_2$ | a | 0.1 | 0.39 | 0.39 |
| $NH_2$ | b | 0.05 | 0.78 | 0.2 |
| $NH_2$ | e | 0.78 | 12.5 | 0.39 |
| $NH_2$ | f | 0.39 | 6.25 | 0.2 |
| $NH_2$ | g | 0.2 | 3.13 | 0.2 |

[a]Data are from reference 42.

microbial properties of ring system variations are increasingly appearing. By structural necessity, some sacrifices are required when the molecules are put together. This often translates, in the analogs discussed below, into deletion of the basic distal nitrogen believed to be needed for orientation of the components of the quinolone stack. Consequently, it is perhaps not too surprising that many of these investigations came up with disappointing results.

In Table i are described the properties of a group of thieno[3,2-*b*]pyridones (47). To a medicinal chemist, as related above, a sulfur atom is often regarded as functionally interchangeable with an olefinic linkage, so that a thiophene ring is often substituted for a benzene ring in drugs. In this sense, the thieno[3,2-*b*]pyridones are bioisosteric with the benzopyridones. The sulfur atom can have three orientations. One is reported in Table i. This variation did not succeed from a microbiological viewpoint.

The pyridobenzodiazines and pyridobenzothiazines of Table j represent yet another annelated tricyclic series (89). They are also not impressively active compared with the CIP standard.

Exploration of the phenanthroline-based ring system (Table k) led to two very weakly active analogs (80).

Thus, these attempts to break out of the pack and start a new synthetic race have not yet led to anything in particular. This area of research is, however, of great importance and must be pursued if this field is not to burn itself out.

## OPTICAL ACTIVITY

The target of the quinolones (the combination of DNA and DNA gyrase) is chiral, and inhibitory drugs would be expected to be most effective if they possessed complementary chirality and made a tight fit. This effect would likely be most pronounced in regions where closeness of approach took place. For technical reasons, it has not yet been possible to place chiral centers directly on the hydrogen-bonding face of the quinolones. In the sections above, however, some chiral analogs in which the asymmetric center was placed in the orienting face (at C-7) or the self-association face (at C-1) were presented. The point has been made, and will now be reinforced with additional examples, that asymmetry because of an attachment to C-7 usually has no profound influence on potency, whereas that caused by an attachment to N-1 is very important. Although this difference may seem anomalous at first glance, the specific way in

**Table i.** MICs of thieno[3,2-*b*]pyridones[a]

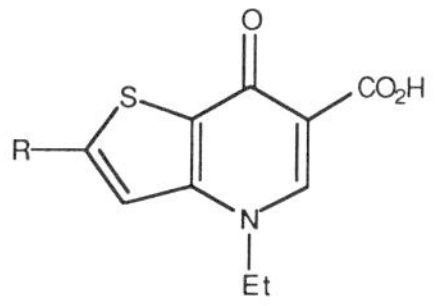

| R | MIC ($\mu$g/ml) for: | | | | | |
|---|---|---|---|---|---|---|
| | Sa | Ec | Kp | Pa | Pv | Mm |
| H | >128 | >128 | >128 | >128 | >128 | >128 |
| CHO | 128 | >128 | >128 | >128 | >128 | >128 |
| $COCH_3$ | >128 | >128 | 8 | >128 | 16 | 4 |
| CH=NPh-pOMe | >128 | >128 | >128 | >128 | >128 | >128 |
| CH=NOH | >128 | >128 | >128 | >128 | >128 | >128 |
| CN | >128 | >128 | >128 | >128 | >128 | >128 |
| CH=NOMe | >128 | >128 | >128 | >128 | 32 | 32 |
| $CH_2OH$ | >128 | >128 | >128 | >128 | >128 | >128 |

[a]Data are from reference 47.

which the molecules self-associate dictates the particular tightness of vertical stacking and the particular orientation of the hydrogen-bonding moieties attached to C-3, C-4, and C-5. In any case, this is used to rationalize the observed effect. The comparatively trivial influence of chirality at C-7 is rationalized as being due to this center being some distance from either the self-association face or the hydrogen-bonding face. Both of these faces are by necessity areas of close contact. Because the orienting face where C-7 lies shows permissive spatial requirements, one infers that closeness of approach is not often seen here. This is also consistent with findings reported in the literature. C-7 substituents may contribute directly to binding with DNA gyrase. The lack of significant enantiopreference at C-7 does not support this view.

The derivatives described above in which chiral centers were attached to N-1 involved rigid, fused, tricyclic ring systems. The analogs reported in Table 1 were prepared in order to see what would happen if the attached group was free to rotate (52, 55). CIP is so

**Table j.** MICs of pyridobenzodiazines and pyridobenzothiazines[a]

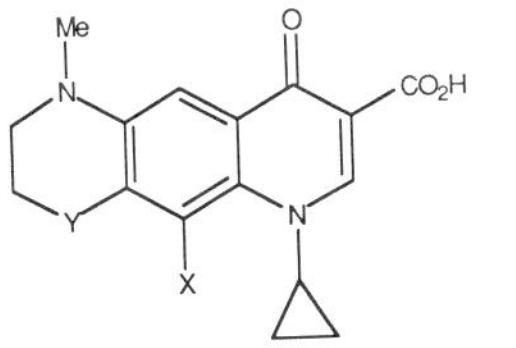

| X | Y | MIC ($\mu$g/ml) for: | | | |
|---|---|---|---|---|---|
| | | Ec | Pa | Sa | Kp |
| Cl | NMe | 12.5 | 100 | 6.25 | 1.56 |
| F | S | 50 | >100 | 100 | 1.56 |
| CIP | | 0.025 | 0.2 | 0.2 | 0.012 |

[a]Data are from reference 89.

**Table k.** MICs of fluorinated phenanthrolinones[a]

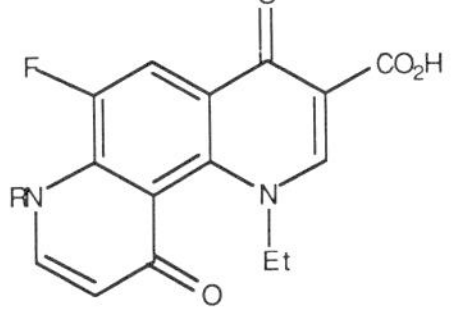

| R | MIC ($\mu$g/ml) for: | | | | |
|---|---|---|---|---|---|
| | Sa | Ef | Ec | Kp | Pa |
| H | >256 | >256 | 64 | 256 | >256 |
| Et | >256 | >256 | >256 | >256 | 256 |

[a]Data are from reference 80.

constructed that chirality is not possible with the exact molecule. Thus, variations in which methyl and aromatic rings were attached to the cyclopropyl moiety were constructed. In all of these derivatives, specific potency suffered even though enzyme potency was encouraging. This suggests a penetration problem. Interestingly, the most potent analogs were the *cis*-methyl pair (Tl;6,7), where the added methyl group would clearly be the smallest in overall size impact. Interestingly, in agreement with this hypothesis, the impact of the chiral center was minimal.

Tables m and n provide additional examples of the small impact of chirality in groups attached to C-7 (18, 75, 76). In both of these series, one with an *N*-1-ethyl substituent and the other with an *N*-1-difluorophenyl, the C-7 and N-1 groups are free to rotate. It is especially interesting that whereas C-7 chirality was unimportant when an aliphatic N-1 substituent was present, there was a comparatively high (10-fold) influence of chirality on enzyme inhibition in the N-1 aryl series (Table n). These data strongly suggest that intercellular concentrations of at least certain quinolones and certain microorganisms are strongly influenced by chirality and that this influence can significantly diminish the influence of enzymatic inhibition.

Very interestingly, and not consistent with the preceding findings, in the diastereomeric pyrrolidinyl series set forth in Table o, high chiral discrimination is seen (10- to 50-fold). This effect is seen both against the enzyme and in intact bacteria. There is no suitable rationale at present for this inconsistent correlation with substituent changes unless this portion of the molecule is close to DNA gyrase in the ternary complex.

With newly introduced TEM (Table p), by contrast, no influence of chirality was observed (14).

Thus, newer work, with certain notable exceptions (Table o), is generally consistent with experience. The points of particular interest are the lesser effect seen when chiral substituents are allowed to rotate and the surprising data in Table o.

## SOME INVESTIGATIONAL QUINOLONES OF CONTEMPORARY INTEREST

Table q lists a number of the more important investigational quinolones from the literature of the last 2 years and gives their structures and extended in vitro antimicrobial spectra. A number of these have been seen

**Table l.** MICs of optical isomers at of N-1 in CIP analogs

R= a, X=Ph; c, X=Me; b, X=Ph; d, X=Me; e; f

| R | MIC (μg/ml) for: Ec | Pa | Sa | DNA gyrase $IC_{50}$ (μg/ml) | Reference(s) |
|---|---|---|---|---|---|
| CIP | 0.025 | 0.2 | 0.2 | | 89 |
| a | 50 | >100 | 3.10 | 14.2 | 52, 54 |
| b | 12.5 | >50 | 0.78 | 12.1 | 52, 54 |
| c | >100 | >100 | >100 | 34.0 | 52, 54 |
| d | 25 | 0.78 | 25 | 19.0 | 52, 54 |
| e | 0.1 | 3.1 | 1.56 | 2.6 | 52, 54 |
| f | 0.05 | 1.56 | 1.56 | 2.7 | 52, 54 |

**Table m.** MICs of optical isomers at C-7 in the alkylamino alkylpyrrolidinyl series[a]

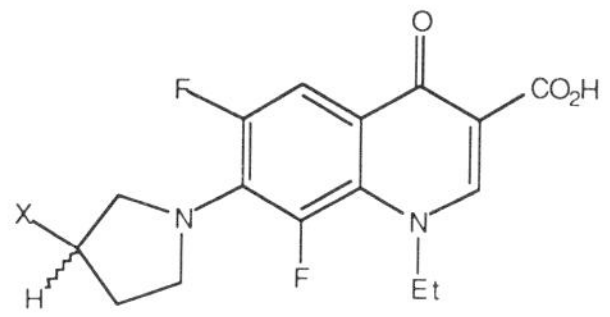

| X[b] | MIC (μg/ml) for: | | | DNA gyrase cleavage (μg/ml) |
|---|---|---|---|---|
| | Ec | Pa | Sa | |
| ~ $CH_2NHEt$ | 0.1 | 1.6 | 0.1 | 2.5 |
| -$CH_2NHEt$ | 0.1 | 3.1 | 0.1 | 2.5 |
| --$CH_2NHEt$ | 0.2 | 3.1 | 0.2 | 2.5 |

[a]Data are from reference 18.
[b]~ , -, and --, refer to the racemate, β-orientation, and α-orientation of the C-3′ substituent, respectively.

**Table n.** MICs of optical isomers at C-7 in the aminopyrrolidinyl series[a]

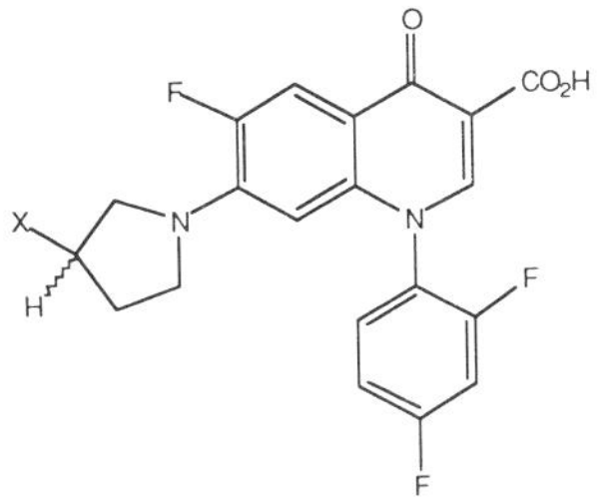

| X[b] | MIC (μg/ml) for: | | | DNA gyrase $IC_{50}$ (μg/ml) |
|---|---|---|---|---|
| | Ec | Pa | Sa | |
| ~ $NH_2$ | 0.02 | 0.1 | 0.02 | 0.4 |
| -$NH_2$ | 0.05 | 0.2 | 0.05 | 1.2 |
| --$NH_2$ | 0.02 | 0.05 | 0.02 | 0.16 |

[a]Data are from references 75 and 76.
[b]See Table m, footnote *b*.

before in this review, embedded in various tables. The importance of this group is that the quinolones of the near future may well emerge from it, and the members of the group represent the culmination of the structure-activity studies detailed in this review. Being the cream of the cream, so to speak, they represent a comparative consensus of what it takes molecularly to be competitive in the quinolone field in 1991 to 1992. Compared with the classical quinolones or with NOR itself, some of these are remarkable substances indeed.

## DUAL-ACTION HYBRID QUINOLONE-CEPHALOSPORINS

One of the more novel avenues of recent quinolone exploration involves the artful coupling of a suitable quinolone and a cephalosporin. Simultaneous coadministration of drugs is occasionally done in the anti-infective field in order to broaden the spectrum of activity or to deal with resistance. The first-day administration of an expanded-spectrum cephalosporin and an aminoglycoside to treat overwhelming sepsis of unknown etiology

**Table o.** MICs of optical isomers at C-7 in the diastereomeric pyrrolidinyl series[a]

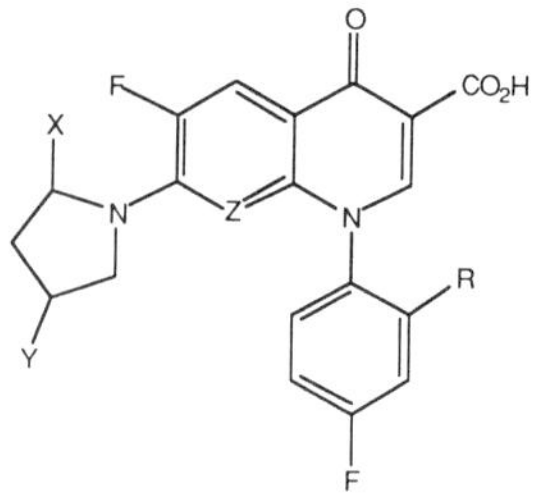

| R | X[b] | Y | Z | MIC ($\mu$g/ml) for: Ec | Pa | Sa | DNA gyrase $IC_{50}$ ($\mu$g/ml) |
|---|---|---|---|---|---|---|---|
| H | --$CH_2OH$ | H | CH | 0.78 | 3.1 | 0.1 | |
| H | -$CH_2OH$ | H | CH | 50 | >100 | 3.1 | |
| F | --$CH_3$ | $NH_2$ | CH | 0.05 | 3.1 | 0.02 | 0.9 |
| F | -$CH_3$ | $NH_2$ | CH | 0.78 | 5.0 | 0.39 | 18 |
| F | --$CH_3$ | $NH_2$ | N | 0.02 | 0.78 | 0.02 | 0.6 |
| F | -$CH_3$ | $NH_2$ | N | 0.39 | 12.5 | 0.2 | 7.5 |

[a]Data are from references 75 and 76.
[b]See Table m, footnote *b*.

**Table p.** MICs of optical isomers at C-7 in the methylpiperazinyl series[a]

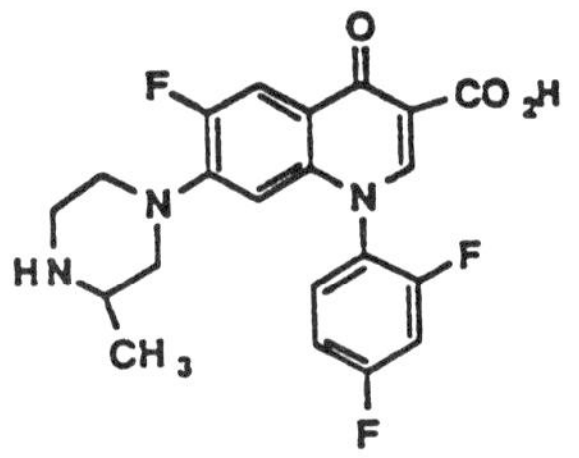

| Drug | Enantiomer | MIC ($\mu$g/ml) for: Ec | Pa | Sa | Kp |
|---|---|---|---|---|---|
| TEM | *R,S* | 0.05 | 0.39 | 0.1 | 0.05 |
| | *S*(−) | 0.05 | 0.20 | 0.1 | 0.1 |
| | *R*(+) | 0.05 | 0.39 | 0.1 | 0.1 |

[a]Data are from reference 14.

and the use of trimethoprim-sulfamethoxazole combinations spring readily to mind. Combinations are generally disfavored, although combinations of two different bacteriostatic or two different bactericidal agents are allowed. The combination in a single molecule of the molecular features of two different drugs, however, rarely works. It is often impossible to join such molecules in a way that allows each to be fully active at a different receptor or enzyme. Another problem lies in different potencies. The optimal ratio of the two drugs to one another is often not 1:1, and some flexibility in dosing is lost by linking the two together. The higher molecular weight usually required often results in lower levels in blood after oral administration. Finally, the cost is usually dramatically

**Table q.** MICs of some recently prominent investigational quinolone analogs

| Drug | | MIC ($\mu$g/ml) for: | | | | | | Reference(s) |
|---|---|---|---|---|---|---|---|---|
| Name | Structure | Ec | Pa | Sa | Sp | Kp | Bf | |
| BMY-40062 | 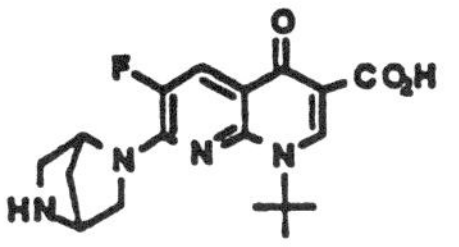 | 0.03 | 0.5 | 0.13 | 0.5 | 0.13 | 4.0 | 27 |
| AM-1091 | 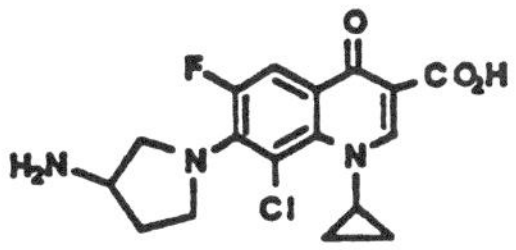 | 0.008 | 0.25 | 0.03 | 0.06 | 0.03 | 0.25 | 66 |
| AT-4140 | 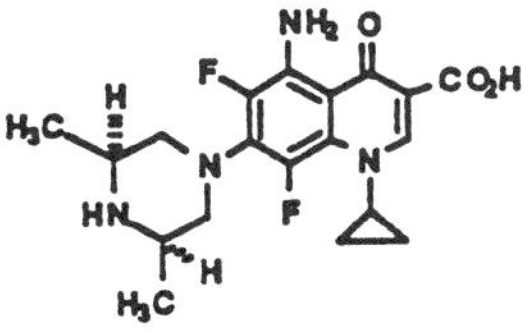 | 0.01 | 0.039 | 0.05 | 0.39 | 0.025 | | 60 |
| QA-241 | 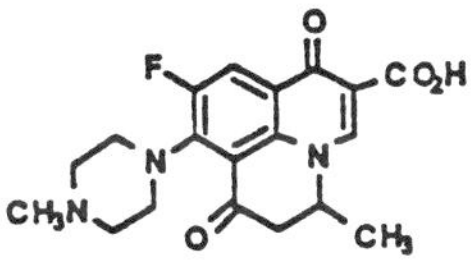 | 0.19 | 6.25 | 0.78 | 6.25 | 0.39 | 6.25 | 3 |
| KB-5246 | 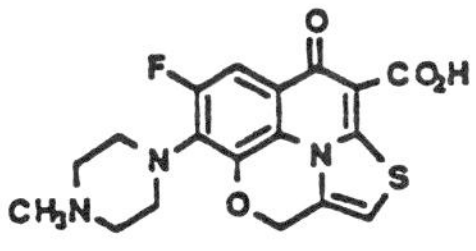 | 0.05 | 0.39 | 0.10 | 0.39 | 0.05 | 3.13 | 46 |
| WIN-57273 | | 0.125 | 2 | 0.002 | 0.03 | 0.25 | 0.25 | 78 |
| | | 0.125 | 2 | 0.002 | 0.03 | 0.5 | 0.5 | 25 |
| E-3846 | 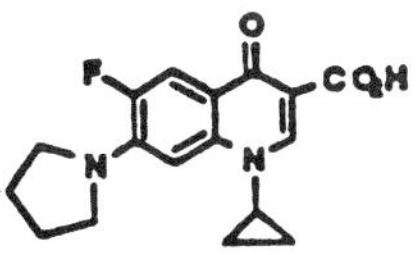 | 0.12 | 4 | 0.12 | 0.5 | 0.5 | 4 | 28 |

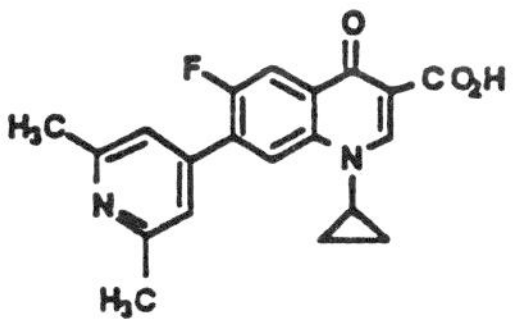

*Continued on following page*

**Table q.** *Continued*

| Drug | | MIC ($\mu$g/ml) for: | | | | | | Reference(s) |
|---|---|---|---|---|---|---|---|---|
| Name | Structure | Ec | Pa | Sa | Sp | Kp | Bf | |
| PD-117,596 | 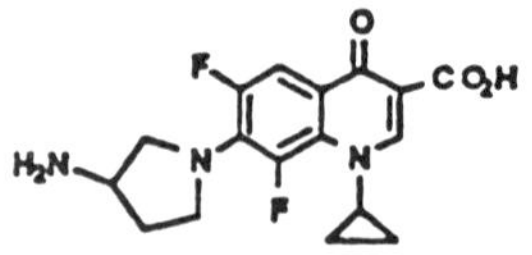 | 0.03 | 0.6 | 0.03 | 0.25 | 0.03 | | 74 |
| AT-4140 (SPA) | 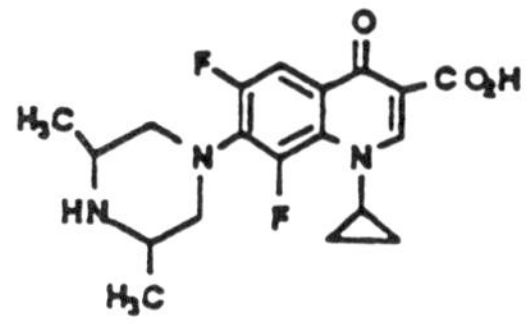 | 0.03 | 0.5 | 0.12 | 0.25 | 0.06 | 0.5 | 16, 17 |
| PD-131,628 | 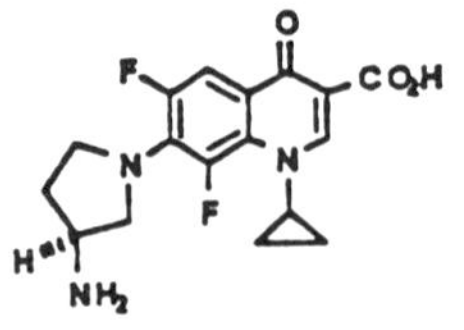 | 0.03 | 0.125 | 0.06 | 0.125 | 0.03 | 2 | 15 |
| E-4497 | 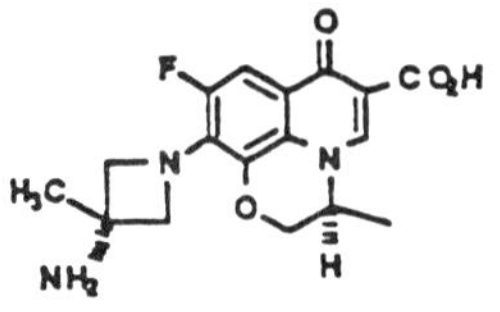 | 0.06 | 0.5 | 0.6 | 0.5 | 0.06 | 4 | 29 |
| NM-394 | 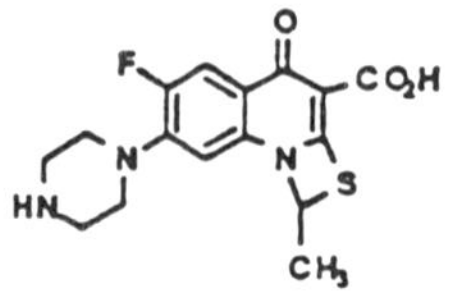 | 0.10 | 0.39 | 0.78 | 1.56 | 0.10 | | 71a |

higher than the cost of administering the two agents separately. The instances when the combination is distinctly superior to the two agents individually are few. The artful combination of certain quinolones with certain cephalosporins has recently been studied. Details of the results follow.

The basic science underlying the work is very interesting. It has been posited for some time, and there is significant chemical evidence to support the idea, that nucleophilic opening of the $\beta$-lactam ring of a cephalosporin containing a suitable C-3 substituent can result in ejection of the substituent at C-3, with the double bond acting as a conductor for the electrons. These novel compounds are stable enough for practical handling but are sufficiently unstable in the presence of biochemical nucleophiles to show usefully enhanced potency. Some biochemical nucleophiles relevant to this discussion are the β-lactamases and the β-lactam-binding proteins. This is illustrated in structure 4 (Fig. 3). The normal cephalosporin substituents that are ejected in this way are acetyl, pyridyl, and a variety of sulfur-linked tetrazoles and related heterocycles. These ejected units are not active as antibacterial agents. If, however, the ejected unit is antimicrobial, the possibility of a synergistic effect exists. Since the cephalosporins as well as the quinolones are bactericidal and since their comparative potencies are in the same general range, this combination appears suitable for the purpose. The best-understood way to make the connection is hydrolysis of the ester group of the cephalosporin under conditions that do not lead to lactonization and then formation of an ester with the quinolone carboxyl group. Since the simple esters of the quinolones are prodrugs and are not intrinsically biologically active, the theory is that the quinolone component would not directly contribute until it was released by a nucleophile. Of course, since the better its nucleofugic properties, the more potent the β-lactam, the quinolone would have an indirect effect on potency. With this theory in mind, what is the reality?

In Table r1, seven such hybrids are compared with the starting cephalosporin, which bears a standard acetyloxy moiety at C-3 (1). Against *E. coli,* all of the agents showed intenser activity, some of them strikingly so. The results against the other organisms, with the possible exception of *S. pneumoniae,* were about what would be expected from the cephalosporin alone. Table r2 lists a collection of similar analogs with C-7 cephalosporin side chains likely to convey resistance to β-lactamases. Here, retention of activity is comforting, but there is no significant enhancing effect of the quinolone component except against the anaerobe *Bacteroides faecalis* (1). If a classical thienylacetic acid amide C-7 side chain is used, some significantly active combination drugs appear. These are shown in Table r3 (Tr3;5,6). It is difficult to sort out trends, as more than one thing is being varied as one goes along. Nonetheless, the fifth entry shows rather nice potency across the board (1, 20). Table r4 shows a small selection of FLE analogs in which the cephalosporin component is varied. Clearly, this matters, but the variations in potency with different microorganisms follow idiosyncratic trends (1). Table r5 illustrates the findings with Ro 23-9424 (a combination of desacetylcefotaxime and FLE, one of the best of the codrugs described to date (43). Unfortunately, its potency against *Pseudomonas, Staphylococcus,* and *Bacteroides* spp. is comparatively low.

The work described in Table r6 attempts to address the question of whether the combination has intrinsic activity or whether it acquires its activity following β-lactam cleavage. The evidence is suggestive but not compelling, because the comparator (deacetylcephalothin [structure C]) has a hydroxyl group to eject from C-3, whereas the quinolone combinations all have esters, which would be expected to be considerably more

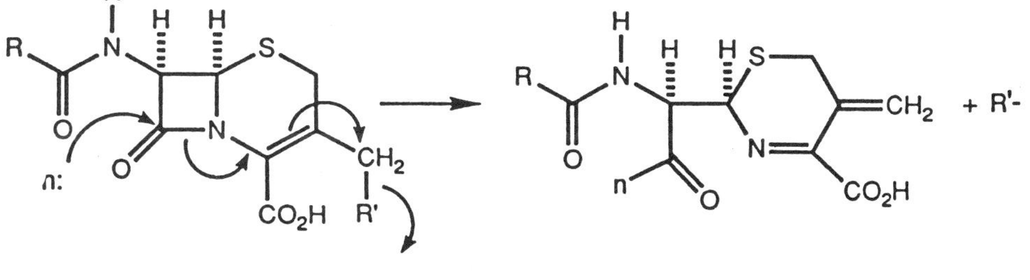

**Figure 3.** Structure 4.

**Table r1.** MICs of dual-action cephalosporin-quinolone hybrids[a]

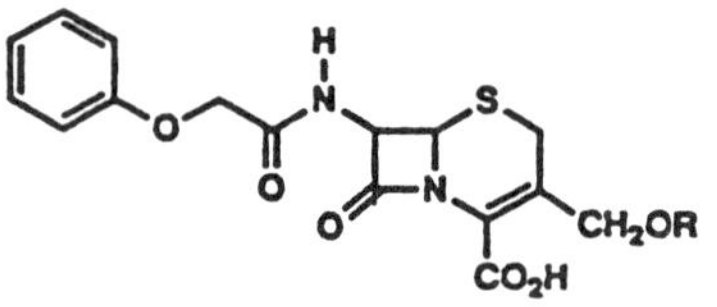

| $R^b$ | MIC ($\mu$g/ml) for: | | | | | |
|---|---|---|---|---|---|---|
| | Ec | Pa | Sa | Sp | Spy | Bf |
| $COCH_3$ | 128 | > 128 | 0.5 | 0.25 | 0.06 | 64 |
| A | | | | < 0.008 | 0.06 | |
| B | 2 | > 256 | 0.25 | | | 64 |
| C | 8 | 128 | 0.5 | | | 64 |
| D | 64 | > 128 | 0.5 | < 0.008 | | 32 |
| E | 8 | > 128 | 0.25 | 2 | 2 | 64 |
| F | 4 | > 128 | 0.5 | 1 | 2 | 128 |
| G | 1 | 128 | 0.125 | 2 | 4 | 64 |

[a]Data are from reference 1.

[b]

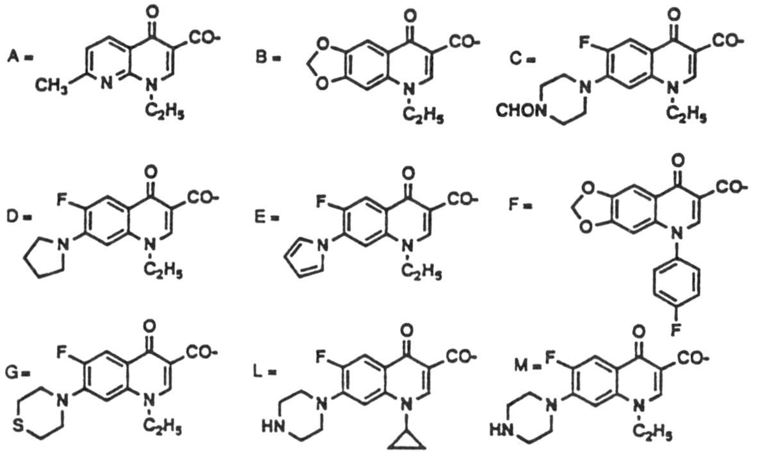

nucleofugic. The combination, therefore, would be more active. A 1:1 mixture of CIP and deacetylcephalothin is already more active on a molar basis than the individual components, suggesting some synergism. The molecular combination (structure A) is sometimes more active than the mixture and sometimes (more often) somewhat less active.

The question is not settled decisively by these data.

The clinical future of the cephalosporin-quinolone hybrids is not yet clear.

## CONCLUSIONS

The classical structure-activity correlations of Albrecht (2) have held up remarkably well with the exception of the surprising activity of certain substituents at N-1 and C-5. The recent revision largely still stands (50). Even though only a comparatively brief time has passed since that revision, a fairly large number of new compounds have been made and tested (50). Their properties have, by and large, fallen into place. The search for a

**Table r2.** MICs of dual-action cephalosporin-quinolone hybrids[a]

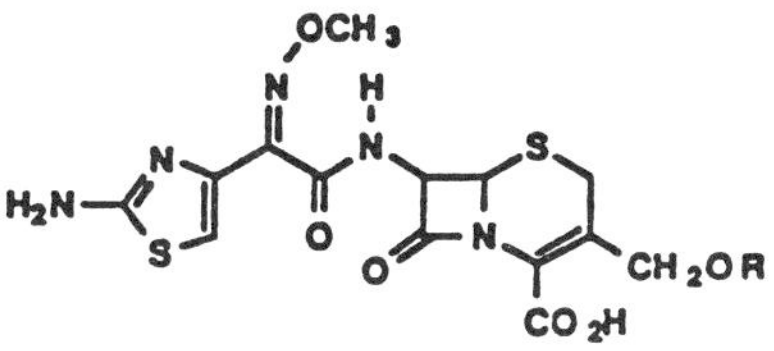

| $R^b$ | MIC (μg/ml) for: | | | | | |
|---|---|---|---|---|---|---|
| | Ec | Pa | Sa | Sp | Spy | Bf |
| $COCH_3$ | 0.063 | 64 | 2 | 0.016 | <0.008 | >128 |
| A | 1 | >128 | 2 | | | >128 |
| B | 0.5 | 128 | 2 | | | 32 |
| C | 1 | >128 | 4 | | | 32 |
| D | 2 | >128 | 0.25 | <0.008 | 1 | 32 |
| G | 0.5 | 128 | 0.5 | 0.016 | <0.008 | 4 |
| H | 0.125 | 8 | 1 | <0.008 | 0.031 | 8 |

[a]Data are from reference 1.
[b]See Table r1, footnote *b*, for structures A to G.

H =

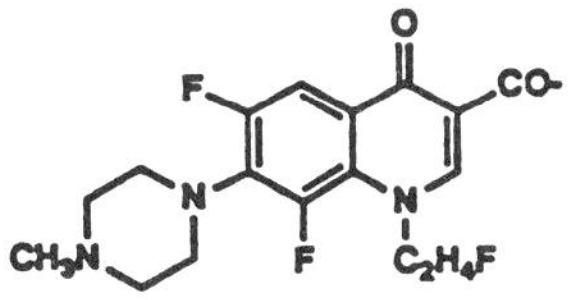

**Table r3.** MICs for dual-action cephalosporin-quinolone hybrids[a]

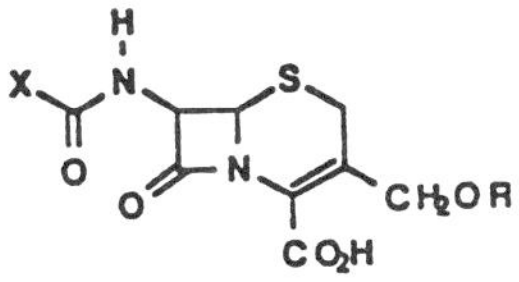

| X | R | MIC (μg/ml) for: | | | | | | Reference |
|---|---|---|---|---|---|---|---|---|
| | | Ec | Pa | Sa | Sp | Spy | Bf | |
| I | B | 1 | >128 | 0.5 | | | 32 | 1 |
| I | C | 8 | >128 | 0.5 | 0.06 | | >128 | 1 |
| J | H | 1 | >128 | 2 | 0.25 | 0.25 | 128 | 1 |
| K | G | 64 | 64 | 1 | 0.125 | 0.016 | 16 | 1 |
| I | L | 0.25 | 2 | 0.5 | 0.06 | <0.008 | 8 | 20 |
| I | M | 1 | 8 | 1 | 0.12 | <0.06 | 8 | 20 |

[a]See Table r1, footnote *b*, for structures A to G and Table r2, footnote *b*, for structure H.

I =    J = Hydrogen    K =

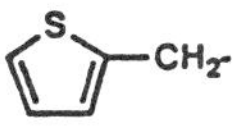

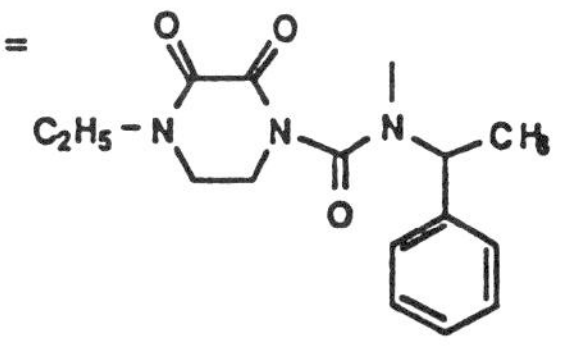

**Table r4.** MICs of dual-action cephalosporin-quinolone hybrids[a]

| R | MIC (μg/ml) for: | | | | | |
|---|---|---|---|---|---|---|
| | Ec | Pa | Sa | Sp | Spy | Bf |
| $CH_3$ | 0.125 | 8 | 1 | <0.008 | 0.03 | 8 |
| $CMe_2CO_2H$ | 0.25 | 8 | 1 | 0.5 | 0.5 | >128 |
| $CH_2CO_2H$ | 0.125 | 32 | 2 | 0.5 | 0.5 | 8 |

[a]Data are from reference 1.

**Table r5.** MICs of quinolone-containing codrugs[a]

| Drug | MIC (μg/ml) for: | | | | | |
|---|---|---|---|---|---|---|
| | Ec | Pa | Sa | Sp | Kp | Bf |
| Ro 23-9424[b] | 0.12 | 8 | 1 | ≤0.06 | 0.12 | 32 |

[a]Data are from reference 43.
[b]Desacetylcephalotaxine plus FLE.

novel ring system that will have a spectrum of activity and a potency analogous to those of the fluoroquinolones is intense but has yet to produce a clear contender.

*Acknowledgments.* We are pleased to acknowledge The National Institute of Allergy and Infectious Diseases for partial support of this effort under grant AI-13155. R.Z. acknowledges stipend support from GM-01341, and R.Z. and P.D. acknowledge support from the Wesley Foundation of Wichita.

## REFERENCES

1. **Albrecht, H. A., G. Beskid, K. Chan, J. G. Christenson, R. Cleeland, K. H. Deitcher, N. H. Georgopapadakou, D. D. Keith, D. L. Pruess, J. Sepinwall, A. C. Specian, Jr., R. L. Then, M. Weigele, K. F. West, and R. Yang.** 1990. Cephalosporin 3′-quinolone esters with a dual mode of action. *J. Med. Chem.* **33:**77–85.
2. **Albrecht, R.** 1977. Development of antibacterial agents of the nalidixic acid type. *Prog. Drug Res.* **21:**9–104.
3. **Asahara, M., A. Tsuji, S. Goto, M. Kazuo, and A. Kiuchi.** 1989. In vitro and in vivo activities of QA-241, a new tricyclic quinolone derivative. *Antimicrob. Agents Chemother.* **33:**1144–1152.
4. **Atarashi, S., H. Tsurumi, T. Fujiwara, and I. Hayakawa.** 1991. Asymmetric reduction of 7,8-difluoro-3-methyl-2H-1,4-benzoxazine. Synthesis of a key intermediate of (S)-(−)-ofloxacin (DR-3355). *J. Heterocyclic Chem.* **28:**329–331.
5. **Atarashi, S., S. Yokohama, K. Yamazaki, K., K. Sakano, K., M. Imamura, and I. Hayakawa.**

**Table r6.** MICs of dual-action cephalosporin-quinolone hybrids[a]

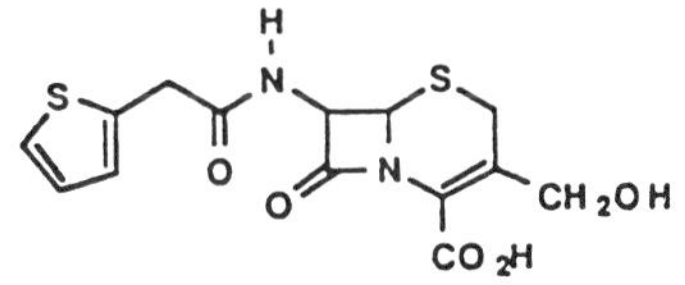

Deacetylcephalothin

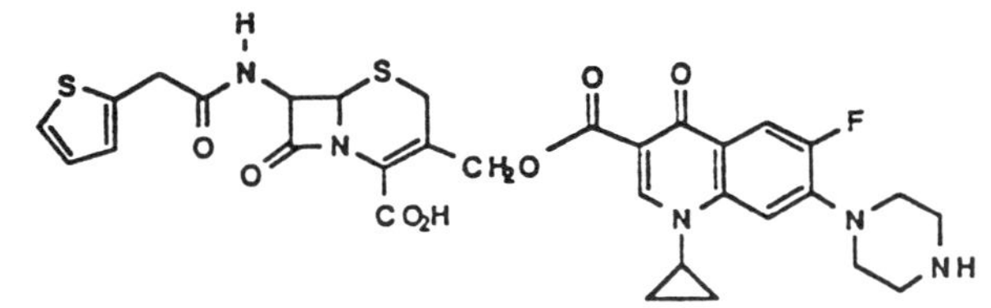

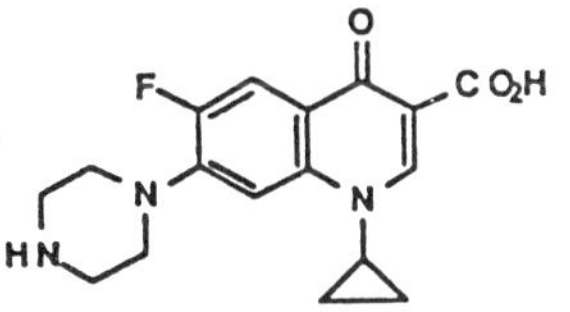

| Structure | MIC (μmol/liter) for: | | | | | |
|---|---|---|---|---|---|---|
| | Ec | Pa | Sa | Sp | Spy | Bf |
| A | 0.37 | 3 | 6 | 0.09 | <0.01 | 12 |
| B+C (1:1) | <0.02 | 3 | 0.36 | 1.5 | 0.36 | 0.73 |
| B | <0.02 | 6 | 0.75 | 3.0 | 1.5 | 1.5 |
| C | 180 | >180 | 2.8 | 2.8 | 0.34 | 90 |

[a]Data are from reference 20.


1987. Synthesis and antibacterial activities of optically active ofloxacin and its fluoromethyl derivative. *Chem. Pharm. Bull.* **35:**1896–1902.

6. **Augeri, D. J., A. H. Fray, and E. F. Kleinman.** 1990. Synthesis and antibacterial activity of 2,3-dehydroofloxacin. *J. Heterocyclic Chem.* **27:**1509–1511.
7. **Bouzard, D., P. Di Cesare, M. Essiz, J. P. Jacquet, J. R. Kiechel, P. Remuzon, A. Weber, T. Oki, M. Masuyoshi, R. E. Kessler, J. Fung-Tomc, and J. Desiderio.** 1990. Fluoronaphthyridines and quinolones as antibacterial agents. 2. Synthesis and structure-activity relationships of new 1-tert-butyl-substituted derivatives. *J. Med. Chem.* **32:**537–542.
8. **Bouzard, D., P. Di Cesare, M. Essiz, J. P. Jacquet, P. Remuzon, A. Weber, T. Oki, and M. Masuyoshi.** 1989. Fluoronaphthyridines and quinolones as antibacterial agents. 1. Synthesis and structure-activity relationships of new 1-substituted derivatives. *J. Med.Chem.* **32:**537–542.
9. **Cecchetti, V., A. Fravolini, R. Fringuelli, G. Mascellani, P. Pagella, M. Palmioli, G. Segre, and P. Terni.** 1987. Quinolonecarboxylic acids. 2. Synthesis and antibacterial evaluation of 7-oxo-2,3-dihydro-7H-pyrido[1,2,3-de][1,4]benzothiazine-6-carboxylic acids. *J. Med. Chem.* **30:**465–473.
10. **Chu, D. T. W., P. B. Fernandes, A. K. Claiborne, E. H. Gracey, and A. G. Pernet.** 1986. Synthesis and structure-activity relationships of new arylfluoronaphthyridine antibacterial agents. *J. Med. Chem.* **29:**2363–2369.
11. **Chu, D. T. W., P. B. Fernandes, A. K. Claiborne, E. Pihuleac, C. W. Nordeen, R. E. Maleczka, Jr., and A. G. Pernet.** 1985. Synthesis and structure-activity relationships of novel arylfluoroquinolone antibacterial agents. *J. Med. Chem.* **28:**1558–1564.
12. **Chu, D. T. W., P. B. Fernandes, A. K. Claiborne, L. Shen, and A. G. Pernet.** 1989. Structure-activity relationships in quinolone antibacterials: replacement of the 3-carboxylic acid group, p. 37–46. *In* P. B. Fernandes (ed.), *International Telesymposium on Quinolones.* M. Prious Science Publishers, Barcelona, Spain.
13. **Chu, D. T. W., P. B. Fernandes, and A. G. Pernet.** 1986. Synthesis and biological activity of benzothiazolo[3,2-a]quinolone antibacterial agents. *J. Med. Chem.* **29:**1531–1534.
14. **Chu, D. T. W., C. W. Nordeen, D. J. Hardy, R. N. Swanson, W. J. Giardina, A. G. Pernet, and J. J. Plattner.** 1991. Synthesis, antibacterial activities, and pharmacological properties of enantiomers of temafloxacin hydrochloride. *J. Med. Chem.* **34:**168–174.
15. **Cohen, M. A., M. D. Huband, G. B. Mailloux, S. L. Yoder, G. E. Roland, J. M. Domagala, and C. L. Heifetz.** 1991. In vitro antibacterial activities

of PD-131628, a new 1,8-naphthyridine anti-infective agent. *Antimicrob. Agents Chemother.* **35:**:141–146.

16. **Cooper, C. S., P. L. Klock, D. T. W. Chu, and P. B. Fernandes.** 1990. The synthesis and antibacterial activities of quinolones containing five and six membered heterocyclic substituents at the 7-position. *J. Antimicrob. Chemother.* **33:**1246–1251.
17. **Cooper, M. A., J. M. Andrews, J. P. Ashby, R. S. Matthews, and R. Wise.** 1990. In vitro activity of sparfloxacin, a new quinolone antimicrobial agent. *J. Antimicrob. Chemother.* **26:**667-676.
18. **Culbertson, T. P., J. M. Domagala, J. B. Nichols, S. Priebe, and R. W. Skeean.** 1987. Enantiomers of 1-ethyl-7-[3-](ethylamino)methyl]-1-pyrrolidinyl]-6,8-difluoro-1,4-dihydro-4-oxo-3-quinoline-carboxylic acid: preparation and biological activity. *J. Med. Chem.* **30:**1711–1715.
19. **Culbertson, T. P., J. P. Sanchez, L. Gambino, and J. A. Sesnie.** 1990. Quinolone antibacterial agents substituted at the 7-position with spiroamines—synthesis and structure activity relationships. *J. Med. Chem.* **33:**2270–2275.
20. **Demuth, T. P., R. E. White, R. A. Tietjen, R. J. Storrin, J. R. Skuster, J. A. Andersen, C. C. McOsker, R. Freedman, and F. J. Rourke.** 1991. Synthesis and antibacterial activity of new C-10 quinolonyl-cephemesters. *J. Antibiot.* **44:**200–209.
21. **Domagala, J. M., A. J. Bridges, T. P. Culbertson, L. Gambino, S. E. Hagen, G. Karrick, K. Porter, J. P. Sanchez, J. A. Sesnie, F. G. Spense, D. Szotek, and J. Wemple.** 1991. Synthesis and biological activity of 5-aminooxy-quinolene and 5-hydroxyquinolone, and the overwhelming influence of the remote N1-substituent in determining the structure activity relationship. *J. Med. Chem.* **34:**1142–1154.
22. **Domagala, J. M., S. E. Hagen, C. L. Heifetz, M. P. Hutt, T. F. Mich, J. P. Sanchez, and A. K. Trehan.** 1988. 7-Substituted 5-amino-1-cyclopropyl-6,8-difluoro-1,4-dihydro-4-oxo-3-quinolinecarboxylic acids: synthesis and biological activity of a new class of quinolone antibacterials. *J. Med. Chem.* **31:**503–506.
23. **Domagala, J. M., L. D. Hanna, C. L. Heifetz, M. P. Hutt, T. F. Mich, J. P. Sanchez, and M. Solomon.** 1986. New structure-activity relationships of the quinolone antibacterials using the target enzyme. The development and application of a DNA gyrase essay. *J. Med. Chem.* **29:**394-403.
24. **Domagala, J. M., C. L. Heifetz, M. P. Hutt, T. F. Mich, J. B. Nichols, M. Solomon, and D. F. Worth.** 1988. 1-Substituted 7-[3[(ethylamino)methyl]-1-pyrrolidinyl]-6,8-difluoro-1,4-dihydro-4-oxo-3-quinolinecarboxylic acids. New quantitative structure-activity relationships at N-1 for the quinolone antibacterials. *J. Med. Chem.* **31:**991–1001.
25. **Eliopoulos, G. M., K. Klimm, L. B. Rice, M. J. Ferraro, and R. C. Moellering.** 1990. Comparative in vitro activity of Win-57273, a new fluoroquinolone antimicrobial agent. *Antimicrob. Agents Chemother.* **34:**1154–1159.
26. **Felmingham, D., M. D. O'Hare, M. J. Robbins, R. A. Wall, A. H. Williams, A. W. Cremer, G. L. Ridgeway, and R. N. Grueneberg.** 1985. Comparative in vitro studies with 4-quinolone antimicrobials. *Drugs Exp. Clin. Res.* **11:**317–329.
27. **Fung-Tomc, J., J. V. Desederio, Y. H. Tsai, G. Warr, and R. E. Kessler.** 1989. In vitro and in vivo antibacterial activities of BMY 40062, a new fluoronaphthyridone. *Antimicrob. Agents Chemother.* **33:**906–914.
28. **Garcia-Rodriquez, J. A., J. E. G. Sanchez, J. L. M. Bellido, and I. Trujillano.** 1990. In vitro activites of irloxacin and E-3846, two new quinolones. *Antimicrob. Agents Chemother.* **34:**1262–1267.
29. **Gargallo-Viola, D., M. Esteve, S. Llovera, X. Roca, and J. Guinea.** 1991. In vitro and in vivo antibacterial activities of E-4497, a new 3-amine-3-methyl-azetidinyl tricyclic fluoroquinolone. *Antimicrob. Agents Chemother.* **35:**442–447.
30. **Gerster, J. F., S. R. Rohlfing, S. E. Pecore, R. M. Winandy, R. M. Stern, J. E. Landmesser, R. A. Olsen, and W. B. Gleason.** 1987. Synthesis, absolute configuration, and antibacterial activity of 6,7-dihydro-5,8-dimethyl-9-fluoro-1-oxo-1*H*,5*H*-benzo[ij]quinolizine-2-carboxylic acid. *J. Med. Chem.* **30:**839–843.
31. **Gerster, J. F., S. R. Rohlfing, N. J. Rustad, M. J. Reiter, S. E. Pecore, R. M. Winandy, and J. E. Landmesser.** 1989. The synthesis and pharmacological profile of the stereoisomers of a tricyclic quinolone antibacterial, p. 85–98. *In* P. B. Fernandes (ed.), *International Telesymposium on Quinolones.* M. Prious Science Publishers, Barcelona, Spain.
32. **Grohe, K., and H. Heitzer.** 1987. Cycloaralierung von Enaminen. I. Synthese von 4-Chinolon-3-carbonsaeuren. *Justus Liebigs Ann. Chem.*, p. 29–37.
33. **Hagen, S. E., J. M. Domagala, C. L. Heifetz, and J. Johnson.** 1991. Synthesis and biological activity of 5-alkyl-1,7,8-trisubstituted-6-fluoroquinoline-3-carboxylic acids. *J. Med. Chem.* **34:**1155–1161.
34. **Hagen, S. E., J. M. Domagala, C. L. Heifetz, J. P. Sanchez, and M. Solomon.** 1991. New quinolone antibacterial agents. Synthesis and biological activity of 7-(3,3- or 3,4-disubstituted-1-pyrrolidinyl)quinoline-3-carboxylic acids. *J. Med. Chem.* **33:**849–853.
35. **Hardy, D. J., R. N. Swanson, D. M. Hensey, N. R. Ramer, R. R. Bower, C. W. Hanson,**

**D. T. W. Chu, and P. B. Fernandes.** 1987. Comparative antibacterial activities of temafloxacin hydrochloride (A-62254) and two reference fluoroquinolones. *Antimicrob. Agents Chemother.* **31:**1768–1774.

36. **Hayakawa, I., T. Hiramitsu, and Y. Tanaka.** 1984. Synthesis and antibacterial activities of substituted 7-oxyo-2,3-dihydro-7H-pyrido[1,2,3-de] [1,4]benzoxazine-6-carboxylic acids. *Chem. Pharm. Bull. Jpn.* **32:**4907–4913.
37. **Hirai, K., H. Aoyama, M. Hosaka, Y. Oomori, Y. Niwata, S. Suzue, and T. Irikura.** 1986. In vitro and in vivo antibacterial activity of AM-833, a new quinolone derivative. *Antimicrob. Agents Chemother.* **29:**1059–1066.
38. **Hogberg, T., I. Khanna, S. D. Drake, L. A. Mitscher, and L. L. Shen.** 1984. Structure-activity relationships among DNA gyrase inhibitors. Synthesis and biological evaluation of 1,2-dihydro-4,4-dimethyl-1-oxo-2-naphthalenecarboxylic acids as 1-carba bioisosteres of oxolinic acid. *J. Med. Chem.* **27:**306-310.
39. **Hogberg, T., M. Vora, S. D. Drake, L. A. Mitscher, and D. T. W. Chu.** 1984. Structure-activity relationships among DNA-gyrase inhibitors. Synthesis and antimicrobial evaluation of chromones and coumarins related to oxolinic acid. *Acta Chem. Scand.* **38:**359–366.
40. **Hoshino, K., K. Sato, K. Akahane, A. Yoshida, I. Hayakawa, M. Sato, T. Une, and Y. Osada.** 1991. Significance of the methyl group on the oxazine ring of ofloxacin derivatives in the inhibition of bacterial and mammalian type II topoisomerases. *Antimicrob. Agents Chemother.* **35:**309–312.
41. **Ishikawa, G., F. Tabusa, H. Miyamoto, M. Kano, H. Ueda, H. Tamaoka, and K. Nakagawa.** 1989. Studies on antibacterial agents. I. Synthesis of substituted 6,7-dihydro-1-oxo-1H,5H-benzo[ij]quinolizine. *Chem. Pharm. Bull. Tokyo* **37:**2103–2108.
42. **Ishikawa, H., H. Uno, H. Miyamoto, H. Ueda, H. Tamaoka, M. Tominaga, and K. Nakagawa.** 1990. Studies on antibacterial agents. II. Synthesis and antibacterial activities of substituted 1,2-dihydro-6-oxo-6H-pyrrolo[3,2,1-ij]quinoline-5-carboxylic acids. *Chem. Pharm. Bull. Tokyo* **38:**2459.
43. **Jones, R. N., A. L. Barry, and C. Thornsberry.** 1989. Antimicrobial activity of Ro 23-9424, a novel ester-linked codrug of fleroxacin and desacetylcefotaxime. *Antimicrob. Agents Chemother.* **33:**944–950.
44. **Koga, H., A. Itoh, S. Murayama, S. Suzue, and T. Irikura.** 1980. Structure-activity relationships of antibacterial 6,7- and 7,8-disubstituted 1-alkyl-1,4-dihydro-4-oxoquinoline-3-carboxylic acids. *J. Med. Chem.* **23:**1358–1363.
45. **Kondo, H., M. Taguchi, Y. Inoue, F. Sakamoto, and G. Tsukamoto.** 1990. Synthesis and antibacterial activity of thiazolo[3,2-A][1,8]naphthyridinecarboxylic, oxazolo[3,2-A][1,B]naphthyridinecarboxylic, and imidazolo[3,2-A][1,8]-naphthyridine-carboxylic acids. *J. Med. Chem.* **33:**2012–2015.
46. **Kotera, Y., and S. Mitsuhashi.** 1989. In vitro and in vivo antibacterial activities of KB-5246, a new tetracyclic quinolone. *Antimicrob. Agents Chemother.* **33:**1896–1900.
47. **Malicorne, G., J. Bompart, L. Giral, and E. Despaux.** 1991. Synthesis and antibacterial activity of 4,7-dihydro-4-ethyl-7-oxothieno(3,2-b)pyridine-6-carboxylic acids. *Eur. J. Med. Chem.* **26:**3–12.
48. **Matsumoto, J., and T. Miyamoto.** 1989. Cinoxacin analogues as potential antibacterial agents: synthesis and antibacterial activity, p. 109–118. *In* P. B. Fernandes (ed.), *International Telesymposium on Quinolones.* M. Prious Science Publishers, Barcelona, Spain.
49. **Matsumoto, J., T. Miyamoto, A. Minamida, Y. Nishimura, H. Egawa, and H. Nishimura.** 1984. Pyridonecarboxylic acids as antibacterial agents. 2. Synthesis and structure-activity relationships of 1,6,7-trisubstituted 1,4-dihydro-4-oxo-1,8-naphthyridine-3-carboxylic acids, including enoxacin, a new antibacterial agent. *J. Med. Chem.* **27:**292–301.
50. **Mitscher, L. A., P. V. Devasthale, and R. M. Zavod.** 1990. Structure-activity relationships of fluoro-4-quinolones, p. 115–146. *In* G. C. Crumplin (ed.), *The 4-Quinolones, Antibacterial Agents in Vitro.* Springer-Verlag, New York.
51. **Mitscher, L. A., H. E. Gracey, G. W. Clark, and T. Suzuki.** 1978. Quinolone antimicrobial agents. 1. Versatile new synthesis of 1-alkyl-1,4-dihydro-4-oxo-3-quinoline-carboxylic acids. *J. Med. Chem.* **21:**485–489.
52. **Mitscher, L. A., P. N. Sharma, D. T. W. Chu, L. L. Shen, and A. G. Pernet.** 1986. Chiral DNA gyrase inhibitors. 1. Synthesis and antimicrobial activity of the enantiomers of 6-fluoro-7(1-piperazinyl)-1(2′-trans-phenyl-1′-cyclo-propyl)-1,4-dihydro-4-oxoquinoline-3-carboxylic acid. *J. Med. Chem.* **29:**2044–2047.
53. **Mitscher, L. A., P. N. Sharma, D. T. W. Chu, L. L. Shen, and A. G. Pernet.** 1987. Chiral DNA gyrase inhibitors. 2. Asymmetric synthesis and biological activity of the enantiomers of 9-fluoro-3-methyl-10-(4-methyl-1-piperazinyl)-7H-pyrido [1,2,3-de]-1,4-benzoxazine-6-carboxylic acid (ofloxacin). *J. Med. Chem.* **30:**2283–2286.
54. **Mitscher, L. A., and L. L. Shen.** A cooperative quinolone-DNA binding model for DNA gyrase inhibition—implications in drug design, in press. *In* T. Perun and C. Propst (ed.), *Nucleic Acid Tar-*

*geted Drug Design.* Marcel Dekker, Inc., New York.

55. **Mitscher, L. A., L. L. Shen, and P. N. Sharma.** Unpublished results.
56. **Miyamoto, H., H. Ueda, T. Otsuka, S. Aki, H. Tamaoka, and K. Nakagawa.** 1990. Studies on antibacterial agents. III. Synthesis and antibacterial activities of substituted 1,4-dihydro-8-methyl-4-oxoquinoline-3-carboxylic acids. *Chem. Pharm. Bull. Tokyo* **38:**2472–2478.
57. **Miyamoto, T., J. Matsumoto, K. Chiba, H. Egawa, K. Shibamori, A. Minamida, Y. Nishimura, H. Okada, M. Katasoka, M. Fujita, T. Hirose, and J. Nakano.** 1990. Pyridonecarboxylic acids as antibacterial agents. 14. Synthesis and structure-activity relationships of 5-substituted 6,8-difluoroquinolones, including sparfloxacin, a new quinolone antibacterial agent with improved potency. *J. Med. Chem.* **33:**1645–1656.
58. **Moran, D. B., C. B. Ziegler, T. S. Dunne, N. A. Kuck, and Y.-I. Lin.** 1989. Synthesis of novel 5-fluoro analogues of norfloxacin and ciprofloxacin. *J. Med. Chem.* **32:**1313.
59. **Morita, S., K. Otsubo, M. Uchida, S. Kawabata, H. Tamaoka, and T. Shimizu.** 1990. Synthesis and antibacterial activity of the metabolites of 9-fluoro-6,7-dihydro-8-(4-hydroxy-1-piperidyl)-5-methyl-1-oxo-1H,5H-benzo[i.j]quinolizine-2-carboxylic acid (OPC-7251). *Chem. Pharm. Bull. Tokyo* **38:**2027.
60. **Nakamura, S., A. Minami, K. Nakata, N. Kurobe, K. Kouno, Y. Sakaguchi, S. Kashimoto, H. Yoshida, T. Kojima, T. Ohue, K. Fujimoto, M. Nakamura, M. Hashimoto, and M. Shimizu.** 1989. In vitro and in vivo antibacterial activities of AT-4140, a new broad-spectrum quinolone. *Antimicrob. Agents Chemother.* **33:**1167–1173.
61. **Narita, H., Y. Konishi, J. Nitta, I. Kitayama, M. Miyazime, Y. Watanabe, A. Yotsuji, and I. Saikawa.** 1986. Pyridone carboxylic acids as antibacterial agents. V. Synthesis and structure-activity relationship of 7-amino-6-fluoro-1-(fluorophenyl)-4-oxo-1,8-naphthyridine-3-carboxylic acids. Yakugaku Zasshi **106:**802–807.
62. **Narita, H., Y. Konishi, J. Nitta, Y. Kobayashi, Y. Watanabe, S. Minami, and I. Saikawa.** 1986. Pyridone carboxylic acids as antibacterial agents. II. Synthesis and structure-activity relationship of 1-(4-hydroxyphenyl)-6-substituted-4-pyridone-3-carboxylic acids. *Yakugaku Zasshi* **106:**782–787.
63. **Narita, H., Y. Konishi, J. Nitta, M. Miyazima, Y. Watanabe, A. Yotsuji, and I. Saikawa.** 1986. Pyridone carboxylic acids as antibacterial agents. III. Synthesis and structure-activity relationship of 1-(4-fluorophenyl)- and 1-(2,4-difluorophenyl)-6-substituted-4-pyridone-3-carboxylic acids. *Yakugaku Zasshi* **106:**788–794.
64. **Narita, H., Y. Konishi, J. Nitta, H. Nagaki, I. Kitayama, Y. Watanabe, and I. Saikawa.** 1986. Pyridone carboxylic acids as antibacterial agents. I. Synthesis and structure-activity relationship of 1-aryl-6-(4-dimethylaminophenyl)-4-pyridone-3-carboxylic acids. *Yakugaku Zasshi* **106:**775–781.
65. **Narita, H., Y. Konishi, J. Nitta, H. Nagaki, Y. Kobayashi, Y. Watanabe, S. Minami, and I. Saikawa.** 1986. Pyridone carboxylic acids as antibacterial agents. IV. Synthesis and structure-activity relationships of 7-amino-1-aryl-6-fluoro-4-quinolone-3-carboxylic acids. *Yakugaku Zasshi* **106:**795–801.
66. **Neu, H. C., A. Novelli, and N. Chin.** 1989. Comparative in vitro activity of a new quinolone, AM-1091. *Antimicrob. Agents Chemother.* **33:**1036–1041.
67. **Nishimura, Y., T. Hirose, H. Okada, K. Shibamori, J. Nakano, and J. Matsumoto.** 1990. Synthesis of 7-thio-substituted 4-oxoquinoline-3-carboxylic acids with antibacterial activity. *Chem. Pharm. Bull. Tokyo* **38:**2190–2198.
68. **Nishimura, Y., and J. Matsumoto.** 1987. Pyridone carboxylic acids as antibacterial agents. 9. Synthesis and antibacterial activity of 1-substituted 6-fluoro-1,4-dihydro-4-oxo-7-(4-pyridyl)-1,8-naphthyridine-3-carboxylic acids. *J. Med. Chem.* **30:**1622–1625.
69. **Nishimura, Y., A. Minamida, and J. Matsumoto.** 1987. Pyridone carboxylic acids as antibacterial agents. XII. Synthesis and antibacterial activity of enoxacin analogues with a variant at position 1. *Chem. Pharm. Bull.* **36:**1223–1228.
70. **Okada, T., T. Tsuji, T. Tsushima, K. Ezumi, T. Yoshida, and S. Matsuura.** 1991. Synthesis and antibacterial activities of novel oxazine and thiazine ring-fused tricyclic quinolonecarboxylic acids: 10-(alicyclic amino)-9-fluoro-7-oxo-7H-pyrido[1,2,3-de][1,4]benzoxazine-6-carboxylic acids and the corresponding 1-thia congeners. *J. Heterocyclic Chem.* **28:**1067–1074.
71. **Okada, T., T. Tsuji, T. Tsushima, T. Yoshida, and S. Matsuura.** 1991. Synthesis and antibacterial activities of novel dihydrooxazine and dihydrothiazine ring-fused tricyclic quinolenecarboxylic acids: 9-fluoro-3-methylene-10-(4-methylpiperazin-1-yl)-7-oxo-2,3-dihydro-7H-pyrido [1,2,3-de][1,4]benzoxazine-6-carboxylic acid and its 1-thia congener. *J. Heterocyclic Chem.* **28:**1061–1065.

71a. **Ozaki, M., M. Matsuda, Y. Tomii, K. Kimura, K. Kazuno, M. Kitano, M. Kise, K. Shibata, M. Otsuki, and T. Nishino.** 1991. In vitro antibacterial activity of a new quinolone, NM394. *Antimicrob. Agents Chemother.* **35:**2490–2495.

72. **Pfeiffer, C. C.** 1956. Optical isomerism and pharmacological action, a generalization. *Science* **124:**29–31.

73. **Remuzon, P., D. Bouzard, P. DiCesare, M. Essiz, J. P. Jacquet, J. R. Kiechel, B. LeDoussal, R. E. Kessler, and J. Fungtomc.** 1991. Fluoronaphthyridines and fluoroquinolones as antibacterial agents. 3. Synthesis and structure activity relationships of new 1-(1,1-dimethyl-2-fluoroethyl), 1-[1-methyl-1-(fluoromethyl)-2-fluoroethyl], and 1-[1,1-(difluoromethyl)-2-fluoroethyl] substituted derivatives. *J. Med. Chem.* **34:**29–37.

74. **Rolston, K. V. I., B. Leblanc, D. H. Ho, and G. P. Bodey.** 1990. In vitro activity of PD-117596, a new quinolone, against bacterial isolates from cancer patients. *J. Antimicrob. Chemother.* **26:**39–44.

75. **Rosen, T., D. T. W. Chu, I. M. Lico, P. B. Fernandes, K. Marsh, L. L. Shen, V. G. Cepa, and A. G. Pernet.** 1988. Design, synthesis and properties of (4S)-7-(4-amino-2-substituted-pyrrolidin-1-yl)quinolone-3-carboxylic acids. *J. Med. Chem.* **31:**1598.

76. **Rosen, T., D. T. W. Chu, I. M. Lico, P. B. Fernandes, L. L. Shen, S. Borodkin, and A. G. Pernet.** 1988. Asymmetric synthesis and properties of the enantiomers of the antibacterial agent 7-(3-aminopyrrolidin-1-yl)-1-(2,4-difluorophenyl)-1,4-dihydro-6-fluoro-4-oxo-1,8-naphthyridine-3-carboxylic acid hydrochloride. *J. Med. Chem.* **31:**1586–1589.

77. **Sanchez, J. P., J. M. Domagala, S. E. Hagen, C. L. Heifetz, M. P. Hutt, J. B. Nichols, and A. K. Trehan.** 1988. Quinolone antibacterial agents. Synthesis and structure-activity relationships of 8-substituted quinoline-3-carboxylic acids and 1,8-naphthyridine-3-carboxylic acids. *J. Med. Chem.* **31:**983–991.

78. **Sedlock, D. M., R. A. Dobson, D. M. Deuel, G. Y. Lesher, and J. B. Rake.** 1990. In vitro and in vivo activities of a new quinolone, WIN 57273, possessing potent activity against gram-positive bacteria. *Antimicrob. Agents Chemother.* **34:**568–575.

79. **Shen, L. L., M. G. Bures, D. T. W. Chu, and J. J. Plattner.** 1990. Quinolone-DNA interaction: how a small drug molecule acquires high DNA binding affinity and specificity, p. 495–512. *In* B. Pullman and J. Jortner (ed.), *Molecular Basis of Specificity in Nucleic Acid-Drug Interactions.* Kluwer Academic Publishers, Amsterdam.

80. **Stotnicki, J. S., B. A. Steinbaugh, and D. P. Strike.** 1988. Tricyclic fluoroquinolones as potential antimicrobial agents. *Drug Design Delivery* **3:**257–261.

81. **Uno, T., H. Kondo, Y. Inoue, Y. Kawahata, M. Sotomura, K. Iuchi, and G. Tsukamoto.** 1990. Synthesis of antimicrobial agents. 3. Syntheses and antibacterial activities of 7-(4-hydroxypiperazin-1-yl) quinolones. *J. Med. Chem.* **33:**2929–2932.

82. **Uno, T., M. Takamatsu, Y. Inoue, Y. Kawahata, K. Iuchi, and G. Tsukamoto.** 1987. Synthesis of antimicrobial agents. I. Syntheses and antibacterial activities of 7-(azole substituted)quinolones. *J. Med. Chem.* **30:**2163–2168.

83. **Venezia, R. A., L. A. Prymas, A. Shayegani, and D. M. Yocum.** 1989. In vitro activities of amifloxacin and two of its metabolites. *Antimicrob. Agents Chemother.* **33:**762–766.

84. **Wentland, M. P., D. M. Bailey, J. B. Cornett, R. A. Dobson, R. G. Powles, and R. B. Wagner.** 1984. Novel amino-substituted 3-quinolinecarboxylic acid antibacterial agents: synthesis and structure-activity relationships. *J. Med. Chem.* **27:**1103–1108.

85. **Wentland, M. P., R. B. Perni, P. H. Dorff, and J. B. Rake.** 1988. Synthesis and bacterial DNA gyrase inhibitory properties of a spirocyclopropylquinolone derivative. *J. Med. Chem.* **31:**1694–1697.

86. **Wise, R., J. M. Andrews, J. P. Ashby, and R. S. Matthews.** 1988. In vitro activity of lomefloxacin, a new quinolone antimicrobial agent, in comparison with those of other agents. *Antimicrob. Agents Chemother.* **32:**617–622.

87. **Yanagisawa, H., H. Nakao, and A. Ando.** 1973. Studies on chemotherapeutic agents. I. Syntheses of quinoline and naphthyridine sulfonamide or phosphonic acid derivatives. *Chem. Pharm. Bull. Jpn.* **21:**1080–1089.

88. **Yoshida, T., Y. Yamamoto, N. Yagi, Y. Takahashi, S. Yasuda, H. Katoh, and Y. Itoh.** 1991. Studies on quinolone antibiotics. 2. Synthesis and antibacterial activity of 7-aminoalkoxy-1-cyclopropyl-6-fluoro-1,4-dihydro-4-oxoquinoline-3-carboxylic acids and their derivatives. *J. Pharm. Soc. Jpn.* 111:19–31.

89. **Yoshida, T., Y. Yamamoto, N. Yagi, S. Yasuda, H. Katoh, and Y. Itoh.** 1990. Studies on quinolone antibacterials. I. Synthesis and antibacterial activity of 7-(2-aminoethoxy)-, 7-(2-aminoethylthio)-, and 7-(2-aminoethylamino)-1-cyclopropyl-6-fluoro-1,4-dihydro-4-oxoquinoline-3-carboxylic acids and their derivatives. *Yakugaku Zasshi* **110:**258–267.

90. **Zhang, M. Q., A. Haemers, D. Van den Berghe, S. R. Pattyn, W. Bollaert, and I. Levshin.** 1991. Quinolone antibacterials. 1. 7-(2-Substituted-4-thiazolyl and thiazolidinyl)quinolones. *J. Heterocyclic Chem.* **28:**673–683.

91. **Zhang, M. Q., A. Haemers, D. Van den Berghe, S. R. Pattyn, W. Bollaert, and I. Levshin.** 1991. Quinolone antibacterials. 2. 6-Substituted-7-(2-thiazolyl and thiazolidinyl)quinolones. *J. Heterocyclic Chem.* **28:**685–695.

92. **Ziegler, C. B., Jr., P. Bitha, N. A. Kuck, T. J. Fenton, P. J. Petersen, and Y.-I. Lin.** 1990. Synthesis and structure-activity relationships of new 7-[3-(fluoromethyl)piperazinyl]- and -(fluorohomopiperazinyl)quinolone antibacterials. *J. Med. Chem.* **33:**142–146.

*Quinolone Antimicrobial Agents, 2nd ed.*
Edited by David C. Hooper and John S. Wolfson


*Chapter 3*

# Mechanisms of Quinolone Action and Bacterial Killing

*David C. Hooper and John S. Wolfson**

In recent years, there has been considerable interest in the development and clinical use of the newer quinolone agents (46, 71, 73, 76, 132, 139, 216, 217). These agents include norfloxacin, ciprofloxacin, ofloxacin, enoxacin, amifloxacin, fleroxacin, temafloxacin, lomefloxacin, and others, many of which are designated only by compound numbers. Nalidixic acid and oxolinic acid were the first quinolone agents marketed. In contrast to these earlier drugs, the newer agents are more potent, have broader spectra of activity in vitro, and are less prone to selection of resistant strains (216).

In this chapter we review information on the mechanisms of action of and bacterial killing by quinolone agents. Mechanisms of bacterial resistance to quinolones will be reviewed in chapter 5. Topics to be discussed here include problems with the structure of DNA, topoisomerases and how they solve these problems, the structure and functions of DNA gyrase, effects of quinolone agents on DNA gyrase and viable bacteria, and determinants of bacterial killing by quinolones.

A number of detailed reviews covering these topics have been published (40, 51, 77, 78, 80, 124, 145, 161, 188, 204, 205, 218).

*David C. Hooper and John S. Wolfson* • Infectious Disease Unit, Massachusetts General Hospital, 14 Fruit Street, Boston, Massachusetts 02114-2696.
*Deceased.

Structural analogs of quinolones, such as the 1,8-naphthyridines nalidixic acid and enoxacin, will for simplicity be referred to as quinolones in this chapter.

## COMMENTS ON THE STRUCTURE OF DNA

The linear, double-helix structure of DNA (208) in a beautiful way encodes genetic information, allows mutation and recombination, and serves as a template for semiconservative replication and transcription (209).

The configuration of the DNA molecule, however, leads to certain difficulties. One problem arises from the condensed state of DNA within the cell. For the bacterium *Escherichia coli,* the chromosome is a circular DNA molecule 1,100 μm long (14) present in a cell only 1 to 2 μm long. This DNA molecule, despite its 1,000-fold-condensed state, must be able to replicate, segregate into daughter chromosomes, and allow transcription of individual genes without becoming lethally entangled.

A second problem occurs because of the helical nature of the DNA duplex. With each turn of the helix, which occurs on the average every 10.4 bp, two single strands are wrapped around each other. In the *E. coli* chromosome, which contains 4 million bp, strands are intertwined about 400,000 times, thus generating a linking number of 400,000. The two DNA strands must then unwind 400,000 times to allow semiconservative replication. In 1963, John Cairns (14) recognized the magnitude of the unwinding problem when he first visualized the replicating chromosome of *E. coli* and deduced that a swivel was required to permit untwisting of the DNA double helix during strand separation.

A third special situation exists for prokaryotes, because negative supercoils are present in DNA isolated from bacteria (6, 51). These negative supercoils result in bacterial DNA that contains slightly less than one helical turn for each 10.4 bp (51) and therefore has a linking number lower than that of eukaryotic DNA. This slightly underwound state of intracellular bacterial DNA is thought to facilitate strand separation required for DNA replication and initiation of transcription. Negative supercoils are energetically unfavorable, and therefore an energy-consuming process within the bacterial cell is needed for their generation.

A fourth, more recently recognized problem in DNA topology arises during transcription of certain genes by RNA polymerase (206). For membrane-bound, looped, or otherwise constrained segments of DNA, tracking of RNA polymerase along the helical DNA template generates positive DNA supercoils ahead of and negative supercoils behind the enzyme (116, 155, 222, 223). If not resolved, accumulation of supercoils of opposite polarities in these domains would likely limit the efficiency of transcription.

Each of these problems is either known or likely to be resolved by one or another member of the class of enzymes called topoisomerases.

## TYPES OF TOPOISOMERASES

For prokaryotic DNA, the problems of entanglement, strand unwinding, and supercoiling are solved, at least in part, by topoisomerases (40, 51, 204, 205) (Table 1). Topoisomerases are enzymes that alter the number of times one single strand of a DNA duplex winds around its complementary strand; that is, topoisomerases selectively alter the linking number of a double-stranded DNA molecule. DNA molecules that differ only in linking numbers are called topological isomers or topoisomers.

Topoisomerases may be categorized into three groups: type II topoisomerases (represented by DNA gyrase and topoisomerase IV in prokaryotes), type I topoisomerases (represented by topoisomerases I and III in prokaryotes), and special topoisomerases (such as enzymes catalyzing transposition or integration into and excision of bacteriophage DNA from the bacterial chromosome).

Type II and type I topoisomerases differ in their mechanisms of action. Type II enzymes transiently cleave both strands of the double helix and pass another double-helical segment through this break, while type I enzymes transiently break one strand of a double helix and pass through another single strand. As was originally demonstrated by Brown and

**Table 1.** Topoisomerases identified in *E. coli*

| Topoisomerase | Type | Subunit(s) | Gene(s) | Gene location(s) (min) |
|---|---|---|---|---|
| I | I | TopA | *topA* | 28 |
| II (DNA gyrase) | II | GyrA | *gyrA* | 48 |
| | | GyrB | *gyrB* | 83 |
| III | I | TopB | *topB* | 39 |
| IV | II | ParC | *parC* | 65 |
| | | ParE | *parE* | 65 |

Cozzarelli (11), DNA topoisomers are altered in linking number in steps of two by type II enzymes and in steps of one by type I enzymes.

Type II and type I topoisomerases have been isolated from many species by bacteria and eukaryotes, including human cells. Presumably, every living organism encodes at least one of each type of topoisomerase. For further discussion of eukaryotic topoisomerases and their inhibition by quinolones, see chapter 7.

### Bacterial Topoisomerase I

James Wang (203) in 1969 isolated the first topoisomerase, topoisomerase I, from *E. coli*. This type I enzyme is a 110-kDa protein and is encoded by the *topA* gene (194), which is located at 28 min on the genetic map of the *E. coli* chromosome. Topoisomerase I from both prokaryotic and eukaryotic sources catalyzes removal of negative supercoils from DNA in the absence of ATP (203). Eukaryotic topoisomerase I has the additional ability to remove positive supercoils from DNA (see chapter 7). The DNA relaxation activity of *E. coli* topoisomerase I is inhibited only by high concentrations of quinolones (133, 190). Within bacteria, topoisomerase I, along with DNA gyrase, regulates the level of negative supercoiling of intracellular DNA (34, 41) and is required for transcription of certain operons (182). A direct role for the enzyme in transcription is also suggested by the accumulation of negative supercoils in plasmid pBR322 DNA in *topA* mutants (153). This accumulation of excessive negative supercoils is dependent on transcription of the plasmid-encoded *tet* gene, suggesting that removal of negative supercoils developing behind RNA polymerase as it moves along the *tet* gene requires topoisomerase I.

Deletion mutants lacking *topA* exist (182), but viability requires compensating mutations in the genes for DNA gyrase (34), reduced gyrase activity resulting from treatment with novobiocin (62), or duplication of a region of the chromosome that includes the genes for topoisomerase IV and an outer membrane protein, TolC (38). These findings suggest that excess negative supercoiling of DNA occurring in the absence of topoisomerase I impairs cell viability and that this impairment can be ameliorated by reduced supercoiling by DNA gyrase.

Novel type I topoisomerases called reverse gyrases have been found in thermophilic archaebacteria (129, 136) and eubacteria (10). Although they relax negatively supercoiled DNA at high temperatures (129), these enzymes differ from the *E. coli* enzyme in that they convert relaxed or negatively supercoiled DNA into positively supercoiled DNA and are ATP dependent (136). Activity of the archaebacterial enzyme was only poorly inhibited by the quinolones oxolinic acid and pefloxacin (129).

### Bacterial Topoisomerase III

More recently, a second type I topoisomerase, topoisomerase III, was identified in *E. coli* (179). Like topoisomerase I, it is able to remove negative but not positive superhelical twists without a requirement for ATP (179), but this activity of topoisomerase III is much less efficient than its ability to decatenate nicked daughter DNA circles of plasmid pBR322 that are multiply interlinked following a cycle of DNA replication (30). This decatenase activity was unaffected by norfloxacin (30). Topoisomerase III can bind RNA as well as DNA and can induce cleavage of both nucleic acids at identical nucleotide sequences although with different site preferences (32).

Topoisomerase III is encoded by the *topB* gene located at 38.7 min on the *E. coli* genetic map (31). The role of the enzyme in intact cells is unclear, but the recent determination that a *mutR* mutant, which has an increased frequency of spontaneous DNA deletions, is a *topB* mutant (170) supports an earlier suggestion that the enzyme may have a role in DNA recombination (207). Survival of mutants with chromosomal deletions encompassing 38.4 to 39 min suggests that the *topB* gene is not an essential gene (31).

## DNA Gyrase (Bacterial Topoisomerase II)

### Gyrase protein structure

Martin Gellert and associates (54) in 1976 isolated the first type II topoisomerase, DNA gyrase from *E. coli* (40, 51, 161, 204, 205). DNA gyrase is a multisubunit enzyme that contains two A subunits (GyrA) and two B subunits (GyrB) (102, 107). The GyrA subunits, which are encoded by the *gyrA* gene (48 min), each contain 875 amino acids totaling 97 kDa in mass, and the GyrB subunits, encoded by the *gyrB* gene (83 min), each contain 804 amino acids and are 90 kDa in mass. The holoenzyme is thus 374 kDa, a mass consistent with a value of 353 kDa, determined by small-angle neutron scattering (107). All activities of the enzyme appear to require both subunits, but certain domains mediate different functions.

GyrA mediates DNA strand breakage and reunion with the tyrosine residue at position 122 (Tyr-122), forming a transient phosphotyrosine linkage with a broken DNA strand. GyrB mediates the ATPase activity of the enzyme. Studies using fragments of GyrA and GyrB have also suggested functional subdomains of these polypeptides. For GyrA, a 59-kDa amino-terminal (N-terminal) tryptic fragment complexed with GyrB was sufficient to support weak DNA supercoiling activity. Addition of the carboxy-terminal (C-terminal) 33-kDa GyrA fragment improved enzyme efficiency and was thought to stabilize the complex (160).

For GyrB, a 47-kDa C-terminal fragment complexed with GyrA supports DNA relaxation but not supercoiling or ATP hydrolysis. The N-terminal domain of GyrB (amino acids 2 through 220) is now known to contain the ATP-binding site, according to X-ray analysis of the structure of a crystal of an N-terminal fragment of GyrB with an ATP analog (213). This information is consistent with earlier studies in which lysines at position 103 and 110 were selectively labeled with a reactive ATP analog (191).

The ATPase activity of DNA gyrase is competitively inhibited by novobiocin and other coumarin derivatives, which are structurally unrelated to quinolones (186). The findings that novobiocin resistance mutations were clustered in the 5′ (N-terminal) region of the *gyrB* gene of an archaebacterium (74) and *E. coli* (at arginine 136 and glycine 164) (21) and that the N-terminal portion of the *E. coli* GyrB binds novobiocin equivalently to intact GyrB (161) suggest that novobiocin, like ATP, also binds to the N-terminal domain of GyrB.

The structure of the complex of DNA gyrase and DNA has been studied by electric dichroism and electron microscopy (101, 158). These observations suggest that a single turn of DNA is wrapped around the enzyme, with DNA entry and exit points in proximity. Addition of ATP or a nonhydrolyzable ATP analog induces a structural change in the complex, suggesting increased wrapping of DNA around the enzyme (158). High-resolution electron microscopy further suggested that the gyrase holoenzyme was a heart-shaped structure with DNA wrapped between the upper portions of the heart (101). Recently, the crystal structure of the N-terminal fragment of GyrB has been resolved at the 2.5-Å (0.25-nm) level (213). As noted above, one of the two domains identified (amino acids 2 through 220) contained the ATP-binding site. The GyrB fragments also formed compact dimers that contained a central 20-Å (2.0-nm) hole lined by positively charged arginine residues, suggesting that this region might be involved in DNA binding and strand passing. Preliminary structural information on a crystal of an N-terminal GyrA fragment (amino acids 1 through 572) complexed with GyrB has also been obtained at lower resolution (159).

## Gyrase genes

The *gyrA* and *gyrB* genes from *E. coli* (1,189) and a number of other species (*Klebsiella pneumoniae gyrA* [33], *Pseudomonas putida gyrB* [146], *Proteus mirabilis gyrB* [172], *Neisseria gonorrhoeae gyrB* [181], *Haloferax* sp. *gyrB* [74], *Mycoplasma pneumoniae gyrB* and *gyrA* [20], *Bacillus subtilis gyrB* and *gyrA* [134], and *Staphylococcus aureus gyrB* and *gyrA* [86]) have been cloned and sequenced. In contrast to the genes of *E. coli*, the *gyrB* and *gyrA* genes of *B. subtilis*, *S. aureus*, and *M. pneumoniae* are contiguous. The expression of *gyrA* and *gyrB* in *E. coli* is known to be induced by DNA relaxation (126), and a 20-bp segment within the *gyrA* promoter region is necessary for this induction (127).

## Activities of gyrase in vitro

Reactions catalyzed by purified DNA gyrase (Table 2) include introduction of negative supercoils into DNA, formation and resolution (catenation and decatenation) of covalently closed circular DNA molecules interlocked like links in a chain, and formation and removal of knots within a duplex DNA molecule. These reactions each require ATP, which the enzyme hydrolyzes to ADP and $P_i$ (48). DNA gyrase also requires a divalent cation (optimally magnesium, although manganese will suffice) for activity. Replacement of magnesium by calcium results in an abortive DNA breakage reaction with each GyrA subunit covalently linked to a DNA strand (160), as occurs after treatment with quinolones and protein denaturants (see below). DNA gyrase also has the abilities to remove positive DNA supercoils catalytically in the presence of a nonhydrolyzable ATP analog (52) and to remove negative supercoils in the absence of ATP. The enzyme is less efficient in relaxing than in supercoiling DNA.

## Functions of gyrase in vivo

Reactions catalyzed by DNA gyrase within living bacteria (Table 2) include introduction of negative supercoils and separation of interlocked replicated daughter chromosomes.

**Table 2.** Activities of *E. coli* DNA gyrase

| Form of enzyme | Activity |
|---|---|
| Purified | Negative supercoiling of DNA[a,b,c] |
| | Removal of negative and positive DNA supercoils[b] |
| | Catenation and decatenation of interlinked DNA circles[a,b,c] |
| | Knotting and unknotting of DNA[a,b,c] |
| | ATP hydrolysis (DNA dependent) |
| | (DNA cleavage stabilized by quinolones or calcium, and gyrase-DNA complex trapped by protein denaturants) |
| Within viable bacteria | Negative supercoiling of DNA[b,c] |
| | Resolution of interlocked DNA recombination intermediates[b] |
| | DNA replication (initiation and elongation)[b,c] |
| | Segregation of replicated chromosomes[b] |
| | Transcription (supercoil-dependent promoters, removal of positive supercoils)[b] |
| | Integrative phage recombination and transposition (Tn*5*) (requirement for supercoiling)[c] |
| | Essential (conditional lethal mutuants) |

[a]Coupled to ATP hydrolysis.
[b]Inhibited by quinolones.
[c]Inhibited by coumarins.

The activities of DNA gyrase and topoisomerase I within living bacteria determine the net level of negative supercoiling of DNA (154), with negative supercoils introduced by DNA gyrase and removed by topoisomerase I. The amounts of intracellular DNA gyrase and topoisomerase I are regulated at the transcriptional level in response to the superhelicity of DNA: decreasing the negative supercoiling of intracellular DNA stimulates transcription of the *gyrA* and *gyrB* genes (126, 127) and suppresses transcription of the *topA* gene (195).

DNA gyrase is essential for DNA replication and is involved in both initiation and elongation (growing-point propagation) as judged by the patterns of replication arrest of, respectively, *gyrB* (144) and *gyrA* (105) conditional lethal mutants. DNA gyrase likely functions to satisfy the requirement for negative supercoils to facilitate binding of initiation proteins to DNA and to enhance DNA strand unwinding during fork propagation. DNA gyrase may also be involved in the termination phase of DNA replication by virtue of its ability to decatenate interlocked daughter DNA molecules resulting from completion of a cycle of DNA replication. In support of this role is the observation that dividing bacteria in which DNA gyrase has been inactivated accumulate partially segregated nucleoids that can fully segregate upon addition of purified DNA gyrase (180). Furthermore, *parA* and *parD* mutants isolated for defects in chromosome partitioning have been found to contain mutant alleles of *gyrB* (97) and *gyrA* (88, 89), respectively.

DNA gyrase is also involved in transcription at least indirectly, because negative supercoiling of DNA can increase expression of some operons and decrease expression of others (164, 173). In addition, the enzyme may also be involved more directly in the removal of positive supercoils accumulating ahead of RNA polymerase as it progresses along constrained DNA templates. This effect is suggested by the accumulation of positive supercoils in plasmid pBR322 DNA in cells treated with gyrase inhibitors (3, 118).

DNA gyrase may also be involved in aspects of DNA recombination (199) and DNA repair (65). Its role in the integrative recombination of bacteriophage lambda appears to be that of providing a required supercoiled DNA substrate (131). In eukaryotes, relaxation of DNA by topoisomerases may suppress recombination and contribute to genome stability (207), and DNA supercoiling may facilitate recombination. Thus, DNA gyrase may facilitate recombination in prokaryotes by virtue of its supercoiling activity. Transposition of transposon Tn*5* also appears to be dependent on DNA supercoiling in the recipient DNA and is affected by reduction in gyrase activity by coumarin inhibitors or *gyrA* mutations (95). A special circumstance of nonhomologous (illegitimate) plasmid recombination facilitated by DNA gyrase in the presence of quinolone inhibitors is discussed in the section "Effects of Quinolones on Plasmids and Illegitimate Recombination in Plasmid Systems" below.

## Bacterial Topoisomerase IV

Recent cloning and DNA sequencing of the *parC* locus, mutations in which cause defects in chromosome partitioning, have revealed homology (36%) between the ParC protein and GyrA (98). In addition, the deduced product of a nearby gene termed *parE* was found to have homology (40%) with GyrB. *parC* encodes a 75-kDa protein (99, 100), and *parE* encodes a 70-kDa protein (98). ParC is associated with the bacterial cell membrane, and this association is enhanced in the presence of magnesium and reduced by treatment with DNase I, suggesting that association of the enzyme with the membrane is dependent on the presence of DNA (100). Purified topoisomerase IV (ParC and ParE together but not alone) catalyzes ATP-dependent relaxation of negatively and positively supercoiled DNAs and unknotting of unnicked duplex DNA. This latter activity classifies topoisomerase IV as a type II enzyme. Unlike DNA gyrase, topoisomerase IV has shown no DNA supercoiling activity. The DNA relaxation activity of topoisomerase IV is inhibited by novobiocin and oxolinic acid (100). Purified GyrA and ParC and purified GyrB and ParE appear not to be interchangeable in vitro.

The functions of topoisomerase IV in vivo are not yet fully defined. Overexpression of *parC* and *parE* resulted in increased DNA relaxation activity in cell lysates and complementation of a *topA* mutant, suggesting that *parC* and *parE* may in some circumstances have a role in removal of DNA supercoils. Plasmid catenanes resulting from plasmid DNA replication accumulate in *parC* and *parE* thermosensitive mutants at nonpermissive temperature, an accumulation not found in *gyrA* and *gyrB* thermosensitive mutants under similar conditions (2). Temperature downshift in these mutants results in reductions in plasmid catenanes, reductions that are not inhibited by norfloxacin. Thus, topoisomerase IV may have a particular role in plasmid decatenation. For decatenation of the replicating bacterial chromosome, topoisomerase IV may share this function with DNA gyrase (117), because some mutants of *gyrA* and *gyrB* have a Par phenotype with defective chromosome segregation (88, 89, 97). Conditional lethal mutants of *parC* and *parE* indicate that these genes are essential, although *gyrA* and *gyrB* together, but not alone, in increased gene dosage on plasmids can complement both *parC* and *parE* mutants (100).

## QUINOLONE ACTIONS ON DNA GYRASE AND VIABLE BACTERIA

### Early Studies

Quinolones have marked effects on DNA gyrase and the bacterial cell. Many of the consequences of exposure of bacteria to quinolones were determined for nalidixic acid and oxolinic acid prior to the discovery of DNA gyrase. Goss et al. (22, 28, 58, 59) reported in the mid-1960s that nalidixic acid selectively antagonized DNA synthesis, caused DNA degradation, and induced filamentation of bacteria. The drug was rapidly bactericidal, but this killing effect was blocked in the presence of chloramphenicol, dinitrophenol, or amino acid starvation, three conditions that have in common inhibition of protein synthesis. Crumplin and Smith (26) additionally found that in the presence of nalidixic acid, intermediate-sized DNA fragments accumulated within the cell.

### DNA Gyrase Is a Primary Target of the Quinolones

In 1977, Gellert (53), Cozzarelli (187), and their associates reported genetic and biochemical experiments that defined the GyrA subunit as a primary target of nalidixic and oxolinic acids. Purified DNA gyrase reconstituted with wild-type GyrB subunits and GyrA subunits isolated from a *gyrA* (formerly *nalA*) mutant resistant to nalidixic acid was active in the presence of drug concentrations that inhibited the wild-type enzyme. More recently, similar findings using mixtures of purified mutant and wild-type GyrA and GyrB subunits from other bacterial species, including *B. subtilis* (185), *Enterococcus faecalis* (138), *S. aureus* (143), *Campylobacter jejuni* (57), *Serratia marcescens* (122), *Pseudomonas aeruginosa* (94, 121, 128, 162), *Haemophilus influenzae* (171), and *Citrobacter freundii* (4), have indicated that the GyrA subunit is also a target of quinolone action. Purified gyrase holoenzyme from a resistant isolate of *Enterobacter cloacae* was also shown to be resistant (120). The activities of newer quinolones, including norfloxacin (24, 68, 69, 84), ofloxacin (166, 167, 220), ciprofloxacin (82, 162), and others, against DNA gyrase are reduced by a mutant GyrA subunit. For *B. subtilis* (185) and *P. aeruginosa* (162), as for *E. coli*, the inferences drawn from studies with purified enzyme subunits from resistant strains have also been complemented by genetic studies in which mutations that confer resistance have mapped in the *gyrA* gene (see below). In *S. aureus* (177) and *Staphylococcus epidermidis* (178), the cloned *gyrA* gene from resistant strains had mutations highly similar to those that cause resistance in *E. coli* (see chapter 5).

Two mutations encoding nalidixic acid resistance have also been identified in the *gyrB* gene (93, 224, 225). One of these mutations, *nalD*, causes increased resistance to newer quinolone agents, while interestingly, the other, *nalC*, produces increased susceptibility to those drugs containing a piperazine substituent at position 7 on the quinolone nucleus (175) (see chapter 5). Thus, the GyrB subunit as well as the GyrA subunit is a target of quinolones, perhaps by direct interaction of the drug with the GyrB subunit or alternatively by indirect interactions that affect the GyrA subunit.

The actions of quinolones on topoisomerase IV in vitro (100) suggest the possibility that this enzyme is also a drug target in vivo. A new quinolone resistance locus, *nfxD*, found in a multiply resistant mutant has been shown to map in the region of the *parC* and *parE* genes (140). The quinolone resistance of *nfxD* appears to be conditional and requires the presence of a quinolone resistance *gyrA* mutation (140). If *nfxD* is an allele of *parC* or *parE*, then its conditional phenotype may reflect the dominant lethality of the interaction of quinolones with wild-type DNA gyrase and would further suggest that the interaction of quinolones with topoisomerase IV alone may have a lesser consequence.

## Actions of Quinolones on Purified DNA Gyrase

Nalidixic acid, oxolinic acid, and other quinolone agents antagonize all of the activities of purified DNA gyrase, including introduction of negative supercoils, catenation-decatenation, and unknotting (40, 51, 204, 205) (Table 2). In addition, quinolones stabilize gyrase-mediated double-strand breaks in DNA at specific sites as revealed by exposure to detergent (sodium dodecyl sulfate) and proteinase K (53, 187). Breaks on opposite DNA strands staggered by 4 bp are generated, and the GyrA subunit protein is covalently attached to the protruding 5′ ends of DNA at the Tyr-122 (87) at what is thought to be the active site of the enzyme. Breakage occurs at preferred DNA sites that fit into a broadly defined consensus sequence and are found within the 120- to 150-bp DNA segment that binds to the enzyme. This cleavage likely results from stabilization of a reaction intermediate before DNA religation and completion of the catalytic cycle and is likely involved in the DNA damage induced by quinolones within viable bacteria (see below).

In recent studies of the structure of DNA gyrase-DNA complexes using electric dichroism (158), the addition of ATP or a nonhydrolyzable analog induced a structural change in the complex that suggested increased wrapping of DNA around the enzyme. This ATP-induced structural change does not occur in the presence of norfloxacin. It was postulated that norfloxacin might stabilize the enzyme-DNA complex in the less-wrapped configuration and block supercoiling by preventing structural transition. This possibility is consistent with previous studies showing that DNA gyrase-DNA complexes are more stable in the presence of quinolone agents (66). An alternative interpretation is that norfloxacin might uncouple double-strand cleavage and the binding of unwrapped DNA segments to the enzyme.

Direct molecular studies of quinolone binding to complexes of DNA gyrase and DNA are discussed in detail in chapter 4, and quinolone structure-activity relationships are considered in detail in chapter 2.

## Actions of Quinolones on Bacterial Metabolism and Bacteriophage Growth

Treatment of bacteria with quinolones decreases introduction of negative supercoils into DNA (3,53) and produces damage to DNA (8, 22, 24, 28, 40, 51, 58, 59, 93, 105, 119, 142, 158, 174, 176, 204, 205, 224) (Table 3). These effects require higher drug concentrations in quinolone-resistant *gyrA* mutants, indicating involvement of DNA gyrase. DNA cleavage can be demonstrated in vivo in cells treated with quinolones and then detergents (119, 176). The nucleotide sequence of the consensus cleavage site in vivo was similar to that found in vitro and had considerable degeneracy (119). The sites of cleavage may be altered by changes in DNA supercoiling (49) and by transcription and translation of the genes at or near a cleavage site (103).

The rapid cessation of DNA synthesis after exposure to quinolones involves DNA gyrase and suggests interference with propagation of the DNA replication fork. In addition, cells treated with fleroxacin at around growth inhibitory concentrations develop large nucleoids at the midpositions of filamenting cells, suggesting inhibition of chromosome decatenation after completion of a round of DNA replication (55). It is not known whether this effect is mediated by antagonism of DNA gyrase or topoisomerase IV or by another drug action. At high quinolone concentrations, RNA and protein synthesis are also inhibited. Cell filamentation occurs, at least in part because of antagonism of DNA synthesis and induction of the SOS DNA repair system (148, 150) (see below). This repair system is error prone, and its induction by quinolones may thus increase rates of mutagenesis in the surviving bacteria (56, 226). In addition, expression of *groEL* and *dnaK,* two genes that are part of the generalized heat shock protein system, which protects the cell against adverse conditions, is also induced by quinolones (106, 197).

**Table 3.** Effects of quinolones on viable bacteria

| |
|---|
| Decrease in introduction of negative supertwists into DNA |
| Impairment of decatenation of interlocked DNA circles |
| Damage to DNA |
| Inhibition of DNA synthesis |
| Antagonism of RNA and protein synthesis (at high drug concentrations) |
| Filamentation of cells |
| Induction of SOS DNA repair system and certain heat shock proteins |
| Rapid cell death |

Quinolone action in bacteria appears to involve more than inhibition of DNA gyrase catalytic activity. Kreuzer and Cozzarelli (105) found that growth of bacteriophage T7 was unaffected when the phage was grown at an elevated temperature that was nonpermissive for bacterial growth of the *E. coli* host strain containing a thermosensitive GyrA subunit, suggesting a reduced or absent requirement for gyrase function for phage replication. Addition of nalidixic acid, however, reduced T7 phage burst size at permissive temperature but not at nonpermissive temperature, suggesting that the inhibitory action of the drug on phage T7 involves DNA gyrase even though gyrase function is not required for phage growth. Thus, quinolone inhibition of phage growth is not simply explained by antagonism of DNA gyrase enzymatic activity but may involve, as suggested by Kreuzer and Cozzarelli (105), the formation of an irreversible complex of drug, DNA, and enzyme that functions as a "poison."

Marked variations in antibacterial potencies of different quinolones have been well documented. In many cases, these variations parallel differences in the inhibitory potencies of individual quinolones against DNA gyrase, as has been demonstrated for *Micrococcus luteus* (229) and *E. coli* (36, 82). Antibacterial activity does not always correlate exactly with antagonism of DNA gyrase, however, indicating that other factors, such as differences in permeation, may affect drug potency (36, 229).

Quinolone concentrations that inhibit the DNA supercoiling and decatenating activities of purified DNA gyrase are often 10- to 100-fold higher than concentrations that inhibit bacterial growth. Quinolones are not thought to be concentrated within bacterial cells, and quinolone inhibition of intracellular supercoiling of bacteriophage lambda DNA exhibited a similar discrepancy (54). These discrepancies have suggested that there might exist an intracellular target of quinolones other than DNA gyrase. There remain, however, possible alternative explanations. First, conditions used to evaluate inhibition of purified enzyme may not reflect the intracellular environment. Second, the growth inhibitory event within a cell may be a subtle perturbation of enzymatic activity, such as one or a few DNA cleavage events or a slight reduction of negative supercoiling of DNA. Related to this latter possibility, a series of quinolones has been shown to inhibit enzyme supercoiling activity by 10% at concentrations of drug similar to those that inhibit cell growth (77). The genetic and biochemical studies described above indicate that DNA gyrase is an intracellular target of quinolone agents. Thus, if other drug targets exist, they must occur in addition to DNA gyrase.

Quinolones inhibit purified *E. coli* topoisomerase I but only at concentrations that are 10-fold more than those inhibiting purified DNA gyrase (133,193), and quinolone-resistant *topA* mutants have not been reported. As noted above, the recent report of inhibition of topoisomerase IV by oxolinic acid and the conservation of sequences in the region of *parC* that are homologous to those that affect quinolone susceptibility in *gyrA* (98, 100) suggest the possibilities that *parC* or *parE* mutants that confer quinolone resistance occur and that topoisomerase IV is a secondary drug target. Further studies are needed.

## Actions of Quinolones on the Bacterial Cell Surface

In order to interact with DNA gyrase in the gram-negative bacterial cell cytoplasm, quinolones must traverse both the outer and the inner membranes (12). The routes of penetration of the outer membrane are not fully understood, but they appear to involve diffusion through porin channels (19, 67, 79). For many quinolone analogs, their sizes (275 to 400 Da) and zwitterionic charge configurations at neutral pH are consistent with the properties known to facilitate diffusion of molecules across the major porins of *E. coli*, OmpF and the slightly smaller OmpC (141). Resistant mutants with reduced drug accumulation and reduced porins have also been reported (see chapter 5).

Lipopolysaccharide (LPS) in the outer membrane appears to be a barrier to more-hydrophobic quinolones because mutants of *Salmonella typhimurium* with defects in LPS structure (deep rough mutants) show increased susceptibility to quinolones with higher hydrophobicity (67). It has been suggested that because they chelate magnesium (193), which is necessary for LPS integrity, quinolones may promote their own diffusion across the outer membrane by disrupting LPS (16), a process analogous to the "self-promoted" pathway of aminoglycoside permeation proposed by Hancock and Raffle (63). When used at high concentrations, fleroxacin, a more-hydrophobic congener, accumulates progressively in *E. coli* cells (16), an effect not seen with the more-hydrophilic congeners norfloxacin (83) and enoxacin (7), which reach a stable steady-state level of accumulation. Magnesium reduces quinolone activity and accumulation and appears to affect the activities of hydrophobic analogs more than those of hydrophilic analogs (16). It remains possible, however, that magnesium-quinolone complexes diffuse less well across the outer membrane or differ at other steps in permeation, and the contribution of a self-promoted pathway to quinolone permeation at drug concentrations around the MIC remains undefined. The reason for the reported loss of the effect of magnesium on quinolone activity in stationary-phase cells is as yet unclear (147).

Treatment of bacteria with subinhibitory concentrations of quinolones may alter the cell surface. Growth of an encapsulated strain of *K. pneumoniae* at concentrations of ciprofloxacin below the MIC resulted in cell complement binding and unmasking of outer membrane antigens, possibly as a result of nonhomogeneity of capsule distribution in filamenting cells (214). K1 capsular polysaccharide production by *E. coli* was also reduced by ciprofloxacin (184). Growth in the presence of low concentrations of quinolones reduces the capacity of some uropathogenic strains of *E. coli* to agglutinate erythrocytes and to adhere to uroepithelial cells (29, 61) and of other *E. coli* strains to adhere to small-bowel cells (43). In other uroadherence assays, however, several quinolones had no effect (104), and nalidixic acid increased *E. coli* adherence to an intestinal monolayer (200). Adherence of some *S. aureus* strains to buccal cells and of *E. faecalis* to platelet-fibrin matrices was also reduced by low concentrations of pefloxacin (29), but *S. epidermidis* adherence to vascular prostheses was unaffected (169). It is not known whether these effects are mediated by inhibition of DNA gyrase and effects on DNA supercoiling, which may alter expression of certain genes, or whether they are mediated by other drug actions.

Changes in the cell envelope associated with cell lysis and bactericidal activity are discussed in the section "Morphological changes associated with cell killing" below.

## Effects of Quinolones on Plasmids and Illegitimate Recombination in Plasmid Systems

Some plasmids are eliminated from their bacterial host cells at subinhibitory quinolone concentrations (81, 152, 210, 211), but the effect is highly dependent on the concentration of quinolone used, the plasmid, and the bacterial host. Coumarin analogs may be more effective than quinolones in some circumstances (81). Plasmid elimination suggests that at certain drug concentrations, plasmid DNA replication or segregation may be more sensitive to drug action than chromosomal DNA replication is.

Plasmid conjugation is inhibited by quinolones (13, 85, 137, 212), as is Hfr-mediated transfer of the bacterial chromosome (5, 9, 47, 64, 72, 85). Although coumermycin and nalidixic acid both inhibit Hfr-mediated transfer of the bacterial chromosome, they differ in the reversibility of the inhibition (85). After removal of coumermycin, transfer resumes from the point of inhibition, but after removal of nalidixic acid, transfer restarts at the origin of transfer, suggesting disruption of the transfer replication fork by nalidixic acid.

Nonhomologous (illegitimate) recombination between plasmid pBR322 and bacteriophage lambda in wild-type cell extracts is stimulated by oxolinic acid (90). Recombination in this system is augmented by the addition of purified DNA gyrase and abolished by coumermycin, and stimulation by oxolinic acid is reduced when extracts from quinolone-resistant *gyrA* mutants are used (91, 92). The recombination sites are also similar to gyrase cleavage sites on DNA (91). A model in which exchange of GyrA subunits that are covalently linked to cleaved DNA strands mediates recombination has been proposed (92). In such a model, the role of quinolones may be to stimulate or stabilize the complex of gyrase and linked cleaved DNA to allow exchange of GyrA-DNA between different $GyrB_2GyrA_2$-DNA complexes to occur. The stimulation by oxolinic acid of gyrase-mediated deletion of pBR322 sequences integrated into the bacterial chromosome may also occur by a similar process (130).

## Characteristics of Bacterial Killing by Quinolones

Exposure of most susceptible bacterial species to quinolone agents results in rapid cell death (24, 25, 28, 40, 58, 96, 174, 218, 227). Although bacterial killing appears to require drug interaction with DNA gyrase, our understanding of the other molecular events involved in this phenomenon is incomplete. Some common characteristics of bacterial killing by quinolones, particularly for *E. coli*, have emerged, however.

## Killing kinetics

Killing is initially rapid but slows or reaches a plateau at a viable cell count about $10^4$-fold below the initial inoculum (15, 22, 24, 28, 35, 44, 58, 174, 221). Those cells persisting at this plateau do not appear to represent a mutant subpopulation, because they exhibit neither resistance to growth inhibition nor reduced killing on reexposure to quinolones. Such a subpopulation may, however, represent cells in a stage of the cell cycle that renders them refractory to the lethal effects of quinolones, as has been found for persisting cells exposed to bactericidal β-lactam antibiotics (70, 75, 123). The possibility of cell cycle-specific alterations in quinolone bactericidal activity is suggested by the finding that nascent *E. coli* daughter cells released from adherent biofilms were killed more often by ciprofloxacin than were cells from the resuspended parent biofilm culture or cells grown in a chemostat, despite comparable growth rates (45). Further studies of quinolone killing of synchronized cell populations will likely be needed to clarify this relationship. In chemostat cultures, bactericidal activity is reduced as growth rates decrease (45).

Nondividing *E. coli* (157, 227, 228) and *Enterococcus faecalis* (113) starved by incubation in phosphate-buffered saline are less effectively killed by quinolones than are exponentially growing cells. Reduced killing of *P. aeruginosa* in the stationary phase of growth by quinolones has also been reported (27).

The rate and magnitude of bacterial killing tend to increase with increasing quinolone concentrations, reaching a maximum at 30- to 60-fold above concentrations that inhibit bacterial growth (148, 174). Above this maximal (or optimal) concentration, killing is reduced (25, 174), and thus the quinolones can exhibit a paradoxical or "Eagle" effect (42) (see below), as has been documented for some bacterial strains exposed to penicillin.

## Relation of killing to inhibition of DNA synthesis and DNA gyrase and conditions that reduce killing

Killing by quinolones involves DNA gyrase, because resistance mutations mapping in *gyrA* result in proportional increases in the concentrations of drug needed to inhibit growth and kill bacteria (18, 183). In addition, in some *gyrA* mutants (e.g., *E. coli* MH5), there appears to be a more selective decrease in quinolone killing relative to bacteriostatic activity (24, 183). These findings, however, fail to differentiate between direct involvement of DNA gyrase (e.g., induction of nonrepairable DNA damage by the enzyme) or indirect involvement as a necessary initial event for a subsequent cascade of events leading to bacterial cell death.

MBCs of quinolones correlate with those concentrations that inhibit bacterial DNA synthesis (18), but inhibition of DNA synthesis alone appears insufficient to effect bacterial killing. Treatment of bacteria with chloramphenicol, rifampin, dinitrophenol, or amino acid starvation (24, 28, 157, 227, 228) reduces quinolone killing but does not affect quinolone inhibition of DNA synthesis (28, 149, 215). These treatments have in common the inhibition of protein synthesis, further suggesting that new synthesis of a protein(s) may also be required for cell lethality. The paradoxical effect of reduced killing with increasing quinolone concentrations may thus result from the partial inhibition of protein synthesis known to occur at high drug concentrations (24).

Other conditions have also been reported to selectively affect bacterial killing by quinolones. Increasing concentrations of magnesium appear to antagonize the bactericidal activities of quinolones to a greater extent than their bacteriostatic activities (156). Growth under strict anaerobic conditions has been associated with reduction in bacterial killing by quinolones, which is reversed by oxygen (112). The molecular mechanisms that underlie these effects remain unclear, however, and the contribution of slower growth rates under anaerobic conditions to reduced quinolone killing has not been fully defined.

## DNA damage and involvement of DNA repair systems

Antagonism of purified and intracellular DNA gyrases by quinolones stabilizes a complex with DNA that is cleaved in both strands, with each strand linked to Tyr-122 of GyrA, although this DNA cleavage is usually not detectable until after the addition of protein denaturants (40, 51). Damage to bacterial DNA is suggested by the potent induction of the RecA (SOS) DNA repair system by quinolones (23, 60, 148, 150). Solubilization of radiolabeled precursors incorporated into DNA occurs after quinolone treatment (22, 114) but may represent induction of lytic bacteriophage (22) or the action of DNA repair mechanisms (114) rather than direct DNA degradation produced by quinolones. This solubilization of DNA appears unrelated to the bactericidal activities of quinolones because it occurs under conditions in which bacterial killing is blocked, and killing occurs in the absence of such solubilization in *recB recC* mutants (114) (see below). Increasing concentrations of quinolones result in increased bacterial killing and increasing induction of the RecA system as measured by expression of *recA-lacZ* gene fusions (148, 151). Maximum killing and induction of RecA synthesis occur at similar quinolone concentrations, above which secondary inhibition of protein synthesis by quinolones may limit both effects.

Induction of the RecA DNA repair system by quinolones requires an active DNA replication fork (60) and a functional exonuclease V encoded by the *recB* and *recC* genes (17). It is thought that the RecA protein is activated by DNA damage (115), possibly by exposure of single-stranded regions of DNA (165). Thus, quinolones may act on DNA gyrase molecules at the replication fork to produce a lesion that is converted by exonuclease V to an activating signal for RecA. Activation of RecA stimulates its protease activity, resulting in cleavage of LexA, the repressor of a set of SOS genes including the *recA* gene itself. Conversion of RecA to its active protease form following treatment with nalidixic acid does not require new protein synthesis (165). Binding of multiple RecA molecules to regions of single-stranded DNA may promote DNA repair (115, 165).

Bacterial strains with defects in the RecA-SOS system exhibit increased killing by quinolones (110, 125, 202), suggesting that components of this system repair or reverse rather than contribute to quinolone killing. In *recB recC* mutants, which are hypersusceptible to quinolone killing, RecA is not activated, resulting in no induction of SOS proteins under control of the *lexA* gene (165). Thus, induction of the SOS proteins in the aggregate is not necessary for quinolone killing. Furthermore, a *lexA3* mutant, which encodes a LexA protein that is resistant to cleavage by activated RecA protease, was shown to be killed by nalidixic acid, similarly to its wild-type parent strain (110), while *recA* (defective) mutants were hypersusceptible (125). *recA gyrA* double mutants also have increased quinolone susceptibility relative to quinolone-resistant *gyrA* single mutants (196). The *recA142* (defective) mutation did not appear to affect the abilities of quinolones to stabilize gyrase-DNA cleavage complexes. Thus, the role of the RecA protein itself appears to be protective or reparative. Also consistent with this inference is the reduced quinolone killing by a *recAoC* mutant, which constitutively expresses RecA protein (202).

It is noteworthy, however, that *recA*-defective mutants have also been shown to have increased susceptibility to other agents thought not to damage DNA or activate RecA, suggesting that RecA might be necessary for normal cell membrane integrity (192). Thus, quinolone hypersusceptibility in some *recA* mutants might result in part from altered drug permeation through the cell membrane. There is as yet no direct evidence to support this possibility.

## Morphological changes associated with cell killing

Filamentation of cells following treatment with quinolones (24, 35, 39, 44, 58, 174) likely occurs at least in part from induction of the SOS system, which includes the *sulA (sfiA)* gene, whose product antagonizes the *sulB (ftsZ)* gene product, which is necessary for cell division (37, 201). After exposure of the cell to norfloxacin or ciprofloxacin, filamentation begins by 30 min, continues for 2 to 4 h, and is followed by formation of polar vacuoles and then cell lysis (39, 44). Under these conditions, loss of cell viability occurs primarily within the first 30 to 90 min. Maximal filamentation appears to occur at quinolone concentrations below those producing maximal killing (35). Thus, the role of filamentation per se in quinolone-induced bacterial lethality remains unclear. Quinolone-induced cell lysis has also been associated with decreases in the average peptidoglycan chain length, suggesting a role for autolysin activity in the final events of cell death (198).

## Differences among quinolones

Quinolones differ in their abilities to kill bacteria (174). Ofloxacin and ciprofloxacin, for instance, reduce the viable counts of *E. coli* KL16 more rapidly than does norfloxacin or nalidixic acid. In addition, conditions that substantially reduce the bactericidal effects of some quinolones have lesser effects on killing by other quinolones. Treatment with rifampin or chloramphenicol, which abolishes the bactericidal activity of norfloxacin and nalidixic acid, has only a partial effect on ciprofloxacin, ofloxacin, lomefloxacin, pefloxacin, and fleroxacin (108, 109, 112, 157, 174). This phenomenon has been interpreted to indicate that the latter group of quinolones possess a mechanism of killing (termed mechanism B) in addition to that possessed by all quinolones (termed mechanism A). The ability of some quinolones (such as norfloxacin and enoxacin) to retain bactericidal activity under conditions of starvation in phosphate-buffered saline has been used as a definition of killing mechanism C. The molecular events underlying these mechanisms remain to be completely defined. A *gyrA* mutation eliminates mechanism B for ciprofloxacin (111), but as noted above, a direct or indirect role for DNA gyrase in killing by mechanism B cannot yet be distinguished.

## Differences among species and analysis of mutants

Killing of some bacterial species, such as *Staphylococcus saprophyticus* (50) and *E. faecalis* (113), may be slower than killing of *E. coli,* but the reasons for these differences remain undefined.

Analysis of mutants with selective reductions in killing by bactericidal agents may provide insight into the genetic loci necessary for bacterial killing (135, 163). Such mutants have been described as "tolerant" to killing or as "high persisters" because of the increase in the persisting subpopulation after drug exposure. Enrichment for such mutants has been accomplished by cyclic exposure to high concentrations of $\beta$-lactams or quinolones, often following mutagenesis (135, 221).

In *E. coli* KL16 following nitrosoguanidine mutagenesis, cyclic exposure to high concentrations of norfloxacin resulted in strain DS1, which exhibited a 2-fold increase in the MIC of norfloxacin but a 1,000-fold reduction in killing by norfloxacin. The differences in killing by norfloxacin between DS1 and KL16 were seen at similar growth rates and extended to other quinolones such as ciprofloxacin and ofloxacin and to the GyrB antagonists coumermycin and novobiocin but not to gentamicin and rifampin (221). A locus necessary for this phenotype was localized to the region around 1 to 2 min on the *E. coli* chromosome and was termed *hipQ* (219), because of the *hi*gh-*p*ersister phenotype. It is noteworthy that 15 genes involved in cell division are clustered around min 2 on the *E. coli* chromosome.

Enrichment by cyclic exposure to high concentrations of ampicillin resulted in identification of the *hipA* locus (34 min), mutations in which exhibited high persistence in the presence of ampicillin (135) and nalidixic acid (168). Killing by norfloxacin and ofloxacin was also reduced in *hipA* mutants, and DS1 (*hipQ*) exhibits reduced killing by ampicillin and other β-lactams (219). These findings suggest that there is overlap in the pathways that are important for killing of bacteria by quinolones and β-lactams. HipA appears to be involved in cell division 168), but the function of HipQ is unknown.

One *gyrA* mutation, which causes quinolone resistance in strain MH5, has also been reported to cause a disproportionate reduction in killing by quinolones (24, 183), suggesting that it may be possible to distinguish interactions of quinolones with the complex of DNA gyrase and DNA that are necessary for bacteriostatic and bactericidal activity. Further work is needed.

## Possible mechanisms of bacterial killing by quinolones

Many details of the mechanism(s) of bacterial killing by quinolones remain unclear (22, 40, 148, 150, 174). One working model envisions as an initial event an interaction of quinolones with a complex of DNA gyrase and DNA that results in damage to DNA by induction of a lesion that either is nonrepairable or is rendered nonrepairable when altered by repair enzymes. Observations that quinolones (i) promote gyrase-mediated DNA cleavage in certain settings, (ii) induce the SOS DNA repair system, and (iii) have increased potency against bacteria with mutations in SOS repair genes are consistent with this hypothesis.

Subsequent (and consequent) to this initial event, other events appear to be necessary, and some of them may involve the mechanisms of cell division and may overlap with pathways required for bactericidal action after treatment with β-lactams. Genetic and molecular analysis of *hip*-type mutants will likely be most useful in dissecting these events.

## REFERENCES


1. **Adachi, T., M. Mizuuchi, E. A. Robinson, E. Appella, M. H. O'Dea, M. Gellert, and K. Mizuuchi.** 1987. DNA sequence of the *E. coli gyrB* gene: application of a new sequencing strategy. *Nucleic Acids Res.* **15:**771–784.
2. **Adams, D. E., E. M. Shekhtman, E. L. Zechiedrich, M. B. Schmid, and N. R. Cozzarelli.** 1992. The role of topoisomerase IV in partitioning bacterial replicons and the structure of catenated intermediates in DNA replication. *Cell* **71:**277–288.
3. **Aleixandre, V., G. Herrera, A. Urios, and M. Blanco.** 1991. Effects of ciprofloxacin on plasmid DNA supercoiling of *Escherichia coli* topoisomerase I and gyrase mutants. *Antimicrob. Agents Chemother.* **35:**20–23.
4. **Aoyama, H., K. Sato, T. Fujii, K. Fujimaki, M. Inoue, and S. Mitsuhashi.** 1988. Purification of *Citrobacter freundii* DNA gyrase and inhibition by quinolones. *Antimicrob. Agents Chemother.* **32:**104–109.
5. **Barbour, S. D.** 1967. Effect of nalidixic acid on conjugational transfer and expression of episomal *lac* genes in *Escherichia coli* K12. *J. Mol. Biol.* **28:**373–376.
6. **Bauer, W. R.** 1987. Structure and reactions of closed duplex DNA. *Annu. Rev. Biophys. Bioeng.* **7:**287–313.
7. **Bedard, J., S. Wong, and L. E. Bryan.** 1987. Accumulation of enoxacin by *Escherichia coli* and *Bacillus subtilis. Antimicrob. Agents Chemother.* **31:**1348–1354.
8. **Bliska, J. B., and N. R. Cozzarelli.** 1987. Use of site-specific recombination as probe of DNA structure and metabolism in vivo. *J. Mol. Biol.* **194:**205–218.
9. **Bouck, N., and E. A. Adelberg.** 1970. Mechanisms of action of nalidixic acid on conjugating bacteria. *J. Bacteriol.* **102:**688-701.
10. **Bouthier de la Tour, C., C. Portemer, R. Huber, P. Forterre, and M. Duguet.** 1991. Reverse gyrase in thermophilic eubacteria. *J. Bacteriol.* **173:**3921–3923.
11. **Brown, P. O., and N. R. Cozzarelli.** 1979. A sign inversion mechanism for enzymatic supercoiling of DNA. *Science* **206:**1081–1083.

12. **Bryan, L. E., and J. Bedard.** 1991. Impermeability to quinolones in gram-positive and gram-negative bacteria. *Eur. J. Clin. Microbiol. Infect. Dis.* **10:**232–239.
13. **Burman, L. G.** 1977. R-plasmid transfer and its response to nalidixic acid. *J. Bacteriol.* **131:**76–81.
14. **Cairns, J.** 1963. The chromosome of *Escherichia coli.* Cold Spring Harbor Symp. Quant. Biol. **28:**43–46.
15. **Carret, G., J. P. Flandrois, and J. R. Lobry.** 1991. Biphasic kinetics of bacterial killing by quinolones. *J. Antimicrob. Chemother.* **27:**319–327.
16. **Chapman, J. S., and N. Georgopapadakou.** 1988. Routes of quinolone permeation in *Escherichia coli. Antimicrob. Agents Chemother.* **32:**438–442.
17. **Chaudhury, A. M., and G. R. Smith.** 1985. Role of *Escherichia coli* RecBC enzyme in SOS induction. *Mol. Gen. Genet.* **201:**525–528.
18. **Chow, R. T., T. J. Dougherty, H. S. Fraimow, E. Y. Bellin, and M. H. Miller.** 1988. Association between early inhibition of DNA synthesis and the MICs and MBCs of carboxyquinolone antimicrobial agents for wild-type and mutant [*gyrA nfxB*(*ompF*) *acrA*] *Escherichia coli* K-12. *Antimicrob. Agents Chemother.* **32:**1113–1118.
19. **Cohen, S. P., D. C. Hooper, J. S. Wolfson, K. S. Souza, L. M. McMurry, and S. B. Levy.** 1988. Endogenous active efflux of norfloxacin in susceptible *Escherichia coli. Antimicrob. Agents Chemother.* **32:**1187–1191.
20. **Colman, S. D., P.-C. Hu, and K. F. Bott.** 1990. *Mycoplasma pneumoniae* DNA gyrase genes. *Mol. Microbiol.* **4:**1129–1134.
21. **Contreras, A., and A. Maxwell.** 1992. *gyrB* mutations which confer coumarin resistance also affect DNA supercoiling and ATP hydrolysis by *Escherichia coli* DNA gyrase. *Mol. Microbiol.* **6:**1617–1624.
22. **Cook, W. A., W. H. Deitz, and W. A. Goss.** 1966. Mechanism of action of nalidixic acid on *Escherichia coli.* IV. Effects on stability of cellular constituents. *J. Bacteriol.* **91:**774–779.
23. **Courtright, J. B., D. A. Turowski, and S. E. Sonstein.** 1988. Alteration of bacterial DNA structure, gene expression, and plasmid encoded antibiotic resistance following exposure to enoxacin. *J. Antimicrob. Chemother.* **21**(Suppl. B):1–18.
24. **Crumplin, G. C., M. Kenwright, and T. Hirst.** 1984. Investigations into the mechanisms of action of the antibacterial agent norfloxacin. *J. Antimicrob. Chemother.* **13**(Suppl. B):9–23.
25. **Crumplin, G. C., and J. T. Smith.** 1975. Nalidixic acid: an antibacterial paradox. *Antimicrob. Agents Chemother.* **8:**251–261.
26. **Crumplin, G. C., and J. T. Smith.** 1976. Nalidixic acid and bacterial chromosome replication. *Nature* (London) **260:**643–645.
27. **Davey, P., M. Barza, and M. Stuart.** 1988. Tolerance of *Pseudomonas aeruginosa* to killing by ciprofloxacin, gentamicin, and imipenem *in vitro* and *in vivo. J. Antimicrob. Chemother.* **21:**395–404.
28. **Deitz, W. H., T. M. Cook, and W. A. Goss.** 1966. Mechanism of action of nalidixic acid on *Escherichia coli.* III. Conditions required for lethality. *J. Bacteriol.* **91:**768–773.
29. **Desnottes, J. F., N. Diallo, C. Loubeyre, and N. Moreau.** 1990. Effect of pefloxacin on microorganism: host cell interaction. *J. Antimicrob. Chemother.* **26**(Suppl. B):17–26.
30. **DiGate, R. J., and K. J. Marians.** 1988. Identification of a potent decatenating enzyme from *Escherichia coli. J. Biol. Chem.* **263:**13366–13373.
31. **DiGate, R. J., and K. J. Marians.** 1989. Molecular cloning and DNA sequence analysis of *Escherichia coli topB,* the gene encoding topoisomerase III. *J. Biol. Chem.* **264:**17924–17930.
32. **DiGate, R. J., and K. J. Marians.** 1992. *Escherichia coli* topoisomerase III-catalyzed cleavage of RNA. *J. Biol. Chem.* **267:**20532–20535.
33. **Dimri, G. P., and H. K. Das.** 1990. Cloning and sequence analysis of *gyrA* gene of *Klebsiella pneumoniae. Nucleic Acids Res.* **18:**151–156.
34. **Dinardo, S., K. A. Voelkel, R. Sternglanz, A. E. Reynolds, and A. Wright.** 1982. *Escherichia coli* DNA topoisomerase I mutants have compensatory mutations in DNA gyrase genes. *Cell* **31:**43–51.
35. **Diver, J. M., and R. Wise.** 1986. Morphological and biochemical changes in *Escherichia coli* after exposure to ciprofloxacin. *J. Antimicrob. Chemother.* **18**(Suppl. D.):31–41.
36. **Domagala, J. M., L. D. Hanna, C. L. Heifetz, M. P. Hutt, T. F. Mich, J. P. Sanchez, and M. Solomon.** 1986. New structure-activity relationships of the quinolone antibacterials using the target enzyme. The development and application of a DNA gyrase assay. *J. Med. Chem.* **29:**394–404.
37. **Donachie, W., and A. Robinson.** 1987. Cell division: parameter values and the process, p. 1578–1593. *In* F. C. Neidhardt, J. L. Ingraham, K. B. Low, B. Magasanik, M. Schaechter, and H. E. Umbarger (ed.), *Escherichia coli and Salmonella typhimurium: Cellular and Molecular Biology,* vol. 2. American Society for Microbiology, Washington, D.C.
38. **Dorman, C. J., A. S. Lynch, N. Ni Bhriain, and C. F. Higgins.** 1989. DNA supercoiling in *Escherichia coli: topA* mutations can be suppressed by DNA amplifications involving the *tolC* locus. *Mol. Microbiol.* **3:**531–540.
39. **Dougherty, T. J., and J. J. Saukkonen.** 1985. Membrane permeability changes associated with DNA gyrase inhibitors in *Escherichia coli. Antimicrob. Agents Chemother.* **28:**200–206.

40. **Drlica, K.** 1984. Biology of bacterial deoxyribonucleic acid topoisomerases. *Microbiol. Rev.* **48:**273–289.
41. **Drlica, K.** 1992. Control of bacterial DNA supercoiling. *Mol. Microbiol.* **6:**425–433.
42. **Eagle, H., and A. D. Musselman.** 1948. The rate of bactericidal action of penicillin in vitro as a function of its concentration, and its paradoxically reduced activity at high concentrations against certain organisms. *J. Exp. Med.* **88:**99–131.
43. **Edmiston, C. E., and M. P. Goheen.** 1989. Impact of subinhibitory concentrations of quinolones on adherence of Enterobacteriaceae to cells of the small bowel. *Rev. Infect. Dis.* **11**(Suppl. 5):S948–S949.
44. **Elliott, T. S. J., A. Shelton, and D. Greenwood.** 1987. The response of *Escherichia coli* to ciprofloxacin and norfloxacin. *J. Med. Microbiol.* **23:**83–88.
45. **Evans, D. J., D. G. Allison, M. R. W. Brown, and P. Gilbert.** 1991. Susceptibility of *Pseudomonas aeruginosa* and *Escherichia coli* biofilms towards ciprofloxacin: effect of specific growth rate. *J. Antimicrob. Chemother.* **27:**177–184.
46. **Fass, R. J.** 1985. Quinolones. *Ann. Intern. Med.* **102:**400–401.
47. **Fenwick, R. G., Jr., and R. Curtiss III.** 1973. Conjugal deoxyribonucleic acid replication by *Escherichia coli* K-12: effect of nalidixic acid. *J. Bacteriol.* **116:**1236–1246.
48. **Fisher, L. M., C. A. Austin, R. Hopewell, E. E. C. Margerrison, M. Oram, S. Patel, K. Plummer, J.-H. Sng, and S. Sreedharan.** 1992. DNA supercoiling and relaxation by ATP-dependent DNA topoisomerases. *Phil. Trans. R. Soc. Lond. B* **336:**83–91.
49. **Franco, R. J., and K. Drlica.** 1988. DNA gyrase on the bacterial chromosome. Oxolinic acid-induced DNA cleavage in the *dnaA-gyrB* region. *J. Mol. Biol.* **201:**229- 233.
50. **Garlando, F., S. Rietiker, M. G. Täuber, M. Flepp, B. Meier, and R. Lüthy.** 1987. Single-dose ciprofloxacin at 100 versus 250 mg for treatment of uncomplicated urinary tract infections in women. *Antimicrob. Agents Chemother.* **31:**354–356.
51. **Gellert, M.** 1981. DNA topoisomerases. *Annu. Rev. Biochem.* **50:**879–910.
52. **Gellert, M., L. M. Fisher, H. Ohmori, M. H. O'Dea, and K. Mizuuchi.** 1981. DNA gyrase: site-specific interactions and transient double-strand breakage of DNA. *Cold Spring Harbor Symp. Quant. Biol.* **45:**391–398.
53. **Gellert, M., K. Mizuuchi, M. H. O'Dea, T. Itoh, and J. Tomizawa.** 1977. Nalidixic acid resistance: a second genetic character involved in DNA gyrase activity. *Proc. Natl. Acad. Sci. USA* **74:**4772–4776.
54. **Gellert, M., K. Mizuuchi, M. H. O'Dea, and H. A. Nash.** 1976. DNA gyrase: an enzyme that introduces superhelical turns into DNA. *Proc. Natl. Acad. Sci. USA* **73:**3872–3876.
55. **Georgopapadakou, N. H., and A. Bertasso.** 1991. Effects of quinolones on nucleoid segregation in *Escherichia coli. Antimicrob. Agents Chemother.* **35:**2645–2648.
56. **Gocke, E.** 1991. Mechanism of quinolone mutagenicity in bacteria. *Mutat. Res.* **248:**135–143.
57. **Gootz, T. D., and B. A. Martin.** 1991. Characterization of high level quinolone resistance in *Campylobacter jejuni. Antimicrob. Agents Chemother.* **35:**840–845.
58. **Goss, W. A., W. H. Deitz, and T. M. Cook.** 1964. Mechanism of action of nalidixic acid on *Escherichia coli. J. Bacteriol.* **88:**1112–1118.
59. **Goss, W. A., W. H. Deitz, and T. M. Cook.** 1965. Mechanism of action of nalidixic acid on *Escherichia coli.* II. Inhibition of deoxyribonucleic acid synthesis. *J. Bacteriol.* **89:**1068–1074.
60. **Gudas, L. J., and A. B. Pardee.** 1976. DNA synthesis inhibition and the induction of protein X in *Escherichia coli. J. Mol. Biol.* **101:**459–477.
61. **Hammani, A., L. Agueda, M. Archambaud, N. Marty, L. Lapchine, and G. Chabanon.** 1987. Etude in vitro des effects de l'acide oxolinique à concentrations sub-inhibitrices sur l'activité des hémagglutinines et de l'adhésion aux cellules uroéphithéliales des *Escherichia coli* isolés des urines. *Pathol. Biol.* **35:**545–550.
62. **Hammond, G. G., P. J. Cassidy, and K. M. Overbye.** 1991. Novobiocin-dependent *topA* deletion mutants of *Escherichia coli. J. Bacteriol.* **173:**5564–5567.
63. **Hancock, R. E. W., and V. J. Raffle.** 1981. Involvement of the outer membrane in gentamicin and streptomycin uptake and killing in *Pseudomonas aeruginosa. Antimicrob. Agents Chemother.* **19:**777–785.
64. **Hane, M. W.** 1971. Some effects of nalidixic acid on conjugation in *Escherichia coli* K-12. *J. Bacteriol.* **105:**46–56.
65. **Hays, J. B., and S. Boehmer.** 1978. Antagonists of DNA gyrase inhibit repair and recombination of UV-irradiated phage lambda. *Proc. Natl. Acad. Sci. USA* **75:**4125–4129.
66. **Higgins, N. P., and N. R. Cozzarelli.** 1982. The binding of gyrase to DNA: analysis by retention by nitrocellulose filters. *Nucleic Acids Res.* **10:**6833–6847.
67. **Hirai, K., H. Aoyama, T. Irikura, S. Iyobe, and S. Mitsuhashi.** 1986. Differences in susceptibility to quinolones of outer membrane mutants of *Salmonella typhimurium* and *Escherichia coli. Antimicrob. Agents Chemother.* **29:**535–538.
68. **Hirai, K., H. Aoyama, S. Suzue, T. Irikura, S. Iyobe, and S. Mitsuhashi.** 1986. Isolation and

characterization of norfloxacin-resistant mutants of *Escherichia coli* K-12. *Antimicrob. Agents Chemother.* **30**:248–253.

69. **Hirai, K., S. Suzue, T. Irikura, S. Iyobe, and S. Mitsuhashi.** 1987. Mutations producing resistance to norfloxacin in *Pseudomonas aeruginosa*. *Antimicrob. Agents Chemother.* **31**:582–586.
70. **Hoffmann, B., W. Messer, and U. Schwarz.** 1972. Regulation of polar cap formation in the life cycle of *Escherichia coli*. *J. Supramol. Struct.* **1**:29–37.
71. **Hoiby, N.** 1986. Clinical uses of nalidixic acid analogues: the fluoroquinolones. *Eur. J. Clin. Microbiol.* **5**:138–140.
72. **Hollom, S., and R. H. Pritchard.** 1965. Effect of inhibition of DNA synthesis on mating in *Escherichia coli* K12. *Genet. Res.* **6**:479–483.
73. **Holmes, B., R. N. Brogden, and D. M. Richards.** 1985. Norfloxacin. A review of its antibacterial activity, pharmacokinetic properties, and therapeutic use. *Drugs* **30**:482–513.
74. **Holmes, M. L., and M. L. Dyall-Smith.** 1991. Mutations in DNA gyrase result in novobiocin resistance in halophilic archaebacteria. *J. Bacteriol.* **173**:642–648.
75. **Holzhoffer, S., R. Sussmuth, and R. Haag.** 1985. Oscillating tolerance in synchronized cultures of *Staphylococcus aureus*. *Antimicrob. Agents Chemother.* **28**:456–457.
76. **Hooper, D. C., and J. S. Wolfson.** 1985. The fluoroquinolones: pharmacology, clinical uses, and toxicities in humans. *Antimicrob. Agents Chemother.* **28**:716–721.
77. **Hooper, D. C., and J. S. Wolfson.** 1988. Mode of action of quinolone antimicrobial agents. *Rev. Infect. Dis.* **10**(Suppl. 1):S14–S21.
78. **Hooper, D. C., and J. S. Wolfson.** 1989. Mode of action of the quinolone antimicrobial agents: review of recent information. *Rev. Infect. Dis.* **11**(Suppl. 5):S902–S911.
79. **Hooper, D. C., and J. S. Wolfson.** 1991. The quinolones: mode of action and bacterial resistance, p. 665–690. *In* V. Lorian (ed.), *Antibiotics in Laboratory Medicine*, 3rd ed. The Williams & Wilkins Co., Baltimore.
80. **Hooper, D. C., and J. S. Wolfson.** 1991. Mode of action of the new quinolones: new data. *Eur. J. Clin. Microbiol. Infect. Dis.* **10**:223–231.
81. **Hooper, D. C., J. S. Wolfson, G. L. McHugh, M. D. Swartz, C. Tung, and M. N. Swartz.** 1984. Elimination of plasmid pMG110 from *Escherichia coli* by novobiocin and other inhibitors of DNA gyrase. *Antimicrob. Agents Chemother.* **25**:586–590.
82. **Hooper, D. C., J. S. Wolfson, E. Y. Ng, and M. N. Swartz.** 1987. Mechanisms of action of and resistance to ciprofloxacin. *Am. J. Med.* **82**(Suppl. 4A):12–20.
83. **Hooper, D. C., J. S. Wolfson, K. S. Souza, E. Y. Ng, G. L. McHugh, and M. N. Swartz.** 1989. Mechanisms of quinolone resistance in *Escherichia coli:* characterization of *nfxB* and *cfxB*, two mutant resistance loci decreasing norfloxacin accumulation. *Antimicrob. Agents Chemother.* **33**:283–290.
84. **Hooper, D. C., J. S. Wolfson, K. S. Souza, C. Tung, G. L. McHugh, and M. N. Swartz.** 1986. Genetic and biochemical characterization of norfloxacin resistance in *Escherichia coli. Antimicrob. Agents Chemother.* **29**:639–644.
85. **Hooper, D. C., J. S. Wolfson, C. Tung, K. S. Souza, and M. N. Swartz.** 1989. Effects of inhibition of the B subunit of DNA gyrase on conjugation in *Escherichia coli*. *J. Bacteriol.* **171**:2235–2237.
86. **Hopewell, R., M. Oram, R. Briesewitz, and L. M. Fisher.** 1990. DNA cloning and organization of the *Staphylococcus aureus gyrA* and *gyrB* genes: close homology among gyrase proteins and implications for 4-quinolone action and resistance. *J. Bacteriol.* **172**:3481–3484.
87. **Horowitz, D. S., and J. C. Wang.** 1987. Mapping the active site tyrosine of *Escherichia coli* DNA gyrase. *J. Biol. Chem.* **262**:5339–5344.
88. **Hussain, K., K. J. Begg, G. P. C. Salmond, and W. D. Donachie.** 1987. *parD:* a new gene coding for a protein required for chromosome partitioning and septum localization in *Escherichia coli*. *Mol. Microbiol.* **1**:73–81.
89. **Hussain, K., E. J. Elliott, and G. P. C. Salmond.** 1987. The *parD*− mutant of *Escherichia coli* also carries a $gyrA_{am}$ mutation. The complete sequence of *gyrA*. *Mol. Microbiol.* **1**:259–273.
90. **Ikeda, H., K. Aoki, and A. Naito.** 1982. Illegitimate recombination mediated *in vitro* by DNA gyrase of *Escherichia coli:* structure of recombinant DNA molecules. *Proc. Natl. Acad. Sci. USA* **79**:3724–3728.
91. **Ikeda, H., I. Kawasaki, and M. Gellert.** 1984. Mechanism of illegitimate recombination: common sites for recombination and cleavage mediated by *E. coli* DNA gyrase. *Mol. Gen. Genet.* **196**:546–549.
92. **Ikeda, H., and M. Shiozaki.** 1984. Nonhomologous recombination mediated by *Escherichia coli* DNA gyrase: possible involvement of DNA replication. *Cold Spring Harbor Symp. Quant. Biol.* **49**:401–409.
93. **Inoue, S., T. Ohue, J. Yamagishi, S. Nakamura, and M. Shimizu.** 1978. Mode of incomplete cross-resistance among pipemidic, piromidic, and nalidixic acids. *Antimicrob. Agents Chemother.* **14**:240–245.
94. **Inoue, Y., K. Sato, T. Fujii, K. Hirai, M. Inoue, S. Iyobe, and S. Mitsuhashi.** 1987. Some properties of subunits of DNA gyrase from *Pseu-*

*domonas aeruginosa* PAO1 and its nalidixic acid-resistant mutant. *J. Bacteriol.* **169:**2322–2325.

95. **Isberg, R. R., and M. Syvanen.** 1982. DNA gyrase is a host factor required for transposition of Tn*5*. *Cell* **30:**9–18.
96. **Ito, A., K. Hirai, M. Inoue, H. Koga, S. Suzue, T. Irikura, and S. Mitsuhashi.** 1980. In vitro antibacterial activity of AM-715, a new nalidixic acid analog. *Antimicrob. Agents Chemother.* **17:**103–108.
97. **Kato, J., Y. Nishimura, and H. Suzuki.** 1989. *Escherichia coli parA* is an allele of the *gyrB* gene. *Mol. Gen. Genet.* **217:**178–181.
98. **Kato, J.-I., Y. Nishimura, R. Imamura, H. Niki, S. Hiraga, and H. Suzuki.** 1990. New topoisomerase essential for chromosome segregation in *E. coli. Cell* **63:**393–404.
99. **Kato, J.-I., Y. Nishimura, M. Yamada, H. Suzuki, and Y. Hirota.** 1988. Gene organization in the region containing a new gene involved in chromosome partition in *Escherichia coli. J. Bacteriol.* **170:**3967–3977.
100. **Kato, J.-I., H. Suzuki, and H. Ikeda.** 1992. Purification and characterization of DNA topoisomerase IV in *Escherichia coli. J. Biol. Chem.* **267:**25676–25684.
101. **Kirchhausen, T., J. C. Wang, and S. C. Harrison.** 1985. DNA gyrase and its complexes with DNA: direct observations by electron microscopy. *Cell* **41:**933–943.
102. **Klevan, L., and J. C. Wang.** 1980. DNA gyrase-DNA complex containing 140 bp of DNA and an $\alpha_2\beta_2$ protein core. *Biochemistry* **19:**5229–5234.
103. **Koo, H.-S., H.-Y. Wu, and L. F. Liu.** 1990. Effects of transcription and translation on gyrase-mediated DNA cleavage in *Escherichia coli. J. Biol. Chem.* **265:**12300–12305.
104. **Kovarick, J. M., I. M. Hoepelman, and J. Verhoef.** 1989. Influence of fluoroquinolones on expression and function of P-fimbriae in uropathogenic *Escherichia coli. Antimicrob. Agents Chemother.* **33:**684–688.
105. **Kreuzer, K. N., and N. R. Cozzarelli.** 1979. *Escherichia coli* mutants thermosensitive for deoxyribonucleic acid gyrase subunit A: effects on deoxyribonucleic acid replication, transcription, and bacteriophage growth. *J. Bacteriol.* **140:**424–435.
106. **Krueger, J. H., and G. C. Walker.** 1984. *groEL* and *dnaK* genes of *Escherichia coli* are induced by UV irradiation and nalidixic acid in an *htpR*$^+$-dependent fashion. *Proc. Natl. Acad. Sci. USA* **81:**1499–1503.
107. **Krueger, S., G. Zaccai, A. Wlodawer, J. Langowski, M. O'Dea, A. Maxwell, and M. Gellert.** 1990. Neutron and light-scattering studies of DNA gyrase and its complex with DNA. *J. Mol. Biol.* **211:**211–220.
108. **Lewin, C. S., and S. G. B. Amyes.** 1990. Conditions required for the bactericidal activity of pefloxacin and fleroxacin against *Escherichia coli* KL16. *J. Med. Microbiol.* **32:**83–86.
109. **Lewin, C. S., S. G. B. Amyes, and J. T. Smith.** 1989. Bactericidal activity of enoxacin and lomefloxacin against *Escherichia coli* KL16. *Eur. J. Clin. Microbiol. Infect. Dis.* **8:**731–733.
110. **Lewin, C. S., B. M. A. Howard, N. T. Ratcliffe, and J. T. Smith.** 1989. 4-Quinolones and the SOS response. *J. Med. Microbiol.* **29:**139–144.
111. **Lewin, C. S., B. M. A. Howard, and J. T. Smith.** 1991. Protein- and RNA-synthesis independent bactericidal activity of ciprofloxacin that involves the A subunit of DNA gyrase. *J. Med. Microbiol.* **34:**19–22.
112. **Lewin, C. S., I. Morrissey, and J. T. Smith.** 1991. The mode of action of quinolones: the paradox in activity of low and high concentrations and activity in the anaerobic environment. *Eur. J. Clin. Microbiol. Infect. Dis.* **10:**240–248.
113. **Lewin, C. S., I. Morrissey, and J. T. Smith.** 1991. The fluoroquinolones exert a reduced rate of kill against *Enterococcus faecalis. J. Pharm. Pharmacol.* **43:**492–494.
114. **Lewin, C. S., and J. T. Smith.** 1990. DNA breakdown by the 4-quinolones and its significance. *J. Med. Microbiol.* **31:**65–70.
115. **Little, J. W., and D. W. Mount.** 1982. The SOS regulatory system of *Escherichia coli. Cell* **29:**11–22.
116. **Liu, L. F., and J. C. Wang.** 1987. Supercoiling of the DNA template during transcription. *Proc. Natl. Acad. Sci. USA* **84:**7024–7027.
117. **Lobner-Olesen, A., and P. L. Kuempel.** 1992. Chromosome partitioning in *Escherichia coli. J. Bacteriol.* **174:**7883–7889.
118. **Lockshon, D., and D. R. Morris.** 1983. Positively supercoiled plasmid DNA is produced by treatment of *Escherichia coli* with DNA gyrase inhibitors. *Nucleic Acids Res.* **11:**2999–3017.
119. **Lockshon, D., and D. R. Morris.** 1985. Sites of reaction of *Escherichia coli* DNA gyrase on pBR322 *in vivo* as revealed by oxolinic acid-induced plasmid linearization. *J. Mol. Biol.* **181:**63–74.
120. **Lucain, C., P. Regamey, F. Bellido, and J.-C. Pechère.** 1989. Resistance emerging after pefloxacin therapy of experimental *Enterobacter cloacae* peritonitis. *Antimicrob. Agents Chemother.* **33:**937–943.
121. **Masecar, B. L., R. A. Celesk, and N. J. Robillard.** 1990. Analysis of acquired ciprofloxacin resistance in a clinical strain of *Pseudomonas aeruginosa. Antimicrob. Agents Chemother.* **34:**281–286.
122. **Masecar, B. L., and N. J. Robillard.** 1991. Spontaneous quinolone resistance in *Serratia mar-*

*cescens* due to a mutation in *gyrA*. *Antimicrob. Agents Chemother.* **35:**898–902.

123. **Mathison, G. E.** 1968. Kinetics of death induced by penicillin and chloramphenicol in synchronous cultures of *Escherichia coli*. *Nature* (London) **219:**405–407.

124. **Maxwell, A.** 1992. The molecular basis of quinolone action. *J. Antimicrob. Chemother.* **30:**409–416.

125. **McDaniel, L. S., L. H. Rogers, and W. E. Hill.** 1978. Survival of recombination-deficient mutants of *Escherichia coli* during incubation with nalidixic acid. *J. Bacteriol.* **134:**1195–1198.

126. **Menzel, R., and M. Gellert.** 1983. Regulation of the genes for *E. coli* DNA gyrase: homeostatic control of DNA supercoiling. *Cell* **34:**105–113.

127. **Menzel, R., and M. Gellert.** 1987. Modulation of transcription by DNA supercoiling: a deletion analysis of the *Escherichia coli gyrA* and *gyrB* promoters. *Proc. Natl. Acad. Sci. USA* **84:**4185–4189.

128. **Miller, R. V., and T. R. Scurlock.** 1983. DNA gyrase (topoisomerase II) from *Pseudomonas aeruginosa*. *Biochem. Biophys. Res. Commun.* **110:**694–700.

129. **Mirambeau, G., M. Duguet, and P. Forterre.** 1984. ATP-dependent DNA topoisomerase from the archaebacterium *Sulfolobus acidocaldarius*. *J. Mol. Biol.* **179:**559–563.

130. **Miura-Masuda, A., and H. Ikeda.** 1990. The DNA gyrase of *Escherichia coli* participates in the formation of a spontaneous deletion by *recA*-independent recombination in vivo. *Mol. Gen. Genet.* **220:**345–352.

131. **Mizuuchi, K., M. Gellert, and H. A. Nash.** 1978. Involvement of super-twisted DNA in integrative recombination of bacteriophage lambda. *J. Mol. Biol.* **121:**375–392.

132. **Monk, J. P., and D. M. Campoli-Richards.** 1987. Ofloxacin. A review of its antibacterial activity, pharmacokinetic properties, and therapeutic use. *Drugs* **33:**346–391.

133. **Moreau, N. J., H. Robaux, L. Baron, and X. Tabary.** 1990. Inhibitory effects of quinolones on prokaryotic and eukaryotic DNA topoisomerases I and II. *Antimicrob. Agents Chemother.* **34:**1955–1960.

134. **Moriya, S., N. Ogasawara, and H. Yoshikawa.** 1985. Structure and function of the region of the replication origin of the *Bacillus subtilis* chromosome. III. Nucleotide sequence of some 10,000 base pairs in the origin region. *Nucleic Acids Res.* **13:**2251–2264.

135. **Moyed, H. S., and K. P. Bertrand.** 1983. *hipA*, a newly recognized gene of *Escherichia coli* K-12 that affects frequency of persistence after inhibition of murein synthesis. *J. Bacteriol.* **155:**768–777.

136. **Nadal, M., G. Mirambeau, P. Forterre, W.-D. Reiter, and M. Duguet.** 1986. Positively supercoiled DNA in a virus-like particle of an archaebacterium. *Nature* (London) **321:**256–258.

137. **Nakamura, S., S. Inoue, M. Simizu, S. Iyobe, and S. Mitsuhashi.** 1976. Inhibition of conjugal transfer of R plasmids by pipemidic acid and related compounds. *Antimicrob. Agents Chemother.* **10:**779–785.

138. **Nakanishi, N., S. Yoshida, H. Wakebe, M. Inoue, and S. Mitsuhashi.** 1991. Mechanisms of clinical resistance to fluoroquinolones in *Enterococcus faecalis*. *Antimicrob. Agents Chemother.* **35:**1053–1059.

139. **Neu, H. C.** 1987. Clinical use of the quinolones. Lancet **ii:**1319–1322.

140. **Ng, E. Y., G. L. McHugh, J. S. Wolfson, and D. C. Hooper.** 1992. Other genetic loci involved in quinolone resistance in *Escherichia coli*, abstr. 1546. *Program Abstr. 32nd Intersci. Conf. Antimicrob. Agents Chemother.*

141. **Nikaido, H.** 1985. Role of permeability barriers in resistance to $\beta$-lactam antibiotics. *Pharmacol. Ther.* **27:**197–231.

142. **O'Connor, M. B., and M. H. Malamy.** 1985. Mapping of DNA gyrase cleavage sites in vivo. Oxolinic acid induced cleavages in plasmid pBR322. *J. Mol. Biol.* **181:**545–550.

143. **Okuda, J., S. Okamoto, M. Takahata, and T. Nishino.** 1991. Inhibitory effects of ciprofloxacin and sparfloxacin on DNA gyrase purified from fluoroquinolone-resistant strains of methicillin-resistant *Staphylococcus aureus*. *Antimicrob. Agents Chemother.* **35:**2288–2293.

144. **Orr, E., and W. L. Staudenbauer.** 1981. An *Escherichia coli* mutant thermosensitive in the B subunit of DNA gyrase: effect on the structure and replication of the colicin E1 plasmid *in vitro*. *Mol. Gen. Genet.* **181:**52–56.

145. **Osheroff, N., E. L. Zechiedrich, and K. C. Gale.** 1991. Catalytic function of DNA topoisomerase II. *Bioessays* **13:**269–275.

146. **Parales, R. E., and C. S. Harwood.** 1990. Nucleotide sequence of the *gyrB* gene of *Pseudomonas putida*. *Nucleic Acids Res.* **18:**5880.

147. **Pérez-Giraldo, C., C. Hurtado, F. J. Morán, and M. T. Blanco.** 1990. The influence of magnesium on ofloxacin activity against different growth phases of *Escherichia coli*. *Antimicrob. Agents Chemother.* **25:**1021–1026.

148. **Phillips, I., E. Culebras, F. Moreno, and F. Baquero.** 1987. Induction of the SOS response by new 4-quinolones. *J. Antimicrob. Chemother.* **20:**631–638.

149. **Piddock, L. J. V., R. N. Walters, and J. M. Diver.** 1990. Correlation of quinolone MIC and inhibition of DNA, RNA, and protein synthesis and induction of SOS response in *Escherichia*

*coli. Antimicrob. Agents Chemother.* **34:**2331–2336.

150. **Piddock, L. J. V., and R. Wise.** 1987. Induction of the SOS response in *Escherichia coli* by 4-quinolone antimicrobial agents. *FEMS Microbiol. Lett.* **41:**289–294.
151. **Piddock, L. J. V., and M. Zhu.** 1991. Mechanism of action of sparfloxacin against and mechanism of resistance in gram-negative and gram-positive bacteria. *Antimicrob. Agents Chemother.* **35:**2423–2427.
152. **Platt, D. J., and A. C. Black.** 1987. Plasmid ecology and the elimination of plasmids by 4-quinolones. *J. Antimicrob. Chemother.* **20:**137–142.
153. **Pruss, G. J., and K. Drlica.** 1986. Topoisomerase I mutants: the gene on pBR322 that encodes resistance to tetracycline affects DNA supercoiling. *Proc. Natl. Acad. Sci. USA* **83:**8952–8956.
154. **Pruss, G. J., S. H. Manes, and K. Drlica.** 1982. *Escherichia coli* DNA topoisomerase I mutants: increased supercoiling is corrected by mutations near gyrase genes. *Cell* **31:**35–42.
155. **Rahmouni, A. R., and R. D. Wells.** 1992. Direct evidence for the effect of transcription on local DNA supercoiling *in vivo*. *J. Mol. Biol.* **223:**131–144.
156. **Ratcliffe, N. T., and J. T. Smith.** 1984. The mechanism of reduced activity of 4-quinolone agents in urine, p. 563–569. *In* D. Adam, W. Stille, G. Ruckdeschel, H. Knothe, H. Lode, and H. V. Eikenberg (ed.), *Gyrase Hemmer, Forschritte der antimikrobiellen und antineoplastischen Chemotherapie FAC 3-5.* Futuramed Verlage, Munich.
157. **Ratcliffe, N. T., and J. T. Smith.** 1985. Norfloxacin has a novel bactericidal mechanism unrelated to that of other 4-quinolones. *J. Pharm. Pharmacol.* **37:**92P.
158. **Rau, D. C., M. Gellert, F. Thoma, and A. Maxwell.** 1987. Structure of the DNA gyrase-DNA complex as revealed by transient electric dichroism. *J. Mol. Biol.* **193:**555–569.
159. **Reece, R. J., Z. Dauter, K. S. Wilson, A. Maxwell, and D. B. Wigley.** 1990. Preliminary crystallographic analysis of the breakage-reunion domain of *Escherichia coli* DNA gyrase A protein. *J. Mol. Biol.* **215:**493–495.
160. **Reece, R. J., and A. Maxwell.** 1989. Tryptic fragments of the *Escherichia coli* DNA gyrase A protein. *J. Biol. Chem.* **264:**19648–19653.
161. **Reece, R. J., and A. Maxwell.** 1991. DNA gyrase: structure and function. *Crit. Rev. Biochem. Mol. Biol.* **26:**335–375.
162. **Robillard, N. J., and A. L. Scarpa.** 1988. Genetic and physiological characterization of ciprofloxacin resistance in *Pseudomonas aeruginosa* PAO. *Antimicrob. Agents Chemother.* **32:**535–539.
163. **Ronda, C., J. L. Garcia, E. Garcia, J. M. Sanchez-Puelles, and R. Lopez.** 1987. Biological role of pneumococcal amidase. Cloning of the *lytA* gene in *Streptococcus pneumoniae. Eur. J. Biochem.* **164:**621–624.
164. **Sanzey, B.** 1979. Modulation of gene expression by drugs affecting deoxyribonucleic acid gyrase. *J. Bacteriol.* **138:**40–47.
165. **Sassanfar, M., and J. W. Roberts.** 1990. Nature of the SOS-inducing signal in *Escherichia coli.* The involvement of DNA replication. *J. Mol. Biol.* **212:**79–96.
166. **Sato, K., Y. Inoue, T. Fujii, H. Aoyama, M. Inoue, and S. Mitsuhashi.** 1986. Purification and properties of DNA gyrase from a fluoroquinolone-resistant strain of *Escherichia coli. Antimicrob. Agents Chemother.* **30:**777–780.
167. **Sato, K., Y. Inoue, T. Fujii, H. Aoyama, and S. Mitsuhashi.** 1986. Antibacterial activity of ofloxacin and its mode of action. *Infection* **14**(Suppl. 4):S226–S230.
168. **Scherrer, R., and H. S. Moyed.** 1988. Conditional impairment of cell division and altered lethality in *hipA* mutants of *Escherichia coli* K-12. *J. Bacteriol.* **170:**3321–3326.
169. **Schmitt, D. D., D. F. Bandyk, C. E. Edmiston, M. F. Levy, G. R. Seabrook, and J. B. Towne.** 1989. The in vitro effect of subinhibitory concentrations of quinolones and vancomycin on adherence of slime-producing *Staphylococcus epidermidis* to vascular prostheses. *Rev. Infect. Dis.* **11**(Suppl. 5):S947–S948.
170. **Schofield, M. A., R. Agbunag, M. L. Michaels, and J. H. Miller.** 1992. Cloning and sequencing of *Escherichia coli mutR* shows its identity to *topB*, encoding topoisomerase III. *J. Bacteriol.* **174:**5168–5170.
171. **Setlow, J. K., E. Cabrera-Juárez, W. L. Albritton, D. Spikes, and A. Muschler.** 1985. Mutations affecting gyrase in *Haemophilus influenzae. J. Bacteriol.* **164:**525–534.
172. **Skovgaard, O.** 1990. Nucleotide sequence of a *Proteus mirabilis* DNA fragment homologous to the *60K-rnpA-rpmH-dnaA-dnaN-recF-gyrB* region of *Escherichia coli. Gene* **93:**27–34.
173. **Smith, G. R.** 1981. DNA supercoiling: another level for regulating gene expression. *Cell* **24:**599–600.
174. **Smith, J. T.** 1984. Awakening the slumbering potential of the 4-quinolone antibacterials. *Pharm. J.* **233:**299–305.
175. **Smith, J. T.** 1984. Mutational resistance to 4-quinolone antibacterial agents. *Eur. J. Clin. Microbiol.* **3:**347–350.
176. **Snyder, M., and K. Drlica.** 1979. DNA gyrase on the bacterial chromosome: DNA cleavage in-

duced by oxolinic acid. *J. Mol. Biol.* **131:**287–302.

177. **Sreedharan, S., M. Oram, B. Jensen, L. R. Peterson, and L. M. Fisher.** 1990. DNA gyrase *gyrA* mutations in ciprofloxacin-resistant strains of *Staphylococcus aureus:* close similarity with quinolone resistance mutations in *Escherichia coli. J. Bacteriol.* **172:**7260–7262.
178. **Sreedharan, S., L. R. Peterson, and L. M. Fisher.** 1991. Ciprofloxacin resistance in coagulase-positive and -negative staphylococci: role of mutations at serine 84 in the DNA gyrase A protein of *Staphylococcus aureus* and *Staphylococcus epidermidis. Antimicrob. Agents Chemother.* **35:**2151–2154.
179. **Srivenugopal, K. S., D. Lockshon, and D. R. Morris.** 1984. *Escherichia coli* DNA topoisomerase III: purification and characterization of a new type I enzyme. *Biochemistry* **23:**1899–1906.
180. **Steck, T. R., and K. Drlica.** 1984. Bacterial chromosome segregation: evidence for DNA gyrase involvement in decatenation. *Cell* **36:**1081–1088.
181. **Stein, D. C., R. J. Danaher, and T. M. Cook.** 1991. Characterization of a *gyrB* mutation responsible for low-level nalidixic acid resistance in *Neisseria gonorrhoeae. Antimicrob. Agents Chemother.* **35:**622–626.
182. **Sternglanz, R., S. DiNardo, K. A. Voelkel, Y. Nishimura, Y. Hirota, K. Becherer, L. Zumstein, and J. C. Wang.** 1981. Mutations in the gene coding for *Escherichia coli* DNA topoisomerase I affect transcription and transposition. *Proc. Natl. Acad. Sci. USA* **78:**2747–2751.
183. **Stevens, P. J. E.** 1980. Bactericidal effect against *Escherichia coli* of nalidixic acid and four structurally related compounds. *J. Antimicrob. Chemother.* **6:**535–542.
184. **Suerbaum, S., H. Leying, H.-P. Kroll, J. Gmeiner, and W. Offerkuch.** 1987. Influence of $\beta$-lactam antibiotics and ciprofloxacin on cell envelope of *Escherichia coli. Antimicrob. Agents Chemother.* **31:**1106–1110.
185. **Sugino, A., and K. F. Bott.** 1980. *Bacillus subtilis* deoxyribonucleic acid gyrase. *J. Bacteriol.* **141:**1331–1339.
186. **Sugino, A., N. P. Higgins, P. O. Brown, C. L. Peebles, and N. R. Cozzarelli.** 1978. Energy coupling in DNA gyrase and the mechanism of action of novobiocin. *Proc. Natl. Acad. Sci. USA* **75:**4838–4842.
187. **Sugino, A., C. L. Peebles, K. N. Kruezer, and N. R. Cozzarelli.** 1977. Mechanism of action of nalidixic acid: purification of *Escherichia coli nalA* gene product and its relationship to DNA gyrase and a novel nicking-closing enzyme. *Proc. Natl. Acad. Sci. USA* **74:**4767–4771.
188. **Sutcliffe, J. A., T. D. Gootz, and J. F. Barrett.** 1989. Biochemical characteristics and physiological significance of major DNA topoisomerases. *Antimicrob. Agents Chemother.* **33:**2027–2033.
189. **Swanberg, S. L., and J. C. Wang.** 1987. Cloning and sequencing of the *Escherichia coli gyrA* gene coding for the A subunit of DNA gyrase. *J. Mol. Biol.* **197:**729–736.
190. **Tabary, X., N. Moreau, C. Dureuil, and F. Le Goffic.** 1987. Effect of DNA gyrase inhibitors pefloxacin, five other quinolones, novobiocin, and clorobiocin on *Escherichia coli* topoisomerase I. *Antimicrob. Agents Chemother.* **31:**1925–1928.
191. **Tamura, J. K., and M. Gellert.** 1990. Characterization of the ATP binding site on *Escherichia coli* DNA gyrase. *J. Biol. Chem.* **265:**21342–21349.
192. **Tessman, E. S., and P. K. Peterson.** 1985. Isolation of protease-proficient, recombinase-deficient *recA* mutants of *Escherichia coli* K-12. *J. Bacteriol.* **163:**688–695.
193. **Timmers, K., and R. Sternglanz.** 1978. Ionization and divalent cation dissociation constants of nalidixic and oxolinic acids. *Bioinorg. Chem.* **9:**145–155.
194. **Trucksis, M., E. I. Golub, D. J. Zabel, and R. E. Depew.** 1981. *Escherichia coli* and *Salmonella typhimurium supX* genes specify deoxyribonucleic acid topoisomerase I. *J. Bacteriol.* **147:**679–681.
195. **Tse-Dinh, Y.-C.** 1985. Regulation of the *Escherichia coli* DNA topoisomerase I gene by DNA supercoiling. *Nucleic Acids Res.* **13:**4751–4763.
196. **Urios, A., G. Herrera, V. Aleixandre, and M. Blanco.** 1991. Influence of *recA* mutations on *gyrA* dependent quinolone resistance. *Biochimie* **73:**519–521.
197. **VanBogelen, R. A., P. M. Kelley, and F. C. Neidhardt.** 1987. Differential induction of heat shock, SOS, and oxidation stress regulons and accumulation of nucleotides in *Escherichia coli. J. Bacteriol.* **169:**26–32.
198. **Vincent, S., B. Glauner, and L. Gutmann.** 1991. Lytic effect of two fluoroquinolones, ofloxacin and pefloxacin, on *Escherichia coli* W7 and its consequences on peptidoglycan composition. *Antimicrob. Agents Chemother.* **35:**1381–1385.
199. **von Wright, A., and B. A. Bridges.** 1981. Effect of *gyrB*-mediated changes in chromosome structure on killing *Escherichia coli* by ultraviolet: experiments with strains differing in deoxyribonucleic acid repair capacity. *J. Bacteriol.* **146:**18–23.
200. **Vosbeck, K., H. Hanschin, E. B. Menge, and O. Zak.** 1979. Effects of subminimal inhibitory concentrations of antibiotics on adhesiveness of *Escherichia coli* in vitro. *Rev. Infect. Dis.* **1:**845–851.

201. **Walker, G. C.** 1984. Mutagenesis and inducible responses to DNA damage in *Escherichia coli*. *Microbiol. Rev.* **48:**60–93.

202. **Walters, R. N., L. J. V. Piddock, and R. Wise.** 1989. The effect of mutations in the SOS response on the kinetics of quinolone killing. *J. Antimicrob. Chemother.* **24:**863–873.

203. **Wang, J. C.** 1971. Interaction between DNA and an *Escherichia coli* protein omega. *J. Mol. Biol.* **55:**523–533.

204. **Wang, J. C.** 1985. DNA topoisomerases. *Annu. Rev. Biochem.* **54:**655–697.

205. **Wang, J. C.** 1987. Recent studies of DNA topoisomerases. *Biochim. Biophys. Acta* **909:**1–9.

206. **Wang, J. C.** 1991. DNA topoisomerases: why so many? *J. Biol. Chem.* **266:**6659–6662.

207. **Wang, J. C., P. R. Caron, and R. A. Kim.** 1990. The role of DNA topoisomerases in recombination and genome stability: a double-edged sword? *Cell* **62:**403–406.

208. **Watson, J. D., and F. H. C. Crick.** 1953. The structure of DNA. *Cold Spring Harbor Symp. Quant. Biol.* **18:**123–131.

209. **Watson, J. D., N. H. Hopkins, J. W. Roberts, J. A. Steitz, and A. M. Weiner (ed.).** 1987. *Molecular Biology of the Gene,* 4th ed., vol. 1. *General Principles.* Benjamin/Cummings Publishing Co. Inc., Menlo Park, Calif.

210. **Weisser, J., and B. Wiedemann.** 1985. Elimination of plasmids by new 4-quinolones. *Antimicrob. Agents Chemother.* **28:**700–702.

211. **Weisser, J., and B. Wiedemann.** 1986. Elimination of plasmids by enoxacin and ofloxacin at near inhibitory concentrations. *J. Antimicrob. Chemother.* **18:**575–583.

212. **Weisser, J., and B. Wiedemann.** 1987. Inhibition of R-plasmid transfer in *Escherichia coli* by 4-quinolones. *Antimicrob. Agents Chemother.* **31:**531–534.

213. **Wigley, D. B., G. J. Davies, E. J. Dodson, A. Maxwell, and G. Dodson.** 1991. Crystal structure of an N-terminal fragment of the DNA gyrase B protein. *Nature* (London) **351:**624–629.

214. **Williams, P.** 1987. Sub-MICs of cefuroxime and ciprofloxacin influence interaction of complement and immunoglobulins with *Klebsiella pneumoniae*. *Antimicrob. Agents Chemother.* **31:**758–762.

215. **Winshell, E. B., and H. S. Rosenkranz.** 1970. Nalidixic acid and the metabolism of *Escherichia coli*. *J. Bacteriol.* **104:**1168–1175.

216. **Wolfson, J. S., and D. C. Hooper.** 1985. The fluoroquinolones: structures, mechanisms of action and resistance, and spectra of activity in vitro. *Antimicrob. Agents Chemother.* **28:**581–586.

217. **Wolfson, J. S., and D. C. Hooper.** 1988. Norfloxacin: a targeted fluoroquinolone antimicrobial agent. *Ann. Intern. Med.* **108:**238–251.

218. **Wolfson, J. S., and D. C. Hooper.** 1990. Mechanisms of killing of bacteria by 4-quinolones, p. 69–85. *In* G. C. Crumplin (ed.), *The 4-Quinolones. Antibacterial Agents In Vitro.* Springer-Verlag, London.

219. **Wolfson, J. S., D. C. Hooper, G. L. McHugh, M. A. Bozza, and M. N. Swartz.** 1990. Mutants of *Escherichia coli* K-12 exhibiting reduced killing by both quinolone and $\beta$-lactam antimicrobial agents. *Antimicrob. Agents Chemother.* **34:**1938–1943.

220. **Wolfson, J. S., D. C. Hooper, E. Y. Ng, K. S. Souza, G. L. McHugh, and M. N. Swartz.** 1987. Antagonism of wild-type and resistant *Escherichia coli* and its DNA gyrase by the tricyclic 4-quinolone analogs ofloxacin and S-25930 stereoisomers. *Antimicrob. Agents Chemother.* **31:**1861–1863.

221. **Wolfson, J. S., D. C. Hooper, D. J. Shih, G. L. McHugh, and M. N. Swartz.** 1989. Isolation and characterization of an *Escherichia coli* strain exhibiting partial tolerance to quinolones. *Antimicrob. Agents Chemother.* **33:**705–709.

222. **Wu, H.-Y., and L. F. Liu.** 1991. DNA looping alters local DNA conformation during transcription. *J. Mol. Biol.* **219:**615–622.

223. **Wu, H.-Y., S. Shyy, J. C. Wang, and L. F. Liu.** 1988. Transcription generates positively and negatively supercoiling domains in the template. *Cell* **53:**433–440.

224. **Yamagishi, J., Y. Furutami, S. Inoue, T. Ohue, S. Nakamura, and M. Shimizu.** 1981. New nalidixic acid resistance mutations related to deoxyribonucleic acid gyrase activity. *J. Bacteriol.* **148:**450–458.

225. **Yamagishi, J., H. Yoshida, M. Yamayoshi, and S. Nakamura.** 1986. Nalidixic acid-resistant mutations of the *gyrB* gene of Escherichia coli. *Mol. Gen. Genet.* **204:**367–373.

226. **Ysern, P., B. Clerch, M. Castano, I. Gilbert, J. Barbé, and M. Llagostera.** 1990. Induction of SOS genes in *Escherichia coli* and mutagenesis in *Salmonella typhimurium* by fluoroquinolones. *Mutagenesis* **5:**63–66.

227. **Zeiler, H.-J.** 1985. Evaluation of the in vitro bactericidal action of ciprofloxacin on cells of *Escherichia coli* in the logarithmic and stationary phases of growth. *Antimicrob. Agents Chemother.* **28:**524–527.

228. **Zeiler, H.-J., and K. Grohe.** 1984. The *in vitro* and *in vivo* activity of ciprofloxacin. *Eur. J. Clin. Microbiol.* **3:**339–343.

229. **Zweerink, M. M., and A. Edison.** 1986. Inhibition of *Micrococcus luteus* DNA gyrase by norfloxacin and 10 other quinolone carboxylic acids. *Antimicrob. Agents Chemother.* **29:**598–601.

*Quinolone Antimicrobial Agents, 2nd ed.*
Edited by David C. Hooper and John S. Wolfson


*Chapter 4*

# Quinolone-DNA Interaction

***Linus L. Shen***

Quinolones are a group of low-molecular-weight, synthetic, extremely potent antibacterial agents. The functional target of these drugs is the enzyme DNA gyrase, an essential type II DNA topoisomerase that exists only in bacteria (reviewed in references 5, 10, 29, 40, and 44). DNA gyrase is a tetramer composed of two A subunits, the 105-kDa proteins encoded by the *gyrA* gene, and two B subunits, the 95-kDa proteins encoded by the *gyrB* gene. Biochemical mechanistic studies have revealed that the functions of the two subunits are responsible for direct DNA cutting and resealing and for the ATP-driven energy transduction process, respectively. The enzyme catalyzes the supercoiling reaction via reduction of the DNA linking number of a covalently closed circular DNA carried out by a concerted strand-breaking-passing-resealing process. The end product of the sequential enzyme-catalyzed reactions is an underwound DNA molecule that spontaneously adopts a negatively supercoiled form as a result of its tendency to take the lowest-energy double-helical configuration. A complete run of supercoiling involves the following four steps: (i) binding of gyrase to DNA substrate to stabilize a positive DNA node, (ii) cleavage of DNA at 4-bp-staggered sites at the node to forming covalent linkages between a tyrosine group on the gyrase A subunit and the 5′ end of the DNA chain, (iii) passage of the intact DNA segment at the node through the opened DNA gate and thus inversion of the sign of the node, and (iv) resealing of the DNA break and release of the enzyme to start a new supercoiling run (2, 24). Quinolone-type drugs such as oxolinic acid trap the cut intermediate (the DNA gate) by stabilizing the enzyme-DNA complex, thus preventing enzyme turnover. The complex is termed a "cleavable complex," since upon addition of a protein denaturant, the complex yields a double-stranded break in DNA with the A subunit attached covalently to the revealed 5′ ends. These observations provide key evidence that the target of the drug is the A subunit of DNA gyrase. Such drug-induced gyrase-dependent damage to chromosomal DNA is believed to be the source of the effects of quinolones on bacterial viability (17; reviewed in reference 8). Investigations of quinolone resistance mutants reveal a much more complex mechanism than was anticipated. The conclusion that *gyrA* is the exclusive target of quinolones has been complicated by the finding that some mutations leading to quinolone resistance are also found in *gyrB* (46, 47, 49).

Studies of direct binding of quinolones to DNA or DNA gyrase have been carried out. The accumulated data indicate that quinolones are nucleic acid-targeted drugs. This

***Linus L. Shen*** • Anti-infective Research Division, Abbott Laboratories, Abbott Park, Illinois 60064.

review summarizes the properties of quinolone-DNA interaction and elucidates the role of this interaction in the inhibition of DNA gyrase and, on the negative side, its possible role in creating adverse effects.

## EARLY STUDIES

The earliest attempt at investigating quinolone-DNA interaction occurred in 1972, when the binding of radiolabeled nalidixic acid to calf thymus DNA was studied by an equilibrium dialysis method (1). No binding was detected in these single-point binding experiments. Two other preliminary reports in the early 1980s (6, 7) also indicated that nalidixic acid does not bind to double-stranded DNA or supercoiled DNA but does bind to single-stranded DNA, though only in the presence of excess copper ions. The absence of drug binding to native DNA could be due to the low binding affinity of nalidixic acid and the low sensitivity of the UV spectroscopic method used in these studies.

In an attempt to explore the mechanism of action of quinolones at the molecular level, my coworkers and I (39) initiated our investigation by having [$^3$H]norfloxacin synthesized, and a series of radioligand binding experiments using a membrane ultrafiltration technique was carried out. The initial finding, published in 1985, was surprising; [$^3$H]norfloxacin does not bind to DNA gyrase but instead binds to pure DNA, with the extent of binding depending on DNA topological forms (39).

The finding that norfloxacin, a zwitterion, binds to the negatively charged DNA molecule was somewhat unexpected. A few preliminary reports from the binding experiments that used equilibrium dialysis, fluorescence measurements, and nuclear magnetic resonance (NMR) opposed the existence of an interaction between the drug and DNA (19, 27). Without experimental details, one of these reports (19) concluded that quinolones bind to the enzyme, not to DNA. The negative results shown in the other report (27) can be accounted for after detailed examinations (26, 32), and the absence of binding is attributed to the fluorescence-quenching phenomenon of the bound ligand. On the other side, the interaction of quinolone with DNA was supported by the results obtained by Tornaletti and Pedrini (42), who demonstrated that quinolones in the presence of magnesium ions unwind DNA. This phenomenon was confirmed by later studies on the same subject (26, 31). Some direct effects of certain selected quinolones on DNA were also observed. In addition to the quenching of the drugs' intrinsic fluorescence, some quinolones cause fluorine-19 NMR spectroscopic changes and DNA cleavage (31). These direct actions of quinolones on DNA will be discussed below.

## INVESTIGATIONS ON THE SPECIFICITY OF QUINOLONE BINDING TO PURE DNA

### Quinolones Prefer to Bind to Single-Stranded DNA

The finding that quinolones bind to DNA but not to DNA gyrase (39) has stimulated more-detailed investigations on the specificity of binding to DNA and on the role of such an interaction in DNA gyrase inhibition. A radioligand-binding method was used to demonstrate that quinolones prefer to bind to single-stranded DNA rather than to double-stranded DNA. This property constitutes the single most important characteristic of the drugs' actions, explaining many intriguing phenomena related to drug-DNA interaction, as will be discussed below. The experimental results showing this unique property of DNA binding of quinolones are illustrated in Fig. 1, which shows the binding of [$^3$H]norfloxacin to different structural forms of ColE1 DNA in a drug concentration range near their supercoiling inhibition constant. It is clear

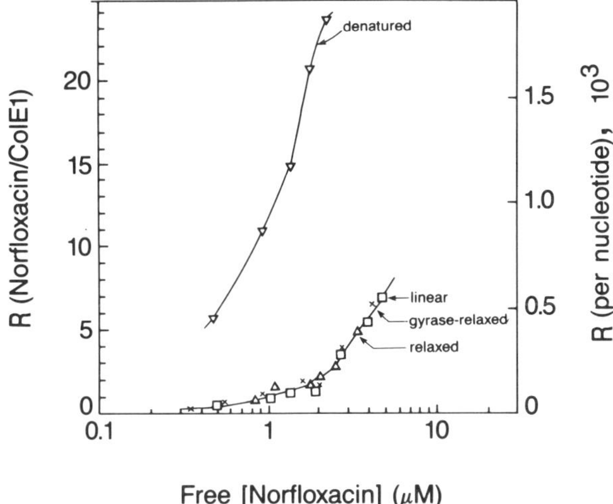


**Figure 1.** Binding of [$^3$H]norfloxacin to linear (□) or relaxed (△) DNA, to complex formed of gyrase and relaxed DNA (×), and to heat-denatured single-stranded ColE1 DNA (▽). R, molar binding ratio. Data are from reference 39 with permission.

that the binding affinity is greater for single-stranded (heat-denatured) DNA than for either linear or covalently closed relaxed double-stranded DNA. Figure 1 also shows that the amount of drug binding to the complex formed between relaxed DNA substrate and DNA gyrase in the absence of ATP is indistinguishable from that binding to the DNA alone, again suggesting the absence of drug binding to DNA gyrase in this drug concentration range.

## Binding to Double-Stranded DNA Is Weak and Shows No Base Specificity

Although norfloxacin binding to relaxed or linear forms of double-stranded DNA is weak compared with binding to single-stranded DNA, it would be interesting to know whether such a low level of drug binding shows any base-binding preference with double-stranded DNA fragments. Three native double-stranded DNA preparations of various G+C contents were selected and studied for this purpose, and the results showed that the amount of drug binding did not correlate with the G+C content of the native DNA (34). These results suggest that when DNA double strands are intact, the binding not only is restricted but also shows no base preference. Norfloxacin binding to pBR322 DNA cellulose was investigated by the fluorescence-quenching method and found to be noncooperative (26); this result is consistent with the lack of cooperativity noted when linear or relaxed DNA was used in the radioligand-binding technique (34). It is conceivable that the pBR322 DNA covalently linked to cellulose resin was cleaved and did not retain its superhelical form after the UV irradiation step for immobilization.

## When Strands Are Separated, Drug Prefers Guanine to Other Bases

When DNA strands are separated, the amount of quinolone binding increases, and consequently, the second level of binding specificity, i.e., the binding preference at the nucleotide level, is revealed. Information concerning the binding preference at this level was obtained mainly from studies using the single-stranded DNA homopolymers (34). Results illustrated in Fig. 2A show a sequence of binding preference to poly(dG), poly(dA), poly(dT), and poly(dC) in decreas-

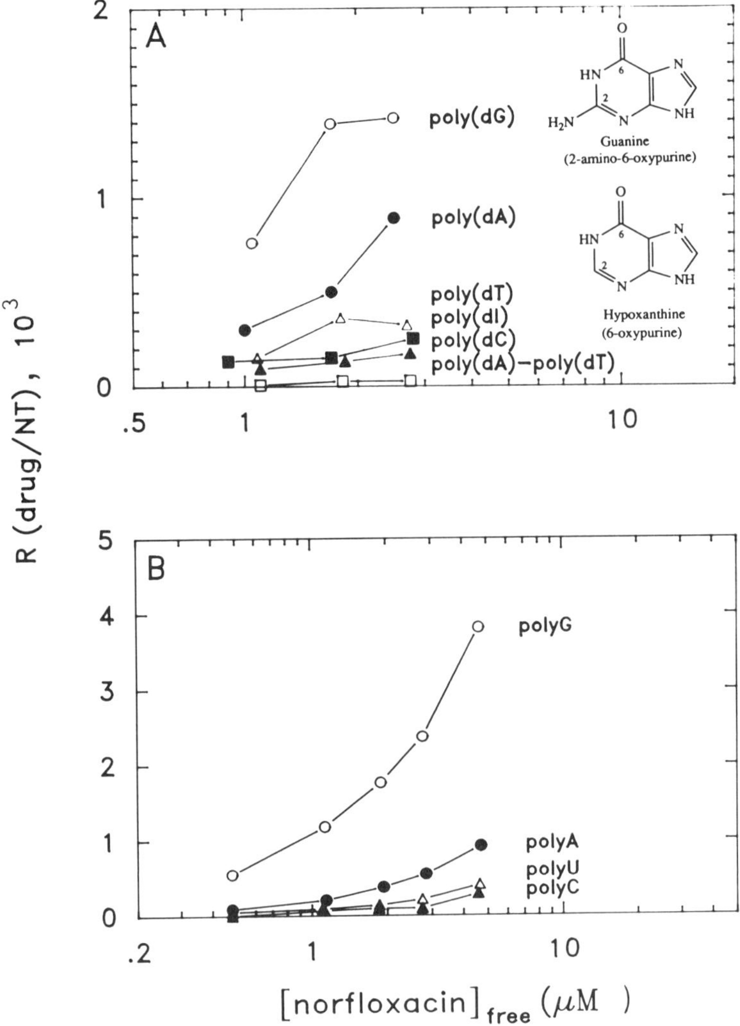


**Figure 2.** Binding of [$^3$H]norfloxacin to synthetic model homopolymers. (A) Membrane filtration method was used to measure the amounts of drug binding to polydeoxyribonucleotides poly(dG) (○), poly(dA) (●), poly(dT) (△), poly(dI) (■), poly(dC) (▲), and poly(DA)-poly(dT) duplex (□) at three drug concentrations. (B) The same membrane filtration method was used to determine the amounts of drug binding to polyribonucleotides poly(G) (○), poly(A) (●), poly(U) (△), and poly(C) (▲) at five drug concentrations. Inserts in panel A show chemical structures of the bases making up poly(dG) and poly(dI), i.e., guanine and hypoxanthine, respectively. NT, nucleotide. Data are from reference 34 with permission.

ing order, while binding to the double-stranded poly(dA)-poly(dT) is virtually nondetectable. Binding to poly(dG) is distinctly greater than that to the other three polydeoxyribonucleotides. One unique structural feature of the guanine base is that it has two common hydrogen bond donors, while every other base has only one. These results suggest that hydrogen bonds are involved with drug binding, presumably between the hydrogen bond donor groups on the base and the 4-keto and/or 3-carboxyl group on the quinolone ring. Also shown in Fig. 2A is the level of drug binding to poly(dI), which is about fivefold lower than that to poly(dG). The structural difference between guanosine and inosine is an extra amino group on the purine ring of the former (Fig. 2A, inset). This group is an important hydrogen bond donor when complementary strands are pairing. Similar results are obtained with synthetic polyribonucleotides (Fig. 2B). The results given above suggest that quinolones bind to DNA bases (preferentially to guanine groups) in a single-stranded DNA region through hydrogen bonds.

### Specific Type of Binding Can Be Observed Only with Supercoiled DNA

Though the binding of quinolones to the native double-stranded forms of DNA is weak, there is one exception: binding to the supercoiled form of covalently closed circular DNA shows a characteristic enhanced pattern (Fig. 3). The binding of [$^3$H]norfloxacin to supercoiled ColE1 DNA has been described as a specific type of drug binding on the basis of the following three observations: (i) the binding is saturable and takes place at a drug's supercoiling inhibitory concentration (39), (ii) the binding affinities of some selected quinolones to this DNA site are directly proportional to their supercoiling inhibition constants (39), and (iii) binding to this saturable site is highly cooperative (34). The observation that specific binding can be seen only with the supercoiled form but not with the relaxed or linear form is consistent with the observation that the drugs prefer to bind to single-stranded DNA and with the fact that supercoiled DNA is underwound. A remnant single-stranded "bubble" retained in the supercoil may serve as a denatured DNA pocket for the drug to bind to securely.

### Role of DNA Gyrase in Quinolone Binding to DNA Substrate

The next key question that needed to be answered before an inhibition model could be proposed was how the specific mode of drug binding observed with the supercoiled DNA (the product of the catalytic reaction) could be used to accommodate a drug inhibition mechanism of DNA gyrase that requires relaxed DNA as its substrate to which quinolone binds only weakly and nonspecifically. The answer to this puzzling question was obtained from studies of quinolone binding to enzyme-DNA complexes (37). To prevent the conversion of relaxed DNA in the presence of ATP to the supercoiled form that gives specific binding as mentioned above, only a nonhydrolyzable triphosphate nucleotide was used in these binding experiments involving DNA gyrase. The results showed that the extent of drug binding to relaxed DNA substrate may be induced by the addition of DNA gyrase, which alone possessed no drug-binding sites. Furthermore, induced binding to the gyrase-DNA complex showed a saturable phase that highly resembles the pattern of binding to supercoiled DNA in terms of the amount and cooperativity of binding (34). It was also interesting to observe that a similar cooperative drug-binding site may be induced by the enzyme without the need of a nucleotide energy source when linearized DNA was used. This induction was presumably due to the free DNA ends, which do not restrict conformational change or DNA unwinding during the enzyme-wrapping and gate-opening steps that follow DNA cleavage. Moreover, there was a close relation between the appearance of such a characteristic binding and drug-induced DNA breakage (37), which is considered the central event responsible for cell killing (18). These results provided key evidence suggesting that the binding of DNA gyrase to the DNA substrate creates a site that allows the drug to bind in a cooperative manner.

## COOPERATIVE QUINOLONE-DNA BINDING MODEL FOR GYRASE INHIBITION

The absence of binding of norfloxacin to DNA gyrase and the high level of specific binding to DNA described above have led to the proposal of a quinolone-DNA cooperative

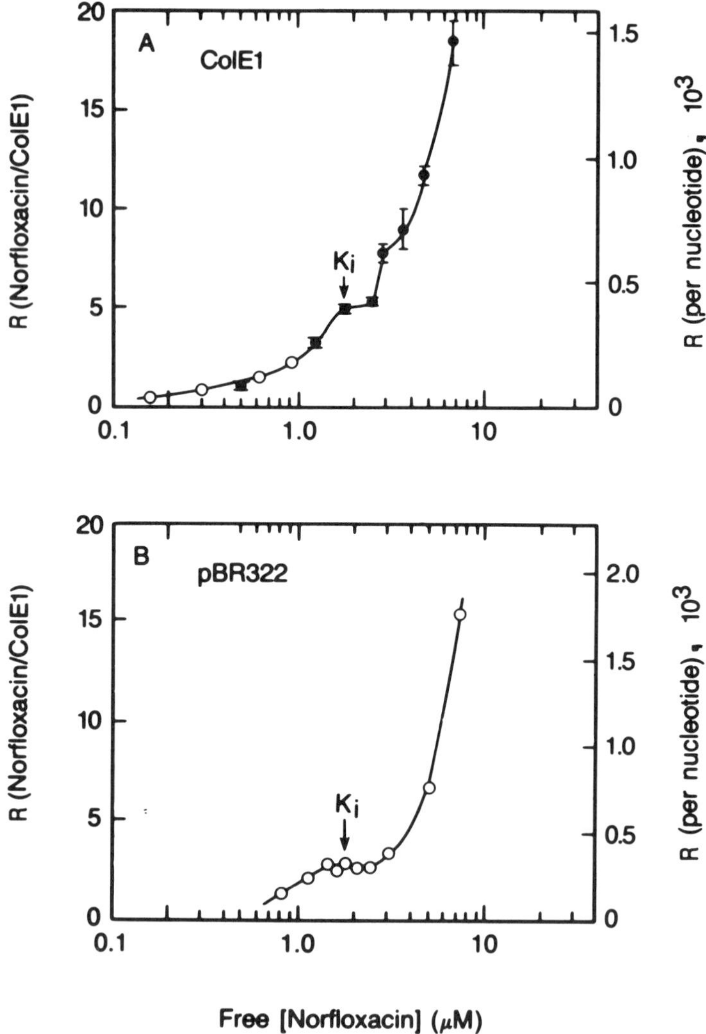


**Figure 3.** Binding of norfloxacin to supercoiled plasmid DNA. R, molar binding ratio. Vertical bars represent standard deviations. Different symbols indicate results obtained from different experiments. Values of supercoiling $K_i$ (inhibition constant against *E. coli* DNA gyrase) are marked with arrows for comparison. Reprinted from reference 39 with permission.

binding model for the inhibition of DNA gyrase (38). Experimental evidence favors the notion that the bound enzyme induces a drug-binding site on the relaxed DNA substrate. My colleagues and I proposed (38) that the binding site is formed during the gate-opening step, which requires the binding of ATP. The separated, short, single-stranded DNA segments between the 4-bp-staggered cuts form a simulated denatured DNA bubble that is an ideal site for the drug to bind to (Fig. 4). Drug molecules acquire high binding affinity through a cooperative binding mechanism achieved via self-association of the drug molecules. Two types of interactions, seen in the nalidixic acid crystal structure, are feasible: $\pi$-$\pi$ stacking between the quinolone rings and tail-to-tail hydrophobic interactions between the N-1 substitution groups (Fig. 4, inset). Such interactions result in the forma-

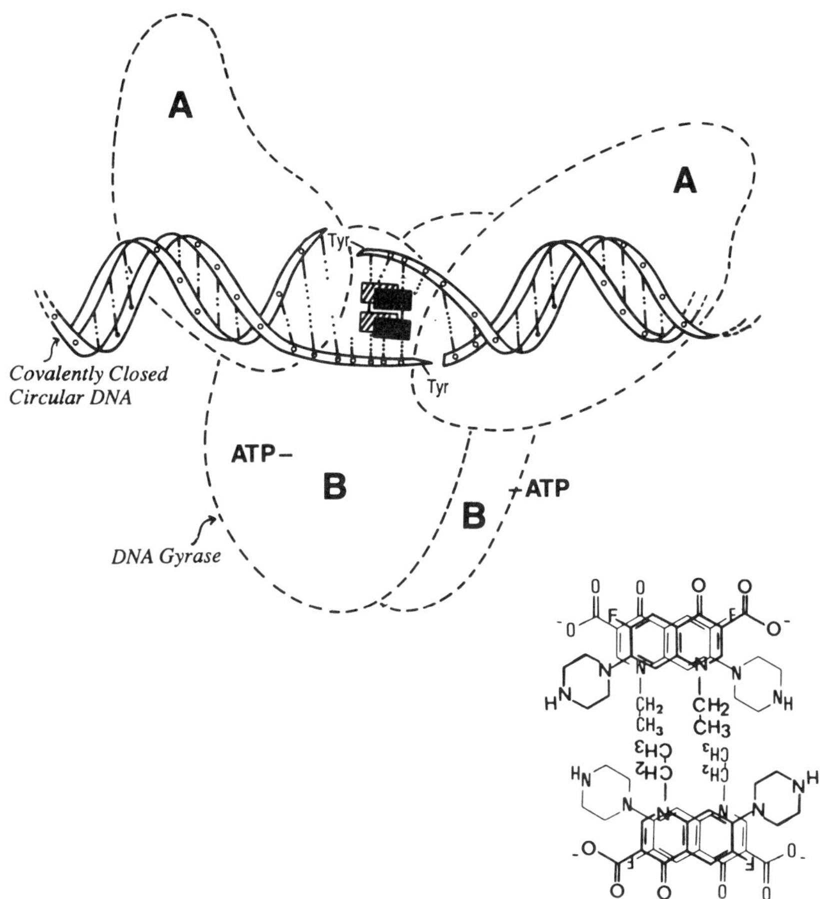


**Figure 4.** Proposed quinolone-DNA cooperative binding model for DNA gyrase inhibition. Filled and hatched boxes denote the quinolone molecules that self-assemble to form a supermolecule inside the gyrase-induced DNA pocket; the drug binds to the unpaired bases via hydrogen bonds (dotted lines). Details of the proposed mode of self-association are illustrated at lower right. The binding pocket is believed to be induced during the intermediate gate-opening step of the DNA supercoiling process. Gyrase A subunits form covalent bonds between tyrosine 122 and the 5′ end of the DNA chain (12), and the subsequent opening of the DNA chains along the 4-bp-staggered cuts results in a locally denatured DNA bubble that is an ideal site for the drug to bind to. When relaxed DNA substrate (represented by the double-helical ribbon in the diagram) is used, ATP is required for the induction of this specific drug-binding site. Dashed curves mimic the shape of the DNA gyrase, a tetramer composed of two A subunits and two B subunits, as revealed by the electron microscopic image of the *Micrococcus luteus* enzyme (17). Reprinted partly from reference 38 with permission.

tion of a supermolecule with a set of multiple hydrogen bond acceptors in a consolidated unit, thus extending the binding beyond a unidimensional domain; i.e., the assembled drug molecules can act together to saturate the DNA binding pocket with the functional binding groups distributed in a multidimensional space.

This working model has two important features: (i) the geometry of the drug-binding site on DNA induced by the action of DNA gyrase and (ii) the unique abilities of the drug molecules to occupy such a site. The two aspects are equally important in determining drug-binding affinity and specificity. It is evident that DNA binding specificity at the enzyme inhibition level is controlled by the binding of the enzyme, which creates a favorable DNA site with a specific configuration to accommodate drug binding. This may be viewed as a third level of drug-binding specificity.

An alternative model favoring an intercalative mode of quinolone binding to DNA has been proposed (26). This model suggested that quinolone binds to a DNA site through stacking with the nearby base and through a magnesium bridge between the DNA phosphate group and the carbonyl and carboxyl groups of the norfloxacin molecule. The model, however, deserves some further discussion. First, the model cannot accommodate the binding cooperativity phenomenon, which was observed with supercoiled DNA and the gyrase-DNA complex. The conclusion that binding of norfloxacin to supercoiled DNA lacks cooperativity when pBR322 DNA cellulose is used as a model (26) is invalid, as the reported negative result may be due to loss of DNA supercoiling during the UV irradiation immobilization process. Second, it is doubtful that the two bonding modes, the magnesium bridge and ring stacking, can account for the strong binding affinity of the quinolone to a site on pure DNA (a dissociation constant in the range of 1 to 2 $\mu$M) (39). Third, the model does not satisfactorily explain the observation that quinolones bind with greater preference to single-stranded DNA. In addition, if as one of the two bonding modes responsible for the high binding affinity, stacking with the unpaired base is important for drug binding to DNA, then why do quinolones prefer to bind to guanosine rather than adenosine or inosine when all of these have purine rings? Fourth, the model fits the current structure-activity relationships of quinolone antibacterial agents less satisfactorily (see chapter 2). The model, for instance, cannot explain why the N-1 and C-8 substituents have to be hydrophobic for good potency. While the actual role of magnesium ions in quinolone binding to DNA still remains obscure, it may be a magnesium-induced DNA conformational change (9) that promotes formation of a specific drug-binding site. Whether magnesium ions play a catalytic role in quinolone binding to DNA, as suggested for nalidixic acid (6), deserves further investigation. The catalytic role was proposed when it was found that metal ions are required for nalidixic acid binding to DNA but are not retained in the drug-DNA complex.

The cooperative quinolone-DNA binding model in general agrees with the current structure-activity relationships of quinolones (3, 21, 23, 30, 45) and has provided a general guideline for efforts at synthesizing active quinolones with novel structures (4, 15, 22). The proposed model suggests three functional domains on the quinolone molecule (Fig. 5): the DNA-binding domain, the drug self-association domain, and the drug-enzyme interaction domain. The hypothetical quinolone-enzyme interaction domain, i.e., the space occupied by the substituents at C-7, was proposed as a possible location of functional groups for further strengthening binding of the drug to the complex, and this proposal is consistent with the observed potency increase of new amphoteric quinolones with piperazinyl or other basic substituents located at this position. Studies of quinolone-resistant mutants support such a hypothesis and will be discussed in the next section.

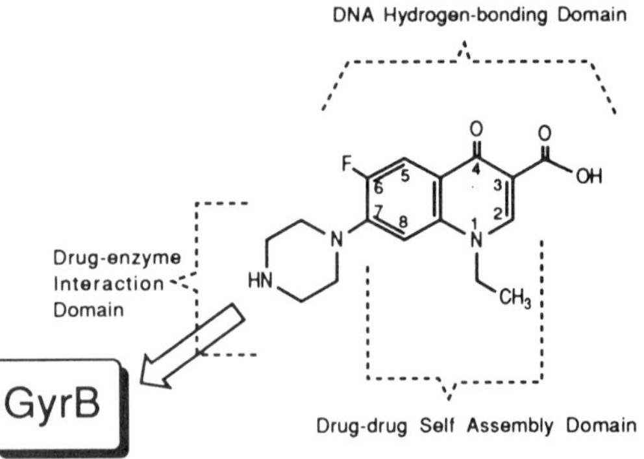


**Figure 5.** Functional domains of quinolone antibacterial agents. The original proposal was published in reference 38. Recent evidence (49) showed that the interaction site with C-7 substituents is the gyrase B subunit. See the text for details.

## QUINOLONE RESISTANCE MECHANISM RESULTING FROM DNA GYRASE MUTATION

The cooperative drug-DNA binding model suggests an indirect interaction between quinolone and the enzyme. Consequently, there have been some concerns about how such a model can explain quinolone resistance mutations that were mapped on the structural genes of DNA gyrase. The cooperative binding model provides a solution to this question. In fact, when the model was proposed in 1989, it was predicted that any mutation, either in *gyrA* or in *gyrB*, that altered the geometry of the enzyme-induced drug-binding pocket on DNA could lead to drug resistance (26). Such a mutation is more likely to occur in *gyrA*, since the A subunit is directly involved in forming the DNA gate, i.e., the drug-binding site. The gyrase B subunit, the energy transduction machinery that provides a conformational change to assist the DNA gate opening and strand passing, is obviously also important to the formation of such a site. This hypothesis offers an explanation of why quinolone resistance mutations indeed occur in both A and B subunits. In the remaining part of this section, properties of quinolone-resistant gyrase mutations will be examined in more detail in conjunction with the proposed model.

As mentioned above, the C-7 substituents were proposed as the domain that interacts with the enzyme for further strengthening drug binding (Fig. 5). Recent results with quinolone resistance mutants suggest that the C-7 substituent interaction site on the enzyme may be the "quinolone pocket" on the B subunit. This proposal is based on the differential activity responses of quinolones with charged and noncharged C-7 substituents to two different types of *gyrB* mutations that have altered charge properties at the quinolone pocket (49). It is evident that such a direct interaction would not provide sufficient bond strength to account for drug binding; such an interaction is thus more likely to play a supporting role. According to this quinolone pocket hypothesis (49), bound quinolones are in close contact with two oppositely charged amino acids in the B subunit pocket: Asp-426 and Lys-447. Two types of mutations related to the change of the two amino acids have been isolated: the type I mutant, which renders the pocket more positively charged by replacing Asp-426 with Asn (defined here as I[+]-type mutation because it gains a net charge), and the type II mutant, which has the positively charged Lys-447 replaced by a negatively charged Glu (designated as II[−]-type mutation by the same definition). Amphoteric quinolones having a positive charge at the C-7 substituent (such as norfloxacin and ciprofloxacin) are resistant to the type I[+] mutation but are hypersensitive to type II[−] mutations. Those "acidic quinolones," such as nalidixic acid and oxolinic acid, that have no charged substituent at C-7 are equally resistant to these two types of mutations. These observations fit the simple model that these two amino acids are in direct contact with the bound drug through either electrostatic interactions (for amphoteric quinolones) or hydrophobic interactions (for acidic quinolones), though the model does not rule out the possibility that the mutations also cause a conformational alteration of the pocket on the enzyme molecule and so affect the fitting of drug molecules. The proposal of a quinolone ionic interaction site on the B subunit is plausible, since it is consistent with the fact that a positively charged substituent, such as piperazine or aminopyrrolidine groups, has to be included at the C-7 position in order to have high potency. The hypothesis of the direct interaction of the B subunit with a C-7 substituent is oversimplified as a binding model per se because it neglects consideration of other important factors, but it fits nicely with the previous prediction (38) that the C-7 substituents function as possible secondary interaction sites with the enzyme for further strengthening the binding of the more potent amphoteric quinolones (Fig. 5). The validity of this proposal could be assessed in the future by chemical approaches, i.e., synthesizing novel quinolone probes with systematically varied structural and charge properties on the C-7 substituents.

In contrast to *gyrB* mutations, an overwhelming number of quinolone resistance mutations are found in *gyrA*. These mutations all result from single-point mutations but occur at a variety of sites distributed in the region between amino acids 67 and 106, the so-called "quinolone resistance-determining region" (48). High-level quinolone resistance normally involves no change in charge property in this region. Several quinolone-resistant *Escherichia coli* clinical isolates, for example, have been shown to have Ser-83 replaced by Leu or Trp (25) and gave rise to a higher level of resistance to nalidixic acid than did the new quinolones with piperazinyl substituents. Other lower-level resistance mutations in *gyrA* are reported to involve changes of Asp-87 to Asn, Gly-81 to Cys, Ala-67 to Ser, and Gln-106 to His (48). Among them, only the change of Asp-87 to Asn involved a change in the charge property in this region. The mutation is identical to the type I[+] mutation defined above and shows a resistance pattern similar to that shown by the corresponding *gyrB* mutation. It may therefore be argued that C-7 substituents interact with Asp-87, but this proposal contradicts the observation that nalidixic acid, which lacks a positive charge at the C-7 position, gave an even higher level of resistance to this mutant (64-fold increase in MIC) than, for example, norfloxacin did (8-fold increase). In contrast, a recent preliminary publication (2a) reported the isolation of a novel mutation in *gyrA* that involves a change in the charge property (Gly-81 to Asp) and results in a high degree of resistance to the new fluoroquinolones but not to nalidixic acid. Such a *gyrA* mutation mimics the type II[−] *gyrB* mutation defined above. This mutation, however, renders a resistance pattern opposite to that of the *gyrB* type II[−] mutation: no hypersensitivity but an exceedingly high level of resistance (more than 1,000-fold increase in MIC) to the new amphoteric quinolone (ciprofloxacin) was observed. The results thus suggest the absence of an interaction between the C-7 substituent and the amino acid in the A subunit. The fact that the introduction of a negative charge in this region in the mutant enzyme does not reduce sensitivity to the acidic quinolone (nalidixic acid) also suggests the absence of an ionic interaction between the amino acid and the carboxylic group of the drug. In summary, no evidence from these mutation studies supports the notion that subunit A of DNA gyrase interacts electrostatically with quinolone at either the C-3 or the C-7 position.

The high-level quinolone resistance of *gyrA* Ser-83 mutants and the weaker binding of quinolone to the complex of DNA and mutant gyrase than to that of DNA and the wild-type gyrase have prompted the proposal that Ser-83 is a direct quinolone-binding site mediated through a hydrogen bond (20). Such a binding model would entirely ignore the high DNA-binding capability of the drug and the high degree of similarity between binding to supercoiled DNA and to the enzyme-DNA complex. From the discussion above, it seems certain that the interaction site with the C-7 substituents is the quinolone resistance-determining region on gyrase subunit B. If the C-4 keto and C-3 carboxyl groups sites interact further with the A subunit, then at least some trace amount of drug binding to the enzyme alone should be detected, but so far no such binding has been found. In fact, the reduced binding of norfloxacin to the complex of DNA and mutant DNA gyrase is predictable from the proposed cooperative binding model, and the result supports the quinolone resistance hypothesis based on the model.

The lack of direct binding of drug to gyrase, the uniquely characteristic binding of drug to DNA,and the lack of specificity in *gyrA* mutations favor a model in which quinolone molecules are not in direct contact with the gyrase A subunit. However, definitive evidence deciding in favor of either of these proposals or requiring postulation of a still different model will probably come from X-ray crystallography of the ternary complex, which is at present not forthcoming.

## A MODEL FOR THE DIFFERENTIAL ANTIGYRASE ACTIVITIES OF OFLOXACIN ENANTIOMERS

An intriguing question has been raised: how may the model be used to interpret the large activity differences of ofloxacin enantiomers that have chiral centers located in the drug self-assembly domain? In this section, it will be demonstrated that the proposed stacking model can be used to explain the large activity differences between the ofloxacin enantiomers with nonfunctional chiral groups located near their N-1 positions (Fig. 6).

Ofloxacin, synthesized in the early 1980s at Daiichi Seiyaku Co., has an antibacterial potency roughly equal to that of norfloxacin against *E. coli* (43) and a supercoiling inhibition activity slightly less than that of norfloxacin (38). The compound has a unique tricyclic structure with a methyl group at the asymmetric C-3 position in the oxazine ring (Fig. 6). The *S*-(−)-ofloxacin isomer is approximately 8 to 128 times more potent than *R*-(+)-ofloxacin against selected laboratory bacterial strains (11). The stereochemistry evidently affects the enzyme activity rather than other factors such as the drug transport process, since inhibitory activities against purified DNA gyrase also differ in the same proportion in these two enantiomers (13, 16).

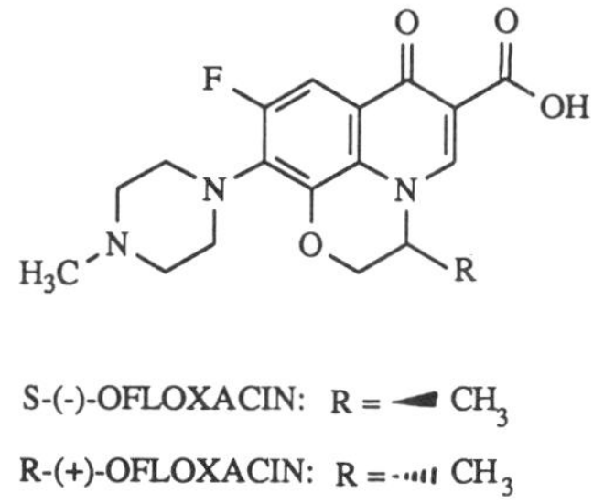

S-(-)-OFLOXACIN: R = $CH_3$

R-(+)-OFLOXACIN: R = $CH_3$

**Figure 6.** Structures of ofloxacin enantiomers.

As shown in Fig. 7, with *S*-ofloxacin as an example, the six-membered oxazine ring is not planar. Instead, the ring is puckered in two different ways, namely, the *endo* (front) pucker and the *exo* (back) pucker conformations (defined in Fig. 7). Molecular orbital calculations indicate that the two puckered-ring forms have approximately equivalent energies. The ring puckering, however, affects the projection of the methyl group from the plane of the quinolone ring system. As our model indicates, the ring-ring stacking mechanism shown in Fig. 4 is an important determinant of the affinity of drug binding to the DNA site. The ability of the molecule to stack properly to fit the binding site is therefore crucial in determining its inhibitory potency. Molecular modeling was therefore used to analyze possible stacking orientations for the enantiomers of ofloxacin (36). As shown in Fig. 8, for each enantiomer, four orientations were investigated: (i) the *endo* form stacked with the ring puckers facing outside (A and a), (ii) the *endo* form with the ring puckers facing inside (B and b), (iii) the *exo* form with the ring puckers facing inside (C and c), and (iv) the *exo* form with the ring puckers facing outside (D and d). In this preliminary model (36), my colleagues and I attempted to stack the pairs directly on top of each other such that the planes of the quinolone rings were essentially parallel. The close contacts between the two stacked rings determine the distance between the rings, which, in turn, relates to the $\pi$–$\pi$ stacking energy present. Thus, the orientations that place both the pucker and the methyl group outside the complex result in the shortest ring-ring distance, about 3.5 Å (0.35 nm) for orientations A and d. The largest ring-ring distance, about 5.4 Å (0.54 nm) for orientations D and a, was observed when the methyl groups were facing inside and the puckers were facing outside. As indicated in Fig. 8, the most favorable stacking orientation for either enantiomer is the pair with both the ring pucker and the methyl group located on the outside of the

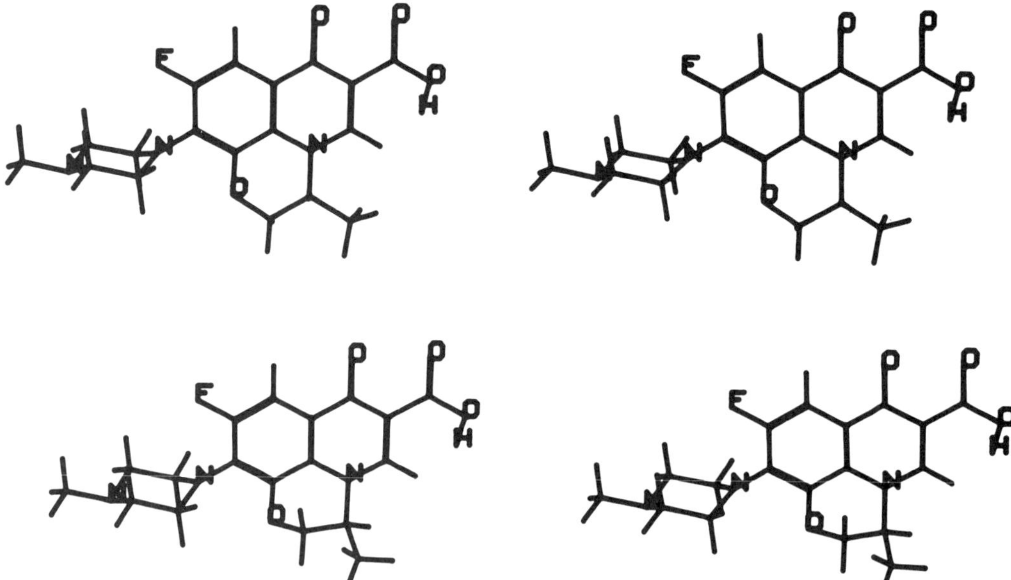

**Figure 7.** Stereo view of the conformation of *S*-ofloxacin with different oxazine ring puckers: *endo* form (top) and *exo* form (bottom). The terms *endo* and *exo* refer to the projection in space of the methyl group on the oxazine ring as a result of ring puckering. Reprinted from reference 36 with permission.

stacked complex, i.e., configurations A and d for *S*- and *R*-ofloxacins, respectively.

A key finding of this exercise is that the most favorable orientation of *S*-ofloxacin (A) is stacked in a different manner than the best orientation of *R*-ofloxacin (d). Specifically, the *S* isomer prefers to stack with the key hydrogen bond acceptors (3-carboxyl and 4-keto) located to the "northwest" and "southeast," while the best *R*-isomer orientation has these functional groups located to the "southwest" and "northeast." In our proposed cooperative binding model, the carbonyl groups are important hydrogen-bonding acceptors interacting with the DNA. Though the actual stacking orientation may not be exactly what the model shows in A and d, the important message obtained from this modeling is that the two ofloxacin enantiomers cannot stack in the same way to fit an asymmetric DNA site because of steric hindrance of the methyl groups located in chiral positions.

For proof of this chirality transformation model, it is of utmost importance to investigate the binding of ofloxacin enantiomers to supercoiled DNA. Preliminary results of this study have been reported by Hoshino et al. (14). Unexpectedly, the two enantiomers demonstrated a similar pattern of specific binding with nearly identical binding affinities and binding cooperativities. The only difference was the maximum molar binding ratio at the saturation plateau. More precisely, their results showed that about four *S* isomers bind to the DNA receptor, but only two of the less active *R* isomers bind. Interpretation of how such a binding difference in the number of bound drugs could be translated into a difference in antigyrase activity was not available at that time.

I have just described the specific forms of drug binding with DNA that take place at a relatively lower drug concentration near the drug $K_i$s, e.g., 1 $\mu$M for norfloxacin. Another form of drug binding takes place at relatively higher drug concentrations. Because of its lack of binding saturation and cooperativity, this form of binding may be viewed as the nonspecific type of drug binding and is described below.

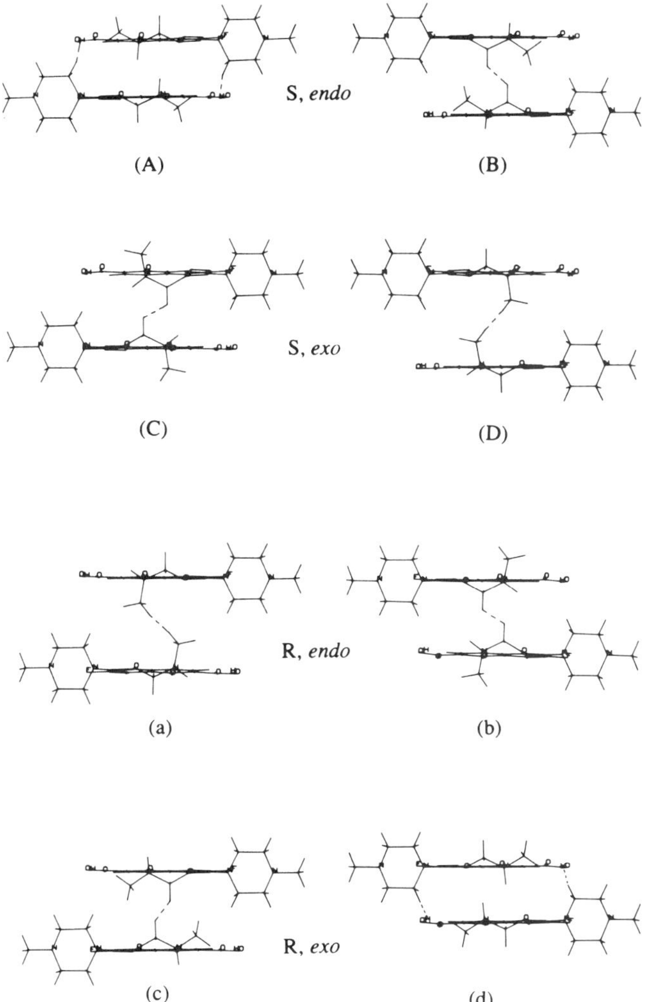


**Figure 8.** The eight stacking orientations of ofloxacin enantiomers *S*-ofloxacin (A through D), *R*-ofloxacin (a through d), and their conformers investigated in this model. The stacked molecular pairs were viewed in the 4-keto-to-N-1 direction. Reprinted from reference 36 with permission.

## NONSPECIFIC TYPE OF DNA-QUINOLONE INTERACTION AND SOME DIRECT EFFECTS OF QUINOLONE BINDING TO DNA

### Nonspecific Type of Binding

I have observed various forms of drug binding with different forms of DNA throughout a wide range of drug concentrations. In addition to the specific form of binding described above, a nonspecific mode of binding is observed particularly at higher drug concentrations. The binding of [$^3$H]norfloxacin to single-stranded (heat-denatured) DNA and to relaxed or linear DNA as illustrated in Fig. 2 is typical of this type of binding, since it lacks binding cooperativity and demonstrates no binding saturation. The binding of [$^3$H]norfloxacin to supercoiled ColE1 DNA at high concentrations (up to the drug's solubility limit of 1 mM) also fits this type of binding (34).

## DNA-Unwinding Effect of Quinolones

Quinolones at high concentrations bind to native DNA nonspecifically and reversibly (35). The fact that the drug binds preferentially to single-stranded DNA rather than to double-stranded DNA implies that quinolones are not DNA intercalators. Tornaletti and Pedrini (41) have demonstrated that quinolones at high concentration unwind DNA in the presence of magnesium ions, though these quinolones are not DNA intercalators. Using a different method for testing DNA unwinding (28), my colleagues and I confirmed their results by showing that major quinolones at 50 μg/ml or more do not show a DNA-unwinding effect in the absence of magnesium (35). In the presence of magnesium, quinolones at high concentrations do unwind DNA to various degrees. Norfloxacin at about 100 μM, for example, unwinds DNA. Such magnesium-dependent DNA unwinding by quinolones, however, may be antagonized by polyamines at physiological intracellular concentrations (31). This implies that in intact cells, where numerous DNA-binding components are present, such drug-dependent DNA unwinding may not take place after all.

## Spectroscopic Changes in Quinolone-DNA Interaction

### Quenching of drug's intrinsic fluorescence

It may be expected that ligand-DNA interaction would cause spectroscopic changes. Quinolones possess strong fluorescence chromophores (34), while DNA is essentially a nonfluorescent molecule. As shown in Fig. 9A, when increasing amounts of single-stranded DNA were added to norfloxacin solution, the drug's intrinsic fluorescence intensity was progressively quenched. The extent of quenching is proportional to the amount of drug bound to DNA as determined by a filter binding method (Fig. 9B), indicating a nearly complete fluorescence quenching of the DNA-bound drug. The phenomenon explains the negative results obtained by some investigators (27), who showed an absence of norfloxacin binding to DNA by utilizing equilib-

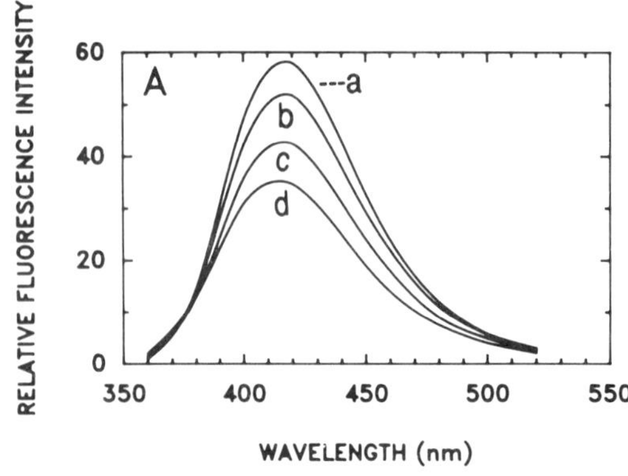


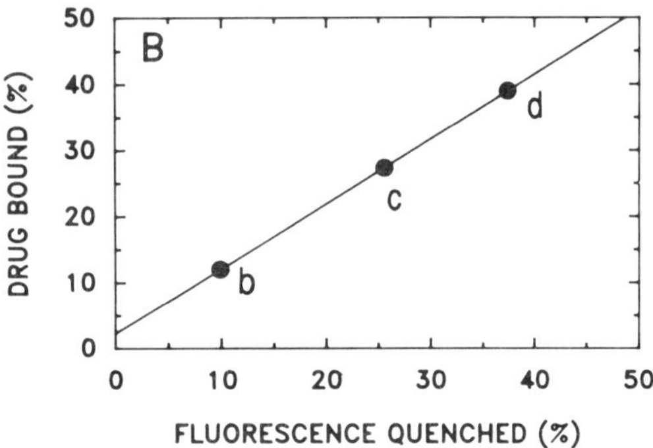


**Figure 9.** Quenching effect of DNA on the intrinsic fluorescence of norfloxacin. (A) Emission spectra of norfloxacin (1.2 μM) excited at 340 nm. Curves from top to bottom correspond to the spectra of norfloxacin (1.5 ml) with 0, 10, 30, and 60 μl of thermally denatured calf thymus DNA (3.65 mg/ml) added to give nucleotide/drug ratios of 0 (a), 6 (b), 18 (c), and 36 (d), respectively. The addition of DNA caused no more than a 4% volume change. (B) Correlation of the amount of drug bound and the percentage of fluorescence quenching. The percentage of drug bound at the same experimental conditions as for panel A was determined by an ultrafiltration technique using [$^3$H]norfloxacin. Both parameters shown have been corrected by dilution factors. Reprinted from reference 33 with permission.

rium dialysis and fluorescence measurement as a method of quantification. In fact, the extent of fluorescence quenching shown in Fig. 9A is sufficient to indicate the existence of quinolone-DNA interaction (32).

### Fluorine-19 NMR spectral changes

The fluorine-19 NMR spectrum of difloxacin in a phosphate buffer at pH 7 exhibits two sharp resonances that correspond to the two fluorine atoms of the compound (Fig. 10, spectrum A). When denatured DNA is added to the drug solution, a down-field shift for both resonances and a dramatic broadening of both fluorine signals are observed (Fig. 10). Though it is not possible to determine the exact nature of the drug-DNA interaction from this experiment, results indicate that the drug indeed binds to the denatured DNA at high concentration.

### Direct DNA Cleavage

The interaction of certain quinolone congeners with DNA causes direct single-stranded DNA nicking or breaking under ambient laboratory lights. These quinolones were synthesized as part of the effort to modify the 3-carboxyl group for improving antibacterial potency (4). Figure 11a shows the dose-response of the nicking of supercoiled

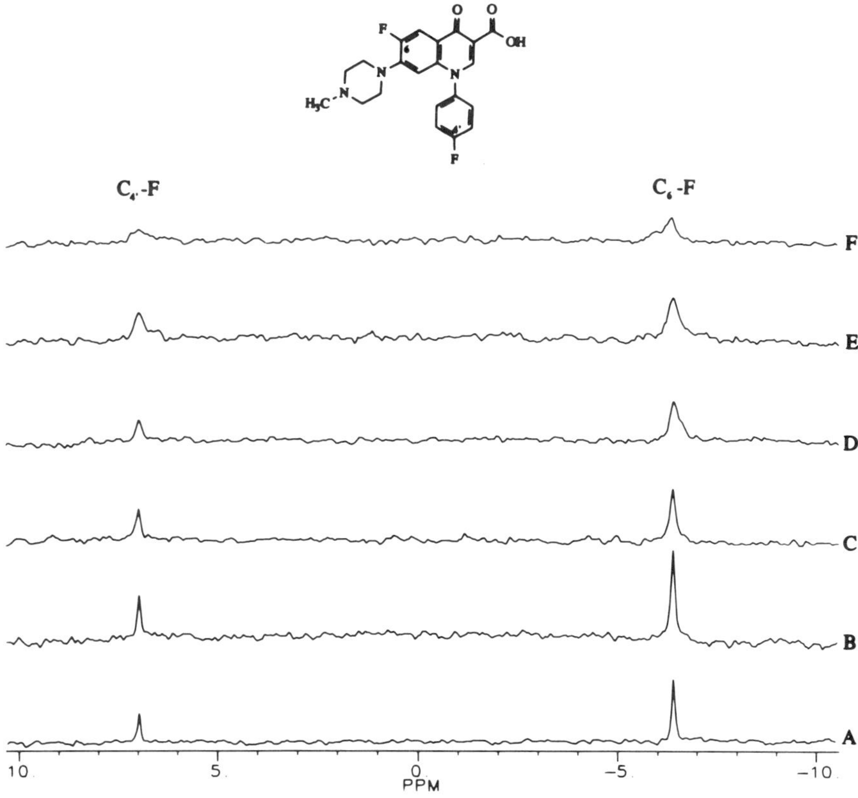


**Figure 10.** Fluorine-19 NMR spectra of difloxacin and difloxacin-DNA complex. (A) Difloxacin (0.1 mM) in phosphate buffer (pH 7.4); (B through F) mixtures of difloxacin (0.1 mM) and denatured calf thymus DNA in the same buffer. The molar ratios of nucleotide to drug in the mixtures are 1.4, 3.6, 7, 10.7, and 14 for spectra B through F, respectively. Inset shows the structure of difloxacin. Reprinted from reference 33 with permission.

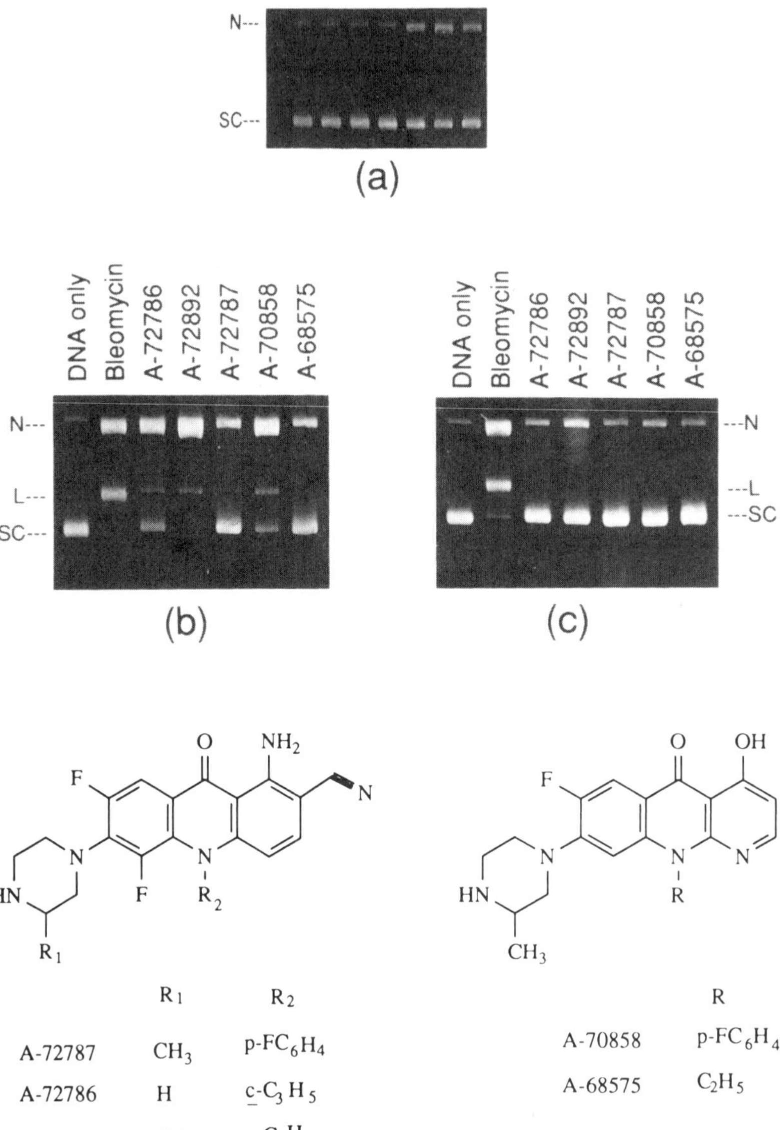


**Figure 11.** Intrinsic DNA-nicking activities of some selected quinolone derivatives in the absence of topoisomerases. (a) Dose dependence of DNA nicking by A-72786. Supercoiled ColE1 DNA (0.2 $\mu$g) was incubated with increasing amounts of the compound (number at top of each lane indicates the drug concentration in micrograms per milliliter) in 20 $\mu$l of Tris-HCl (150 mM, pH 7.4) for 60 min under ambient laboratory lighting. The nicking activity is visualized by the conversion of the supercoiled band (SC) to the nicked band (N) in a 1% agarose gel stained with ethidium bromide after the run. (b) DNA-nicking activities of a number of derivatives at 64 $\mu$g/ml. To amplify the effect, the reaction mixture was placed about 6 in. (ca. 15 cm) below a 60-W fluorescent light tube. The increase in light intensity apparently caused more-extensive DNA nicking, as evidenced by the appearance of the linear-DNA band (L). Bleomycin at the same concentration was included for comparison. (c) Same as gel b except that the reaction mixture was shielded from the light. Reprinted from reference 33 with permission.

ColE1 DNA after incubation with increasing amounts of A-72786. Direct DNA-nicking activities of this compound are evident, as is shown by conversion of the supercoiled band to the nicked-DNA band. The nicking activities of a number of other similar derivatives, with bleomycin as a positive control, are shown in Fig. 11b. All these tricyclic quinolones (structures also shown in Fig. 11) evidently cause single-stranded DNA nicking in a light-dependent manner, as the reaction did not take place when experiments were performed in test tubes shielded from the light (Fig. 11c). Preirradiation of the compounds followed by incubation with DNA under low light did not cause DNA nicking, indicating that the compounds were not converted to a new DNA-nicking species by the light.

## CONCLUDING REMARKS

Quinolones may be classified as DNA-targeted drugs. Binding specificities and criteria for the classification of quinolone-DNA interactions have been summarized in this chapter. The specific type of quinolone-DNA interaction is strong and takes place at relatively low drug concentrations, e.g., 1 $\mu$M for norfloxacin, and this type of binding results in an inhibition of DNA gyrase according to my model. The specific quinolone-binding site is believed to be a single-stranded DNA pocket induced by the target enzyme. The higher binding affinity of quinolones for this site is achieved through a cooperative drug self-association process, as proposed above. Nonspecific binding to DNA takes place at relatively high drug concentrations. Some direct effects of this nonspecific interaction are presented here. In general, the nonspecific interaction is weak, and the binding of drug to native DNA is limited by the base pairing of the double-helical strands. The drug causes DNA unwinding only at a high drug concentration in the presence of magnesium ions; however, such an effect demonstrated in vitro is less likely to be significant in vivo, since this interaction may be counteracted by other DNA-interacting components such as histones and polyamines. Not all quinolones show such adverse in vitro effects, but testing the DNA-unwinding activity and the direct DNA nicking or breaking activity is strongly recommended as a precautionary measure for new quinolones under development.

## REFERENCES


1. **Bourguignon, G. J., M. Levitt, and R. Sternglanz.** 1973. Studies on the mechanism of action of nucleic acid. *Antimicrob. Agents Chemother.* **4:**479–486.
2. **Brown, P. O., and N. R. Cozzarelli.** 1979. A sign inversion mechanism for enzymatic supercoiling of DNA. *Science* **206:**1081–1083.

2a. **Cambau, E., F. Bordon, E. Collatz, and L. Gutmann.** 1992. *Abstr. Gen. Meet. Am. Soc. Microbiol. 1992,* abstr. A-96.

3. **Chu, D. T., and P. B. Fernandes.** 1989. Structure-activity relationships of the fluoroquinolones. *Antimicrob. Agents Chemother.* **33:**131–135.
4. **Chu, D. T. W., P. B. Fernandes, A. K. Claiborne, L. L. Shen, and A. G. Pernet.** 1988. Structure-activity relationships in quinolone antibacterials: design, synthesis and biological activities of novel isothiazoloquinolones. *Drugs Exp. Clin. Res.* **14:**379–383.
5. **Cozzarelli, N. R.** 1980. DNA gyrase and the supercoiling of DNA. *Science* **207:**953–960.
6. **Crumplin, G. C., J. M. Midgley, and J. T. Smith.** 1980. Mechanisms of action of nalidixic acid and its congeners. *Antibiot. Chem.* **8:**13–35.
7. **Dreyfuss, J. M., and J. M. Midgley.** 1983. Structure-activity relationships in aromatic ring fused 4-pyrridones substituted at position 3. *J. Pharm. Pharmacol.* **35:**75P.
8. **Drlica, K.** 1984. Biology of bacterial deoxyribonucleic acid topoisomerases. *Microbiol. Rev.* **48:**273–289.
9. **Eichhorn, G. L.** 1962. Metal ions as stabilizers or destabilizers of the deoxyribonucleic acid structure. *Nature* (London) **194:**474–475.
10. **Gellert, M.** 1981. DNA topoisomerases. *Annu. Rev. Biochem.* **50:**879–910.
11. **Hayakawa, I., S. Atarashi, S. Yokohoma, M. Imamura, K.-I. Sakano, and M. Furukawa.** 1986. Synthesis and antibacterial activities of optically active ofloxacin. *Antimicrob. Agents Chemother.* **29:**163–164.
12. **Horowitz, D. S., and J. C. Wang.** 1987. Mapping the active site tyrosine of *Escherichia coli* DNA gyrase. *J. Biol. Chem.* **262:**5339–5344.

13. **Hoshino, K., K. Sato, K. Akahane, A. Yoshida, I. Hayakawa, M. Sato, T. Une, and Y. Osada.** 1991. Significance of the methyl group on the oxazine ring of ofloxacin derivatives in the inhibition of bacterial and mammalian type II topoisomerases. *Antimicrob. Agents Chemother.* **35:**309–312.
14. **Hoshino, K., K. Sato, I. Hayakawa, M. Sato, and Y. Osada.** 1990. Mechanism of action of optically active isomers of ofloxacin against bacteria, abstr. 11. *Program Abstr. Third Conf. DNA Topoisomerases Ther.*
15. **Hubschwerlen, C., P. Pflieger, J.-L. Speckin, K. Gubernator, H. Gmunder, P. Angehrn, and I. Kompis.** 1992. Pyrimido[1,6-a]benzimidazoles: a new class of DNA gyrase inhibitors. *J. Med. Chem.* **35:**1385–1392.
16. **Imamura, M., S. Shibamura, I. Hayakawa, and Y. Osada.** 1987. Inhibition of DNA gyrase by optically active ofloxacin. *Antimicrob. Agents Chemother.* **31:**325–327.
17. **Kirchhausen, T., J. C. Wang, and S. C. Harrison.** 1985. DNA gyrase and its complexes with DNA: direct observation by electron microscopy. *Cell* **41:**933–943.
18. **Kreuzer, K. N., and N. R. Cozzarelli.** 1979. *Escherichia coli* mutants thermosensitive for deoxyribonucleic acid gyrase subunit A: effect of deoxyribonucleic acid replication, transcription, and bacteriophage growth. *J. Bacteriol.* **140:**424–435.
19. **Le Goffic, F.** 1985. Les quinolones, mecanisme d'action, p. 15–23. *In* J. J. Pocidalo, F. Vachon, and B. Regnier (ed.), *Les Nouvelles Quinolones.* Editiones Arnette, Paris.
20. **Maxwell, A.** 1992. The molecular basis of quinolone action. *J. Antimicrob. Chemother.* **30:**409–416.
21. **Mitscher, L. A., P. V. Devasthale, and R. M. Zavod.** 1990. Structure-activity relationships of fluoro-4-quinolones, p. 115–146. *In* G. C. Crumplin (ed.), *The 4-Quinolones: Antibacterial Agents In Vitro.* Springer-Verlag, New York.
22. **Mitscher, L. A. R. M. Zavod, P. V. Devasthale, D. T. W. Chu, L. L. Shen, P. N. Sharma, and A. G. Pernet.** 1991. Microbes beware: quinolones. Parts 1 and 2. *Chemtech* **21:**50–56, 249–255.
23. **Mitscher, L. A., R. M. Zavod, and P. N. Sharma.** 1989. Structure-activity relationships of the newer quinolone antibacterial agents, p. 3–22. *In* P. B. Fernandes (ed.), *International Telesymposium on Quinolones.* J. R. Prous Science Publishers, Barcelona, Spain.
24. **Morrison, A., and N. R. Cozzarelli.** 1981. Contacts between DNA gyrase and its binding site on DNA: features of symmetry and asymmetry revealed by protection from nucleases. *Proc. Natl. Acad. Sci. USA* **78:**1416–1420.
25. **Oram, M., and L. M. Fisher.** 1991. 4-Quinolone resistance mutations in the DNA gyrase of *Escherichia coli* clinical isolates identified by using the polymerase chain reaction. *Antimicrob. Agents Chemother.* **35:**387–389.
26. **Palu', G., S. Valisena, G. Ciarrocchi, B. Gatto, and M. Palumbo.** 1992. Quinolone binding to DNA is mediated by magnesium ions. *Proc. Natl. Acad. Sci. USA* **89:**9671–9675.
27. **Palu', G., S. Valisena, M. Peracchi, and M. Palumbo.** 1988. Do quinolones bind DNA? *Biochem. Pharmacol.* **37:**1887–1888.
28. **Pommier, Y., J. M. Covey, D. Kerrigan, J. Markovits, and R. Pharm.** 1987. DNA unwinding and inhibition of mouse leukemia L1210 DNA topoisomerase I by intercalation. *Nucleic Acids Res.* **15:**6713–6731.
29. **Reece, R. J., and A. Maxwell.** 1991. DNA gyrase: structure and function. *Crit. Rev. Biochem. Mol. Biol.* **26:**335–375.
30. **Rosen, T.** 1990. The fluoroquinolone antibacterial agents, p. 235–295. *In* G. P. Ellis and G. B. West (ed.), *Progress in Medicinal Chemistry.* Elsevier Science Publishers, Amsterdam.
31. **Shen, L., J. Baranowski, D. T. W. Chu, and A. G. Pernet.** 1989. DNA unwinding properties of new quinolones—the antagonizing effect of polyamines, abstr. 29. *Program Abstr. 29th Intersci. Conf. Antimicrob. Agents Chemother.*
32. **Shen, L. L.** 1989. A reply: "do quinolones bind to DNA?"—yes. *Biochem. Pharmacol.* **38:**2042–2044.
33. **Shen, L. L., J. Baranowski, M. Nuss, J. Tadanier, C. Lee, D. T. W. Chu, and J. J. Plattner.** 1990. Aspects of quinolone-DNA interactions, p. 147–158. *In* G. Crumpin (ed.), *The 4-Quinolones: Antibacterial Agents In Vitro.* Springer-Verlag London Ltd., London.
34. **Shen, L. L., J. Baranowski, and A. G. Pernet.** 1989. Mechanism of inhibition of DNA gyrase by quinolone antibacterials: specificity and cooperativity of drug binding to DNA. *Biochemistry* **28:**3879–3885.
35. **Shen, L. L., J. Baranowski, T. Wai, D. T. W. Chu, and A. G. Pernet.** 1989. The binding of quinolones to DNA: should we worry about it?, p. 159–170. *In* P. B. Fernandes (ed.), *International Telesymposium on Quinolones.* J. R. Prous Science Publishers, Barcelona, Spain.
36. **Shen, L. L., M. G. Bures, D. T. W. Chu, and J. J. Plattner.** 1990. Quinolone-DNA interaction: how a small drug molecule acquires high DNA binding affinity and specificity, p. 495–512. *In* B. Pullman (ed.), *Molecular Basis of Specificity in Nucleic Acid-Drug Interaction.* Kluwer Academic Publishers, Dordrecht, The Netherlands.
37. **Shen, L. L., W. E. Kohlbrenner, D. Weigl, and J. Baranowski.** 1989. Mechanism of quinolone inhibition of DNA gyrase. Appearance of unique norfloxacin binding sites in enzyme-DNA complexes. *J. Biol. Chem.* **264:**2973–2978.

38. **Shen, L. L., L. A. Mitscher, P. N. Sharma, T. J. O'Donnell, D. W. T. Chu, C. S. Cooper, T. Rosen, and A. G. Pernet.** 1989. Mechanism of inhibition of DNA gyrase by quinolone antibacterials. A cooperative drug-DNA binding model. *Biochemistry* **28:**2886–2894.

39. **Shen, L. L., and A. G. Pernet.** 1985. Mechanism of inhibition of DNA gyrase by analogues of nalidixic acid: the target of the drugs is DNA. *Proc. Natl. Acad. Sci USA* **82:**307–311.

40. **Sutcliffe, J. A., T. D. Gootz, and J. F. Barrett.** 1989. Biochemical characteristics and physiological significance of major DNA topoisomerases. *Antimicrob. Agents Chemother.* **33:**2027–2033.

41. **Tornaletti, S., and A. M. Pedrini.** 1986. Effect of nalidixic acid on DNA conformation, abstr. 54. *Cold Spring Harbor Meet. Biol. Effect DNA Topol.*

42. **Tornaletti, S., and A. M. Pedrini.** 1988. Studies on the interaction of 4-quinolones with DNA by DNA unwinding experiments. *Biochim. Biophys. Acta* **949:**279–287.

43. **Une, T., T. Fujimoto, K. Sato, and Y. Osada.** 1988. In vitro activity of DR-3355, an optically active ofloxacin. *Antimicrob. Agents Chemother.* **32:**1336–1340.

44. **Wang, J. C.** 1982. DNA topoisomerases. *Sci. Am.* **247:**94–109.

45. **Wentland, M. P.** 1990. Structure-activity relationships of fluoroquinolones, p. 1–43. *In* C. Siporin, C. L. Heifetz, and J. M. Domagala (ed.), *The New Generation of Quinolones.* Marcel Dekker, Inc., New York.

46. **Yamagishi, J., Y. Furutani, S. Inoue, T. Ohue, S. Nakamura, and M. Shimizu.** 1981. New nalidixic acid resistance mutations related to deoxyribonucleic acid gyrase activity. *J. Bacteriol.* **148:**450–458.

47. **Yamagishi, J., H. Yoshida, M. Yamayoshi, and S. Nakamura.** 1986. Nalidixic acid-resistant mutations of the *gyrB* gene of *Escherichia coli. Mol. Gen. Genet.* **204:**367–373.

48. **Yoshida, H., M. Bogaki, M. Nakamura, and S. Nakamura.** 1990. Quinolone resistance-determining region in the DNA gyrase *gyrA* gene of *Escherichia coli. Antimicrob. Agents Chemother.* **34:**1271–1272.

49. **Yoshida, H., M. Bogaki, M. Nakamura, L. M. Yamanaka, and S. Nakamura.** 1991. Quinolone resistance-determining region in the DNA gyrase *gyrB* gene of *Escherichia coli. Antimicrob. Agents Chemother.* **35:**1647–1650.

*Quinolone Antimicrobial Agents, 2nd ed.*
Edited by David C. Hooper and John S. Wolfson


*Chapter 5*

# Mechanisms of Bacterial Resistance to Quinolones

*David C. Hooper and John S. Wolfson**

With the increasing use of quinolones in clinical settings has come increasing recognition of the potential for development of resistance among bacteria to compromise drug utility (69, 174) (see chapter 8). Understanding of the mechanisms by which resistance is effected is important not only in general clinical procedures but also in devising strategies by which to circumvent resistance and in understanding drug action in susceptible bacteria (see chapter 3).

## SELECTION OF RESISTANT BACTERIA

The spontaneous occurrence of preexisting resistant mutant bacteria at low frequency in a bacterial population may be detected by selection of such mutants by plating large numbers of bacteria on quinolone-containing agar. Resistant mutants contain mutations in chromosomal genes that reduce quinolone susceptibility. Acquisition by susceptible bacteria of new resistance genes on plasmids, as commonly occurs in bacteria acquiring resistance to ß-lactams and aminoglycosides, has not yet been documented for quinolone-resistant bacteria in clinical settings but has been demonstrated in the laboratory (see Paucity of Plasmid-Mediated Resistance below).

The frequency of selection of chromosomal mutants in the laboratory depends on the selecting quinolone, the drug concentration used for selection, and the bacterium. As the selection concentration increases above the MIC, the number of resistant mutants identified in the bacterial population decreases (29, 72). This decrease presumably reflects the observation (see below) that mutations differ in the level of resistance conferred; thus, on exposure to higher drug concentrations on the selecting agar, mutants causing lower levels of resistance are unable to grow. It may be that at very high drug concentrations, no single spontaneous mutation is sufficient to cause resistance.

Selection frequencies also differ among quinolones. For example, mutant *Escherichia coli* cells are selected with nalidixic acid (at 8- to 16-fold above the MIC) 100 - to 1,000-fold more frequently than with ciprofloxacin, ofloxacin, or other fluoroquinolones (at comparable factors above their MICs) (19, 27, 37, 72, 74, 154, 175). Differences of this type likely result at least in part from differences in the effects of particular mutations or resistance mechanisms on susceptibility to the different drugs. For example, a particular amino acid change in the DNA gyrase A protein (GyrA) may cause a 128-fold increase in resistance to nalidixic

---

*David C. Hooper and John S. Wolfson* • Infectious Disease Unit, Massachusetts General Hospital, 14 Fruit Street, Boston, Massachusetts 02114-2696.
*Deceased.

acid but only a 16- to 32-fold increase in resistance to ciprofloxacin. Other examples are discussed in more detail below.

For a given quinolone and selecting drug concentration (at the same level above the MIC), bacterial species also differ in the frequency of selection of mutants. In particular, resistant mutants of *Pseudomonas aeruginosa* and to some extent of *Staphylococcus aureus* can be selected more frequently than resistant mutants of *E. coli* (1, 18, 29, 32, 38, 39, 88, 146). A higher frequency of resistance selection may also occur with some strains of *Enterobacter cloacae* and *Serratia marcescens* (171). For streptococci, the frequencies of resistant mutants selected at sixfold above the MIC were somewhat higher for norfloxacin than for ciprofloxacin, ofloxacin, and enoxacin (130).

Certain mutations also exhibit an unexpected and puzzling phenomenon. *marA* mutants, which confer pleiotropic resistance to quinolones, tetracycline, and chloramphenicol, may be selected with any of these antimicrobial agents (23). The frequency of selection, however, is at least 100-fold higher with tetracycline and chloramphenicol than with norfloxacin. Although it is possible that different mutant alleles of the same or closely linked genes in the *marA* region are selected by the different drugs, such a substantial difference in the spontaneous occurrence of such putative alleles would be surprising. Susceptible bacteria exposed to norfloxacin are killed rapidly, but exposure to tetracycline or chloramphenicol results in inhibition of bacterial growth without bacterial cell death. Because *marA* mutants selected on agar containing these latter two bacteriostatic drugs appear only after prolonged incubation, it is possible that events occurring in the nongrowing bacteria exposed to tetracycline contribute to the increased frequency of resistant mutant bacteria, but the mechanism of such an effect has not been defined.

Highly resistant bacteria containing multiple mutations may be selected for many species by serial passage in media containing increasing concentrations of quinolones (8, 72, 74, 94, 161). In such bacteria, multiple mutations may contribute additively to resistance (58, 74).

## BACTERIAL RESISTANCE TO QUINOLONES RESULTING FROM ALTERATIONS IN DNA GYRASE

The principal target of quinolone action is the essential bacterial enzyme DNA gyrase, which is composed of two A (GyrA) and two B (GyrB) subunits, products of the *gyrA* and *gyrB* genes, respectively (see chapter 3). Mutations in both genes have been shown to cause quinolone resistance.

### Alterations in GyrA

A role for alterations of the GyrA protein subunit in quinolone resistance has now been determined for a large number of species by several methods (Table 1). Mutations in the *gyrA* gene that confer resistance to quinolones have been directly identified by genetic mapping or DNA sequencing in *E. coli* (26, 28, 45, 58, 65, 72, 74, 159, 175), *P. aeruginosa* (66, 78, 134, 136), *Haemophilus influenzae* (148), and *Bacillus subtilis* (158). Also in *S. aureus*, mutations in *gyrA* analogous to those causing resistance in *E. coli* have been found in resistant members of pairs of strains isolated from patients before and after treatment with ciprofloxacin (156). Such changes appear to be relatively common in highly resistant clinical isolates (36, 48), but the level of resistance conferred by a particular change in GyrA has yet to be determined for *S. aureus*.

Indirect evidence for the presence of *gyrA* mutations in resistant strains based on increased in quinolone susceptibility following introduction of plasmids containing a wild-type *E. coli* $gyrA^+$ gene has been found in *S. marcescens* (100), *Klebsiella pneumoniae*, *Providencia stuartii*, *Acinetobacter cal-*

**Table 1.** Species of bacteria in which quinolone resistance has been linked to altered DNA gyrase

| Species | Subunit altered | Method | Reference(s) |
|---|---|---|---|
| *Haemophilus influenzae* | A | Subunit mixing | 148 |
| *Neisseria gonorrhoeae* | B | (DNA sequencing) | 157 |
| *Campylobacter jejuni* | A | Subunit mixing | 47, 147 |
| *Serratia marcescens* | A | Subunit mixing | 42, 100 |
| | | *gyrA*$^+$ complementation | 100 |
| *Enterobacter cloacae* | | Purified enzyme | 96 |
| *Citrobacter freundii* | A | Subunit mixing | 5 |
| *Klebsiella pneumoniae* | A | *gyrA*$^+$ complementation | 60 |
| *Providencia stuartii* | A | *gyrA*$^+$ complementation | 60 |
| *Acinetobacter calcoaceticus* | A | *gyrA*$^+$ complementation | 60 |
| *Pseudomonas aeruginosa* | A | Subunit mixing | 78, 99, 136 |
| | | Genetic mapping | 66, 134 |
| | | *gyrA*$^+$ complementation | 135 |
| *Enterococcus faecalis* | A | Subunit mixing | 109 |
| *Staphylococcus aureus* | A | Subunit mixing | 110, 121 |
| | | (DNA sequencing) | 155 |
| *Staphylococcus epidermidis* | A | (DNA sequencing) | 156 |
| *Bacillus subtilis* | A | Subunit mixing | 158 |
| | | Genetic mapping | 158 |

*coaceticus*, and *P. aeruginosa* (60, 135). This complementation or dominance test is based on the dominance of the susceptibility of *gyrA*$^+$ over quinolone-resistent *gyrA* in merodiploid strains, which contain both genes. This dominance likely results from the ability of wild-type GyrA to mediate quinolone-induced bacterial DNA damage in hybrid (GyrA$^+$/GyrA$^{QR}$-GyrB$_2$) DNA gyrase molecules and from a requirement for only a small number of such DNA lesions per chromosome for antibacterial effect. With this test, negative results and small decrements in resistance (131) cannot be considered evidence for the absence of chromosomal *gyrA* mutations because plasmid instability, poor plasmid gene expression, and failure of heterologous Gyr subunits to form a functional enzyme in some host strains may also produce negative results.

In addition, resistance attributable to alterations in GyrA has been shown for *E. coli* (6, 72, 143, 175), *P. aeruginosa* (78, 99, 136), *Citrobacter freundii* (4, 5), *Serratia marcescens* (42, 100), *Campylobacter jejuni* (47), *Enterococcus faecalis* (109), and *S. aureus* (110, 121) by purification of GyrA subunits from resistant and susceptible strains, mixing with purified wild-type GyrB subunits, and comparison of quinolone inhibition of DNA supercoiling activity reconstituted with the different subunits in vitro. In three other studies, resistance was associated with quinolone resistance of purified DNA gyrase supercoiling activity in pefloxacin-resistant *Enterobacter cloacae* selected in an animal model (96) and ciprofloxacin-resistant *C. jejuni* isolated from patients after ciprofloxacin treatment (147). Quinolone resistance of DNA synthesis was also found in EDTA-permeabilized pefloxacin-resistant *P. aeruginosa* selected in an animal model (102). In these last three studies, the contribution of GyrA or GyrB to resistance was not determined.

The largest amount of information on the changes in protein structure responsible for drug resistance has been acquired from nucleotide sequencing of resistant *gyrA* mutants of *E. coli*. In almost all cases studied, single changes in amino acid sequence were responsible (Table 2). These changes were clustered in the amino-terminal portions of the poly-

**Table 2.** Amino acid substitutions in *E. coli* DNA gyrase A protein that alter quinolone susceptibility

| Position | Change | Type of change[a] | n | Increase in MIC (fold) | |
|---|---|---|---|---|---|
| | | | | Nalidixic acid | Ciprofloxacin |
| 67 | Ala → Ser[b] | NP → P | 1 | 8 | 4 |
| 81 | Gly → Cys[b] | P → lg P | 1 | 16 | 8 |
| | Gly → Asp[c] | P → −1 | 1 | 1 | 8 |
| 83 | Ser → Leu[b,d] | P → lg NP | 9 | 128 | 32 |
| | Ser → Trp[b,d,e] | P → lg NP | 4 | 128 | 32 |
| | Ser → Ala[f] | P → NP | (1) | 20 | 10 |
| 84 | Ala → Pro[b] | NP → lg NP | 1 | 8 | 8 |
| 87 | Asp → Asn[b] | −1 → P | 1 | 64 | 16 |
| | Asp → Val[d] | −1 → NP | 1 | | |
| 106 | Gln → His[b] | P → +1 | 1 | 4 | 4 |
| | Gln → Arg[f] | P → +1 | (1) | 2.5 | 10 |

[a]NP, nonpolar; P, polar, lg, large; −1, negative charge; +1, positive charge; Ala, alanine; Ser, serine; Gly, glycine; Cys, cysteine; Asp, aspartic acid; Leu, leucine; Trp, tryptophan; Pro, proline; Asn, asparagine; Val, valine; Gln, glutamine; His, histidine; Arg, arginine.
[b]Nalidixic or pipemidic acid selection (178).
[c]Norfloxacin selection in vivo (15).
[d]Resistant clinical isolate (122).
[e]Enoxacin selection in vivo (one isolate) (28).
[f]Site-directed mutagenesis (56).

peptide sequence near tyrosine 122, the amino acid that is covalently linked to DNA following exposure of gyrase-DNA complexes to quinolones and protein denaturants (178, 181) and thus is presumed to be in the active site of the enzyme. Particularly notable is the occurrence of alterations at position 83, which occurred in 19 of 26 independent spontaneous resistant mutants from both laboratory (178, 181) and clinical (28, 122) sources. In all of these mutants, the wild-type serine 83 (Ser-83), a polar amino acid, was changed to either leucine (Leu) or tryptophan (Trp), both of which have nonpolar, bulky side chains. These changes resulted in a 128-fold increase in resistance to nalidixic acid and a lesser increase in resistance to ciprofloxacin (32-fold) and other fluoroquinolones. Change of Ser-83 to alanine (Ala), which contains a small, nonpolar side group, by mutagenesis in vitro resulted in increases in resistance of 20- and 10-fold for nalidixic acid and ciprofloxacin, respectively, indicating that both nonpolarity and bulk in amino acid side groups interfere with quinolone action on DNA gyrase. These amino acid changes have also been correlated with the binding of norfloxacin to a complex of DNA gyrase and DNA, with the complex of the resistant GyrA(Trp-83)-containing enzyme binding 60-fold less drug than that of the wild-type GyrA(Ser-83)-containing enzyme (172). In the absence of DNA, levels of binding to both enzymes were equivalently low, confirming earlier data that indicate that quinolones interact specifically with the complex of DNA and DNA gyrase rather than with the enzyme alone (see chapter 4).

Strikingly similar changes have been found among resistant *S. aureus* strains (Table 3). In GyrA, changes of Ser-84, which is equivalent to Ser-83 in *E. coli* (98), to Leu were found in 19 of 28 independent mutants (36, 48). In three other mutants, Ser-84 was changed to Ala. Distinct from the sequence of *E. coli*, a change in Ser-85 to proline (Pro) was also identified alone and in combination with Leu-84 (155), and in six mutants, a lysine at position 88 (Lys-88) was found instead of the wild-type glutamic acid (Glu) residue (48). Ciprofloxacin resistance in *Staphylococcus epidermidis* has also been associated with a change of Ser-84 to phenylalanine (Phe) (156). Proof of the contribu-

**Table 3.** Amino acid substitutions in *S. aureus* DNA gyrase A protein associated with quinolone resistance in clinical isolates[a]

| Position | Change[b] | Type of change[c] | *n* | Ciprofloxacin MIC (μg/ml) |
|---|---|---|---|---|
| 84 | Ser → Leu | P → lg NP | 16 | 16–128 |
| | Ser → Ala | P → NP | 3 | 16 |
| 84 | Ser → Leu | P → lg NP | 3 | 64–128 |
| 85 | Ser → Pro | P → NP | | |
| 88 | Glu → Lys | −1 → +1 | 6 | 16–32 |

[a]Clinical isolates were from Minnesota, Tennessee, and Indiana (36,48).
[b]Ser, serine; Leu, leucine; Ala, alanine; Pro, proline; Glu, glutamic acid; Lys, lysine.
[c]P, polar; NP, nonpolar; lg, large; −1, negative charge; +1, positive charge.

tion of these amino acid changes to resistance awaits further genetic studies.

Other changes in the region of GyrA between amino acids 67 and 106 in *E. coli* GyrA have been shown to effect quinolone resistance but at a lower level (Table 2). The level of resistance caused by a change of aspartic acid, a negatively charged amino acid, at position 87 (Asp-87) to asparagine (Asn), an uncharged, polar amino acid, was, however, only slightly below that caused by Leu-83 or Trp-83. In general, the increments in resistance to nalidixic acid were greater than or equal to the increments for fluoroquinolones. Two exceptions have been reported. A change of glycine at position 81 (Gly-81) (polar) to Asp (−1 charge) (15, 105) and a change of glutamine at position 106 (Gln-106) (polar) to arginine (Arg) (+1 charge), which was constructed by in vitro mutagenesis (56), both conferred greater increases in resistance to fluoroquinolones than to nalidixic acid.

The effects of these amino acid changes on the secondary and tertiary structures of the gyrase A protein and the means by which these changes confer resistance are not yet known, although the simplest explanation is that these alterations affect the affinities of quinolones for the DNA gyrase-DNA complex. An alternative possibility based on the data of Shen and associates suggesting that quinolones bind cooperatively to single-stranded-DNA pockets created by DNA gyrase (150, 151) (see chapter 4) is that the resistant DNA gyrase blocks access of the quinolones to the pocket or produces a pocket in which quinolone binding is decreased without alteration in drug binding to the protein itself.

## Alterations in GyrB

*E. coli* resistance loci *nalC* and *nalD*, which were selected for resistance to nalidixic acid (77), were shown to be alleles of *gyrB* (176, 177). Both mutant alleles encoded single amino acid changes in the midportion of GyrB (Table 4). The *nalD* allele, which encodes a change of Asp-426 (−1 charge) to Asn (uncharged, polar), also caused modest increases in resistance to other quinolones as well as to nalidixic acid, whereas the *nalC* allele, which encodes a change of lysine at position 447 (Lys) (+1 charge) to Glu (−1 charge), caused hypersusceptibility to quinolones that, unlike nalidixic acid, have a positively charged piperazinyl substituent at position 7 (153). Eleven independent additional resistant *gyrB* mutants have either Asn-426 ($n = 8$) or Glu-447 ($n = 3$) (179). On the basis of these findings and the hydrophobicity profile of the GyrB amino acid sequence, which suggested that these amino acid residues may be near one another on the surface of GyrB, Yoshida and associates have proposed a model in which the negative charge of GyrB (Glu-447) causes a direct electrostatic attraction of the positively charged piperazinyl

**Table 4.** Amino acid substitutions in *E. coli* DNA gyrase B protein that alter quinolone susceptibility[a]

| Position | Change | Type of change | *n* | Change in MIC (fold) | |
|---|---|---|---|---|---|
| | | | | Nalidixic acid | Ciprofloxacin |
| 426 | Asp → Asn | −1 → P | 9 | 16 | 8 |
| 447 | Lys → Glu | +1 → −1 | 4 | 16 | 0.25 |

[a]Selected on nalidixic acid or enoxacin at fourfold MIC (179). For abbreviations, see Table 2, footnote *a*.

group, thereby increasing enzyme sensitivity to piperazinylated quinolones (179). Proof of a direct or indirect interaction of quinolones with GyrB awaits further structural studies.

For species other than *E. coli*, there is little information on the role of GyrB in quinolone resistance. In *Neisseria gonorrhoeae*, low-level resistance to nalidixic acid has been transferred with DNA containing the *N. gonorrhoeae* homolog of *E. coli gyrB* (67% amino acid identity). The resistant *gyrB* was also found to encode Asn-419, which corresponds to Asn-426 in resistant *E. coli* GyrB (157).

### Relative Occurrence of *gyrA* and *gyrB* Mutations

In an analysis of independent *E. coli* mutants selected with nalidixic acid (at fourfold above the MIC), equal numbers appeared to have *gyrA* and *gyrB* mutations, as determined by complementation with *gyrA*$^+$- and *gyrB*$^+$-containing plasmids, respectively (108). A similar distribution was found among five enoxacin-selected mutants (at fourfold above the MIC). The highest levels of resistance were in *gyrA* mutants, and among the small number of clinical isolates studied, *gyrA* mutants predominated. In *P. aeruginosa*, *gyrA*-type mutations (determined by phenotype) were selected more frequently with nalidixic acid, and mutations with pleiotropic resistance were selected more frequently with enoxacin (182). Thus, the relative frequency of *gyrA* and *gyrB* mutants depends on the level of resistance selected, the selecting drug, and the bacterial strain. Selection for higher levels of resistance may favor *gyrA* mutants in *E. coli*.

## BACTERIAL RESISTANCE RESULTING FROM CHANGES IN OTHER TOPOISOMERASES

No mutations in the genes for *E. coli* topoisomerase I, topoisomerase III, and topoisomerase IV have been shown to cause quinolone resistance (see chapter 3). A resistance locus, *nfxD* (114), isolated from a highly resistant strain serially passaged on increasing concentrations of norfloxacin, however, is located in the region of the *parC* and *parE* genes, which encode topoisomerase IV (84). This locus appears to express quinolone resistance conditionally in the presence of a *gyrA* resistance mutation. The recessivity of *nfxD* to *gyrA*$^+$ suggests that *nfxD* may contribute to resistance only additively in strains that have already acquired at least one mutation. If *nfxD* is an allele of one of the genes of topoisomerase IV, its recessivity to *gyrA*$^+$ might suggest the possibility of exchange of subunits between DNA gyrase and topoisomerase IV. Reconstitution of topoisomerase activities by using purified heterologous subunits has not, however, been possible (85).

In *S. aureus*, a resistance locus, termed *flqA*, has been shown to be distinct from the genes for DNA gyrase and from the *norA* gene, which likely affects drug permeation (167). The function of FlqA is unknown, but mutant FlqA alters the expression of novobiocin resistance from the *nov* locus, likely an allele of *gyrB*, suggesting the possibility that it is a topoisomerase that interacts with DNA gyrase. Interestingly, *flqA* was the only mutant locus found in each of 12 mutants selected independently with ciprofloxacin or ofloxacin.

## BACTERIAL RESISTANCE TO QUINOLONES ASSOCIATED WITH CHANGES IN DRUG PERMEATION

In order to reach their principal intracellular target, DNA gyrase, the quinolones must traverse the outer and inner membranes of gram-negative bacteria. Quinolones differ in hydrophobicity (Table 5), as determined by their partition coefficient between octanol and aqueous phosphate buffer (20, 64), and these differences may affect their interactions with both membranes.

### Penetration of the Gram-Negative Outer Membrane

The means by which quinolones traverse the bacterial outer membrane have been inferred from studies with mutants that have specific defects in outer membrane components or that were selected for resistance to quinolones and, more recently, by direct studies with proteoliposomes.

Hydrophilic quinolones (and other small molecules) appear to cross the outer membranes of gram-negative bacilli through water-filled porin protein channels, which provide direct pathways between the cell exterior and the periplasmic space (57, 118). Studies of reconstituted lipid vesicles containing purified porin proteins (proteoliposomes) have identified the size limits and most favorable charge configurations for diffusion of substances through these channels (115) and have recently documented the diffusion of nalidixic acid and ofloxacin through the OmpF general diffusion porin of *E. coli* at rates greater than those of several cephalosporins (144). The size of many quinolone analogs (232 to 400 Da) and the presence in some of a zwitterionic configuration at neutral pH (138) are compatible with diffusion through OmpF and the slightly smaller channel of OmpC (115, 118). Expression of these proteins is regulated reciprocally by the bacterial cell in part in response to environmental signals such as osmolarity of the growth medium and temperature (40, 55, 87, 97, 145).

**Table 5.** Hydrophobicity of quinolones and activity against *S. typhimurium* deep rough mutants[a]

| Compound | Hydrophobicity[b] | Ionic type[c] | Ratio of MIC of indicated mutant/MIC of wild-type strain | | |
|---|---|---|---|---|---|
| | | | *rfaG* | *rfaF* | *rfaE* |
| Enoxacin | 0.007 | Amphoteric | 1 | 1 | 1 |
| Norfloxacin | 0.01 | Amphoteric | 1 | 1 | 1 |
| Ciprofloxacin | 0.02 | Amphoteric | 1 | 1 | 1 |
| Pipemidic acid | 0.03 | Amphoteric | 1 | 1 | 1 |
| Cinoxacin | 0.03 | Acidic | 1 | 1 | 1 |
| Fleroxacin | 0.08 | Amphoteric | 0.5 | 0.5 | 0.5 |
| Ofloxacin | 0.33 | Amphoteric | 0.5 | 0.5 | 0.5 |
| Miloxacin | 1.12 | Acidic | 0.5 | 0.5 | 0.5 |
| Pefloxacin | 1.32 | Amphoteric | 0.5 | 0.5 | 0.5 |
| Oxolinic acid | 2.23 | Acidic | 0.25 | 0.25 | 0.13 |
| Nalidixic acid | 8.92 | Acidic | 0.25 | 0.13 | 0.06 |
| Rosoxacin | 10.7 | Acidic | 0.13 | 0.13 | 0.06 |
| Piromidic acid | 11.7 | Acidic | 0.13 | 0.06 | 0.03 |
| Flumequine | 13.0 | Acidic | 0.13 | 0.13 | 0.06 |

[a]Data were taken from reference 64 with permission.
[b]Partition coefficient in *n*-octanol–0.1 M phosphate buffer (pH 7.2).
[c]Amphoteric, contains negatively charged carboxyl group at position 3 and positively charged piperazinyl group at position 7; acidic, contains negatively charged carboxyl group at position 3.

For hydrophobic antimicrobial agents, the outer membrane has paradoxically been observed to be a barrier to drug diffusion despite the presumed greater solubility of hydrophobic compounds in membrane phospholipid bilayers (116). This barrier property has been attributed to lipopolysaccharides (LPS) on the external surface of the outer membrane, which block drug access to the underlying phospholipid layer. Consistent with this concept, studies with mutants of *Salmonella typhimurium* with defects in LPS structure (deep rough mutants) have shown increased susceptibility to quinolones with higher hydrophobicity (Table 5) (64), but the extent to which quinolones enter the wild-type cell by diffusing across the phospholipid bilayer of the outer membrane remains uncertain. It has been suggested that quinolones (particularly the more hydrophobic congeners) may promote their own diffusion across the phospholipid layer (20) because they are capable of chelating magnesium (20, 162), which is necessary for stabilizing LPS in the outer membrane (116). This concept has arisen from three observations. (i) Increases in magnesium concentration (from 1 to 14 mM [73] or from 0.2 to 5 mM [20]) result in decreases in quinolone activity and decreases in accumulation of norfloxacin (73) and fleroxacin (20) by *E. coli* cells. (ii) The reduction in quinolone activity by magnesium was greatest with the most hydrophobic quinolones (20). (iii) Fleroxacin, a relatively hydrophobic analog, at a high concentration accumulated progressively in *E. coli* cells (20), an effect not seen with the more hydrophilic analogs norfloxacin (73) and enoxacin (12). An alternative explanation for such findings is that drug-magnesium complexes penetrate porin channels less well. Noteworthy also is the finding that hydrophobicity affects the penetration of zwitterionic cephalosporins less than the penetration of monoanionic cephalosporins in liposomes reconstituted with *E. coli* OmpF porin (115); thus, for quinolones, a zwitterionic configuration may also affect drug permeation more strongly than hydrophobicity.

## Resistance Mutations Associated with Changes in the Outer Membrane in *E. coli*

*E. coli ompF* null (transposon-inactivated) (22) and missense (12, 19, 20, 64, 72) mutants exhibit only about a twofold increment in resistance to many hydrophilic quinolones (Table 6), possibly because of a compensatory increase in the OmpC porin (23). *ompC*

**Table 6.** Effect of mutations that alter porin outer membrane proteins on quinolone and other resistances in *E. coli*[a]

| Mutation (reference) | Location on map (min) | Phenotype | Selecting agent(s)[b] | MIC (μg/ml) | | | | |
|---|---|---|---|---|---|---|---|---|
| | | | | NAL[c] | NFX | CFX | TC | CM |
| None (wild type) (72) | | OmpF$^+$ OmpC$^+$ | None | 4.0 | 0.08 | 0.02 | 4.0 | 8.0 |
| *ompF* (72) | 21 | OmpF$^-$ OmpC$^+$ | | 8.0 | 0.16 | | 4.0 | 8.0 |
| *ompC* (72) | 48 | OmpF$^+$ OmpC$^-$ | | 4.0 | 0.08 | | | 8.0 |
| *nfxB* (72) | 19 | OmpF$^-$ OmpC$^+$ | NFX | 16.0 | 0.32 | 0.04 | 16.0 | 32.0 |
| *norB* (65) | 34 | OmpF$^-$ OmpC$^+$ | NFX | 16.0[d] | 0.32 | 0.08 | | 16.0 |
| *norC*[e] (65) | 8 | OmpF$^-$ OmpC$^+$ | NFX | 1.0[d] | 0.32 | 0.04 | | 4.0 |
| *cfxB* (74) | 34 | OmpF$^-$ OmpC$^+$ | CFX | 16.0 | 0.32 | 0.08 | 8.0 | 32.0 |
| *marA* (23) | 34 | OmpF$^-$ OmpC$^+$ | TC, CM | 16.0[d] | 0.32 | 0.16 | 32.0 | 32.0 |

[a]Data were taken from reference 70 with permission.
[b]NFX, norfloxacin; CFX, ciprofloxacin; TC, tetracycline; CM, chloramphenicol.
[c]NAL, nalidixic acid.
[d]MICs of parent wild-type strain differed slightly from that listed; values for the mutants are adjusted to reflect the observed factor increment in MIC above the wild-type strain.
[e]The *norC* mutant also has alterations in LPS.

mutants, in contrast, have virtually no detectable change in quinolone resistance (19, 20, 64, 72).

A class of *E. coli* mutants selected for resistance to hydrophilic quinolones and distinct from *gyrA* and *gyrB* mutants has several features consistent with resistance caused at least in part by decreased permeation through OmpF. These mutations (designated *nfxB* [19 min on the *E. coli* genetic map] [72], *norB* [34 min] [65], *norC* [8 min] [65], *nfxC* [34 min] [71], and *cfxB* [34 min] [73]) are genetically distinct from *ompF* and confer (i) pleiotropic resistance to quinolones and structurally unrelated agents such as tetracycline, chloramphenicol, and some ß-lactams; (ii) substantial decreases in OmpF porin; and (iii) reduced accumulation of quinolones.

*marA* mutants (23, 24) selected for resistance to tetracycline and chloramphenicol and *soxQ* mutants (50, 51) selected for resistance to the naphthoquinone menadione also express resistance to quinolones and have reduced OmpF, and the *marA*, *cfxB*, and *soxQ* mutations (all located at 34 min on the *E. coli* genetic map) are closely linked, if not allelic (50, 71, 73, 74). *marA* mutants also exhibit reduced accumulation of [$^3$H]norfloxacin and changes in other as yet unidentified outer membrane proteins (23).

Recent cloning and sequencing of the 34-min region of the *E. coli* chromosome has identified a potentially complex operon of at least three genes, which have altered expression in *mar* mutants (21, 54) and in response to environmental insults (137). Decreased *ompF* expression seen in *marA* (24), *cfxB* (71, 73), and *soxQ* (50) mutants is effected after transcription and is dependent on the *micF* locus, which encodes a 96-base antisense RNA species that is complementary to the 5′ end of *ompF* mRNA (104). Increased *micF* expression, which has been shown to reduce *ompF* translation likely from destabilization of *ompF* mRNA binding to the ribosome (3, 104), is also seen in these mutants (24, 71). The inferred amino acid sequence of MarA has homology with those of other proteins in *E. coli* that act as positive transcriptional regulators (21), suggesting that MarA acts directly to increase *micF* transcription, thereby reducing *ompF* translation.

*soxQ* and *cfxB* mutants also have altered expression of endonuclease IV, glucose-6-phosphate dehydrogenase, and other proteins of unknown function (50). Thus, the *marA*, *cfxB*, *nfxC*, and *soxQ* mutations appear to be in genes that are components of overlapping networks of genes that allow the cell to respond to a variety of environmental insults, which include, interestingly, the synthetic quinolone agents.

Other mutants with a similar pleiotropic resistance phenotype, but not genetically characterized, have been reported (12, 19); some of these mutants had decreases in both OmpF and OmpC porins (19).

Although reductions in OmpF contribute to resistance to hydrophilic quinolones in *E. coli*, factors in addition to changes in porin pathways are also involved (23). The details of the mechanism(s) of quinolone resistance in the *nfxB*, *norB*, and *cfxB* mutants are complex and not fully defined. The level of resistance in these mutants is two- to fourfold greater than that in *ompF* mutants (Table 6), suggesting that other factors are contributing. In addition, although *nfxB* (and *cfxB*) mutants at steady state accumulate less [$^3$H]norfloxacin than do wild-type cells (73) by a factor similar to the increment in resistance between mutant and wild-type cells, the reduction in the initial rate of drug accumulation is insufficient to account for a reduced steady-state level of drug in mutant cells whose mass doubles every 40 min.

Energy is an additional factor that appears to be necessary for the reduced norfloxacin accumulation found in *nfxB*, *cfxB* (73), and *marA* (23) (see below) mutants, as was first recognized for wild-type and *ompF E. coli* (22). Energy inhibitors such as dinitrophenol, carbonyl cyanide *m*-chlorophenylhydrazone (CCCP), and azide all produce increases in [$^3$H]norfloxacin accumulation and abolish the differences between mutant and wild-type cells (73). The demonstration of energy-dependent and saturable accumulation of [$^3$H]-norfloxacin in everted (inside-out) inner membrane vesicles from either *marA* or wild-type cells suggested that there is at the inner membrane (even in wild-type *E. coli*) an energy-requiring transporter mediating norfloxacin efflux (22) (see below). For such an efflux mechanism to contribute to resistance, however, the drug must be transported across both the inner and the outer membranes (22), perhaps at zones of adherence between the two membranes (10). No mutants that affect the putative efflux carrier have been identified, however, and direct assessment of the role of such a carrier in the resistance phenotype is thus not yet possible. NorA, a candidate fluoroquinolone efflux protein, has, however, been identified in *S. aureus* (see below).

Among mutants of *E. coli* selected for resistance to the more hydrophobic quinolone analog nalidixic acid, *nalB* (57.5 min on the *E. coli* map) mutants were thought to have resistance due to decreased permeation, because after treatment with the chelating agent EDTA, the concentrations of nalidixic acid required to inhibit DNA synthesis returned to wild-type levels (14, 58). No such effect of EDTA treatment was seen with similarly selected *gyrA* mutants resistant to nalidixic acid (14). More recently, the *emr* locus, which is located at 57.5 min and may be related to *nalB*, has been cloned and shown to confer resistance to nalidixic acid and other hydrophobic compounds but not to hydrophilic fluoroquinolones (95). *emr* contains two open reading frames, one of which, *emrB*, encodes a hydrophobic protein predicted to contain 14 membrane-spanning helices. EmrB thus appears to belong to a family of multidrug efflux pumps, which includes the Qac and NorA proteins of *S. aureus* and the Bmr protein of *B. subtilis* (see below).

Mutants in the *nalD* locus (89.5 min; distinct from the *gyrB* mutation originally designated *nalD* [176]) were also more susceptible to the action of nalidixic acid on DNA synthesis after EDTA treatment and accumulated less nalidixic acid and glycerol than the parent strain at 37°C but not at 30°C, suggesting a defect in nalidixic acid uptake at 37°C (75). Some quinolone-resistant mutants also exhibit alterations in LPS profiles (65), but the direct contribution of LPS alterations to resistance is uncertain because of possible secondary effects on porin protein diffusion channels (123).

A number of other mutations (*crp* [89], *cya* [89, 90], *icd* [62, 90], *purB* [61, 90], and *ctr* [61]) also confer low-level resistance to nalidixic acid by uncertain mechanisms. Some nalidixic acid-resistant mutants of *E. coli* K-12 have been found to produce a new hemolysin similar to $\tau$-hemolysin (170), but the nature of the mutation was not defined.

### Quinolone Resistance Associated with Changes in the Outer Membrane in Species Other Than *E. coli*

In species of gram-negative bacilli other than *E. coli*, resistance selected with quinolones has also been associated with resistance to other classes of antimicrobial agents and in many instances with changes in outer membrane proteins. *P. aeruginosa* has been studied most extensively, and resistance selected with quinolones has been found to be pleiotropic and associated with both reductions and increases in outer membrane proteins (Table 7) (80). The *nalB* gene of *P. aeruginosa* causes resistance to quinolones and structurally unrelated antimicrobial agents, suggesting decreases in drug permeation (134, 136).

In addition, a mutation in another gene, *nfxB* (66), selected with norfloxacin causes resistance to newer quinolone agents, hypersusceptibility to ß-lactams and aminoglycosides, and reduced accumulation of norfloxacin, suggesting decreased drug permeation. *nfxB* mutants have a new 54-kDa outer membrane protein rather than a decrease in the amount of a previously existing protein. Introduction of cloned *nfxB*$^+$ re-

**Table 7.** Quinolone resistance mutations in *P. aeruginosa* PAO thought to affect drug permeation[a]

| Gene | Drug susceptibility pattern | | Associated changes in outer membrane |
|---|---|---|---|
| | Drug(s) | Response | |
| *nalB* | Quinolone | R | New 49-kDa OMP |
| | β-Lactam | R | |
| | Chloramphenicol | R | |
| *nfxB* | Quinolone | R | New 54-kDa OMP |
| | β-Lactam | S | |
| | Aminoglycosides | S | |
| *nfxC* | Quinolone | R | Increase in 50-kDa OMP |
| | Imipenem | R | Decrease in 46-kDa OMP |
| | Chloramphenicol | R | |
| | β-Lactam | S | |
| | Aminoglycosides | S | |

[a]Adapted from reference 80 with permission. R, resistant; S, hypersusceptible; OMP, outer membrane protein.

verses the resistance, the changes in the 54-kDa outer membrane protein (120), and the reduced drug accumulation in *nfxB* mutants (81), and the nucleotide sequence of *nfxB* indicates its similarity to regulatory genes (63). Thus, *nfxB* may be similar to *marA* in *E. coli* in regulating outer membrane proteins, although the types of outer membrane protein changes effected will likely differ in *P. aeruginosa* and *E. coli*.

A third quinolone resistance locus in *P. aeruginosa*, *nfxC*, was associated with cross-resistance to chloramphenicol and the carbapenem imipenem but hypersusceptibility to ß-lactams and aminoglycosides (43). *nfxC* mutants also exhibited decreases in a 46-kDa protein and increases in a 50-kDa outer membrane protein as well as reduced norfloxacin accumulation. Imipenem-selected mutants, which also had reductions in a 46-kDa protein, were not cross-resistant to quinolones, suggesting that this protein may be involved in imipenem resistance. The pleiotropic phenotype of the *nfxC* mutants suggests that like *nfxB*, *nfxC* will probably be a regulatory locus.

Other mutants of *P. aeruginosa* selected with quinolones and characterized phenotypically but not genetically have shown cross-resistance to chloramphenicol, ß-lactams, and imipenem (7, 102, 127, 132). Selection for resistance with another carbapenem, meropenem, but not imipenem (7, 43, 132) also produced mutants with pleiotropic resistance that included resistance to quinolones and overproduction of outer membrane protein OprM (101). Reductions in outer membrane protein OprF have also been seen in enoxacin- and lomefloxacin-selected resistant mutants (59, 127), and reductions in OprD have been seen in pefloxacin-selected resistant mutants (102). Overexpression of another outer membrane protein, OprH, resulted in increased quinolone susceptibility by an unknown mechanism (183). Reduced accumulation of new quinolones has also been reported in some mutants of *P. aeruginosa* (17, 66, 91). The variability in the changes in outer membrane proteins among resistant strains of *P. aeruginosa* leaves uncertain the role of particular membrane proteins in quinolone resistance.

Additional examples of pleiotropic drug resistance that include quinolone agents have been reported for *Enterobacter* sp., *K. pneumoniae*, *Salmonella paratyphi*, *Serratia marcescens*, *C. freundii*, and other bacterial species (4, 9, 46, 52, 53, 106, 126, 128, 129, 140, 141, 163, 164), and for some strains, changes in outer membranes that suggest a decrease in porin-like proteins have been documented (30). The role of these membrane changes in resistance and whether the proteins involved are porins, however, are uncertain. In some cases, selection with other agents involved in pleiotropic resistance has been reported (31, 140). Reduced accumulation of new quinolones was also seen in some mutants of *Proteus vulgaris* (79). Isolates identified before and after therapy of human infections with quinolones also acquire pleiotropic resistance associated with changes in outer membrane proteins and altered drug accumulation. In *Bacteroides fragilis*, an interesting association between increased resistance to norfloxacin and increased resistance to ß-lactam antibiotics has been reported, but the mechanism has not yet been defined (86).

## Transport across the Inner Membrane and Drug Efflux Mechanisms

Little is known about the interaction of quinolones with the bacterial inner membrane. In studies with everted inner membrane vesicles of *E. coli*, lactate or NADH energized the uptake of norfloxacin, which corresponds to the efflux of norfloxacin in an intact cell with a normal membrane orientation (22, 23). This uptake in everted vesicles was saturable, with an apparent $K_m$ of 200 $\mu$M, and was inhibited by CCCP and dinitrophenol and partially inhibited by nigericin and valinomycin, which, respectively, collapse the proton and electrochemical gradients across the membrane. Thus, in wild-type *E. coli*, there appears to be a low-affinity efflux transporter of norfloxacin that is driven by the proton motive force. In the absence of an energy substrate, the concentrations of drug within these vesicles were estimated to be equivalent to the external drug concentration and were suggested to result from passive diffusion. *E. coli* mutants with altered efflux transport of fluoroquinolones have not yet been identified, and the role of this putative efflux transporter in fluoroquinolone resistance thus remains undefined.

No studies have assessed quinolone transport in the opposite direction by use of right-side-out inner membrane vesicles. In artificial vesicles prepared with negatively charged phospholipids, hydrophilic quinolones exhibit increased binding at pHs at which the quinolone either is positively charged or has a minimum charge (and minimum aqueous solubility) (11).

Information on the role of efflux in quinolone resistance in other gram-negative bacilli is also limited. The reduced accumulation of quinolones seen in some mutants of *P. aeruginosa* (17, 66, 91, 92) and *Proteus vulgaris* (79) was eliminated by treatment with CCCP, suggesting the presence of an efflux mechanism in these organisms (16, 17, 79). Caution should be used in interpreting results that rely solely on the effects of CCCP, however, because CCCP facilitated the uptake of pefloxacin into artificial liposomes, which lack specific transporters (44). The extent to which protonophores other than CCCP and quinolones other than pefloxacin have this effect is not clear. In one study, an OprF-deficient strain of *P. aeruginosa* was plated on ofloxacin (92). Two resistant mutants selected had reduced drug accumulation and a reduction in MIC (not seen in the parent strain) when the pH of the medium was raised from 6.5 to 8.5. The dependence of the resistance phenotype on low external pH led those authors to suggest that this dependence may result from drug efflux coupled to a pH gradient across the cell membrane.

In gram-positive bacteria, which lack an outer membrane, resistance by altered permeation will affect the inner membrane predominantly. The *norA* gene present on the chromosome of *S. aureus* encodes a hydrophobic protein thought to contain 12 membrane-spanning domains (180). *norA* cloned on a high-copy-number plasmid confers resistance to hydrophilic more than hydrophobic quinolones in *E. coli* and *S. aureus* (82, 167, 180). *S. aureus* and *E. coli* cells containing clones *norA* exhibit reduced accumulation of enoxacin (180) and norfloxacin (82, 166), a reduction that is abolished by treatment with CCCP. Everted vesicles prepared from *E.*

*coli* cells containing cloned *norA* also exhibit *norA*-dependent, lactate-energized uptake of norfloxacin, a measure of efflux in the right-side-out membrane orientation (166). This uptake is saturable, with an apparent $K_m$ of 6 $\mu$M, a drug concentration around the MIC of norfloxacin for *S. aureus* (68) and substantially below the $K_m$ reported for *E. coli*. Uptake is inhibited by nigericin but not valinomycin, indicating that *norA*-mediated norfloxacin transport is coupled to the proton gradient across the cell membrane (166). Interestingly, this uptake was also inhibited by reserpine and verapamil, calcium channel blockers that inhibit the ATP-dependent efflux of chemotherapeutic agents mediated by the Mdr (P-glycoprotein) protein in mammalian cells (119) and the apparent efflux of quinolones and unrelated compounds by the Bmr protein of *B. subtilis* (111, 112). Although Mdr has no homology with NorA, Bmr is highly homologous (44% amino acid identity with NorA), and cloned *bmr* in *B. subtilis* causes increases in fluoroquinolone resistance that are reversed by reserpine (111). A quinolone resistance locus, *flqB*, on the *S. aureus* chromosome is linked to *norA*, and the resistance of this mutant is greater for hydrophilic than for hydrophobic quinolones (165, 166) and is reversed by reserpine (166, 167), suggesting that *flqB* is an allele of *norA*, possibly with augmented expression. Thus, NorA is a strong candidate for a quinolone efflux secondary transporter driven by the proton gradient across the cell membrane, and it appears, on the basis of its amino acid sequence and hydropathy profile, to be a member of a larger group of transporters (93, 117) that includes Bmr and the plasmid-encoded Tet (152) and Qac (139) proteins, the last two of which mediate active efflux of tetracycline and quaternary ammonium compounds, respectively. The chromosomal location of *norA* and the synthetic nature of quinolone agents indicate that NorA likely functions in *S. aureus* for purposes other than quinolone transport. *norA* cloned in *B. subtilis*, like *bmr*, also confers resistance to rhodamine 6G, ethidium bromide, chloramphenicol, and other compounds (113), but the normal function of NorA in *S. aureus* remains to be defined.

The differential effect of *flqB* on resistance to hydrophilic over hydrophobic compounds may account in part for the greater increment in resistance to ciprofloxacin relative to ofloxacin in a strain selected for high-level resistance by serial passage on norfloxacin (165).

## FITNESS OF RESISTANT MUTANTS

Alterations in chromosomal genes that cause quinolone resistance may impair bacterial function. *E. coli* and *P. aeruginosa* strains with several resistance mutations tend to grow more slowly on conventional laboratory media than their wild-type parent strains (59, 67). Some quinolone-resistant strains of *P. aeruginosa* also have reduced virulence properties (133). In contrast, strains with *gyrA* mutations conferring the highest level of resistance appear to have little alteration in DNA supercoiling in contrast to those *gyrA* mutants conferring lower levels of resistance (2). Quinolone-resistant strains of *S. aureus* also appear to be stable and capable of dissemination in the hospital environment (13). Thus, it may not be possible to reliably predict the effect of quinolone resistance mutations on other bacterial properties.

## PAUCITY OF PLASMID-MEDIATED RESISTANCE

There have been a few reports of plasmid-mediated resistance to quinolones among clinical bacterial isolates (107, 125, 160), but none has yet been confirmed, and the mechanisms have not been defined (25). This scarcity of plasmid-mediated resistance may result in part from the abilities of quinolones to inhibit plasmid conjugation and to eliminate some plasmids from their host cells (see chapter 3). In addition, the dominance of the susceptible wild-type *gyr*$^+$ genes to the resistant mutant *gyr* alleles in cells containing both wild-type and mutant genes (58) predicts that introduction of a plasmid containing a resistant *gyr* allele into a susceptible (*gyr*$^+$) recipient cell would not result in phenotypic resistance. Also, for *ompF* mutations, which affect quinolone permeation, introduction into wild-type cells may result only in delayed expression of low-level resistance because of the requirement to dilute out the many copies of wild-type OmpF protein in the outer membrane (41).

Plasmid-mediated quinolone resistance is, however, possible at least under certain laboratory conditions. (i) Resistant *gyrA* genes on plasmids are able to confer resistance to the host bacterial cell if the amount of chromosomally encoded gyrase protein is reduced, as occurs in certain thermosensitive *gyrA* mutant hosts at intermediate and nonpermissive temperatures (28, 181). (ii) An exception to the dominance of wild-type over mutant quinolone resistance loci in *E. coli* may be the *cfxB* mutation, which appears to be dominant to *cfxB*$^+$ (73) and thus might be expressed if introduced on a plasmid. (iii) In addition, as described above, the *norA* gene of *S. aureus* when cloned on a high-copy-number plasmid confers quinolone resistance in both *E. coli* and *S. aureus* (180).

## INTRINSIC RESISTANCE

With the synthesis of increasing numbers of quinolone congeners, the spectrum of bacterial species inhibited by quinolones has increased and now includes strict anaerobic species as well as aerobic gram-positive and gram-negative bacteria (173). Thus, among bacterial species, intrinsic resistance to a broad range of quinolone congeners appears to be rare, perhaps reflecting conservation of DNA gyrase structure in prokaryotes (homology between the inferred amino acid sequences of the *E. coli* and *B. subtilis* enzymes is 50% for the gyrase A protein [181] and 60% for the gyrase B protein [177]).

Fungi, in contrast, appear to be inhibited poorly by many quinolone congeners alone, although quinolones may augment the activity of amphotericin B (35, 169). The fungi that have been studied, *Saccharomyces cerevisiae* (49) and *Schizosaccharomyces pombe* (168), like other eukaryotes, contain topoisomerases structurally and functionally distinct from DNA gyrase (see chapter 7). Yeast (49) and other eukaryotic type II topoisomerases are usually more than 100-fold less sensitive to the originally identified quinolones than are wild-type bacterial DNA gyrases (33, 76, 103, 124, 142). Recent newer quinolone analogs with markedly enhanced activity against eukaryotic topoisomerase II have been identified, however (see chapter 7), and fungal topoisomerases are now being investigated as drug targets (34, 149). The contribution of impermeability to intrinsic quinolone resistance among fungi is unknown. Quinolone derivatives active against fungi might also be expected to be those with increased activity against mammalian topoisomerases because of structural similarities in the yeast and mammalian enzymes (49, 103) and thus may prove more toxic for human use.

## REFERENCES


1. **Aldridge, K. E., A. Henderberg, and C. V. Sanders**. 1989. Mutational frequency of gram-positive and gram-negative bacteria to resistance to lomefloxacin and other quinolones. *Rev. Infect. Dis.* **11**(Suppl. 5):S974–S975.
2. **Aleixandre, V., G. Herrera, A. Urios, and M. Blanco**. 1991. Effects of ciprofloxacin on plasmid DNA supercoiling of *Escherichia coli* topoisomerase I and gyrase mutants. *Antimicrob. Agents Chemother.* **35**:20-23.
3. **Andersen, J., and N. Delihas**. 1990. *micF* RNA binds to the 5′ end of *ompF* mRNA and to a protein from *Escherichia coli*. *Biochemistry* **29**: 9249-9256.
4. **Aoyama, H., K. Fujimaki, K. Sato, T. Fujii, M. Inoue, K. Hirai, and S. Mitsuhashi**. 1988. Clinical isolate of *Citrobacter freundii* highly resistant to new quinolones. *Antimicrob. Agents Chemother.* **32**:922-924.
5. **Aoyama, H., K. Sato, T. Fujii, K. Fujimaki, M. Inoue, and S. Mitsuhashi**. 1988. Purification

of *Citrobacter freundii* DNA gyrase and inhibition by quinolones. *Antimicrob. Agents Chemother.* **32:**104-109.

6. **Aoyama, H., K. Sato, T. Kato, K. Hirai, and S. Mitsuhashi**. 1987. Norfloxacin resistance in a clinical isolate of *Escherichia coli*. *Antimicrob. Agents Chemother.* **31:**1640-1641.
7. **Aubert, G., B. Pozzetto, and G. Dorche**. 1992. Emergence of quinolone-imipenem cross-resistance in *Pseudomonas aeruginosa* after fluoroquinolone therapy. *J. Antimicrob. Chemother.* **29:**307-312.
8. **Barry, A. L., and R. N. Jones**. 1984. Cross-resistance among cinoxacin, ciprofloxacin, DJ-6783, enoxacin, nalidixic acid, norfloxacin, and oxolinic acid after in vitro selection of resistant populations. *Antimicrob. Agents Chemother.* **25:**775-777.
9. **Bayer, A. S., L. Hirano, and J. Yih**. 1988. Development of ß-lactam resistance and increased quinolone MICs during therapy of experimental *Pseudomonas aeruginosa* endocarditis. *Antimicrob. Agents Chemother.* **32:**231–235.
10. **Bayer, M. H., G. P. Costello, and M. E. Bayer**. 1982. Isolation and partial characterization of membrane vesicles carrying markers of the membrane adhesion sites. *J. Bacteriol.* **149:**758-767.
11. **Bedard, J., and L. E. Bryan**. 1989. Interaction of the fluoroquinolone antimicrobial agents ciprofloxacin and enoxacin with liposomes. *Antimicrob. Agents Chemother.* **33:**1379-1382.
12. **Bedard, J., S. Wong, and L. E. Bryan**. 1987. Accumulation of enoxacin by *Escherichia coli* and *Bacillus subtilis*. *Antimicrob. Agents Chemother.* **31:**1348-1354.
13. **Blumberg, H. M., D. Rimland, J. A. Kiehlbauch, P. M. Terry, and I. K. Wachsmuth**. 1992. Epidemiologic typing of *Staphylococcus aureus* by DNA restriction fragment length polymorphisms of rRNA genes: elucidation of the clonal nature of a group of bacteriophage-nontypeable, ciprofloxacin-resistant, methicillin-susceptible *S. aureus* isolates. *J. Clin. Microbiol.* **30:**362-369.
14. **Bourguignon, G. J., M. Levitt, and R. Sternglanz**. 1973. Studies on the mechanism of action of nalidixic acid. *Antimicrob. Agents Chemother.* **4:**479-486.
15. **Cambau, E., F. Bordon, E. Collatz, and L. Gutmann**. 1992. A novel *gyrA* mutation confers resistance to fluoroquinolones but not to nalidixic acid in *Escherichia coli*. *Abstr. 92nd Gen. Meet. Am. Soc. Microbiol. 1992*, p. 17, abstr. A-96.
16. **Celesk, R. A., and N. J. Robillard**. 1989. Factors influencing the accumulation of ciprofloxacin in *Pseudomonas aeruginosa*. *Antimicrob. Agents Chemother.* **33:**1921–1926.
17. **Chamberland, S., A. S. Bayer, T. Schollaardt, S. A. Wong, and L. E. Bryan**. 1989. Characterization of mechanisms of quinolone resistance in *Pseudomonas aeruginosa* strains isolated in vitro and in vivo during experimental endocarditis. *Antimicrob. Agents Chemother.* **33:**624-634.
18. **Chantot, J. F., and A. Bryskier**. 1985. Antibacterial activity of ofloxacin and other 4-quinolone derivatives: *in-vitro* and *in-vivo* comparison. *J. Antimicrob. Chemother.* **16:**475-484.
19. **Chapman, J. S., A. Bertasso, and N. H. Georgopapadakou**. 1989. Fleroxacin resistance in *Escherichia coli*. *Antimicrob. Agents Chemother.* **33:**239-241.
20. **Chapman, J. S., and N. H. Georgopapadakou**. 1988. Routes of quinolone permeation in *Escherichia coli*. *Antimicrob. Agents Chemother.* **32:**438-442.
21. **Cohen, S. P., H. Hächler, and S. B. Levy**. 1993. Genetic and functional analysis of the multiple antibiotic resistance (*mar*) locus in *Escherichia coli*. *J. Bacteriol.* **175:**1484–1492.
22. **Cohen, S. P., D. C. Hooper, J. S. Wolfson, K. S. Souza, L. M. McMurry, and S. B. Levy**. 1988. An endogenous active efflux of norfloxacin in susceptible *Escherichia coli*. *Antimicrob. Agents Chemother.* **32:**1187-1191.
23. **Cohen, S. P., L. M. McMurry, D. C. Hooper, J. S. Wolfson, and S. B. Levy**. 1989. Cross-resistance to fluoroquinolones in multiple antibiotic resistant (Mar) *Escherichia coli* selected by tetracycline and chloramphenicol: decreased drug accumulation associated with membrane changes in addition to OmpF reduction. *Antimicrob. Agents Chemother.* **33:**1318–1325.
24. **Cohen, S. P., L. M. McMurry, and S. B. Levy**. 1988. *marA* locus causes decreased expression of OmpF porin in multiple-antibiotic-resistant (Mar) mutants of *Escherichia coli*. *J. Bacteriol.* **170:**5416-5422.
25. **Courvalin, P**. 1990. Plasmid-mediated 4-quinolone resistance: a real or apparent absence? *Antimicrob. Agents Chemother.* **34:**681-684.
26. **Crumplin, G. C., M. Kenwright, and T. Hirst**. 1984. Investigations into the mechanisms of action of the antibacterial agent norfloxacin. *J. Antimicrob. Chemother.* **13**(Suppl. B):9-23.
27. **Crumplin, G. C., and M. Odell**. 1987. Development of resistance to ofloxacin. *Drugs* **34**(Suppl. 1):1-8.
28. **Cullen, M. E., A. W. Wyke, R. Kuroda, and L. M. Fisher**. 1989. Cloning and characterization of a DNA gyrase A gene from *Escherichia coli* that confers clinical resistance to 4-quinolones. *Antimicrob. Agents Chemother.* **33:**886-894.
29. **Cullman, W., M. Stieglitz, B. Baars, and W. Opferkuch**. 1985. Comparative evaluation of recently developed quinolone compounds—with a note on the frequency of resistant mutants. *Chemotherapy* (Basel) **31:**19-28.

30. **Daikos, G. L., V. T. Lolans, and G. G. Jackson.** 1988. Alterations in outer membrane proteins of *Pseudomonas aeruginosa* associated with selective resistance to quinolones. *Antimicrob. Agents Chemother.* **32:**785–787.
31. **Dang, P., L. Gutmann, C. Quentin, R. Williamson, and E. Collatz.** 1988. Some properties of *Serratia marcescens*, *Salmonella paratyphi* A, and *Enterobacter cloacae* with non-enzyme-dependent multiple resistance to ß-lactam antibiotics, aminoglycosides, and quinolones. *Rev. Infect. Dis.* **10:**899-904.
32. **Duckworth, G. J., and J. D. Williams.** 1984. Frequency of appearance of resistant variants to norfloxacin and nalidixic acid. *J. Antimicrob. Chemother.* **13**(Suppl. B):33-38.
33. **Duguet, M., C. Lavenot, F. Harper, G. Miranbeau, and A.-M. De Recondo.** 1983. DNA topoisomerases from rat liver: physiological variations. *Nucleic Acids Res.* **11:**1059-1075.
34. **Elsea, S. H., N. Osheroff, and J. L. Nitiss.** 1992. Cytotoxicity of quinolones towards eukaryotic cells: identification of topoisomerase II as the primary cellular target for the quinolone CP-115,953 in yeast. *J. Biol. Chem.* **267:**13150-13153.
35. **Eng, R. H. K., S. M. Smith, M. L. Corrado, and H. H. Gadebusch.** 1982. Antifungal activity of norfloxacin (MK 0366) and amphotericin B in combination, abstr. 479. *Program Abstr. 22nd Intersci. Conf. Antimicrob. Agents Chemother.*
36. **Fasching, C. E., F. C. Tenover, T. G. Slama, L. M. Fisher, S. Sreedharan, M. Oram, K. Willard, L. M. Sinn, D. M. Gerding, and L. R. Peterson.** 1991. *gyrA* mutations in ciprofloxacin-resistant, methicillin-resistant *Staphylococcus aureus* from Indiana, Minnesota, and Tennessee. *J. Infect. Dis.* **164:**976-979.
37. **Felmingham, D., P. Foxall, M. D. O'Hare, G. Webb, G. Ghosh, and R. N. Grüneberg.** 1988. Resistance studies with ofloxacin. *J. Antimicrob. Chemother.* **22**(Suppl. C):27–34.
38. **Felmingham, D., M. J. Robbins, P. Foxall, M. D. O'Hare, G. L. Ridgway, and R. N. Grüneberg.** 1989. In vitro activity, postantibiotic effect, and resistance studies with amifloxacin. *Rev. Infect. Dis.* **11**(Suppl. 5):S952-S954.
39. **Fernandes, P. B., C. W. Hanson, J. M. Stamm, C. Vojtko, N. L. Shipkowitz, and E. St. Martin.** 1987. The frequency of in-vitro resistance development to fluoroquinolones and the use of murine pyelonephritis model to demonstrate selection of resistance in vivo. *J. Antimicrob. Chemother.* **19:**449-465.
40. **Forst, S., D. Comeau, S. Norioka, and M. Inouye.** 1987. Localization and membrane topology of EnvZ, a protein involved in osmoregulation of OmpF and OmpC in *Escherichia coli. J. Biol. Chem.* **262:**16433-16438.
41. **Foulds, J.** 1976. *tolF* locus in *Escherichia coli*: chromosomal location and relationship of loci *cmlB* and *tolD*. *J. Bacteriol.* **128:**604-608.
42. **Fujimaki, K., T. Fujii, H. Aoyama, K.-I. Sato, Y. Inoue, M. Inoue, and S. Mitsuhashi.** 1989. Quinolone resistance in clinical isolates of *Serratia marcescens. Antimicrob. Agents Chemother.* **33:**785–787.
43. **Fukuda, K., M. Hosaka, K. Hirai, and S. Iyobe.** 1990. New norfloxacin resistance gene in *Pseudomonas aeruginosa* PAO. *Antimicrob. Agents Chemother.* **34:**1757-1761.
44. **Furet, Y. X., J. Deshusses, and J.-C. Pechère.** 1992. Transport of pefloxacin across the bacterial cytoplasmic membrane in quinolone-susceptible *Staphylococcus aureus. Antimicrob. Agents Chemother.* **36:**2506-2511.
45. **Gellert, M., K. Mizuuchi, M. H. O'Dea, T. Itoh, and J. Tomizawa.** 1977. Nalidixic acid resistance: a second genetic character involved in DNA gyrase activity. *Proc. Natl. Acad. Sci. USA* **74:**4772-4776.
46. **George, A. M., and S. B. Levy.** 1983. Gene in the major cotransduction gap of the *Escherichia coli* K-12 linkage map required for the expression of chromosomal resistance to tetracycline and other antibiotics. *J. Bacteriol.* **155:**541–548.
47. **Gootz, T. D., and B. A. Martin.** 1991. Characterization of high-level quinolone resistance in *Campylobacter jejuni. Antimicrob. Agents Chemother.* **35:**840–845.
48. **Goswitz, J. J., K. E. Willard, C. E. Fasching, and L. R. Peterson.** 1992. Detection of *gyrA* gene mutations associated with ciprofloxacin resistance in methicillin-resistant *Staphylococcus aureus*: analysis by polymerase chain reaction and automated direct DNA sequencing. *Antimicrob. Agents Chemother.* **36:**1166–1169.
49. **Goto, T., P. Laipis, and J. C. Wang.** 1984. The purification and characterization of DNA topoisomerases I and II of the yeast *Saccharomyces cerevisiae. J. Biol. Chem.* **259:**10422–10429.
50. **Greenberg, J. T., J. H. Chou, P. A. Monach, and B. Demple.** 1991. Activation of oxidative stress genes by mutations at the *soxQ/cfxB/marA* locus of *Escherichia coli. J. Bacteriol.* **173:**4433–4439.
51. **Greenberg, J. T., and B. Demple.** 1989. A global response induced in *Escherichia coli* by redox-cycling agents overlaps with that induced by peroxide stress. *J. Bacteriol.* **171:**3933–3939.
52. **Gutmann, L., D. Billot-Klein, R. Williamson, F. W. Goldstein, J. Mounier, J. F. Acar, and E. Collatz.** 1988. Mutation of *Salmonella paratyphi* A conferring cross-resistance to several groups of antibiotics by decreased permeability and loss of invasiveness. *Antimicrob. Agents Chemother.* **32:**195–201.

53. **Gutmann, L., R. Williamson, N. Moreau, M.-D. Kitzis, E. Collatz, J. F. Acar, and F. W. Goldstein**. 1985. Cross-resistance to nalidixic acid, trimethoprim, and chloramphenicol associated with alterations in outer membrane proteins of Klebsiella, Enterobacter, and Serratia. *J. Infect. Dis.* **151:**501–507.
54. **Hächler, H., S. P. Cohen, and S. B. Levy**. 1991. *marA*, a regulated locus which controls expression of chromosomal multiple antibiotic resistance in *Escherichia coli. J. Bacteriol.* **163:**5532–5538.
55. **Hall, M. N., and T. J. Silhavey**. 1981. The *ompB* locus and the regulation of the major outer membrane porin proteins of *Escherichia coli* K12. *J. Mol. Biol.* **146:**23–43.
56. **Hallett, P., and A. Maxwell**. 1991. Novel quinolone resistance mutations of the *Escherichia coli* DNA gyrase A protein: enzymatic analysis of the mutant proteins. *Antimicrob. Agents Chemother.* **35:**335–340.
57. **Hancock, R. E. W.** 1987. Role of porins in outer membrane permeability. *J. Bacteriol.* **169:**929–933.
58. **Hane, M. W., and T. H. Wood**. 1969. *Escherichia coli* K-12 mutants resistant to nalidixic acid: genetic mapping and dominance studies. *J. Bacteriol.* **99:**238–241.
59. **Hashmi, Z. S., and J. M. B. Smith**. 1991. Outer membrane changes in quinolone resistant *Pseudomonas aeruginosa. J. Antimicrob. Chemother.* **28:**465–469.
60. **Heisig, P., and B. Wiedemann**. 1991. Use of a broad-host-range *gyrA* plasmid for genetic characterization of fluoroquinolone-resistant gram-negative bacteria. *Antimicrob. Agents Chemother.* **35:**2031–2036.
61. **Helling, R. B., and B. S. Adams.** 1970. Nalidixic acid-resistant auxotrophs of *Escherichia coli. J. Bacteriol.* **104:**1027–1029.
62. **Helling, R. B., and J. S. Kukora**. 1971. Nalidixic acid-resistant mutants of *Escherichia coli* deficient in isocitrate dehydrogenase. *J. Bacteriol.* **105:**1224–1226.
63. **Hirai, K.** Personal communication.
64. **Hirai, K., H. Aoyama, T. Irikura, S. Iyobe, and S. Mitsuhashi**. 1986. Differences in susceptibility to quinolones of outer membrane mutants of *Salmonella typhimurium* and *Escherichia coli. Antimicrob. Agents Chemother.* **29:**535–538.
65. **Hirai, K., H. Aoyama, S. Suzue, T. Irikura, S. Iyobe, and S. Mitsuhashi**. 1986. Isolation and characterization of norfloxacin-resistant mutants of *Escherichia coli* K-12. *Antimicrob. Agents Chemother.* **30:**248–253.
66. **Hirai, K., S. Suzue, T. Irikura, S. Iyobe, and S. Mitsuhashi**. 1987. Mutations producing resistance to norfloxacin in *Pseudomonas aeruginosa. Antimicrob. Agents Chemother.* **31:**582–586.
67. **Hooper, D. C.** Unpublished observations.
68. **Hooper, D. C., M. Trucksis, E. Ng, and J. Wolfson**. 1992. Genetic studies of 4-quinolone action in *Escherichia coli* and *Staphylococcus aureus*, abstr. 19. *Program Abstr. 4th Conf. DNA Topoisomerases Ther.*
69. **Hooper, D. C., and J. S. Wolfson.** 1989. Bacterial resistance to the quinolone antimicrobial agents. *Am. J. Med.* **87**(Suppl. 6C)**:**17S-23S.
70. **Hooper, D. C., and J. S. Wolfson**. 1991. The quinolones: mode of action and bacterial resistance, p. 665–690. *In* V. Lorian (ed.), *Antibiotics in Laboratory Medicine*, 3rd ed. The Williams & Wilkins Co., Baltimore.
71. **Hooper, D. C., J. S. Wolfson, M. A. Bozza, and E. Y. Ng**. 1992. Genetics and regulation of outer membrane protein expression by quinolone resistance loci *nfxB*, *nfxC*, and *cfxB*. *Antimicrob. Agents Chemother.* **36:**1151–1154.
72. **Hooper, D. C., J. S. Wolfson, E. Y. Ng, and M. N. Swartz**. 1987. Mechanisms of action of and resistance to ciprofloxacin. *Am. J. Med.* **82**(Suppl. 4A)**:**12–20.
73. **Hooper, D. C., J. S. Wolfson, K. S. Souza, E. Y. Ng, G. L. McHugh, and M. N. Swartz**. 1989. Mechanisms of quinolone resistance in *Escherichia coli*: characterization of *nfxB* and *cfxB*, two mutant resistance loci decreasing norfloxacin accumulation. *Antimicrob. Agents Chemother.* **33:**283–290.
74. **Hooper, D. C., J. S. Wolfson, K. S. Souza, C. Tung, G. L. McHugh, and M. N. Swartz**. 1986. Genetic and biochemical characterization of norfloxacin resistance in *Escherichia coli. Antimicrob. Agents Chemother.* **29:**639–644.
75. **Hrebenda, J., H. Heleszko, K. Brzostek, and J. Bielecki**. 1985. Mutation affecting resistance of *Escherichia coli* K12 to nalidixic acid. *J. Gen. Microbiol.* **131:**2285–2292.
76. **Hussy, P., G. Maass, B. Tümmler, F. Gorsse, and U. Schomburg**. 1986. Effects of 4-quinolones and novobiocin on calf thymus DNA polymerase $\alpha$ primase complex, topoisomerases I and II, and growth of mammalian lymphoblasts. *Antimicrob. Agents Chemother.* **29:**1073–1078.
77. **Inoue, S., T. Ohue, J. Yamagishi, S. Nakamura, and M. Shimizu**. 1978. Mode of incomplete cross-resistance among pipemidic, piromidic, and nalidixic acids. *Antimicrob. Agents Chemother.* **14:**240–245.
78. **Inoue, Y., K. Sato, T. Fujii, K. Hirai, M. Inoue, S. Iyobe, and S. Mitsuhashi**. 1987. Some properties of subunits of DNA gyrase from *Pseudomonas aeruginosa* PAO1 and its nalidixic acid-resistant mutant. *J. Bacteriol.* **169:**2322–2325.
79. **Ishii, H., K. Sato, K. Hoshino, M. Sato, A. Yamaguchi, T. Sawai, and Y. Osada**. 1991. Active efflux of ofloxacin by a highly quinolone-

resistant strain of *Proteus vulgaris*. *J. Antimicrob. Chemother.* **28:**827–836.

80. **Iyobe, S., K. Hirai, and H. Hashimoto**. 1991. Drug resistance of *Pseudomonas aeruginosa* with special reference to new quinolones. *Antibiot. Chemother.* (Basel) **44:**202–214.
81. **Jakics, E. B., S. Iyobe, K. Hirai, H. Fukuda, and H. Hashimoto**. 1992. Occurrence of the *nfxB* type mutation in clinical isolates of *Pseudomonas aeruginosa*. *Antimicrob. Agents Chemother.* **36:**2562–2565.
82. **Kaatz, G. W., S. M. Seo, and C. A. Ruble**. 1991. Mechanisms of fluoroquinolone resistance in *Staphylococcus aureus*. *J. Infect. Dis.* **163:**1080–1086.
83. **Kato, J., Y. Nishimura, and H. Suzuki**. 1989. *Escherichia coli parA* is an allele of the *gyrB* gene. *Mol. Gen. Genet.* **217:**178–181.
84. **Kato, J.-I., Y. Nishimura, R. Imamura, H. Niki, S. Hiraga, and H. Suzuki**. 1990. New topoisomerase essential for chromosome segregation in *E. coli*. *Cell* **63:**393–404.
85. **Kato, J.-I., H. Suzuki, and H. Ikeda**. 1992. Purification and characterization of DNA topoisomerase IV in *Escherichia coli*. *J. Biol. Chem.* **267:**25676–25684.
86. **Kato, N., M. Miyauchi, Y. Muto, K. Watanabe, and K. Ueno**. 1988. Emergence of fluoroquinolone resistance in *Bacteroides fragilis* accompanied by resistance to ß-lactam antibiotics. *Antimicrob. Agents Chemother.* **32:**1437–1438.
87. **Kawaji, H., T. Mizuno, and S. Mizushima**. 1979. Influence of molecular size and osmolarity of sugars and dextrans on the synthesis of outer membrane proteins O-8 and O-9 of *Escherichia coli* K-12. *J. Bacteriol.* **140:**843–847.
88. **Kumada, T., and H. C. Neu**. 1985. *In-vitro* activity of ofloxacin, a quinolone carboxylic acid compared to other quinolones and other antimicrobial agents. *J. Antimicrob. Chemother.* **16:**563–574.
89. **Kumar, S**. 1976. Properties of adenyl cyclase and cyclic adenosine 3′,5′-monophosphate receptor protein-deficient mutants of *Escherichia coli*. *J. Bacteriol.* **125:**545–555.
90. **Kumar, S**. 1980. Types of spontaneous nalidixic acid resistant mutants of *Escherichia coli*. *Indian J. Exp. Biol.* **18:**341–343.
91. **Legakis, N. J., L. S. Tzouvelekis, A. Makris, and H. Kotsifaki**. 1989. Outer membrane alterations in multiresistant mutants of *Pseudomonas aeruginosa* selected with ciprofloxacin. *Antimicrob. Agents Chemother.* **33:**124–127.
92. **Lei, Y., K. Sato, and T. Nakae**. 1991. Ofloxacin-resistant *Pseudomonas aeruginosa* mutants with elevated drug extrusion across the inner membrane. *Biochem. Biophys. Res. Commun.* **178:**1043–1048.
93. **Levy, S. B**. 1992. Active efflux mechanisms for antimicrobial resistance. *Antimicrob. Agents Chemother.* **36:**695–703.
94. **Limb, D. I., D. J. W. Dabbs, and R. C. Spencer**. 1987. In-vitro selection of bacteria resistant to the 4-quinolone agents. *J. Antimicrob. Chemother.* **19:**65–71.
95. **Lomovskaya, O., and K. Lewis**. 1992. *emr*, an *Escherichia coli* locus for multidrug resistance. *Proc. Natl. Acad. Sci. USA* **89:**8938–8942.
96. **Lucain, C., P. Regamey, F. Bellido, and J.-C. Pechère**. 1989. Resistance emerging after pefloxacin therapy of experimental *Enterobacter cloacae* peritonitis. *Antimicrob. Agents Chemother.* **33:**937–943.
97. **Lugtenberg, B., R. Peters, H. Bernheimer, and W. Berendsen**. 1976. Influence of cultural conditions and mutations on the composition of the outer membrane proteins of *Escherichia coli*. *Mol. Gen. Genet.* **147:**251–262.
98. **Margerrison, E. E. C., R. Hopewell, and L. M. Fisher**. 1992. Nucleotide sequence of the *Staphylococcus aureus gyrB-gyrA* locus encoding the DNA gyrase A and B proteins. *J. Bacteriol.* **174:**1596–1603.
99. **Masecar, B. L., R. A. Celesk, and N. J. Robillard**. 1990. Analysis of acquired ciprofloxacin resistance in a clinical strain of *Pseudomonas aeruginosa*. *Antimicrob. Agents Chemother.* **34:**281–286.
100. **Masecar, B. L., and N. J. Robillard**. 1991. Spontaneous quinolone resistance in *Serratia marcescens* due to a mutation in *gyrA*. *Antimicrob. Agents Chemother.* **35:**898–902.
101. **Masuda, N., and S. Ohya**. 1992. Cross-resistance to meropenem, cephems, and quinolones in *Pseudomonas aeruginosa*. *Antimicrob. Agents Chemother.* **36:**1847–1851.
102. **Michea-Hamzehpour, M., C. Lucain, and J.-C. Pechère**. 1991. Resistance to pefloxacin in *Pseudomonas aeruginosa*. *Antimicrob. Agents Chemother.* **35:**512–518.
103. **Miller, K. G., L. F. Liu, and P. T. Englund**. 1981. A homogeneous type II DNA topoisomerase from HeLa cell nuclei. *J. Biol. Chem.* **256:**9334–9339.
104. **Mizuno, T., M.-Y. Chou, and M. Inouye**. 1984. A unique mechanism regulating gene expression: translational inhibition by a complementary RNA transcript (micRNA). *Proc. Natl. Acad. Sci. USA* **81:**1966–1970.
105. **Moniot-Ville, N., J. Guibert, N. Moreau, J. F. Acar, E. Collatz, and L. Gutmann**. 1991. Mechanisms of quinolone resistance in a clinical isolate of *Escherichia coli* highly resistant to fluoroquinolones but susceptible to nalidixic acid. *Antimicrob. Agents Chemother.* **35:**519–523.
106. **Mouton, R. P., and S. T. A. Mulders**. 1987. Combined resistance to quinolones and beta-lac-

tams after in vitro transfer on single drugs. *Chemotherapy* (Basel) **33:**189-196.

107. **Munshi, M. H., K. Haider, M. M. Rahaman, D. A. Sack, Z. U. Ahmed, and M. G. Morshed.** 1987. Plasmid-mediated resistance to nalidixic acid in *Shigella dysenteriae* type 1. *Lancet* **ii:**419-421.
108. **Nakamura, S., M. Nakamura, T. Kojima, and H. Yoshida.** 1989. *gyrA* and *gyrB* mutations in quinolone-resistant strains of *Escherichia coli. Antimicrob. Agents Chemother.* **33:**254-255.
109. **Nakanishi, N., S. Yoshida, H. Wakebe, M. Inoue, and S. Mitsuhashi.** 1991. Mechanisms of clinical resistance to fluoroquinolones in *Enterococcus faecalis. Antimicrob. Agents Chemother.* **35:**1053-1059.
110. **Nakanishi, N., S. Yoshida, H. Wakebe, M. Inoue, T. Yamaguchi, and S. Mitsuhashi.** 1991. Mechanisms of clinical resistance to fluoroquinolones in *Staphylococcus aureus. Antimicrob. Agents Chemother.* **35:**2562-2567.
111. **Neyfakh, A. A.** 1992. The multidrug efflux transporter of *Bacillus subtilis* is a structural and functional homolog of the *Staphylococcus* NorA protein. *Antimicrob. Agents Chemother.* **36:**484-485.
112. **Neyfakh, A. A., V. E. Bidnenko, and L. B. Chen.** 1991. Efflux-mediated multidrug-resistance in *Bacillus subtilis*: similarities and dissimilarities with the mammalian system. *Proc. Natl. Acad. Sci. USA* **88:**4781-4785.
113. **Neyfakh, A. A., C. M. Borsch, and G. W. Kaatz.** 1993. Fluoroquinolone resistance protein NorA of *Staphylococcus aureus* is a multidrug efflux transporter. *Antimicrob. Agents Chemother.* **37:**128-129.
114. **Ng, E. Y., G. L. McHugh, J. S. Wolfson, and D. C. Hooper.** 1992. Other genetic loci involved in quinolone resistance in *Escherichia coli*, abstr. 1546. *Program Abstr. 32nd Intersci. Conf. Antimicrob. Agents Chemother.*
115. **Nikaido, H.** 1985. Role of permeability barriers in resistance to ß-lactam antibiotics. *Pharmacol. Ther.* **27:**197-231.
116. **Nikaido, H., and T. Nakae.** 1979. The outer membrane of gram-negative bacteria. *Adv. Microb. Physiol.* **20:**163-250.
117. **Nikaido, H., and M. H. Saier, Jr.** 1992. Transport proteins in bacteria: common themes in their design. *Science* **258:**936-942.
118. **Nikaido, H., and M. Vaara.** 1985. Molecular basis of bacterial outer membrane permeability. *Microbiol. Rev.* **49:**1-32.
119. **Nooter, K., and H. Herweijer.** 1991. Multidrug resistance (*mdr*) genes in human cancer. *Br. J. Cancer* **63:**663-669.
120. **Okazaki, T., S. Iyobe, H. Hashimoto, and K. Hirai.** 1991. Cloning and characterization of a DNA fragment that complements the *nfxB* mutation in *Pseudomonas aeruginosa* PAO. *FEMS Microbiol. Lett.* **79:**31-36.
121. **Okuda, J., S. Okamoto, M. Takahata, and T. Nishino.** 1991. Inhibitory effects of ciprofloxacin and sparfloxacin on DNA gyrase purified from fluoroquinolone-resistant strains of methicillin-resistant *Staphylococcus aureus. Antimicrob. Agents Chemother.* **35:**2288-2293.
122. **Oram, M., and L. M. Fisher.** 1991. 4-Quinolone resistance mutations in the DNA gyrase of *Escherichia coli* clinical isolates identified by using the polymerase chain reaction. *Antimicrob. Agents Chemother.* **35:**387-389.
123. **Osborn, M. J., and H.C.P. Wu.** 1980. Proteins of the outer membrane of gram-negative bacteria. *Annu. Rev. Microbiol.* **34:**369-422.
124. **Osheroff, N., E. R. Shelton, and D. L. Brutlag.** 1983. DNA topoisomerase II from *Drosophila melanogaster*. Relaxation of supercoiled DNA. *J. Biol. Chem.* **258:**9536-9543.
125. **Panhotra, B. R., B. Desai, and P. L. Sharma.** 1985. Nalidixic-acid-resistant *Shigella dysenteriae* I. *Lancet* **i:**763.
126. **Piddock, L. J. V., M. Hall, D. J. Griggs, and R. Wise.** 1989 Selection and phenotypic characterization of the mechanism of resistance of enterobacteriaceae to quinolones. *Rev. Infect. Dis.* **11**(Suppl. 5)**:**S977-S978.
127. **Piddock, L. J. V., M. C. Hall, F. Bellido, M. Bains, and R. E. W. Hancock.** 1992. A pleiotropic, posttherapy, enoxacin-resistant mutant of *Pseudomonas aeruginosa. Antimicrob. Agents Chemother.* **36:**1057-1061.
128. **Piddock, L. J. V., M. C. Hall, and R. N. Walters.** 1991. Phenotypic characterization of quinolone-resistant mutants of Enterobacteriaceae selected from wild type, *gyrA* type and multiply-resistant (*marA*) type strains. *J. Antimicrob. Chemother.* **28:**185-198.
129. **Piddock, L. J. V., W. J. A. Wijnands, and R. Wise.** 1987. Quinolone/ureidopenicillin cross-resistance. *Lancet* **ii:**907.
130. **Piddock, L. J. V., and R. Wise.** 1988. The selection and frequency of streptococci with decreased susceptibility to ofloxacin compared to other quinolones. *J. Antimicrob. Chemother.* **22**(Suppl. C)**:**45-51.
131. **Power, E. G. M., J. L. Muñoz Bellido, and I. Phillips.** 1992. Detection of ciprofloxacin resistance in gram-negative bacteria due to alterations in *gyrA. J. Antimicrob. Chemother.* **29:**9-17.
132. **Rådberg, G., L. E. Nilsson, and S. Svensson.** 1990. Development of quinolone-imipenem cross-resistance in *Pseudomonas aeruginosa* during exposure to ciprofloxacin. *Antimicrob. Agents Chemother.* **34:**2142-2147.
133. **Ravizzola, G., F. Pirali, A. Paolucci, L. Terlenghi, L. Peroni, A. Colombi, and A. Turano.**

1987. Reduced virulence in ciprofloxacin-resistant variants of *Pseudomonas aeruginosa* strains. *J. Antimicrob. Chemother.* **20:**825-829.

134. **Rella, M., and D. Haas**. 1982. Resistance of *Pseudomonas aeruginosa* PAO to nalidixic acid and low levels of ß-lactam antibiotics: mapping of chromosomal genes. *Antimicrob. Agents Chemother.* **22:**242-249.
135. **Robillard, N. J.** 1990. Broad-host-range gyrase A gene probe. *Antimicrob. Agents Chemother.* **34:**1889-1894.
136. **Robillard, N. J., and A. L. Scarpa**. 1988. Genetic and physiological characterization of ciprofloxacin resistance in *Pseudomonas aeruginosa* PAO. *Antimicrob. Agents Chemother.* **32:**535-539.
137. **Rosner, J. L., T.-J. Chai, and J. Foulds**. 1991. Regulation of OmpF porin expression by salicylate in *Escherichia coli. J. Bacteriol.* **173:**5631-5638.
138. **Ross, D. L., and C. M. Riley.** 1990. Aqueous solubilities of some variously substituted quinolone antimicrobials. *Int. J. Pharm.* **63:**237-250.
139. **Rouch, D. A., D. S. Cram, D. DiBerardino, T. G. Littlejohn, and R. A. Skurray.** 1990. Efflux-mediated antiseptic resistance gene *qacA* from *Staphylococcus aureus*: common ancestry with tetracycline- and sugar-transport proteins. *Mol. Microbiol.* **4:**2051-2062.
140. **Sanders, C. C., W. E. Sanders, R. V. Goering, and V. Werner**. 1984. Selection of multiple antibiotic resistance by quinolones, ß-lactams, and aminoglycosides with special reference to cross-resistance between unrelated drug classes. *Antimicrob. Agents Chemother.* **26:**797-801.
141. **Sanders, C. C., and C. Watanakunakorn**. 1986. Emergence of resistance to ß-lactams, aminoglycosides, and quinolones during combination therapy for infection due to *Serratia marcescens. J. Infect. Dis.* **153:**617-619.
142. **Sato, K., K. Hoshino, T. Une, and Y. Osada**. 1989. Inhibitory effects of ofloxacin on DNA gyrase of *Escherichia coli* and topoisomerase II of bovine calf thymus. *Rev. Infect. Dis.* **11**(Suppl. 5):S915-S916.
143. **Sato, K., Y. Inoue, T. Fujii, H. Aoyama, M. Inoue, and S. Mitsuhashi**. 1986. Purification and properties of DNA gyrase from a fluoroquinolone-resistant strain of *Escherichia coli. Antimicrob. Agents Chemother.* **30:**777-780.
144. **Sawai, T., A. Yamaguchi, A. Saiki, and K. Hoshino**. 1992. OmpF channel permeability of quinolones and their comparison with ß-lactams. *FEMS Microbiol. Lett.* **95:**105-108.
145. **Schnaitman, C. A., and G. A. McDonald**. 1984. Regulation of outer membrane protein synthesis in *Escherichia coli* K-12: deletion of *ompC* affects expression of the OmpF protein. *J. Bacteriol.* **159:**555-563.
146. **Scribner, R. K., D. F. Welch, and M. I. Marks**. 1985. Low frequency of bacterial resistance to enoxacin *in vitro* and in experimental pneumonia. *J. Antimicrob. Chemother.* **16:**597-603.
147. **Segreti, J., T. D. Gootz, L. J. Goodman, G. W. Parkhurst, J. P. Quinn, B. A. Martin, and G. M. Trenholme**. 1992. High-level quinolone resistance in clinical isolates of *Campylobacter jejuni. J. Infect. Dis.* **165:**667-670.
148. **Setlow, J. K., E. Cabrera-Juárez, W. L. Albritton, D. Spikes, and A. Muschler**. 1985. Mutations affecting gyrase in *Haemophilus influenzae. J. Bacteriol.* **164:**525-534.
149. **Shen, L. L., J. Baranowski, J. Fostel, D. A. Montgomery, and P. A. Lartey**. 1992. DNA topoisomerases from pathogenic fungi: targets for the discovery of antifungal drugs. *Antimicrob. Agents Chemother.* **36:**2778-2784.
150. **Shen, L. L., W. E. Kohlbrenner, D. Weigl, and J. Baranowski.** 1989. Mechanism of quinolone inhibition of DNA gyrase. Appearance of unique norfloxacin binding sites in enzyme-DNA complexes. *J. Biol. Chem.* **264:**2973-2978.
151. **Shen, L. L., L. A. Mitscher, P. N. Sharma, T. J. O'Donnell, D. W. T. Chu, C. S. Cooper, T. Rosen, and A. G. Pernet**. 1989. Mechanism of inhibition of DNA gyrase by quinolone antibacterials: a cooperative drug-DNA binding model. *Biochemistry* **28:**3886-3894.
152. **Sheridan, R. P., and I. Chopra**. 1991. Origin of tetracycline efflux proteins: conclusions from nucleotide sequence analysis. *Mol. Microbiol.* **5:**895-900.
153. **Smith, J. T.** 1984. Mutational resistance to 4-quinolone antibacterial agents. *Eur. J. Clin. Microbiol.* **3:**347-350.
154. **Smith, J. T.** 1986. Frequency and expression of mutational resistance to the 4-quinolone antibacterials. *Scand. J. Infect. Dis.* **49:**115-123.
155. **Sreedharan, S., M. Oram, B. Jensen, L. R. Peterson, and L. M. Fisher**. 1990. DNA gyrase *gyrA* mutations in ciprofloxacin-resistant strains of *Staphylococcus aureus*: close similarity with quinolone resistance mutations in *Escherichia coli. J. Bacteriol.* **172:**7260-7262.
156. **Sreedharan, S., L. R. Peterson, and L. M. Fisher.** 1991. Ciprofloxacin resistance in coagulase-positive and -negative staphylococci: role of mutations at serine 84 in the DNA gyrase A protein of *Staphylococcus aureus* and *Staphylococcus epidermidis. Antimicrob. Agents Chemother.* **35:**2151-2154.
157. **Stein, D. C., R. J. Danaher, and T. M. Cook.** 1991. Characterization of a *gyrB* mutation responsible for low-level nalidixic acid resistance in *Neisseria gonorrhoeae. Antimicrob. Agents Chemother.* **35:**622-626.
158. **Sugino, A., N. P. Higgins, P. O. Brown, C. L. Peebles, and N. R. Cozzarelli.** 1978. Energy

coupling in DNA gyrase and the mechanism of action of novobiocin. *Proc. Natl. Acad. Sci. USA* **75:**4838-4842.

159. **Sugino, A., C. L. Peebles, K. N. Kruezer, and N. R. Cozzarelli.** 1977. Mechanism of action of nalidixic acid: purification of *Escherichia coli nalA* gene product and its relationship to DNA gyrase and a novel nicking-closing enzyme. *Proc. Natl. Acad. Sci. USA* **74:**4767-4771.
160. **Tanaka, M., H. Ishii, K. Sato, Y. Osada, and T. Nishino.** 1991. Characterization of high-level quinolone resistance in methicillin-resistant *Staphylococcus aureus*, abstr. 308. *Program Abstr. 31st Intersci. Conf. Antimicrob. Agents Chemother.*
161. **Tenney, J. H., R. W. Maack, and G. R. Chippendale.** 1983. Rapid selection of organisms with increasing resistance on subinhibitory concentrations of norfloxacin on agar. *Antimicrob. Agents Chemother.* **23:**188-189.
162. **Timmers, K., and R. Sternglanz.** 1978. Ionization and divalent cation dissociation constants of nalidixic and oxolinic acids. *Bioinorg. Chem.* **9:**145-155.
163. **Traub, W. H.** 1985. Incomplete cross-resistance of nalidixic and pipemidic acid-resistant variants of *Serratia marcescens* against ciprofloxacin, enoxacin, and norfloxacin. *Chemotherapy* (Basel) **31:**34-39.
164. **Traub, W. H., and I. Kleber.** 1977. Selected and spontaneous variants of *Serratia marcescens* with combined resistance against chloramphenicol, nalidixic acid, and trimethoprim. *Chemotherapy* (Basel) **23:**436-451.
165. **Trucksis, M., D. C. Hooper, and J. S. Wolfson.** 1991. Emerging resistance to fluoroquinolones in staphylococci: an alert. *Ann. Intern. Med.* **114:**424-426.
166. **Trucksis, M., E. Ng, M. Bozza, and D. Hooper.** 1992. Quinolone resistance mutation in *Staphylococcus aureus* linked to *norA* and conditions affecting *norA*-mediated quinolone efflux in *Escherichia coli*, abstr. A-98, p. 17. *Abstr. 92nd Gen. Meet. Am. Soc. Microbiol. 1992.*
167. **Trucksis, M., J. S. Wolfson, and D. C. Hooper.** 1991. A novel locus conferring fluoroquinolone resistance in *Staphylococcus aureus*. *J. Bacteriol.* **173:**5854-5860.
168. **Uemura, T., K. Morikawa, and M. Yanagida.** 1986. The nucleotide sequence of the fission yeast DNA topoisomerase II gene: structural and functional relationships to other DNA topoisomerases. *EMBO J.* **5:**2355-2361.
169. **Vangdal, M., and T. Bergan.** 1984. *In vitro* synergistic activity of nalidixic acid and amphotericin B against fungi. *Drugs Exp. Clin. Res.* **X:**443-444.
170. **Walton, J. R., and D. H. Smith.** 1969. New hemolysin ($\tau$) produced by *Escherichia coli. J. Bacteriol.* **98:**304-305.
171. **Watanabe, M., Y. Kotera, K. Yosue, M. Inoue, and S. Mitsuhashi.** 1990. In vitro emergence of quinolone-resistant mutants of *Escherichia coli, Enterobacter cloacae,* and *Serratia marcescens. Antimicrob. Agents Chemother.* **34:**173-175.
172. **Willmott, C. J. R., and A. Maxwell.** 1993. A single point mutation in the DNA gyrase A protein greatly reduces binding of fluoroquinolones to the gyrase-DNA complex. *Antimicrob. Agents Chemother.* **37:**126-127.
173. **Wolfson, J. S., and D. C. Hooper.** 1989. Fluoroquinolone antimicrobial agents. *Clin. Microbiol. Rev.* **2:**378-424.
174. **Wolfson, J. S., and D. C. Hooper.** 1989. Bacterial resistance to quinolones: mechanisms and clinical importance. *Rev. Infect. Dis.* **11**(Suppl. 5):S960-S968.
175. **Wolfson, J. S., D. C. Hooper, E. Y. Ng, K. S. Souza, G. L. McHugh, and M. N. Swartz.** 1987. Antagonism of wild-type and resistant *Escherichia coli* and its DNA gyrase by the tricyclic 4-quinolone analogs ofloxacin and S-25930 stereoisomers. *Antimicrob. Agents Chemother.* **31:**1861-1863.
176. **Yamagishi, J., Y. Furutami, S. Inoue, T. Ohue, S. Nakamura, and M. Shimizu.** 1981. New nalidixic acid resistance mutations related to deoxyribonucleic acid gyrase activity. *J. Bacteriol.* **148:**450-458.
177. **Yamagishi, J., H. Yoshida, M. Yamayoshi, and S. Nakamura.** 1986. Nalidixic acid-resistant mutations of the *gyrB* gene of *Escherichia coli. Mol. Gen. Genet.* **204:**367-373.
178. **Yoshida, H., M. Bogaki, M. Nakamura, and S. Nakamura.** 1990. Quinolone resistance-determining region in the DNA gyrase *gyrA* gene of *Escherichia coli. Antimicrob. Agents Chemother.* **34:**1271-1272.
179. **Yoshida, H., M. Bogaki, M. Nakamura, L. M. Yamanaka, and S. Nakamura.** 1991. Quinolone resistance-determining region of the DNA gyrase *gyrB* gene of *Escherichia coli. Antimicrob. Agents Chemother.* **35:**1647-1650.
180. **Yoshida, H., M. Bogaki, S. Nakamura, K. Ubukata, and M. Konno.** 1990. Nucleotide sequence and characterization of the *Staphylococcus aureus norA* gene, which confers resistance to quinolones. *J. Bacteriol.* **172:**6942-6949.
181. **Yoshida, H., T. Kojima, J. Yamagishi, and S. Nakamura.** 1988. Quinolone-resistant mutations of the *gyrA* gene of *Escherichia coli. Mol. Gen. Genet.* **211:**1-7.
182. **Yoshida, H., M. Nakamura, M. Bogaki, and S. Nakamura.** 1990. Proportion of DNA gyrase mutants among quinolone-resistant strains of *Pseu-*

*domonas aeruginosa. Antimicrob. Agents Chemother.* **34:**1273–1275.

183. **Young, M., and R. E. W. Hancock.** 1992. Fluoroquinolone supersusceptibility mediated by outer membrane protein OprH overexpression in *Pseudomonas aeruginosa*: evidence for involvement of a nonporin pathway. *Antimicrob. Agents Chemother.* **36:**2365–2369.

*Quinolone Antimicrobial Agents, 2nd ed.*
Edited by David C. Hooper and John S. Wolfson


*Chapter 6*

# Quinolone Resistance in Clinical Practice: Occurrence and Importance

*Lance R. Peterson*

The new fluoroquinolone agents are important additions to the medical treatment of infectious diseases in many diverse settings. Their use has been well summarized in recent reviews (60, 141). These new agents have a potent, broad-spectrum in vitro activity that makes them potentially useful as therapeutic agents for a wide variety of serious infections (5, 44, 46). How these valuable antimicrobial agents are administered in clinical practice may well determine whether they will be useful for many years or whether the rapid development of bacterial resistance will shorten their therapeutic lifetimes (134).

By mid-1992, five fluoroquinolone agents were available for clinical use in the United States and one had been voluntarily withdrawn. Norfloxacin, the first of the available new agents, is approved for use in the therapy of complicated and uncomplicated urinary tract infections (138). Ciprofloxacin (approved for use in December 1987), ofloxacin (approved in 1990), and lomefloxacin (approved in 1992) extend the clinical applicability of these new agents to additional sites and kinds of infection, including infectious diarrhea, infections involving the lower respiratory tract, infections of skin and skin structures, infections of bones and joints, prostatitis, and some sexually transmitted diseases (129, 130). Temafloxacin was withdrawn from use because of adverse effects.

The purpose of this chapter is to (i) review the clinical settings in which bacterial resistance to fluoroquinolones has been a problem, (ii) discuss the possible reasons for this development of resistance, and (iii) propose approaches that can be used to minimize the future development of bacterial resistance to this important class of antimicrobial agents.

## HISTORICAL ASPECTS OF QUINOLONE RESISTANCE

Evaluation of the ongoing clinical utility of quinolone antimicrobial agents has primarily taken two approaches. One common approach has been to describe the development of resistant isolates during a period of high-volume use of quinolone antibacterial agents (92, 105). These reports have demonstrated the potential for development of resistance in many diverse isolates, each of which will be discussed in later sections. The other general approach has been to compare, over time, the in vitro activities of these agents against large numbers of bacterial pathogens with those of other compounds (38, 60, 75). In this setting, the tested fluoroquinolones usually continue to show excellent activity, although the report

*Lance R. Peterson* • Clinical Microbiology, Northwestern Memorial Hospital, and Departments of Pathology and Medicine, Northwestern University Medical School, Chicago, Illinois 60611.

by Dornbusch et al. demonstrated increased resistance of *Pseudomonas aeruginosa* to several agents, including ciprofloxacin (38). This apparent dichotomy can be explained if we consider that the reports of development of resistance in individual practice settings are valid demonstrations that significant resistance to these new agents can occur and that while most microorganisms still exhibit susceptibility to the fluoroquinolone agents (conclusions demonstrated by large in vitro studies), the potential for widespread resistance at some time in the future does exist if these antimicrobial agents are misused.

Useful lessons may be learned from experience with the first available quinolone antibiotic, nalidixic acid, which was introduced into general clinical use in the United States in 1964. Initial reports found this new agent to be well tolerated and very effective in the treatment of urinary tract infections (17). In 1966, Ronald et al. reported on a series of 50 patients with chronic urinary tract infections treated with nalidixic acid. Thirty-two of 54 strains from these patients were eradicated during treatment. However, 13 strains from 13 individuals developed resistance during therapy with nalidixic acid (115). Resistance appeared within 48 h in these patients and apparently led to clinical failure in all of them (115). This article led to a general skepticism about the utility of quinolone antimicrobial agents. It is noteworthy that subsequent reports did not confirm such a high rate of resistance development and have raised speculation that the high level of resistance development seen by Ronald et al. was due to underdosing (at least one type of inappropriate use) of the drug (18, 126). Other instances of the development of a high percentage of nalidixic acid-resistant isolates also appeared to occur during the treatment of patients with complicated urinary tract infections (111). It is this background of experience with nalidixic acid and the more recent development of fluoroquinolone resistance in certain bacteria (most notably *P. aeruginosa* and staphylococci) that makes it important to develop strategies for the clinical use of fluoroquinolone antimicrobial agents (60, 131).

## TREATMENT ISSUES IN BACTERIAL RESISTANCE

Three major issues involving bacterial resistance arise when any class of antimicrobial agents is used in clinical practice. These issues are (i) the spectrum of activity (or lack of initial resistance in vitro) of the compound in question, (ii) the development of superinfections during therapy with any extended-spectrum antibiotic, and (iii) the development of new resistance to the antibiotic class and subsequent spread of this resistance with the widespread use of the new agent(s). The antimicrobial spectrum of fluoroquinolone agents has been excellent, which makes the initial enthusiasm for and widespread use of these drugs understandable. Similarly, there have been no excess problems of superinfections associated with use of these compounds compared with other extended-spectrum agents (141). Superinfections have usually occurred at a low incidence ($\leq 5\%$) for ciprofloxacin and, as expected, have involved microorganisms with marginal to no intrinsic susceptibility to ciprofloxacin (139).

Emergence of resistant bacteria during the early treatment trials of the new fluoroquinolone agents was also low (58, 141). Fewer than 2% of patients treated for uncomplicated urinary tract infections developed resistant isolates during therapy (2, 116, 141). Single-step (a common measure of in vitro resistance) resistance in *Escherichia coli* rarely develops ($\leq 10^{-10}$) when the quinolone concentration is at least eightfold greater than the MIC for the test organism. This condition is usually fulfilled in the urine during the clinical treatment of urinary tract infection (30, 43, 58).

Other bacterial species have also been studied, and most exhibit this (low) level of resistance development at frequencies of $\leq 10^{-9}$ (31, 81, 124, 137). While these numbers (in vitro mutational frequencies) are somewhat difficult to interpret clinically, they approximate the frequency with which resistance develops in vitro when aminoglycosides are tested in similar experiments, implying that clinical resistance development directed toward the new fluoroquinolones may approximate that seen with the use of aminoglycosides. An interesting review by Milatovic and Braveny surmised that the likelihood of resistance developing (during therapy) was 9.2% for broad-spectrum penicillins, 8.6% for third-generation cephalosporins, 11.8% for ciprofloxacin, and 13.4% for aminoglycosides (88). The older quinolone, nalidixic acid, had in vitro resistance frequencies 2 or 3 orders of magnitude higher than those of the new fluoroquinolones and developed higher levels of resistance (up to 64-fold increases in MIC) when the same laboratory measures were used to test for resistance development. With the newer compounds, the expression of bacterial resistance was, as noted above, generally considered an infrequent event, occurring with a mutational frequency of $10^{-7}$ to $10^{-11}$ CFU. This implies that a bacterial infection would need to involve at least $10^7$ to $10^{11}$ bacterial cells for there to be a chance that 1 resistant bacterium would develop. Even at this low rate of resistance development, the level of resistance (the new MIC required for activity against the resistant microbe) is such that the concentration of quinolone antimicrobial agent present at sites such as urine would still exceed the MIC for most of the resistant (mutant) bacteria, thus allowing a successful clinical outcome (81, 124, 137). Therefore, the expectation has been that less resistance would be seen with the newer agents. However, later experiments found that serial passage of bacteria on agar (or in broth) containing concentrations of a fluoroquinolone slightly above the MIC of the drug for the organism can produce strains that are highly resistant to the new compound (61, 63, 123). Such a selection process likely results in several mutational changes that lead to the development of stable, high-level resistance. These events presumably can occur in vivo during treatment of various infections.

The fluoroquinolone antimicrobial agents are rapidly bactericidal. They effect cell death through an interaction with DNA gyrase (59). Recognized mechanisms by which bacteria develop resistance to fluoroquinolones generally fall into three categories: a mutational change(s) in the bacterial DNA gyrase; selected changes in outer membrane proteins of the bacterial cell; and development of a highly active, energy-dependent efflux system capable of excluding a significant quantity of the drug from the bacterial cell. This last mechanism is generally felt to occur in association with changes in outer membrane protein(s) of gram-negative bacteria, although this may not necessarily be true for staphylococci, which lack an outer membrane (19, 62, 96). All three mechanisms have recently been reviewed (15, 70, 72, 96, 140). Chapter 5 contains an in-depth discussion of these resistance mechanisms.

The use of antimicrobial agents is often associated with an anticipation that some resistance directed toward the agent(s) being used will develop in microorganisms. Møller reported an evaluation of this concept over a 7-year period (89). He found that such an assumption was not true for *Staphylococcus aureus* or *E. coli* but that a correlation between antibiotic use and the emergence of resistance could be shown for *Staphylococcus epidermidis*. Therefore, it appears that the clinical use of any new compound(s) should be accompanied by careful monitoring for the development of resistance in important pathogenic microbes as a measure of the development of bacterial resistance that may be clinically significant. During the early period of ciprofloxacin use, occasional resistance in pathogenic bacteria was observed (22, 29, 65). Of note is the recent report by Muder et al., who associated the use of ciprofloxacin with the development of quinolone resistance in several gram-negative isolates, particularly *Serratia marcescens* and *Proteus mirabilis* (92). Should more reports of this latter type appear, there will be an increasingly urgent need to develop strategies for the appropriate clinical use of these new compounds, lest we lose the utility of the entire quinolone class of antimicrobial agents.

Many reports of bacterial resistance to the new fluoroquinolones have appeared, and these will be reviewed below. They can be divided into reports describing specific sites of infections that are more prone to permit the emergence of resistant bacteria when these infections are treated and reports describing certain bacterial species that are more likely to develop resistance when exposed to quinolone agents. Table 1 contains a description of the clinical situations in which the development of microbial resistance is more common, and Table 2 lists the various pathogens that have been reported as developing resistance to quinolones during clinical therapy. As can be seen, patients with severe underlying disease (cystic fibrosis, malignancy, etc.), those with structural alterations (foreign-body infections, complicated urinary tract infections, and burn and surgical wound infections), those with difficult-to-heal lesions (infected decubitus ulcers or diabetic foot ulcerations), and those colonized with problem pathogens (methicillin-resistant *S. aureus* [MRSA]) all share certain characteristics. The clinical situations occur in patients with diminished host defenses due to malignancy, foreign bodies, debility, impaired circulation, or other local immune dysfunction. Also, while many organisms are capable of developing resistance to the quinolone compounds, the resistant bacterial pathogens reported with greatest frequency are the staphylococci, streptococci, and pseudomonads (3, 78, 139, 141).

**Table 1.** Clinical settings for resistance[a]

| Clinical setting | % of infections where resistance may develop during treatment |
|---|---|
| Cystic fibrosis | 10–15 |
| Colonization states | 27 |
| Malignancy prophylaxis | ±15 |
| Foreign bodies | NE[b] |
| Complicated urinary tract infection | 10 |
| Bone and joint infections | 15 |
| Foot infections in diabetics | NE |
| Skin and soft tissue infections | 13 |
| Burn infections | NE |

[a]Data were compiled from reference 141.
[b]NE, percentage not estimated.

## IN VIVO DEVELOPMENT OF RESISTANCE WITH QUINOLONE THERAPY IN ANIMAL MODELS OF INFECTION

Animal models have played an important role in the evaluation of potential in vivo efficacy during the development of quinolone antimicrobial agents (104). Such models have also been used to demonstrate that resistance to the quinolones can develop during treatment of infections caused by both gram-negative and gram-positive bacteria (4, 20, 42, 71). Similarly, they have been used to evaluate the mechanisms by which resistance to the fluoroquinolones develop and to demonstrate that exposure to quinolone antimicrobial agents can result in either increased resistance or increased susceptibility to other classes of antimicrobial agents (20, 91). While these animal studies have contributed to our understanding in the use of quinolones, the extensive clinical trials and human experience with the quinolones provide more-valuable insights into the problems (resistance development) we can expect with these agents and with potential strategies to avoid widespread resistance development.

## CLINICAL INFECTIONS ASSOCIATED WITH RESISTANCE DEVELOPMENT

### Reports Based on Site of Infection

#### Lower respiratory tract infections

Several publications have dealt with the development of bacterial resistance during the therapy of lower respiratory tract infections with fluoroquinolones (6, 10, 11, 21,

**Table 2.** Selected bacteria reported as developing resistance during therapy with fluoroquinolone antimicrobial agents

| Frequently develop resistance | Occasionally to rarely develop resistance |
|---|---|
| *Staphylococcus aureus* | *Escherichia coli* |
| MRSA | *Haemophilus parainfluenzae* |
| *Pseudomonas aeruginosa* | *Serratia marcescens* |
| *Streptococcus pneumoniae* | *Enterobacter aerogenes* |
| *Xanthomonas maltophilia* | *Citrobacter freundii* |
| Enterococci | *Shigella dysenteriae* |
| *Staphylococcus epidermidis* | *Corynebacterium* spp. |
| *Helicobacter pylori* | *Moraxella catarrhalis* |
| *Campylobacter jejuni* | *Acinetobacter* spp. |

37, 51, 57, 68, 77, 78, 103, 118, 119, 122). The focus of the reports has been the development of resistance by *P. aeruginosa* in patients with cystic fibrosis who were treated for prolonged periods (6, 10, 11, 21, 37, 51, 57, 68, 77, 78, 103, 118, 119, 122) and in patients undergoing treatment with one of these agents who experienced the emergence of resistant *Streptococcus pneumoniae* as a significant pathogen (34, 78, 83, 103). These reports highlight the problems encountered in treating patients with an uncorrectable underlying disease (cystic fibrosis), particularly one that impairs host immune response, as well as the potential difficulty in treating infections whose pathogens are only modestly susceptible to the antimicrobial agent being used (*S. pneumoniae*).

Several observations should be noted, however. Despite the development of quinolone resistance in *P. aeruginosa*, clinical success was quite good in these studies, and the appearance of resistant isolates was not always associated with clinical failure (57). Resistance that develops in this setting tends to be unstable and to disappear after therapy is stopped (21). Scully et al. found that four of six isolates that had developed resistance to ciprofloxacin during therapy reverted to a susceptible state during posttreatment follow-up (118). Furthermore, in a comparative study reported by Hodson et al., the frequency of isolates developing resistance to ciprofloxacin was no greater than that of isolates developing resistance to the conventional intravenous agents used in the investigation (57).

The reported resistance and superinfections observed with infections due to *S. pneumoniae* have appeared as isolated cases outside of formal clinical trials so that no data on the true prevalence of problems associated with the use of quinolones for infections involving this pathogen are available. Other than these two problem areas, the development of quinolone resistance during treatment of lower respiratory tract infections has been infrequent. Wolfson and Hooper summarized nine reported studies and found that 17 (6%) of 302 patients harbored diverse pathogens that developed resistance to ciprofloxacin (141).

## Gastrointestinal infections

The emergence of resistance to fluoroquinolones in bacterial enteropathogens had been somewhat unanticipated because of the high concentrations these agents achieved in the gastrointestinal tract coupled with the excellent in vitro activity of fluoroquinolones against the likely enteropathogens (14, 27, 39, 67, 94, 97, 102, 141). However, resistance, particularly in *Campylobacter* spp., has developed during treatment and has been associated with bacteriologic failure (52). A recent report found that 2 of 54 soldiers treated with ciprofloxacin for *Campylobacter jejuni* enteritis had a bacteriologic and clinical relapse associated with the development of resistance in their *Campylobacter* isolates (106). These two patients were also coinfected with *Salmonella* spp., which were eradicated by quinolone therapy. Resistance in *C. jejuni* and *Campylobacter coli* in Finland has been reported, with no strains resistant to ciprofloxacin in 1980 and 10% resistant in 1990 (112). A similar increase in quinolone resistance from poultry-derived strains of *Campylobacter* spp. was reported from The Netherlands coincident with the use of a new fluoroquinolone (enrofloxacin, a derivative of ciprofloxacin) in veterinary medicine (40) (see chapter 25). Use of enrofloxacin in the veterinary arena for treatment of domestic animals has begun in the United States (127a). This particular use for the new fluoroquinolone agents seems to take unnecessary risks that might lead to the emergence of widespread resistance to the quinolone class of antibiotics.

Salmonellae have been reported as developing resistance to new quinolones (16, 64). In a report by Calderøn et al., the resistance was accompanied by therapeutic failure of enoxacin treatment (16). Even in the absence of resistance development, therapy of enteric infections with quinolones has occasionally had an unexpectedly high relapse rate (98). The reasons for these clinical observations are unclear. A recent report by Gootz and Martin demonstrated that a single-step mutation leading to high-level resistance can occur in *C. jejuni*, which is unique compared with other gram-negative enteric pathogens (53). This observation may explain at least some of the unexpected (negative) results seen in the treatment of enteropathogens with these new compounds.

## Skin, soft tissue, and bone infections or colonization

The newer fluoroquinolones do not appear to be immune from the emergence of bacterial resistance in settings where chronic infections and debilitating underlying diseases are present. The development of bacterial resistance during drug treatment has been reported by many authors. Here, too, the predominant pathogens have been *P. aeruginosa* and staphylococci (3, 36, 41, 45, 49, 54, 80, 93, 105, 119, 127, 133). The infections during which resistance has developed usually occurred in patients with underlying diseases such as diabetes mellitus, vascular insufficiency, or chronic osteomyelitis or when a foreign body was present. My own experience was particularly distressing in that resistance to both ciprofloxacin and rifampin emerged during combination therapy (105). When oral ciprofloxacin plus rifampin was used for a 2-week treatment of 11 patients colonized with MRSA, isolates from three patients developed resistance to ciprofloxacin and isolates from two patients developed resistance to rifampin. This development of resistance was associated with failure to eradicate the target organism (105). Similarly alarming, during the study period, resistance to ciprofloxacin in MRSA emerged throughout the medical center, and 36% of 115 MRSA isolates recovered were found to be resistant to rifampin. The resistance to ciprofloxacin persisted after the clinical trial was terminated, while that to rifampin disappeared 1 year after the clinical study was halted (105). It appeared from this study that not only would quinolone resistance in MRSA likely develop if the agent were used in an attempt to eradicate MRSA colonization but that resistance to the fluoroquinolones would become permanently associated with the MRSA isolates endemic within the institution (Table 3).

## Urinary tract infections

Use of the new quinolone agents for treatment of urinary tract infections has been well studied. The results in uncomplicated urinary tract infection have been very favorable, with only 1.7% of patients receiving norfloxacin and 2.9% of those given ciprofloxacin developing subsequent infections with quinolone-resistant bacteria (141). The reasons for the success of these agents in the treatment of

**Table 3.** Percent ciprofloxacin susceptibility at the Department of Veterans Affairs Center, Minneapolis, Minn.

| Organism | % Ciprofloxacin susceptibility (no. of isolates) | | |
|---|---|---|---|
| | Dec. 1987 | Sept. 1988 | Sept. 1991 |
| *S. aureus* | 98 (64) | 100 (75) | 89 (55) |
| MRSA | 100 (14) | 50 (2) | 0 (24) |
| *S. epidermidis* | 97 (103) | 98 (83) | 70 (113) |
| *P. aeruginosa* | 100 (55) | 98 (47) | 96 (51) |
| Enterococci | 98 (86) | 96 (59) | 62 (81) |
| *Enterobacteriaceae* | 100 (184) | 100 (192) | 99 (190) |

urinary tract infections is at least partially understood. During therapy of any urinary tract infection, changes in the fecal and periurethral microflora are noted. This is particularly important in the therapy of urinary tract infection, as the areas involved in these infections are the likely sources of reinfecting organisms. Studies evaluating changes in this flora have demonstrated that quinolones (norfloxacin) are able to eradicate the infecting pathogen from the periurethral area in 93% of patients compared with only 57% of those treated with trimethoprim-sulfamethoxazole and that resistant bacteria rarely emerge (56, 94, 120). In general, these investigations have demonstrated that quinolones exert a major impact on reducing the gram-negative facultative flora from these areas, cause some reduction of the gram-positive flora, and have little effect on the anaerobic fecal flora. In most circumstances, it appears that the successful use of these agents in eradicating pathogenic bacteria during the therapy of urinary tract infection does not lead to the development or dissemination of resistant bacteria (141).

The two settings in which resistance has emerged are (i) situations in which too low a dose of quinolone has been used (13, 79) and (ii) complicated urinary tract infections such as chronic pyelonephritis or prostatitis or in the presence of renal calculi (9, 36, 55).

### Infections in the immunocompromised host

Fluoroquinolones have been used in immunocompromised hosts both for treatment of documented (or suspected) infections and for prophylaxis (12, 35, 73, 84). While most reports have demonstrated a reduction in gram-negative bacteremias through the use of quinolone prophylaxis, such prophylaxis selects for quinolone-resistant bacterial strains in the fecal flora, most strikingly seen as an increase in the numbers of quinolone-resistant staphylococci in the gastrointestinal tract (50). More-serious clinical problems have also been seen. Kotilainen et al. reported seven neutropenic patients who developed bacteremia with ciprofloxacin-resistant coagulase-negative staphylococci soon after the introduction of ciprofloxacin in their hospital in Finland (74). Classen et al. also reported the occurrence of bacteremia due to *Streptococcus mitis* in five of nine bone marrow transplant recipients receiving oral norfloxacin (26). The MICs of norfloxacin for all these isolates ranged from 2 to 4 $\mu$g/ml (26).

These reports demonstrate two primary disadvantages associated with the use of the quinolone agents for prophylaxis in compromised patients. First is the potential during prophylaxis for the development or selection of resistant isolates, which may then persist and spread within the institutional environment. Second is the problem of a physician faced with a seriously infected patient who is receiving a fluoroquinolone as a prophylactic agent: it will not be possible to use a fluoroquinolone in subsequent treatment of the patient, as the patient will likely be infected with a quinolone-resistant pathogen.

## Resistance during and after Fluoroquinolone Therapy

The observations that resistant bacterial

isolates can occur in the setting of fluoroquinolone therapy are not unexpected, and such isolates have occurred for all the available fluoroquinolones. Løpez-Brea and Alarcon recently isolated fluoroquinolone-resistant *E. coli* and *Klebsiella pneumoniae* from an infected Hickman catheter in a patient who was receiving intravenous ciprofloxacin at a dose of 200 mg every 12 h (82). Both isolates were highly resistant to all six quinolones tested. A particularly well done report documented the emergence of imipenem, norfloxacin, and ciprofloxacin resistance in individual strains of *P. aeruginosa* associated with bacteriologic failure of antibiotic treatment. These investigators employed an exotoxin A gene probe to type their sensitive and resistant bacterial isolates to ensure that the observations made were associated with the development of bacterial resistance rather than being due to superinfection with unrelated antibiotic-resistant strains (100). Similar reports of resistant bacteria appearing during treatment have involved ofloxacin (23) and norfloxacin (90). It should be noted that infection with isolates resistant to the therapeutic agents that a patient is receiving or has received is not unique to the quinolone class of antimicrobial agents. Chow et al. reported a large series evaluating the phenomenon in association with use of broad-spectrum cephalosporins (25). They found that 69% of blood culture isolates of *Enterobacter* spp. were resistant to the extended-spectrum cephalosporins if the patients had previously received a third-generation cephalosporin compared with only 20% resistance in isolates from patients who had not received one of these compounds. They also noted that the development of resistance in *Enterobacter* spp. was much higher for the third-generation cephalosporins than it was for other cephalosporins or for aminoglycosides (25). While similar data for the fluoroquinolones are not available, it appears that the overall development of resistance in isolates during therapy should be comparable to that of other potent, extended-spectrum agents (88).

## Specific Microorganisms Prone to Develop Resistance to the Fluoroquinolones

### *Enterobacteriaceae*

Development of resistance among members of the *Enterobacteriaceae* has not been a frequent occurrence. In fact, the first isolation of a fluoroquinone-resistant *E. coli* strain from Scandinavia was so unique that it warranted a published report in 1990 (69). However, the observation by Muder et al. associating widespread use of ciprofloxacin with a significant increase in quinolone-resistant isolates of *P. mirabilis* and *S. marcescens* indicates that development of such resistance is possible and that the (mis)use of these agents has the potential to lead to development of bacterial resistance, even in highly sensitive bacterial species (92). Those authors studied patients in both acute- and chronic-care settings. In the chronic-care setting, most isolates of ciprofloxacin-resistant bacteria were cultured from patients who had previously received a fluoroquinolone (81%), suggesting that selection of resistant bacteria was a primary factor. However, only 32% of patients harboring a ciprofloxacin-resistant bacterium in the acute-care setting had prior therapy with the quinolone, suggesting that a clone of resistant microbes can persist and horizontally spread within the institutional environment once the organisms become established (92). This latter phenomenon has been well described with MRSA and points to the problem that can occur once fluoroquinolone resistance develops beyond a certain threshold within an institution (8, 105).

### Pneumococci

Pneumococci are only modestly susceptible to such agents as ciprofloxacin and ofloxacin. There is a growing concern that *S. pneumoniae* will be a major pathogen responsible for therapeutic failures with many fluoroquinolone agents. Serious failures or infections due to pneumococci have occurred in patients receiving ciprofloxacin (78, 103, 114), and caution in the treatment of patients whose infections may be due to *S. pneumoniae* is advised. Two investigations used relatively low doses of ciprofloxacin (78, 103). Four of six patients reported by Lee et al. received no more than 500 mg twice daily as their initial therapeutic regimen (78). Using less than maximal dosing may be a significant risk factor leading to therapeutic failure and the emergence of bacterial resistance, particularly when an antimicrobial agent only moderately active against the infecting pathogen is used. Newer fluoroquinolones, such as the recently withdrawn temafloxacin, had improved activity against *S. pneumoniae*, demonstrating that the potential role of selected fluoroquinolone agents for these infections remains but that clinical utility needs to be determined.

### *P. aeruginosa*

The gram-negative bacillus *P. aeruginosa* is one of the important clinical targets for the fluoroquinolone agents (ciprofloxacin), as this drug provides the only effective oral agent against this difficult-to-treat pathogen. Resistance to fluoroquinolones and other agents has been seen in *P. aeruginosa* (3, 24). The difficulty with *P. aeruginosa* has been widely (geographically) observed. Kresken and Wiedemann have reported problems with *P. aeruginosa* in Germany (75), and Parry et al. have found problems with *P. aeruginosa* in their institution in the United States (101). The potential for these (and other) bacteria resistant to the fluoroquinolones to be cross-resistant to other classes of antimicrobial agents is also a concern. Chow et al. have demonstrated that such cross-resistance occurs, particularly in isolates obtained from patients with severe burns (24). However, while this cross-resistance between the quinolones and other antipseudomonal agents can occur, at present it appears infrequently (24).

## Staphylococci

Staphylococci, particularly MRSA, currently are the principal pathogenic bacterial species that should be expected to rapidly express resistance to the new fluoroquinolones during clinical use. Reports describing this event have appeared worldwide (3, 8, 32, 66, 85, 109, 113, 117, 121, 125, 131). My own experience confirms the problem but is not unique. In my medical center, in January 1988, we began an intensive effort to eradicate MRSA colonization from patients by using ciprofloxacin combined with rifampin. Our general use of the new fluoroquinolone also increased at that time, following U.S. Food and Drug Administration approval of ciprofloxacin. Over the ensuing 2 years, the percentage of MRSA susceptible to ciprofloxacin went from 100 to 0%, as shown in Table 3 (105). Many of these MRSA strains are highly resistant to ciprofloxacin, with MICs in excess of 256 $\mu$g/ml. Our experience was mirrored by the observations of Blumberg et al., which emphasize the stability of quinolone resistance in MRSA and the potential for horizontal spread of this multiresistant pathogen within an institutional environment (8). Additionally, neither our experience (105) nor that of Tebas et al. (128) suggests that combining a new fluoroquinolone with another agent (rifampin) will prevent the emergence of resistance in staphylococci. We have also seen a reduction in the number of coagulase-negative staphylococcal and enterococcal strains susceptible to ciprofloxacin (Table 1), indicating diminishing susceptibility of most of our gram-positive cocci to ciprofloxacin. This is of special concern because many patients harboring the resistant strains have never received a fluoroquinolone. When such strains become frequent within any institution, the benefit of the new fluoroquinolones as single-agent empiric therapy for patients potentially infected with those bacterial pathogens is lost.

## Other microorganisms

A few other microorganisms that appear to have a propensity for the development of resistance to the new fluoroquinolones have appeared (58). Hooper and Wolfson tabulated reports of ciprofloxacin resistance among organisms including *Helicobacter pylori*, *Enterobacter* and *Klebsiella* spp., and *Corynebacterium* strain JK. Similarly, they found reports of *H. pylori* and *Citrobacter freundii* resistant to ofloxacin, *Enterobacter* spp. resistant to pefloxacin, and *Neisseria gonorrhoeae* resistant to enoxacin (58). The most common microbes in these clinical case-type reports of resistance development involve *Brucella melitensis* (1, 76) and mycobacteria (132, 136).

## STRATEGIES FOR MINIMIZING QUINOLONE RESISTANCE

The bacterial species prone to development of quinolone resistance include strains whose initial MICs are close to the maximal achievable concentrations for these antimicrobial agents in blood and many body fluids. Blaser et al. (7) and Felmingham et al. (43) have reported that the development of resistance to fluoroquinolone antibiotics can be eliminated or markedly reduced if the concentration of antibiotic to which the organism is exposed exceeds the MIC by at least 8- to 10-fold. Therefore, by examining the achievable drug levels at any site and comparing this information with in vitro susceptibility data, it is possible to estimate which infection sites (as well as which microbes) may be best treated with these agents. Typical concentrations of norfloxacin, ciprofloxacin, and ofloxacin taken from recent reviews of the extravascular distribution of fluoroquinolones are listed in Table 4 (47, 48, 95). Combining the information from this table with in vitro susceptibility test data makes it possible to construct a list of drug level/susceptibility ratios, i.e., a therapeutic index, which is one potential measure for predicting possible emergence of resistance during therapy of infection. Examples of this are in Table 5. It is readily apparent from the data that for treating many infections outside the urinary tract, it is important to avoid using too low a dosage of antimicrobial agent in order to maintain as favorable a therapeutic index as possible. For ciprofloxacin use in therapy of infections outside the urinary or gastrointestinal tract, the maximal daily dose (1,500 mg) should routinely be used. When ofloxacin is used in these settings, a maximal daily dose of 800 mg should be used. As noted above, the concept of underdosing when quinolone antimicrobial agents are used has been applied to nalidixic acid in the past. Stamey and Bragonje suggested that too low a dosage of nalidixic acid in the therapy of urinary tract infection was likely the cause of the emergence of large numbers of resistant clinical isolates (126). As part of a strategy to avoid underdosing, the prescriber should also remember to caution the patient against taking concomitant medications that can chelate the quinolones in the gut (particularly aluminum- or magnesium-containing antacids and zinc- or iron-containing vitamins) and therefore impair systemic absorption of the compound, effectively leading to underdosing (33, 110) (see chapter 11). Continued observation for other conditions that might interfere with the therapeutic activity of these agents is necessary (107).

Similarly, it is important to realize that the development of resistance during therapy does not always correlate with actual treatment failure (87) and that information such as that in Table 5 is more useful in predicting how to prevent the development of resistance than in predicting when it will develop or when therapeutic failure will occur. Clinical treatment trials are invaluable in helping determine which therapy settings most predispose to the development of bacterial resistance (140).

Voss and Braveny recently presented an interesting observation relating to the development of resistance and clinical failure in intensive care unit patients infected with *P. aeruginosa* who were treated with various antimicrobial agents (135). They found that treatment with ceftazidime resulted in devel-

**Table 4.** Distribution of norfloxacin, ciprofloxacin, and ofloxacin at selected tissue sites[a]

| Site | Concn (μg/ml) or ratio of: | | | | | |
|---|---|---|---|---|---|---|
| | Norfloxacin | | Ciprofloxacin | | Ofloxacin | |
| | Serum | Tissue (%) | Serum | Tissue (%) | Serum | Tissue (%) |
| Blister fluid | 1.5 | 1.0 (67) | 2.3 | 1.4 (61) | 10.7 | 5.2 (49) |
| PMN | Ratio = 224% | | Ratio = 349% | | Ratio = 815% | |
| Bone | | | 2.9 | 1.6 (55) | 2.0 | 1.22 (61) |
| Prostatic tissue | 1.5 | 1.7 (113) | 1.6 | 4.5 (281) | 1.9 | 4.0 (210) |
| Prostatic fluid | 1.4 | 0.14 (10) | 1.44 | 2.4 (154) | | 2.5 |
| Urine | | 422–58 | | 150–51 | | 458–93 |

[a]Data are from references 47, 48, and 95. PMN, polymorphonuclear leukocyte.

**Table 5.** Therapeutic index of quinolone for selected sites and microorganisms

| Site | Therapeutic index of quinolone for: | | | | |
|---|---|---|---|---|---|
| | *Escherichia coli* | *Proteus* spp. | *Pseudomonas aeruginosa* | *Staphylococcus aureus* | *Enterococcus faecalis* |
| Bone | 15 | 3 | 1 | 2 | 1 |
| Soft tissue | 15 | 3 | 1 | 2 | 1 |
| Prostatic tissue | 30 | 6 | 2 | 4 | 2 |
| Urine | >900 | >180 | >60 | >120 | >60 |

opment of resistant isolates in 14.3% of the patients and pathogen eradication in 28.6%. Of imipenem-treated patients, 15.4% developed resistance and 46.1% showed eradication of *P. aeruginosa*. Of ciprofloxacin-treated patients, on the other hand, 27.3% developed resistant isolates and 72.7% showed pathogen eradication (135). In this particular series, it appeared that for the quinolone used in treating infections due to *P. aeruginosa*, there was a good correlation between the development of bacterial resistance (or lack thereof) and clinical treatment outcome. While the highest percentage of resistant isolates was associated with ciprofloxacin use, the greatest rate of pathogen eradication was also associated with fluoroquinolone therapy. However, the close correlation between susceptibility or resistance and clinical outcome was seen only with ciprofloxacin, and this close a direct relationship between in vitro and in vivo results is not typical of most studies.

The use of combination therapy has often been suggested as one means of avoiding the development of resistant microbes during antimicrobial agent therapy, although not all authors are optimistic about this approach (118, 139). Preliminary reports have indicated that combined therapy may be useful in patients with cystic fibrosis (77). Milatovic and Braveny evaluated the concept for several agents in their review and found that while combination therapy may lower the incidence of resistance development, it does not eliminate the possibility of such an event (88). My own experience reinforces the concept that this approach may not always be successful in that the addition of rifampin as part of the treatment regimen (in my medical center) did not appear to slow the emergence of quinolone resistance in MRSA when the combination was used for patients colonized with MRSA (105).

Table 1 lists the types of infections during which resistance is most likely to develop. As can be seen, patients with severe underlying disease (cystic fibrosis and malignancy) and those with structural alterations (foreign-body infections, burns, and complicated urinary tract infections), those with difficult-to-heal lesions (decubitus ulcers and diabetic foot ulcerations), and those colonized with problem pathogens (MRSA) all share certain characteristics. The infections occur in patients with diminished host defenses due to malignancy, foreign bodies, debility, impaired circulation, or local immune dysfunction. They also often require prolonged therapy, such as that for bone and joint infections. Also, patients with these infections are often treated in an institutional setting. When all these described factors are present, the possibility for the development of antibacterial resistance during a given treatment episode is greatest. When such resistance occurs in an institutional setting, the potential for spread of a resistant clone of pathogens from one patient to another exists. The spread of quinolone-resistant isolates has occurred, and it appears to take place even though bacteria are unable to pass quinolone resistance to one another via a plasmid-mediated process (28).

Successful prevention of the development of nosocomial bacterial clones resistant to fluoroquinolone antibacterial agents or elimination of this resistance once it occurs within an institutional setting has not been reported and will require innovative approaches to the use of these agents. Using a "targeted" approach for extended-spectrum agents within institutions or in other settings where the development of resistance is of concern might be one such approach. Targeting for quinolone use has been suggested for norfloxacin (138). Targeting implies the use of an agent primarily in therapy of infections when a high likelihood of clinical success is anticipated and when little possibility of resistance development is expected. It also implies using agents in ways that maximize these desired outcomes. The information contained in Table 5 combined with the reports of clinical studies suggests that as an example of targeting, a clinical approach to the use of fluoroquinolones would be to use them for urinary tract infections. Clinical results with these new agents in the treatment of urinary tract infections have been very impressive, and the therapeutic index within the urinary collecting system is well in excess of 10-fold, indicating that development of resistance would be minimal. Restricting the use of orally administered fluoroquinolones only (or predominantly) to these types of infections in institutional settings where bacterial resistance to quinolones is prevalent in pathogenic bacterial species may be one way to allow for the reestablishment of a more sensitive bacterial population within the institution. This same approach also could be considered, as a preventive measure, in hospitals where bacterial resistance to other classes of antimicrobial agents has been a problem and where there is a desire to avoid the development of resistance toward the fluoroquinolones. Such use of these agents would mean that few hospitalized patients (other than those with a urinary tract infection) would receive an oral fluoroquinolone while they are inpatients and that they would not be given such therapy except when they are discharged with an infection needing continued extended-spectrum antibiotic treatment on an outpatient basis. However, this approach to the use of fluoroquinolones is likely not practical in most settings (108).

It appears that a group of selected clinical settings, particularly within institutions, may predispose to the development of resistant bacterial isolates and that use of the fluoroquinolone agents in these clinical settings should be avoided or at least markedly curtailed. Doing so is especially difficult with a class of antibacterial agents as easily used as the orally administered fluoroquinolone antibiotics, but the effort may be important to the long-term utility of these agents. These settings include prolonged use (beyond 2 to 4 weeks) in individual institutionalized patients; therapy of lesions unlikely to respond, such as ischemic skin ulcerations; attempts at eradication of colonization states, particularly in debilitated patients; and attempted therapy of infections at the site of major (uncorrectable) structural abnormalities or (unremovable) foreign bodies, again where the possibility of success is remote. When infections occurring in such settings are treated with any antimicrobial agent, the probability of resistance development is high, and when this occurs within an institution, the potential for dissemination of a resistant bacterial clone is great.

The use of ciprofloxacin inpatients with cystic fibrosis exemplifies the strategy for reducing the likelihood of the development of bacterial resistance to fluoroquinolones. Resistant *P. aeruginosa* emerges more frequently as therapy continues over several weeks, so the current recommendation for use of quinolones in these patients is to avoid therapeutic courses more than 2 to 4 weeks in duration and to alternate use of fluoroquinolones and other agents (77).

The new fluoroquinolone antibacterial agents show promise for a long, useful future because of their broad spectrum of activity and ease of use. However, prescribers must remember that these drugs are not more potent than some other classes of extended-spectrum parenteral antibacterial agents, only easier to use. Their successful application to the therapy of difficult and serious infections still requires the good ancillary medical care (such as adequate debridement of infected pressure sores or surgical revascularization when infection takes place in the presence of vascular insufficiency) that would be given if any other class of antibiotic were chosen for treatment.

The continued development of additional quinolone-class antimicrobial agents presents the potential for compounds that are active against microorganisms that have already developed resistance to currently available agents (99). However, such development is not immediately in sight for the most troublesome pathogens. Maple et al. have demonstrated that at least for MRSA, it is likely there will be cross-resistance between most, if not all, quinolone agents now under study (86).

Finally, the potential for bacteria that develop quinolone resistance during treatment with a fluoroquinolone to simultaneously develop cross-resistance to other classes of antimicrobial agents is of concern, as these pathogens would then be very difficult to treat. Chow et al. have demonstrated that such cross-resistance can occasionally occur, particularly in isolates obtained from burn patients (24). They suggested that combination therapy may be useful in treating the resultant infections. Using an animal model, my laboratory has found that this approach can be successful for treating highly resistant isolates, including those that develop resistance to the new quinolones (ciprofloxacin) during initial therapy (42). Therefore, when isolates become resistant to the newer fluoroquinolones during therapy, these isolates would probably remain responsive to other classes of extended-spectrum antimicrobial agents administered either alone or in combination.

## CONCLUSIONS

The new fluoroquinolones offer all medical practitioners a potent class of antibacterial agents that can remain useful for many years to come, provided care is exercised in their application to appropriate infectious disease therapy. There appears to be little justification for the use of these agents in the practice of veterinary medicine, as it has already been demonstrated that such use appears linked to an increase in the isolation of quinolone-resistant bacteria.

The use of these agents in the institutional setting demands particular attention, as it is here that resistant isolates, emerging during previous exposure to these compounds, have the best opportunity to spread from one patient to another. Several recommendations for limiting the development of quinolone resistance within institutions can be made. (i) Avoid long-term use with inpatients for most infections. (ii) Do not use quinolones either for trivial infections or in an attempt to treat colonizing bacteria in patients with severe underlying disease. (iii) Avoid underdosing when using quinolones (and make certain that other concomitantly administered agents do not interfere with the absorption of orally administered quinolones). (iv) Attempt to focus on therapy of infections with high therapeutic indices (infection site drug level/MIC ratio of ≥8). (v) Do not use currently available agents for treatment of infections involving MRSA.

Appropriate clinical use of these potent new agents can help preserve them as important antibiotics for serious and difficult-to-treat infections for many years to come.

## REFERENCES


1. **Al-Sibai, M. B., and S. M. H. Qadri.** 1990. Development of ciprofloxacin resistance in *Brucella melitensis*. *J. Antimicrob. Chemother.* **25:**302–303.
2. **Arcieri, G., E. Griffith, G. Gruenwaldt, A. Heyd, A. O'Brien, N. Becker, and R. August.** 1987. Ciprofloxacin: an update on clinical experience. *J. Med.* **82**(Suppl. 4A)**:**381–386.
3. **Ball, P.** 1990. Emergent resistance to ciprofloxacin amongst *Pseudomonas aeruginosa* and *Staphylococcus aureus*: clinical significance and therapeutic approaches. *J. Antimicrob. Chemother.* **26**(Suppl. F)**:**165–179.
4. **Bamberger, D. M., L. R. Peterson, D. N. Gerding, J. A. Moody, and C. E. Fasching.** 1986. Ciprofloxacin, azlocillin, ceftizoxime and amikacin alone and in combination against gram-negative bacilli in an infected chamber model. *J. Antimicrob. Chemother.* **18:**51–63.
5. **Barry, A. L., R. N. Jones, C. Thornsberry, L. W. Ayers, E. H. Gerlach, and H. M. Sommers.** 1984. Antibacterial activities of ciprofloxacin, norfloxacin, oxolinic acid, cinoxacin, and nalidixic acid. *Antimicrob. Agents Chemother.* **25:**644–647.
6. **Bender, S. W., H. G. Posselt, R. Wonne, R. Strehl, P. M. Shah, and A. Bauernfeind.** 1986. Ciprofloxacin treatment of patients with cystic fibrosis and pseudomonas bronchopneumonia, p. 272–278. *In* H. C. Neu and H. Weuta (ed.), *1st Int. Ciprofloxacin Workshop*. Excerpta Medica, Amsterdam.
7. **Blaser, J., B. B. Stone, M. C. Groner, and S. H. Zinner.** 1987. Comparative study with enoxacin and netilmicin in a pharmacodynamic model to determine importance of ratio of antibiotic peak concentration to MIC for bactericidal activity and emergence of resistance. *Antimicrob. Agents Chemother.* **31:**1054–1060.
8. **Blumberg, H. M., D. Rimland, D. J. Carroll, P. Terry, and I. K. Wachsmuth.** 1991. Rapid development of ciprofloxacin resistance in methicillin-susceptible and -resistant *Staphylococcus aureus*. *J. Infect. Dis.* **163:**1279–1285.
9. **Boerema, J. B. J., and H. K. van Saene.** 1987. Norfloxacin treatment in complicated urinary tract infections. *Scand. J. Infect. Dis.* **48**(Suppl.)**:**20–26.
10. **Bosso, J. A., J. E. Allen, and J. M. Matsen.** 1989. Changing susceptibility of *Pseudomonas aeruginosa* isolates from cystic fibrosis patients with the clinical use of newer antibiotics. *Antimicrob. Agents Chemother.* **33:**526–528.
11. **Bosso, J. A., P. G. Black, and J. M. Matsen.** 1987. Ciprofloxacin versus tobramycin plus azlocillin in pulmonary exacerbations in adult patients with cystic fibrosis. *Am. J. Med.* **82**(Suppl. 4A)**:**180–184.
12. **Bow, E. J., E. Rayner, and T. J. Louie.** 1988. Comparison of norfloxacin with cotrimoxazole for infection prophylaxis in acute leukemia. The trade-off for reduced gram-negative sepsis. *Am. J. Med.* **84:**847–854.
13. **Brown, E. M., R. Morris, and T. P. Stephenson.** 1986. The efficacy and safety of ciprofloxacin in the treatment of chronic *Pseudomonas aeruginosa* urinary tract infection. *J. Antimicrob. Chemother.* **18**(Suppl. D)**:**123–127.
14. **Brumfitt, W., I. Franklin, D. Grady, J. M. T. Hamilton-Miller, and A. Iliffe.** 1984. Changes in the pharmacokinetics of ciprofloxacin and fecal flora during administration of a 7-day course to human volunteers. *Antimicrob. Agents Chemother.* **26:**757–761.
15. **Bryan, L. E., J. Bedard, S. Wong, and S. Chamberland.** 1989. Quinolone antimicrobial agents: mechanism of action and resistance development. *Clin. Invest. Med.* **12:**14–19.
16. **Calderøn, E., A. Cruz, H. Rangel, A. Coronel, and E. Zorrilla.** 1991. Treatment of acute diarrhea in adults. *Curr. Ther. Res.* **49:**792–800.
17. **Campbell, J. L., M. W. Thomley, and R. I. Parsons.** 1964. Clinical evaluation of nalidixic acid: NeGram. *J. Urol.* **92:**549–551.
18. **Cederberg, A., T. Denneberg, M. Ekberg, and I. Juhlin.** 1974. Nalidixic acid in urinary tract infections with particular reference to the emergence of resistance. *Scand. J. Infect. Dis.* **6:**259–264.
19. **Celesk, R. A., and N. J. Robillard.** 1989. Factors influencing the accumulation of ciprofloxacin in *Pseudomonas aeruginosa*. *Antimicrob. Agents Chemother.* **33:**1921–1926.
20. **Chamberland, S., A. S. Bayer, T. Schollaardt, S. A. Wong, and L. E. Bryan.** 1989. Characterization of mechanisms of quinolone resistance in *Pseudomonas aeruginosa* strains isolated in vitro and in vivo during experimental endocarditis. *Antimicrob. Agents Chemother.* **33:**624–634.
21. **Chamberland, S., F. Malouin, T. Schollaardt, T. R. Parr, Jr., and L. E. Bryan.** 1990. Persis-

tence of *Pseudomonas aeruginosa* during ciprofloxacin therapy of a cystic fibrosis patient: transient resistance to quinolones and protein *F*− deficiency. *J. Antimicrob. Chemother.* **25**:995–1010.

22. **Chapman, S. T., D. C. E. Speller, and D. S. Reeves.** 1985. Resistance to ciprofloxacin. *Lancet* **ii**:39.
23. **Cheng, A. F., M. K. W. Li, T. K. W. Ling, and G. L. French.** 1987. Emergence of ofloxacin-resistant *Citrobacter freundii* and *Pseudomonas maltophilia* after ofloxacin therapy. *J. Antimicrob. Ther.* **20**:283–285.
24. **Chow, A. W., J. Wong, K. H. Bartlett, S. D. Shafran, and H. G. Stiver.** 1989. Cross-resistance of *Pseudomonas aeruginosa* to ciprofloxacin, extended-spectrum ß-lactams, and aminoglycosides and susceptibility to antibiotic combinations. *Antimicrob. Agents Chemother.* **33**:1368–1372.
25. **Chow, J. W., M. J. Fine, D. M. Shales, J. P. Quinn, D. C. Hooper, M. P. Johnson, R. Ramphal, M. M. Wagener, D. K. Miyashiro, and V. L. Yu.** 1991. *Enterobacter* bacteremia: clinical features and emergence of antibiotic resistance during therapy. *Ann. Intern. Med.* **115**:585–590.
26. **Classen, D. C., J. P. Burke, C. D. Ford, S. Evershed, M. R. Aloia, J. K. Wilfahrt, and J. A. Elliott.** 1990. *Streptococcus mitis* sepsis in bone marrow transplant patients receiving oral antimicrobial prophylaxis. *Am. J. Med.* **89**:441–446.
27. **Cofsky, R. D., L. duBouchet, and S. H. Landesman.** 1984. Recovery of norfloxacin in feces after administration of a single oral dose to humans. *Antimicrob. Agents Chemother.* **26**:110–111.
28. **Courvalin, P.** 1990. Plasmid mediated 4-quinolone resistance: a real or apparent absence? *Antimicrob. Agents Chemother.* **34**:681–684.
29. **Crook, S. M., J. B. Selkon, and P. D. McLardy Smith.** 1985. Clinical resistance to long-term oral ciprofloxacin. *Lancet* **i**:1275.
30. **Crumplin, G. C., and M. Odell.** 1987. Development of resistance to ofloxacin. *Drugs* **34**(Suppl. 1):1–8.
31. **Cullmann, W., M. Steiglitz, B. Baars, and W. Opferkuch.** 1985. Comparative evaluation of recently developed quinolone compounds—with a note on the frequency of resistant mutants. *Chemotherapy* (Basel) **31**:19–28.
32. **Daum, T. E., D. R. Schaberg, M. S. Terpenning, W. S. Sottile, and C. A. Kauffman.** 1990. Increasing resistance of *Staphylococcus aureus* to ciprofloxacin. *Antimicrob. Agents Chemother.* **34**:1862–1863.
33. **Davies, B. I., and F. P. V. Maesen.** 1989. Drug interactions with quinolones. *Rev. Infect. Dis.* **11**(Suppl. 5):S1083–S1090.
34. **Davies, B. I., F. P. Maesen, and C. Bauer.** 1986. Ciprofloxacin in the treatment of acute and chronic bronchitis. *Eur. J. Clin. Microbiol.* **5**:226–231.
35. **Dekker, A. W., M. Rozenberg-Arska, and J. Verhoef.** 1987. Infection prophylaxis in acute leukemia: a comparison of ciprofloxacin with trimethoprim-sulfamethoxazole and colistin. *Ann. Intern. Med.* **106**:7–12.
36. **Desplaces, N., L. Gutmann, J. Carlet, J. Guibert, and J. F. Acar.** 1986. The new quinolones and their combination with other agents for therapy of severe infections. *J. Antimicrob. Chemother.* **17**(Suppl. A):25–39.
37. **Diver, J. M., T. Schollaardt, H. R. Rabin, C. Thorson, and L. E. Bryan.** 1991. Persistence mechanisms in *Pseudomonas aeruginosa* from cystic fibrosis patients undergoing ciprofloxacin therapy. *Antimicrob. Agents Chemother.* **35**:1538–1546.
38. **Dornbusch, K., and the European Study Group on Antibiotic Resistance.** 1990. Resistance to ß-lactam antibiotics and ciprofloxacin in Gram-negative bacilli and staphylococci isolated from blood: a European collaborative study. *J. Antimicrob. Chemother.* **26**:269–278.
39. **Edlund, C., A. Lidbeck, L. Kager, and C. F. Nord.** 1987. Comparative effects of enoxacin and norfloxacin on human colonic microflora. *Antimicrob. Agents Chemother.* **31**:1846–1848.
40. **Endtz, H. P., G. J. Ruijs, B. van Klingeren, W. H. Jansen, T. van der Reyden, and R. P. Mouton.** 1991. Quinolone resistance in campylobacter isolated from man and poultry following the introduction of fluoroquinolones in veterinary medicine. *J. Antimicrob. Chemother.* **27**:199–208.
41. **Eron, L. J.** 1987. Therapy of skin and skin structure infections with ciprofloxacin: an overview. *Am. J. Med.* **82**(Suppl. 4A):224–226.
42. **Fasching, C. E., D. N. Gerding, and L. R. Peterson.** 1987. Treatment of ciprofloxacin- and ceftizoxime-induced resistant gram-negative bacilli. *Am. J. Med.* **82**(Suppl. 4A):80–86.
43. **Felmingham, D., P. Foxall, M. D. O'Hare, G. Webb, G. Ghosh, and R. N. Gruuneberg.** 1988. Resistance studies with ofloxacin. *J. Antimicrob. Chemother.* **22**(Suppl. C):27–34.
44. **Fernandes, P. B.** 1988. Mode of action, and *in vitro* and *in vivo* activities of the fluoroquinolones. *J. Clin. Pharmacol.* **28**:156–168.
45. **Follath, F., M. Bindschedler, M. Wenk, R. Frei, H. Stalder, and H. Reber.** 1986. Use of ciprofloxacin in the treatment of *Pseudomonas aeruginosa* infections. *Eur. J. Clin. Microbiol.* **5**:236–240.
46. **Forward, K. R., G. K. M. Harding, G. J. Gray, B. A. Urias, and A. R. Ronald.** 1983.

Comparative activities of norfloxacin and fifteen other antipseudomonal agents against gentamicin-susceptible and -resistant *Pseudomonas aeruginosa* strains. *Antimicrob. Agents Chemother.* **24:**602–604.

47. **Gerding, D. N., and J. A. Hitt.** 1989. Tissue penetration of the new quinolones in humans. *Rev. Infect. Dis.* **11**(Suppl. 5):S1046–1057.
48. **Gerding, D. N., L. R. Peterson, C. E. Hughes, D. M. Bamberger, and T. A. Larson.** 1991. Extravascular antimicrobial distribution and the respective blood concentrations in man, p. 880–961. *In* V. Lorian (ed.), *Antibiotics in Laboratory Medicine*, 3rd ed. The Williams & Wilkins Co., Baltimore.
49. **Gilbert, D. N., A. D. Tice, P. K. Marsh, P. C. Kraven, and L. C. Preheim.** 1987. Oral ciprofloxacin for chronic contiguous osteomyelitis caused by aerobic gram-negative bacilli. *Am. J. Med.* **82**(Suppl. 4A):254–258.
50. **Giuliano, M., A. Pantosti, G. Gentile, W. Acrese, and P. Martino.** 1989. Selective decontamination with the new fluorinated quinolones in bone marrow transplant patients: the effects on oral and intestinal microflora. *Microecol. Ther.* **18:**69–71.
51. **Goldfarb, J., R. C. Stern, M. D. Reed, T. S. Yamashita, C. M. Myers, and J. L. Blumer.** 1987. Ciprofloxacin monotherapy for acute pulmonary exacerbations of cystic fibrosis. *Am. J. Med.* **82**(Suppl. 4A):174–179.
52. **Goodman, L. J., G. M. Trenholme, R. L. Kaplan, J. Segreti, D. Hines, R. Petrak, J. A. Nelson, K. W. Mayer, W. Landau, G. W. Parkhurst, and S. Levin.** 1990. Empiric antimicrobial therapy of domestically acquired acute diarrhea in urban adults. *Arch. Intern. Med.* **150:**541–546.
53. **Gootz, T. D., and B. A. Martin.** 1991. Characterization of high-level quinolone resistance in *Campylobacter jejuni*. *Antimicrob. Agents Chemother.* **35:**840–845.
54. **Greenberg, R. N., D. J. Kennedy, R. M. Relly, K. L. Luppen, W. J. Weinandt, M. R. Bollinger, F. Aguirre, F. Kodesch, and A. M. K. Saeed.** 1987. Treatment of bone, joint and soft-tissue infections with oral ciprofloxacin. *Antimicrob. Agents Chemother.* **31:**151–155.
55. **Guiber, J. M., D. M. Destree, and J. F. Acar.** 1987. Ciprofloxacin (Bay o 9867): clinical evaluation in urinary tract infections due to *Pseudomonas aeruginosa*. *Chemioterapia* **6**(Suppl. 2):524–525.
56. **Haase, D. A., G. L. M. Harding, M. J. Thompson, J. K. Kennedy, B. A. Urias, and A. R. Ronald.** 1984. Comparative trial of norfloxacin and trimethoprim-sulfamethoxazole in the treatment of women with localized, acute, symptomatic urinary tract infections and antimicrobial effect on periurethral and fecal microflora. *Antimicrob. Agents Chemother.* **26:**481–484.
57. **Hodson, M. E., C. M. Roberts, R. J. A. Butland, M. J. Smith, and J. C. Batten.** 1987. Oral ciprofloxacin compared with conventional intravenous treatment for *Pseudomonas aeruginosa* infection in adults with cystic fibrosis. *Lancet* **i:**235–237.
58. **Hooper, D. C., and J. S. Wolfson.** 1989. Bacterial resistance to the quinolone antimicrobial agents. *Am. J. Med.* **87**(Suppl. 6C):17S–23S.
59. **Hooper, D. C., and J. S. Wolfson.** 1991. Mode of action of the new quinolones: new data. *Eur. J. Clin. Microbiol. Infect. Dis.* **10:**223–231.
60. **Hooper, D. C., and J. S. Wolfson.** 1991. Fluoroquinolone antimicrobial agents. *N. Engl. J. Med.* **324:**384–394.
61. **Hooper, D. C., J. S. Wolfson, E. Y. Ng, K. S. Souza, G. L. McHugh, and M. N. Swartz.** 1987. Antagonism of wild-type and resistant *Escherichia coli* and its DNA gyrase by the tricyclic 4-quinolone analogs ofloxacin and S-25930 stereoisomers. *Antimicrob. Agents Chemother.* **31:**1861–1863.
62. **Hooper, D. C., J. S. Wolfson, K. S. Souza, E. Y. Ng, G. L. McHugh, and M. L. Swartz.** 1989. Mechanisms of quinolone resistance in *Escherichia coli:* characterization of *nfxB* and *cfxB*, two mutant resistant loci decreasing norfloxacin accumulation. *Antimicrob. Agents Chemother.* **33:**283–290.
63. **Hooper, D. C., J. S. Wolfson, K. S. Souza, C. Tung, G. L. McHugh, and M. N. Swartz.** 1986. Genetic and biochemical characterization of norfloxacin resistance in *Escherichia coli*. *Antimicrob. Agents Chemother.* **29:**639–644.
64. **Howard, A. J., T. D. Joseph, L. L. O. Bloodworth, J. A. Frost, H. Chart, and B. Rowe.** 1990. The emergence of ciprofloxacin resistance in *Salmonella typhimurium*. *J. Antimicrob. Chemother.* **26:**296–298.
65. **Humphreys, H., and E. Mulvihill.** 1985. Ciprofloxacin-resistant *Staphylococcus aureus*. *Lancet* **ii:**383.
66. **Isaacs, R. D., P. J. Kunke, R. L. Cohen, and J. W. Smith.** 1988. Ciprofloxacin resistance in epidemic methicillin-resistant *Staphylococcus aureus*. *Lancet* **ii:**843.
67. **Janin, N., H. Meugnier, J. F. Desnottes, R. Woehrle, and J. Fleurette.** 1987. Recovery of pefloxacin in saliva and feces and its action on oral and fecal floras in healthy volunteers. *Antimicrob. Agents Chemother.* **31:**1665–1668.
68. **Jensen, T., S. S. Pedersen, C. H. Neilsen, N. Høiby, and C. Koch.** 1987. The efficacy and safety of ciprofloxacin and ofloxacin in chronic *Pseudomonas aeruginosa* infection in cystic fibrosis. *J. Antimicrob. Chemother.* **20:**585–594.

69. **Jonsson, M., M. Walder, and A. Forsgren.** 1990. First clinical isolate of highly fluoroquinolone-resistant *Escherichia coli* in Scandinavia. *Eur. J. Clin. Microbiol. Infect. Dis.* **9:**851–853.
70. **Kaatz, G. W., and S. M. Seo.** 1988. Mechanism of ciprofloxacin resistance in *Pseudomonas aeruginosa*. *J. Infect. Dis.* **158:**537–541.
71. **Kaatz, G. W., S. M. Seo, S. L. Barriere, L. M. Albrecht, and M. J. Rybak.** 1991. Development of resistance to fleroxacin during therapy of experimental methicillin-susceptible *Staphylococcus aureus* endocarditis. *Antimicrob. Agents Chemother.* **35:**1547–1550.
72. **Kaatz, G. W., S. M. Seo, and C. A. Ruble.** 1991. Mechanisms of fluoroquinolone resistance in *Staphylococcus aureus*. *J. Infect. Dis.* **163:**1080–1086.
73. **Kern, W., E. Kurrie, and E. Vanek.** 1987. Ofloxacin for prevention of bacterial infections in granulocytopenic patients. *Infection* **15:**427–432.
74. **Kotilainen, P., J. Nikoskelainen, and P. Huovinen.** 1990. Emergence of ciprofloxacin-resistant coagulase-negative staphylococcal skin flora in immunocompromised patients receiving ciprofloxacin. *J. Infect. Dis.* **161:**41–44.
75. **Kresken, M., and B. Wiedemann.** 1988. Development of resistance to nalidixic acid and the fluoroquinolones after the introduction of norfloxacin and ofloxacin. *Antimicrob. Agents Chemother.* **32:**1285–1288.
76. **Lang, R., R. Raz, T. Sacks, and M. Shapiro.** 1990. Failure of prolonged treatment with ciprofloxacin in acute infections due to *Brucella melitensis*. *J. Antimicrob. Chemother.* **26:**841–846.
77. **LeBel, M.** 1991. Fluoroquinolones in the treatment of cystic fibrosis: a critical appraisal. *Eur. J. Clin. Microbiol. Infect. Dis.* **10:**316–324.
78. **Lee, B. L., A. M. Padula, R. C. Kimbrough, S. R. Jones, R. E. Chaisson, J. Mills, and M. A. Sande.** 1991. Infectious complications with respiratory pathogens despite ciprofloxacin therapy. *N. Engl. J. Med.* **325:**520–521.
79. **Leigh, D. A., F. X. S. Emmanuel, and V. J. Petch.** 1986. Ciprofloxacin therapy in complicated urinary tract infections caused by *Pseudomonas aeruginosa* and other resistant bacteria. *J. Antimicrob. Chemother.* **18**(Suppl. D)**:**117–121.
80. **Licitra, C. M., R. G. Brooks, and B. E. Sieger.** 1987. Clinical efficacy and levels of ciprofloxacin in tissue in patients with soft tissue infection. *Antimicrob. Agents Chemother.* **31:**805–807.
81. **Limb, D. I., D. J. W. Dabbs, and R. C. Spencer.** 1987. *In vitro* selection of bacteria resistant to the 4-quinolone agents. *J. Antimicrob. Chemother.* **19:**65–71.
82. **Løpez-Brea, M., and T. Alarcon.** 1990. Isolation of fluoroquinolone resistant *Escherichia coli* and *Klebsiella pneumonia* from an infected Hickman catheter. *Eur. J. Clin. Microbiol. Infect. Dis.* **9:**345–347.
83. **Maesen, F. P. V., B. I. Davies, and J. P. Teengs.** 1986. Pefloxacin in acute exacerbations of chronic bronchitis. *J. Antimicrob. Chemother.* **16:**379–388.
84. **Maiche, A. G.** 1991. Use of fluoroquinolones in the immunocompromised host. *Eur. J. Clin. Microbiol. Infect. Dis.* **10:**361–367.
85. **Maple, P., J. Hamilton-Miller, and W. Brumfitt.** 1989. Ciprofloxacin resistance in methicillin- and gentamicin-resistant *Staphylococcus aureus*. *Eur. J. Clin. Microbiol. Infect. Dis.* **9:**622–624.
86. **Maple, P., J. M. T. Hamilton-Miller, and W. Brumfitt.** 1991. Differing activities of quinolones against ciprofloxacin-susceptible and ciprofloxacin-resistant, methicillin-resistant *Staphylococcus aureus*. *Antimicrob. Agents Chemother.* **35:**345–350.
87. **Mehtar, S., Y. Drabu, and P. Blakemore.** 1986. Ciprofloxacin in the treatment of infections caused by gentamicin-resistant gram-negative bacteria. *Eur. J. Clin. Microbiol.* **5:**248–251.
88. **Milatovic, D., and I. Braveny.** 1987. Development of resistance during antibiotic therapy. *Eur. J. Clin. Microbiol.* **6:**234–244.
89. **Møller, J. K.** 1989. Antimicrobial usage and microbial resistance in a university hospital during a seven-year period. *J. Antimicrob. Chemother.* **24:**983–992.
90. **Moniot-Ville, N., J. Guibert, N. Moreau, J. F. Acar, E. Collatz, and L. Gutmann.** 1991. Mechanisms of quinolone resistance in a clinical isolate of *Escherichia coli* highly resistant to fluoroquinolones but susceptible to nalidixic acid. *Antimicrob. Agents Chemother.* **35:**519–523.
91. **Moody, J. A., C. E. Fasching, D. N. Gerding, and L. R. Peterson.** 1990. Association between changes in plasmid content or outer membrane proteins and increased susceptibility to beta-lactam or aminoglycoside antibiotics among *Pseudomonas aeruginosa* after *in vitro* and *in vivo* exposure to ciprofloxacin. *Curr. Ther. Res.* **48:**427–433.
92. **Muder, R. R., C. Brennen, A. M. Goetz, M. M. Wagener, and J. D. Rihs.** 1991. Association with prior fluoroquinolone therapy of widespread ciprofloxacin resistance among gram-negative isolates in a Veterans Affairs medical center. *Antimicrob. Agents Chemother.* **35:**256–258.
93. **Mulligan, M. E., P. J. Ruane, L. Johnston, P. Wong, J. P. Wheelock, K. MacDonald, J. F. Reinhardt, C. C. Johnson, B. Statner, I. Blomquist, J. McCarthy, W. O'Brien, S. Gardner, L. Hammer, and D. M. Citron.** 1987. Ciprofloxacin for eradication of methicillin-resistant *Staphylococcus aureus* colonization. *Am. J. Med.* **82**(Suppl. 4A)**:**215–219.

94. **Murray, B. E.** 1989. Impact of fluoroquinolones on the gastrointestinal flora. *Rev. Infect. Dis.* **11**(Suppl. 5):S1372–1378.
95. **Naber, K. G.** 1989. Use of quinolones in urinary tract infections and prostatitis. *Rev. Infect. Dis.* **11**(Suppl. 5):S1321–S1337.
96. **Nakanishi, N., S. Yoshida, H. Wakebe, M. Inoue, T. Yamaguchi, and S. Mitsuhashi.** 1991. Mechanisms of clinical resistance to fluoroquinolones in *Staphylococcus aureus*. *Antimicrob. Agents Chemother.* **35:**2562–2567.
97. **Nakashima, M., M. Kanamaru, T. Uematsu, A. Takiguchi, A. Mizuno, T. Itaya, F. Kawahara, T. Ooie, S. Saito, H. Uchida, and K. Masuzawa.** 1988. Clinical pharmacokinetics and tolerance of fleroxacin in healthy male volunteers. *J. Antimicrob. Chemother.* **22**(Suppl. D):133–144.
98. **Neill, M. A., S. M. Opal, J. Heelan, R. Giusti, J. E. Cassidy, R. White, and K. H. Mayer.** 1991. Failure of ciprofloxacin to eradicate convalescent fecal excretion after acute salmonellosis: experience during an outbreak in health care workers. *Ann. Intern. Med.* **114:**195–199.
99. **Neuman, M., and A. Esanu.** 1988. Gaps and perspectives of new fluoroquinolones. *Drugs Exp. Clin. Res.* **14:**385–391.
100. **Ogle, J. W., L. B. Reller, and M. L. Vasil.** 1988. Development of resistance in *Pseudomonas aeruginosa* to imipenem, norfloxacin, and ciprofloxacin during therapy: proof provided by typing with a DNA probe. *J. Infect. Dis.* **157:**743–748.
101. **Parry, M. F., K. B. Panzer, and M. E. Yukna.** 1989. Quinolone resistance: susceptibility data from a 300-bed community hospital. *Am. J. Med.* **87**(Suppl. 5A):12S–15S.
102. **Pecquet, S. S., T. Jensen, and E. F. Hvidberg.** 1987. Effect of oral ofloxacin on fecal bacteria in human volunteers. *Antimicrob. Agents Chemother.* **31:**124–125.
103. **Peréz-Trallero, E., J. M. Garcia-Arenzana, J. A. Jimenez, and A. Peris.** 1990. Therapeutic failure and selection of resistance to quinolones in a case of pneumococcal pneumonia treated with ciprofloxacin. *Eur. J. Clin. Microbiol. Infect. Dis.* **9:**905–906.
104. **Peterson, L. R.** 1986. Animal models: the *in vivo* evaluation of ciprofloxacin. *J. Antimicrob. Chemother.* **18**(Suppl. D.):55–64.
105. **Peterson, L. R., J. N. Quick, B. Jensen, S. Homann, S. Johnson, J. Tenquist, C. Shanholtzer, R. A. Petzel, L. Sinn, and D. N. Gerding.** 1990. Emergence of ciprofloxacin resistance in nosocomial methicillin-resistant *Staphylococcus aureus* (MRSA) isolates during ciprofloxacin plus rifampin therapy for MRSA colonization. *Arch. Intern. Med.* **150:**2151–2155.
106. **Petruccelli, B. P., G. S. Murphy, J. L. Sanchez, S. Walz, R. DeFraites, J. Gelnett, R. L. Haberberger, P. Echeverria, and D. N. Taylor.** 1992. Treatment of traveler's diarrhea with ciprofloxacin and loperamide. *J. Infect. Dis.* **165:**557–560.
107. **Phillips, G., B. E. Johnson, and J. Ferguson.** 1990. The loss of antibiotic activity of ciprofloxacin by photodegradation. *J. Antimicrob. Chemother.* **26:**783–789.
108. **Piddock, L. J. V., and R. Wise.** 1989. Mechanisms of resistance to quinolones and clinical perspectives. *J. Antimicrob. Chemother.* **23:**475–483.
109. **Piercy, E. A., D. Barbaro, J. P. Luby, and P. A. Mackowiak.** 1989. Ciprofloxacin for methicillin-resistant *Staphylococcus aureus* infections. *Antimicrob. Agents Chemother.* **33:**128–130.
110. **Polk, R. E., D. P. Healy, J. Sahai, L. Drwal, and E. Racht.** 1989. Effect of ferrous sulfate and multivitamins with zinc on absorption of ciprofloxacin in normal volunteers. *Antimicrob. Agents Chemother.* **33:**1841–1844.
111. **Preiksaitis, J. K., L. Thompson, G. K. M. Harding, T. J. Marrie, S. Hoban, and A. R. Ronald.** 1981. A comparison of the efficacy of nalidixic acid and cephalexin in bacteriuric women and their effect on fecal and periurethral carriage of *Enterobacteriaceae*. *J. Infect. Dis.* **143:**603–608.
112. **Rautelin, H., O.-V. Renkonen, and T. U. Kosunen.** 1991. Emergence of fluoroquinolone resistance in *Campylobacter jejuni* and *Campylobacter coli* in subjects from Finland. *Antimicrob. Agents Chemother.* **35:**2065–2069.
113. **Raviglione, M. C., J. F. Boyle, P. Mauriuz, A. Paublos-Mendez, H. Cortes, and A. Merlo.** 1990. Ciprofloxacin-resistant methicillin-resistant *Staphylococcus aureus* in an acute-care hospital. *Antimicrob. Agents Chemother.* **34:**2050–2054.
114. **Righter, J.** 1990. Pneumococcal meningitis during intravenous ciprofloxacin therapy. *Am. J. Med.* **88:**548.
115. **Ronald, A. R., M. Turck, and R. G. Petersdorf.** 1966. A critical evaluation of nalidixic acid in urinary-tract infections. *N. Engl. J. Med.* **275:**1081–1089.
116. **Rylander, M., S. R. Norrby, and R. Svard.** 1987. Norfloxacin versus cotrimoxazole for treatment of urinary tract infections in adults: microbiological results of a coordinated multicentre study. *Scand. J. Infect. Dis.* **19:**551–557.
117. **Schaefler, S.** 1989. Methicillin-resistant strains of *Staphylococcus aureus* resistant to quinolones. *J. Clin. Microbiol.* **27:**335–336.
118. **Scully, B. E., M. Nakatomi, C. Ores, S. Davidson, and H. C. Neu.** 1987. Ciprofloxacin therapy in cystic fibrosis. *Am. J. Med.* **82**(Suppl. 4A):196–201.

119. **Scully, B. E., H. C. Neu, M. F. Parry, and W. Mandell.** 1986. Oral ciprofloxacin therapy of infections due to *Pseudomonas aeruginosa. Lancet* **ii:**819–822.
120. **Shah, P. M.** 1988. Influence of quinolones on human microflora. *Quin. Bull.* **4:**15–20.
121. **Shalit, I., S. A. Berger, A. Gorea, and H. Frimerman.** 1989. Widespread quinolone resistance among methicillin-resistant *Staphylococcus aureus* isolates in a general hospital. *Antimicrob. Agents Chemother.* **33:**593–594.
122. **Shalit, I., H. R. Stutman, M. I. Marks, S. A. Chartrand, and B. C. Hilman.** 1987. Randomized study of two dosage regimens of ciprofloxacin for treating chronic bronchopulmonary infection in patients with cystic fibrosis. *Am. J. Med.* **82**(Suppl. 4A)**:**189–195.
123. **Sinn, L. M., B. Jensen, L. R. Peterson, and C. E. Fasching.** 1990. In vitro development of high-level resistance to ciprofloxacin in methicillin-resistant *Staphylococcus aureus,* p. 9, abstr. A-51. *Abstr. 90th Annu. Meet. Am. Soc. Microbiol. 1990.*
124. **Smith, J. T.** 1986. Frequency and expression of mutational resistance to the 4-quinolone antibacterials. *Scand. J. Infect. Dis. Suppl.* **49:**115–123.
125. **Smith, S. M., R. H. K. Eng, P. Bais, P. Fan-Havard, and F. Tecson-Tumang.** 1990. Epidemiology of ciprofloxacin resistance among patients with methicillin-resistant *Staphylococcus aureus. J. Antimicrob. Chemother.* **26:**567–572.
126. **Stamey, T. A., and J. Bragonje.** 1976. Resistance to nalidixic acid: a misconception due to underdosage. *J. Am. Med. Assoc.* **236:**1857–1860.
127. **Swedish Study Group.** 1988. Therapy of acute and chronic gram-negative osteomyelitis with ciprofloxacin. *J. Antimicrob. Chemother.* **22:**221–228.
127a. **Tauxe, R. V.** 1993. Growing threat of multiply resistant *Salmonella, Shigella*, and cholera, session 135. *Program 93rd Gen. Meet. Am. Soc. Microbiol. 1993.*
128. **Tebas, P., R. Martinez Ruiz, F. Roman, P. Mendaza, J. C. Rodriguez Diaz, R. Daza, and J. M. L. de Letona.** 1991. Early resistance to rifampin and ciprofloxacin in the treatment of right-sided *Staphylococcus aureus* endocarditis. *J. Infect. Dis.* **163:**204–205.
129. **The Medical Letter on Drugs and Therapeutics.** 1988. Ciprofloxacin. *Med. Lett. Drug Ther.* **30:**11–13.
130. **The Medical Letter on Drugs and Therapeutics.** 1991. Ofloxacin. *Med. Lett. Drug Ther.* **33:**71–73.
131. **Trucksis, M., D. C. Hooper, and J. S. Wolfson.** 1991. Emerging resistance to fluoroquinolones in staphylococci: an alert. *Ann. Intern. Med.* **114:**424–425.
132. **Tsukamura, M., E. Nakamura, S. Yoshi, and H. Amano.** 1985. Therapeutic effect of a new antibacterial substance ofloxacin (DL8280) on pulmonary tuberculosis. *Am. Rev. Respir. Dis.* **131:**352–356.
133. **Valtonen, V., L. Karppinen, and A.-L. Kariniemi.** 1989. A comparative study of ciprofloxacin and conventional therapy in the treatment of patients with chronic lower leg ulcers infected with *Pseudomonas aeruginosa* and other gram-negative rods. *Scand. J. Infect. Dis. Suppl.* **60:**79–83.
134. **Van Landuyt, H. W., K. Magerman, and B. Gordts.** 1990. The importance of the quinolones in antibacterial therapy. *J. Antimicrob. Chemother.* **26**(Suppl. D)**:**1–6.
135. **Voss, A., and I. Braveny.** 1990. Development of resistance to new ß-lactams and ciprofloxacin during therapy: a prospective study, abstr. 977. *Program Abstr. 30th Intersci. Conf. Antimicrob. Agents Chemother.*
136. **Wallace, R. J., Jr., G. Bedsole, G. Sumter, C. V. Sanders, L. C. Steere, B. A. Brown, J. Smith, and D. R. Graham.** 1990. Activities of ciprofloxacin and ofloxacin against rapidly growing mycobacteria with demonstration of acquired resistance following single-drug therapy. *Antimicrob. Agents Chemother.* **34:**65–70.
137. **Watanabe, M., Y. Kotera, K. Yosue, M. Inoue, and S. Mitsuhashi.** 1990. In vitro emergence of quinolone-resistant mutants *Escherichia coli, Enterobacter cloacae,* and *Serratia marcescens. Antimicrob. Agents Chemother.* **34:**173–175.
138. **Wolfson, J., and D. C. Hooper.** 1988. Norfloxacin: a new targeted fluoroquinolone antimicrobial agent. *Ann. Intern. Med.* **108:**238–251.
139. **Wolfson, J. S.** 1989. Quinolone antimicrobial agents: adverse effects and bacterial resistance. *Eur. J. Clin. Microbiol. Infect. Dis.* **8:**1080–1092.
140. **Wolfson, J. S., and D. C. Hooper.** 1989. Bacterial resistance to quinolones: mechanisms and clinical importance. *Rev. Infect. Dis.* **11**(Suppl. 5)**:**S960–S968.
141. **Wolfson, J. S., and D. C. Hooper.** 1989. Fluoroquinolone antimicrobial agents. *Clin. Microbiol. Rev.* **2:**378–424.

*Quinolone Antimicrobial Agents, 2nd ed.*
Edited by David C. Hooper and John S. Wolfson


*Chapter 7*

# Quinolones and Eukaryotic Topoisomerases

***Thomas D. Gootz and Neil Osheroff***

An extensive body of evidence indicates that DNA gyrase is the primary target through which quinolones exert their antibacterial activities. However, relatively little work has been done to examine the effects of quinolones on other types of topoisomerases in bacteria or eukaryotes. Topoisomerases fall into two general categories (types I and II) based on the biochemical mechanism responsible for DNA strand passage. Type I enzymes characteristically catalyze single-stranded-DNA cleavage and strand passage in the absence of ATP, while type II topoisomerases mediate double-strand breakage with passage of another helix through the transient break by a process requiring energy from the hydrolysis of ATP (102, 135, 146). The DNA strand passage reactions mediated by topoisomerases are essential for maintaining the appropriate state of DNA supercoiling in the cell, for efficient replication of DNA, and for separation of daughter DNA molecules during cell division (6, 38, 61, 135). Type I and II topoisomerases are found in all cells and act in concert to maintain the optimal DNA conformation in the cell.

***Thomas D. Gootz*** • Department of Immunology and Infectious Diseases, Central Research Division, Pfizer Inc., Groton, Connecticut 06340. ***Neil Osheroff*** • Department of Biochemistry, School of Medicine, Vanderbilt University, Nashville, Tennessee 37232-0146.

Eukaryotic topoisomerase II can catenate, relax, and unknot DNA by a duplex strand passage mechanism that is analogous to that conducted by the bacterial enzyme (135). In addition to their similar biochemical mechanisms, bacterial DNA gyrase and eukaryotic topoisomerase II (referred to simply as topoisomerase II) also share significant homology at the amino acid level (49, 52, 88, 139, 141). Studies have shown that regions in the N terminus and the middle portion of the eukaryotic type II monomer share significant homology with the B and A subunits, respectively, of DNA gyrase (88). This conservation of sequence homology suggests that a gene fusion event between the prokaryotic A and B subunits occurred during the course of evolution to produce the single gene encoding the eukaryotic type II monomer (88). These high degrees of homology, which appear to be common among the type II topoisomerases, are not found with the type I enzymes (30, 140).

Given the similarities in biochemical mechanisms and amino acid sequences between bacterial DNA gyrase and topoisomerase II, it is reasonable to question whether quinolone antibacterial agents demonstrate inhibitory activity against topoisomerase II from higher organisms. It has been generally accepted that quinolones at concentrations routinely achieved in vivo do not affect the latter enzyme (11, 62, 73). The high selectivity of nalidixic acid and the newer fluoroquinolones for DNA gyrase compared with that of the eukaryotic enzyme has been cited in numerous reports (62, 73, 91, 105). More recently, however, several studies have described new quinolones that appear to have lost this selectivity for DNA gyrase and show significant effects against eukaryotic topoisomerase II in vitro at concentrations that are clinically relevant. These quinolones come from several different structural series, and classical structure-activity relationships characterizing their interaction with topoisomerase II are beginning to emerge. In addition, several studies have investigated the effects of fluoroquinolones on cultured eukaryotic cells. Some results have correlated the cytotoxic effects obtained with these newer quinolones to their inhibition of topoisomerase II in vitro. It has been suggested (7) that such studies are relevant in assessing the potential toxicity of new quinolone antibacterial agents in order to advance only those agents with potent DNA gyrase inhibitory activity and no effect on mammalian topoisomerase II.

This chapter reviews the literature with respect to the reported effects of quinolones on topoisomerase II in vitro and considers those reports relevant to the effects of quinolones on whole cells. The initial part of the chapter will describe in more detail some of the enzymatic properties of topoisomerase II and the consequences to the cell of the actions of known inhibitors of this important enzyme.

## EUKARYOTIC DNA TOPOISOMERASE II

### Physiological Roles and Regulation

DNA topoisomerase II is a highly conserved enzyme (102, 107, 135, 146) that is essential to the survival of eukaryotic cells (35, 52, 61, 143). It is required for the unlinking (i.e., segregation) of daughter chromosomes during mitosis (35, 61, 144) and meiosis (119) and plays necessary roles in chromosome condensation (3, 97, 142, 151) and the maintenance of proper chromosome structure (12, 38, 39, 46, 47). In addition, considerable evidence points to important functions for the enzyme in DNA replication, transcription, and recombination (6, 24, 34, 77, 102, 107, 119, 135, 146).

The physiological concentration and activity of topoisomerase II vary over cell and growth cycles in a manner that reflects the enzyme's fundamental involvement in DNA replication and chromosome segregation. First, enzyme levels fluctuate throughout the cell cycle, increasing more than twofold and peaking at the time of mitosis (22, 55). In addition, topoisomerase II concentration and activity are sensitive to the proliferative state of cells and are in some cases increased in rapidly growing cells >100-fold over levels in slow-growing, quiescent, or differentiated cells (14, 37, 54, 59, 70, 96, 132, 133). Finally, enzyme levels and/or activities increase 3- to 20-fold following the treatment of cells with serum, mitogens, or transforming viruses (27, 48, 70, 92, 137).

Little is known concerning the processes that are responsible for the physiological regulation of topoisomerase II. Alterations in the level of transcription of the gene for the type II enzyme (41) and changes in the enzyme's stability (55) have been reported. Phosphorylation also may play a role in the cellular modulation of topoisomerase II. The enzyme exists as a phosphoprotein in vivo (2, 56, 80, 121), and modification by either casein kinase II (1) or protein kinase C (123) stimulates its activity two- to threefold in vitro. Metabolic labeling studies have implicated both of these kinases in the enzyme's physiological modifications (2, 121).

### Catalytic Cycle

All of the cellular activities of topoisomerase II stem directly from the mechanism by which it alters DNA topology (102, 107). Thus, before the enzyme's physiological functions can be effectively dissected or its drug interactions fully exploited, it is imperative to understand the pathway by which this important enzyme carries out its catalytic cycle.

Topoisomerase II alters the topological state of nucleic acids by passing an intact helix of DNA through a transient break that it generates in a separate helix. As a consequence of its double-stranded DNA passage reaction, the enzyme can relax (i.e., remove superhelical twists) from supercoiled DNA as well as knot-unknot or catenate-decatenate double-stranded nucleic acids (102, 107, 135, 146). Unlike its prokaryotic counterpart, DNA gyrase (135, 146), purified eukaryotic topoisomerase II has no intrinsic ability to introduce superhelical twists into DNA. The double-stranded DNA passage reaction of topoisomerase II takes place at the expense of ATP hydrolysis and requires the presence of magnesium (107, 146). Although the enzyme's mechanism appears to be concerted and quite complex in nature, it can be broken down into a series of discrete and straightforward steps (107). The reaction steps that make up the catalytic cycle of topoisomerase II are shown in Fig. 1, which depicts one round of enzyme-mediated DNA relaxation. Two points should be mentioned before the catalytic cycle is discussed. First, as a result of its double-stranded DNA passage mechanism, topoisomerase II removes two superhelical twists per reaction cycle. Second, only the topological state of DNA is altered by the enzyme's actions; both the nucleic acid sequence and the chemical structure of the relaxed DNA product are identical to those of the original supercoiled substrate.

The catalytic cycle of topoisomerase II comprises at least six steps. A brief description follows. (i) Topoisomerase II binds to DNA at points of helix-helix juxtaposition (67, 156). Presumably, one of these helices is the DNA segment that the enzyme cleaves (i.e., cleavage helix) and the other is the segment that it passes through the break (i.e., passage helix). Neither DNA recognition nor enzyme DNA binding requires cofactors of any kind (101, 156). (ii) In the presence of a

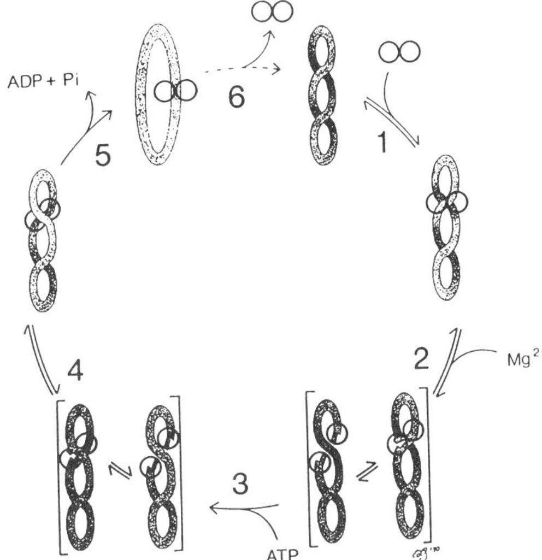


**Figure 1.** Catalytic cycle of topoisomerase II. The homodimeric enzyme is represented by paired circles. The double-stranded DNA passage reaction of topoisomerase II comprises the following six steps: (1) substrate recognition and binding, (2) pre-strand passage DNA cleavage and religation, (3) double-stranded DNA passage, (4) post-strand passage DNA cleavage and religation, (5) ATP hydrolysis, and (6) enzyme turnover. Transient DNA cleavage complexes are shown in brackets.

divalent cation (magnesium is used in vivo) (101, 106, 124), topoisomerase II transiently cuts and religates the cleavage helix (102, 107). This DNA cleavage-religation equilibrium can be readily reversed by the removal of the divalent cation (101), the addition of salt (85, 106), or a shift to suboptimal temperatures (68, 69, 85, 118). Cleavage takes place at preferred sequences within the nucleic acid backbone (4, 85, 94, 106, 124, 125). During cleavage, the enzyme forms a covalent linkage with the newly generated DNA 5′ termini via a phosphotyrosyl bond (122). Each cleaved DNA strand is complexed with a separate subunit of the homodimeric type II enzyme (155). This covalent topoisomerase II-DNA complex is referred to as the cleavage complex (45). (iii) Upon ATP binding, the enzyme-DNA complex undergoes a structural reorientation (102, 105, 107). During this reorientation, the passage helix is translocated through the transient double-stranded break made in the cleavage helix. (iv) Following DNA strand passage, topoisomerase II once again establishes a DNA cleavage-religation equilibrium (107). Hence, the enzyme generates cleavage complexes both prior to and following strand passage. While the properties of these complexes are similar, the post-strand passage cleavage complex is intrinsically approximately fourfold more stable than its pre-strand passage counterpart (100, 118). (v) Topoisomerase II hydrolyzes its ATP cofactor to ADP and $P_i$ (102, 107), which in turn triggers (vi) enzyme turnover (i.e., recycling). As described in the following section, the ability to analyze the individual steps of the enzyme's catalytic cycle has contributed greatly to our understanding of the actions of topoisomerase II-targeted drugs.

## TOPOISOMERASE II-TARGETED ANTINEOPLASTIC DRUGS

Beyond its critical physiological functions, topoisomerase II is the target for some of the most potent antineoplastic drugs currently used for the treatment of human cancers. Among the topoisomerase II-targeted drugs in clinical use are the epipodophyllotoxins (etoposide and teniposide), 4′-(9-acridinylamino)methane-sulfon-*m*-anisidide (*m*-AMSA), adriamycin, and mitoxantrone (83, 86, 127, 159).

Although all of these compounds inhibit the enzyme's overall catalytic activity, their clinical efficacies correlate with their ability to stabilize covalent topoisomerase II-DNA cleavage complexes (83, 86). (In other words, they shift the enzyme's DNA cleavage-religation equilibria toward the cleavage event.) At least in vitro, both the enzyme's pre-strand passage (19, 103, 110, 117) and post-strand passage (118) DNA cleavage complexes are targets for these drugs. For several years, the tight coupling of the DNA cleavage and religation reactions of topoisomerase II proved to be a formidable stumbling block to describing the detailed mechanism of drug action. While it generally was assumed that antineoplastic agents enhanced enzyme-mediated breakage by inhibiting DNA religation (83, 127), it was impossible to confirm this assumption until assays that uncoupled religation from the enzyme's DNA cleavage reaction were developed. Recently, three different assays specific for religation have been established. The first takes advantage of the fact that topoisomerase II-DNA cleavage complexes established in the presence of calcium (rather than magnesium) can be trapped in a kinetically competent form following chelation of the divalent cation (106, 155). The other two take advantage of the finding that the enzyme's religation reaction is less sensitive to extremes of temperature (either high or low) than is its DNA cleavage reaction (68, 69, 85, 106, 118). By determining the effects of etoposide and *m*-AMSA on the apparent first-order rate constant for topoisomerase II-mediated DNA religation in the assay systems described above, it was demonstrated experimentally that these two structurally disparate antineoplastic drugs stabilize enzyme-DNA cleavage complexes primarily by impairing the ability of topoisomerase II to religate cleaved nucleic acids (103, 117, 118).

Despite the fact that structure-activity relationships have been established within individual drug series (9, 87), the common features that link these structurally disparate agents are not yet known. Even the site of drug action has yet to be characterized. All of the topoisomerase II-targeted antineoplastic drugs discussed above interact with DNA, but there is no common mode of binding (the first two are nonintercalative, while the last three are intercalative [21, 120, 147, 150]). Moreover, there is no correlation between drug potency and either drug-DNA binding affinity (21, 150) or binding thermodynamics (145). Fluorescence-quenching data suggest that etoposide may be able to interact with topoisomerase II in the absence of DNA (104). However, if parallels with gyrase-targeted (129) or topoisomerase I-targeted (57) drugs prevail, it is likely that the site of drug action is the enzyme-DNA complex.

Because of the mechanism of drug action, cells that are treated with topoisomerase II-targeted agents accumulate high levels of protein-associated breaks in their genetic material (83, 86, 127, 157). The pathway that leads from increased concentrations of cleavage complexes to cell death has not been fully elucidated. However, topoisomerase II-mediated illegitimate recombination (5, 33, 82, 109, 111, 127) and cellular events resembling apoptosis (76) both have been implicated. In addition, the lethal processing of these cleavage complexes appears to require ATP (81), calcium (13), and protein synthesis (20, 128) and is exacerbated by DNA transcription (60, 127, 157) and replication (127, 157). In support of a role for DNA replication in drug-induced cell death, topoisomerase II-targeted agents appear to be considerably more lethal in S phase (during which DNA synthesis takes place) than in any other phase of the cell cycle (40, 89, 127). Treated cells generally progress until $G_2$ phase, dying prior to mitosis (40, 127).

Since topoisomerase II-targeted drugs act primarily by converting the type II enzyme into a cellular poison (79), the higher the physiological content of topoisomerase II, the more sensitive the cell is towards these agents (14, 133, 159). Enzyme levels are usually elevated in rapidly proliferating or neoplastic cells (14, 37, 54, 59). Thus, clinically aggressive tumors appear to be most sensitive to these drugs (14, 133). Hypersensitivity to topoisomerase II-targeted agents has been associated with an overexpression of the enzyme or mutations in genes that encode DNA repair systems (31, 75, 79, 98, 133). Drug resistance has been correlated with decreased drug accumulation (10), decreased expression of topoisomerase II (18, 32, 44, 112), or mutations in topoisomerase II that decrease its sensitivity towards these agents (83, 86, 127, 159). Only three drug-resistant mammalian cell lines containing altered type II topoisomerase have been characterized to the extent that the mutant enzyme and/or gene has been isolated (17, 29, 134, 160). While two of the lines display broad resistance to different classes of topoisomerase II-targeted drugs (29, 134), one line (HL-60/AMSA) is capable of distinguishing between intercalative and nonintercalative agents (160). Therefore, the interaction domains for different classes of antineoplastic drugs appear to be similar but not identical. Thus far, the genetic alteration for only one mutant type II topoisomerase has been identified. Drug resistance in the enzyme from human leukemic CCRF-CEM cells correlates with the substitution of glutamine for arginine at position 449 (17). This residue in the eukaryotic enzyme is homologous to arginine 413 in the B subunit of *Escherichia coli* DNA gyrase (152).

## REPORTED EFFECTS OF QUINOLONES ON THE CATALYTIC ACTIVITY OF EUKARYOTIC TOPOISOMERASE II IN VITRO

As in the case of the classical antineoplastic agents, the effects of quinolones on topoisomerase II have been assessed by employing assays that measure either catalytic activity or the potential of the drugs to stimulate enzyme-mediated DNA cleavage. The methods employed for measuring catalytic relaxation, catenation, or unknotting activity with purified topoisomerase II and various DNA substrates have been reviewed elsewhere (8). Such assays are most useful when performed in a manner that allows quantitation of the effects of a test agent, as shown in Fig. 2 and 3 (7). In Fig. 2, a time course is established, in this instance measuring the conversion of knotted phage P4 DNA to its simple circular unknotted form by purified calf thymus topoisomerase II. Because of its less compact structure, the unknotted form fails to migrate into agarose gels during electrophoresis. In this example, the time course of the unknotting reaction in the absence of drug allows the definition of assay parame-

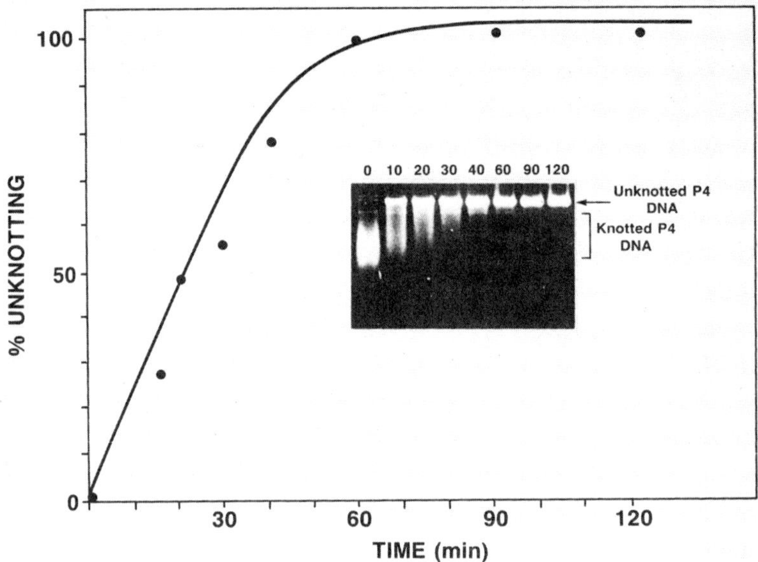


**Figure 2.** Time course study illustrating the unknotting of P4 head DNA to its simple circular form by calf thymus topoisomerase II. The inset is a photograph of the ethidium bromide-stained DNA (after electrophoresis) time course study indicating relative positions of the unknotted and knotted P4 DNAs at the indicated times (in minutes). Reproduced from reference 7 with permission.

ters that provide linear reaction kinetics, where 50% of the DNA has been converted to the unknotted form, as determined from photographs of ethidium bromide-stained gels. Using these conditions, the inhibitory effects of test agents on the catalytic activity of topoisomerase II can be determined quantitatively by measuring a 50% completion point in the presence of each drug ($IC_{50}$). As shown in Fig. 3, the inhibitory effects of quinolones on the unknotting activity of calf thymus topoisomerase II can be determined in this quantitative manner. In this example, the relatively higher inhibitory potency of the antitumor agent ellipticine compared with the potencies of ciprofloxacin, norfloxacin, and quinolone CP-67,015 is evident (7).

Several investigators have assessed the effects of quinolones on the various catalytic activities of topoisomerase II. As reviewed previously (51), most of these studies have found that the quinolones developed for clinical use are not potent inhibitors of these activities in vitro.

Miller et al. found that nalidixic and oxolinic acids had $IC_{50}$s of 500 and 100 $\mu$g/ml, respectively, for decatenation mediated by topoisomerase II isolated from HeLa cell nuclei (91). A similar degree of activity was found by Hussy et al., who used topoisomerase II isolated from calf thymus nuclei (73). These investigators determined the following $IC_{50}$s for ciprofloxacin, norfloxacin, ofloxacin, and nalidixic acid by using a catenation reaction: 150, 300, 1,300, and 1,000 $\mu$g/ml, respectively. Such studies also suggested that there was no correlation between the potencies of quinolones against bacterial DNA gyrase and their relative levels of inhibition of topoisomerase II (73). Using an assay for measuring the relaxation activity of topoisomerase II isolated from *Drosophila melanogaster* nuclei, Osheroff et al. found $K_i$s for nalidixic and oxolinic acids of 625 and 340 $\mu$g/ml, respectively (105). These relatively high drug levels required for inhibition may explain the failure of earlier studies to demonstrate any inhibi-

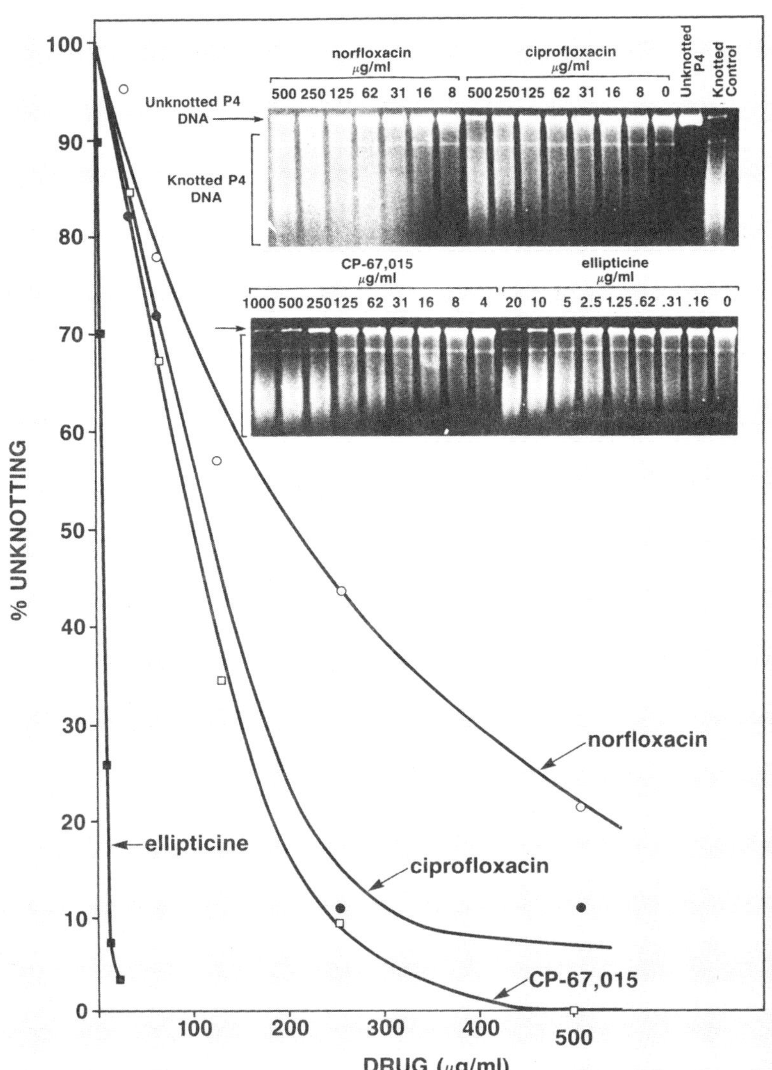


**Figure 3.** Comparative inhibitory effects of different quinolones in the P4 unknotting assay. Norfloxacin, ciprofloxacin, and CP-67,015 are representative of the quinolones tested; levels of these drugs needed to inhibit unknotting are much higher than the level of ellipticine (representative of the antitumor compounds) required. The inset is a photograph of the ethidium bromide-stained DNA agarose gel after electrophoresis of reactions inhibited by norfloxacin, ciprofloxacin, CP-67,015, and ellipticine, from which the percentage of inhibition of unknotting versus that of the drug-free control was calculated after densitometric analysis. To the right of the ciprofloxacin data are data for the knotted (enzyme-free P4 DNA substrate) and completely unknotted DNA controls. Reproduced from reference 7 with permission.

tion of *D. melanogaster* and rat liver topoisomerase II by low levels of nalidixic acid analogs (73, 84, 105, 108). In contrast, coumermycin A1 and novobiocin, two DNA gyrase B subunit inhibitors, are 10- to 100-fold more potent at inhibiting topoisomerase II relaxation activity in vitro than are quinolones (105).

A number of investigators have characterized the inhibitory effects of quinolones on topoisomerase II relative to the drugs' inhibition of DNA gyrase and expressed results in terms of a selectivity ratio. Hoshino et al. (65) studied the inhibition of *E. coli* DNA gyrase supercoiling activity compared with the DNA relaxation activity of calf thymus topoisomerase II by nalidixic acid and fluoroquinolones. The data obtained indicate that $IC_{50}$s generated against gyrase with ofloxacin, ciprofloxacin, lomefloxacin, enoxacin, CI-934, and nalidixic acid ranged between 0.13 and 23.0 $\mu$g/ml (Table 1). The $IC_{50}$s against topoisomerase II-mediated relaxation varied considerably, with ofloxacin being the least inhibitory and CI-934 having the lowest $IC_{50}$. These results confirmed earlier studies indicating that there is no direct correlation between inhibitory potencies against bacterial and mammalian enzymes for the quinolones studied. Those authors also expressed their results in terms of a selectivity ratio by dividing the $IC_{50}$ obtained for topoisomerase II by 3he $IC_{50}$ generated against DNA gyrase. By means of this exercise, it was concluded that ofloxacin and ciprofloxacin demonstrated a high selectivity for DNA gyrase, while enoxacin, CI-934, and nalidixic acid possessed poor selectivity (65). Such calculations may prove misleading when the relative inhibitory potencies of quinolones against these enzymes are compared, and it should be kept in mind that the absolute inhibitory levels against topoisomerase II are also important to consider. For example, while nalidixic acid had the lowest selectivity ratio of the quinolones in this study (Table 1), it also had one of the highest $IC_{50}$s against topoisomerase II.

This type of selectivity analysis has been reported for various quinolones in other studies (73), which in general agree that relatively high concentrations of compound are required to inhibit the catalytic activity of topoisomerase II in vitro.

While it has been established that some quinolones are more active than others at inhibiting the catalytic activity of topoisomerase II, very few studies have attempted to probe the structure-activity relationship of quinolones that may account for these differences. Recently, however, Hoshino et al. (64) studied several structurally related analogs of ofloxacin for their inhibitory effects on DNA gyrase supercoiling and calf thymus topoisomerase II relaxation activities. Their study presents some of the most direct evidence that the structural features of quinolones that confer potency against DNA gyrase do not necessarily impart increased inhibition of topoisomerase II. As illustrated in Table 2, the stereochemistry at the 3 position of the oxazine ring significantly influenced the relative potency against each enzyme (64). The pure S isomer of ofloxacin, DR-3355, was twofold more potent than ofloxacin against DNA gyrase, and it was severalfold more inhibitory than either

**Table 1.** Selectivities of quinolones

| Compound | $IC_{50}$ ($\mu$g/ml)[a] | | Selectivity ratio[b] |
|---|---|---|---|
| | DNA gyrase from *E. coli* KL-16[c] | Topoisomerase II from calf thymus[d] | |
| Ofloxacin | 0.76 | 1,870 | 2,461 |
| Ciprofloxacin | 0.13 | 155 | 1,192 |
| Lomefloxacin | 0.78 | 280 | 359 |
| Enoxacin | 1.72 | 93 | 54 |
| CI-934 | 3.55 | 64 | 18 |
| Nalidixic acid | 23.0 | 385 | 17 |

[a]Data are from Hoshino et al. (65).
[b]Determined by dividing $IC_{50}$ for topoisomerase II by $IC_{50}$ for DNA gyrase.
[c]Measured by DNA supercoiling assay.
[d]Measured by DNA relaxation assay.

**Table 2.** Influence of stereochemistry on the inhibitory activities of ofloxacin derivatives for DNA gyrase and topoisomerase II[a]

| Quinolone | | | $IC_{50}$[b] (μg/ml) | |
|---|---|---|---|---|
| | R[1] | R[2] | DNA gyrase | Topoisomerase II |
| Ofloxacin | $CH_3$ | H | 0.76 | 1,870 |
| DR-3355 | $CH_3$ | H | 0.38 | 1,380 |
| DR-3354 | H | $CH_3$ | 4.7 | 2,550 |
| DL-8165 | H | H | 3.1 | 178 |
| DN-9494 | $CH_2$ | $CH_2$ | 0.70 | 64 |

[a]Data are from Hoshino et al. (64).
[b]Concentration of drug that inhibits 50% of *E. coli* KL-16 DNA gyrase supercoiling activity or calf thymus topoisomerase II relaxation activity.

the corresponding pure R isomer (DR-3354), or the desmethyl derivative (DL-8165) in this regard. Interestingly, the desmethyl derivative was 10 times more active at inhibiting topoisomerase II than the corresponding methylated analogs. The exomethylene derivative (DN-9494) was the most potent analog against calf thymus topoisomerase II relaxation activity ($IC_{50}$ of 64 μg/ml), yet it was twofold less potent than the S isomer against gyrase. This divergence in potency with regard to stereochemistry and substitution on the oxazine ring for these ofloxacin derivatives implies that the active sites for DNA gyrase and topoisomerase II recognize different spatial characteristics of quinolones.

Given the relatively weak inhibition of the catalytic activity of topoisomerase II exhibited by quinolones in vitro, the relevance of this activity for the eukaryotic cell remains uncertain. Very few studies have attempted to establish whether there is a relationship between the topoisomerase II inhibition observed in vitro and cell viability. Oomori et al. (99), however, studied the cytotoxicities of several fluoroquinolones for HeLa cells in relation to their relative potencies against the relaxation activity of topoisomerase II purified from the same cell line. These investigators found the $IC_{50}$s for cell growth after 48 h of exposure to the drugs to be 253, 204, 140, 113, and 230 μg/ml for fleroxacin, ofloxacin, norfloxacin, ciprofloxacin, and nalidixic acid, respectively (99). $IC_{50}$s for relaxation inhibition were 193, 169, 132, 87.3, and 34.4 μg/ml for fleroxacin, nalidixic acid, ofloxacin, norfloxacin, and ciprofloxacin, respectively (99). The relationship between the inhibitory potencies of these agents against the enzyme and their cytotoxicities was linear. Interestingly, ciprofloxacin was also the most inhibitory quinolone against DNA, RNA, and protein synthesis as measured in this HeLa cell line (99). Those authors pointed out, however, that the inhibitory potencies observed with these quinolones were 2 orders of magnitude above the levels required for antibacterial activity.

## IN VITRO EFFECTS OF QUINOLONES ON TOPOISOMERASE I

A limited number of studies that evaluate the interactions of quinolones with eukaryotic topoisomerase I are available. Quinolones have been shown to be less inhibitory for *E. coli* topoisomerase I than for DNA gyrase. Tabary et al. (136) found that the $IC_{50}$s of pefloxacin, ciprofloxacin, norfloxacin, and ofloxacin against prokaryotic topoisomerase I ranged between 35 and 50 $\mu$g/ml in the relaxation assay. This level of relaxation inhibition was approximately 10-fold lower than what was observed against DNA gyrase supercoiling activity. It is not surprising, therefore, that little inhibition of eukaryotic topoisomerase I has been observed with quinolones (136). In one study (73), nalidixic acid and ofloxacin at concentrations of up to 1,000 $\mu$g/ml showed no inhibitory activities against calf thymus nuclear topoisomerase I relaxation activity. Norfloxacin and ciprofloxacin exhibited limited inhibition in these tests, with $IC_{50}$s between 300 and 400 $\mu$g/ml (73).

## ENHANCEMENT OF TOPOISOMERASE II-MEDIATED DNA CLEAVAGE BY QUINOLONES

The majority of studies in the literature that have investigated the effects of quinolones on eukaryotic topoisomerase II have studied inhibition of catalytic activity. While this is a valid approach that has also been used with the antitumor topoisomerase II inhibitors, it is not necessarily the most relevant parameter with which to correlate the cytotoxic potentials of these agents. As pointed out above, topoisomerase II-targeted drugs such as the epipodophyllotoxins stabilize a cleavage intermediate formed between double-stranded DNA and topoisomerase II in vitro. Formation of this cleavage complex also has been observed in DNA breakage assays using whole cells cultured in the presence of topoisomerase II inhibitors. A direct correlation between cell toxicity and cleavage complex stabilization by drug has been established for many topoisomerase II inhibitors and is a central theme of the "poison hypothesis" accounting for the cytotoxic effects of these drugs (79).

Given the relevance of cleavage complex formation to the mechanism of action of known topoisomerase II inhibitors, some studies have evaluated quinolones for their abilities to stimulate topoisomerase II-mediated DNA cleavage in vitro. As described above, the generation of linear DNA in the presence of topoisomerase II and drug is a stoichiometric process: the amount of linear DNA formed is dependent on the concentrations of enzyme, DNA, and drug (45, 103, 117, 118). These double-stranded-DNA breaks can be observed following treatment of the complexes with denaturing agents and protease, with subsequent electrophoresis of the DNA in agarose gels (7, 45). By quantitating the linear DNA cleavage products, the relative potency of topoisomerase II inhibitors can be assessed.

Nelson et al. (95) were the first to report that oxolinic acid stimulates DNA cleavage in vitro in the presence of T4 phage topoisomerase II (which has many characteristics in common with the eukaryotic enzyme). Barrett et al. (7) more thoroughly studied the effects of some newer quinolones on topoisomerase II purified from calf thymus. They found that ciprofloxacin, norfloxacin, oxolinic acid, and nalidixic acid were weak inhibitors of the catalytic unknotting and catenation activities of this enzyme. These quinolones also were not very active at inducing topoisomerase II-mediated DNA cleavage compared with the antitumor agent etoposide (7). Barrett et al. used two types of cleavage assays: one utilizing a nonradiolabeled DNA substrate and a second, which was more sensitive, employing a linearized DNA substrate end labeled with $^{32}P$. In the assay with radiolabeled substrate, ciprofloxacin stimulated enzyme-mediated DNA cleavage ($CC_{50}$ [concentration of drug that produces half-maximal DNA cleavage] of 120 $\mu$g/ml) but was 27-fold less potent than etoposide in this regard. That study, however, identified a novel 6,8-difluoro-7-pyridyl-4-quinolone, CP-67,015 (Fig. 4), that was significantly more potent than other quinolones

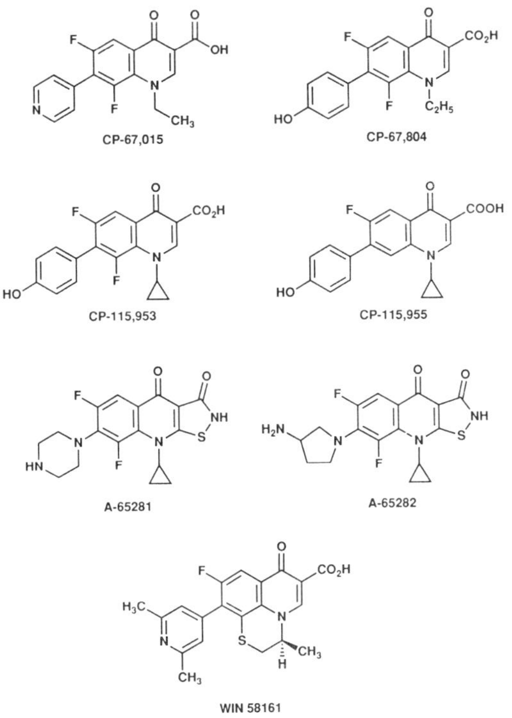

CP-67,015 CP-67,804

CP-115,953 CP-115,955

A-65281 A-65282

WIN 58161

**Figure 4.** Structures of novel quinolones that act against topoisomerase II.

in stimulating DNA cleavage. In the radiolabeled- and nonradiolabeled-DNA cleavage assays, CP-67,015 demonstrated $CC_{50}$s of 33 and 73 $\mu$g/ml, respectively (7). The linear DNA cleavage patterns generated in the presence of CP-67,015 in the assay with radiolabeled DNA showed qualitative and quantitative differences from those generated by etoposide (7). These results are consistent with previously published results, which indicate that different structural families of topoisomerase II inhibitors generate unique cleavage patterns with enzyme in vitro and therefore likely recognize different DNA cleavage sites in the presence of the enzyme (19, 95, 138, 153).

An important aspect of the study with CP-67,015 was that both catalytic (unknotting and catenation) and cleavage activities obtained with calf thymus topoisomerase II were compared. As in the case with etoposide, the $CC_{50}$s for the cleavage assays run with CP-67,015 were usually lower than the corresponding $IC_{50}$s obtained for inhibition of catalytic activity (7). This was particularly true for the cleavage assay using $^{32}$P-radiolabeled DNA as substrate. This suggests that cleavage assays may be more sensitive for detecting the effects of quinolones on topoisomerase II. It is interesting that a similar observation has been made by Domagala and colleagues (36) with DNA gyrase; for a number of quinolones, they observed a better correlation between the generation of gyrase-mediated DNA cleavage and the MIC than between the MIC and the $IC_{50}$s for gyrase supercoiling. While CP-67,015 was shown to be a potent antibacterial agent and highly inhibitory for DNA gyrase (7), its increase in potency against topoisomerase II was an important finding, distinguishing this compound from other quinolones. This activity was also a critical consideration in determining the overall safety of CP-67,015, as will be discussed below in the section describing the genotoxic effects of this quinolone.

While CP-67,015 was one of the first quinolones shown to have potent activity against topoisomerase II, other quinolone analogs have recently been shown to enhance enzyme-mediated DNA cleavage. Kohlbrenner et al. examined the activities of novel isothiazolo-quinolones for stimulating calf thymus topoisomerase II-mediated DNA breakage in vitro (78). Two of these quinolones, A-65281 and A-65282 (Fig. 4), had $IC_{50}$s in the DNA-unknotting assay of 8 $\mu$g/ml and showed strong DNA cleavage activities, i.e., down to 4 $\mu$g/ml in the presence of the enzyme (78). The structure-activity relationship in this series revealed that both the 6,8-difluoro substitution and an N-9 cyclopropyl group were important in determining potency for enhancing topoisomerase II-mediated DNA cleavage (78). Both A-65281 and A-65282 were nearly as potent as the antitumor agent etoposide with respect to this activity. Thus, studies with the isothiazoloquinolone derivatives add to the information generated with CP-67,015, indicating that specific substitutions on the quinolone nucleus can lead to compounds that have significant activities against both DNA gyrase and eukaryotic topoisomerase II in vitro.

Another series of studies described the topoisomerase II activity of several 10-(3′,5′-dimethyl-4′pyridinyl)-6-pyridobenzothiazinyl (oxazine) carboxylic acids (26, 149). The most potent of these quinolones, WIN 58161 (Fig. 4), formed covalent complexes between purified HeLa cell topoisomerase II and DNA with a 50% effective concentration ($EC_{50}$) of 9.4 $\mu$M ($\sim$4 $\mu$g/ml). WIN 58161 was about 12-fold less potent than etoposide in these in vitro cleavage assays. Additional in vitro studies indicated that the compound did not intercalate into DNA and established that protein-associated DNA strand breaks were produced when P388 cells were exposed to WIN 58161 (26). Enantiomeric specificity was again demonstrated to influence potency against topoisomerase II, since the pure 3-*S*-methyl enantiomer was over 2 orders of magnitude more active at inducing cleavage than the *R*-methyl enantiomer.

Evidence that quinolones and antitumor inhibitors of topoisomerase II show both a common inhibitor-binding site and a common mechanism of action comes from studies using mutants of the T4 phage enzyme. While the mammalian enzyme is a homodimer, T4 phage topoisomerase II contains three subunits, designated by their sizes as 39 (catalyzes ATP hydrolysis), 52 (conducts DNA breakage and resealing), and 60 (confers structural stability) (71, 72). T4 topoisomerase II is involved in phage DNA replication and has many properties in common with the mammalian enzyme; it is normally inhibited by *m*-AMSA, ellipticine, teniposide, and etoposide but is insensitive to oxolinic acid (71). Mutant T4 phage were isolated under selection with *m*-AMSA, and one drug-resistant mutant was found to contain topoisomerase II with an alteration in the 39-kDa subunit (71). The enzyme from this mutant demonstrated *m*-AMSA-resistant DNA relaxation activity and was insensitive to *m*-AMSA-enhanced DNA cleavage. Interestingly, this mutation conferred a DNA gyrase-like sensitivity to oxolinic acid, as measured in a cleavage assay. The mutant enzyme was also ultrasensitive to the epipodophyllotoxins etoposide and teniposide (71). Those authors hypothesized that the mutant topoisomerase II had an altered binding site that decreased the binding of some antitumor agents while favoring binding of other compounds, including the quinolone antibiotic oxolinic acid. These results suggest that the binding sites on T4 topoisomerase II for some antitumor drugs and oxolinic acid are either the same or overlapping. If the sites for these two classes of drugs are similar, it might be expected that minor structural modifications on the quinolone nucleus could significantly increase their affinities for topoisomerase II. This conclusion is consistent with the observations reported above for some quinolones discussed in this review.

These corroborating observations cause us to reconsider the previously held doctrine that all quinolones are highly selective for bacterial DNA gyrase. Studies using purified topoisomerase II have also led to important new observations addressing the biochemical mechanism by which these novel quinolones interact with topoisomerase II.

## MECHANISTIC STUDIES OF C-7-HYDROXYPHENYL-SUBSTITUTED QUINOLONES: THE CP-115,953 SERIES

As already described, most quinolone antimicrobial agents are poor effectors of eukaryotic topoisomerase II (51, 63, 158). While all antibacterial quinolones in clinical use contain an aliphatic group at the C-7 position (25, 148), compounds with aromatic C-7 groups (pyridine, 2,6-dimethylpyridine, and quinoline) also have been reported (7, 74, 149). These latter compounds are distinguished from quinolone antimicrobial agents by their increased activity toward the eukaryotic enzyme (7, 74, 149). However, in all cases, potency was still considerably lower than that of a topoisomerase II-targeted antineoplastic drug such as etoposide.

To further assess the influence of aromatic C-7 substituents on the activities of quinolones, the effects of quinolone derivative CP-115,953 and analogous compounds (all of which contain a hydroxyphenyl ring at C-7) on eukaryotic topoisomerase II were examined (114–116). Structures of these quinolones are shown in Fig. 4. All members of the CP-115,953 series are nonintercalative with respect to DNA (116). Furthermore, in addition to their activities against eukaryotic topoisomerase II, all are extremely effective against bacterial DNA gyrase (114, 116). In fact, CP-115,953 is approximately fourfold more effective than ciprofloxacin at inducing gyrase-mediated DNA cleavage (116). Finally, CP-115,953 is the most potent of these compounds in all respects and therefore will be the primary focus of this section.

Initial studies employed topoisomerase II from *D. melanogaster* (114, 116). As shown in Fig. 5A, CP-115,953 is a potent enhancer of enzyme-mediated DNA breakage. As calculated from the linear portion ($\leq$50 $\mu$M drug) of the drug concentration curves, CP-115,953 is approximately two times more potent than etoposide. Similar results were found for the quinolone's effects on both the pre-strand passage (Fig. 5) and post-strand passage DNA cleavage-religation equilibria (116). In addition, CP-115,953 was considerably more potent (relative to etoposide) against the mammalian type II enzyme (115). Thus, CP-115,953 is the first quinolone reported to have greater activity against eukaryotic topoisomerase II than does an antineoplastic drug in clinical use.

Substitution of an ethyl group for the cyclopropyl at N-1 (CP-67,804) or removal of the fluorine at C-8 (CP-115,955) reduced quinolone activity to $\sim$40% that of CP-115,953 (114, 116). It should be noted, however, that despite their decreased activities, CP-67,804 and CP-115,955 were still considerably more potent against the *Drosophila* type II enzyme than any other quinolone previously reported (except CP-115,953). Previously proposed models for quinolone action suggest that the C-7 substituent is important for drug-gyrase interactions (130, 154). In this regard, CP-115,955 differs from ciprofloxacin only at its C-7 position yet is $\sim$20-fold more potent at enhancing *Drosophila* topoisomerase II-mediated DNA cleavage (114). Thus, the presence of the hydroxyphenyl ring at position C-7 appears to be critical to the dramatic activities of quinolones in the CP-115,953 series.

As previously mentioned, two different topoisomerase II-targeted antineoplastic drugs enhanced enzyme-mediated DNA breakage primarily by inhibiting DNA religation (103, 117, 118). This was not the case for CP-115,953. As seen in the heat-induced DNA religation assay of Fig. 5B, the quinolone displayed little ability to inhibit DNA religation (116). These findings, which are in marked contrast to those with etoposide, were confirmed by using the other two religation assays described earlier (116). Furthermore, comparable results were obtained when religation was carried out in the presence of either CP-67,804 or CP-115,953 (114, 116). Since these quinolones have little effect on DNA religation, it is likely that they enhance topoisomerase II-mediated DNA breakage primarily by stimulating the enzyme's forward rate of nucleic acid cleavage. Therefore, quinolones in the CP-115,953 series appear to represent a novel mechanistic class of potent topoisomerase II-targeted drugs.

## RELEVANT EFFECTS ON WHOLE CELLS

Numerous effects of quinolones on mammalian cells have been reported in the literature (15, 16, 28, 51, 66, 113; see also chapter 28). Quinolones have been shown to stimulate thymidine incorporation in

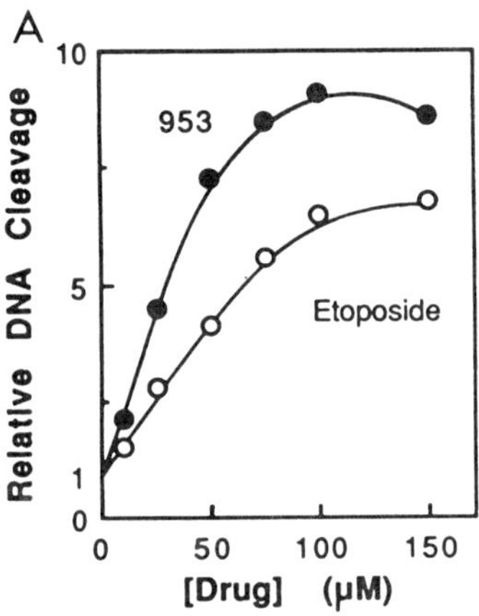


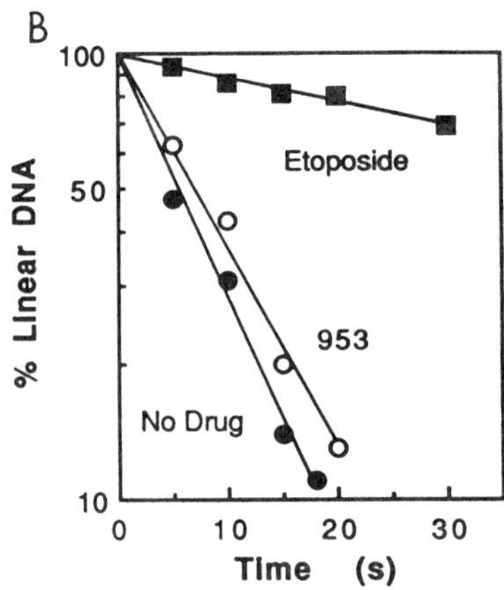


**Figure 5.** Effects of CP-115,953 on the DNA cleavage (A) and religation (B) reactions of *Drosophila* topoisomerase II. (A) Results are plotted as the relative amount of double-stranded DNA cleavage versus drug concentration. The relative level of DNA cleavage was set arbitrarily at 1 in the absence of drug. An etoposide cleavage titration is shown for comparison. Data represent averages of two independent experiments (standard error, ≤0.9). (B) Religation was initiated by shifting assay mixtures from 30 to 55°C. Results obtained with 50 μM CP-115,953 are compared with those obtained in the absence of drug or in the presence of 100 μM etoposide. The drug concentrations employed generated similar levels of enzyme-mediated DNA breakage. Data are plotted in a semilogarithmic fashion as the loss of linear DNA versus time. The percent linear DNA for each assay was set arbitrarily to 100% at time zero. Plots represent the averages of three independent experiments (average standard error, ≤5%). Data are reproduced from reference 116 with permission.

phytohemagglutinin-stimulated lymphocytes and inhibit cell cycle progression, mitogen-induced mononuclear cell proliferation, and immunoglobulin secretion in vitro (16, 42, 43). The synthesis of interleukin-1 was reported to be inhibited at high concentrations of ciprofloxacin, while the production of interleukin-2 was up-regulated at the mRNA level (113).

Two recent reviews have described the reported genotoxic effects of quinolones in various in vitro cell systems (28, 51). Ciprofloxacin, norfloxacin, ofloxacin, and pefloxacin have been claimed to be mutagenic in the mouse lymphoma cell assay and also to produce a positive response in the rat hepatocyte unscheduled DNA synthesis (UDS) assay (126). These quinolones, however, did not show abnormal effects in either the Ames or the Chinese hamster V-79 cell tests for gene mutagenicity or in micronucleus and dominant lethal tests in mice (126, 131). The activity of ciprofloxacin in the UDS assay was confirmed in a separate study in which the compound produced a UDS response in human lymphocytes in vitro when tested at 5 μg/ml (16). A recent study indicates that ciprofloxacin induces double-stranded DNA breaks in human lymphoblastoid cells exposed to 80 μg of drug per ml in vitro (15). Tests with norfloxacin and fleroxacin (AM-833) indicated that these two drugs are not mutagenic, do not induce DNA strand breakage, and do not elicit a UDS response in either human or mouse skin fibroblasts (66).

While all of the in vitro effects described above are of potential medical interest, no direct evidence indicates that they result from inhibition of topoisomerase II. In addition, the literature contains much debate concerning the relevance of positive in vitro genotoxicity results observed in a single test system, since quinolones appear not to induce the same responses in in vivo test systems (23, 90, 93, 131). This position is consistent with the good overall safety record that has been achieved for quinolones approved for clinical use. From this experience, it has been generally accepted that the safety of new quinolone antibacterial agents can be reliably determined by establishing their lack of genotoxic activities in a standard battery of in vitro and in vivo tests.

Much less is known, however, concerning the toxicity of the quinolones described in this chapter, which have demonstrated significantly increased potency toward topoisomerase II. One of the first quinolones described for its activity against topoisomerase II, the 6,8-difluoro-7-pyridyl-4-quinolone CP-67,015, has been characterized with regard to its genotoxic activity (58). CP-67,015 was not mutagenic in the Ames test but was a directly acting mutagen in the mouse lymphoma cell assay, the Chinese hamster ovary cell hypoxanthine-guanine phosphoribosyl transferase gene (HGPRT) assay, and the V-79 cell–HGPRT forward mutation assay (58). This quinolone also induced chromosome aberrations in cultured human lymphocytes at concentrations of $\geq 50$ $\mu$g/ml and produced genetically abnormal bone marrow cells in mice given five daily parenteral doses of 500 mg/kg of body weight per day. Surprisingly, sister chromatid exchange was only marginally stimulated with CP-67,015 in human lymphocytes or CHO cells in vitro, even at levels that produced severe chromosome breakage (58). As described above, this quinolone was only 7- to 10-fold less potent than the antitumor agent etoposide for stimulating topoisomerase II-mediated DNA cleavage in vitro, thus establishing a probable link with topoisomerase II and its reported genotoxic activity in cells.

The cytotoxic activity of the potent topoisomerase II-acting quinolones CP-115,953 and CP-67,804 also have been investigated (116). Two tissue culture lines were employed for this purpose: a wild-type CHO cell line and its Vpm$^R$-5 mutant, which was derived because of its resistance to epipodophyllotoxins (50, 53, 134). The mutant line is 10- to 20-fold more resistant than its wild type to etoposide and is cross-resistant to a number of other topoisomerase II-targeted antineoplastic drugs (50). Drug resistance in the Vpm$^R$-5 cell line results from a mutant, resistant form of topoisomerase II and not from reduced drug accumulation (134).

CP-115,953 and etoposide were equally cytotoxic to the wild-type CHO cells, with an $EC_{50}$ of 9 $\mu$M (116). CP-67,804, which was less potent at enhancing topoisomerase II-mediated DNA cleavage than either CP-115,953 or etoposide, demonstrated an $EC_{50}$ of 70 $\mu$M against wild-type CHO cells. While the Vpm$^R$-5 mutant cell line showed some degree of cross-resistance to CP-67,804 and CP-115, 953 (3.7- and 1.3-fold increases in $EC_{50}$s, respectively), resistance was not as pronounced as that observed with etoposide (12-fold increase in $EC_{50}$ over that of wild type). Regardless of the magnitude of the increase in resistance against the Vpm$^R$-5 cell line, the cytotoxicity results obtained considered along with the activities of these quinolones against purified topoisomerase II (described above) strongly suggest that this enzyme is a target for these quinolones in mammalian cells.

The cytotoxic effects of another topoisomerase II-active quinolone, WIN 58161, also have been studied. As mentioned above, WIN 58161 at 9 $\mu$M induced significant amounts of topoisomerase II-mediated DNA cleavage in vitro (26, 149). It also generated intracellular protein-associated DNA strand breaks in P388 cells at this concentration, as measured in an alkaline elution assay. Furthermore, this quinolone was cytotoxic to cells in vitro and displayed activity in vivo against a broad spectrum of murine leukemia and solid tumors (P388, B16, Colo 38, and Maw 16C) at high doses of drug (26).

Recent results generated with the topoisomerase II-active quinolones CP-67,015, CP-67,804, CP-115,953, and WIN 58161 indicate that increased potency against this enzyme confers cytotoxic and DNA strand-breaking activities in whole cells in a manner that is representative of classical antineoplastic topoisomerase II-targeted drugs. These compounds are clearly different from all other quinolones with respect to the potency exhibited against both the eukaryotic enzyme and whole cells. Further studies with resistant mutants should more clearly establish the relationship of activity against topoisomerase II and cell cytotoxicity.

## SUMMARY

In recent years, quinolones have been optimized for their activities against DNA gyrase, leading to compounds with potent antibacterial activities. While a homologous topoisomerase II exists in eukaryotic cells, quinolones developed to date for medical use have demonstrated inhibition of this enzyme only at concentrations that are 2 to 3 orders of magnitude above that required for antibacterial activity. However, the doctrine that all quinolones are impotent antagonists of topoisomerase II needs to be changed in light of the recently reported effects of some quinolones from structurally diverse series. These quinolones induce significant topoisomerase II-mediated DNA cleavage in vitro and produce potent cytotoxic effects in cultured cells. In addition, WIN 58161 has demonstrated DNA strand breakage in whole cells by alkaline elution. Preliminary evidence suggests that some of these quinolones demonstrate antitumor effects in experimental animal models. Mechanistic studies with CP-115,953 indicate that it is nonintercalating and, unlike the epipodophyllotoxins, fails to block DNA religation mediated by this enzyme. Quinolones such as CP-67,015, CP-115,953, A-65281, A-65282, and WIN 58161 are clearly different from quinolones developed so far for clinical use with respect to their potency against topoisomerase II. These observations underscore the importance of carefully testing new quinolones in standard systems for genotoxicity in order to ensure their safety for future use as antibacterial agents.

## REFERENCES

1. **Ackerman, P., C. V. C. Glover, and N. Osheroff.** 1985. Phosphorylation of DNA topoisomerase II by casein kinase II: modulation of eukaryotic topoisomerase II activity *in vitro*. *Proc. Natl. Acad. Sci. USA* **82:**3164–3168.
2. **Ackerman, P., C. V. C. Glover, and N. Osheroff.** 1988. Phosphorylation of DNA topoisomerase II *in vivo* and in total homogenates of *Drosophila* Kc cells. *J. Biol. Chem.* **263:**12653–12660.
3. **Adachi, Y., M. Luke, and U. K. Laemmli.** 1991. Chromosome assembly *in vitro:* topoisomerase II is required for condensation. *Cell* **64:**137–148.
4. **Andersen, A. H., K. Christiansen, E. L. Zechiedrich, P. S. Jensen, N. Osheroff, and O. Westergaard.** 1989. Strand specificity of the topoisomerase II-mediated double-stranded DNA cleavage reaction. *Biochemistry* **28:**6237–6244.
5. **Andersson, H. C., and B. A. Kihlman.** 1989. The production of chromosomal alterations in human lymphocytes by drugs known to interfere with the activity of DNA topoisomerase II. I. *m*-AMSA. *Carcinogen* **10:**123–130.
6. **Bae, Y.-S., I. Kawasaki, H. Ikeda, and L. F. Liu.** 1988. Illegitimate recombination mediated by calf thymus DNA topoisomerase II *in vitro*. *Proc. Natl. Acad. Sci. USA* **85:**2076–2080.
7. **Barrett, J. F., T. D. Gootz, P. R. McGuirk, C. A. Farrell, and S. A. Sokolowski.** 1989. Use of *in vitro* topoisomerase II assays for studying quinolone antibacterial agents. *Antimicrob. Agents Chemother.* **33:**1697–1703.
8. **Barrett, J. F., J. A. Sutcliffe, and T. D. Gootz.** 1990. *In vitro* assays used to measure the activity of topoisomerases. *Antimicrob. Agents Chemother.* **34:**1–7.
9. **Baugley, B. C.** 1990. The possible role of electron-transfer complexes in the antitumor action of amsacrine analogues. *Biophys. Chem.* **35:**203–212.
10. **Beck, W. T., and M. K. Danks.** 1991. Characterization of multidrug resistance in human tumor cells, p. 3–55. *In* I. G. Robinson (ed.), *Molecular and Cellular Biology of Multidrug Resistance in Tumor Cells.* Plenum Publishing Corp., New York.
11. **Bergan, T.** 1988. Pharmacokinetics of fluorinated quinolones, p. 119–154. *In* V. T. Andriole (ed.), *The Quinolones.* Academic Press, Inc., New York.
12. **Berrios, M., N. Osheroff, and P. A. Fisher.** 1985. *In situ* localization of DNA topoisomerase II, a major polypeptide component of the *Drosophila* nuclear matrix fraction. *Proc. Natl. Acad. Sci. USA* **82:**4142–4146.
13. **Bertrand, R., D. Kerrigan, M. Sarang, and Y. Pommier.** 1991. Cell death induced by topoisomerase II inhibitors: role of calcium in mammalian cells. *Biochem. Pharmacol.* **42:**77–85.

14. **Bodley, A. L., H.-Y. Wu, and L. F. Liu.** 1987. Regulation of DNA topoisomerases during cellular differentiation. *NCI Monogr.* **4:**31–35.
15. **Bredberg, A., M. Brant, and M. Jaszyk.** 1991. Ciprofloxacin-induced inhibition of topoisomerase II in human lymphoblastoid cells. *Antimicrob. Agents Chemother.* **35:**448–450.
16. **Bredberg, A., M. Brant, K. Riesbeck, Y. Azou, and A. Forsgren.** 1989. 4-Quinolone antibiotics: positive genotoxic screening tests despite an apparent lack of mutation induction. *Mutat. Res.* **211:**171–180.
17. **Bugg, B. Y., M. K. Danks, W. T. Beck, and D. P. Suttle.** 1991. Expression of a mutant DNA topoisomerase II in CCRF-CEM human leukemic cells selected for resistance to teniposide. *Proc. Natl. Acad. Sci. USA* **88:**7654–7658.
18. **Charcosset, J.-Y., J.-M. Saucier, and A. Jacquemin-Sablon.** 1988. Reduced DNA topoisomerase II activity and drug-stimulated DNA cleavage in 9-hydroxyellipticine-resistant cells. *Biochem. Pharmacol.* **37:**2145–2149.
19. **Chen, G. L., L. Yang, T. C. Rowe, B. D. Halligan, K. M. Tewey, and L. F. Liu.** 1984. Nonintercalative antitumor drugs interfere with the breakage-reunion reaction of mammalian DNA topoisomerase II. *J. Biol. Chem.* **259:**13560–13566.
20. **Chow, K.-C., C. K. King, and W. E. Ross.** 1988. Abrogation of etoposide-mediated cytotoxicity by cycloheximide. *Biochem. Pharmacol.* **37:**1117–1122.
21. **Chow, K.-C., T. L. MacDonald, and W. E. Ross.** 1988. DNA binding by epipodophyllotoxins and N-acetyl anthracyclines: implications for mechanism of topoisomerase II inhibition. *Mol. Pharmacol.* **34:**467–473.
22. **Chow, K.-C., and W. E. Ross.** 1987. Topoisomerase-specific drug sensitivity in relation to cell cycle progression. *Mol. Cell. Biol.* **7:**3119–3123.
23. **Christ, W., T. Lehnert, and V. Ulbrich.** 1988. Specific toxicologic aspects of the quinolones. *Rev. Infect. Dis.* **10**(Suppl. 1):S141–S146.
24. **Christman, M. F., F. S. Dietrich, and G. R. Fink.** 1988. Mitotic recombination in the rDNA of *S. cerevisiae* is suppressed by the combined action of DNA topoisomerases I and II. *Cell* **55:**413–425.
25. **Chu, D. T. W., and P. B. Fernandes.** 1989. Structure-activity relationships of the fluoroquinolones. *Antimicrob. Agents Chemother.* **33:**131–135.
26. **Coughlin, S. A., D. W. Danz, R. G. Robinson, P. S. Moskwa, M. P. Wentland, G. Y. Lesher, and J. B. Rake.** 1991. Mechanism of action of WIN-58161. *Proc. Am. Assoc. Cancer Res.* **32:**337.
27. **Crespi, M. D., A. G. Mladovan, and A. Baldi.** 1988. Increment of DNA topoisomerases in chemically and virally transformed cells. *Exp. Cell Res.* **175:**206–215.
28. **Crumplin, G. C.** 1990. *In vitro* genotoxicity assessment and the effects of 4-quinolones upon human cells, p. 173–200. *In* G. C. Crumplin (ed.), *The 4-Quinolones: Antibacterial Agents In Vitro.* Springer-Verlag, London.
29. **Danks, M. K., C. A. Schmidt, M. C. Cirtain, D. P. Suttle, and W. T. Beck.** 1988. Altered catalytic activity of and DNA cleavage by DNA topoisomerase II from human leukemic cells selected for resistance to VM-26. *Biochemistry* **27:**8861–8869.
30. **D'Arpa, P., P. S. Machlin, H. Ratrie III, N. F. Rothfield, D. W. Cleveland, and W. C. Earnshaw.** 1988. cDNA cloning of human DNA topoisomerase I: catalytic activity of a 67.7-kDa carboxyl-terminal fragment. *Proc. Natl. Acad. Sci. USA* **85:**2543–2547.
31. **Davies, S. M., C. N. Robson, S. L. Davies, and I. D. Hickson.** 1988. Nuclear topoisomerase II levels correlate with the sensitivity of mammalian cells to intercalating agents and epipodophyllotoxins. *J. Biol. Chem.* **263:**17724–17729.
32. **Deffie, A. M., J. K. Batra, and G. J. Goldenberg.** 1989. Direct correlation between DNA topoisomerase II activity and cytotoxicity in adriamycin-sensitive and -resistant p388 leukemia cell lines. *Cancer Res.* **48:**58–62.
33. **DeVore, R., J. Whitlock, J. D. Hainsworth, and D. H. Johnson.** 1989. Therapy-related acute nonlymphocytic leukemia with monocytic features and rearrangement of chromosome 11q. *Ann. Intern. Med.* **110:**740–742.
34. **Dillehay, L. E., D. Jacobson-Kram, and J. R. Williams.** 1989. DNA topoisomerases and models of sister-chromatid exchange. *Mutat. Res.* **215:**15–23.
35. **DiNardo, S., K. Voelkel, and R. Sternglanz.** 1984. DNA topoisomerase II mutant *Saccharomyces cerevisiae:* topoisomerase II is required for segregation of daughter molecules at the termination of DNA replication. *Proc. Natl. Acad. Sci. USA* **81:**2616–2620.
36. **Domagala, J. M., L. D. Hanna, C. L. Heifetz, M. P. Hutt, T. F. Mich, J. P. Sanchez, and M. Solomon.** 1986. New structure-activity relationships of the quinolone antibacterials using the target enzyme. The development and application of a DNA gyrase assay. *J. Med. Chem.* **29:**394-404.
37. **Duget, M., C. Lavenot, F. Harper, G. Mirambeau, and A. De Recondo.** 1983. DNA topoisomerases from rat liver: physiological variations. *Nucleic Acids Res.* **11:**1059-1075.
38. **Earnshaw, W. C., B. Halligan, C. A. Cooke, M. M. S. Heck, and L. F. Liu.** 1985. Topoisomerase II is a structural component of mitotic chromosome scaffolds. *J. Cell Biol.* **100:**1706–1715.

39. **Earnshaw, W. C., and M. M. S. Heck.** 1985. Localization of topoisomerase II in mitotic chromosomes. *J. Cell Biol.* **100:**1716–1725.
40. **Estey, E., R. C. Adlakha, W. N. Hittelman, and L. A. Zwelling.** 1987. Cell cycle dependent variations in drug-induced topoisomerase II-mediated DNA cleavage and cytotoxicity. *Biochemistry* **26:**4338–4344.
41. **Fairman, R., and D. L. Brutlag.** 1988. Expression of the *Drosophila* type II topoisomerase is developmentally regulated. *Biochemistry* **27:**560–565.
42. **Forsgren, A., A. Bredberg, A. B. Pardee, S. F. Schlossman, and T. F. Tedder.** 1987. Effects of ciprofloxacin on eucaryotic pyrimidine nucleotide biosynthesis and cell growth. *Antimicrob. Agents Chemother.* **31:**774–779.
43. **Forsgren, A., S. F. Schlossman, and T. F. Tedder.** 1987. 4-Quinolone drugs affect cell cycle progression and function of human lymphocytes in vitro. *Antimicrob. Agents Chemother.* **31:**768–773.
44. **Friche, E., M. K. Danks, C. A. Schmidt, and W. T. Beck.** 1991. Decreased DNA topoisomerase II in daunorubicin-resistant Ehrlich ascites tumor cells. *Cancer Res.* **51:**4213–4218.
45. **Gale, K. C., and N. Osheroff.** 1990. Uncoupling the DNA cleavage and religation activities of topoisomerase II with a single-stranded nucleic acid substrate: evidence for an active enzyme-cleaved DNA intermediate. *Biochemistry* **29:**9538–9545.
46. **Gasser, S. M., and U. K. Laemmli.** 1986. The organization of chromatin loops: characterization of a scaffold attachment site. *EMBO J.* **5:**511–518.
47. **Gasser, S. M., T. Laroche, J. Falquet, E. Boy de la Tour, and U. K. Laemmli.** 1986. Metaphase chromosome structure: involvement of topoisomerase II. *J. Mol. Biol.* **188:**613–629.
48. **Genovese, J. A., M. D. Crespi, G. Castro, F. H. Medina, and A. Baldi.** 1988. Effects of human transforming growth factors on topoisomerases from normal fibroblasts. *Life Sci.* **43:**2137–2143.
49. **Giaever, G., R. Lynn, T. Goto, and J. C. Wang.** 1986. The complete nucleotide sequence of the structural gene *TOP2* of yeast DNA topoisomerase II. *J. Biol. Chem.* **261:**12448–12454.
50. **Glisson, B., R. Gupta, S. Smallwood-Kentro, and W. Ross.** 1986. Characterization of acquired epipodophyllotoxin resistance in a Chinese hamster ovary cell line: loss of drug-stimulated DNA cleavage activity. *Cancer Res.* **46:**1934–1938.
51. **Gootz, T. D., J. F. Barrett, and J. A. Sutcliffe.** 1990. Inhibitory effects of quinolone antibacterial agents on eucaryotic topoisomerases and related test systems. *Antimicrob. Agents Chemother.* **34:**8–12.
52. **Goto, T., and J. C. Wang.** 1984. Yeast DNA topoisomerase II is encoded by a single-copy, essential gene. *Cell* **36:**1073–1080.
53. **Gupta, R. S.** 1983. Genetic, biochemical, and cross-resistance studies with mutants of Chinese hamster ovary cells resistant to the anticancer drugs, VM-26 and VP-16-213. *Cancer Res.* **43:**1568–1574.
54. **Heck, M. M. S., and W. C. Earnshaw.** 1986. Topoisomerase II: a specific marker for cell proliferation. *J. Cell Biol.* **103:**2569–2581.
55. **Heck, M. M. S., W. N. Hittelman, and W. C. Earnshaw.** 1988. Differential expression of DNA topoisomerases I and II during the eukaryotic cell cycle. *Proc. Nat. Acad. Sci. USA* **85:**1086–1090.
56. **Heck, M. M. S., W. N. Hittelman, and W. C. Earnshaw.** 1989. *In vivo* phosphorylation of the 170-kDa form of eukaryotic DNA topoisomerase II. *J. Biol. Chem.* **264:**15161–15164.
57. **Hertzberg, R. P., R. W. Busby, M. J. Caranfa, K. G. Holden, R. K. Johnson, S. M. Hecht, and W. D. Kingsbury.** 1990. Irreversible trapping of the DNA-topoisomerase I covalent complex: affinity labeling of the camptothecin binding site. *J. Biol. Chem.* **265:**19287–19295.
58. **Holden, H. E., J. F. Barrett, C. M. Huntington, P. A. Muehlbauer, and M. G. Wahrenburg.** 1989. Genetic profile of a nalidixic acid analog: a model for the mechanism of sister chromatid exchange induction. *Environ. Mol. Mutagen.* **13:**238–252.
59. **Holden, J. A., D. H. Rolfson, and C. T. Wittwer.** 1990. Human DNA topoisomerase II: evaluation of enzyme activity in normal and neoplastic tissues. *Biochemistry* **29:**2127–2134.
60. **Holm, C., J. M. Covey, D. Kerrigan, and Y. Pommier.** 1989. Differential requirement of DNA replication for the cytotoxicity of DNA topoisomerase I and II inhibitors in Chinese hamster DC3F cells. *Cancer Res.* **49:**6365–6368.
61. **Holm, C., T. Goto, J. C. Wang, and D. Botstein.** 1985. DNA topoisomerase II is required at the time of mitosis in yeast. *Cell* **41:**553–563.
62. **Hooper, D. C., and J. S. Wolfson.** 1989. Adverse effects of quinolone antimicrobial agents, p. 249–271. *In* J. S. Wolfson and D. C. Hooper (ed.), *Quinolone Antimicrobial Agents.* American Society for Microbiology, Washington, D.C.
63. **Hooper, D. C., and J. S. Wolfson.** 1991. Fluoroquinolone antimicrobial agents. *N. Engl. J. Med.* **324:**384–394.
64. **Hoshino, K., K. Sato, K. Akahane, A. Yoshida, I. Hayakawa, M. Sato, T. Une, and Y. Osada.** 1991. Significance of the methyl group on the oxazine ring of ofloxacin derivatives in the inhibition of bacterial and mammalian type II topoisomerases. *Antimicrob. Agents Chemother.* **35:**309–312.

65. **Hoshino, K., K. Sato, T. Une, and Y. Osada.** 1989. Inhibitory effects of quinolones on DNA gyrase of *Escherichia coli* and topoisomerase II of fetal calf thymus. *Antimicrob. Agents Chemother.* **33:**1816–1818.
66. **Hosomi, J., A. Maeda, Y. Oomori, T. Irikura, and T. Yokota.** 1988. Mutagenicity of norfloxacin and AM-833 in bacteria and mammalian cells. *Rev. Infect. Dis.* **10**(Suppl.1):S148–S149.
67. **Howard, M. T., M. P. Lee, T.-S. Hsieh, and J. D. Griffith.** 1990. *Drosophila* topoisomerase II-DNA interactions are affected by DNA structure. *J. Mol. Biol.* **217:**53–62.
68. **Hsiang, Y.-H., J. B. Jiang, and L. F. Liu.** 1989. Topoisomerase II-mediated DNA cleavage by amonafide and its structural analogs. *Mol. Pharmacol.* **36:**371–376.
69. **Hsiang, Y.-H., and L. F. Liu.** 1989. Evidence for the reversibility of cellular DNA lesions induced by mammalian topoisomerase II poisons. *J. Biol. Chem.* **264:**9713–9715.
70. **Hsiang, Y.-H., H.-Y. Wu, and L. F. Liu.** 1988. Proliferation-dependent regulation of DNA topoisomerase II in cultured cells. *Cancer Res.* **48:**3230–3235.
71. **Huff, A. C., and K. N. Kreuzer.** 1990. Evidence for a common mechanism of action for antitumor and antibacterial agents that inhibit type II DNA topoisomerases. *J. Biol. Chem.* **265:**20496–20505.
72. **Huff, A. C., J. K. Leatherwood, and K. N. Kreuzer.** 1989. Bacteriophage T4 DNA topoisomerase is the target of antitumor agent 4′-(9-acridinylamino) methane sulfon-*m*-anisidide (*m*-AMSA) in T4-infected *Escherichia coli. Proc. Natl. Acad. Sci. USA* **86:**1307–1311.
73. **Hussy, P., G. Maass, B. Tümmler, F. Grosse, and U. Schomburg.** 1986. Effect of 4-quinolones and novobiocin on calf thymus DNA polymerase a primase complex, topoisomerase I and II, and growth of mammalian lymphoblasts. *Antimicrob. Agents Chemother.* **29:**1073–1078.
74. **Jefson, M. R., P. R. McGuirk, A. E. Girard, T. D. Gootz, and J. F. Barrett.** 1989. The synthesis and properties of optically pure C10-heteroaryl quinolones structurally related to ofloxacin, abstr. 1190. *Program Abstr. 29th Intersci. Conf. Antimicrob. Agents Chemother.*
75. **Jeggo, P. A., K. Caldecott, S. Pidsley, and G. R. Banks.** 1989. Sensitivity of Chinese hamster ovary mutants defective in DNA double-strand break repair to topoisomerase II inhibitors. *Cancer Res.* **49:**7057–7063.
76. **Kaufman, S. H.** 1989. Induction of endonucleolytic DNA cleavage in human acute myelogenous leukemia cells by etoposide, camptothecin, and other cytotoxic anticancer drugs: a cautionary note. *Cancer Res.* **49:**5870–5878.
77. **Kim, R. A., and J. C. Wang.** 1989. A subthreshold level of DNA topoisomerases leads to the excision of yeast rDNA as extrachromosomal rings. *Cell* **57:**975–985.
78. **Kohlbrenner, W. E., N. Wideburg, D. Weigl, A. Saldivar, and D. T. W. Chu.** 1992. Induction of calf thymus topoisomerase II-mediated DNA breakage by the antibacterial isothiazoloquinolones A-65281 and A-65282. *Antimicrob. Agents Chemother.* **36:**81–86.
79. **Kreuzer, K. N., and N. R. Cozzarelli.** 1979. *Escherichia coli* mutants thermosensitive for deoxyribonucleic acid gyrase subunit A: effects on deoxyribonucleic acid replication, transcription, and bacteriophage growth. *J. Bacteriol.* **140:**424–435.
80. **Kroll, D. J., and T. C. Rowe.** 1991. Phosphorylation of DNA topoisomerase II in a human tumor cell line. *J. Biol. Chem.* **266:**7957–7961.
81. **Kupfer, F., A. L. Bodley, and L. F. Liu.** 1987. Involvement of intracellular ATP in cytotoxicity of topoisomerase II-targeting antitumor drugs. *NCI Monogr.* **4:**37–40.
82. **Lin, M., L. F. Liu, D. Jacobson-Kram, and J. R. Williams.** 1986. Induction of sister chromatid exchanges by inhibitors of topoisomerases. *Cell Biol. Toxicol.* **2:**485–494.
83. **Liu, L. F.** 1989. DNA topoisomerase poisons as antitumor drugs. *Annu. Rev. Biochem.* **58:**351–375.
84. **Liu, L. F., J. L. Davis, and R. Calendar.** 1981. Novel topologically knotted DNA from bacteriophage P4 capsids: studies with DNA topoisomerases. *Nucleic Acids Res.* **9:**3979–3989.
85. **Liu, L. F., T. C. Rowe, L. Yang, K. M. Tewey, and G. L. Chen.** 1983. Cleavage of DNA by mammalian DNA topoisomerase II. *J. Biol. Chem.* **258:**15365–15370.
86. **Lock, R. B., and W. E. Ross.** 1987. DNA topoisomerases in cancer therapy. *Anti-Cancer Drug Design* **2:**151–154.
87. **Long, B. H.** 1987. Structure-activity relationships of podophyllin congeners that inhibit topoisomerase II. *NCI Monogr.* **4:**123–127.
88. **Lynn, R., G. Giaever, S. L. Swanberg, and J. C. Wang.** 1986. Tandem regions of yeast DNA topoisomerase II share homology with different subunits of bacterial gyrase. *Science* **233:**647–649.
89. **Markovits, J., Y. Pommier, D. Kerrigan, J. M. Covey, E. J. Tilden, and K. W. Kohn.** 1987. Topoisomerase II-mediated DNA breaks and cytotoxicity in relation to cell proliferation and the cell cycle in NIH 3T3 fibroblasts and L1210 leukemia cells. *Cancer Res.* **47:**2050–2055.
90. **McQueen, C. A., and G. M. Williams.** 1987. Effects of quinolone antibiotics in tests for genotoxicity. *Am. J. Med.* **82**(Suppl. 4A):94–96.

91. **Miller, K. G., L. F. Liu, and P. T. Englund.** 1981. A homogeneous type II DNA topoisomerase from HeLa cell nuclei. *J. Biol. Chem.* **256:**9334–9339.
92. **Miskimins, R., W. K. Miskimins, H. Bernstein, and N. Shimizu.** 1983. Epidermal growth factor-induced topoisomerase(s): intercellular translocation and relation to DNA synthesis. *Exp. Cell Res.* **146:**53–62.
93. **Mitelman, F., A.-M. Kolnig, B. Strömbeck, R. Norrby, B. Kromann-Andersen, P. Sommer, and J. Wadstein.** 1988. No cytogenetic effects of quinolone treatment in humans. *Antimicrob. Agents Chemother.* **32:**936–937.
94. **Muller, M. T., J. R. Spitzner, J. A. DiDonato, V. B. Mehta, K. Tsutsui, and K. Tsutsui.** 1988. Single-strand DNA cleavages by eukaryotic topoisomerase II. *Biochemistry* **27:**8369–8379.
95. **Nelson, E. M., K. M. Tewey, and L. F. Liu.** 1984. Mechanism of antitumor drug action: poisoning of mammalian DNA topoisomerase II on DNA by 4′-(9-acridinylamino) methane-sulfon-*m*-anisidide. *Proc. Natl. Acad. Sci. USA* **81:**1361–1365.
96. **Nelson, W., K. Cho, Y. Hsiang, L. F. Liu, and D. S. Coffey.** 1987. Growth-related elevations of DNA topoisomerase II levels found in Dunning R3327 rat prostatic adenocarcinomas. *Cancer Res.* **47:**3246–3250.
97. **Newport, J., and T. Spann.** 1987. Disassembly of the nucleus in mitotic extracts: membrane vesicularization, lamin disassembly, and chromosome condensation are independent processes. *Cell* **48:**219–230.
98. **Nitiss, J., and J. C. Wang.** 1988. DNA topoisomerase-targeting antitumor drugs can be studied in yeast. *Proc. Natl. Acad. Sci. USA* **85:**7501–7505.
99. **Oomori, Y., T. Yasue, H. Aoyama, K. Hirai, S. Suzue, and T. Yokota.** 1988. Effects of fleroxacin on HeLa cell functions and topoisomerase II. *J. Antimicrob. Chemother.* **22**(Suppl. D)**:**91–97.
100. **Osheroff, N.** 1986. Eukaryotic topoisomerase II: characterization of enzyme turnover. *J. Biol. Chem.* **261:**9944–9950.
101. **Osheroff, N.** 1987. Role of the divalent cation in topoisomerase II-mediated reactions. *Biochemistry* **26:**6402-6406.
102. **Osheroff, N.** 1989. Biochemical basis for the interactions of type I and type II topoisomerases with DNA. *Pharmacol. Ther.* **41:**223–241.
103. **Osheroff, N.** 1989. Effect of antineoplastic agents on the DNA cleavage/religation equilibrium of eukaryotic topoisomerase II: inhibition of DNA religation by etoposide. *Biochemistry* **28:**6157-6160.
104. **Osheroff, N., and K. C. Gale.** 1988. Effect of etoposide on the DNA cleavage/religation reaction of topoisomerase II: analysis of drug action. *FASEB J.* **2:**A1761.
105. **Osheroff, N., E. R. Shelton, and D. L. Brutlag.** 1983. DNA topoisomerase II from *Drosophila melanogaster:* relaxation of supercoiled DNA. *J. Biol. Chem.* **258:**9536–9543.
106. **Osheroff, N., and E. L. Zechiedrich.** 1987. Calcium-promoted DNA cleavage by eukaryotic topoisomerase II: trapping the covalent enzyme-DNA complex in an active form. *Biochemistry* **26:**4303–4309.
107. **Osheroff, N., E. L. Zechiedrich, and K. C. Gale.** 1991. Catalytic function of DNA topoisomerase II. *BioEssays* **13:**269–275.
108. **Phillips, I.** 1987. Bacterial mutagenicity and the 4-quinolones. *J. Antimicrob. Chemother.* **20:**771–773.
109. **Pommier, Y., D. Kerrigan, J. M. Covey, C.-S. Kao-Shan, and J. Whang-Peng.** 1988. Sister chromatid exchanges, chromosomal aberrations, and cytotoxicity produced by antitumor topoisomerase II inhibitors in sensitive (DC3F) and resistant (DC3F/9-OHE) Chinese hamster cells. *Cancer Res.* **48:**512–516.
110. **Pommier, Y., J. K. Minford, R. E. Schwartz, L. A. Zwelling, and K. W. Kohn.** 1985. Effects of the intercalators 4′-(9-acridinylamino) methane sulfon-*m*-anisidide (*m*-AMSA, amsacrine) and 2-methyl-9-hydrozyellipticinium (2-Me-9-OH-E+) on topoisomerase II-mediated DNA strand cleavage and strand passage. *Biochemistry* **24:**6410–6416.
111. **Pommier, Y., L. A. Zwelling, C.-S. Kao-Shan, J. Whang-Peng, and M. O. Bradley.** 1985. Correlations between intercalator-induced DNA strand breaks and sister chromatid exchanges, mutations, and cytotoxicity in Chinese hamster ovary cells. *Cancer Res.* **45:**3143–3149.
112. **Potmesil, M., Y.-H. Hsiang, L. F. Liu, B. Bank, H. Grossberg, S. Kirschenbaum, T. J. Forlenzar, A. Penziner, D. Kanganis, D. Knowles, F. Tranganos, and R. Silber.** 1988. Resistance of human leukemic and normal lymphocytes to drug-induced DNA cleavage and low levels of DNA topoisomerase II. *Cancer Res.* **48:**3537–3543.
113. **Riesbeck, K., J. Andersson, M. Gullberg, and A. Forsgren.** 1989. Fluorinated 4-quinolones induce hyperproduction of interleukin 2. *Proc. Natl. Acad. Sci. USA* **86:**2809–2813.
114. **Robinson, M. J., B. A. Martin, T. D. Gootz, P. R. McGuirk, and N. Osheroff.** 1992. Effects of novel fluoroquinolones on the catalytic activities of eukaryotic topoisomerase II: influence of the C-8 fluorine group. *Antimicrob. Agents Chemother.* **36:**751–756.
115. **Robinson, M. J., S. H. Elsea, B. A. Martin, T. D. Gootz, P. R. McGuirk, J. A. Sutcliffe, and N. Osheroff.** *In* T. Andoh, H. Ikeda, and M. Oguro (ed.), *DNA Topoisomerases in Chemotherapy*, in press. CRC Press, Boca Raton, Fla.

116. **Robinson, M. J., B. A. Martin, T. D. Gootz, P. R. McGuirk, M. Moynihan, J. A. Sutcliffe, and N. Osheroff.** 1991. Effects of quinolone derivatives on eukaryotic topoisomerase II: a novel mechanism for enhancement of enzyme-mediated DNA cleavage. *J. Biol. Chem.* **266:**14585–14592.

117. **Robinson, M. J., and N. Osheroff.** 1990. Stabilization of the topoisomerase II-DNA cleavage complex by antineoplastic drugs: inhibition of enzyme-mediated DNA religation by 4′-(9-acridinyl-amino) methane sulfon-*m*-anisidide. *Biochemistry* **29:**2511–2515.

118. **Robinson, M. J., and N. Osheroff.** 1991. Effects of antineoplastic drugs on the post-strand passage DNA cleavage/religation equilibrium of topoisomerase II. *Biochemistry* **30:**1807–1813.

119. **Rose, D., W. Thomas, and C. Holm.** 1990. Segregation of recombined chromosomes in meiosis I required DNA topoisomerase II. *Cell* **60:**1009–1017.

120. **Ross, W. E., T. Rowe, B. Glisson, J. Yalowich, and L. Liu.** 1984. Role of topoisomerase II in mediating epipodophyllotoxin-induced DNA cleavage. *Cancer Res.* **44:**5857–5860.

121. **Rottman, M., H. C. Schröder, M. Gramzow, K. Renneisen, B. Kurelec, A. Dorn, U. Friese, and E. G. Müller.** 1987. Specific phosphorylation of proteins in pore complex-laminae from the sponge *Geodia cydonium* by the homologous aggregation factor and phorbol ester. Role of protein kinase C in the phosphorylation of topoisomerase II. *EMBO J.* **6:**3939–3944.

122. **Rowe, T. C., G. L. Chen, Y.-H. Hsiang, and L. F. Liu.** 1986. DNA damage by antitumor acridines mediated by mammalian DNA topoisomerase II. *Cancer Res.* **46:**2021–2026.

123. **Sahyoun, N., M. Wolf, J. Besterman, T.-S. Hsieh, M. Sander, H. LeVine III, K.-J. Chang, and P. Cuatrecasas.** 1986. Protein kinase C phosphorylates topoisomerase II: topoisomerase II activation and its possible role in phorbol ester-induced differentiation of HL-60 cells. *Proc. Natl. Acad. Sci. USA* **83:**1603–1607.

124. **Sander, M., and T.-S. Hsieh.** 1983. Double-strand DNA cleavage by type II DNA topoisomerase from *Drosophila melanogaster. J. Biol. Chem.* **258:**8421–8428.

125. **Sander, M., and T.-S. Hsieh.** 1985. *Drosophila* topoisomerase II double-strand DNA cleavage: analysis of DNA sequence homology at the cleavage site. *Nucleic Acids Res.* **13:**1057–1072.

126. **Schluter, G.** 1986. Toxicology of ciprofloxacin, p. 61–70. *In* H. C. Neu and H. Wenta (ed.), *Proceedings of the First International Ciprofloxacin Workshop.* Elsevier Science Publishing Inc., Amsterdam.

127. **Schneider, E., Y.-H. Hsiang, and L. F. Liu.** 1990. DNA topoisomerases as anticancer drug targets. *Adv. Pharmacol.* **21:**149–183.

128. **Schneider, E., P. A. Lawson, and R. K. Ralph.** 1989. Inhibition of protein synthesis reduces the cytotoxicity of 4′-(9-acridinylamino)methane sulfon-*m*-anisidide without affecting DNA breakage and DNA topoisomerase II in murine mastocytoma cell line. *Biochem. Pharmacol.* **38:**263–269.

129. **Shen, L. L., W. E. Kohlbrenner, D. Weigl, and J. Baranowski.** 1989. Mechanism of quinolone inhibition of DNA gyrase: appearance of unique norfloxacin binding sites in enzyme-DNA complexes. *J. Biol. Chem.* **264:**2973–2978.

130. **Shen, L. L., L. A. Mitscher, P. N. Sharma, T. J. O'Donnell, D. W. T. Chu, C. S. Cooper, T. Rosen, and A. G. Pernet.** 1989. Mechanism of inhibition of DNA gyrase by antibacterials: a cooperative drug-DNA binding model. *Biochemistry* **28:**3886–3894.

131. **Stahlmann, R., and H. Lode.** 1988. Safety overview: toxicity adverse effects and drug interactions, p. 201–233. *In* V. T. Andriole (ed.), *The Quinolones.* Academic Press, Inc., New York.

132. **Sullivan, D. M., K.-C. Chow, B. S. Glisson, and W. E. Ross.** 1987. Role of proliferation in determining sensitivity to topoisomerase II-active chemotherapy agents. *NCI Monogr.* **4:**73–78.

133. **Sullivan, D. M., M. D. Latham, and W. E. Ross.** 1987. Proliferation-dependent topoisomerase II content as a determinant of antineoplastic drug action in human, mouse, and Chinese hamster ovary cells. *Cancer Res.* **47:**3973–3979.

134. **Sullivan, D. M., M. D. Latham, T. C. Rowe, and W. E. Ross.** 1989. Purification and characterization of an altered topoisomerase II from a drug-resistant Chinese hamster ovary cell line. *Biochemistry* **28:**5680–5687.

135. **Sutcliffe, J. A., T. D. Gootz, and J. F. Barrett.** 1989. Biochemical characteristics and physiological significance of major DNA topoisomerases. *Antimicrob. Agents Chemother.* **33:**2027–2033.

136. **Tabary, X., N. Moreau, C. Dureuil, and F. Le Goffic.** 1987. Effect of DNA gyrase inhibitors pefloxacin, five other quinolones, novobiocin, and clorobiocin on *Escherichia coli* topoisomerase I. *Antimicrob. Agents Chemother.* **31:**1925–1928.

137. **Taudou, G., G. Mirambeau, C. Lavenot, A. den Garabedian, J. Vermeersch, and M. Duget.** 1984. DNA topoisomerase activities in concanavalin A-stimulated lymphocytes. *FEBS Lett.* **176:**431–435.

138. **Tewey, K. M., G. L. Chen, E. M. Nelson, and L. F. Liu.** 1984. Intercalative antitumor drugs interfere with the breakage-reunion reaction of mammalian topoisomerase II. *J. Biol. Chem.* **259:**9182–9187.

139. **Tsai-Pflugfelder, M., L. F. Liu, A. A. Liu, K. M. Tewey, J. Whang-Peng, T. Knutsen, K. Huebner, C. M. Croce, and J. C. Wang.** 1988. Cloning and sequencing of cDNA encoding hu-

man DNA topoisomerase II and localization of the gene to chromosome region 17q21-22. *Proc. Natl. Acad. Sci. USA* **85:**7177–7181.

140. **Tse-Ding, Y.-C., and J. C. Wang.** 1986. Complete nucleotide sequence of the *topA* gene encoding *Escherichia coli* DNA topoisomerase I. *J. Mol. Biol.* **191:**321–331.

141. **Uemura, T., K. Morikawa, and M. Yanagida.** 1986. The nucleotide sequence of the fission yeast DNA topoisomerase II gene; structural and functional relationships to other DNA topoisomerases. *EMBO J.* **5:**2355–2361.

142. **Uemura, T., H. Ohkuru, Y. Adachi, K. Morino, K. Shiozaki, and M. Yanagida.** 1987. DNA topoisomerase II is required for condensation and separation of mitotic chromosomes in *S. pombe*. *Cell* **50:**917–925.

143. **Uemura, T., and M. Yanagida.** 1984. Isolation of type I and II DNA topoisomerase mutants from fission yeast; single and double mutants show different phenotypes in cell growth and chromatin organization. *EMBO J.* **3:**1737–1744.

144. **Uemura, T., and M. Yanagida.** 1986. Mitotic spindle pulls but fails to separate chromosomes in type II DNA topoisomerase mutants: uncoordinated mitosis. *EMBO J.* **5:**1003–1010.

145. **Wadkins, R. M., and D. E. Graves.** 1991. Interactions of anilinoacridines with nucleic acids: effects of substituent modifications on DNA binding properties. *Biochemistry* **30:**4278–4283.

146. **Wang, J. C.** 1985. DNA topoisomerases. *Annu. Rev. Biochem.* **54:**665–697.

147. **Waring, M. J.** 1981. DNA modification and cancer. *Annu. Rev. Biochem.* **50:**159–192.

148. **Wentland, M. P.** 1990. Structure-activity relationships of fluoroquinolones, p. 1–43. *In* C. Siporin, C. L. Heifetz, and J. M. Domagala (ed.), *The New Generation of Quinolones.* Marcel Dekker, Inc., New York.

149. **Wentland, M. P., G. Y. Lesher, M. Reuman, G. M. Pilling, M. T. Saindane, R. B. Perni, M. A. Eissenstat, J. D. Weaver III, J. B. Rake, and S. A. Coughlin.** 1991. Mammalian topoisomerase II inhibitory activity of 1,8-bridged-7-(2,6-dimethyl-4-pyridinyl)-3-quinolone carboxylic acids. *Proc. Am. Assoc. Cancer Res.* **32:**336.

150. **Wilson, W. R., B. C. Baugley, L. P. G. Wakelin, and M. J. Waring.** 1981. Interaction of the antitumor drug 4′-(9-acridinylamino) methane sulfon-*m*-anisidide and related acridines with nucleic acids. *Mol. Pharmacol.* **20:**404–414.

151. **Wood, E. R., and W. C. Earnshaw.** 1990. Mitotic chromatin condensation *in vitro* using somatic cell extracts and nuclei with variable levels of endogenous topoisomerase II. *J. Cell Biol.* **111:**2839–2850.

152. **Wyckoff, E., D. Natalie, J. M. Nolan, M. Lee, and T.-S. Hsieh.** 1989. Structure of the *Drosophila* DNA topoisomerase II gene: nucleotide sequence and homology among topoisomerase II. *J. Mol. Biol.* **205:**1–13.

153. **Yang, L., T. C. Rowe, E. M. Nelson, and L. F. Liu.** 1985. *In vivo* mapping of DNA topoisomerase II-specific cleavage sites on SV40 chromatin. *Cell* **41:**127–132.

154. **Yoshida, H., M. Bogaki, M. Nakamura, L. M. Yamanaka, and S. Nakamura.** 1991. Quinolone resistance-determining region in the DNA gyrase *gyrB* gene of *Escherichia coli. Antimicrob. Agents Chemother.* **35:**1647–1650.

155. **Zechiedrich, E. L., K. Christiansen, A. H. Andersen, O. Westergaard, and N. Osheroff.** 1989. Double-stranded DNA cleavage/religation reaction of eukaryotic topoisomerase II: evidence for a nicked DNA intermediate. *Biochemistry* **28:**6229–6236.

156. **Zechiedrich, E. L., and N. Osheroff.** 1990. Eukaryotic topoisomerases recognize nucleic acid topology by preferentially interacting with DNA crossovers. *EMBO J.* **9:**4555–4562.

157. **Zhang, H., P. D'Arpa, and L. F. Liu.** 1990. A model for tumor cell killing by topoisomerase poisons. *Cancer Cells* **2:**23–27.

158. **Zimmer, C., K. Storl, and J. Storl.** 1990. Microbial DNA topoisomerases and their inhibition by antibiotics. *J. Basic Microbiol.* **30:**209–224.

159. **Zwelling, L. A.** 1989. Topoisomerase II as a target of antileukemia drugs: a review of controversial areas. *Hematol. Pathol.* **3:**101–112.

160. **Zwelling, L. A., M. Hinds, D. Chan, J. Mayes, K. L. Sie, E. Parker, L. Silberman, A. Radcliffe, M. Beran, and M. Blick.** 1989. Characterization of an amsacrine-resistant line of human leukemia cells. *J. Biol. Chem.* **264:**16411–16420.

*Quinolone Antimicrobial Agents, 2nd ed.*
Edited by David C. Hooper and John S. Wolfson


*Chapter 8*

# Activity In Vitro of the Quinolones

*G. M. Eliopoulos and C. T. Eliopoulos*

Development of the fluoroquinolone antimicrobial agents represents a major advance in antimicrobial chemotherapy. In comparison with the early quinolones such as nalidixic acid, the newer agents not only demonstrate greater potency against common gram-negative bacteria but also provide activity against *Pseudomonas aeruginosa* and various gram-positive organisms, including *Staphylococcus aureus* (67). The broad spectrum of these antimicrobial agents' activities against other pathogens, including mycobacteria, *Chlamydia* species, rickettsiae, and even plasmodia, has also generated considerable interest, especially considering the limited options currently available for treatment of infections caused by these microorganisms. Nevertheless, since the introduction of the fluoroquinolones, the potential limitations of these agents (primarily the emergence of resistant strains within some institutions) have been increasingly appreciated.

This chapter reviews the in vitro antimicrobial activities of the currently available fluoroquinolones and the technical factors that influence determination of drug activities. Representative agents presently under investigation are discussed to illustrate the possibilities for future development of fluoroquinolones with greater potency against gram-positive bacteria, anaerobes, and other microbes against which the currently available agents provide relatively weak activity. Neither specific mention nor omission of individual drugs is intended to reflect an assessment of their ultimate clinical roles. As in our previous review (67), our primary purpose is to explore the potential antimicrobial spectrum of the fluoroquinolones as a class of therapeutic agents.

## ANTIMICROBIAL ACTIVITY

### Gram-Negative Bacteria

#### *Enterobacteriaceae*

The clinical utility of nalidixic acid and other older quinolone antimicrobial agents derived principally from their activities against bacteria of the family *Enterobacteriaceae.* Against this group of organisms, concentrations of nalidixic acid required to inhibit 90% of isolates ($MIC_{90}$) generally equaled or exceeded 8 $\mu$g/ml (67). The increased potency of the fluoroquinolones against these organisms is evident from the data presented in Tables 1 and 2 (most of these data are derived from studies published since 1988). Ciprofloxacin, the most active of the currently available drugs of this class,

*G. M. Eliopoulos and C. T. Eliopoulos* • Department of Medicine, New England Deaconess Hospital, Boston, Massachusetts 02215, and Harvard Medical School, Boston, Massachusetts 02115.

**Table 1.** Susceptibilities of common *Enterobacteriaceae* to earlier quinolones based on data collected since 1988

| Organism | Representative $MIC_{90}$ (range) ($\mu$g/ml) of[a]: | | | | |
|---|---|---|---|---|---|
| | CPX | NFX | ENX | OFX | PFX |
| *Escherichia coli* | ≤0.06 (≤0.01–0.25) | 0.12 (0.01–0.5) | 0.25 (0.03–2) | 0.12 (0.02–1) | 0.12 (0.12–0.25) |
| *Klebsiella pneumoniae* | 0.12 (0.02–1) | 0.5 (0.2–2) | 1 (0.5–2) | 0.25 (0.12–1) | 2 (0.5–2) |
| *Klebsiella oxytoca* | 0.12 (≤0.01–0.25) | 0.25 (0.1–0.5) | 0.5 (0.5) | 0.5 (0.12–2) | 1 (1) |
| *Klebsiella* spp. | 0.25 (≤0.03–3.13) | 0.5 (0.25–4) | 2 (0.5–4) | 1 (0.25–6.25) | 0.5 (0.5) |
| *Hafnia alvei* | 0.03 (0.02–0.06) | 0.12 (0.12) | 0.12 (0.12) | 0.25 (0.06–0.25) | |
| *Serratia marcescens* | 0.25 (0.06–12.5) | 1 (≤0.25–50) | 2 (1–25) | 1 (0.5–25) | 1 (1–8) |
| *Serratia* spp. | 0.25 (0.03–2) | 2 (0.25–8) | 4 (0.5–8) | 1 (0.5–4) | [1.0][b] |
| *Enterobacter cloacae* | 0.12 (≤0.03–0.5) | 0.5 (≤0.25–2) | 0.5 (0.1–1) | 0.25 (0.1–1) | 0.5 (0.5) |
| *Enterobacter aerogenes* | 0.06 (≤0.03–0.25) | 0.5 (0.2–2) | 0.25 (0.25–0.39) | 0.25 (0.12–1) | [0.25] |
| *Enterobacter agglomerans* | 0.06 (≤0.01–0.06) | 0.25 (0.25) | 0.25 (0.25) | 0.25 (0.06–0.25) | [0.5] |
| *Enterobacter* spp. | 0.12 (≤0.03–2) | 0.25 (0.125–8) | 0.5 (0.5) | 1 (0.1–1.56) | |
| *Citrobacter freundii* | 0.12 (≤0.03–6.25) | 0.5 (≤0.25–50) | 0.5 (0.25–1.56) | 0.5 (0.1–25) | (0.4–1) |
| *Citrobacter diversus* | ≤0.03 (≤0.01–0.25) | ≤0.12 (≤0.06–0.12) | ≤0.12 (≤0.12) | ≤0.06 (≤0.06–1) | |
| *Proteus mirabilis* | 0.06 (≤0.03–0.39) | 0.1 (0.12–0.5) | 0.5 (0.25–1.56) | 0.5 (0.12–1) | 0.25 (0.25) |
| *Proteus vulgaris* | 0.06 (0.01–0.25) | 0.1 (0.12–0.5) | 0.5 (0.25–2) | 0.25 (0.06–0.5) | 0.25 (0.25) |
| *Morganella morganii* | 0.06 (0.01–6.25) | 0.12 (≤0.06–0.25) | 0.5 (≤0.12–1.56) | 0.25 (0.1–12.5) | 0.25–4 |
| *Providencia rettgeri* | 1.0 (0.03–2) | 2 (0.25–3.1) | 1 (0.5–6.25) | 1.0 (0.5–8) | [0.5] |
| *Providencia stuartii* | 0.5 (0.125–2) | 2 (≤0.25–2) | 2 (1–2) | 1 (1–8) | [4] |

[a]Abbreviations: CPX, ciprofloxacin; NFX, norfloxacin; ENX, enoxacin; OFX, ofloxacin; PFX, pefloxacin. Data were derived from the following references: for ciprofloxacin, 1a, 4, 6, 22, 25, 38, 44, 45, 48, 50, 53, 61, 69, 74, 80, 87, 88, 91, 93, 108, 124, 128, 129, 139, 140, 144, 145, 152, 168, 173, 176, 177, 180, 204, 205, 207, 213, 220, 227, 231, 235, 241, 243, 253, 256; for norfloxacin, 4, 6, 25, 32, 45, 91, 93, 128, 144, 145, 152, 177, 241, 243; for enoxacin, 1a, 4, 6, 32, 45, 91, 128, 139, 140, 180; for ofloxacin, 1a, 4, 6, 38, 44, 45, 74, 88, 91, 108, 124, 128, 139, 144, 145, 152, 168, 173, 177, 180, 213, 231, 235, 238, 253, 256; for pefloxacin, 91, 152, 238, 243.

[b]Derived from data collected prior to 1988 (67).

**Table 2.** Susceptibilities of common *Enterobacteriaceae* to newer fluoroquinolone antimicrobial agents

| Organism | Representative $MIC_{90}$ (range) ($\mu$g/ml) of[a]: | | | | | |
|---|---|---|---|---|---|---|
| | TMX | LMX | FLX | TOS | SPX | L-OFX |
| *Escherichia coli* | 0.12 (≤0.02–1.0) | 0.2 (0.06–1.0) | 0.1 (0.03–2) | ≤0.03 (≤0.02–0.5) | ≤0.06 (≤0.03–0.1) | ≤0.06 (0.03–0.1) |
| *Klebsiella* spp. | 1.0 (0.12–2) | 1.0 (0.2–6.25) | 0.5 (0.12–6.25) | 0.12 (0.06–0.5) | 0.12 (≤0.03–1) | 0.25 (0.06–3.1) |
| *Serratia* sp. | 2 (0.5–2) | 2 (0.25–25) | 0.5 (0.25–25) | 0.5 (0.25–0.5) | 1 (0.12–12.5) | 3.1 (0.12–12.5) |
| *Enterobacter cloacae* | 0.5 (0.5) | 0.5 (≤0.25–1) | 0.25 (0.12–0.25) | 0.12 (0.12) | 0.25 (0.12–0.5) | 0.2 (0.06–0.2) |
| *Enterobacter aerogenes* | 0.25 (0.25) | 0.5 (≤0.25–1) | 0.12 (≤0.12–0.25) | 0.12 (0.06–0.12) | 0.12 (0.12–0.5) | 0.12 (0.12) |
| *Citrobacter* spp. | 0.5 (0.5) | 0.5 (0.12–25) | 0.12 (≤0.06–25) | 0.12 (0.03–0.25) | 0.5 (0.6–2) | 0.5 (0.06–6.2) |
| *Proteus mirabilis* | 0.5(0.5–1) | 1(0.5–1) | 0.5 (≤0.12–0.25) | 0.12(0.12–0.25) | 0.5(0.25–1) | 0.2 (0.2–8) |
| *Proteus vulgaris* | 1 (1) | 0.5 (0.25–1) | 0.12 (≤0.12–0.25) | 0.25 (0.25) | 0.5 (0.5–1) | 0.2 (0.2–0.5) |
| *Morganella morganii* | 2 (2) | 0.25 (0.25–12.5) | 0.12 (≤0.6–12.5) | 0.25 (0.12–0.5) | 0.5 (0.25–1) | 0.5 (0.06–6.2) |
| *Providencia rettgeri* | 0.5 (0.25–1) | 4 (1.6–6.2) | 0.5 (0.12–1) | 0.25 (0.12–0.5) | 0.5 (0.25–2) | 1 (1) |
| *Providencia stuartii* | 2 (0.5–2) | 1 (1–4) | 1 (0.5–2) | 1 (1) | 0.5 (0.2–2) | 1 (1) |

[a]Abbreviations: TMX, temafloxacin; LMX, lomefloxacin; FLX, fleroxacin; TOS, tosufloxacin; SPX, sparfloxacin; L-OFX, *S*-(−)-ofloxacin. Data were derived from the following references: for temafloxacin, 25, 50, 139, 140, 177, 227; for lomefloxacin, 32, 45, 152, 213, 235, 238, 241, 243, 253; for fleroxacin, 22, 108, 128, 129, 177, 204, 207, 235, 253; for tosufloxacin, 4, 25, 44, 74, 80, 140; for sparfloxacin, 38, 50, 61, 87, 144, 168, 207, 243; for *S*-(−)-ofloxacin, 93, 124, 171, 231, 235.

inhibits 90% of all isolates at concentrations of ≤0.25 $\mu$g/ml for almost all of the species represented. Strains of *Providencia stuartii*, *Providencia rettgeri*, and *Serratia marcescens* tend to be less exquisitely susceptible to the fluoroquinolones, but occasional isolates of other species that show reduced susceptibility to these agents are encountered. For example, ciprofloxacin-resistant strains of *Escherichia coli* (MIC, 32 $\mu$g/ml) (139, 140), *Klebsiella pneumoniae*, (MIC, 8 $\mu$g/ml) (253), and *Enterobacter cloacae* (MIC, 16 to 25 $\mu$g/ml) (145, 213) are included among isolates examined in the studies cited in Table 1. Activities of ciprofloxacin and fleroxacin against uncommon clinical isolates of the family *Enterobacteriaceae* were reported by Hohl et al. (120). The two fluoroquinolones inhibited all strains at concentrations of ≤0.125 and ≤0.5 $\mu$g/ml, respectively.

Activities of several newer fluoroquinolones are shown in Table 2. One of these, designated DR-3355, is the *S*-(−)-optical isomer of ofloxacin (124, 231, 235). It is generally twice as active as ofloxacin and substantially more active than the *R*-(+)-isomer of ofloxacin (231). None of these is intrinsically more active than ciprofloxacin against the *Enterobacteriaceae*.

### *Pseudomonas* spp. and other gram-negative organisms

Activity against *P. aeruginosa* is a feature of the fluoroquinolones that distinguishes them from the older quinolone antimicrobial agents. $MIC_{90}$s of several of these agents against *P. aeruginosa*, as derived from recent studies, are shown in Table 3. Although the ranges of $MIC_{90}$s for the various drugs are quite broad, reflecting significant numbers of resistant isolates in several strain collections, most studies calculate $MIC_{90}$s that fall within somewhat narrower ranges: ciprofloxacin, 0.5 to 2 $\mu$g/ml; enoxacin, 4 to 16 $\mu$g/ml; ofloxacin, 2 to 8 $\mu$g/ml; temafloxacin, fleroxacin, and lomefloxacin, 4 to 8 $\mu$g/ml; and tosufloxacin, 1 to 4 $\mu$g/ml (references cited in footnote *a* of Table 3). In only 6 of 44 studies did $MIC_{90}$s of ciprofloxacin exceed 1 μg/ml.

In contrast, *Pseudomonas cepacia* and *Xanthomonas maltophilia* are often resistant to the fluoroquinolones. Against these isolates, $MIC_{90}$s of ciprofloxacin fell below 4 μg/ml in only 2 of 14 studies of *P. cepacia* and in 4 of 24 studies of *X. maltophilia* (Table 3). Several of the newer agents appear to be more potent than ciprofloxacin against the latter species. These newer agents include sparfloxacin, tosufloxacin, and the newest investigational agents WIN 57273 ($MIC_{90}$, 2 to 4 μg/ml) (44, 69), PD 127,391 ($MIC_{90}$, 0.25 to 2 μg/ml) (87, 173, 206), PD 117,558 ($MIC_{90}$, 0.5 μg/ml) (204), PD 117,596 ($MIC_{90}$, 0.25 μg/ml) (205, 206), and BMY 40062 (88). Most isolates of *Pseudomonas pseudomallei* are resistant to clinically achievable concentrations of the fluoroquinolones. Greater degrees of susceptibility are observed among strains of *Pseudomonas fluorescens* and *Pseudomonas putida* (Table 3), *Pseudomonas acidovorans* (140), *Pseudomonas stutzeri* (3), and *Pseudomonas putrefaciens* (52). For the last three species, $MIC_{90}$s of ciprofloxacin were 0.12, 0.5, and 1 μg/ml, respectively.

As illustrated in Table 4, *Aeromonas* spp., *Eikenella corrodens,* and *Pasturella multocida* are quite susceptible to this class of antimicrobial agents ($MIC_{90}$s, ≤0.06 μg/ml). Seventy-two isolates of *Plesiomonas shigelloides* isolated from patients with diarrhea proved susceptible to both ciprofloxacin and norfloxacin at concentrations of ≤1 μg/ml (132). Among isolates recovered from bite wounds, species designated EF-4 and M-5 as well as *Moraxella* spp. were susceptible to ciprofloxacin (MIC, <0.25 μg/ml), ofloxacin (MIC, ≤0.125 μg/ml) and enoxacin (MIC, ≤0.5 μg/ml) (100). Against 18 strains of *Flavobacterium* sp. II B examined in that study, MICs of these agents ranged from 0.5 to 1, 0.25 to 2, and 0.5 to 4 μg/ml, respectively (100). Susceptibilities of *Acinetobacter* spp. to any of the fluoroquinolones vary over a broad range, with some isolates proving highly resistant (Table 4). Tosufloxacin appears to be consistently more active than ciprofloxacin against strains of this genus (16, 44, 74, 140). Based on comparisons of MICs of ciprofloxacin, norfloxacin, and ofloxacin for 50% of strains ($MIC_{50}$s), there did not appear to be significant differences in intrinsic susceptibilities of four *Acinetobacter* spp. to fluoroquinolones; however, all of the highly resistant strains belonged to the species *Acinetobacter baumannii* and ge-

**Table 3.** Susceptibilities of pseudomonads to fluoroquinolones

| Drug | Range of $MIC_{90}$s (μg/ml) against[a]: | | | | |
|---|---|---|---|---|---|
| | *P. aeruginosa* | *P. cepacia* | *X. maltophilia* | *P. pseudomallei* | *P. fluorescens-P. putida* |
| Ciprofloxacin | 0.25–8 | 0.5–16 | 2–25 | 3.1–8 | 0.12–>2 |
| Norfloxacin | 2–16 | 25–50 | 25–>64 | 8–64 | |
| Enoxacin | 3.1–32 | 16–25 | 3.1–16 | 6.3–32 | 1.0 |
| Ofloxacin | 2–>50 | 8–32 | 3.1–>25 | 6.3–32 | 4 |
| Temafloxacin | 2–16 | 16 | 2–16 | 6.3–16 | 1.8 |
| Lomefloxacin | 4–>50 | 16 | 8–>25 | 6.3 | |
| Fleroxacin | 2–>50 | 8–16 | 8–25 | 6.3 | 4.8 |
| Tosufloxacin | 0.5–>16 | 1–8 | 1–4 | 3.1 | 0.2 |
| Sparfloxacin | 1.56–8 | 1.0 | 0.5–>2 | | 1–2 |

[a]Data were derived from the following references: for ciprofloxacin, 1a, 4, 6, 7, 16, 18, 22, 28, 38, 44, 45, 47, 48, 50, 61, 69, 74, 80, 87, 88, 91, 93, 108, 128, 139, 140, 144, 145, 157, 168, 173, 176, 177, 180, 204–207, 213, 220, 223, 231, 235, 241, 243, 252, 253, 256, 260; for norfloxacin, 1a, 4, 6, 7, 32, 45, 47, 91, 93, 128, 144, 145, 177, 223, 241, 243, 252, 260; for enoxacin, 1a, 4, 6, 18, 32, 45, 91, 128, 139, 180, 206, 252, 260; for ofloxacin, 1a, 4, 6, 18, 38, 44, 45, 74, 88, 91, 108, 128, 139, 144, 145, 157, 168, 173, 177, 180, 213, 231, 235, 238, 252, 253, 256, 260; for temafloxacin, 18, 37, 50, 139, 140, 177, 206, 223, 260; for lomefloxacin, 32, 45, 233, 235, 238, 241, 243, 252, 260; for fleroxacin, 1a, 16, 18, 22, 108, 128, 129, 177, 206, 207, 235, 253, 260; for tosufloxacin, 4, 16, 18, 44, 74, 140, 260; for sparfloxacin, 16, 38, 50, 61, 87, 144, 157, 168, 206, 207, 243.

**Table 4.** Activities of fluoroquinolones against miscellaneous gram-negative bacteria

| Organism | Representative $MIC_{90}$ ($MIC_{max}$) (μg/ml) of[a]: | | | | | |
|---|---|---|---|---|---|---|
| | CPX | OFX | TMX | FLX | TOS | SPX |
| *Acinetobacter* spp. | 0.25–2 (>128) | 0.25–1 (>128) | 0.25–2 (2) | 0.5–4 (32) | 0.03–0.25 (1) | 0.06–1 (16) |
| *Aeromonas* spp. | ≤0.06 (0.25) | 0.03–0.5 (1) | 0.03–0.12 (0.5) | 0.12–0.25 (1) | ≤0.06 (0.06) | ≤0.12 (1) |
| *Alcaligenes* spp. | 4–>25 (64) | ≥25 (64) | | 4–>25(>25) | | 4 (8) |
| *Brucella* spp. | 0.25–1.25 (2.5) | 0.02–0.25 (1) | 0.25 (0.5) | 0.5–1 (1) | | 0.25–1.5 (1.5) |
| *Eikenella corrodens* | 0.06 (0.06) | 0.06 (0.12) | | | | 0.03 |
| *Pasteurella multocida* | ≤0.03 | 0.06 (0.25) | | | | |

[a]$MIC_{max}$, maximum MIC. For other abbreviations, see Table 1, footnote *a*, and Table 2, footnote *a*. For references, see Table 3, footnote *a*, as well as the following: for ciprofloxacin, 25, 98, 100, 138, 233, 238; for ofloxacin, 92, 98, 100, 138, 207, 208, 233; for temafloxacin, 25, 37, 92; for fleroxacin, 92, 98, 204, 208; for tosufloxacin, 25; for sparfloxacin, 68, 92.

nospecies 3 (233). *Alcaligenes* spp. tend to be relatively resistant to the fluoroquinolone antimicrobial agents (3, 8, 98, 121, 123, 207, 235). Although only limited data are available, *Francisella tularensis* has been found to be susceptible to killing by ciprofloxacin at concentrations of ≤0.15 μg/ml (229). Although ofloxacin and pefloxacin were also highly active against most isolates, occasional isolates required 5 μg of these agents per ml to demonstrate a 99.9% reduction in viable cells.

## Gastrointestinal pathogens

Considerable interest has focused on the use of fluoroquinolones as potential agents in the treatment of gastrointestinal tract infections. Most species of gram-negative bacteria associated with diarrheal syndromes are highly susceptible to this class of antimicrobial agents (Table 5). Various fluoroquinolones have shown potent activity against enterotoxigenic, enteropathogenic, and enteroinvasive strains of *E. coli* (25, 103, 124). Activity against *Salmonella* spp. extends to include *Salmonella typhi,* which is inhibited by ciprofloxacin and several other agents at concentrations of ≤0.12 μg/ml (45, 103), but resistant salmonellae have been encountered (118). Among the *Vibrio* spp., both *Vibrio cholerae* and *Vibrio parahaemolyticus* are typically highly susceptible to the fluoroquinolones (25, 124, 165, 217). Although activities of these agents are somewhat lower against *Campylobacter jejuni* than against the other enteropathogens mentioned, most isolates are fully susceptible. In studies comparing temafloxacin (25, 139, 217) or tosufloxacin (25, 74, 80) with ciprofloxacin and other agents directly, the two new drugs have shown activities at least comparable to and sometimes superior to those of the latter agents. *Campylobacter fetus* strains, which are resistant to nalidixic acid, are inhibited by ciprofloxacin at 1.0 μg/ml (82). A group of organisms designated *Campylobacter upsaliensis,* which were recovered from cultures of blood and feces, were studied by

**Table 5.** Susceptibilities of gastrointestinal tract pathogens to fluoroquinolone antimicrobial agents

| Drug | Range of $MIC_{90}$s ($\mu$g/ml) against[a]: | | | | | |
|---|---|---|---|---|---|---|
| | *Salmonella* spp. | *Shigella* spp. | *Campylobacter jejuni* | *Yersinia enterocolitica* | *Vibrio* spp. | *Helicobacter pylori* |
| Ciprofloxacin | ≤0.06 | ≤0.03 | 0.12–0.78 | ≤0.06 | ≤0.008–0.2 | 0.25–8 |
| Norfloxacin | ≤0.06–0.25 | ≤0.06–0.12 | 0.25–2 | ≤0.12 | 0.03–0.12 | 0.25–8 |
| Ofloxacin | 0.12–0.25 | 0.06–0.78 | 0.12–2 | 0.06–0.25 | 0.78 | 1.0 |
| Enoxacin | 0.25 | 0.06–0.25 | 1–32 | 0.12–0.25 | | 16 |
| Temafloxacin | 0.12–0.25 | 0.03–0.12 | 0.125 | 0.06–0.5 | 0.06–0.25 | 4 |
| Lomefloxacin | 0.25 | 0.06–0.25 | 0.125–1 | ≤0.06–0.25 | ≤0.06–0.25 | 2–4 |
| Fleroxacin | ≤0.12–0.25 | ≤0.125 | 0.5 | ≤0.06–2 | 0.125–0.5 | 4 |
| Sparfloxacin | ≤0.06 | ≤0.06 | 0.12–0.25 | ≤0.06 | | 0.5–4 |
| Tosufloxacin | 0.03 | ≤0.03 | 0.06 | 0.125 | ≤0.015 | |

[a]References: for ciprofloxacin, 22, 25, 38, 44, 45, 50, 68, 69, 74, 80, 88, 91, 93, 107, 108, 124, 128, 129, 144, 145, 156, 168, 173, 176, 177, 205, 207, 213, 217, 218, 220, 238, 243, 253, 256; for norfloxacin, 25, 45, 91, 93, 128, 144, 145, 159, 177, 217, 243; for ofloxacin, 37, 38, 44, 45, 74, 88, 91, 107, 108, 124, 128, 139, 144, 145, 156, 168, 173, 177, 213, 238, 253, 256; for enoxacin, 45, 67, 91, 128, 139, 144, 218; for temafloxacin, 25, 37, 50, 139, 177, 217; for lomefloxacin, 45, 159, 201, 217, 218, 238, 243, 253; for fleroxacin, 22, 108, 128, 129, 177, 218, 253; for sparfloxacin, 38, 50, 68, 144, 243; for tosufloxacin, 25, 44, 74.

Preston et al. (188). Ninety percent of strains were killed at the following concentrations: sparfloxacin, ≤0.12 $\mu$g/ml; ofloxacin and ciprofloxacin, 0.25 $\mu$g/ml; pefloxacin, lomefloxacin, and fleroxacin, 0.5 $\mu$g/ml; norfloxacin, 2 $\mu$g/ml (188). Most studies report $MIC_{90}$s of ciprofloxacin against *Helicobacter pylori* between 0.25 and 0.5 $\mu$g/ml (68, 107, 168, 218, 243), although more-resistant strains are occasionally encountered (50). There is not yet enough evidence to suggest a significant advantage in potency of any other fluoroquinolone over ciprofloxacin against these isolates.

## Respiratory tract pathogens

Several gram-negative pathogenic bacteria of respiratory tract origin are highly susceptible to the fluoroquinolones. Several of these were discussed above (Table 4). Susceptibilities of *Haemophilus influenzae, Neisseria meningitidis,* and *Moraxella catarrhalis* are indicated in Table 6. Occasional isolates of *M. catarrhalis* with reduced susceptibilities, i.e., with MICs of ciprofloxacin between 0.5 and 2 $\mu$g/ml, are encountered (69, 74, 219). Strains of *Haemophilus parainfluenzae* are exquisitely susceptible to ciprofloxacin ($MIC_{90}$, 0.008 to 0.032 $\mu$g/ml) and several other fluoroquinolones (189, 220). $MIC_{90}$s of ciprofloxacin and ofloxacin against *Capnocytophaga* spp. were 0.12 and 0.25 $\mu$g/ml, respectively, in one study (5). Most strains of *Bordetella* spp. are fully susceptible to ciprofloxacin ($MIC_{90}$s, ≤0.12 $\mu$g/ml), ofloxacin ($MIC_{90}$s, ≤0.5 $\mu$g/ml), and several of the newer agents of this class. The upper range of $MIC_{90}$s against these strains reflects reduced activity against *Bordetella bronchiseptica* (MIC ranges, 1 to 4 $\mu$g of ciprofloxacin and 2 to 8 $\mu$g of ofloxacin per ml) (150). *Nocardia* spp. (included here for convenience) are generally resistant to the currently available fluoroquinolones. The investigational agent PD 117,558 appears to have more-promising activity ($MIC_{90}$, 2 $\mu$g/ml) against *Nocardia asteroides* (20).

**Table 6.** Susceptibilities of gram-negative respiratory pathogens *M. pneumoniae* and *C. pneumoniae* to fluoroquinolone antimicrobial agents

| Organism | Range of $MIC_{90}$s (μg/ml) against[a]: | | | | | | |
|---|---|---|---|---|---|---|---|
| | CPX | OFX | TMX | LMX | FLX | SPX | TOS |
| *Haemophilus influenzae* | ≤0.008–≤0.06 | ≤0.06–0.5 | ≤0.06 | ≤0.06–0.12 | ≤0.06–1 | ≤0.06 | ≤0.06 |
| *Moraxella catarrhalis* | ≤0.03–0.25 | 0.06–0.5 | 0.03–0.5 | ≤0.1–1 | 0.25–2 | 0.01–0.12 | ≤0.01–0.5 |
| *Neisseria meningitidis* | ≤0.008–0.12 | ≤0.06–0.4 | 0.015–0.06 | ≤0.06–0.4 | ≤0.03–0.25 | ≤0.06 | ≤0.03 |
| *Bordetella* spp. | ≤0.06–4 | 0.12–8 | ≤0.06 | 0.25 | 0.125–0.5 | | |
| *Legionella* spp.[b] | ≤0.12(1–2) | ≤0.06–(1) | ≤0.03(0.25) | ≤0.06 | ≤0.06 | ≤0.06(1) | (0.25) |
| *Nocardia* spp | 1.4–>25 | 2.6–>25 | 32 | | 64 | | 0.6–18 |
| *Mycoplasma pneumoniae* | 1–8 | 0.78[c] | 2 | 4–8 | 4 | 0.1–0.25 | |
| *Chlamydia pneumoniae*[d] | 1–2 | 1 | 0.5 | 4 | 2 | | |

[a]See Table 1, footnote *a*, and Table 2, footnote *a*, for abbreviations. Data were derived from the following references: for ciprofloxacin, 1a, 4, 6, 16, 18, 22, 30, 38, 44–46, 48, 50, 62, 64, 65, 69, 74, 78, 80, 88, 91, 108, 122, 127, 128, 135, 139, 140, 144, 145, 150, 168, 173, 176, 177, 180, 189, 204, 205, 207, 213, 219, 220, 227, 231, 235, 243, 248, 253, 256, 261; for ofloxacin, 1a, 4, 6, 18, 38, 44, 45, 74, 78, 88, 91, 108, 122, 128, 135, 139, 144, 145, 150, 168, 173, 177, 180, 189, 219, 227, 231, 235, 238, 253, 256, 262; for temafloxacin, 18, 20, 37, 50, 78, 122, 139, 140, 177, 219, 227, 245; for lomefloxacin, 30, 45, 78, 122, 135, 201, 219, 238, 243, 253; for fleroxacin, 1a, 16, 18, 20, 22, 78, 108, 122, 128, 129, 135, 173, 177, 204, 207, 219, 253; for sparfloxacin, 16, 38, 50, 65, 127, 135, 144, 168, 219, 243; for tosufloxacin, 4, 16, 18, 44, 74, 80, 140, 207, 261.

[b]Values in parentheses were derived in charcoal-containing media.

[c]$MIC_{50}$.

[d]Too few strains were tested to compute the $MIC_{90}$. Range of MICs shown.

Inhibitory concentrations of the fluoroquinolones against *Legionella* spp. appear to vary widely, but this variation is largely attributable to differences in the compositions of growth media utilized for testing (127). Markedly lower activities have been noted in studies employing media containing charcoal, which also adversely affects activities of fluoroquinolones against other bacteria such as *Staphylococcus epidermidis* (71). In other media, *Legionella* spp. are highly susceptible to the fluoroquinolones (Table 6). The validity of results obtained in charcoal-free media is supported by studies that have examined the abilities of fluoroquinolones to inhibit or kill *Legionella* spp. within cultured macrophages and in human monocytes. In such studies, several fluoroquinolones, including ofloxacin, ciprofloxacin, sparfloxacin, and fleroxacin, have proven highly effective (143, 186, 210).

It is convenient to consider here the susceptibilities of *Mycoplasma pneumoniae* and *Chlamydia pneumoniae* to fluoroquinolones. Ofloxacin inhibited each of 48 isolates of *M. pneumoniae* at a concentration of 1.56 μg/ml in a 1983 study by Osada and Ogawa (179). In a more recent study, the $MIC_{50}$ of this drug against 11 isolates was 0.78 μg/ml, which is identical to that of ciprofloxacin (168). Roughly comparable activities can be surmised for temafloxacin (227, 245) and ciprofloxacin (135, 168, 227, 246); however, higher $MIC_{90}$s have been reported for ciprofloxacin and lomefloxacin (30). Fortunately, several of the newer investigational agents, including sparfloxacin ($MIC_{90}$, 0.125 μg/ml) (246), WIN 57273 ($MIC_{90}$, 0.125 μg/ml) (135), and PD 127,391 ($MIC_{90}$, 0.031 μg/ml) (246), appear to be substantially more active against *M. pneumoniae.* In each instance, the $MIC_{90}$ of ciprofloxacin was 2 μg/ml.

The type strain TW183 of *Chlamydia pneumoniae* was subjected to antimicrobial susceptibility testing in cell culture by Fenelon et al. (78). Temafloxacin (MIC, 0.5 μg/ml) and A-56620 (MIC, 0.125 μg/ml)

**Table 7.** Susceptibilities of gram-positive bacteria to fluoroquinolone antimicrobial agents

| Organism | Representative $MIC_{90}$ (range) (μg/ml) of[a]: | | | |
|---|---|---|---|---|
| | CPX | NFX | ENX | OFX |
| *Staphylococcus aureus* | 0.5 (0.25–2) | 2 (1–4) | 2 (2–4) | 0.5 (0.1–2) |
| Coagulase-negative staphylococci | 0.5 (≤0.1–>2) | 2 (0.5–>4) | 2 (0.5–4) | 1 (0.25–2) |
| *Streptococcus pneumoniae* | 2 (0.78–6.2) | 16 (4–>16) | 16 (8–16) | 2 (1–8) |
| *Streptococcus pyogenes* | 1 (0.5–4) | 4 (2–16) | >8 (>8) | 2 (1–4) |
| *Streptococcus agalactiae* | 2 (0.5–4) | 16 (4–16) | >8 (>8) | 2 (2–4) |
| *Streptococcus bovis* | 4 (1–4) | >8 | >8 | 4 (2–4) |
| *Streptococcus* spp.[b] | 2 (0.5–4) | 16 (4–32) | 32 (8–32) | 4 (1–6.2) |
| *Enterococcus faecalis* | 2 (0.5–4) | 8 (4–32) | 8 (8–16) | 4 (2–6.2) |
| *Enterococcus faecium* | 4 (2–8) | ≥12.5 | 32 | 6.2 (2–16) |
| *Listeria monocytogenes* | 2 (0.5–2) | 8 (4–16) | 8 (8–16) | 2 (2–4) |
| *Corynebacterium* spp. | 1 (0.05–128) | 4 (4–>128) | 8 (4–>128) | 1 (0.5–64) |
| *Bacillus* spp. | 0.25 (0.12–1) | 1 (1) | 1 (0.5–1) | 0.5 (0.5) |

[a]See Table 1, footnote *a*, and Table 2, footnote *a*, for abbreviations. Data were derived from the following references: for ciprofloxacin, 1a, 4, 6, 15, 16, 18, 22, 35, 37, 38, 44, 45, 48, 50, 58, 68, 69, 74, 80, 87, 88, 90, 91, 93, 100, 105, 108, 114, 128, 130, 139, 140, 144, 145, 161, 162, 168, 173, 176–178, 181, 201, 204, 205, 207, 209, 213, 219, 220, 227, 231, 235, 241, 243, 250, 253, 256; for norfloxacin, 1a, 4, 6, 32, 45, 90, 91, 93, 114, 128, 144, 145, 161, 177, 209, 241, 243; for enoxacin, 1a, 4, 6, 18, 32, 45, 90, 91, 100, 128, 161, 162, 178, 209; for ofloxacin, 1a, 4, 6, 15, 18, 35, 37, 38, 44, 45, 50, 74, 88, 90, 91, 100, 108, 128, 130, 139, 144, 145, 161, 162, 168, 173, 177, 178, 201, 213, 219, 227, 231, 235, 238, 253, 256; for pefloxacin, 58, 90, 91, 161, 238, 243; for temafloxacin, 18, 37, 50, 58, 90, 139, 140, 162, 177, 219, 227; for lomefloxacin, 32, 45, 90, 152, 162, 201, 219, 235, 238, 241, 243, 253; for fleroxacin, 1a, 12, 16, 18, 22, 58, 90, 108, 128, 129, 161, 162, 177, 181, 204, 207, 219, 235, 253; for tosufloxacin, 4, 16, 18, 44, 74, 80, 140, 161; for sparfloxacin, 15, 16, 35, 38, 50, 68, 87, 90, 144, 168, 207, 219, 243; for *S*-(−)-ofloxacin, 93, 171, 231, 235.
[b]Includes streptococci of groups B, C, F, G, and viridans.

were the most active fluoroquinolones tested, followed by ofloxacin (MIC, 1 μg/ml) and ciprofloxacin, perfloxacin, and fleroxacin (MICs, 2 μg/ml). Against this strain and two additional clinical isolates, MICs of ciprofloxacin of 1 μg/ml were reported by Chirgwin et al. (46).

## GRAM-POSITIVE BACTERIA

### Staphylococci

Activities of several fluoroquinolones against staphylococci and other gram-positive bacteria are shown in Table 7. Most isolates of *S. aureus*, including most methicillin-resistant strains, are susceptible to ciprofloxacin and ofloxacin at concentrations of approximately 0.5 μg/ml (15, 207, 238). Some studies suggest a modest decrease in susceptibility to these drugs among methicillin-resistant strains (243), but other studies do not (15, 35, 69, 130, 238). However, fluoroquinolone resistance is now increasingly encountered, particularly among methicillin-resistant strains; MICs against some of these strains may exceed 100 μg/ml (178). Data from collections specifically assembled on the basis of resistance to these agents have been excluded in compiling Table 7 (15, 35, 38, 161, 178, 213, 243). Although several of the newest agents demonstrate substantially greater activities against staphylococci than do older drugs of this class (Tables 7 and 8), strains resistant to the earlier agents show diminished susceptibilities to the newer drugs as well (15, 35, 161, 243).

Coagulase-negative staphylococci are typically inhibited by concentrations of fluoroquinolones comparable to those active against *S. aureus*. Isolates resistant to fluoroquinolones are occasionally encountered among this group as well (35). Strains of *Staphylococcus saprophyticus* are modestly more resistant to fluoroquinolone antimicrobial agents than are strains of *S. epidermidis*. Examination of 15 recent studies reveals that the median $MIC_{90}$ of ciprofloxacin falls between 0.5 and 1 μg/ml for the former and between

Table 7. *Continued*

| Representative $MIC_{90}$ (range) ($\mu$g/ml) of[a]: | | | | | | |
|---|---|---|---|---|---|---|
| PFX | TMX | LMX | FLX | TOS | SPX | L-OFX |
| 0.5 (0.1–2) | 0.25 (0.1–0.5) | 2 (0.5–4) | 1 (0.125–4) | 0.06 (0.02–0.1) | 0.12 (0.06–0.25) | 0.25 (0.1–1) |
| 1 (0.5–4) | 0.25 (0.1–2) | 2 (0.5–4) | 1 (0.5–8) | 0.12 (.03–0.25) | 0.12 (0.03–>4) | 0.5 (0.1–1) |
| 12 (8–16) | 1 (0.5–1) | 8 (4–16) | 8 (8–25) | 0.25 (0.06–0.5) | 0.5 (0.25–1) | 2 (1–4) |
| 8 (8–16) | 0.5 (0.5–4) | 8 (4–12.5) | 8 (4–12.5) | 0.12 (0.06–0.25) | 1 (0.5–2) | 1 (0.5–1.56) |
| 32 | 2 (0.5–2) | 16 (8–32) | 8 (≥8) | 0.25 (0.12–0.5) | 0.5 (0.5–2) | 2 |
| | 2 (2) | | >8 | 0.25 (0.25) | | |
| >12.5 | 2 (0.5–4) | 8 (4–16) | 8 (4–8) | 0.5 (0.06–0.5) | 1 (0.25–1) | 1 (1) |
| 8 (4–8) | 2 (2) | 8 (4–16) | 8 (8–>16) | 0.5 (0.5) | 1 (0.25–1) | 2 (1.56–3.1) |
| | 12.5 | 8 (8) | 8 (8) | 1.0 (1.0) | 1 (0.5–4) | 3.1 (3.1) |
| 8 (6–8) | 2 (1–2) | 8 (6.2–8) | 8 (4–>16) | 0.25 (0.12–0.25) | 2 (1–4) | 1 |
| 8 (8–>128) | 2 (1–32) | >12.5 | 2 (1–32) | 0.25 (0.25) | 0.25 (0.25–64) | 1 |
| | 0.5 (0.5) | | 0.5 (0.5–1) | 0.06 (0.06) | 0.25 (0.25) | |

0.25 and 0.5 $\mu$g/ml for the latter species (15, 22, 50, 87, 88, 105, 140, 177, 200, 207, 219, 235, 243, 253, 256). Mean $MIC_{90}$s of ciprofloxacin, norfloxacin, and fleroxacin for *S. saprophyticus* have also been reported to be approximately 2 to 3 times higher than those for *S. epidermidis* (181). Activities of several fluoroquinolones against various other species of coagulase-negative staphylococci have also been examined (12, 15, 86, 87, 105).

## Streptococci

Activities of the earliest fluoroquinolones against streptococci are substantially lower than those against staphylococci. Temafloxacin demonstrates approximately twofold-greater potency than ciprofloxacin or ofloxacin against pneumococci and group A streptococci (Table 7), a small but consistent difference. Several of the newer agents still under development, including tosufloxacin, sparfloxacin, WIN 57273, and others shown in Table 8, show even greater activities against various streptococcal isolates. Tosufloxacin, WIN 57273, and PD 127,391 are highly active against *Streptococcus bovis* ($MIC_{90}$s, ≤0.25 $\mu$g/ml), against which ciprofloxacin and ofloxacin provide only weak activity (37, 44, 128, 173).

Enhanced activity against streptococci has also been obtained in a novel way through the linkage of the cephalosporin desacetylcefotaxime by an ester bond with either fleroxacin or ciprofloxacin. The resulting compounds have been designated Ro 23-9424 (22) and Ro 24-6392 (126), respectively. Detailed studies of the former indicate both binding to the penicillin-binding proteins of the bacterial cell membrane by the cephem and inhibition of replicative-DNA synthesis subsequent to the release of the fleroxacin moiety (95). Inhibitory activities of Ro 23-9424 against pneumococci and group A streptococci ($MIC_{90}$s, ≤0.25 $\mu$g/ml) are substantially greater than those of fleroxacin ($MIC_{90}$s, 8 $\mu$g/ml) (108, 129). Ro 24-6392 inhibited 90% of these organisms at a concentration of

**Table 8.** Activities of the newest quinolones

| Organism | $MIC_{90}$ range ($MIC_{max}$) (μg/ml)[a] | | | |
|---|---|---|---|---|
| | PD 117558 | E4497 | WIN 57273 | NM394 |
| *Staphylococcus aureus*[b] | ≤0.03 | 0.12 (1) | ≤0.03 (0.03) | 1.5 (3.1) |
| Coagulase-negative staphylococci | ≤0.03 | 0.12 (0.12) | 0.008–0.03 (0.5) | 0.8 (1.6) |
| *Streptococcus pyogenes* | 0.06 | | 0.03–0.12 (0.12) | 0.8 (1.6) |
| *Streptococcus pneumoniae* | 0.06 | 0.5 (1) | 0.03–0.06 (0.06) | 6.2 (6.2) |
| *Enterococcus faecalis* | 0.12 | 1 (4) | 0.06–0.16 (0.16) | 1.6 (3.1) |
| *Escherichia coli* | ≤0.03 | 0.12 (2) | 0.12–0.25 (2) | 0.1 (0.4) |
| *Klebsiella* spp. | 0.06–0.12 | 0.12 (0.25) | 0.5–1 (2) | 0.39 (0.78) |
| *Enterobacter* spp. | ≤0.06 | 0.12 (0.5) | 0.25–1 (32) | 0.05 (0.1) |
| *Serratia* spp. | 0.5 | 0.25 (0.5) | 2–16 (32) | 6.25 (6.25) |
| *Providencia stuartii* | | | 0.5–4 (4) | |
| *Pseudomonas aeruginosa* | 4 (16) | 2 (2) | 2–8 (>32) | 0.78 (1.56) |
| *Xanthomonas maltophilia* | 0.5 (1) | | 2–4 (8) | |

[a]Abbreviations: $MIC_{max}$, upper limit of MIC range. Data were derived from the following sources: for PD 117,558, 204; for E4497, 93; for WIN 57273, 44, 69, 128, 213; for NM394, 180; for PD 127,391, 87, 173, 176, 206, 256; for PD 131,628, 15, 48, 87; for E3846, 91; for PD 117,596, 205, 206, 220; for KB-5246, 145; for QA-241, 6, 174.
[b]Excludes strains selected for fluoroquinolone resistance.

≤0.06 μg/ml (126). Such results clearly reflect the contribution of the cephalosporin to in vitro activity of the dual-action compounds against streptococci.

### *Listeria monocytogenes* and enterococci

Ciprofloxacin and the other earlier fluoroquinolones demonstrate only modest activity against *L. monocytogenes* (Table 7). Although several of the newer agents, including tosufloxacin (16, 18, 44, 74), WIN 57273 (69, 128, 213), PD 117,558 (204), and PD 127,391 (173), inhibit 90% of isolates at concentrations of ≤0.25 μg/ml, the central nervous system tropisms of these organisms challenge the utility of quinolones in the treatment of listerial infections.

Most studies report $MIC_{90}$s of ciprofloxacin between 2 and 4 μg/ml for *Enterococcus faecalis*. Neither ofloxacin nor temafloxacin offers any advantage against this group of organisms. *Enterococcus faecium* demonstrates modestly greater levels of resistance to these drugs, with $MIC_{90}$s of ciprofloxacin generally 4 μg/ml (16, 68, 88, 144, 209, 231). Strains of enterococci that are resistant to ampicillin, vancomycin, and synergism by traditional combinations are now being encountered. Quinolone antimicrobial agents with potent activities against such organisms would be highly desirable. Several of the agents under investigation inhibit *E. faecalis* at concentrations of ≤0.25 μg/ml (Table 8), but *E. faecium* tends to be more resistant, with $MIC_{90}$s of 0.5 to 4 μg/ml (69, 87, 205).

### Other gram-positive bacteria

Ciprofloxacin ($MIC_{90}$, 0.06 μg/ml) and pefloxacin ($MIC_{90}$, 0.5 μg/ml) were highly active against *Erysipelothrix rhusiopathiae* in one study that examined only 10 strains (240). Activities of fluoroquinolones against *Bacillus* spp. have been reported as follows ($MIC_{90}$s): ciprofloxacin, 0.12 to 1.0 μg/ml (18, 128, 204, 205, 207, 249); ofloxacin and temafloxacin, 0.5 μg/ml (18, 128); fleroxacin, 0.5 to 1.0 μg/ml (18, 128, 204, 207); sparfloxacin, 0.25 μg/ml (207); tosufloxacin, 0.06 μg/ml (18); PD 117,558 and PD 117,596, ≤0.03 μg/ml (18, 205). Most strains of *Corynebacterium jeikeium* are at least moderately susceptible to several quinolones, including ciprofloxacin (18, 37, 68, 69, 74, 128, 173, 205, 207), ofloxacin (18,

Table 8. *Continued*

| MIC$_{90}$ range (MIC$_{max}$) ($\mu$g/ml)[a] | | | | | |
|---|---|---|---|---|---|
| PD 127,391 | PD 131,628 | E3846 | PD 117,596 | KB-5246 | QA-241 |
| 0.03–0.12 (>2) | 0.12 (>2) | 0.12 (0.12) | ≤0.03–0.06 (.06) | 0.1 (0.4) | 1–2 (3.1) |
| ≤0.06 (0.1) | 0.03–>2 (>2) | 0.25 (0.25) | 0.03–0.06 (0.06) | 0.2 (0.2) | 1–2 (2) |
| 0.06–0.25 (1) | 0.25 (0.25) | | 0.25 (0.25) | 0.2 (0.2) | 8 (12.5) |
| 0.12 (0.12) | 0.25 (0.25) | 1 (1) | 0.06–0.25 (0.25) | 0.4 (0.4) | 4–6.2 (12.5) |
| 0.12–0.25 (2) | 0.5 (>2) | | 0.25 (0.25) | | 4–6.2 (6.2) |
| ≤0.3 (0.25) | ≤0.03 (0.5) | 0.25 (1) | ≤0.03 (0.06) | 0.05 (6.25) | 0.2 (1.56) |
| ≤0.02–0.1 (0.25) | ≤0.06 (4) | 0.5–4 (16) | ≤0.03 (0.12) | 0.03–0.1 (0.78) | 0.5–1 (3–13) |
| ≤0.03–0.1 (0.5) | ≤0.03–0.5(1) | 1 (8) | ≤0.06 (0.25) | 0.2 (2.5) | 0.5 (1) |
| 0.12 (0.5) | 0.5 (8) | 4 (8) | ≤0.06 (0.12) | 6.25 (50) | 2–6.2 (50) |
| 0.12 (1) | | | | | 2 (4) |
| 0.5–1 (>2) | 0.5–1 (8) | 64 (≥128) | 0.12–0.25 (2) | 3.13 (6.25) | 4–12.5 (50) |
| 0.25–2 (>2) | >2 | | 0.25 (0.5) | 6.25 (25) | 6.25–8 (12.5) |

74, 128, 173), temafloxacin (18, 37), and fleroxacin (18, 128, 129, 204, 207), with MIC$_{90}$s between 0.5 and 2 $\mu$g/ml. WIN 57273 is the most active of the investigational agents (MIC$_{90}$, ≤0.03 $\mu$g/ml) (69, 128), although others also show excellent activity (18, 74, 204, 205, 220). *Leuconostoc* spp. and *Lactobacillus* spp. (MIC$_{90}$s, 4 $\mu$g/ml) are more resistant to ciprofloxacin, and *Pediococcus* spp. are even more resistant (MIC$_{90}$, 16 $\mu$g/ml) (228).

## Anaerobic Bacteria

Ciprofloxacin and ofloxacin demonstrate relatively weak activities against most anaerobic bacteria (Table 9), and norfloxacin, enoxacin, and pefloxacin are even less potent (67). Temafloxacin was four- to eightfold more active than ciprofloxacin against *Bacteroides fragilis* in several studies, but inhibitory concentrations are still relatively high (MIC$_{90}$s, 1 to 4 $\mu$g/ml) (37, 50, 140, 177). Other *Bacteroides* spp. are no more susceptible to these agents than are *B. fragilis*. Although *Clostridium perfringens* tends to be somewhat more susceptible to these agents than are *Bacteroides* spp., the currently or soon-to-be available fluoroquinolones cannot, as a class, be considered particularly active against anaerobic bacteria. Nevertheless, the investigational agents sparfloxacin, WIN 57273 (Table 9), and PD 127,391 (256) promise considerably greater activities against both gram-positive and gram-negative anaerobes.

Ciprofloxacin inhibits 90% of *Propionibacterium* spp. and *Eubacterium* spp. at concentrations between 2 and 16 $\mu$g/ml (13, 81, 99, 141, 187, 226, 251), of *Mobiluncus* spp. at between 1 and 4 $\mu$g/ml (125, 142), and of *Actinomyces* spp. at 8 $\mu$g/ml (13, 187, 251).

## Genital Pathogens

### Bacterial pathogens

Routine isolates of *Neisseria gonorrhoeae* are exquisitely susceptible to several of the fluoroquinolones. Ciprofloxacin inhibits most strains at concentrations of ≤0.015 $\mu$g/ml, with a range of MIC$_{90}$s between 0.002 and 0.12 $\mu$g/ml (6, 22, 38, 44, 45, 48, 50, 69, 74, 80, 88, 91, 108, 128, 139, 140, 144, 145, 151, 168, 173, 177, 213, 215, 220,

**Table 9.** Susceptibilities of anaerobic bacteria to fluoroquinolone antimicrobial agents

| Organism | Range of $MIC_{90}$s (μg/ml)[a] | | | | | | | |
|---|---|---|---|---|---|---|---|---|
| | CPX | OFX | TMX | LMX | FLX | TOS | SPX | WIN |
| *Bacteroides fragilis* | 4–128 | 2–12.5 | 1–4 | 8–64 | ≥16 | 1–4 | 1–2 | 0.25–1.0 |
| *Bacteroides* spp. | 1–32 | 2–32 | 4 | 8–32 | 2–64 | 1–8 | 4 | 0.25–1.0 |
| *Fusobacterium* spp. | 2–8 | 2–16 | 1 | 16 | 16 | 0.5–8 | | |
| *Clostridium* spp. | 1–16 | 1–8 | 2–32 | 16 | 2–32 | 0.25–8 | 4 | 0.12–0.25 |
| *Clostridium perfringens* | 0.5–8 | 0.5–8 | 0.5 | 2–8 | 1–4 | 0.25 | 0.5–2 | |
| *Clostridium difficile* | 8–25 | 12.5–16 | 4 | ≥32 | 16–32 | 4 | 6.25 | |
| Gram-positive cocci | 2–6.25 | 2–8 | 1–4 | 4–25 | 8–12.5 | 0.25–2 | 1–4 | 0.03–0.12 |

[a]For abbreviations, see Table 1, footnote *a*, and Table 2, footnote *a*. WIN, WIN 57273. Data were derived from the following sources: for ciprofloxacin, 6, 16, 37, 38, 44, 45, 48, 50, 69, 74, 80, 88, 91, 100, 108, 133, 140, 144, 145, 173, 177, 181, 201, 213, 217, 235, 243, 253; for ofloxacin, 6, 37, 38, 44, 45, 74, 88, 91, 100, 101, 108, 133, 144, 145, 173, 177, 201, 213, 235, 253, 256; for temafloxacin, 37, 50, 140, 177, 217; for lomefloxacin, 45, 133, 201, 217, 235, 243, 253; for fleroxacin, 22, 108, 177, 181, 235, 253; for tosufloxacin, 2, 16, 44, 74, 80, 133, 140, 213; for sparfloxacin, 16, 38, 50, 144, 243; for WIN 57273, 44, 69, 128, 213.

235, 243, 253, 256). However, MICs of 1.0 μg/ml have been recorded (151). A median MIC of ≤0.03 μg/ml can also be estimated for ofloxacin (6, 18, 38, 44, 45, 74, 88, 91, 108, 140, 144, 145, 168, 173, 235, 238, 256), temafloxacin (18, 50, 139, 140, 177, 215), and tosufloxacin (18, 44, 74, 80, 140, 215). Other investigational agents demonstrate very high potency against gonococci (44, 48, 69, 91, 128, 145, 173, 213, 220, 256).

Ninety percent of 122 strains of *Haemophilus ducreyi* were inhibited by ciprofloxacin at a concentration of 0.03 μg/ml (53). The $MIC_{90}$ of ciprofloxacin against *Gardnerella vaginalis* is 2 μg/ml, but some strains are resistant (139, 140, 151).

### *Chlamydia trachomatis*

A number of studies have examined activities of fluoroquinolones against *C. trachomatis*. Most of these show ciprofloxacin to inhibit isolates at concentrations of ≤2 μg/ml (Table 10), although inhibitory concentrations of up to 4 μg/ml have been recorded (50). Ofloxacin was at least as active in all studies and was twofold more active than ciprofloxacin in several studies (88, 158, 166). Temafloxacin, sparfloxacin, tosufloxacin, BMY 40062, and difloxacin are substantially more active than the older compounds, with $MIC_{90}$s of ≤0.25 μg/ml (50, 88, 158, 168, 177, 215, 216). Potencies at these levels are comparable to those of doxycycline and tetracycline against *C. trachomatis* (9, 10).

### Mycoplasmas and ureaplasmas

Several of the fluoroquinolones inhibit *Mycoplasma hominis* at $MIC_{90}$s between 0.5 and 2 μg/ml, including ciprofloxacin (137, 151, 246), ofloxacin (136, 137), fleroxacin (137), and lomefloxacin (137) (Table 10). Several of the newest agents display markedly greater activities. WIN 57273 inhibited 37 isolates at a concentration of 0.004 μg/ml (136). Sparfloxacin and PD 127,391 $MIC_{90}$s were each 0.03 μg/ml when tested against 30 isolates of *M. hominis* (246), while another study reported an $MIC_{90}$ of the former to be 0.06 μg/ml (136). *Ureaplasma urealyticum* strains are generally less susceptible to these agents than is *M. hominis* (Table 10), with ofloxacin being two- to eightfold more active than ciprofloxacin in several but not all (201) studies. Sparfloxacin and PD 127,391 inhibited 90% of strains at concentrations of 0.5 and 0.25 μg/ml, respectively, when studied with 30 isolates; the ciprofloxacin $MIC_{90}$ against the same isolates was 4 μg/ml (246).

**Table 10.** Expected susceptibilities of genital pathogens to representative fluoroquinolone antimicrobial agents

| Drug | Range of $MIC_{90}$s (μg/ml) against[a] | | |
|---|---|---|---|
| | *C. trachomatis* | *M. hominis* | *U. urealyticum* |
| Ciprofloxacin | 1.0–3.1 | 0.5–2 | 1–16 |
| Norfloxacin | ≥16 | 8 | 16 |
| Ofloxacin | 0.5–1.6 | 1–2 | 2–4 |
| Temafloxacin | 0.25 | 0.12–8 (2)[b] | 4–32 (4)[b] |
| Fleroxacin | 1.5–6.3 | 2 | 4 |
| Lomefloxacin | 2–3.1 | 2 | 4–8 |
| Sparfloxacin | 0.06 | ≤0.06 | 0.5 |
| PD 127,391 | 0.06 | 0.03 | 0.25 |

[a]Data were derived from the following references: for ciprofloxacin, 50, 88, 135, 137, 151, 158, 166, 168, 181, 201, 215, 216, 227, 246; for norfloxacin, 137, 158, 166, 168, 216; for ofloxacin, 88, 135–137, 146, 158, 166, 168, 201, 227; for temafloxacin, 177, 214–216, 227, 245; for fleroxacin, 135, 137, 146, 158, 166, 216; for lomefloxacin, 135, 137, 158, 166, 201, 230; for sparfloxacin, 50, 135, 136, 168, 246; for PD 127,391, 246, 256.

[b]The upper values of $MIC_{90}$ ranges for *M. hominis* and *U. urealyticum* are 2 and 4 μg/ml, respectively, if the "initial" MIC (antimicrobial effect at the time the control tube first indicates growth) is used (245).

### *Rickettsiaceae*

Fluoroquinolones have demonstrated activity against members of the family *Rickettsiaceae*. Using a plaque inhibition assay to determine drug susceptibilities of *Rickettsia rickettsii* and *Rickettsia conorii* cultured in Vero cells, Raoult et al. (191) found sparfloxacin to inhibit these species at 0.125 and 0.25 μg/ml, respectively. MICs were twofold higher in a neutral red dye uptake assay. Ciprofloxacin inhibited *R. conorii* at 0.25 μg/ml and was rickettsiacidal at 0.5 μg/ml with the plaque assay technique; at 1 μg/ml, the drug prevented a lethal effect in embryonated chicken eggs (192). This group has also shown inhibitory activity by pefloxacin and ofloxacin against both species at concentrations of 0.5 to 1.0 μg/ml (191).

Sparfloxacin at 1.0 μg/ml (191), like pefloxacin at 1.0 μg/ml and ofloxacin at 0.5 μg/ml (193), was effective against *Coxiella burnetii* in multiplying, persistently infected cell lines; however, the drug did not lead to eradication of organisms in cells that were blocked from multiplying.

### Mycobacteria

Various fluoroquinolones have demonstrated activities against several species of mycobacteria that cause infections in humans. Both ciprofloxacin and ofloxacin inhibited *Mycobacterium tuberculosis* at concentrations of ≤2 μg/ml for 90% of isolates in numerous studies (21, 57, 79, 94, 111, 116, 194, 236, 262), but more-resistant strains have also been encountered (49, 106, 234). Several *N*-alkyl analogs of ciprofloxacin have shown greater activity against *M. tuberculosis* than the parent compound. For example, *N*-isopropylciprofloxacin ($MIC_{90}$, 0.125 μg/ml) was eightfold more active than ciprofloxacin against 74 strains of this organism (111). Sparfloxacin is approximately two to three times more potent than ciprofloxacin or ofloxacin against *M. tuberculosis* (194).

Inhibitory activities of fluoroquinolones against rapidly growing mycobacteria vary over a wide range. Strains of *Mycobacterium fortuitum* tend to be more susceptible to these antimicrobial agents than is *Mycobacterium chelonei*. $MIC_{90}$s of ciprofloxacin for the former range from 0.125 to 1.0 μg/ml (111, 236, 247). Temafloxacin activity is comparable to that of ciprofloxacin (236), and ofloxacin is only twofold less active (236, 247). *M. fortuitum* biovar *fortuitum* strains ($MIC_{90}$ of ciprofloxacin, 0.125 μg/ml) are more susceptible than those of two other biovariants of this species ($MIC_{90}$, 1.0 μg/ml) (247). In contrast, $MIC_{90}$s of ciprofloxacin for *M.*

*chelonei* equal or exceed 8 μg/ml (94, 111, 236, 247). Resistance to other fluoroquinolones parallels resistance to ciprofloxacin.

At concentrations of 2 μg/ml or less, ciprofloxacin inhibits 90% of strains of *Mycobacterium xenopi* (49), *Mycobacterium malmoense* (111, 244), *Mycobacterium smegmatis,* and pigmented rapid growers (247). *Mycobacterium kansasii* is inhibited by the drug at concentrations from 1 to 4 μg/ml (94). Strains of the *Mycobacterium avium-Mycobacterium intracellulare* complex are relatively resistant to the quinolones. $MIC_{90}$s of ≥ 8 μg/ml are typical (29, 49, 94, 111, 116, 234, 236, 259). The other currently available agents offer no advantage against ciprofloxacin-resistant strains (116, 236). However, WIN 57273 and sparfloxacin appear to be two- to fourfold more active than ciprofloxacin (68, 69, 116, 183, 196, 259). In an in vitro radiorespirometric method, several fluoroquinolones, including ofloxacin, sparfloxacin, WIN 57273, and a number of other investigational agents, have shown promising activity against *Mycobacterium leprae* (84, 85). The in vitro and in vivo activities of the new quinolones against mycobacteria have been extensively reviewed by Leysen et al. (154).

### *Plasmodium* spp.

Plasmodia of either human or animal origin have proven susceptible to some fluoroquinolones at clinically achievable concentrations (26). Using reduction of [$^3$H]hypoxanthine incorporation as a measure of drug inhibitory effects against two strains of *Plasmodium falciparum,* Divo et al. (60) found 50% inhibitory concentrations of ciprofloxacin equal to 0.52 μg/ml against one and 1.4 μg/ml against the other at a 96-h time point. The 50% inhibitory concentrations of enoxacin were 0.2 and 0.8 μg/ml, respectively. Several other drugs show potentially useful activities in such test systems (26, 60), and some activity in vivo has been reported with pefloxacin (59) and norfloxacin (211). However, clinical responses of patients with falciparum malaria to norfloxacin (162a) have been inconsistent, while responses to ciprofloxacin (249a) have been poor, indicating that currently available fluoroquinolones are not likely candidates for first-line therapy of falciparum malaria (162a).

## FACTORS AFFECTING ASSESSMENT OF QUINOLONE ANTIMICROBIAL ACTIVITY

### Media and Techniques

Correlation between measurements of fluoroquinolone antimicrobial activity as determined by agar and microdilution broth techniques is generally good. Macrodilution broth methods sometimes yield slightly higher MICs (102, 134, 175). Use of various agar media usually yields comparable results (173, 235). A significant exception to this is encountered when susceptibilities of *Legionella* spp. are tested in charcoal-based media, which yield higher MICs than starch-based media (64, 127). This effect is not specific to *Legionella* spp., because charcoal antagonizes fluoroquinolone activities against other bacteria as well. However, not all *Legionella* spp. grow well in starch media (64).

Although occasional discrepancies are encountered, supplementation of media with human serum usually has minimal (less than fourfold) effects on fluoroquinolone activity. Activities of ciprofloxacin (23, 41, 255), norfloxacin (224), enoxacin (23, 167, 254), and ofloxacin (33, 148) were little affected by the addition of 40 to 50% serum to test media. Human serum minimally influences the activities of WIN 57273 (44), sparfloxacin (50), QA-241 (6), BMY 40062 (88), PD 127,391 (256), lomefloxacin (253), fleroxacin (119), or DR-3355 (235). Addition of serum reduced up to eightfold the activity of S-25930, which is approximately 95% protein bound (185). Activities of temafloxacin and tosufloxacin against some isolates were adversely affected by serum, although against most strains, activities were not significantly different from those in unsupplemented media (74, 80, 113). Studies employing high concentrations of serum should take into account the tendency of such media to become quite alkaline when incubated in room air (119). As discussed below, changes in medium pH alone may affect activities of fluoroquinolones.

## Activity in Urine and Effect of pH and Magnesium

Because quinolone antimicrobial agents are widely used for the treatment of urinary tract infections, tests of in vitro activity have also been carried out in urine or in urine-supplemented media. Activities of these agents are substantially reduced in such media, with MICs up to 64-fold higher than those obtained in standard laboratory media (40, 41, 80, 104, 117, 119, 148, 160, 224, 235). High urinary concentrations of magnesium, which are commonly in the range of 8 to 10 mM, account in large part for this reduction in activity. Supplementation of standard media with magnesium to levels present in human urine results in 2- to 16-fold increases in MICs of fluoroquinolones for various bacteria (36, 45, 80, 93, 173). Numerous other examples of this effect have been cited (257).

Reduced potencies of these drugs in urine can also be ascribed in part to diminished activities of many fluoroquinolones at low pH levels prevailing in this medium. For example, activities of ciprofloxacin or norfloxacin against *E. coli* and *S. aureus* are eightfold lower at pH 4.8 than at pH 6.8 (19). Decreased activities in standard media adjusted to acidic pHs can also be demonstrated for several quinolones, including enoxacin (167), ofloxacin (148), fleroxacin (36), tosufloxacin (74), lomefloxacin (45), PD 127,391 (173), QA-241 (6), sparfloxacin (38), and temafloxacin (37). Activities of such fluoroquinolones are also lower in acid urine than in urine at pH 7.0 to 7.2. Thus, both the high magnesium concentrations and the low pH of normal urine contribute to the reduced activities of these antimicrobial agents when they are tested in this medium.

In contrast, activities of some fluoroquinolones, such as difloxacin (13, 117) and BMY 40062 (88), are not adversely affected to a significant degree at lower pHs, while those of S-25930 and S-25932 (170), WIN 57273 (69, 128), and others (257) are actually greater at acidic pH levels. Our own studies found the activity of WIN 57273 against gram-negative bacilli to be two to five times greater at pH 5.4 than at pH 7.4, whereas activity against gram-positive cocci was unaffected or slightly decreased at the lower pH (69).

## Effect of Inoculum Size

Although increases in MICs of fluoroquinolones are observed with increases in the inoculum size of test organisms, these effects are usually small in comparison with those seen with other antimicrobial agents. For 2-$\log_{10}$ increases in inoculum (generally $10^4$ to $10^6$ or $10^5$ to $10^7$ CFU/ml), several studies indicate decreases in drug activities of fourfold or less for various fluoroquinolones (19, 36, 148, 160, 175, 224), including newer agents such as sparfloxacin (38), WIN 57273 (44), PD 127,391 (173), BMY 40062 (88), and DR-3355 (235). In some cases, however, inoculum effects of greater importance have been observed. For example, while MICs of fleroxacin against *E. coli* ATCC 25922 were identical (0.06 $\mu$g/ml) at inocula of $10^4$ and $10^6$ CFU/ml, MICs of the drug against *S. aureus* ATCC 29213 increased from 0.5 to $>32$ $\mu$g/ml between $6 \times 10^4$ and $6 \times 10^6$ CFU/ml (119). For ciprofloxacin, 10-fold increases in MICs against *S. aureus* and 100-fold increases against enterococci have been observed when inocula were increased from $10^5$ to $10^7$ CFU/ml (134). Other specific examples of significant inoculum effects for fluoroquinolones are provided elsewhere (67, 257).

It is important to note that even the modest inoculum effects generally reported for fluoroquinolone antimicrobial agents may contribute to significant reductions in activity when combined with other factors influencing drug potency. For example, against *Brucella* spp., an increase in inoculum from $10^3$ to $10^6$ CFU/ml and a decrease in pH from 7 to 5 each diminished activities of ciprofloxacin and ofloxacin by only 1 dilution. However, activities of both drugs were reduced fourfold (to MICs of 2 and 4 μg/ml, respectively) when the two test conditions were changed simultaneously (92).

## BACTERICIDAL ACTIVITY

### MBCs

With great consistency, MBCs of the fluoroquinolone antimicrobial agents are usually within 2 dilutions of the MICs when tested at standard inocula. Data pertaining to ciprofloxacin, ofloxacin, norfloxacin, enoxacin, pefloxacin, and fleroxacin have been reviewed previously (67, 257). However, similar observations have been made with the newer members of this class, including sparfloxacin (144, 194, 207), WIN 57273 (128, 130), PD 127,391 (173, 256), QA-241 (6), and DR-3355 [*S*-(−)-ofloxacin] (235). Occasional exceptions to this general observation are encountered with both gram-positive and gram-negative isolates, with MBCs that are sixfold or more above MICs (33, 36, 45, 92, 253). Factors that affect inhibitory activities of fluoroquinolones as noted above usually alter bactericidal activities in the same direction (257).

### Time-Kill Techniques

Studies that examine the bactericidal activities of fluoroquinolone antimicrobial agents over time confirm the excellent activities of these drugs against most gram-negative isolates predicted by MBC results. Exposure of both *Enterobacteriaceae* and *P. aeruginosa* to various fluoroquinolones at concentrations of two to four times the MIC typically reduces viable cell counts by 3 $\log_{10}$ or more by 2 h of incubation (40, 41, 74, 80, 88, 170, 224). Bactericidal effects are sometimes evident even within 1 h of exposure to the drug (31, 88, 173). At twice the MICs of fluoroquinolones, regrowth by 24 h of incubation may occur following an initial reduction in viable cells (74). In laboratory media specifically lacking essential nutrients, fluoroquinolones (ciprofloxacin and ofloxacin) were the only class of antimicrobial agents that exhibited bactericidal activity against nongrowing bacteria of several species (73). However, the bactericidal activity of ciprofloxacin against nongrowing bacteria appears to be strain dependent (264). Bactericidal activities of sparfloxacin and ciprofloxacin against two strains of *E. coli* were comparable under both aerobic and anaerobic conditions in one study (51), but in another study, neither ciprofloxacin nor ofloxacin exhibited bactericidal activity against either *E. coli* or *S. aureus* under anaerobic conditions (153). Ciprofloxacin was effective in sterilizing cultures of *Brucella melitensis* at 48 h of incubation, but streptomycin accomplished this in 12 h (208).

Fluoroquinolones also usually exhibit bactericidal activities against susceptible gram-positive isolates at two- to fourfold multiples of the MIC. There is a general sense that the rate of killing of gram-positive organisms may be slower than that of gram-negative bacteria, even for drugs such as WIN 57273, with enhanced activities against the former (69). These drugs, however, still usually attain 3-$\log_{10}$ reductions in viable cell counts by 4 to 8 h of incubation (88, 130, 161, 227). Most strains of staphylococci show 3- to 4-$\log_{10}$ killing upon exposure to clinically achievable concentrations of ciprofloxacin within 24 h (41, 77, 161, 221), but major strain differences can exist, with some strains showing 5-$\log_{10}$ reduction within 2 h and others lacking a bactericidal effect within that period (41). *S. aureus* exposed to ciprofloxacin or ofloxacin under conditions that do not support growth shows little loss of viability (1.4- to 1.5-$\log_{10}$ killing at 24 h) (73). Although enterococci undergo ≥3-$\log_{10}$ killing upon exposure to fluoroquinolones in some studies (130, 225, 263), this effect is not seen consistently (69), and none of the clinically available agents can be relied upon completely when bactericidal activity is essential to clinical outcome.

## PAE

The postantibiotic effect (PAE) of an antimicrobial agent is measured as the amount of time that elapses between transient exposure of a bacterial culture to the agent and the point at which growth resumes, with this value corrected for any delay in growth observed with unexposed cultures of the same organism (89). This effect is of theoretical clinical interest because drug concentrations may fall below the MIC of an antimicrobial agent during part of the interval between doses. The greater the PAE, the lower the likelihood that bacterial growth will resume during this period of subinhibitory concentrations in serum or tissue (67, 257).

For staphylococci and *P. aeruginosa*, exposure to ciprofloxacin at 2.5 to 3.0 μg/ml for 1 to 2 h resulted in a PAE of approximately 2 h (42, 89). Under similar conditions, PAE against *E. coli* was 4 h, but against *E. faecalis*, no measurable effect was found (42). Exposure to 1 μg of tosufloxacin per ml resulted in PAEs as follows: *E. coli*, 2.3 h; *P. aeruginosa*, 1.7 h; *S. aureus*, 3.4 h; *E. faecalis*, 1 h (74). A number of factors in addition to the species tested appear to affect PAEs, including the concentration of drug used (200, 265) and the duration of exposure (89, 265). Small differences can be ascribed to the drugs themselves: PAEs against *S. aureus* exposed to 10 times the MIC for 2 h were 1.5 h for ciprofloxacin, 1.4 h for norfloxacin, and 1.25 h for pefloxacin (265). Such differences are not likely to be clinically important. Broader ranges of differences can be ascribed to strain variations: exposure of five strains of each species to lomefloxacin at 5 μg/ml for 30 min resulted in PAEs ranging from 0.2 to 2 h for *P. aeruginosa*, 0.75 to 2.4 h for *K. pneumoniae*, and 0 to 3 h for *E. cloacae* (238). Reproducibility of PAE measurements also increases as the multiple of the MIC to which bacteria are exposed increases (265).

PAEs can also be determined in urine at concentrations attainable in that medium. In urine, PAEs of sparfloxacin at 100 μg/ml and tosufloxacin at 80 μg/ml against *E. coli* were both 5.3 h (38, 74). Lomefloxacin PAEs against both a susceptible (MIC, 0.12 μg/ml) and a more-resistant (MIC, 1.0 μg/ml) strain of *E. coli* were each 3 h (45).

Whether such results are directly applicable to clinical practice is open to question. PAEs against *S. aureus* for ciprofloxacin, norfloxacin, and pefloxacin in serum were twice those measured in Mueller-Hinton broth (55). This could be attributed to a heat-sensitive factor, because heating serum for 30 min at 56°C negated this effect. PAEs of norfloxacin against bacterial species determined in vivo (implantation of threads impregnated with bacteria into antibiotic-treated mice) were longer than corresponding PAEs determined in vitro (199), suggesting that commonly used in vitro measurements may underestimate PAEs for some fluoroquinolones. Standard measurements may also be inaccurate in representing events for intracellular bacteria. Although ciprofloxacin, ofloxacin, and pefloxacin each inhibited multiplication of *Legionella pneumophila* within human monocyte-derived macrophages in one study, prolonged inhibition following removal of drugs was noted only for pefloxacin (190).

## RESISTANCE TO QUINOLONES

### Spontaneous Mutants

Frequencies of isolation of single-step, spontaneous mutants resistant to the fluoroquinolones are low in comparison with frequencies of resistance to nalidixic acid, i.e., typically $<10^{-9}$ when the antimicrobial agent is used at eight times the MIC (33, 67, 148, 160, 212, 257). For example, with tosufloxacin, frequencies of resistance to eight times the MIC were $<10^{-10}$ for *S. aureus, E. coli,* and *P. aeruginosa* (74). More-variable results were obtained on media incorporating the drug at four times the MIC: *S. aureus,* $1 \times <10^{-9}$ to $3.4 \times 10^{-7}$; *E. coli,* $1 \times <10^{-9}$; and *P. aeruginosa,* $1 \times <10^{-10}$ to $5.3 \times 10^{-8}$ (74, 80). For various species of gram-negative bacteria, a frequency of resistance to four or eight times the MIC of $<10^{-10}$ has been reported for several newer compounds, including temafloxacin (37), lomefloxacin (45), fleroxacin (34), and PD 127,391 (173). Occasional isolates of various species give rise to resistant mutants at higher frequencies (67). Frequencies of resistance to ciprofloxacin or norfloxacin (four times the MIC) of $\geq 10^{-7}$ are detected more commonly in *E. cloacae* and *S. marcescens* than in *E. coli* (249). For WIN 57273, a drug particularly active against gram-positive organisms, resistance frequencies of $<10^{-10}$ have been reported among gram-positive isolates, including methicillin-resistant *S. aureus* (44), but resistance to eight times the MIC at a frequency of $1.2 \times 10^{-7}$ has also been encountered in *S. aureus* (69). Mutation rates to quinolone resistance at eight times the MIC among *S. aureus* were $\leq 10^{-9}$ for ciprofloxacin, ofloxacin, temafloxacin, sparfloxacin, WIN 57273, and others in one study (83); however, some differences between drugs were noted at four times the MIC. For *S. epidermidis,* at both four and eight times the MIC, resistance frequencies were $\geq$14-fold higher for WIN 57273 than for ofloxacin (83). Such differences may not be clinically significant, however, given the 30-fold-greater potency of the former agent. Particularly high frequencies of resistance to fluoroquinolones have been reported in *M. fortuitum,* with six of seven strains giving rise to ciprofloxacin-resistant colonies (eight times the MIC) at frequencies between $10^{-5}$ and $10^{-7}$ (247).

### Resistance Derived by Serial Passage

By repeated subculture of susceptible isolates through incremental concentrations of a fluoroquinolone antimicrobial agent, colonies with substantial resistance to the drug (often 100-fold or greater increase in MIC) can be obtained (45, 69, 70, 74, 109, 117, 155, 212, 232, 242). Resistance is generally stable on passage in drug-free media and results in relative cross-resistance to other agents of this class (17, 45, 74, 117, 155). The dual mode of action of Ro 23-9424 (fleroxacin-desacetylcefotaxime) does not prevent the development of resistance to the drug upon serial passage through increasing concentrations (108).

### Resistance among Clinical Isolates

A comparison of data shown in Table 1, which are derived from studies published since 1988, with those that we have reviewed previously (67) reveals no significant changes in overall susceptibilities of *Enterobacteriaceae* to the fluoroquinolones. Stability in resistance to quinolones between 1975 and 1986 among members of this family has also been reported from Germany (147). Nevertheless, in a report from a hospital in Madrid, Spain, ciprofloxacin resistance in *E. coli* increased from 0.06% of isolates in 1987 to 2.4% of isolates in the first quarter of 1991 (202). A separate report from the same city documented an increase in norfloxacin resistance among *E. coli* causing community-acquired urinary infections from 0 to 4.3% over a roughly similar period (1). Ciprofloxacin resistance has also increased in *Campylobacter* spp. in The Netherlands and Finland from 0% in the early 1980s to approximately 10% of isolates tested in 1989 to 1990 (72, 197). In Germany, there appears to have been a slight shift toward quinolone resistance in *P. aeruginosa,* as indicated by an increase in the number of strains with MICs fourfold greater than the modal MIC of these drugs for the species (147). Fluoroquinolone resistance among staphylococci has increased dramatically in several centers (24, 54, 184, 198). Rates of ciprofloxacin resistance among methicillin-resistant *S. aureus* (up to 80% or more [24, 198]) are higher than those for methicillin-susceptible isolates (2.5% [54] to 13.6% [24]). These observations predict that resistance to fluoroquinolones among clinical isolates will continue to increase. For further information on resistance to quinolones, see chapter 5.

## ANTIMICROBIAL COMBINATIONS

The in vitro activities of antimicrobial combinations consisting of a quinolone and one or more antibiotics of other classes have received considerable attention (66, 67, 169, 257). Because the site of action of quinolone antimicrobial agents differs from that of other clinically available agents, such combinations may result in synergistic antimicrobial activity or may delay the emergence of subpopulations resistant to one or more of the antimicrobial agents (67).

### *Enterobacteriaceae*

Numerous combinations of fluoroquinolones with various aminoglycosides have been tested against members of the family *Enterobacteriaceae.* Significant interactions have been quite uncommon, with occasional reports of antimicrobial synergism and only rare instances of apparent antagonism. Haller (112) studied ciprofloxacin in combination with five aminoglycosides against 200 *Enterobacteriaceae* by using a checkerboard dilution method and found evidence of synergism or antagonism in <1% of interactions, and even these were not reproducible on repeat testing. Similar results have been noted in studies examining norfloxacin (172), enoxacin (11), and other agents (67). Synergistic inhibitory or bactericidal activities of gentamicin combined with either enoxacin or norfloxacin against 15 to 20% of *Enterobacteriaceae* were observed in one study (237). Convincing demonstrations of bactericidal synergism between fluoroquinolones and aminoglycosides have occasionally been presented (31).

Synergism between fluoroquinolones and various $\beta$-lactams is also observed relatively infrequently. Against 200 strains of *Enterobacteriaceae,* Haller (112) found reproducible synergism between ciprofloxacin and several penicillins and cephalosporins in fewer than 5% of the interactions tested. Other studies confirm the sporadic occurrence of synergism between a number of quinolones and $\beta$-lactam antibiotics against these organisms (11, 31, 39, 63, 148). Ciprofloxacin-imipenem synergism was detected against 22% of *Enterobacter* spp. in one study (43), but others have found that this combination, like other quinolone–$\beta$-lactam combinations, demonstrates synergism against few isolates of the family *Enterobacteriaceae* (27). With such combinations, antagonistic or nearly antagonistic interactions have been reported but are fortunately quite rare (39, 164).

### *P. aeruginosa* and Other Gram-Negative Organisms

Combinations of ciprofloxacin with an aminoglycoside sometimes yield synergistic activity against *P. aeruginosa.* Some studies report favorable interactions against 20 to 30% of isolates (39, 56), while others have found little or no evidence of synergism (76, 112). Studies utilizing time-kill curve methodologies provide examples of both true bactericidal synergism and suppression of the emergence of resistant subpopulations (66). Combination of ciprofloxacin with gentamicin, tobramycin, or amikacin against ciprofloxacin-resistant strains of *X. maltophilia* resulted in clinically relevant synergism in only 8.5% of interactions tested (47). Combinations of ciprofloxacin with streptomycin sterilized cultures of *B. melitensis* substantially faster than either drug alone; however, addition of minocycline to ciprofloxacin resulted in delayed bactericidal activity relative to that observed for either agent alone (208).

Against *P. aeruginosa*, synergistic activity between ciprofloxacin and azlocillin has been observed in 10 to 60% of strains (66, 169). Resistance to azlocillin may reduce but does not necessarily eliminate the possibility that synergism will occur (28, 39). Synergism between ciprofloxacin and other antipseudomonal penicillins and cephalosporins at rates within this broad range have also been reported (66, 169). Ceftazidime-ciprofloxacin combinations have resulted in inhibitory synergism at clinically achievable concentrations against 7.5 to 75% of strains (28, 76). The higher value was observed against ceftazidime-resistant, ciprofloxacin-susceptible strains of *P. aeruginosa* (28). Enoxacin combined with piperacillin or cefsulodin synergistically inhibited 17 and 28.5% of isolates, respectively (11). Several studies have observed synergistic interactions between ciprofloxacin and imipenem against fewer than 10% to more than 40% of *P. aeruginosa* isolates (27, 43, 97). Susceptibility or resistance to imipenem does not consistently affect outcome of interaction studies, but lower rates of synergism have been noted among *P. aeruginosa* resistant to the quinolone (97). There does not appear to be a significant likelihood of antagonism between fluoroquinolones and β-lactam antibiotics (66, 67, 169).

Synergism at clinically achievable concentrations between ciprofloxacin and β-lactams against *X. maltophilia* resistant to both drugs was observed with mezlocillin for five of nine strains, with cefoperazone for four strains, with piperacillin or ceftazadime for three strains, and with aztreonam for one of nine strains (47). Synergism was not observed with imipenem in that study except at more-than-achievable concentrations. In time-kill studies, ciprofloxacin combined with imipenem led to synergistic interactions at clinically achievable concentrations against three of seven ciprofloxacin-resistant *P. cepacia* isolates (149). In high-inoculum broth cultures, addition of erythromycin suppressed the emergence of ciprofloxacin-resistant populations of *L. pneumophila* (14). Combinations of ciprofloxacin with rifampin were effective in mutually suppressing resistance to the other agent. In that study, ciprofloxacin was added at 0.25 μg/ml (four times the MBC). It is not certain that any benefit of such combinations would occur at higher concentrations of the fluoroquinolone or with lower bacterial inocula. In another study, rifampin antagonized the bactericidal activity of ciprofloxacin in broth culture but was indifferent when tested against *L. pneumophila* within monocytes (115).

## Staphylococci

Combinations of ciprofloxacin with an aminoglycoside are generally additive or indifferent against *S. aureus* (222), although synergism has been reported against some isolates (169). Ofloxacin plus oxacillin was additive or indifferent against methicillin-susceptible strains of *S. aureus* and coagulase-negative staphylococci, but inhibitory synergism was observed against some methicillin-resistant isolates, particularly at 30°C (203). Bactericidal synergism was noted against a methicillin-resistant coagulase-negative staphylococcus when ofloxacin at 1 μg/ml was combined with oxacillin at 2 μg/ml (203). Synergistic interactions between ciprofloxacin and azlocillin have been observed against 14 to 40% of *S. aureus* strains (39, 163), but such combinations are not likely to be used in therapy of staphylococcal infections. Combinations of ciprofloxacin with vancomycin are usually indifferent (182, 221). However, addition of vancomycin may reduce the rate of killing of *S. aureus* observed with the fluoroquinolones (182). Several studies demonstrate the potential of rifampin to antagonize the bactericidal activities of fluoroquinolones against *S. aureus* (77, 110, 239), but such combinations do not necessarily result in reduced serum bactericidal activity (110) and can delay the emergency of drug-resistant subpopulations (110, 131). Other work has provided evidence of indifference between ciprofloxacin and rifampin in both inhibitory and bactericidal activities (169).

### Anaerobes

Although several of the newest fluoroquinolones demonstrate enhanced activities against anaerobic bacteria as discussed above, because of the relatively weak anaerobic activities of currently available antimicrobial agents of this class, combinations of these drugs with others possessing greater anaerobic activities are occasionally employed. Fortunately, in studies published to date, antagonism between fluoroquinolones and other agents against anaerobic organisms appears to be quite rare (66, 101, 169, 257). Combinations of ciprofloxacin and mezlocillin, clindamycin, or cefoxitin synergistically inhibited approximately 30 to 40% of *B. fragilis* isolates tested in one study (75). Whiting et al. (251) have observed ciprofloxacin-mezlocillin synergism against 16% of *Bacteroides* spp. (1 of 9 *B. fragilis* and 2 of 10 non-*B. fragilis* group isolates). Ciprofloxacin-cefotaxime inhibited four of nine strains (44%) of *B. fragilis* synergistically. Combined with ciprofloxacin, cefotaxime or clindamycin produced synergism against 3 and 4 isolates, respectively, of 21 gram-positive organisms. An antagonistic interaction between clindamycin and the fluoroquinolones was noted against only one anaerobic streptococcal isolate. Indifferent or additive interactions occur when metronidazole is combined with ciprofloxacin (251) or ofloxacin (101). However, the latter combination has resulted in synergism against a few *C. perfringens* isolates (101).

### Mycobacteria

Inhibitory synergism between ciprofloxacin and amikacin, erythromycin, imipenem, or trimethoprim-sulfamethoxazole has been demonstrated against a minority of strains representing seven species of mycobacteria (96). Inhibitory and bactericidal synergism between ciprofloxacin and ethambutol was observed against 100 and 90%, respectively, of *M. avium* strains (258). However, only 20% of the strains were killed by the combination at clinically achievable concentrations. Combinations of ofloxacin with ethambutol also demonstrated enhanced activity against *M. avium* (195). Combinations of ciprofloxacin with rifampin were less active, and addition of ciprofloxacin to the combination of rifampin plus ethambutol did not further enhance activity. Sparfloxacin combined with ethambutol synergistically inhibited 9 of 10 strains of *M. avium* (259). The triple combination of sparfloxacin, rifampin, and ethambutol showed synergism (fractional inhibitory concentration [FIC] index, $\leq 0.75$) against all 10 isolates, but sparfloxacin combined with rifampin resulted in FIC indices of $\geq 2$ against 3 of 10 strains, possibly indicating a trend towards antagonism.

## CONCLUSIONS

The fluoroquinolones as a class offer excellent in vitro activity against the vast majority of commonly encountered gram-negative bacteria. Resistance is more often observed among *Pseudomonas* spp. and related organisms. Although most staphylococci remain susceptible to ciprofloxacin, the rapid appearance of resistant strains, especially among methicillin-resistant isolates of *S. aureus*, underscores the need for agents with enhanced potency against such organisms, with greater capacity to forestall emergence of drug-resistant mutant strains, or both. Several newer fluoroquinolones that are now under investigation demonstrate activities against gram-positive bacteria superior to those of currently available agents. Among the newest fluoroquinolones are drugs that at low concentrations inhibit a number of other potential pathogens, including mycobacteria, legionellae, chlamydiae, and mycoplasmas, against which presently available therapeutic regimens are quite limited.

## REFERENCES


1. **Aguiar J. M., J. Chacon, R. Canton, and F. Baquero.** 1992. The emergence of highly fluoroquinolone-resistant *Escherichia coli* in community-acquired urinary tract infections. *J. Antimicrob. Chemother.* **29:**349–350.

1a. **Akaniro, J. C., C. E. Vidaurre, H. R. Stutman, and M. I. Marks.** 1990. Comparative in vitro activity of a new quinolone, fleroxacin, against respiratory pathogens from patients with cystic fibrosis. *Antimicrob. Agents Chemother.* **34:**1880–1884.

2. **Appelbaum, P. C., S. K. Spangler, and M. R. Jacobs.** 1991. Susceptibilities of 394 *Bacteroides fragilis*, non-*B. fragilis* group *Bacteroides* species, and *Fusobacterium* species to newer antimicrobial agents. *Antimicrob. Agents Chemother.* **35:**1214–1218.

3. **Appelbaum, P. C., S. K. Spangler, and L. Sollenberger.** 1986. Susceptibility of non-fermentative gram-negative bacteria to ciprofloxacin, norfloxacin, amifloxacin, pefloxacin and cefpirome. *J. Antimicrob. Chemother.* **18:**675–679.

4. **Arguedas, A. G., J. C. Akaniro, H. R. Stutman, and M. I. Marks.** 1990. In vitro activity of tosufloxacin, a new quinolone, against respiratory pathogens derived from cystic fibrosis sputum. *Antimicrob. Agents Chemother.* **34:**2223–2227.

5. **Arlet, G., M.-J. Sanson-LePors, I. M. Cosin, M. Ortenberg, and Y. Perol.** 1987. In vitro susceptibility of 96 *Capnocytophaga* strains, including a beta-lactamase producer, to new beta-lactam antibiotics and six quinolones. *Antimicrob. Agents Chemother.* **31:**1283–1284.

6. **Asahara, M., A. Tsuji, S. Goto, K. Masuda, and A. Kiuchi.** 1989. In vitro and in vivo activities of QA-241, a new tricyclic quinolone derivative. *Antimicrob. Agents Chemother.* **33:**1144–1152.

7. **Ashdown, L. R.** 1988. In vitro activities of the newer beta-lactam and quinolone antimicrobial agents against *Pseudomonas pseudomallei*. *Antimicrob. Agents Chemother.* **32:**1435–1436.

8. **Auckenthaler, R., M. Michea-Hamzehpour, and J. C. Pechere.** 1986. In vitro activity of newer quinolones against aerobic bacteria. *J. Antimicrob. Chemother.* **17**(Suppl. B):29–39.

9. **Aznar, J., M. C. Caballero, M. C. Lozano, C. DeMiguel, J. C. Palomares, and E. J. Perea.** 1985. Activities of new quinolone derivatives against genital pathogens. *Antimicrob. Agents Chemother.* **27:**76–78.

10. **Bailey, J. M. G., C. Heppelston, and S. J. Richmond.** 1984. Comparison of the in vitro activities of ofloxacin and tetracycline against *Chlamydia trachomatis* as assessed by indirect immunofluorescence. *Antimicrob. Agents Chemother.* **26:**13–16.

11. **Baltch, A. L., C. Bassey, G. Fanciullo, and R. P. Smith.** 1987. In vitro antimicrobial activity of enoxacin in combination with eight other antibiotics against *Pseudomonas aeruginosa*, Enterobacteriaceae, and *Staphylococcus aureus*. *J. Antimicrob. Chemother.* **19:**45–48.

12. **Bannerman, T. L., D. L. Wadiak, and W. E. Kloos.** 1991. Susceptibility of *Staphylococcus* species and subspecies to fleroxacin. *Antimicrob. Agents Chemother.* **35:**2135–2139.

13. **Bansal, M. B., and H. Thadepalli.** 1987. Activity of difloxacin (A-56619) and A-56620 against clinical anaerobic bacteria in vitro. *Antimicrob. Agents Chemother.* **31:**619–621.

14. **Barker, J. E., and I. D. Farrell.** 1990. The effects of single and combined antibiotics on the growth of *Legionella pneumophila* using time-kill studies. *J. Antimicrob. Chemother.* **26:**45–53.

15. **Barry, A. L., and P. C. Fuchs.** 1991. Antistaphylococcal activity of the fluoroquinolones CI-960, PD 131628, sparfloxacin, ofloxacin and ciprofloxacin. *Eur. J. Clin. Microbiol. Infect. Dis.* **10:**168–171.

16. **Barry, A. L., and P. C. Fuchs.** 1991. In vitro activities of sparfloxacin, tosufloxacin, ciprofloxacin, and fleroxacin. *Antimicrob. Agents Chemother.* **35:**955–960.

17. **Barry, A. L., and R. N. Jones.** 1984. Cross-resistance among cinoxacin, ciprofloxacin, DJ-6783, enoxacin, nalidixic acid, norfloxacin, and oxolinic acid after in vitro selection of resistant populations. *Antimicrob. Agents Chemother.* **25:**775–777.

18. **Barry, A. L., and R. N. Jones.** 1989. In vitro activities of temafloxacin, tosufloxacin (A-61827) and five other fluoroquinolone agents. *J. Antimicrob. Chemother.* **23:**527–535.

19. **Bauernfeind, A., and C. Petermuller.** 1983. In vitro activity of ciprofloxacin, norfloxacin and nalidixic acid. *Eur. J. Clin. Microbiol.* **2:**111–115.

20. **Berkey, P., D. Moore, and K. Rolston.** 1988. In vitro susceptibilities of *Nocardia* species to newer antimicrobial agents. *Antimicrob. Agents Chemother.* **32:**1078–1079.

21. **Berlin, O. G. W., L. S. Young, and D. A. Bruckner.** 1987. In vitro activity of six fluori-

nated quinolones against *Mycobacterium tuberculosis*. *J. Antimicrob. Chemother.* **19:**611–615.

22. **Beskid, G., V. Fallat, E. R. Lipschitz, D. H. McGarry, R. Cleeland, K. Chan, D. D. Keith, and J. Unowsky.** 1989. In vitro activities of a dual-action antibacterial agent, Ro 23-9424, and comparative agents. *Antimicrob. Agents Chemother.* **33:**1072–1077.
23. **Blaser, J., M. N. Dudley, D. Gilbert, and S. H. Zinner.** 1986. Influence of medium and method on the in vitro susceptibility of *Pseudomonas aeruginosa* and other bacteria to ciprofloxacin and enoxacin. *Antimicrob. Agents Chemother.* **29:**927–929.
24. **Blumberg, H. M., D. Rimland, D. J. Carroll, P. Terry, and I. K. Wachsmuth.** 1991. Rapid development of ciprofloxacin resistance in methicillin-susceptible and -resistant *Staphylococcus aureus*. *J. Infect. Dis.* **163:**1279–1285.
25. **Bryan, J. P., C. Waters, J. Sheffield, R. E. Krieg, P. L. Perine, and K. Wagner.** 1990. In vitro activities of tosufloxacin, temafloxacin, and A-56620 against pathogens of diarrhea. *Antimicrob. Agents Chemother.* **34:**368–370.
26. **Bryskier, A., and M. T. Labro.** 1990. Quinolones and malaria: an avenue for the future. *Quinolones Bull.* **6:**1–4.
27. **Bustamante, C. I., G. L. Drusano, R. C. Wharton, and J. C. Wade.** 1987. Synergism of the combinations of imipenem plus ciprofloxacin and imipenem plus amikacin against *Pseudomonas aeruginosa* and other bacterial pathogens. *Antimicrob. Agents Chemother.* **31:**632–634.
28. **Bustamante, C. I., R. C. Wharton, and J. C. Wade.** 1990. In vitro activity of ciprofloxacin in combination with ceftazidime, aztreonam, and azlocillin against multiresistant isolates of *Pseudomonas aeruginosa*. *Antimicrob. Agents Chemother.* **34:**1814–1815
29. **Byrne, S. K., G. L. Geddes, J. L. Isaac-Renton, and W. A. Black.** 1990. Comparison of in vitro antimicrobial susceptibilities of *Mycobacterium avium-Mycobacterium intracellulare* strains from patients with acquired immunodeficiency syndrome (AIDS), patients without AIDS, and animal sources. *Antimicrob. Agents Chemother.* **34:**1390–1392.
30. **Cassell, G. H., K. B. Waites, M. S. Pate, K. C. Canupp, and L. B. Duffy.** 1989. Comparative susceptibility of *Mycoplasma pneumoniae* to erythromycin, ciprofloxacin, and lomefloxacin. *Diagn. Microbiol. Infect. Dis.* **12:**433–435.
31. **Chalkley, L. J., and H. J. Koornhof.** 1985. Antimicrobial activity of ciprofloxacin against *Pseudomonas aeruginosa, Escherichia coli*, and *Staphylococcus aureus* determined by the killing curve method: antibiotic comparisons and synergistic interactions. *Antimicrob. Agents Chemother.* **28:**331–342.
32. **Chambers, S. T., B. A. Peddie, R. A. Robson, E. J. Begg, and D. R. Boswell.** 1991. Antimicrobial effects of lomefloxacin in vitro. *J. Antimicrob. Chemother.* **27:**481–489.
33. **Chantot, J. F., and A. Bryskier.** 1985. Antibacterial activity of ofloxacin and other 4-quinolone derivatives: in vitro and in vivo comparison. *J. Antimicrob. Chemother.* **16:** 475–484.
34. **Chapman, J. S., A. Bertasso, and N. H. Georgopapadakou.** 1989. Fleroxacin resistance in *Escherichia coli*. *Antimicrob. Agents Chemother.* **33:**239–241.
35. **Chaudhry, A. Z., C. C. Knapp, J. Sierra-Madero, and J. A. Washington.** 1990. Antistaphylococcal activities of sparfloxacin (CI-978; AT-4140), ofloxacin, and ciprofloxacin. *Antimicrob. Agents Chemother.* **34:**1843–1845.
36. **Chin, N.-X., D. C. Brittain, and H. C. Neu.** 1986. In vitro activity of Ro 23-6240, a new fluorinated 4-quinolone. *Antimicrob. Agents Chemother.* **29:**675–680.
37. **Chin, N.-X., V. M. Figueredo, A. Novelli, and H. C. Neu.** 1988. In vitro activity of temafloxacin, a new difluoro quinolone antimicrobial agent. *Eur. J. Clin. Microbiol. Infect. Dis.* **7:**58–63.
38. **Chin, N.-X., J.-W. Gu, K.-W. Yu, Y.-X. Zhang, and H. C. Neu.** 1991. In vitro activity of sparfloxacin. *Antimicrob. Agents Chemother.* **35:**567–571.
39. **Chin, N.-X., K. Jules, and H. C. Neu.** 1986. Synergy of ciprofloxacin and azlocillin in vitro and in a neutropenic mouse model of infection. *Eur. J. Clin. Microbiol.* **5:**23–28.
40. **Chin, N.-X., and H. C. Neu.** 1983. In vitro activity of enoxacin, a quinolone carboxylic acid, compared with those of norfloxacin, new beta-lactams, aminoglycosides, and trimethoprim. *Antimicrob. Agents Chemother.* **24:**754–763.
41. **Chin, N.-X., and H. C. Neu.** 1984. Ciprofloxacin, a quinolone carboxylic acid compound active against aerobic and anaerobic bacteria. *Antimicrob. Agents Chemother.* **25:**319–326.
42. **Chin, N.-X., and H. C. Neu.** 1987. Post-antibiotic suppressive effect of ciprofloxacin against gram-positive and gram-negative bacteria. *Am. J. Med.* **82**(Suppl. 4A)**:**58-62.
43. **Chin, N.-X., and H. C. Neu.** 1987. Synergy of imipenem—a novel carbapenem, and rifampin and ciprofloxacin against *Pseudomonas aeruginosa, Serratia marcescens* and *Enterobacter* species. Chemotherapy **33:**183–188.
44. **Chin, N.-X., and H. C. Neu.** 1991. In-vitro activity of WIN 57273 compared to the activity of other fluoroquinolones and two beta-lactam antibiotics. *J. Antimicrob. Chemother.* **27:**781–791.

45. **Chin, N.-X., A. Novelli, and H. C. Neu.** 1988. In vitro activity of lomefloxacin (SC-47111; NY-198), a difluoroquinolone 3-carboxylic acid, compared with those of other quinolones. *Antimicrob. Agents Chemother.* **32:**656–662.
46. **Chirgwin, K., P. M. Roblin, and M. R. Hammerschlag.** 1989. In vitro susceptibilities of *Chlamydia pneumoniae* (*Chlamydia* sp. strain TWAR). *Antimicrob. Agents Chemother.* **33:**1634–1635.
47. **Chow, A. W., J. Wong, and K. H. Bartlett.** 1988. Synergistic interactions of ciprofloxacin and extended-spectrum beta-lactams or aminoglycosides against multiply drug-resistant *Pseudomonas maltophilia. Antimicrob. Agents Chemother.* **32:**782–784.
48. **Cohen, M. A., M. D. Huband, G. B. Mailloux, S. L. Yoder, G. E. Roland, J. M. Domagala, and C. L. Heifetz.** 1991. In vitro antibacterial activities of PD 131628, a new 1,8-naphthyridine anti-infective agent. *Antimicrob. Agents Chemother.* **35:**141–146.
49. **Collins, C. H., and A. H. C. Uttley.** 1985. In vitro susceptibility of mycobacteria to ciprofloxacin. *J. Antimicrob. Chemother.* **16:**575–580.
50. **Cooper, M. A., J. M. Andrews, J. P. Ashby, R. S. Matthews, and R. Wise.** 1990. In-vitro activity of sparfloxacin, a new quinolone antimicrobial agent. *J. Antimicrob. Chemother.* **26:**667–676.
51. **Cooper, M. A., J. M. Andrews, and R. Wise.** 1991. Bactericidal activity of sparfloxacin and ciprofloxacin under anaerobic conditions. *J. Antimicrob. Chemother.* **28:**399–405.
52. **Cornaglia, G., R. Pompei, B. Dainelli, and G. Satta.** 1987. In vitro activity of ciprofloxacin against aerobic bacteria isolated in a southern European hospital. *Antimicrob. Agents Chemother.* **31:**1651–1655.
53. **Dangor, Y., S. D. Miller, F. da L. Exposto, and H. J. Koornhof.** 1988. Antimicrobial susceptibilities of Southern African isolates of *Haemophilus ducreyi. Antimicrob. Agents Chemother.* **32:**1458–1460.
54. **Daum, T. E., D. R. Schaberg, M. S. Terpenning, W. S. Sottile, and C. A. Kauffman.** 1990. Increasing resistance of *Staphylococcus aureus* to ciprofloxacin. *Antimicrob. Agents Chemother.* **34:**1862–1863.
55. **Davidson, R. J., G. G. Zhanel, R. Phillips, and D. J. Hoban.** 1991. Human serum enhances the postantibiotic effect of fluoroquinolones against *Staphylococcus aureus. Antimicrob. Agents Chemother.* **35:**1261–1263.
56. **Davies, G. S. R., and J. Cohen.** 1985. In vitro study of the activity of ciprofloxacin alone and in combination against strains of *Pseudomonas aeruginosa* with multiple antibiotic resistance. *J. Antimicrob. Chemother.* **16:**713–717.
57. **Davies, S., P. S. Sparham, and R. C. Spencer.** 1987. Comparative in vitro activity of five fluoroquinolones against mycobacteria. *Antimicrob. Agents Chemother.* **19:**605–609.
58. **Decre, D., A. Bure, B. Pangon, A. Philippon, and E. Bergogne-Berezin.** 1991. In vitro susceptibility of *Rhodococcus equi* to 27 antibiotics. *Antimicrob. Agents Chemother.* **28:**311–312.
59. **Deloron, P., J. P. Lepers, L. Raharimalala, B. Dubois, P. Coulanges, and J. J. Pocidalo.** 1991. Pefloxacin for falciparum malaria: only modest success. *Ann. Intern. Med.* **114:**874–875.
60. **Divo, A. A., A. C. Sartorelli, C. L. Patton, and F. J. Bia.** 1988. Activity of fluoroquinolone antibiotics against *Plasmodium falciparum* in vitro. *Antimicrob. Agents Chemother.* **32:**1182–1186.
61. **Doebbeling, B. N., M. A. Pfaller, M. J. Bale, and R. P. Wenzel.** 1990. Comparative in vitro activity of the new quinolone sparfloxacin (CI-978, AT-4140) against nosocomial gram-negative bloodstream isolates. *Eur. J. Clin. Microbiol. Infect. Dis.* **9:**298–301.
62. **Doern, G. V., and T. A. Tubert.** 1988. In vitro activities of 39 antimicrobial agents for *Branhamella catarrhalis* and comparison of results with different quantitative susceptibility test methods. *Antimicrob. Agents Chemother.* **32:**259–261.
63. **Drugeon, H. B., J. Caillon, M. E. Juvin, and J. L. Pirault.** 1987. Dynamics of ceftazidime-pefloxacin interaction shown by a new killing curve-chequer-board method. *Antimicrob. Agents Chemother.* **19:**197–203.
64. **Edelstein, P. H., and M. A. C. Edelstein.** 1989. WIN 57273 is bactericidal for *Legionella pneumophila* grown in alveolar macrophages. *Antimicrob. Agents Chemother.* **33:**2132–2136.
65. **Edelstein, P. H., M. A. C. Edelstein, J. Weidenfeld, and M. B. Dorr.** 1990. In vitro activity of sparfloxacin (CI-978; AT-4140) for clinical *Legionella* isolates, pharmacokinetics in guinea pigs, and use to treat guinea pigs with *L. pneumophila* pneumonia. *Antimicrob. Agents Chemother.* **34:**2122–2127.
66. **Eliopoulos, G. M., and C. T. Eliopoulos.** 1989. Ciprofloxacin in combination with other antimicrobials. *Am. J. Med.* **87**(Suppl. 5A)**:**17S–22S.
67. **Eliopoulos, G. M., and C. T. Eliopoulos.** 1989. Quinolone antimicrobial agents: activity in vitro, p. 35–70. *In* J. S. Wolfson and D. C. Hooper (ed.), *Quinolone Antimicrobial Agents.* American Society for Microbiology, Washington, D.C.
68. **Eliopoulos, G. M., K. Klimm, and M. L. Grayson.** 1990. In vitro activity of sparfloxacin (AT-4140, CI-978, PD 131501), a new quinolone antimicrobial agent. *Diagn. Microbiol. Infect. Dis.* **13:**345–348.
69. **Eliopoulos, G. M., K. Klimm, L. B. Rice, M. J. Ferraro, and R. C. Moellering, Jr.** 1990.

Comparative in vitro activity of WIN 57273, a new fluoroquinolone antimicrobial agent. *Antimicrob. Agents Chemother.* **34:**1154–1159.

70. **Eliopoulos, G. M., A. E. Moellering, E. Reiszner, and R. C. Moellering, Jr.** 1985. In vitro activities of the quinolone antimicrobial agents A-56619 and A-56620. *Antimicrob. Agents Chemother.* **28:**514–520.
71. **Eliopoulos, G. M., E. Reiszner, M. J. Ferraro, C. Wennersten, and R. C. Moellering, Jr.** 1988. Effect of growth medium on the activity of fluoroquinolones and other antimicrobials against *Legionella* species. *Rev. Infect. Dis.* **10**(Suppl. 1):S56.
72. **Endtz, H. P., G. J. Ruijs, B. van Klingeren, W. H. Jansen, T. van der Reyden, and R. P. Mouton.** 1991. Quinolone resistance in campylobacter isolated from man and poultry following the introduction of fluoroquinolones in veterinary medicine. *Antimicrob. Agents Chemother.* **27:**199–208.
73. **Eng, R. H. K., F. T. Padberg, S. M. Smith, E. N. Tan, and C. E. Cherubin.** 1991. Bactericidal effects of antibiotics on slowly growing and nongrowing bacteria. *Antimicrob. Agents Chemother.* **35:**1824–1828.
74. **Espinoza, A. M., N.-X. Chin, A. Novelli, and H. C. Neu.** 1988. Comparative in vitro activity of a new fluorinated 4-quinolone, T-3262 (A-60969). *Antimicrob. Agents Chemother.* **32:**663–670.
75. **Esposito, S., A. Gupta, and H. Thadepalli.** 1987. In vitro synergy of ciprofloxacin and three other antibiotics against *Bacteroides fragilis*. *Drugs Exp. Clin. Res.* **13:**489–492.
76. **Farrag, N. N., J. W. A. Bendig, C. Talboys, and B. S. Azadian.** 1986. In vitro study of the activity of ciprofloxacin combined with amikacin or ceftazidime against *Pseudomonas aeruginosa*. *Antimicrob. Agents Chemother.* **18:**770.
77. **Fass, R. J., and V. L. Helsel.** 1987. In vitro antistaphylococcal activity of pefloxacin alone and in combination with other antistaphylococcal drugs. *Antimicrob. Agents Chemother.* **31:**1457–1460.
78. **Fenelon, L. E., G. Mumtaz, and G. L. Ridgway.** 1990. The in-vitro antibiotic susceptibility of *Chlamydia pneumoniae*. *J. Antimicrob. Chemother.* **26:**763–767.
79. **Fenlon, C. H., and M. H. Cynamon.** 1986. Comparative in vitro activities of ciprofloxacin and other 4-quinolones against *Mycobacterium tuberculosis* and *Mycobacterium intracellulare*. *Antimicrob. Agents Chemother.* **29:**386–388.
80. **Fernandes, P. B., D. T. W. Chu, R. N. Swanson, N. R. Ramer, C. W. Hanson, R. R. Bower, J. M. Stamm, and D. J. Hardy.** 1988. A-61827 (A-60969), a new fluoronaphthyridine with activity against both aerobic and anaerobic bacteria. *Antimicrob. Agents Chemother.* **32:**27–32.
81. **Fernandes, P. B., N. Shipkowitz, R. R. Bower, K. P. Jarvis, J. Weisz, and D. T. W. Chu.** 1986. In vitro and in vivo potency of five new fluoroquinolones against anaerobic bacteria. *Antimicrob. Agents Chemother.* **18:**693–701.
82. **Fliegelman, R. M., R. M. Petrak, L. J. Goodman, J. Segreti, G. M. Trenholme, and R. L. Kaplan.** 1985. Comparative in vitro activities of twelve antimicrobial agents against *Campylobacter* species. *Antimicrob. Agents Chemother.* **27:**429–430.
83. **Forstall, G. J., C. C. Knapp, and J. A. Washington.** 1991. Activity of new quinolones against ciprofloxacin-resistant staphylococci. *Antimicrob. Agents Chemother.* **35:**1679–1681.
84. **Franzblau, S. G.** 1989. Drug susceptibility testing of *Mycobacterium leprae* in the BACTEC 460 system. *Antimicrob. Agents Chemother.* **33:**2115–2117.
85. **Franzblau, S. G., and K. E. White.** 1990. Comparative in vitro activities of 20 fluoroquinolones against *Mycobacterium leprae*. *Antimicrob. Agents Chemother.* **34:**229–231.
86. **Fuchs, P. C.** 1991. In vitro activity of temafloxacin against gram-positive cocci including methicillin-resistant *Staphylococcus aureus*. *Am. J. Med.* **91** (Suppl. 6A):S15–S18.
87. **Fuchs, P. C., A. L. Barry, M. A. Pfaller, S. D. Allen, and E. H. Gerlach.** 1991. Multicenter evaluation of the in vitro activities of three new quinolones, sparfloxacin, CI-960, and PD 131,628, compared with the activity of ciprofloxacin against 5,252 clinical bacterial isolates. *Antimicrob. Agents Chemother.* **35:**764–766.
88. **Fung-Tomc, J., J. V. Desiderio, Y. H. Tsai, G. Warr, and R. E. Kessler.** 1989. In vitro and in vivo antibacterial activities of BMY 40062, a new fluoronaphthyridone. *Antimicrob. Agents Chemother.* **33:**906–914.
89. **Fuursted, K.** 1987. Post-antibiotic effect of ciprofloxacin on *Pseudomonas aeruginosa*. *Eur. J. Clin. Microbiol.* **6:**271–274.
90. **Garcia-Rodriguez, J. A., J. E. Garcia Sanchez, J. L. Munoz Bellido, T. N. Mayoral, E. Garcia Sanchez, and I. Garcia Garcia.** 1991. In vitro activity of 79 antimicrobial agents against *Corynebacterium* group D2. *Antimicrob. Agents Chemother.* **35:**2140–2143.
91. **Garcia-Rodriguez, J. A., J. E. Garcia Sanchez, J. L. Munoz Bellido, and I. Trujillano.** 1990. In vitro activities of irloxacin and E-3846, two new quinolones. *Antimicrob. Agents Chemother.* **34:**1262–1267.
92. **Garcia-Rodriguez, J. A., J. E. Garcia Sanchez, and I. Trujillano.** 1991. Lack of effective bactericidal activity of new quinolones aginst *Brucella* spp. *Antimicrob. Agents Chemother.* **35:**756–759.

93. **Gargallo-Viola, D., M. Esteve, S. Llovera, X. Roca, and J. Guinea.** 1991. In vitro and in vivo antibacterial activities of E-4497, a new 3-amine-3-methyl-azetidinyl tricyclic fluoroquinolone. *Antimicrob. Agents Chemother.* **35:**442–447.
94. **Gay, J. D., D. R. DeYoung, and G. D. Roberts.** 1984. In vitro activities of norfloxacin and ciprofloxacin against *Mycobacterium tuberculosis, M. avium* complex, *M. chelonei, M. fortuitum,* and *M. kansasii. Antimicrob. Agents Chemother.* **26:**94–96.
95. **Georgopapadakou, N. H., A. Bertasso, K. K. Chan, J. S. Chapman, R. Cleeland, L. M. Cummings, B. A. Dix, and D. D. Keith.** 1989. Mode of action of the dual-action cephalosporin Ro 23-9424. *Antimicrob. Agents Chemother.* **33:**1067–1071.
96. **Gevaudan, M. J., M. N. Mallet, C. Guilian, P. Terriou, P. Lagier, and P. deMicco.** 1988. Etude de la sensibilité de sept éspeces de mycobacteries aux nouvelles quinolones. *Pathol. Biol.* **36:**477–481.
97. **Giamarellou, H., and G. Petrikkos.** 1987. Ciprofloxacin interactions with imipenem and amikacin against multiresistant *Pseudomonas aeruginosa. Antimicrob. Agents Chemother.* **31:**959–961.
98. **Glupczynski, Y., W. Hansen, J. Freney, and E. Yourassowsky.** 1988. In vitro susceptibility of *Alcaligenes denitrificans* subsp. *xylosoxidans* to 24 antimicrobial agents. *Antimicrob. Agents Chemother.* **32:**276–278.
99. **Goldstein, E. J. C., and D. M. Citron.** 1985. Comparative activity of the quinolones against anaerobic bacteria isolated at community hospitals. *Antimicrob. Agents Chemother.* **27:**657–659.
100. **Goldstein, E. J. C., and D. M. Citron.** 1988. Comparative activities of cefuroxime, amoxicillin-clavulanic acid, ciprofloxacin, enoxacin, and ofloxacin against aerobic and anaerobic bacteria isolated from bite wounds. *Antimicrob. Agents Chemother.* **32:**1143–1148.
101. **Goldstein, E. J. C., and D. M. Citron.** 1991. Susceptibility of anaerobic bacteria isolated from intra-abdominal infections to ofloxacin and interaction of ofloxacin with metronidazole. *Antimicrob. Agents Chemother.* **35:**2447–2449.
102. **Gombert, M. E., and T. M. Aulicino.** 1985. Comparison of agar dilution, microtitre broth dilution and tube macrodilution susceptibility testing of ciprofloxacin against several pathogens at two different inocula. *J. Antimicrob. Chemother.* **16:**709–712.
103. **Goossens, H., P. DeMol, H. Coignau, J. Levy, O. Grados, G. Ghysels, H. A. Innocent, and J.-P. Butzler.** 1985. Comparative in vitro activities of aztreonam, ciprofloxacin, norfloxacin, ofloxacin, HR 810 (a new cephalosporin), RU28965 (a new macrolide), and other agents against enteropathogens. *Antimicrob. Agents Chemother.* **27:**388–392.
104. **Gordon, R. C., L. I. Stevens, C. E. Edmiston, Jr., and K. Mohan.** 1976. Comparative in vitro studies of cinoxacin, nalidixic acid, and oxolinic acid. *Antimicrob. Agents Chemother.* **10:**918–920.
105. **Gorzynski, E. A., D. Amsterdam, T. R. Beam, Jr., and C. Rotstein.** 1989. Comparative in vitro activities of teicoplanin, vancomycin, oxacillin, and other antimicrobial agents against bacteremic isolates of gram-positive cocci. *Antimicrob. Agents Chemother.* **33:**2019–2022.
106. **Gorzynski, E. A., S. I. Gutman, and W. Allen.** 1989. Comparative antimycobacterial activities of difloxacin, temafloxacin, enoxacin, pefloxacin, reference fluoroquinolones, and a new macrolide, clarithromycin. *Antimicrob. Agents Chemother.* **33:**591–592.
107. **Grayson, M. L., G. M. Eliopoulos, M. J. Ferraro, and R. C. Moellering, Jr.** 1989. Effect of varying pH on the susceptibility of *Campylobacter pylori* to antimicrobial agents. *Eur. J. Clin. Microbiol. Infect. Dis.* **8:**888–889.
108. **Gu, J.-W., and H. C. Neu.** 1990. In vitro activity of Ro 23-9424, a dual-action cephalosporin, compared with activities of other antibiotics. *Antimicrob. Agents Chemother.* **34:**189–195.
109. **Haas, C. E., D. E. Nix, and J. J. Schentag.** 1990. In vitro selection of resistant *Helicobacter pylori. Antimicrob. Agents Chemother.* **34:**1637–1641.
110. **Hackbarth, C. J., H. F. Chambers, and M. A. Sande.** 1986. Serum bactericidal activity of rifampin in combination with other antimicrobial agents against *Staphylococcus aureus. Antimicrob. Agents Chemother.* **29:**611–613.
111. **Haemers, A., D. C. Leysen, W. Bollaert, M. Zhang, and S. R. Pattyn.** 1990. Influence of N substitution on antimycobacterial activity of ciprofloxacin. *Antimicrob. Agents Chemother.* **34:**496–497.
112. **Haller, I.** 1985. Comprehensive evaluation of ciprofloxacin-aminoglycoside combinations against *Enterobacteriaceae* and *Pseudomonas aeruginosa* strain. *Antimicrob. Agents Chemother.* **28:**663–666.
113. **Hardy, D. J., R. N. Swanson, D. M. Hensey, N. R. Ramer, R. R. Bower, C. W. Hanson, D. T. W. Chu, and P. B. Fernandes.** 1987. Comparative antibacterial activities of temafloxacin hydrochloride (A-62254) and two reference fluoroquinolones. *Antimicrob. Agents Chemother.* **31:**1768–1774.
114. **Harnett, N., S. Brown, and C. Krishnan.** 1991. Emergence of quinolone resistance among clinical isolates of methicillin-resistant *Staphylococcus*

*aureus* in Ontario, Canada. *Antimicrob. Agents Chemother.* **35:**1911–1913.

115. **Havlicheck, D., L. Saravolatz, and D. Pohlod.** 1987. Effect of quinolones and other antimicrobial agents on cell-associated *Legionella pneumophila. Antimicrob. Agents Chemother.* **31:**1529–1534.
116. **Heifets, L. B., and P. J. Lindholm-Levy.** 1990. MICs and MBCs of Win 57273 against *Mycobacterium avium* and *M. tuberculosis. Antimicrob. Agents Chemother.* **34:**770–774.
117. **Hirschhorn, L., and H. C. Neu.** 1986. Factors influencing the in vitro activity of two new arylfluoroquinolone antimicrobial agents, difloxacin (A-56619) and A-56620. *Antimicrob. Agents Chemother.* **30:**143–146.
118. **Hof, H., I. Ehrhard, and H. Tschäpe.** 1991. Presence of quinolone resistance in a strain of *Salmonella typhimurium. Eur. J. Clin. Microbiol. Infect. Dis.* **10:**747–749.
119. **Hohl, P., and A. M. Felber.** 1988. Effect of method, medium, pH and inoculum on the in-vitro antibacterial activities of fleroxacin and norfloxacin. *J. Antimicrob. Chemother.* **22**(Suppl. D):71–80.
120. **Hohl, P., J. Luthy-Hottenstein, J. Zollinger-Iten, and M. Altwegg.** 1990. In vitro activities of fleroxacin, cefetamet, ciprofloxacin, ceftriaxone, trimethoprim-sulfamethoxazole, and amoxicillin-clavulanic acid against rare members of the family *Enterobacteriaceae* primarily of human (clinical) origin. *Antimicrob. Agents Chemother.* **34:**1605–1608.
121. **Hohl, P., A. VonGraevenitz, and J. Zollinger-Iten.** 1987. Fleroxacin (Ro23-6240): activity in vitro against 355 enteropathogenic and non-fermentative gram-negative bacilli and *Legionella pneumophila. J. Antimicrob. Chemother.* **20:**373–378.
122. **Hoppe, J., and C. G. Simon.** 1990. In vitro susceptibilities of *Bordetella pertussis* and *Bordetella parapertussis* to seven fluoroquinolones. *Antimicrob. Agents Chemother.* **34:**2287–2288.
123. **Husson, M. O., D. Izard, L. Bouillet, and H. Leclerc.** 1985. Comparative in vitro activity of ciprofloxacin against non-fermenters. *J. Antimicrob. Chemother.* **15:**457–462.
124. **Inagaki, Y., S. Horiuchi, T. Une, and R. Nakaya.** 1989. In-vitro activity of DR-3355, an optically active isomer of ofloxacin, against bacterial pathogens associated with travellers' diarrhea. *J. Antimicrob. Chemother.* **24:**547–549.
125. **Jones, B. M., I. Geary, M. E. Lee, and B. I. Duerden.** 1986. Activity of pefloxacin and thirteen other antimicrobial agents in vitro against isolates from hospital and genitourinary infections. *Antimicrob. Agents Chemother.* **17:**739–746.
126. **Jones, R. N.** 1990. In vitro activity of Ro 24-6392, a novel ester-linked co-drug combining ciprofloxacin and desacetylcefotaxime. *Eur. J. Clin. Microbiol. Infect. Dis.* **9:**435–438.
127. **Jones, R. N.** 1991. Activity of sparfloxacin (AT-4140), PD127391 and PD131628 against *Legionella* spp. *J. Antimicrob. Chemother.* **27:**389–396.
128. **Jones, R. N., and A. L. Barry.** 1990. In vitro evaluation of WIN 57273, a new broad-spectrum fluoroquinolone. *Antimicrob. Agents Chemother.* **34:**306–313.
129. **Jones, R. N., A. L. Barry, and C. Thornsberry.** 1989. Antimicrobial activity of Ro 23-9424, a novel ester-linked codrug of fleroxacin and desacetylcefotaxime. *Antimicrob. Agents Chemother.* **33:**944–950.
130. **Kaatz, G. W., and S. M. Seo.** 1990. WIN 57273, a new fluoroquinolone with enhanced in vitro activity versus gram-positive pathogens. *Antimicrob. Agents Chemother.* **34:**1376–1380.
131. **Kaatz, G. W., S. M. Seo, S. L. Barriere, L. M. Albrecht, and M. J. Rybak.** 1989. Ciprofloxacin and rifampin, alone and in combination, for therapy for experimental *Staphylococcus aureus* endocarditis. *Antimicrob. Agents Chemother.* **33:**1184–1187.
132. **Kain, K. C., and M. T. Kelly.** 1989. Antimicrobial susceptibility of *Plesiomonas shigelloides* from patients with diarrhea. *Antimicrob. Agents Chemother.* **33:**1609–1610.
133. **Kato, N., M. Miyauchi, Y. Muto, K. Watanabe, and K. Ueno.** 1988. Emergence of fluoroquinolone resistance in *Bacteroides fragilis* accompanied by resistance to beta-lactam antibiotics. *Antimicrob. Agents Chemother.* **32:**1437–1438.
134. **Kayser, F. H., and J. Novak.** 1987. In vitro activity of ciprofloxacin against gram-positive bacteria. *Am. J. Med.* **82**(Suppl. 4A):33–39.
135. **Kenny, G. E., and F. D. Cartwright.** 1991. Susceptibility of *Mycoplasma pneumoniae* to several new quinolones, tetracycline, and erythromycin. *Antimicrob. Agents Chemother.* **35:**587–589.
136. **Kenny, G. E., and F. D. Cartwright.** 1991. Susceptibilities of *Mycoplasma hominis* and *Ureaplasma urealyticum* to two new quinolones, sparfloxacin and WIN 27573. *Antimicrob. Agents Chemother.* **35:**1515–1516.
137. **Kenny, G. E., T. M. Hooton, M. C. Roberts, F. D. Cartwright, and J. Hoyt.** 1989. Susceptibilities of genital mycoplasmas to the newer quinolones as determined by the agar dilution method. *Antimicrob. Agents Chemother.* **33:**103–107.
138. **Khan, M. Y., M. Dizon, and F. W. Kiel.** 1989. Comparative in vitro activities of ofloxacin, difloxacin, ciprofloxacin, and other selected antimicrobial agents against *Brucella melitensis. Antimicrob. Agents Chemother.* **33:**1409–1410.

139. **King, A., L. Bethune, and I. Phillips.** 1991. The in-vitro activity of temafloxacin compared with other antimicrobial agents. *J. Antimicrob. Chemother.* **27:**769–779.
140. **King, A., L. Bethune, and I. Phillips.** 1991. The in vitro activity of tosufloxacin, a new fluorinated quinolone, compared with that of ciprofloxacin and temafloxacin. *J. Antimicrob. Chemother.* **28:**719–725.
141. **King, A., and I. Phillips.** 1986. The comparative in vitro activity of pefloxacin. *J. Antimicrob. Chemother.* **17**(Suppl. B)**:**1–10.
142. **King, A., and I. Phillips.** 1986. The comparative in vitro activity of eight newer quinolones and nalidixic acid. *J. Antimicrob. Chemother.* **18**(Suppl. D)**:**1–20.
143. **Kitsukawa, K., J. Hara, and A. Saito.** 1991. Inhibition of *Legionella pneumophila* in guinea pig peritoneal macrophages by new quinolone, macrolide and other antimicrobial agents. *J. Antimicrob. Chemother.* **27:**343–353.
144. **Kojima, T., M. Inoue, and S. Mitsuhashi.** 1989. In vitro activity of AT-4140 against clinical bacterial isolates. *Antimicrob. Agents Chemother.* **33:**1980–1988.
145. **Kotera, Y., and S. Mitsuhashi.** 1989. In vitro and in vivo antibacterial activities of KB-5246, a new tetracycline quinolone. *Antimicrob. Agents Chemother.* **33:**1896–1900.
146. **Krausse, R., and U. Ulmann.** 1988. Comparative in vitro activity of fleroxacin (RO 23-6240) against *Ureaplasma urealyticum* and *Mycoplasma hominis*. *Eur. J. Clin. Microbiol. Infect. Dis.* **7:**67–69.
147. **Kresken, M., and B. Wiedemann.** 1988. Development of resistance to nalidixic acid and the fluoroquinolones after introduction of norfloxacin and ofloxacin. *Antimicrob. Agents Chemother.* **32:**1285–1288.
148. **Kumada, T., and H. C. Neu.** 1985. In vitro activity of ofloxacin, a quinolone carboxylic acid compared to other quinolones and other antimicrobial agents. *J. Antimicrob. Chemother.* **16:**563–574.
149. **Kumar, A., R. Woford-McQueen, and R. C. Gordon.** 1989. Ciprofloxacin, imipenem and rifampicin: in-vitro synergy of two and three drug combinations against *Pseudomonas cepacia*. *J. Antimicrob. Chemother.* **23:**831–835.
150. **Kurzynski, T. A., D. M. Boehm, J. A. Rott-Petri, R. F. Schell, and P. E. Allison.** 1988. Antimicrobial susceptibilities of *Bordetella* species isolated in a multicenter pertussis surveillance project. *Antimicrob. Agents Chemother.* **32:**137–140.
151. **Lefevre, J. C., and R. Bauriaud.** 1989. Comparative in vitro activities of pristinamycin and other antimicrobial agents against genital pathogens. *Antimicrob. Agents Chemother.* **33:**2152–2154.
152. **Leigh, D. A., S. Tait, and B. Walsh.** 1991. Antibacterial activity of lomefloxacin. *J. Antimicrob. Chemother.* **27:**589–598.
153. **Lewin, C. S., I. Morrissey, and J. T. Smith.** 1989. Role of oxygen in the bactericidal action of the 4-quinolones. *Rev. Infect. Dis.* **11**(Suppl. 5)**:**S913–S914.
154. **Leysen, D. C., A. Haemers, and S. A. Pattyn.** 1989. Mycobacteria and the new quinolones. *Antimicrob. Agents Chemother.* **33:**1–5.
155. **Limb, D. I., D. J. W. Dabbs, and R. C. Spencer.** 1987. In vitro selection of bacteria resistant to the 4-quinolone agents. *J. Antimicrob. Chemother.* **19:**65–71.
156. **Ling, J., K. M. Kam, A. W. Lam, and G. L. French.** 1988. Susceptibilities of Hong Kong isolates of multiply resistant *Shigella* spp. to 25 antimicrobial agents, including ampicillin plus sulbactam and new 4-quinolones. *Antimicrob. Agents Chemother.* **32:**20–23.
157. **Louie, A., A. L. Baltch, W. J. Ritz, and R. P. Smith.** 1991. Comparative in-vitro susceptibilities of *Pseudomonas aeruginosa*, *Xanthomonas maltophilia*, and *Pseudomonas* spp. to sparfloxacin (CI-978, AT-4140, PD131501) and reference antimicrobial agents. *J. Antimicrob. Chemother.* **27:**793–799.
158. **Maeda, H., A. Fujii, K. Nakata, S. Arakawa, and S. Kamidono.** 1988. In vitro activities of T-3262, NY-198, fleroxacin (AM-833; Ro 23-6240), and other new quinolone agents against clinically isolated *Chlamydia trachomatis* strains. *Antimicrob. Agents Chemother.* **32:**1080–1081.
159. **Magalhaes, M., L. R. Trabulsi, and A. C. Montelli.** 1989. Lomefloxacin activity against 2,813 clinical isolates: a collaborative study at three medical centers in Brazil. *Diagn. Microbiol. Infect. Dis.* **12:**35S–39S.
160. **Mandell, W., and H. C. Neu.** 1986. In vitro activity of CI-934, a new quinolone, compared with that of other quinolones and other antimicrobial agents. *Antimicrob. Agents Chemother.* **29:**852–857.
161. **Maple, P. A. C., J. M. T. Hamilton-Miller, and W. Brumfitt.** 1991. Differing activities of quinolones against ciprofloxacin-susceptible and ciprofloxacin-resistant, methicillin-resistant *Staphylococcus aureus*. *Antimicrob. Agents Chemother.* **35:**345–350.
162. **Mazzulli, T., A. E. Simor, R. Jaeger, S. Fuller, and D. E. Low.** 1990. Comparative in vitro activities of several new fluoroquinolones and beta-lactam antimicrobial agents against community isolates of *Streptococcus pneumoniae*. *Antimicrob. Agents Chemother.* **34:**467–469.

162a. **McClean, K. L., D. Hitchman, and S. D. Shafran.** 1992. Norfloxacin is inferior to chloroquine for falciparum malaria in northwestern Zambia: a comparative clinical trial. *J. Infect. Dis.* **165:**904–907.

163. **Moody, J. A., D. N. Gerding, and L. R. Peterson.** 1987. Evaluation of ciprofloxacin's synergism with other agents by multiple in vitro methods. *Am. J. Med.* **82**(Suppl. 4A):44–54.
164. **Moody, J. A., L. R. Peterson, and D. N. Gerding.** 1985. In vitro activity of ciprofloxacin combined with azlocillin. *Antimicrob. Agents Chemother.* **28:**849–850.
165. **Morris, J. G., Jr., J. H. Tenney, and G. L. Drusano.** 1985. In vitro susceptibility of pathogenic *Vibrio* species to norfloxacin and six other antimicrobial agents. *Antimicrob. Agents Chemother.* **28:**442–445.
166. **Nagayama, A., T. Nakao, and H. Taen.** 1988. In vitro activities of ofloxacin and four other new quinoline-carboxylic acids against *Chlamydia trachomatis. Antimicrob. Agents Chemother.* **32:**1735–1737.
167. **Nakamura, S., A. Minami, H. Katae, S. Inoue, J. Yamagishi, Y. Takase, and M. Shimizu.** 1983. In vitro antibacterial properties of AT-2266, a new pyridonecarboxylic acid. *Antimicrob. Agents Chemother.* **23:**641–648.
168. **Nakamura, S., A. Minami, K. Nakata, N. Kurobe, K. Kouno, Y. Sakaguchi, S. Kashimoto, et al.** 1989. In vitro and in vivo antibacterial activities of AT-4140, a new broad-spectrum quinolone. *Antimicrob. Agents Chemother.* **33:**1167–1173.
169. **Neu, H. C.** 1989. Synergy of fluoroquinolones with other antimicrobial agents. *Rev. Infect. Dis.* **11:**(Suppl. 5):S1025–S1035.
170. **Neu, H. C., and N.-X. Chin.** 1987. In vitro activity of two new quinolone antimicrobial agents, S-25930 and S-25932 compared with that of other agents. *J. Antimicrob. Chemother.* **19:**175–185.
171. **Neu, H. C., and N.-X. Chin.** 1989. In vitro activity of S-ofloxacin. *Antimicrob. Agents Chemother.* **33:**1105–1107.
172. **Neu, H. C., and P. Labthavikul.** 1982. In vitro activity of norfloxacin, a quinolone-carboxylic acid, compared with that of beta-lactams, aminoglycosides, and trimethoprim. *Antimicrob. Agents Chemother.* **22:**23–27.
173. **Neu, H. C., A. Novelli, and N.-X. Chin.** 1989. Comparative in vitro activity of a new quinolone, AM-1091. *Antimicrob. Agents Chemother.* **33:**1036–1041.
174. **Niu, W.-W., and H. C. Neu.** 1989. Comparative in vitro activity of a new fluorinated 4-quinolone, QA-241. *Diagn. Microbiol. Infect. Dis.* **12:**243–251.
175. **Norrby, S. R., and M. Jonsson.** 1983. Antibacterial activity of norfloxacin. *Antimicrob. Agents Chemother.* **23:**15–18.
176. **Norrby, S. R., and M. Jonsson.** 1988. Comparative in vitro activity of PD 127,391, a new fluorinated 4-quinolone derivative. *Antimicrob. Agents Chemother.* **32:**1278–1281.
177. **Nye, K., Y. G. Shi, J. M. Andrews, J. P. Ashby, and R. Wise.** 1989. The in-vitro activity, pharmacokinetics, and tissue penetration of temafloxacin. *J. Antimicrob. Chemother.* **24:**415–424.
178. **Okuda, J., S. Okamoto, M. Takahata, and T. Nishino.** 1991. Inhibitory effects of ciprofloxacin and sparfloxacin on DNA gyrase purified from fluoroquinolone-resistant strains of methicillin-resistant *Staphylococcus aureus. Antimicrob. Agents Chemother.* **35:**2288–2293.
179. **Osada, Y., and H. Ogawa.** 1983. Antimycoplasmal activity of ofloxacin (DL-8280). *Antimicrob. Agents Chemother.* **23:**509–511.
180. **Ozaki, M., M. Matsuda, Y. Tomii, K. Kimura, K. Kazuno, M. Kitano, M. Kise, et al.** 1991. In vitro antibacterial activity of a new quinolone, NM394. *Antimicrob. Agents Chemother.* **35:**2490–2495.
181. **Paganoni, R., C. Herzog, A. Braunsteiner, and P. Hohl.** 1988. Fleroxacin: in-vitro activity worldwide against 20,807 clinical isolates and comparison to ciprofloxacin and norfloxacin. *J. Antimicrob. Chemother.* **22**(Suppl. D):3–17.
182. **Paton, J. H., and E. W. Williams.** 1987. Interaction between ciprofloxacin and vancomycin against staphylococci. *J. Antimicrob. Chemother.* **20:**251–254.
183. **Perronne, C., A. Gikas, C. Truffot-Pernot, J. Grosset, J.-L. Vilde, and J.-J. Pocidalo.** 1991. Activities of sparfloxacin, azithromycin, temafloxacin, and rifapentine compared with that of clarithyromycin against multiplication of *Mycobacterium avium* complex within human macrophages. *Antimicrob. Agents Chemother.* **35:**1356–1359.
184. **Peterson, L. R., J. N. Quick, B. Jensen, S. Homann, S. Johnson, J. Tenquist, C. Shanholtzer, R. A. Petzel, L. Sinn, and D. N. Gerding.** 1990. Emergence of ciprofloxacin resistance in nosocomial methicillin-resistant *Staphylococcus aureus* isolates. *Arch. Intern. Med.* **150:**2151–2155.
185. **Piddock, L. J. V., J. M. Andrews, J. M. Diver, and R. Wise.** 1986. In vitro studies of S-25930 and S-25932, two new 4-quinolones. *Eur. J. Clin. Microbiol.* **5:**303–310.
186. **Pohlod, D. J., L. S. Saravolatz, and M. M. Somerville.** 1988. Inhibition of *Legionella pneumophila* multiplication within human macrophages by fleroxacin. *J. Antimicrob. Chemother.* **22**(Suppl. D):49–54.
187. **Prabhala, R. H., B. Rao, R. Marshall, M. B. Bansal, and H. Thadapelli.** 1984. In vitro sus-

ceptibility of anaerobic bacteria to ciprofloxacin (Bay o 9867). *Antimicrob. Agents Chemother.* **26:**785–786.

188. **Preston, M. A., A. E. Simor, S. L. Walmsley, S. A. Fuller, A. J. Lastorvica, K. Sandstedt, and J. L. Penner.** 1990. In vitro susceptibility of *"Campylobacter upsaliensis"* to twenty-four antimicrobial agents. *Eur. J. Clin. Microbiol. Infect. Dis.* **9:**822–824.
189. **Quentin, R., N. Koubaa, B. Cattier, M. Gavignet, and A. Goudeau.** 1988. In vitro activities of five new quinolones against 88 genital and neonatal *Haemophilus* isolates. *Antimicrob. Agents Chemother.* **32:**147–149.
190. **Rajagopalan-Levasseur, P. E., Dournon, G. Dameron, J.-L. Vilde, and J.-J. Pocidalo.** 1990. Comparative postantibacterial activities of pefloxacin, ciprofloxacin, and ofloxacin against intracellular multiplication of *Legionella pneumophila* serogroup 1. *Antimicrob. Agents Chemother.* **34:**1733–1738.
191. **Raoult, D., P. Bres, M. Drancourt, and G. Vestris.** 1991. In vitro susceptibilities of *Coxiella burnetti, Rickettsia rickettsii,* and *Rickettsia conorii* to the fluoroquinolone sparfloxacin. *Antimicrob. Agents Chemother.* **35:**88–91.
192. **Raoult, D., P. Rousselier, V. Galicher, R. Perez, and J. Tamalet.** 1986. In vitro susceptibility of *Rickettsia conorii* to ciprofloxacin as determined by suppressing lethality in chicken embryos and by plaque assay. *Antimicrob. Agents Chemother.* **29:**424–425.
193. **Raoult, D., M. R. Yeaman, and O. G. Baca.** 1989. Susceptibility of *Coxiella burnetii* to pefloxacin and ofloxacin in ovo and in persistently infected L929 cells. *Antimicrob. Agents Chemother.* **33:**621–623.
194. **Rastogi, N., and K. S. Goh.** 1991. In vitro activity of the new difluorinated quinolone sparfloxacin (AT-4140) against *Mycobacterium tuberculosis* compared with activities of ofloxacin and ciprofloxacin. *Antimicrob. Agents Chemother.* **35:**1933–1936.
195. **Rastogi, N., K. S. Goh, and H. L. David.** 1990. Enhancement of drug susceptibility of *Mycobacterium avium* by inhibitors of cell envelope synthesis. *Antimicrob. Agents Chemother.* **34:**759–764.
196. **Rastogi, N., V. Labrousse, K. S. Goh, and J. P. Carvalho de Sousa.** 1991. Antimycobacterial spectrum of sparfloxacin and its activities alone and in association with other drugs against *Mycobacterium avium* complex growing extracellularly and intracellularly in murine and human macrophages. *Antimicrob. Agents Chemother.* **35:**2473–2480.
197. **Rautelin, H., O.-V. Renkonen, and T. U. Kosunen.** 1991. Emergence of fluoroquinolone resistance in *Campylobacter jejuni* and *Campylobacter coli* in subjects from Finland. *Antimicrob. Agents Chemother.* **35:**2065–2069.
198. **Raviglione, M. C., J. F. Boyle, P. Mariuz, A. Pablos-Mendez, H. Cortes, and A. Merlo.** 1990. Ciprofloxacin-resistant methicillin-resistant *Staphylococcus aureus* in an acute-care hospital. *Antimicrob. Agents Chemother.* **34:**2050–2054.
199. **Renneberg, J., and M. Walder.** 1989. Postantibiotic effects of imipenem, norfloxacin, and amikacin in vitro and in vivo. *Antimicrob. Agents Chemother.* **33:**1714–1720.
200. **Rescott, D. L., D. E. Nix, P. Holden, and J. J. Schentag.** 1988. Comparison of two methods for determining in vitro postantibiotic effects of three antibiotics on *Escherichia coli. Antimicrob. Agents Chemother.* **32:**450–453.
201. **Robbins, M. J., A. J. Baskerville, M. Sanghrajka, G. Mumtaz, D. Felmingham, G. L. Ridgway, and R. N. Gruneberg.** 1989. Comparative in vitro activity of lomefloxacin, a difluoro-quinolone. *Diagn. Microbiol. Infect. Dis.* **12:**65S–76S.
202. **Rodriguez-Creixems, M., M. Diaz, P. Munoz, J. Baraia, E. Cercenado, and E. Bouza.** 1991. Emergence of clinical isolates of *Escherichia coli* resistant to ciprofloxacin, abstr. 138. *Program Abstr. 31st Intersci. Conf. Antimicrob. Agents Chemother.*
203. **Rohner, P., C. Herter, R. Auckenthaler, J.-C. Pechere, F. A. Waldvogel, and D. P. Lew.** 1989. Synergistic effect of quinolones and oxacillin on methicillin-resistant *Staphylococcus* species. *Antimicrob. Agents Chemother.* **33:**2037–2041.
204. **Rolston, K. V. I., B. LeBlanc, G. Gooch, D. H. Ho, and G. P. Bodey.** 1989. In-vitro activity of PD 117558, a new quinolone against bacterial isolates from cancer patients. *J. Antimicrob. Chemother.* **23:**363–371.
205. **Rolston, K. V. I., B. LeBlanc, D. H. Ho, and G. P. Bodey.** 1990. In-vitro activity of PD 117 596, a new quinolone, against bacterial isolates from cancer patients. *J. Antimicrob. Chemother.* **26:**39–44.
206. **Rolston, K. V. I., M. Messer, and D. H. Ho.** 1990. Comparative in vitro activities of newer quinolones against *Pseudomonas* species and *Xanthomonas maltophilia* isolated from patients with cancer. *Antimicrob. Agents Chemother.* **34:**1812–1813.
207. **Rolston, K. V. I., H. Nguyen, M. Messer, B. LeBlanc, D. H. Ho, and G. P. Bodey.** 1990. In vitro activity of sparfloxacin (CI-978, AT-4140) against clinical isolates from cancer patients. *Antimicrob. Agents Chemother.* **34:**2263–2266.
208. **Rubinstein, E., R. Lang, B. Shasha, B. Hagar, L. Diamanstein, G. Joseph, M. Anderson, and K. Harrison.** 1991. In vitro susceptibility of *Bru-*

*cella melitensis* to antibiotics. *Antimicrob. Agents Chemother.* **35:**1925–1927.

209. **Sahm, D. F., and G. T. Koburov.** 1989. In vitro activities of quinolones against enterococci resistent to penicillin-aminoglycoside synergy. *Antimicrob. Agents Chemother.* **33:**71–77.
210. **Saito, A., K. Sawatari, Y. Fukuda, M. Nagasawa, H. Koga, A. Tomonage, H. Nakazato, et al.** 1985. Susceptibility of *Legionella pneumophila* to ofloxacin in vitro and in experimental *Legionella* pneumonia in guinea pigs. *Antimicrob. Agents Chemother.* **28:**15–20.
211. **Sarma, P. S.** 1989. Norfloxacin: a new drug in the treatment of falciparum malaria. *Ann. Intern. Med.* **111:**336–337.
212. **Scribner, R. K., D. F. Welch, and M. I. Marks.** 1985. Low frequency of bacterial resistance to enoxacin in vitro and in experimental pneumonia. *J. Antimicrob. Chemother.* **16:**597–603.
213. **Sedlock, D. M., R. A. Dobson, D. M. Deuel, G. Y. Lesher, and J. B. Rake.** 1990. In vitro and in vivo activities of a new quinolone, WIN 57273, possessing potent activity against gram-positive bacteria. *Antimicrob. Agents Chemother.* **34:**568–575.
214. **Segreti, J.** 1991. In vitro activities of temafloxacin against pathogens causing sexually transmitted diseases. *Am. J. Med.* **91**(Suppl. 6A):24S–26S.
215. **Segreti, J., D. J. Hirsch, A. A. Harris, K. S. Kapell, H. Orbach, and H. A. Kessler.** 1990. In vitro activity of tosufloxacin (A-61827; T-3262) against selected genital pathogens. *Antimicrob. Agents Chemother.* **34:**971–973.
216. **Segreti, J., H. A. Kessler, K. S. Kapell, and G. N. Trenholme.** 1989. In vitro activities of temafloxacin (A-62254) and four other antibiotics against *Chlamydia trachomatis. Antimicrob. Agents Chemother.* **33:**118–119.
217. **Segreti, J., J. A. Nelson, L. J. Goodman, R. L. Kaplan, and G. M. Trenholme.** 1989. In vitro activities of lomefloxacin and temafloxacin against pathogens causing diarrhea. *Antimicrob. Agents Chemother.* **33:**1385–1387.
218. **Simor, A. E., S. Ferro, and D. E. Low.** 1989. Comparative in vitro activities of six new fluoroquinolones and other oral antimicrobial agents against *Campylobacter pylori. Antimicrob. Agents Chemother.* **33:**108–109.
219. **Simor, A. E., S. A. Fuller, and D. E. Low.** 1990. Comparative in vitro activities of sparfloxacin (CI-978; AT-4140) and other antimicrobial agents against staphylococci, enterococci, and respiratory tract pathogens. *Antimicrob. Agents Chemother.* **34:**2283–2286.
220. **Smith, R. P., A. L. Baltch, M. C. Hammer, and J. V. Conroy.** 1988. In vitro activities of PD 117,596 and reference antibiotics against 448 clinical bacterial strains. *Antimicrob. Agents Chemother.* **32:**1450–1455.
221. **Smith, S. M., and R. H. K. Eng.** 1985. Activity of ciprofloxacin against methicillin-resistant *Staphylococcus aureus. Antimicrob. Agents Chemother.* **27:**688–691.
222. **Smith, S. M., R. H. K. Eng, and E. Berman.** 1986. The effect of ciprofloxacin on methicillin-resistant *Staphylocccus aureus. J. Antimicrob. Chemother.* **17:**287–295.
223. **Sookpranee, T., M. Sookpranee, M. A. Mellencamp, and L. C. Preheim.** 1991. *Pseudomonas pseudomallei*, a common pathogen in Thailand that is resistant to the bactericidal effects of many antibiotics. *Antimicrob. Agents Chemother.* **35:**484–489.
224. **Stamm, J. M., C. W. Hanson, D. T. W. Chu, R. Bailer, C. Vojtko, and P. B. Fernandes.** 1986. In vitro evaluation of A-56619 (difloxacin) and A-56620: new aryl-fluoroquinolones. *Antimicrob. Agents Chemother.* **29:**193–200.
225. **Stratton, C. W., C. Liu, H. B. Ratner, and L. S. Weeks.** 1987. Bactericidal activity of daptomycin (LY146032) compared with those of ciprofloxacin, vancomycin, and ampicillin against enterococci as determined by kill-kinetic studies. *Antimicrob. Agents Chemother.* **31:**1014–1016.
226. **Sutter, V. L., Y. Y. Kwok, and J. Bulkacz.** 1985. Comparative activity of ciprofloxacin against anaerobic bacteria. *Antimicrob. Agents Chemother.* **27:**427–428.
227. **Swanson, R. N., D. J. Hardy, D. T. W. Chu, N. L. Shipkowitz, and J. J. Clement.** 1991. Activity of temafloxacin against respiratory pathogens. *Antimicrob. Agents Chemother.* **35:**423–429.
228. **Swenson, J. M., R. R. Facklam, and C. Thornsberry.** 1990. Antimicrobial susceptibility of vancomycin-resistant *Leuconostoc, Pediococcus*, and *Lactobacillus* species. *Antimicrob. Agents Chemother.* **34:**543–549.
229. **Syrjala, H., R. Schildt, and S. Raisainen.** 1991. In vitro susceptibility of *Francisella tularensis* to fluoroquinolones and treatment of tularemia with norfloxacin and ciprofloxacin. *Eur. J. Clin. Microbiol. Infect. Dis.* **10:**68–70.
230. **Talbot, H., and B. Romanowski.** 1989. In vitro activities of lomefloxacin, tetracycline, penicillin, spectinomycin, and ceftriaxone against *Neisseria gonorrhoeae* and *Chlamydia trachomatis. Antimicrob. Agents Chemother.* **33:**2049–2051.
231. **Tanaka, M., M. Otsuki, T. Une, and T. Nishino.** 1990. In-vitro and in-vivo activity of DR-3355, an optically active isomer of ofloxacin. *J. Antimicrob. Chemother.* **26:**659–666.
232. **Tenney, J. H., R. W. Maack, and G. R. Chippendale.** 1983. Rapid selection of organisms with increasing resistance on subinhibitory concentrations of norfloxacin in agar. *Antimicrob. Agents Chemother.* **23:**188–189.

233. **Traub, W. H., and M. Spohr.** 1989. Antimicrobial drug susceptibility of clinical isolates of *Acinetobacter* species (*A. baumannii, A. haemolyticus*, genospecies 3, and genospecies 6). *Antimicrob. Agents Chemother.* **33:**1617–1619.

234. **Trimble, K. A., R. B. Clark, W. E. Sanders, Jr., J. W. Frankel, R. Cacciatore, and H. Valdez.** 1987. Activity of ciprofloxacin against *Mycobacteria* in vitro: comparison of BACTEC and macrobroth dilution methods. *J. Antimicrob. Chemother.* **19:**617–622.

235. **Une, T., T. Fujimoto, K. Sato, and Y. Osada.** 1988. In vitro activity of DR-3355, an optically active ofloxacin. *Antimicrob. Agents Chemother.* **32:**1336–1340.

236. **Van Caekenberghe, D.** 1990. Comparative in-vitro activities of ten fluoroquinolones and fusidic acid against *Mycobacterium* spp. *J. Antimicrob. Chemother.* **26:**381–386.

237. **Van der Auwera, P.** 1985. Interaction of gentamicin, dibekacin, netilmicin and amikacin with various penicillins, cephalosporins, minocycline and new fluoroquinolones against *Enterobacteriaceae* and *Pseudomonas aeruginosa. J. Antimicrob. Chemother.* **16:**581–587.

238. **Van der Auwera, P., P. Grenier, Y. Glupczynski, and D. Pierard.** 1989. In-vitro activity of lomefloxacin in comparison with pefloxacin and ofloxacin. *J. Antimicrob. Chemother.* **23:**209–219.

239. **Van der Auwera, P., and P. Joly.** 1987. Comparative in vitro activities of teicoplanin, vancomycin, coumermycin and ciprofloxacin, alone and in combination with rifampicin or LM427, against *Staphylococcus aureus. J. Antimicrob. Chemother.* **19:**313–320.

240. **Venditti, M., V. Gelfusa, A. Tarasi, C. Brandimarte, and P. Serra.** 1990. Antimicrobial susceptibilities of *Erysipelothrix rhusiopathiae. Antimicrob. Agents Chemother.* **34:**2038–2040.

241. **Venezia, R. A., L. A. Prymas, A. Shayegani, and D. M. Yocum.** 1989. In vitro activities of amifloxacin and two of its metabolites. *Antimicrob. Agents Chemother.* **33:**762–766.

242. **Verbist, L.** 1987. Comparative in vitro activity of Ro 23-6240, a new trifluorinated quinolone. *J. Antimicrob. Chemother.* **20:**363–372.

243. **Visser, M. R., M. Rozenberg-Arska, H. Beumer, I. M. Hoepelman, and J. Verhoef.** 1991. Comparative in vitro antibacterial activity of sparfloxacin (AT-4140; RP 64206), a new quinolone. *Antimicrob. Agents Chemother.* **35:**858–868.

244. **Wade, W. G.** 1989. In-vitro activity of ciprofloxacin and other agents against oral bacteria. *J. Antimicrob. Chemother.* **24:**683–687.

245. **Waites, K. B., G. H. Cassell, K. C. Canupp, and P. B. Fernandes.** 1988. In vitro susceptibilities of mycoplasmas and ureaplasmas to new macrolides and aryl-fluoroquinolones. *Antimicrob. Agents Chemother.* **32:**1500–1502.

246. **Waites, K. B., L. B. Duffy, T. Schmid, D. Crabb, M. S. Pate, and G. H. Cassell,** 1991. In vitro susceptibilities of *Mycoplasma pneumoniae, Mycoplasma hominis,* and *Ureaplasma urealyticum* to sparfloxacin and PD 127391. *Antimicrob. Agents Chemother.* **35:**1181–1185.

247. **Wallace, R. J., Jr., G. Bedsole, G. Sumter, C. V. Sanders, L. C. Steele, B. A. Brown, J. Smith, and D. R. Graham.** 1990. Activities of ciprofloxacin and ofloxacin against rapidly growing mycobacteria with demonstration of acquired resistance following single-drug therapy. *Antimicrob. Agents Chemother.* **34:**65–70.

248. **Wallace, R. J., Jr., L. C. Steele, G. Sumter, and J. M. Smith,** 1988. Antimicrobial susceptibility patterns of *Nocardia asteroides. Antimicrob. Agents Chemother.* **32:**1776–1779.

249. **Watanabe, M., Y. Kotera, K. Yosue, M. Inoue, and S. Mitsuhashi.** 1990. In vitro emergence of quinolone-resistant mutants of *Escherichia coli, Enterobacter cloacae,* and *Serratia marcescens. Antimicrob. Agents Chemother.* **34:**173–175.

249a. **Watt, G., G. D. Shanks, M. D. Edstein, K. Pavanand, H. K. Webster, and S. Wechgritaya.** 1991. Ciprofloxacin treatment of drug-resistant falciparum malaria. *J. Infect. Dis.* **164:**602–604.

250. **Weber, D. J., S. M. Saviteer, W. A. Rutala, and C. A. Thomann.** 1988. In vitro susceptibility of *Bacillus* spp. to selected antimicrobial agents. *Antimicrob. Agents Chemother.* **32:**642–645.

251. **Whiting, J. L., N. Cheng, and A. W. Chow.** 1987. Interactions of ciprofloxacin with clindamycin, metronidazole, cefoxitin, cefotaxime, and mezlocillin against gram-positive and gram-negative anaerobic bacteria. *Antimicrob. Agents Chemother.* **31:**1379–1382.

252. **Winton, M. D., E. D. Everett, and S. A. Dolan.** 1988. Activities of five new fluoroquinolones against *Pseudomonas pseudomallei. Antimicrob. Agents Chemother.* **32:**928–929.

253. **Wise, R., J. M. Andrews, J. P. Ashby, and R. S. Matthews.** 1988. In vitro activity of lomefloxacin, a new quinolone antimicrobial agent, in comparison with those of other agents. *Antimicrob. Agents Chemother.* **32:**617–622.

254. **Wise, R., J. M. Andrews, and G. Danks.** 1984. In vitro activity of enoxacin (CI-919), a new quinolone derivative, compared with that of other antimicrobial agents. *J. Antimicrob. Chemother.* **17:**69–73.

255. **Wise, R., J. M. Andrews, and L. J. Edwards.** 1983. In vitro activity of Bay 09867, a new quinolone derivative, compared with those of other antimicrobial agents. *Antimicrob. Agents Chemother.* **23:**559–564.

256. **Wise, R., J. P. Ashby, and J. M. Andrews.** 1988. In vitro activity of PD 127,391, an enhanced-spectrum quinolone. *Antimicrob. Agents Chemother.* **32:**1251–1256.

257. **Wolfson, J. S., and D. C. Hooper.** 1989. Fluoroquinolone antimicrobial agents. *Clin. Microbiol. Rev.* **2:**378–424.

258. **Yajko, D. M., J. Kirihara, C. Sanders, P. Nassos, and W. K. Hadley.** 1988. Antimicrobial synergism against *Mycobacterium avium* complex strains isolated from patients with acquired immune deficiency syndrome. *Antimicrob. Agents Chemother.* **32:**1392–1395.

259. **Yajko, D. M., C. A. Sanders, P. S. Nassos, and W. K. Hadley.** 1990. In vitro susceptibility of *Mycobacterium avium* complex to the new fluoroquinolone sparfloxacin (CI-978; AT-4140) and comparison with ciprofloxacin. *Antimicrob. Agents Chemother.* **34:**2442–2444.

260. **Yamamoto, T., P. Naigowit, S. Dejsirilert, D. Chiewsilp, E. Kondo, T. Yokota, and K. Kanai.** 1990. In vitro susceptibilities of *Pseudomonas pseudomallei* to 27 antimicrobial agents. *Antimicrob. Agents Chemother.* **34:**2027–2029.

261. **Yazawa, K., Y. Mikami, and J. Uno.** 1989. In vitro susceptibility of *Nocardia* spp. to a new fluoroquinolone, tosufloxacin (T-3262). *Antimicrob. Agents Chemother.* **33:**2140–2141.

262. **Yew, W. W., S. Y.-L. Kwan, W. K. Ma, M. A. Khin, and P. Y. Chau.** 1990. In-vitro activity of ofloxacin against *Mycobacterium tuberculosis* and its clinical efficacy in multiply resistant pulmonary tuberculosis. *J. Antimicrob. Chemother.* **26:**227–236.

263. **Yourassowsky, E., M. P. van der Linden, M. J. Lismont, F. Crokaert, and Y. Glupczynski.** 1986. Rate of bactericidal activity for *Streptococcus faecalis* of a new quinolone, CI-934, compared with that of amoxicillin. *Antimicrob. Agents Chemother.* **30:**258–259.

264. **Zeiler, H. J.** 1985. Evaluation of the in vitro bactericidal action of ciprofloxacin on cells of *Escherichia coli* in the logarithmic and stationary phases of growth. *Antimicrob. Agents Chemother.* **28:**524–527.

265. **Zhanel, G. G., R. J. Davidson, and D. J. Hoban.** 1990. Reproducibility of the in-vitro postantibiotic effect of fluoroquinolones against *Staphylococcus aureus*. *J. Antimicrob. Chemother.* **26:**724–726.

*Quinolone Antimicrobial Agents, 2nd ed.*
Edited by David C. Hooper and John S. Wolfson


*Chapter 9*

# Pharmacokinetics of the Quinolone Antimicrobial Agents

*Nigahus Karabalut and George L. Drusano*

The past decade has seen breakthroughs in medicinal chemistry resulting in a new series of compounds, the 6-fluoroquinolone carboxylic acids, that exhibit markedly improved activity against major hospital-acquired pathogens, including *Pseudomonas aeruginosa*. In this chapter, the pharmacokinetic properties of the new fluoroquinolones are examined. Because the number of fluoroquinolones is now substantial and continues to grow, a classification system would be useful. One such system used here is classification of these agents by their predominant clearance pathway: renal (ofloxacin, temafloxacin, and lomefloxacin), hepatic (pefloxacin), or both (norfloxacin, ciprofloxacin, enoxacin, fleroxacin, and rufloxacin). Interactions of these agents with other drugs are discussed in chapter 11.

## FLUOROQUINOLONES EXCRETED PREDOMINANTLY BY THE KIDNEYS

### Ofloxacin

Ofloxacin (Fig. 1) is the prototype of a renally cleared fluoroquinolone and is available in both oral and intravenous dosing forms (94).

Verho et al. (80) evaluated the oral pharmacokinetics of ofloxacin in an open randomized crossover study for single doses of 100, 300, and 600 mg. Maximal concentrations in serum were 1 μg/ml for the 100-mg dose, 3.4 μg/ml for the 300-mg dose, and 6.9 μg/ml for the 600-mg dose (Fig. 2). Absorption was rapid, with maximal concentrations occurring at or before 1 h.

Terminal elimination half-lives varied between 5.6 and 6.4 h. Urinary recovery varied between 75 and 81%. Lockley et al. (55) evaluated a 600-mg dose of ofloxacin and found similar results except for higher maximal concentrations in serum. The area under the curve (AUC) of the concentration in serum plotted versus time, a measure of bioavailability, did not differ between the two studies. Lockley et al. (55) also studied the penetration of ofloxacin into inflammatory blister fluid. High peak concentrations of ofloxacin in blister fluid were obtained (5.2 $\pm$ 0.9 μg/ml [mean $\pm$ standard deviation]), with maximal concentrations at 5.3 $\pm$ 0.8 h. The terminal half-life was longer in blister fluid (8.0 $\pm$ 1.7 h) than in serum, and penetration, as judged by the ratios of the AUC for blister fluid to the AUC for serum, was in excess of unity (125%). Similar results were obtained for ofloxacin (300-mg dose) penetration into noninflammatory blister fluid (47).

*Nigahus Karabalut* • Division of Infectious Diseases, University of Maryland School of Medicine, Baltimore, Maryland 21201. *George L. Drusano* • Division of Clinical Pharmacology, Department of Medicine, Albany Medical College, Albany, New York 12208.

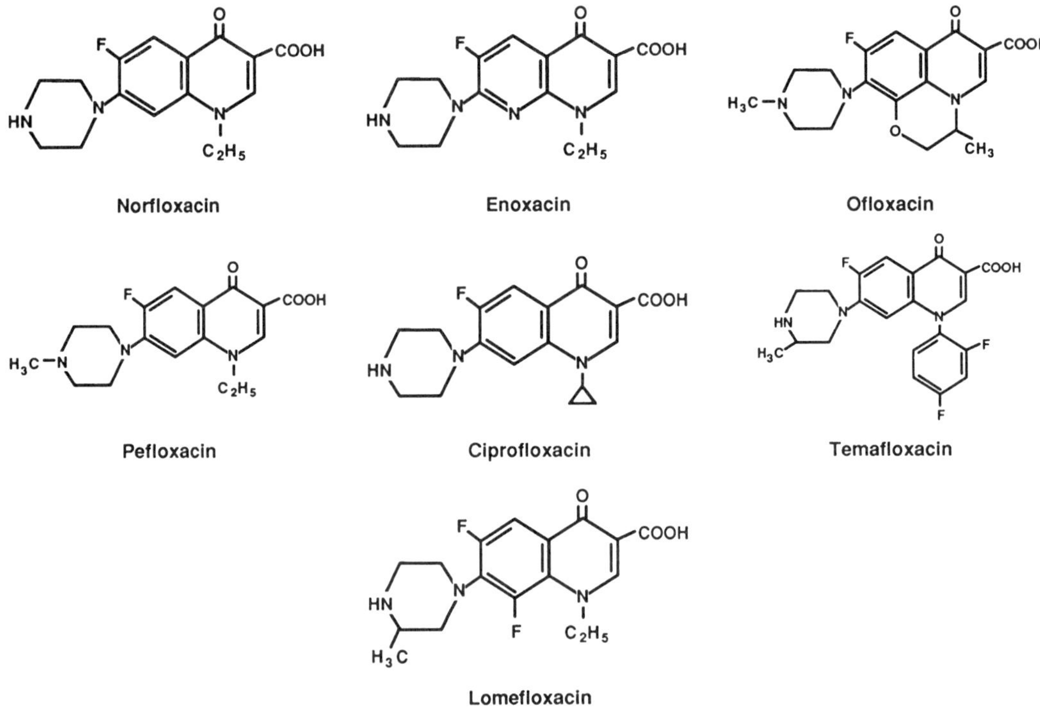

Norfloxacin

Enoxacin

Ofloxacin

Pefloxacin

Ciprofloxacin

Temafloxacin

Lomefloxacin

**Figure 1.** Quinolone structures (taken from reference 63 with permission).

The fluoroquinolones will find substantial use in the outpatient setting. Consequently, it becomes important to examine the effect of concurrent food administration on drug pharmacokinetics. Leroy et al. (52) and Kalager et al. (47) have examined the effect of food on the absorption of ofloxacin and reported similar results. For a 200-mg dose (52), maximum concentrations occurred at 0.83 ± 0.31 h in fasting subjects and at 1.85 ± 1.15 h in fed subjects. AUCs were, however, not statistically significantly different between groups. Half-lives in the study by Leroy et al. (52) were 7.86 ± 1.81 h in fasting subjects and 8.00 ± 1.71 h in nonfasting subjects. Urinary recovery was 74.8% ± 11.6% in fasting subjects and 76.2% ± 7.4% in fed subjects.

Since renal elimination accounts for the majority of ofloxacin clearance, it is clinically important to detail the effect of altered renal function on drug disposition. Fillastre et al. (30) examined the influence of various degrees of renal impairment on the disposition of a single 200-mg oral dose of ofloxacin (Table 1). Renal impairment had a major impact on ofloxacin disposition. Although peak concentrations ($C_{max}$) were relatively unaffected, AUCs increased from 13.8 ± 3.12 μg · h/ml for subjects with normal renal function to 86.05 ± 49.72 μg · h/ml for subjects with severely impaired renal function. Most of the change resulted from an altered terminal-elimination half-life, which increased from 7.86 ± 1.81 to 37.16 ± 23.26 h. Renal clearance and urinary recovery declined as a function of a decreasing glomerular filtration rate (GFR).

Lode et al. (56) examined the pharmacokinetics of ofloxacin after both parenteral and oral administration in single doses of 25, 50, 100, and 200 mg (Table 2). AUCs for serum increased with the dose in a linear fashion over the range examined, paralleling the results in the oral-dose-ranging trials. Volumes of distribution were large, ranging

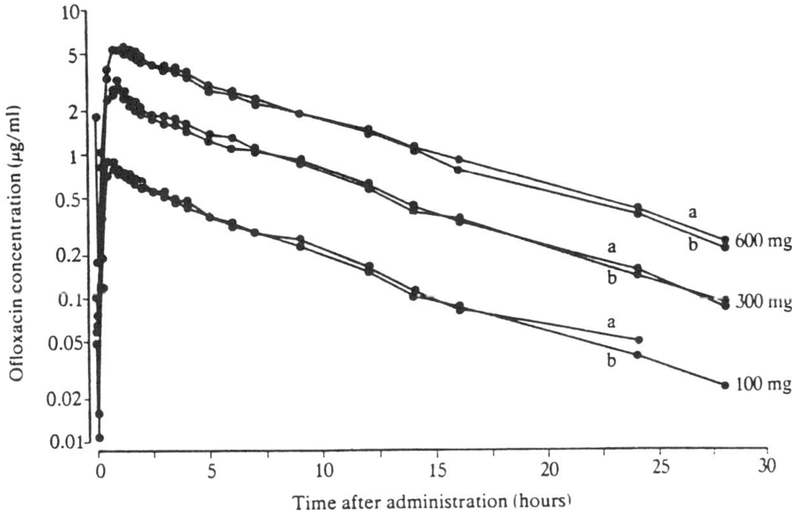


**Figure 2.** Median concentrations of ofloxacin in serum at various times after oral administration of different single doses. (a) Microbiologic assay; (b) high-pressure liquid chromatography assay. (From reference 80.)

from 1.2 to 1.5 liters/kg. Systemic clearances of 0.20 to 0.24 liters/h/kg of body weight were seen, with renal clearances accounting for 75 to 80% of the total serum clearance. Protein binding averaged 25% ± 2.5%, with no dependence on the drug concentration noted within the range of 0.57 to 2.1 μg/ml.

Ofloxacin is less biotransformed than other new fluoroquinolones, with desmethylofloxacin and ofloxacin *N*-oxide being the two major metabolites formed (Table 3). There were no differences between oral and parenteral administration, indicating no first-pass hepatic metabolism after oral administration.

Because both oral and parenteral dosing forms of ofloxacin are available, Lode et al. (56) determined the absolute bioavailability of this agent. For a 200-mg dose, the ratio of the AUC after oral administration to the AUC after intravenous administration was 0.96 for a three-compartment analysis, indicating a virtually complete absorption of the drug when given orally. Despite the excellent absorption of ofloxacin, concentrations in stool are high, i.e., up to 327 ± 274 μg/g after administration of 200 mg orally twice daily for 4 days (51).

## Temafloxacin

Temafloxacin is a new fluoroquinolone with a 7- to 8-h half-life and rapid gastrointestinal absorption. These characteristics make it an ideal antimicrobial agent for once- or twice-daily oral dosing. However, temafloxacin has been withdrawn from the market after reports of a hemolytic syndrome following its use. This decision was implemented by Abbott Pharmaceuticals after the company was notified by the Food and Drug Administration of an excess of serious adverse events involving the drug (see chapter 26).

The chemistry of temafloxacin determines its pharmacokinetic and pharmacodynamic features. The fluorine atom at position 6 enhances the antimicrobial activities of all fluoroquinolone (Fig. 3). The piperazine ring at position 7 further enhances antimicrobial activity, especially against *Pseudomonas* spp. (17). The difluorophenyl group (aryl ring) at position 1 extends temafloxacin's spectrum to include gram-positive bacteria. The difluorophenyl group also improves the water solubility of temafloxacin over that of other quinolones.

**Table 1.** Ofloxacin pharmacokinetic data for subjects with healthy and impaired renal function after a single oral dose of 200 mg[a]

| GFR (ml/min/1.73 m²) | $C_{max}$ (μg/ml) | $T_{max}$ (h) | AUC (μg·h/ml) | $V/F$ (liters/kg) | $t_{1/2}$(h) | CL/$F$ (ml/min/1.73 m²) | $CL_R$ (ml/min/1.73 m²) |
|---|---|---|---|---|---|---|---|
| ≥80 | 2.24 ± 0.90 | 0.83 ± 0.31 | 13.18 ± 3.12 | 2.53 ± 0.78 | 7.86 ± 1.81 | 241.4 ± 53.8 | 196.5 ± 42.9 |
| ≥40, ≥80 | 2.18 ± 0.53 | 1.75 ± 1.66 | 32.33 ± 4.18 | 2.14 ± 0.50 | 15.00 ± 4.40 | 109.4 ± 18.3 | 60.6 ± 9.3 |
| ≥20, <39 | 1.84 ± 0.32 | 2.36 ± 1.60 | 47.48 ± 14.00 | 2.15 ± 0.31 | 25.37 ± 8.56 | 70.8 ± 15.9 | 30.9 ± 7.7 |
| <20 | 1.71 ± 0.62 | 1.60 ± 1.34 | 65.98 ± 15.00 | 2.02 ± 0.26 | 34.84 ± 15.46 | 50.6 ± 14.5 | 13.7 ± 6.2 |
| Hemodialysis | 1.97 ± 0.56 | 3.20 ± 2.59 | 86.05 ± 49.72 | 2.02 ± 0.37 | 37.16 ± 23.26 | 49.2 ± 21.6 | |

[a]Data are from reference 30. Abbreviations: $C_{max}$, maximum concentration of drug in serum; $T_{max}$, time to maximum concentration of drug in serum; $V/F$, volume of distribution divided by bioavailability; $t_{1/2}$, half-life; CL/$F$, total serum clearance divided by bioavailability; $CL_R$, renal clearance. All values are given as means ± standard deviations.

**Table 2.** Pharmacokinetic parameters for ofloxacin in 10 healthy volunteers[a]

| Dose (mg) | Route of administration | $C_{max}$ (mg/liter) | $T_{max}$ (min) | $V_{area}$ (liters) | $t_{1/2\beta}$ (min) | $AUC_{TOT}$ (mg·h/liter) | $CL_{TOT}$ (ml/min) | $CL_R$ (ml/min) | Urinary excretion (% of dose/24 h) |
|---|---|---|---|---|---|---|---|---|---|
| 25 | i.v. | | | 93.9 ± 8.7 | 231 ± 34.5 | 1.5 ± 0.18 | 286 ± 32.6 | 245 ± 29.4 | 82.2 ± 4.5 |
| 50 | i.v. | | | 103.0 ± 31.8 | 260 ± 34.6 | 3.1 ± 0.58 | 276 ± 68.2 | 276 ± 7.0 | 81.1 ± 13.5 |
| 100 | i.v. | | | 89.8 ± 14.7 | 267 ± 36.8 | 7.3 ± 1.2 | 235 ± 37.0 | 185 ± 41.2 | 73.1 ± 10.1 |
| 200 | i.v. | | | 86.0 ± 10.4 | 256 ± 19.8 | 14.4 ± 1.8 | 234 ± 27.8 | 190 ± 27.3 | 77.0 ± 8.2 |
| 200 | Oral | 2.19 ± 0.43 | 76.8 ± 39.2 | 111.0 ± 26.0 | 334 ± 98.9 | 14.6 ± 2.7 | | 197 ± 44.3 | 73.6 ± 7.3 |
| 400 | Oral | 3.51 ± 0.7 | 114.9 ± 38.7 | 102.0 ± 16.3 | 294 ± 45.2 | 28.0 ± 4.9 | | 202 ± 35.0 | 73.3 ± 6.9 |

[a]Data are normalized to a mean body weight of 70 kg and are from reference 56. Abbreviations: $V_{area}$, volume of distribution (per 70 kg of body weight); $t_{1/2\beta}$, half-life at $\beta$ phase; $AUC_{TOT}$, total AUC; $CL_{TOT}$, total clearance; i.v., intravenous. For other abbreviations, see Table 1, footnote $a$. All values are given as means ± standard deviations.

**Table 3.** Mean renal elimination of 200-mg doses of ofloxacin, desmethylofloxacin, and ofloxacin *N*-oxide[a]

| Route of administration | Mean excretion (% of dose/24 h) ± SD | | |
|---|---|---|---|
| | Ofloxacin | Desmethyl-ofloxacin | Ofloxacin *N*-oxide |
| Oral | 73.6 ± 7.3 | 3.0 ± 0.80 | 1.0 ± 0.20 |
| i.v. | 77.0 ± 8.2 | 3.2 ± 0.61 | 1.1 ± 0.18 |

[a]Data are from reference 56. i.v., intravenous.

Because temafloxacin is less lipid soluble, it crosses the blood-brain barrier poorly, reducing the likelihood of central nervous system adverse events. The presence of a methyl group on the piperazine ring at position 7 in temafloxacin relative to an unsubstituted piperazine moiety may also further reduce the risk of central nervous system complications by reducing drug binding to γ-aminobutyric acid receptors in the brain (69).

The pharmacokinetic profile of temafloxacin is quite distinct from that of the other fluoroquinolones because of its 7- to 8-h half-life and high water solubility (38). It is virtually completely absorbed from the gastrointestinal tract, with a bioavailability of approximately 93%, and absorption is not greatly affected by food (40, 41). The time to reach peak concentrations ranges between 2 and 3 h. At doses under 1,200 mg, temafloxacin displays a predictable pharmacokinetic profile, with a linear relationship between levels in serum and dose (38).

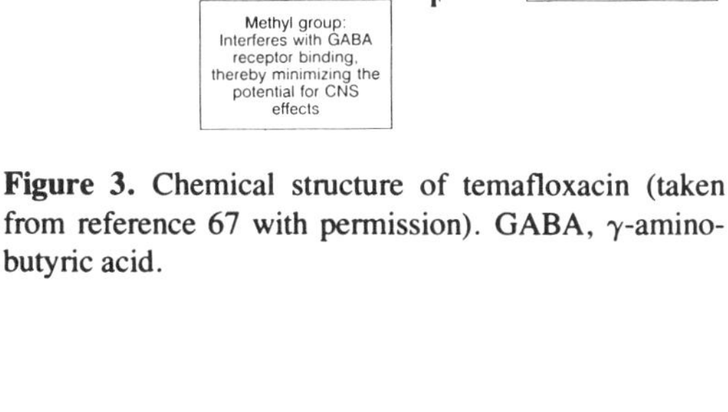

**Figure 3.** Chemical structure of temafloxacin (taken from reference 67 with permission). GABA, γ-aminobutyric acid.

The linear relationship for increasing temafloxacin doses has also been demonstrated for steady-state concentrations in serum in patients given drug twice daily (41). Dosages of 300, 400, and 600 mg twice daily resulted in maximum steady-state concentrations in serum of 3, 4, and 6 μg/ml and corresponding minimum steady-state concentrations of 1.5, 2, and 3 μg/ml, respectively. This relationship predicts that every 100 mg of temafloxacin will result in maximum and minimum steady-state concentrations of 1.0 and 0.5 μg/ml, respectively.

Temafloxacin has good tissue distribution and penetration because of its high water solubility and low protein binding (40), being only 26% bound to protein. In spite of low lipid solubility, temafloxacin is widely distributed in body fluids and tissues, attaining higher levels in bronchial mucosa (14.9 μg/g, after 600 mg twice daily), urine, and prostatic tissue (3.86 μg/g, after 400 mg twice daily) (31, 86) than in plasma following single- and multiple-dose regimens. High intracellular concentrations (79.2 μg/g in alveolar macrophages) and high concentrations in the lung (35.8 μg/g) (76, 86) occur with doses of 600 mg twice daily. Because the ratio of urine to plasma drug concentrations can be as high as 100:1, providing concentrations far above the MICs for 90% of strains of most uropathogens, temafloxacin has excellent activity for treatment of urinary tract infections. Because of its poor penetration into the central nervous system, temafloxacin may not be useful for treating infections at this site.

The major elimination pathway for temafloxacin is renal, principally by glomerular filtration, with tubular secretion playing a minor role. This distribution of renal clearance between glomerular filtration and tubular secretion is different from that with ciprofloxacin, for which tubular secretion substantially exceeds glomerular filtration. About 60% of a given dose of temafloxacin will be recovered unchanged in the urine (38). Urinary recovery of metabolites accounts for up to 6% of the dose, and biliary excretion of both temafloxacin and its metabolites is <2 to 3% of the dose. The clearance of temafloxacin closely correlates with an individual's creatinine clearance ($Cr_{CL}$); consequently, the dosage of temafloxacin should be reduced by at least one-half for patients with a $CR_{CL}$ of <40 ml/min, and no further dosage adjustments are needed in patients undergoing hemodialysis, because temafloxacin is not significantly removed during 4 h of hemodialysis. Dosage adjustment must be considered for the elderly, who may have reductions in lean body mass as well as in renal function. Sörgel and his colleagues (77) were not able to find differences in the peak concentrations of temafloxacin administered to patients with cirrhosis and to healthy controls. Dosage adjustment is not required in cirrhotic patients unless a patient has concomitant impairment of renal function.

Volume of distribution for temafloxacin is between 1.53 and 1.83 liters/kg (41). Hepatic metabolism is no more than 1 to 2% of administered intravenous doses. Only 1% of the administered dose was found in urine as the oxometabolite (piperazine-directed biotransformation). In patients with renal failure, two metabolites resulting from piperazine ring cleavage, desethylene and desmethylene, did not reach levels in plasma of >10 ng/ml (77).

In general, penetration of temafloxacin into body fluids (tears, nasal secretions, saliva, and sweat) is better than that of ciprofloxacin. Unlike ciprofloxacin, temafloxacin has not exhibited in vitro or in vivo effects on methylxanthine metabolism, and its use should not require theophylline drug level monitoring (57).

## Lomefloxacin

By virtue of a methyl substituent on the piperazinyl moiety, lomefloxacin [1-ethyl-6,8-difluoro-1,4-(3-methyl-1-piperazinyl)-4 oxo-3 quinolone carboxylic acid hydrochloride] has virtually complete oral absorption and a long elimination half-life of 7 to 8 h (Fig. 1).

Renal excretion is the most important elimination pathway for lomefloxacin. Pharmacokinetic parameter values from single- and multiple-dose studies are in good agreement. The absorption and distribution of lomefloxacin are not significantly altered, however, by changes in renal function. Lomefloxacin is rapidly absorbed after a single 400-mg oral dose, with $C_{max}$ of 4.5 to 5.3 μg/ml occurring 0.9 to 1.75 h after administration (9). The pharmacokinetics of lomefloxacin given in single and multiple doses in patients with various levels of $CL_{CR}$ are summarized in Table 4. Blum et al. (9) have shown that despite a predominantly renal elimination, lomefloxacin shows a nonrenal clearance that significantly correlates with decreasing renal function.

Concentrations of lomefloxacin in the urine of healthy subjects and in patients with severe renal impairment exceed 18 and 2.5 μg/ml in the 0- to 24-h and 24- to 48-h urine collections, respectively (9). These concentrations are above MICs for susceptible strains of *Escherichia coli*, *Morganella* spp., *Salmonella* spp., *Shigella* spp., *Haemophilus influenzae*, *Neisseria gonorrhoeae*, *Moraxella* spp., and *Legionella* spp. (16). Hemodialysis has no effect on fluoroquinolone pharmacokinetics. Following 4 h of dialysis, <3% of the lomefloxacin dose is recovered in dialysis fluid (9). Thus, no supplementary doses are necessary to compensate for hemodialysis removal.

In a randomized, double-blind, placebo-controlled trial in which single doses of 100, 200, 400, 600, and 800 mg of lomefloxacin were administered to 40 volunteers (62), lomefloxacin was rapidly absorbed after oral administration, achieving maximum concentrations in plasma ranging from 1.0 μg/ml for the 100-mg dose to 6.76 μg/ml for the 800-mg dose approximately 1 h after dosing. Elimination half-lives of 7 to 8 h were noted for all doses. Concentrations in urine at 24 to 32 h after dosing ranged from 9.4 μg/ml for the 100-mg dose to 111.3 μg/ml for the 800-mg dose.

In a randomized, double-blind study in which six different dose regimens (200 mg

**Table 4.** Pharmacokinetic parameters for lomefloxacin from single-dose and multiple-dose studies with renally compromised patients[a]

| Dose | $CL_{CR}$ (ml/min/1.73 m²) | $C_{max}$ (μg/ml) | $T_{max}$ (h) | $CL_T$ (ml/min/1.73 m²) | $CL_R$ (ml/min/1.73 m²) | $CN_{NR}$ (ml/min/1.73 m²) | $t_{1/2}$ (h) |
|---|---|---|---|---|---|---|---|
| 400 mg, oral, once | >80 | 5.22 | 0.9 | 29.2 | 140.4 | 88.7 | 8.1 |
| | 80–<40 | 4.54 | 1.31 | 192.7 | 111.2 | 81.5 | 9.1 |
| | 40–>10 | 4.99 | 1.36 | 77.1 | 28.4 | 48.7 | 20.9 |
| | <10 | 4.48 | 1.75 | 33.8 | 0.6 | 33.2 | 44.2 |
| 200 mg/day for 7 days | >90 | 1.75 | 1.8 | 323.7 | 167.9 | 155.8 | 8.1 |
| | 60–90 | 2.14 | 1.5 | 156.9 | 94.1 | 62.8 | 20.8 |
| | 30–60 | 2.53 | 1.6 | 130.7 | 69.8 | 60.9 | 21.3 |
| | <30 | 3.57 | 1.7 | 68.1 | 24.4 | 43.7 | 32.7 |

[a]$CL_{CR}$, creatinine clearance; $C_{max}$, peak level in serum; $T_{max}$, time to peak; $CL_T$, $CL_R$, and $CL_{NR}$, total, renal, and nonrenal clearances, respectively; $t_{1/2}$, elimination half-life. From reference 8 with permission.

once daily, 400 mg once daily, 400 mg twice daily, 600 mg once daily, 600 mg twice daily, 800 mg once daily) each given for 7 days were compared, Mant (58) showed that at all dose levels, lomefloxacin was rapidly absorbed after oral dosing. On day 1, $C_{max}$ values in plasma, occurring approximately 1 h after dosing, ranged from 1.88 ± 0.29 μg/ml after the 200-mg dose to 5.42 ± 0.68 μg/ml after the 800-mg dose. At day 7, $C_{max}$ values in plasma were significantly higher than on day 1, ranging from 2.01 ± 0.26 μg/ml for the 200-mg dose to 5.99 ± 2.03 μg/ml for the 800-mg dose.

The elimination half-life of lomefloxacin was 7 to 8 h in all six dosage regimens. The half-life at steady state was the same as that observed following the first dose. Coefficients of variation in the ß phase for all half-life values were <20% on both day 1 and day 7. $C_{max}$ increased proportionately with dose. Analysis of trough concentrations in plasma revealed that steady state was reached by day 2 of dosing.

The plasma clearance values were similar for all once-daily dosage regimens at days 1 and 7. The apparent plasma clearance values on day 1 averaged 219 ml/min. Renal clearance was approximately 65% of plasma clearances. In this study, lomefloxacin was well tolerated in single daily doses of up to 800 mg and in twice-daily doses of up to 600 mg (total daily dose, 1,200 mg), confirming its safety.

In summary, with lomefloxacin therapy, steady state is reached on day 2 of dosing, which is consistent with its elimination half-life. $C_{max}$ in plasma, AUC, and urinary excretion demonstrated dose proportionality for single doses and once-daily doses at steady state. Steady-state $C_{max}$ and AUC values for twice-daily regimens were higher than corresponding single-dose values. A 400-mg oral dose of lomefloxacin provides a $C_{max}$ in plasma of 3 μg/ml and a trough concentration of 0.3 μg/ml.

Since available data suggest that there is good tolerance of lomefloxacin over a wide range of concentrations in plasma, dose adjustments appear to be necessary only for patients with $CL_{CR}$ of <40 ml/min. The data show that lomefloxacin can be safely coadministered with methylxanthines (42).

Lebrec et al. (50) showed that liver failure did not affect the pharmacokinetics of lomefloxacin in 12 patients with histologically documented cirrhosis. The changes observed in the clearance of lomefloxacin may be attributed to perturbations of renal function associated with cirrhosis. Thus, no dosage adjustments appear to be necessary for patients with liver failure. In a study employing single oral doses of 400 mg given to patients with different underlying problems, lomefloxacin attained high concentrations in prostate and bone as well as good levels in bronchial secretions (6, 53, 65).

## FLUOROQUINOLONES CLEARED PREDOMINANTLY BY THE LIVER

### Pefloxacin

Pefloxacin is a fluoroquinolone that is primarily cleared by the liver. The structure of pefloxacin differs from that of norfloxacin only in the addition of a methyl group to position 4′ of the piperazinyl substituent at position 7 (Fig. 1). This minor difference in structure markedly alters the half-life and renal handling of pefloxacin, changing it from a compound secreted by the renal tubule to one for which there is net renal tubular reabsorption. Consequently, hepatic extraction and biotransformation dominate the clearance process.

Barre et al. (3) examined the pharmacokinetics of pefloxacin administered orally or intravenously in single doses to volunteers (Table 5). For oral administration (Fig. 4), $C_{max}$ values approximated 1.5 $\mu$g/ml for the 200-mg dose, 3.2 $\mu$g/ml for the 400-mg dose, 5.5 $\mu$g/ml for the 600-mg dose, and slightly less than 7 $\mu$g/ml for the 800-mg dose. $C_{max}$ values increased roughly proportionally with the dose. AUCs were examined for several doses, and no evidence for a saturable clearance pathway was found, although only small numbers of volunteers were examined (three per dosing level). Absorption was rapid at all doses, with $C_{max}$ values occurring at 1 to 2 h. Terminal elimination half-lives ranged from 10.5 ± 2 h (400-mg dose) to 12.6 ± 2.5 h (800-mg dose). Urinary recoveries ranged from 11 to 17% of the administered oral dose. Renal clearances ranged from 12.9 to 21.9 ml/min across doses. Total clearances ranged from 111 ml/min (600-mg dose) to 135 ml/min (200-mg dose). Thus, nonrenal clearance accounted for the vast majority of total drug clearance.

Frydman et al. (33) examined the multiple-dose pharmacokinetics of pefloxacin in 12 healthy subjects who received 400 mg of pefloxacin either orally or intravenously. The pharmacokinetic parameter values observed

**Table 5.** Pharmacokinetic parameters obtained after intravenous infusion and oral administration of pefloxcin[a]

| Parameter[b] | Mean ± SD at dose of: | | | |
|---|---|---|---|---|
| | 200 mg | 400 mg | 600 mg | 800 mg |
| Intravenous infusion | | | | |
| $V_1$ (liters) | 23.2 ± 19.1 | 46.9 ± 8.7 | 68.2 ± 20.0 | 54.6 ± 21.8 |
| $V_B$ (liters) | 100.9 ± 40.9 | 64.8 ± 4.1 | 83.5 ± 14.7 | 65.3 ± 30.9 |
| AUC (mg·h/liter) | 23.4 ± 9.3 | 54.3 ± 4.1 | 82.2 ± 22.5 | 130.9 ± 23.7 |
| CL (ml/min) | 156.4 ± 53.7 | 123.1 ± 9.8 | 27.2 ± 31.0 | 104.8 ± 19.3 |
| $U_\infty$ (mg) | 27.4 ± 13.1 | | 76.2 ± 37.1 | 84.8 ± 19.3 |
| $U_\infty$ (%) | 13.7 ± 6.5 | | 12.5 ± 6.6 | 10.8 ± 2.1 |
| $CL_R$ (ml/min) | 19.6 ± 5.6 | | 15.2 ± 6.6 | 12.0 ± 0.3 |
| Oral administration | | | | |
| Lag time (h) | 0.32 ± 0.14 | 0.48 ± 0.23 | 0.26 ± 0.11 | 0.28 ± 0.22 |
| $t_{1/2\beta}$ (h) | 11.7 ± 3.6 | 10.5 ± 2.0 | 11.3 ± 1.1 | 12.6 ± 2.5 |
| $V$ (liters) | 132.2 ± 26.9 | 112.0 ± 20.5 | 109.9 ± 17.7 | 137.9 ± 2.1 |
| AUC (mg·h/liter) | 25.7 ± 6.3 | 54.5 ± 11.2 | 87.9 ± 8.9 | 105.0 ± 20.7 |
| $CL_T$ (ml/min) | 135.3 ± 35.5 | 125.7 ± 25.7 | 111.3 ± 7.0 | 130.6 ± 28.6 |
| $U_\infty$ (mg) | 23.6 ± 8.0 | 44.3 ± 17.3 | 84.1 ± 23.5 | 136.4 ± 26.7 |
| $U_\infty$ (%) | 11.8 ± 4.0 | 11.1 ± 4.3 | 14.0 ± 3.9 | 17.0 ± 3.3 |
| $CL_R$ (ml/min) | 15.3 ± 3.8 | 12.9 ± 2.6 | 14.7 ± 3.6 | 21.9 ± 4.8 |

[a]Data are from reference 3.
[b]Abbreviations: $V_1$, volume of distribution in the central compartment; $V_B$, volume of distribution of drug in the body; CL, clearance; $U_\infty$ (mg), amount of drug excreted into the urine from time zero to infinity; $U_\infty$ (%), amount of drug excreted into the urine as a percentage of the administered dose from time zero to infinity; $CL_T$, total clearance. For other abbreviations, see Tables 1 and 2, footnotes *a*.

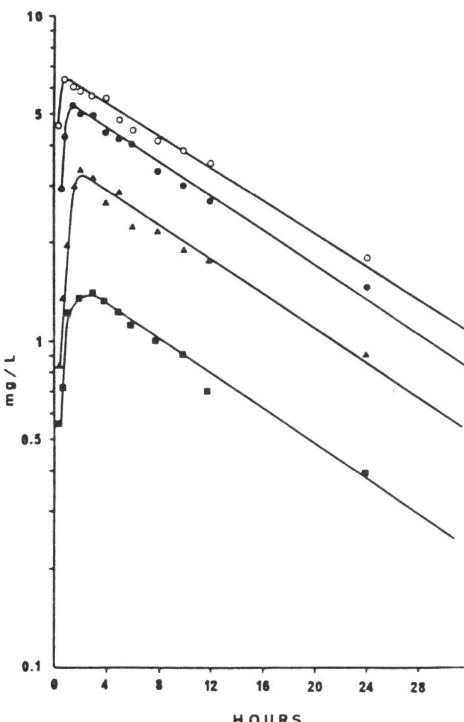


**Figure 4.** Plots of mean concentrations of pefloxacin in plasma versus time obtained in three subjects for each orally administered dose. Lines were generated from best-fit pharmacokinetic parameters. Symbols: ■, 200 mg; ▲, 400 mg; ●, 600 mg; ○, 800 mg. (From reference 3 with permission.)

after the first dose were virtually identical to those of Barre et al. (3). After the last dose (dose 18), however, a major change in pharmacokinetic parameter values was found. Total serum clearance decreased statistically significantly from 123 ml/min for the first dose to 87 ml/min for the last dose and was associated with a significant increase in half-life from 12 to 14.8 h. These data suggested that multiple dosing saturated a nonrenal clearance pathway of pefloxacin.

The disposition of pefloxacin when given intravenously was also examined in dose-ranging (3) and multiple-dosing (33) studies. The dose-ranging study revealed a terminal half-life ranging from 9.7 h (200-mg dose) to 13.8 h (800-mg dose). Total serum clearances were similar to those seen in the oral-dose-ranging study, ranging from 105 ml/min (800-mg dose) to 156 ml/min (200-mg dose). Renal recoveries varied from 11 to 14% of the administered dose.

AUCs were the same as those observed in the oral studies, indicating that pefloxacin absorption was complete and uninfluenced by the dose. Although the mean AUC increased more than in proportion to the increasing dose, the increase was not statistically significant. Although it was concluded that pefloxacin behaved in an approximately dose-linear fashion, significant increases in serum half-life and decreases in serum clearance were observed when first and last doses were compared (Fig. 5). Thus, studies with intravenous pefloxacin, like those with oral pefloxacin, suggest the existence of a saturable nonrenal clearance pathway.

Montay et al. (60) examined the profiles of metabolites in plasma, urine, and bile after the administration of pefloxacin to normal volunteers. The major metabolites in serum were pefloxacin *N*-oxide and *N*-desmethylpefloxacin (norfloxacin). The parent compound, pefloxacin *N*-oxide, norfloxacin, oxonorfloxacin, oxopefloxacin, and traces of pefloxacin glucuronide were recovered in urine (Table 6). Over 72 h after a 800-mg dose, the total urinary recovery of the parent compound plus metabolites accounted for 58.9% ± 3.1% of the administered dose. Pefloxacin concentrations in bile were 10 to 20 $\mu$g/ml at 2 to 12 h after the administration of 800 mg of pefloxacin.

For either oral or intravenous dosing of pefloxacin, a two- or threefold accumulation of the two major metabolites, pefloxacin *N*-oxide and norfloxacin, was found after multiple doses, but the absolute concentrations of the metabolites were low and unlikely to be clinically important. Frydman et al. (33) reported that the terminal half-lives determined for norfloxacin and the *N*-oxide metabolite of pefloxacin were 9.75 and 12 h, respectively. The half-life of norfloxacin, however, is likely artifactually prolonged be-

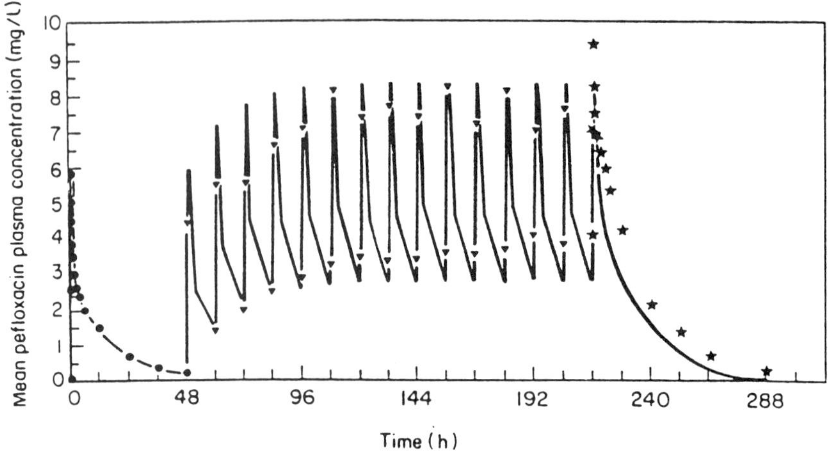


**Figure 5.** Mean pefloxacin concentrations in plasma predicted by superimposition (continuous line) and measured during repeated intravenous administration (400 mg twice a day). Symbols: ●, day 1; ▼, days 3 to 9; ★, day 10. (From reference 33 with permission.)

cause of the relatively slow rate of formation of norfloxacin from pefloxacin.

As with other quinolones, pefloxacin penetrates well into extravascular spaces. Wise et al. (89) examined the concentrations of pefloxacin in serum and blister fluid after 400 mg was given as an intravenous infusion over 1 h. The blisters were induced by an inflammatory method (cantharides plaster application). The penetration, as calculated by the ratio of the AUC for blister fluid to the AUC for serum, was 70%. The penetration of pefloxacin into the cerebrospinal fluid (CSF) of humans, in both the presence and the absence of meningeal inflammation, has been studied by several groups. Dow et al. (21) examined nine subjects with hydrocephalus and external ventricular drains but without meningeal inflammation. CSF and plasma samples were obtained from 1 to 48 h after the infusion of 400 mg of pefloxacin (Fig. 6). Maximum pefloxacin concentrations averaged 8.54 ± 1.53 μg/ml of plasma and 2.97 ± 0.32 μg/ml of CSF. $C_{max}$ values in CSF occurred at 5.44 ± 0.42 h after drug administration. The ratio of drug in CSF to that in

**Table 6.** Urinary recovery of pefloxacin and main metabolites after oral administration[a]

| Compound | Mean recovery (% of dose[b]) ± SE |
|---|---|
| Pefloxacin | 9.3 ± 1 |
| Norfloxacin | 20.2 ± 1 |
| Pefloxacin glucuronide | tr |
| Pefloxacin *N*-oxide | 23.2 ± 1.6 |
| Oxonorfloxacin | 5.4 ± 0.5 |
| Oxopefloxacin | 0.75 ± 0.05 |
| Total | 58.9 ± 3.1 |

[a]Data are from reference 60. A 0- to 72-h urine sample was used.
[b]0.8 g per person ($n$ = 5).

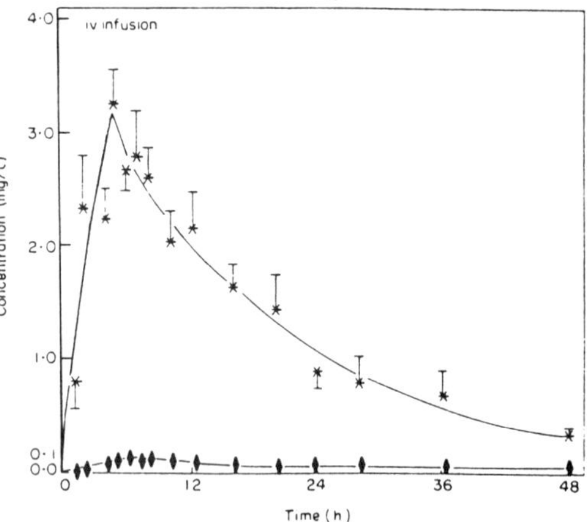


**Figure 6.** Concentrations (mean + standard error of the mean) of pefloxacin (*) and *N*-desmethylpefloxacin (♦) in CSF of humans ($n$ = 9) after a single 1-h intravenous (iv) infusion of 400 mg of pefloxacin. (From reference 21 with permission.)

plasma was relatively stable between 6 and 24 h after the dose (range, 0.57 ± 0.08 to 0.64 ± 0.15).

Wolff et al. (93) examined the penetration of pefloxacin into CSF of 15 patients with meningitis or ventriculitis. Three doses of pefloxacin (either 7.5 or 15 mg/kg) were administered at 12-h intervals to 11 patients intravenously and to 4 patients orally. Concentrations of pefloxacin in CSF measured 2 h after the third intravenous dose and 4 h after the third oral dose ranged from 2.4 to 9 μg/ml in patients receiving 7.5 mg of pefloxacin per kg and from 6.5 to 13 μg/ml in patients receiving 15 mg/kg. These concentrations of pefloxacin in CSF are in excess of the MICs for 90% of the strains of important nonstreptococcal pathogens.

Montay et al. (61) examined the disposition of pefloxacin after a single intravenous infusion of 8 mg/kg in 15 male patients with various degrees of renal failure. No difference in the distribution or elimination of the drug between patients with mild or severe renal impairment was observed, and pharmacokinetic parameter values were similar to those reported for healthy subjects. No accumulation of the *N*-desmethyl metabolite (norfloxacin) occurred.

Hemodialysis (for 4 h) resulted in little removal of pefloxacin from the blood, with an extraction ratio of drug across the dialyzer of 0.28 ± 0.06 and a dialyzer clearance of 62 ± 9 ml/min. Redosing of pefloxacin after hemodialysis may therefore be unnecessary. Thus, overall, renal failure has a minimal effect on the pharmacokinetics of pefloxacin, but studies in which the accumulation of metabolites of pefloxacin in patients with renal failure is evaluated are needed.

Because the major route of total serum clearance of pefloxacin is hepatic biotransformation, it is important to examine the impact of hepatic cirrhosis on pefloxacin pharmacokinetics. In one study (19) (Table 7), the terminal elimination half-life was significantly longer (35.1 ± 19 h) in 16 subjects with histologically proved hepatic cirrhosis than in healthy subjects (11 ± 2.64 h). The total plasma clearance was markedly decreased, from 8.19 + 2.8 liters/h/1.73 m² in healthy subjects to 2.66 ± 1.85 liters/h/1.73 m² in cirrhotic subjects. Urinary excretion of unchanged pefloxacin was higher in the volunteers with cirrhosis than in healthy volunteers, while the excretion of *N*-desmethylpefloxacin (norfloxacin) was lower. A significant correlation between nonrenal clearance and prothrombin time was seen.

**Table 7.** Kinetic parameters of pefloxacin

| Parameter | Mean ± SD in[a]: | |
|---|---|---|
| | Healthy subjects | Patients |
| $t_{1/2}$ (h) | 11.00 ± 2.64 | 35.10 ± 19.00[b] |
| $V_{area}$ (liters/kg) | 1.88 ± 0.37 | 1.54 ± 0.26[c] |
| CL (liters/h/1.73 m²) | 8.19 ± 2.80 | 2.66 ± 1.85[b] |

[a]Twelve healthy subjects each received a single intravenous dose of 400 mg, and 16 patients with cirrhosis received a single intravenous dose of 8 mg/kg. Data are from reference 19. For abbreviations, see Tables 1, 2, and 4, footnotes *a*.
[b]$P < 0.001$.
[c]$P < 0.02$.

Although the clearance of pefloxacin is affected by alterations in hepatic function, the extent to which pefloxacin dosing should be reduced to prevent drug accumulation in patients with hepatic impairment is uncertain. Further investigation into the degree of accumulation with multiple doses and the correlation of clearance with other measures of hepatic function is warranted.

## FLUOROQUINOLONES CLEARED BY BOTH RENAL AND HEPATIC MECHANISMS

### Norfloxacin

Norfloxacin (Fig. 1), the first fluoroquinolone available for clinical use in the United States, is available only as an oral formulation.

Swanson et al. (78) examined the disposition of norfloxacin after sequentially increasing oral doses of 200 to 1,600 mg (Fig. 7). $C_{max}$ values in serum increased linearly with

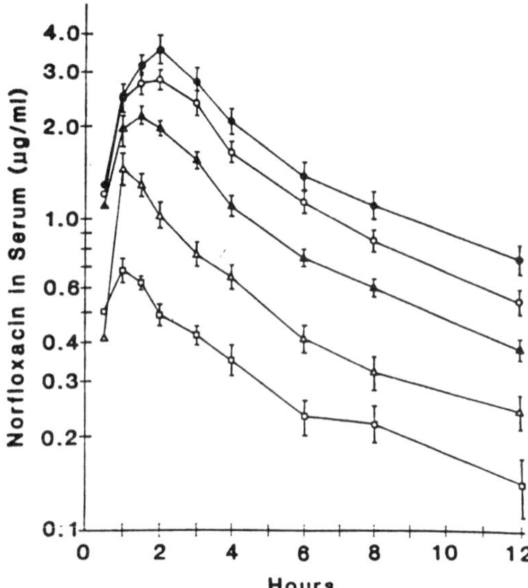


**Figure 7.** Mean concentrations of norfloxacin in serum. Norfloxacin was administered orally at weekly intervals as single doses of 200 (□), 400 (△), 800 (▲), 1,200 (○), or 1,600 (●) mg. Bars indicate standard errors of the means. (From reference 78 with permission.)

increasing doses from 0.75 ± 0.2 μg/ml (200-mg dose) to 3.87 ± 1.3 μg/ml (1,600-mg dose). The time to reach the $C_{max}$ also increased with increasing doses. Serum protein binding was low (14%).

Renal clearances were similar for each dose and ranged from 272 ± 96 to 298 ± 40 ml/min (Table 8). These renal clearances are in excess of GFRs and thus imply net renal tubular secretion of norfloxacin.

Edlund et al. (28) examined the multiple-dose pharmacokinetics of norfloxacin in a study in which 200 mg was administered every 12 h for 7 days. At steady state, the $C_{max}$ and the time to $C_{max}$ were similar to those found by Swanson et al. (78). The half-life was 4.19 ± 0.57 h, and the AUC from 0 to 12 h at steady state (which approximates AUCs extrapolated from zero to infinity for the first dose) was 3.17 ± 0.40 μg · h/ml. Concentrations of norfloxacin in feces at between 3 and 7 days were stable at approximately 950 μg/g of feces. A mean of 28% (range, 8.3 to 53%) of a 400-mg dose of norfloxacin was recovered as the intact parent compound in the feces over 48 h in another study (18).

The coadministration of norfloxacin with food delays the time of attainment of $C_{max}$ values in serum, but recovery in urine over 8 h was little changed (from 28 to 20%) (48), suggesting that the coadministration of food is unlikely to alter the efficacy of norfloxacin in the treatment of urinary tract infections.

Hepatic biotransformation of norfloxacin occurs to some extent. All six metabolites described have modifications in the piperazine ring. The oxo and ethylenediamine derivatives are the two major metabolites recovered in urine, although cumulative recoveries in urine are low relative to that of norfloxacin itself (20% for the oxo form and 4% for the ethylenediamine form). These metabolites have not been detected in serum even after a 1,600-mg dose (66).

**Table 8.** Pharmacokinetic parameters for norfloxacin in 14 healthy men[a]

| Oral dose (mg) | $AUC_{0-12}$ (μg/ml) | $C_{max}$ (μg/ml) | $T_{max}$ (h) | $t_{1/2}{}^{6-12}$ (h) | $CL_R{}^{0-12}$ (ml/min) |
|---|---|---|---|---|---|
| 200 | 3.56 ± 1.13 | 0.75 ± 0.20 | 1.1 ± 0.4 | 7.3 ± 2.9 | 272 ± 96 |
| 400 | 6.26 ± 2.05 | 1.58 ± 0.60 | 1.3 ± 0.4 | 7.4 ± 2.5 | 292 ± 76 |
| 800 | 11.4 ± 2.12 | 2.41 ± 0.43 | 1.5 ± 0.4 | 6.2 ± 1.8 | 273 ± 37 |
| 1,200 | 16.1 ± 4.00 | 3.15 ± 0.76 | 1.8 ± 0.8 | 5.7 ± 1.2 | 288 ± 56 |
| 1,600 | 19.7 ± 6.07 | 3.87 ± 1.27 | 1.9 ± 0.6 | 6.8 ± 1.4 | 298 ± 40 |

[a]Data are from reference 78. Abbreviations: $AUC_{0-12}$, AUC from 0 to 12 h after drug administration; $t_{1/2}{}^{6-12}$, half-life with 6- to 12-h data; $CL_R{}^{0-12}$, ratio of drug excreted/serum AUC (0- to 12-h data). For other abbreviations, see Table 1, footnote *a*. Values are means ± standard deviations.

Adhami et al. (1) examined the penetration of norfloxacin into inflammatory blister fluid after a dose of 400 mg. $C_{max}$ values in blister fluid averaged 1.01 ± 0.27 μg/ml, with $C_{max}$s in serum averaging 1.45 ± 0.09 μg/ml. Serum half-lives and blister fluid half-lives were similar (3.50 ± 0.79 and 3.25 ± 0.52 h, respectively). AUCs from zero to infinity in blister fluid and serum were also similar (5.74 ± 1.6 and 5.4 ± 1.7 μg · h/ml, respectively), indicating an excellent penetration of norfloxacin into the interstitial fluid.

Because norfloxacin is cleared by both renal and hepatic mechanisms, major changes in the profile of the concentration in serum plotted versus time with dysfunction of a single organ system are not expected. Hughes et al. (44) examined the pharmacokinetics of norfloxacin in patients with impaired renal function. Half-lives increased from 3.14 h in the healthy group (GFR, >80 ml/min) to 8.87 h in those with severe renal impairment (GFR, <10 ml/min). AUCs increased from 6.55 to 18.32 μg · h/ml in the patients with the most severe renal dysfunction. Fillastre et al. (29) reported that the mean half-life of norfloxacin was 7.9 h in hemodialyzed patients between dialysis sessions and was not influenced by hemodialysis. Both Hughes et al. (44) and Fillastre et al. (29) recommend altering the administration of norfloxacin for a GFR of 20 to 30 ml/min or less either by halving the dose or by increasing the dosing interval twofold.

Eandi et al. (27) examined the alteration of norfloxacin disposition in patients with liver dysfunction compared with that in healthy volunteers. No change in either serum half-life or AUCs was detected.

## Ciprofloxacin

Ciprofloxacin, like norfloxacin, is cleared by balanced renal and nonrenal mechanisms. This compound is available in both oral and parenteral formulations. While its structure is similar to those of the aforementioned quinolones, it differs in that a cyclopropane ring replaces the ethyl group attached at N-1 (Fig. 1).

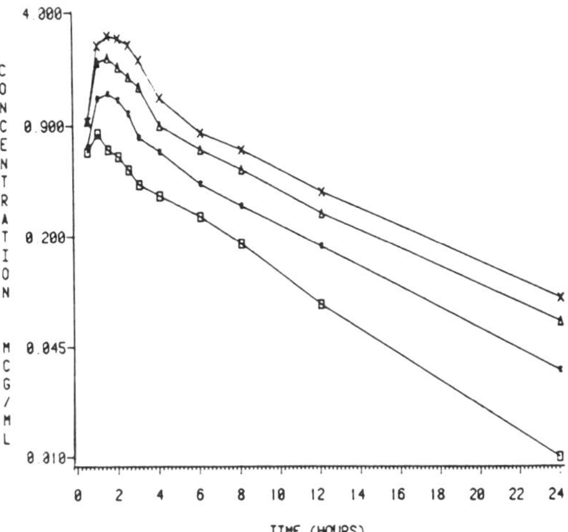


**Figure 8.** Semilogarithmic plot of mean ciprofloxacin concentrations in serum after single doses. Symbols: □, 250-mg dose; ●, 500-mg dose; △, 750-mg dose; ×, 1,000-mg dose. (From reference 79 with permission.)

Tartaglione et al. (79) performed a dose-ranging study for single doses (250 to 1,000 mg) of the oral formulation (Fig. 8, Table 9). $C_{max}$ values were 0.76, 1.60, 2.54, and 3.38 μg/ml for the 250-, 500-, 750-, and 1,000-mg doses, respectively. Absorption was rapid but lengthened from 1.1 h at 250 mg to 1.8 h at 1,000 mg. $C_{max}$ values and AUCs increased proportionally with the dose. Terminal half-lives averaged 4.1 h after the 250- and 500-mg doses but were 6.9 and 6.3 h for the higher doses. Renal clearances were relatively reproducible, ranging from 316 ml/min (1,000 mg) to 477 ml/min (500 mg), and in excess of GFR, indicating a net renal tubular secretion. Consistent with this presumption are the findings of Wingender et al. (85) that probenecid reduces the renal clearance of ciprofloxacin by 46%. Urinary recoveries ranged from 28.5% (1,000 mg) to 44.0% (500 mg).

The pharmacokinetics of orally administered ciprofloxacin have been studied by several investigators. Aronoff et al. (2) examined 250 mg administered every 12 h for 13 doses. Pharmacokinetic parameter values determined on days 1 and 4 were consistent

**Table 9.** Mean values of some pharmacokinetic variables reported for healthy volunteers after single oral doses of ciprofloxacin[a]

| Dose (mg) | $C_{max}$ (mg/liter) | $T_{max}$ (h) | $t_{1/2}$ (h) | AUC (mg/liter·h) | Reference |
|---|---|---|---|---|---|
| 50 | 0.28 | 0.58 | 3.40 | 1.00 | 43 |
| 100 | 0.49 | 0.82 | 4.10 | 1.90 | |
| 250 | 1.45 | 1.00 | 3.97 | 6.37 | 11 |
| 500 | 2.56 | 1.33 | 4.15 | 11.10 | |
| 500 | 2.91 | 1.25 | 4.82 | 12.7 | 20 |
| 750 | 2.65 | 1.10 | 4.75 | 12.20 | 43 |
| 1,000 | 3.38 | 1.80 | 6.30 | 16.60 | 79 |

[a]Data are from reference 13. For abbreviations, see Table 1, footnote *a*.

with those determined during single-dose trials. By day 7, the terminal half-life and apparent serum clearance had both declined significantly, but these changes were small and not likely to be clinically important. LeBel et al. (49) also found changes in the half-life and the nonrenal component of clearance after multiple 500-mg doses of ciprofloxacin. Similar findings have been reported by other investigators, using microbiologic assays, for doses between 250 and 750 mg (12, 37). An additional study in which a 500-mg dose and a high-pressure liquid chromatography assay were used, however, found no alteration in AUC from days 1 to 5 of drug administration (4).

Concentrations of drug in the urine with multiple dosing were quite high for all of the studies cited above. With 250 mg of ciprofloxacin given every 12 h (2), 6- to 12-h urine collections averaged 45 ± 25 to 69 ± 45 μg/ml. In studies with a single 500-mg dose (20), the lowest concentration in urine in the 12- to 24-h collection was 8 μg/ml.

The absolute oral bioavailability of ciprofloxacin is good. In studies with healthy volunteers for doses from 50 to 750 mg, bioavailability ranged from 46 to 84% (7, 24, 43, 71). In some studies (7, 71), a variation in bioavailability was greater with higher doses. As with norfloxacin, the pharmacokinetic parameter values of ciprofloxacin are little affected by administration of the drug with food except for an increase in the time to achieve peak concentrations in serum (51).

The intravenous administration of ciprofloxacin has also been studied. Drusano et al. (23) examined single doses of 100 and 200 mg administered as constant-rate infusions over 30 min (Fig. 9). The total serum clearance averaged 23.0 ± 9.1 liters/h/1.73 m$^2$ for the 100-mg dose and 23.7 ± 5.1 liters/h/1.73 m$^2$ for the 200-mg dose. Clearance was somewhat greater (28.9 ± 2.7 liters/h/1.73 m$^2$), however, when 100 mg was given as a 15-min infusion followed by a 25-mg/h constant infusion for 4 h. Half-lives were 4.7 to 4.8 h, and renal clearance accounted for 65 to 67% of the total clearance. The volumes of distribution were large (2.27 ± 0.85 liters/kg for the 100-mg dose and 2.44 ± 0.51 liters/kg for the 200-mg dose).

Other investigators (7, 26, 43) have examined single doses of intravenously administered ciprofloxacin in this range and have found results with serum clearance similar to the larger value found in the study by Drusano et al. (23) (Table 10). Similar half-lives, volumes of distribution, and dose linearity have also been observed in each of these studies.

Gonzalez et al. (35, 36) used a microbiologic assay to perform two multiple-dose and dose-ranging studies with intravenously administered ciprofloxacin. At doses ranging from 25 to 200 mg given to volunteers every 12 h for 1 week, drug accumulation consistent with the half-life and dosing frequency was seen at each dose. Half-lives were consistently in the range of 3 to 4 h. Serum clearances ranged from 26.9 ± 4.1 liters/h/1.73 m$^2$ (200-mg dose) to 35.4 ± 6.8 liters/h/1.73 m$^2$ (25-mg dose), differences unlikely to be

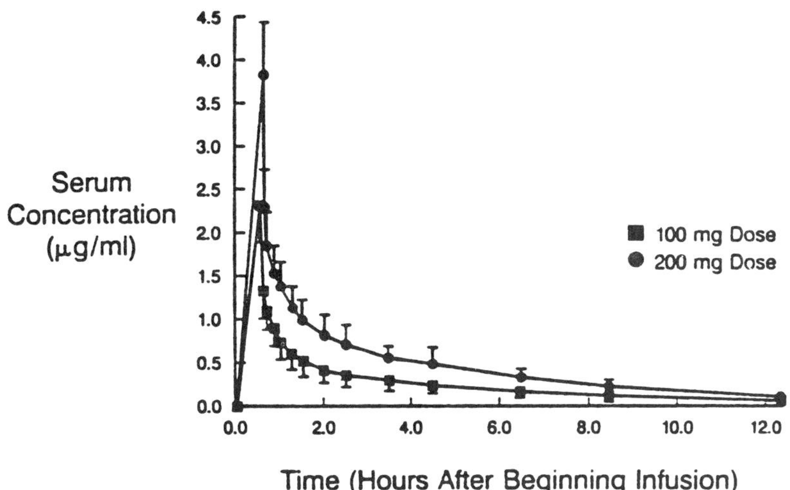


**Figure 9.** Mean concentrations (± standard deviations) in serum after 100- and 200-mg 30-min infusions of ciprofloxacin in six healthy volunteers. (From reference 23 with permission.)

**Table 10.** Plasma clearance, renal clearance, and half-life of ciprofloxacin[a]

| Dose (mg) | $CL_S$ (liters/h/1.73 m²) | $CL_R$ (liters/h/1.73 m²) | $t_{1/2}$ (h) | Reference |
|---|---|---|---|---|
| 100[b,c] | 34.0 ± 5.3[d] | 28.7 ± 4.1[d] | 4.0 ± 0.9 | 91 |
| 25[c,e] | 35.4 ± 6.8 | 20.4[f] | 3.6 ± 0.7 | 35 |
| 50[c,e] | 31.8 ± 3.0 | 21.9[f] | 4.2 ± 0.7 | 35 |
| 75[c,e] | 31.3 ± 5.4 | 24.8[f] | 3.5 ± 0.4 | 35 |
| 100[c,e] | 30.1 ± 3.4 | 18.8[f] | 3.7 ± 0.6 | 36 |
| 150[c,e] | 29.8 ± 4.0 | 18.8[f] | 3.6 ± 0.3 | 36 |
| 200[c,e] | 26.9 ± 4.1 | 18.4[f] | 4.0 ± 0.7 | 36 |
| 50[b,g] | 41.2 ± 7.8 | 25.5 ± 7.0 | 3.0 ± 0.5 | 43 |
| 100[b,g] | 31.8 ± 6.2 | 20.1 ± 4.0 | 3.1 ± 1,9 | 43 |
| 100[b,g] | 23.0 ± 9.1 | 15.5 ± 9.1 | 4.7 ± 0.4 | 23 |
| 200[b,g] | 23.7 ± 5.1 | 15.5 ± 3.0 | 4.8 ± 1.0 | 23 |
| 200[b,g] | 28.5 ± 4.7 | 16.9 ± 3.0 | 4.2 ± 0.8 | 25 |
| 100[b,g] | 42.0 ± 14.2 | NA[h] | 2.90 ± 0.75 | 10 |
| 100[b,g,i] | 9.60 ± 2.09 | 4.61 ± 1.14 | 4.21 ± 0.89 | 26 |
| 150[b,g,i] | 9.57 ± 2.02 | 4.40 ± 1.16 | 4.62 ± 1.19 | 26 |
| 200[b,g,i] | 8.15 ± 1.21 | 3.80 ± 0.87 | 4.22 ± 0.63 | 26 |

[a] $CL_S$, serum clearance. For other abbreviations, see Table 1, footnote *a*. Values are means ± standard deviations.
[b] Single-dose study.
[c] Microbiologic assay.
[d] Not normalized to body surface area.
[e] Multiple-dose study.
[f] Mean of 3 days.
[g] High-pressure liquid chromatography assay.
[h] NA, not available.
[i] Clearance normalized to milliliters per minute per kilogram.

of clinical importance. No significant differences were seen across doses for any of the pharmacokinetic parameter values examined, and clinically important drug accumulation was not seen.

One-third to one-half of the serum clearance of ciprofloxacin is accounted for by nonrenal mechanisms. Four metabolites have been characterized. Each of these compounds has limited microbiologic activity, usually one-quarter to one-half the activity of the parent drug. All metabolism occurs by alterations in the piperazine side chain (Fig. 10). Beermann et al. (4) have quantitated the amounts of metabolites formed after intravenous and oral administration of labeled ciprofloxacin (Table 11). Less than 20% of the administered dose is recoverable as metabolites, even when urine and stool are assayed. Levels of the M2 metabolite are slightly higher after oral administration than after intravenous administration, indicating that limited first-pass hepatic metabolism of ciprofloxacin occurs. After intravenous dosing, 15% of the parent compound is recovered in the stool, suggesting elimination across the intestinal wall, as was proposed by Rohwedder and Bergan (72).

Protein binding for ciprofloxacin has been determined by Joos et al. (46) to be between 16 and 28% and is independent of concentration and pH. Other investigators, using ultracentrifugation techniques (43), have found values in the range of 40%.

As with other fluoroquinolones, tissue penetration of ciprofloxacin is excellent. LeBel et al. (49) studied penetration into blister fluid in a noninflammatory (suction blister) model, and Wise and Donovan (87) examined penetration into an inflammatory (cantharides blister) system after a 500-mg oral dose. In noninflammatory blister fluid, the $C_{max}$ after a single dose was 1.75 ± 0.75 μg/ml, with a concentration after 8 h of 0.45 ± 0.07 μg/ml. The half-life in blister fluid was similar to the half-life in serum. The penetration, calculated as the AUC ratio for blister to serum, was 88.8 ± 26%. The only

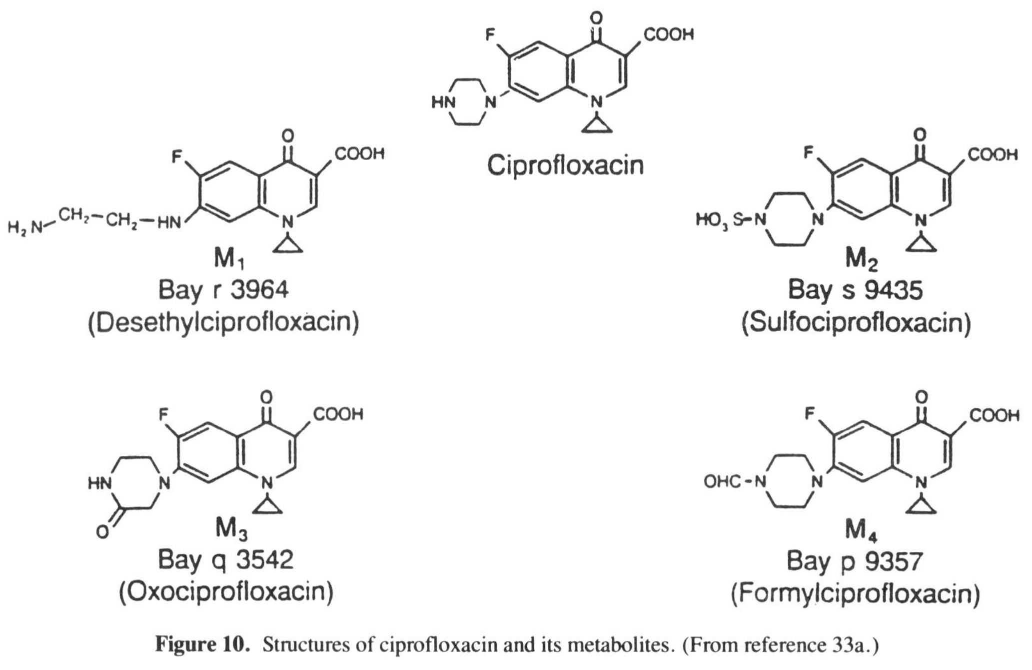

**Figure 10.** Structures of ciprofloxacin and its metabolites. (From reference 33a.)

**Table 11.** Excretion of ciprofloxacin and metabolites after oral and intravenous dosing of $^{14}C$-labeled ciprofloxacin[a]

| Substance[b] | % Excreted | | | |
|---|---|---|---|---|
| | Oral dose (259 mg) | | Intravenous dose (107 mg) | |
| | Urine | Feces | Urine | Feces |
| M1 | 1.4 | 0.5 | 1.3 | 0.5 |
| M2 | 3.7 | 5.9 | 2.6 | 1.3 |
| M3 | 6.2 | 1.1 | 5.6 | 0.8 |
| M4 | ND[c] | ND | ND | ND |
| Ciprofloxacin[d] | 44.7 | 25.0 | 61.5 | 15.2 |

[a]Data are from reference 84a.
[b]M1 is metabolite 1, etc.
[c]ND, not detected.
[d]Detected by high-pressure liquid chromatography.

clinically significant change seen with multiple dosing was an increase in the steady-state concentration of blister fluid at 8 h to 0.97 ± 0.57 μg/ml. In inflammatory blister fluid, penetration was 117% because of the longer half-life of the drug in inflammatory fluid (5.6 h) than in serum (4.4 h).

Wise et al. (87, 91) also examined the penetration of ciprofloxacin into inflammatory blister fluid (as described above) and noninflammatory peritoneal fluid (obtained at an operation) after intravenous administration of drug. Results for the blister fluid again indicated excellent penetration, with an AUC ratio of 1.21. For the peritoneum, the penetration was estimated at 95%, with no differences between the half-lives in peritoneal fluid and serum.

Alterations in ciprofloxacin pharmacokinetics have been studied in patients with various degrees of renal dysfunction. In 32 of these patients, who received single oral doses of 750 mg of ciprofloxacin, significant relationships were found between $CL_{CR}$ and both apparent serum clearance and renal clearance (32). Although no relationship was discernible between the terminal elimination rate constant and $CL_{CR}$, there was a trend toward an increasing terminal elimination half-life with increasing renal dysfunction, with healthy volunteers having a mean half-life of 5.2 ± 0.7 h, while patients maintained on hemodialysis had a mean half-life of 6.9 ± 2.9 h between dialyses. Total apparent serum clearance declined from 43.5 ± 9.0 liters/h/1.73 $m^2$ in healthy volunteers to 25.4 ± 7.8 liters/h/1.73 $m^2$ in patients on hemodialysis. A reduction in dose of approximately one-third was recommended for patients with $CL_{CR}$s of 20 to 30 ml/min/1.73 $m^2$ or less. These findings were reasonably consistent with those of Boelaert et al. (10) and Singlas et al. (74) for doses of 250 and 500 mg, respectively.

Drusano et al. (25) examined the influence of various degrees of renal impairment on the pharmacokinetics of ciprofloxacin (200 mg) administered intravenously (Table 12). Significant relationships were found between normalized $CL_{CR}$ and both normalized serum and renal clearance. A hyperbolic relationship between $CL_{CR}$ and terminal elimination half-life was seen. A dose reduction of 50% was recommended for patients with $CL_{CR}$ of 1.2 to 1.8 liters/h/1.73 $m^2$ (20 to 30 ml/min/1.73 $m^2$) or less. Because of the greater than threefold variability in half-life noted in the anephric patients, it was also recommended that the dose be reduced by half while maintaining a 12-h dosing interval

**Table 12.** Model-independent pharmacokinetic parameters for 200 mg of ciprofloxacin administered to patients with various degrees of renal dysfunction[a]

| $CL_{CR}$ (liters/kg) | $V_{area}$ (liters/h/1.73 $m^2$) | $CL_S$ (liters/h/1.73 $m^2$) | $CL_R$ (liters/h/1.73 $m^2$) | $t_{1/2}$ (h) | % $CL_R/CL_S$ |
|---|---|---|---|---|---|
| >6.0 | 2.49 ± 0.46 | 26.8 ± 5.7 | 16.4 ± 3.5 | 4.27 ± 0.84 | 61.6 ± 8.7 |
| ≥3.6, <6.0 | 3.19 ± 1.26 | 26.3 ± 10.3 | 11.9 ± 5.3 | 6.12 ± 1.61 | 44.9 ± 11.9 |
| ≥0,6, <3.6 | 2.38 ± 0.62 | 15.0 ± 3.8 | 4.5 ± 2.6 | 7.70 ± 1.22 | 29.2 ± 13.2 |
| 0 | 2.73 ± 0.92 | 15.4 ± 4.3 | 0.0 | 8.55 ± 3.27 | 0.0 |

[a]Data are from reference 25. For abbreviations, see Tables 1, 2, and 10, footnotes *a*. Values are means ± standard deviations.

in order to avoid in some patients prolonged periods during which concentrations in serum were below the MIC for less susceptible pathogens. Webb et al. (81) found similar outcomes with a dose of 100 mg administered intravenously but recommended that a 50% reduction in dose for severely impaired patients be accomplished by lengthening the dosing interval to 24 h.

The ability of hemodialysis to clear ciprofloxacin has been examined by Boelaert et al. (10) and Singlas et al. (74). Extraction of ciprofloxacin by hemodialysis was 23 to 31%, and dialysis clearance was 40 to 57 ml/min. In one study (10), the half-life fell from a mean of 5.8 h on an interdialysis day to 3.2 h during dialysis.

Golper et al. (34) found little clearance (6.2 ml/min/1.73 $m^2$) of ciprofloxacin during chronic ambulatory peritoneal dialysis. Considerable dwell times were necessary before attainment of drug concentrations in the dialysate sufficient to inhibit pathogens such as *Staphylococcus aureus*, which may infect these patients. Shalit et al. (73) reported similar findings. Concentrations in dialysate did not exceed 1 μg/ml (the MIC for 90% of the strains of *S. aureus*) until 2.5 h after the dose. Consequently, minimum dwell times of 4 to 6 h will be necessary to attain drug concentrations in dialysis fluid adequate for this or other less susceptible pathogens.

Drusano et al. (22) and Lettieri et al. (54) examined the effect of altered hepatic function on ciprofloxacin disposition. Drusano et al. (22) administered ciprofloxacin (500 mg) to patients with Childs class A and Childs class B cirrhosis and found no alteration in drug disposition based on liver dysfunction. Indocyanine green dye clearance, an index of liver blood flow, was not predictive of ciprofloxacin clearance. Lettieri et al. (54) examined patients with mild to moderate hepatic cirrhosis documented by biopsy. No evidence for an alteration in drug disposition compared with that in normal controls was seen. Both studies concluded that no adjustment in dose was warranted for patients with mild to moderate liver disease. Patients with severe liver disease need to be studied before specific recommendations can be made. Data are also lacking for patients with combined renal and hepatic dysfunctions. A major dose adjustment seems likely to be required, because both major clearance routes are impaired in such patients.

## Enoxacin

Enoxacin, the first of the new fluoroquinolones that is a naphthyridine, differs from norfloxacin only by the substitution of a nitrogen for a carbon at position 8 of the quinolone ring, a difference that improves bioavailability (Fig. 1).

Wolf et al. (92) examined enoxacin given in single and multiple doses to a small number of volunteers. With multiple doses of 400, 600, and 800 mg administered orally twice daily for 2 weeks to four volunteers, $C_{max}$ values in serum were reached rapidly (1.4 to 1.7 h) but did not increase in a linear fashion with the dose (Tables 13 and 14). AUCs also did not increase in a linear fashion with the dose, being 18.47 ± 4.68 for the 400-mg dose, 27.30 ± 6.48 for the 600-mg dose, and 26.99 ± 12.89 for the 800-mg dose. Half-lives during the first dosing interval ranged from 4.9 to 5.4 h. In all groups by the final study day, $C_{max}$ values in serum, half-lives, and AUCs had increased compared with those for day 1 (Table 13).

Chang et al. (15) examined enoxacin doses of 200 and 800 mg administered both intravenously and orally in a four-way randomized crossover design study involving eight subjects (Fig. 11). The doses administered intravenously were given at a constant rate of infusion over 1 h. The half-life, AUC (normalized for dose), and total and renal clearances were dose dependent, confirming the nonlinearity uncovered in the multiple-dose study discussed above. When the doses administered intravenously were examined, mean terminal elimination half-lives were 3.28 h for the 200-mg dose and 4.68 h for the

**Table 13.** Pharmacokinetic parameters of single and multiple doses of enoxacin[a]

| Parameter[b] | Mean ± SD at dose (b.i.d.[c]) of: | | |
|---|---|---|---|
| | 400 mg | 600 mg | 800 mg |
| Single dose (day 1) | | | |
| $C_{max}$ (mg/liter) | 3.09 ± 0.86 | 4.18 ± 0.74 | 3.70 ± 1.30 |
| $T_{max}$ (h) | 1.42 ± 0.67 | 1.67 ± 0.75 | 1.50 ± 0.89 |
| $t_{1/2}$ (h)(harmonic) | 4.90 | 4.74 | 5.44 |
| $AUC_{0-\infty}$ (μg·h/ml) | 18.47 ± 4.68 | 27.30 ± 6.48 | 26.99 ± 12.89 |
| Steady state (day 15) | | | |
| $C_{max}$ (mg/liter) | 4.53 ± 0.81 | 5.90 ± 2.07 | 6.91 ± 2.29 |
| $T_{max}$ (h) | 1.05 ± 0.40 | 2.02 ± 0.72 | 2.49 ± 0.54 |
| $t_{1/2}$ (h)(harmonic) | 5.66 | 5.98 | 6.27 |
| $AUC_{0-12}$ (μg·h/ml) | 25.82 ± 7.18 | 37.30 ± 13.85 | 47.36 ± 15.81 |

[a]Data are from reference 92.
[b]$AUC_{0-\infty}$, AUC for zero time to infinity; for other abbreviations, see Tables 1 and 8, footnotes *a*.
[c]b.i.d., twice a day.

800-mg dose. Somewhat longer half-lives have been reported by other investigators (90). Total serum clearances were 9.25 and 6.85 ml/min/kg, respectively, with renal clearance accounting for approximately 55% of the total (Table 15), indicating that renal tubular secretion occurs.

Approximately 50% of the administered dose was recovered in the urine as enoxacin, with concentrations in urine remaining above the MIC for clinically relevant pathogens for at least 24 h. A substantial amount of the oxo metabolite was also recovered in the urine, averaging 16% of the 200-mg dose and 11% of the 800-mg dose.

**Table 14.** Alteration in drug clearance with repeated administration of enoxacin[a]

| Parameter[b] | Mean value (ml/min/kg) at dose (b.i.d.[c]) of: | | |
|---|---|---|---|
| | 400 mg | 600 mg | 800 mg |
| Single dose (day 1) | | | |
| $CL_{TOT}$ | 5.78 | 6.00 | 9.60 |
| $CL_R$ | 3.60 | 3.83 | 5.42 |
| $CL_{NR}$ | 2.18 | 2.17 | 4.18 |
| Steady state (day 15) | | | |
| $CL_{TOT}$ | 4.17 | 4.41 | 4.85 |
| $CL_R$ | 2.40 | 2.80 | 2.42 |
| $CL_{NR}$ | 1.77 | 1.91 | 2.43 |
| Day 15/day 1 ratio | | | |
| $CL_{TOT}$ | 0.72 | 0.79 | 0.51 |
| $CL_R$ | 0.67 | 0.73 | 0.45 |
| $CL_{NR}$ | 0.81 | 0.88 | 0.58 |

[a]Data are from reference 92.
[b]Abbreviations: $CL_{TOT}$, total body clearance; $CL_R$, renal clearance; $CL_{NR}$, nonrenal clearance.
[c]b.i.d., twice a day.

The absolute oral bioavailability of enoxacin was high (87 to 91%) and independent of dose (15). As with other quinolones examined, the onset of absorption was delayed by a meal, but other pharmacokinetic parameter values were unaltered by food (75).

Protein binding of enoxacin and its 4-oxo metabolite was determined by Wijnands et al. (83) in 8 volunteers receiving 400 mg and in 11 volunteers receiving 600 mg as single doses. The parent compound binding averaged 48% ± 11% for the 400-mg dose and 54% ± 12% for the 600-mg dose. The binding for the metabolite was 58% ± 7% and 69% ± 14%, respectively.

Like other fluoroquinolones, enoxacin penetrates well into tissues. Wise et al. (90) examined penetration into inflammatory blister fluid for enoxacin given as a 600-mg oral dose or a 400-mg intravenous infusion over 1 h. Penetration rates, calculated as a ratio of the AUC in blister fluid to the AUC in serum, were 113 and 133%, respectively.

To evaluate the effect of renal dysfunction on enoxacin disposition, Nix et al. (64) gave single doses of 400 mg to 28 patients with various renal functions. Volumes of distribution and $C_{max}$ values in serum were indepen-

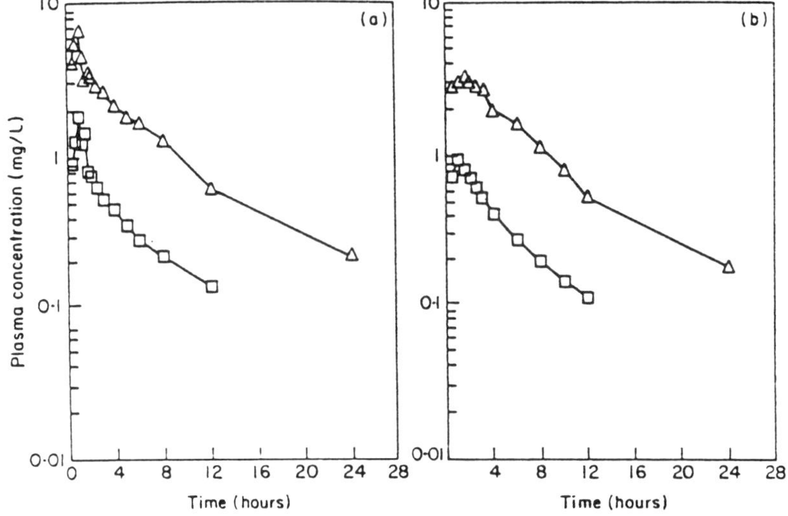


**Figure 11.** Mean concentrations of enoxacin in plasma of human volunteers after 200-mg (□) and 800-mg (△) intravenous (a) and oral (b) doses. (From reference 15 with permission.)

dent of renal function. The apparent clearance, renal clearance, and half-life changed with increasing renal dysfunction (Table 16). A maximum decrease in the apparent clearance of 58% was noted. The half-life increased from 4.9 ± 1.2 to 10.5 ± 3.82 h. Renal clearance was shown to be highly correlated with $CL_{CR}$. These authors concluded that a 50% reduction in the enoxacin dose was appropriate in patients with a $CL_{CR}$ of 30 ml/min or less.

The decrease in serum protein binding of enoxacin (40.1 to 13.5%) seen in patients with renal failure is not expected to be of clinical importance.

## Fleroxacin

Fleroxacin (Ro 23-6240, AM 833) is a trifluorinated quinolone with balanced renal and nonrenal clearances. The drug possesses fluorines attached to positions 6 and 8 of the

**Table 15.** Mean pharmacokinetic parameters in human volunteers after single 200- and 800-mg intravenous and oral doses of enoxacin[a]

| Parameter | Mean RSD (%) | | | |
|---|---|---|---|---|
| | Intravenous dose | | Oral dose | |
| | 200 mg | 800 mg | 200 mg | 800 mg |
| $C_{max}$ (mg/liter) | 1.83 (45) | 6.58 (26) | 1.02 (25) | 3.80 (13) |
| $T_{max}$ (h) | 1.11 (20) | 1.00 (13) | 1.00 (50) | 1.38 (61) |
| $t_{1/2}$ (h) | 3.28 (31) | 4.68 (11) | 3.16 (18) | 4.93 (30) |
| $AUC_{0-\infty}$ (mg·h/liter) | 5.35 (13) | 29.08 (23) | 4.67 (30) | 25.75 (13) |
| Normalized $AUC_{0-\infty}$ (mg·h/liter) | 5.35 (13) | 7.27 (23) | 4.67 (30) | 6.44 (13) |
| $V_b$ (liters/kg) | 2.85 (30) | 2.78 (10) | | |
| CL (ml/min/kg) | 9.25 (14) | 6.85 (18) | | |
| $CL_R$ (ml/min/kg) | 4.96 (20) | 3.78 (22) | 5.30 (21) | 3.81 (16) |
| $CL_{NR}$ (ml/min/kg) | 4.92 (19) | 3.38 (17) | | |

[a]Data are from reference 15. Abbreviations: RSD, relative standard deviation; $CL_{NR}$, nonrenal clearance. For other abbreviations, see Tables 1, 4, and 13, footnotes *a*, and Table 5, footnote *b*.

**Table 16.** Mean pharmacokinetic for nondialysis subjects after oral administration of 400 mg of enoxacin[a]

| Parameter[b] (unit) | Mean ± SD for group with $CL_{CR}$ (ml/min) of: | | | |
|---|---|---|---|---|
| | >60 | ≥30, <60 | ≥15, <30 | <15[c] |
| $C_{max}$ (mg/liter) | 2.25 ± 0.57 | 2.60 ± 0.54 | 2.82 ± 0.78 | 1.93 ± 0.65 |
| $T_{max}$ (h) | 1.6 ± 0.96 | 1.0 ± 0 | 2.1 ± 1.1 | 2.4 ± 1.1 |
| AUC (mg·h/liter)[d] | 16.2 ± 5.3 | 26.2 ± 6.2 | 36.2 ± 11.9 | 28.2 ± 12.2 |
| $t_{1/2}$ (h)[d] | 4.91 ± 1.22 | 7.45 ± 1.84 | 10.5 ± 3.82 | 9.36 ± 3.54 |
| $CL^d/F$ (ml/min) | 466 ± 202 | 264 ± 60 | 197 ± 50 | 286 ± 150 |
| $CL_R{}^d$ (ml/min) | 193 ± 47.3 | 83 ± 27.4 | 30 ± 8.8 | 13 ± 5.2 |
| $V/F$ (liters/kg) | 2.51 ± 0.62 | 2.11 ± 0.37 | 2.30 ± 0.19 | 3.29 ± 1.68 |

[a]Data are from reference 64.
[b]For abbreviations, see Table 1, footnote *a*.
[c]Not on hemodialysis.
[d]Indicates significant difference between groups ($P<0.05$).

quinolone ring as well as a fluoroethyl substituent at position 1.

Weidekamm et al. (82) examined the single-dose pharmacokinetics of 200, 400, and 800 mg given orally as well as of 100 mg given intravenously in a 20-min infusion. In addition, the multiple-dose pharmacokinetics of 800 and 1,200 mg given by mouth daily for 10 days was studied (Fig. 12).

The terminal half-life was 8.6 ± 1.3 h (100 mg given intravenously) to 11.8 ± 2.8 h (1,200 mg given orally at the steady state). The volume of distribution was large, with an average value of 110 ± 36 ml/min for the intravenous dose, with renal clearance accounting for slightly more than 60% of the total clearance (Table 17). Protein binding was 23%. Urinary recovery of the parent compound accounted for 50 to 65% of the dose, with *N*-desmethyl and *N*-oxide metabolites accounting for another 6.5 to 11% of the administered dose. Tubular secretion probably has little to do with the renal handling of the drug, because the coadministration of probenecid had no effect on the parameters examined. The ratio of AUC to the dose for the single-dose oral studies revealed that the drug behaved in a dose-linear fashion over the range of 200 to 800 mg. The AUCs for intravenous and oral doses were similar, indicating virtually complete oral absorption.

For multiple dosing of 800 and 1,200 mg, drug accumulation from days 1 to 10 was in the range predicted from the half-life of the drug and the dosing interval. Ratios of AUC for 800 and 1,200 mg on days 1 and 10 also provided good evidence for dose proportionality. The terminal half-life did show a modest but statistically insignificant increase between days 1 and 10. The total serum

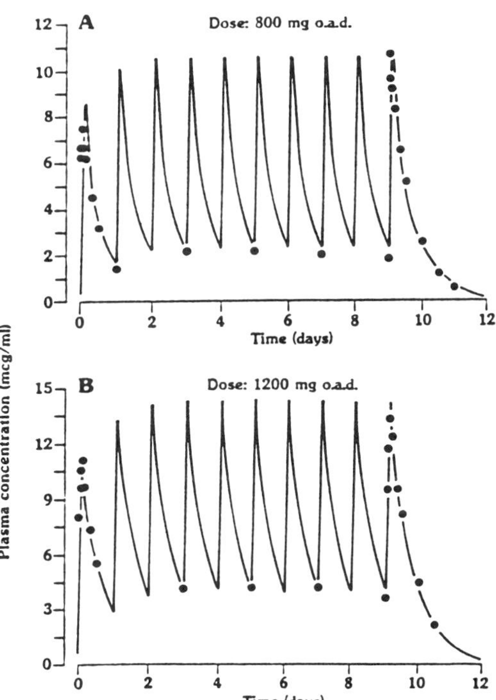


**Figure 12.** Mean fleroxacin concentrations during multiple dosing of 800 (A) and 1,200 (B) mg once daily (o.a.d.) on 10 consecutive days ($n$ = 6). The plasma profiles shown were generated by iteration over all measured concentration points. (From reference 82 with permission.)

**Table 17.** Pharmacokinetic parameters after intravenous and oral administration of fleroxacin[a]

| Parameter[b] | Mean ± SD for dose of[c]: | | | | |
|---|---|---|---|---|---|
| | 100 mg i.v. ($n$ = 6) | 200 mg p.o. ($n$ = 12) | 400 mg p.o. ($n$ = 12) | 800 mg p.o. ($n$ = 12) | 400 mg p.o. + probenecid ($n$ = 5) |
| $C_{max}$ (μg/ml) | 2.85 ± 1.17 | 2.33 ± 0.65 | 4.36 ± 1.15 | 7.04 ± 0.84 | 3.95 ± 0.47 |
| $T_{max}$ (h) | 0.33[d] | 1.1 ± 0.8 | 1.3 ± 1.1 | 1.9 ± 1.0 | 1.2 ± 0.8 |
| $t_{1/2}$ (h)[d] | 8.6 ± 1.3 | 8.9 ± 1.0 | 9.2 ± 1.7 | 10.3 ± 1.4 | 10.9 ± 1.4 |
| AUC (μ·h/ml) | 10.2 ± 1.7 | 20.9 ± 2.4 | 48.3 ± 9.3 | 106.1 ± 16.9 | 61.0 ± 9.1 |
| $V_{ss}$ (liters) | 110.1 ± 25.2 | | | | |
| $CL_S$ (ml/min) | 168.0 ± 36.0 | | | | |
| $CL_R$ (ml/min) | 105.2 ± 27.6 | | | | |
| Urinary excretion (0–60 h) (% of dose) | | | | | |
| Fleroxacin | 62.4 ± 7.1 | 64.6 ± 10.9 | 49.8 ± 9.2 | 51.8 ± 13.8 | 50.1 ± 5.8 |
| *N*-Desmethyl metabolite | 3.6 ± 1.0 | 4.7 ± 1.6 | 5.0 ± 1.3 | 6.5 ± 2.1 | 6.1 ± 1.7 |
| *N*-Oxide metabolite | 2.9 ± 0.9 | 3.1 ± 1.7 | 4.2 ± 1.1 | 5.0 ± 1.5 | 4.7 ± 1.7 |

[a]Data are from reference 82. For abbreviations, see Tables 1, 10, and 13, footnotes *a*.
[b]$V_{ss}$, volume of distribution at steady state.
[c]i.v., intravenous; p.o., peroral.
[d]End point of infusion.

clearance was lower than that seen in the intravenous-dosing study (128 ± 25 versus 168 ± 36 ml/min). Whether this difference represents a trend toward saturability at the higher doses or differences in study populations is unknown. The doses at which potential saturation was observed, however, are larger than those likely to be used clinically.

Fleroxacin has been evaluated by Wise et al. (88) for its ability to penetrate into inflammatory exudate. The AUC for inflammatory fluid averaged 90% ± 6% of the AUC for serum, indicating excellent penetration.

## Rufloxacin

Rufloxacin, a new broad-spectrum fluoroquinolone, has a chemical structure very similar to that of ofloxacin but with a sulfur atom in the thiazide ring (Fig. 13). The pharmacokinetics and safety of rufloxacin were evaluated after repeated oral administration to very small numbers of healthy volunteers, so data are limited.

Mattina and colleagues (59) administered rufloxacin once a day for 6 consecutive days following two different dose schedules. The first group of 11 subjects was given a loading dose of 300 mg on the first day and 150 mg on each subsequent day. The second group of 12 subjects was given a loading dose of 400 mg and 200 mg daily for 5 days. The $C_{max}$ values of rufloxacin in serum after the first administration of drug in the 300/150- and 400/200-mg dose schedules were 2.77 ± 0.24 μg/ml in the 300/150-mg group and 3.62 ± 0.35 μg/ml in the 400/200-mg group and were reached generally after 2 to 4 h. After repeated administration, $C_{max}$ increased to 3.19 ± 0.31 at 3.7 ± 0.7 days and to 4.06 ± 0.33 μg/ml at 4.1 ± 0.3 days in the 300/150- and 400/200-mg groups, respectively. AUC from 0 to 24 h increased with time, being 46.3 ± 4.0 and 58.5 ± 4.4 μg · h/ml for the two regimens after the first dose and increasing after the last administration to 56.4 ± 7.0 and 71.4 ± 5.3 μg · h/ml, respectively (Table 18).

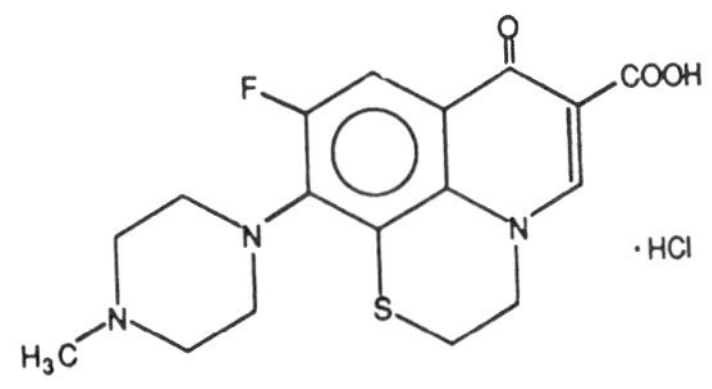

**Figure 13.** Chemical structure of rufloxacin.

The pharmacokinetic analysis shows that after delays of 78 ± 13 min in the 300/150-mg group and 45 ± 16 min in the 400/200-mg dose group, the drug was rapidly absorbed, with an absorption half life of 17 ± 6 min. The initial delay is probably due to dissolution and gastric emptying of the drug. After absorption, the volume of distribution is relatively large, i.e., 118 ± 8 and 136 ± 16 liters for the 300/150- and 400/200-mg groups, respectively. Half-life in plasma was 39.5 ± 2.4 h for the low-dose group and 36 ± 2.8 h for the high-dose group. Mean concentrations of rufloxacin in urine collected 0 to 4 h after the last dose were 46.3 ± 4.6 μg/ml for the low-dose group and 85.4 ± 8.3 μg/ml for the high-dose group. Four days after the last administration, rufloxacin was still clearly detectable in urine, at 10.7 ± 2.9 and 32.7 μg/ml in the two groups, respectively.

Renal clearance of rufloxacin was 20 ml/min, representing about 39% of the total clearance and indicating that some of the drug undergoes renal tubular reabsorption. Preliminary data show that rufloxacin does not have significant pharmacokinetic interaction with methylxanthines (14).

Imbimbo et al. (45) showed that intrasubject variation in the pharmacokinetics of rufloxacin was small, in spite of considerable intersubject variation, when 400 mg of oral rufloxacin was given under controlled conditions at an interval of 2 weeks. The concentrations of rufloxacin in plasma determined by bioassay were higher than those determined by high-pressure liquid chromatography, indicating that one or more active metabolites were formed in humans. This study also showed that 20 to 25% of the drug is

**Table 18.** Individual pharmacokinetic parameters of rufloxacin for subjects on the 400/200-mg dose schedule[a]

| Parameter[b] | Data for subject no.: | | | | | | | | | | | | Mean | SEM |
|---|---|---|---|---|---|---|---|---|---|---|---|---|---|---|
| | 12 | 13 | 14 | 15 | 16 | 17 | 18 | 19 | 20 | 21 | 22 | 23 | | |
| $t_{lag}$ (min) | 2 | 0 | 118 | 1 | 0 | 0 | 115 | 0 | 89 | 0 | 108 | 104 | 45 | 16 |
| $t_{1/2\alpha}$ (min) | 3 | 47 | 5 | 3 | 4 | 4 | 5 | 4 | 47 | 4 | 6 | 5 | 11 | 5 |
| $t_{max}$ (h) | 2 | 4 | 12 | 2 | 2 | 2 | 4 | 2 | 8 | 2 | 4 | 4 | 4.0 | 0.9 |
| $C_{max}$ ($\mu$g/ml) | 3.64 | 2.86 | 1.91 | 5.40 | 5.39 | 3.15 | 2.70 | 3.95 | 5.43 | 3.07 | 2.42 | 3.48 | 3.62 | 0.35 |
| $t_{max,ss}$ (days) | 5.0 | 5.1 | 5.1 | 1.0 | 5.0 | 5.0 | 5.1 | 2.0 | 5.2 | 5.0 | 5.1 | 5.1 | 4.5 | 0.4 |
| $C_{max,ss}$ ($\mu$g/ml) | 4.80 | 3.29 | 2.27 | 5.40 | 5.74 | 3.75 | 3.62 | 5.28 | 4.57 | 2.98 | 2.64 | 4.56 | 4.06 | 0.33 |
| $t_{1/2}$ (h) | 54.5 | 29.4 | 49.2 | 23.8 | 24.8 | 28.8 | 39.5 | 44.6 | 34.7 | 35.6 | 28.5 | 38.4 | 36.0 | 2.8 |
| MRT (h) | 78.6 | 43.5 | 71.0 | 34.3 | 35.9 | 41.6 | 57.2 | 64.4 | 51.2 | 51.4 | 41.3 | 55.5 | 52.2 | 4.0 |
| $V/F$ (liters) | 141 | 129 | 208 | 73 | 70 | 126 | 153 | 99 | 105 | 173 | 167 | 119 | 136 | 16 |
| CL/$F$ (ml/min) | 30 | 51 | 66 | 36 | 33 | 50 | 45 | 26 | 35 | 56 | 68 | 36 | 44 | 4 |
| $CL_R$ (ml/min) | 10 | 14 | 29 | 18 | 12 | 15 | 18 | 8 | 17 | 17 | 28 | | 17 | 2 |
| $CL_{R,ss}$ (ml/min) | 8 | 18 | 25 | 14 | 26 | 25 | 25 | | 25 | 31 | 23 | | 20 | 3 |
| $AUC_{0-24,1st}$ ($\mu$g·h/ml) | 61.0 | 55.9 | 31.9 | 84.8 | 85.7 | 55.8 | 54.4 | 69.8 | 61.6 | 48.6 | 42.2 | 59.7 | 58.5 | 4.4 |
| $AUC_{0-24,6th}$ ($\mu$g·h/ml) | 93.0 | 64.0 | 48.6 | 83.3 | 94.7 | 60.8 | 66.0 | | 82.8 | 51.5 | 50.4 | 89.3 | 71.4 | 5.3 |
| $AUC_{0\infty}$ ($\mu$g·h/ml) | 222.4 | 131.2 | 101.3 | 188.0 | 203.3 | 132.3 | 149.3 | 259.4 | 190.3 | 173.4 | 98.1 | 185.9 | 169.6 | 14.1 |
| $R$ | 3.0 | 2.3 | 3.0 | 2.0 | 2.2 | 2.2 | 2.4 | | 2.7 | 2.1 | 2.4 | 3.0 | 2.5 | 0.1 |
| $f_e$ (%) | 33.9 | 47.8 | 35.7 | 45.4 | 48.2 | 29.0 | 47.1 | | 51.2 | 53.6 | 45.0 | | 43.7 | 2.5 |

[a] Adapted from reference 59.

[b] Abbreviations: $t_{lag}$, lag time; $t_{1/2\alpha}$, half-life at $\alpha$ phase; $t_{max,ss}$, time to maximum steady-state concentration of drug; $C_{max,ss}$, maximum steady-state concentration of drug; MRT, maximum residence time; $CL_{R,ss}$, steady-state renal clearance; $AUC_{0-24,1st}$, $AUC_{0-24}$ on day 1; $f_e$, fraction excreted into urine. For other abbreviations, see Table 1, footnote *a*.

excreted in urine in the first 48 h. These findings indicate that significant hepatic metabolism of norfloxacin occurs, but data are still incomplete.

## SUMMARY

A comparison of the pharmacokinetic properties of the quinolone agents is presented in Table 19. To minimize the variability in approaches between laboratories, data are drawn from a single center (Wise et al. [88, 89]).

Finally, recommendations for dose alteration in patients with renal or hepatic dysfunction are presented in Table 20.

## REFERENCES


1. **Adhami, Z. N., R. Wise, and B. Crump.** 1984. The pharmacokinetics and tissue penetration of norfloxacin. *J. Antimicrob. Chemother.* **13:**87–92.
2. **Aronoff, G. E., C. H. Kenner, R. S. Sloan, and S. T. Pottratz.** 1984. Multiple-dose ciprofloxacin kinetics in normal subjects. *Clin. Pharmacol. Ther.* **36:**384–388.
3. **Barre, J., G. Houin, and J. P. Tillement.** 1984. Dose-dependent pharmacokinetic study of pefloxacin, a new antibacterial agent, in humans. *J. Pharm. Sci.* **73:**1379–1382.
4. **Beermann, D., H. Scholl, W. Wingender, D. Forster, E. Beubler, et al.** 1986. Metabolism of ciprofloxacin in man, p. 141–146. *In* H. C. Neu and H. Weuta (ed.), *1st International Ciprofloxacin Workshop, Leverkusen 1985.* Excerpta Medica, Amsterdam.
6. **Berezin, E. B., and C. M. Serieys.** 1992. Penetration of lomefloxacin into bronchial secretions fol-


**Table 19.** Comparative pharmacokinetics of the new fluoroquinolones[a]

| Fluoroquinolone (dose [mg]) | $C_{max}$ (μg/ml) | $AUC_{0-\infty}$ (μg·h/ml) | $t_{1/2}$ (h) | Urinary recovery (% [24 h]) | Blister fluid penetration (% [$AUC_{serum}$]) |
|---|---|---|---|---|---|
| Ofloxacin (600, p.o.) | 10.7 ± 6.4 | 57.5 ± 11.3 | 7.0 ± 1.1 | 73.0 ± 11.9 | 125 |
| Pefloxacin (400, i.v.) | NA | 56.1 ± 12.1 | 10.5 ± 1.5 | 4.9 ± 0.6 | 69 |
| Norfloxacin (400, p.o.) | 1.45 ± 0.1 | 5.4 ± 1.7 | 3.2 ± 0.5 | 27.0 ± 8.6 | 106 |
| Ciprofloxacin (500, p.o.) | 2.3 ± 0.7 | 9.9 ± 2.4 | 3.9 ± 0.8 | 30.6 ± 9.8 | 117 |
| Enoxacin (600, p.o.) | 3.7 ± 0.5 | 28.8 ± 4.9 | 6.2 ± 1.1 | 61.2 ± 7.4 | 114 |
| Fleroxacin (400, p.o.) | 6.1 ± 2.2 | 78.3 ± 9.4 | 12.0 ± 1.0 | 42.5 ± 3.9[b] | 90 |

[a]Data are summarized from references 88 and 89. Abbreviations: p.o., peroral; i.v., intravenous; $AUC_{serum}$, AUC for concentration in serum; NA, not available. For other abbreviations, see Tables 1 and 13, footnotes *a*. Values are means ± standard deviations.
[b]Urinary recovery at 72 h was 58.6% ± 5.0%.

**Table 20.** Dose alteration with organ system dysfunction[a]

| Quinolone | Dose alteration[b] | |
|---|---|---|
| | Renal | Hepatic[c] |
| Ofloxacin | 50% reduction at GFR of 40–50 ml/min; 75% reduction at 10–20 ml/min | Unnecessary |
| Pefloxacin | Unnecessary | 50% reduction at PT ↑ of 100%; 75% reduction at PT ↑ of 200% |
| Norfloxacin | 33–50% reduction at GFR of 20–30 ml/min | Unnecessary[d] |
| Ciprofloxacin | 33–50% reduction at GFR of 20–30 ml/min | Unnecessary[d] |
| Enoxacin | 33–50% reduction at GFR of 20–30 ml/min | Insufficient data |

[a]Data for the recommendations were drawn from references 19, 25, 27, 29, 30, 61, and 64.
[b]Dose reduction may take place as a dose decrease with maintenance of the dosing interval or as prolongation of the dosing interval with maintenance of the dose. If interval prolongation is chosen, use milligrams per day in the calculation.
[c]Recommendations for pefloxacin in hepatic failure should be regarded with caution because of the large amount of interindividual variation. PT, Prothrombin time.
[d]Data are available for mild to moderate hepatic disease only. Investigation is required for severe hepatic disease.

lowing single and multiple oral administration. *Am. J. Med.* **92**(Suppl. 4A):8–11.

7. **Bergan, T., S. B. Thorsteinsson, R. Solberg, L. Bjornskau, I. M. Kostad, and S. Johnsen.** 1987. Pharmacokinetics of ciprofloxacin: intravenous and increasing oral doses. *Am. J. Med.* **82**(Suppl. 4A):97–102.
8. **Blum, R. A.** 1992. Influence of renal function on the pharmacokinetics of lomefloxacin compared with other fluoroquinolones. *Am. J. Med.* **92**(Suppl. 4A):18S–21S.
9. **Blum, R. A., R. W. Schultz, and J. J. Schentag.** 1990. Pharmacokinetics of lomefloxacin in renally compromised patients. *Antimicrob. Agents Chemother.* **34:**2364–2368.
10. **Boelaert, J., Y. Valcke, M. Schurgers, R. Daneels, M. Rosseneu, M. T. Rosseel, and M. G. Bogaert.** 1985. The pharmacokinetics of ciprofloxacin in patients with impaired renal function. *J. Antimicrob. Chemother.* **16:**87–93.
11. **Brittain, D. C., B. E. Scully, M. J. McElrath, R. Steinman, P. Labthavikul, and H. Neu.** 1985. The pharmacokinetics and serum and urine bactericidal activity of ciprofloxacin. *J. Clin. Pharmacol.* **25:**82–88.
12. **Brumfitt, W., I. Franklin, D. Grady, J. M. T. Hamilton-Miller, and A. Iliffe.** 1984. Changes in the pharmacokinetics of ciprofloxacin and fecal flora during administration of a 7-day course to human volunteers. *Antimicrob. Agents Chemother.* **26:**757–761.
13. **Campoli-Richards, D. M., J. P. Monk, A. Price, P. Benfield, P. A. Todd, and A. Ward.** 1988. Ciprofloxacin: a review of its antibacterial activity, pharmacokinetic properties and therapeutic use. *Drugs* **35:**373–447.
14. **Cesana, M., G. Broccali, B. P. Imbimbo, and A. Crema.** 1991. Effect of single doses of rufloxacin on the disposition of theophylline and caffeine after single administration. *Int. J. Clin. Pharmacol. Ther. Toxicol.* **294:**133–138.
15. **Chang, T., A. Black, A. Dunky, R. Wolf, A. Sedman, J. Latts, and P. G. Welling.** 1988. Pharmacokinetics of intravenous and oral enoxacin in healthy volunteers. *J. Antimicrob. Chemother.* **21**(Suppl. B):49-56.
16. **Chin, N. X., A. Novelli, and H. C. Neu.** 1988. In vitro activity of lomefloxacin (SC-47111; NY-198), a difluoroquinolone carboxylic acid, compared with those of other quinolones. *Antimicrob. Agents Chemother.* **32:**656–662.
17. **Chu, D. T., and P. B. Fernandes.** 1989. Structure-activity relationships of the fluoroquinolones. *Antimicrob. Agents Chemother.* **33:**13–15.
18. **Cofsky, R. D., L. duBouchet, and S. H. Landesman.** 1984. Recovery of norfloxacin in feces after administration of a single oral dose to human volunteers. *Antimicrob. Agents Chemother.* **26:**110–111.
19. **Danan, G., G. Montay, R. Cunci, and S. Erlinger.** 1985. Pefloxacin kinetics in cirrhosis. *Clin. Pharmacol. Ther.* **38:**439–442.
20. **Davis, R. L., J. R. Koup, J. Williams-Warren, A. Weber, and A. L. Smith.** 1985. Pharmacokinetics of three oral formulations of ciprofloxacin. *Antimicrob. Agents Chemother.* **28:**74–77.
21. **Dow, J., J. Chazal, A. M. Frydman, P. Janny, R. Woehrle, F. Djebbar, and J. Gaillot.** 1986. Transfer kinetics of pefloxacin into cerebro-spinal fluid after one hour iv infusion of 400 mg in man. *J. Antimicrob. Chemother.* **17**(Suppl. B):81–87.
22. **Drusano, G., A. Forrest, K. Plaisance, P. Garjian, G. Yuen, M. Egorin, M. Didolkar, and H. C. Standiford.** 1987. *Program Abstr. 27th Intersci. Conf. Antimicrob. Agents Chemother.*, abstr. 1269.
23. **Drusano, G. L., K. I. Plaisance, A. Forrest, and H. C. Standiford.** 1986. Dose ranging study and constant infusion evaluation of ciprofloxacin. *Antimicrob. Agents Chemother.* **30:**440–443.
24. **Drusano, G. L., H. C. Standiford, K. Plaisance, A. Forrest, J. Leslie, and J. Caldwell.** 1986. Absolute oral bioavailability of ciprofloxacin. *Antimicrob. Agents Chemother.* **30:**444–446.
25. **Drusano, G. L., M. Weir, A. Forrest, K. Plaisance, T. Emm, and H. C. Standiford.** 1987. Pharmacokinetics of intravenously administered ciprofloxacin in patients with various degrees of renal function. *Antimicrob. Agents Chemother.* **31:**860–864.
26. **Dudley, M. N., J. Ericson, and S. H. Zinner.** 1987. Effect of dose on serum pharmacokinetics of intravenous ciprofloxacin with identification and characterization of extravascular compartments using noncompartmental and compartmental pharmacokinetic models. *Antimicrob. Agents Chemother.* **31:**1782–1786.
27. **Eandi, M., I. Viano, F. DiNola, L. Leone, and E. Genazzani.** 1983. Pharmacokinetics of norfloxacin in healthy volunteers and patients with renal and hepatic damage. *Eur. J. Clin. Microbiol.* **2:**253–259.
28. **Edlund, C., T. Bergan, K. Josefsson, R. Solberg, and C. E. Nord.** 1987. Effect of norfloxacin on human oropharyngeal and colonic microflora and multiple-dose pharmacokinetics. *Scand. J. Infect. Dis.* **19:**113–121.
29. **Fillastre, J. P., T. Hannedouche, A. Leroy, and G. Humbert.** 1984. Pharmacokinetics of norfloxacin in renal failure. *J. Antimicrob. Chemother.* **14:**439.
30. **Fillastre, J. P., A. Leroy, and G. Humbert.** 1987. Ofloxacin pharmacokinetics in renal failure. *Antimicrob. Agents Chemother.* **31:**156–160.
31. **Fornara, P., E. Schollmayer, R. Seelmann, et al.** 1990. The penetration of temafloxacin into prostatic tissue, abstr. 339. *Book Abstr. 3rd Int. Symp. New Quinolones.*

32. **Forrest, A., M. Weir, K. I. Plaisance, G. L. Drusano, J. Leslie, and H. C. Standiford.** 1988. Relationships between renal function and disposition of oral ciprofloxacin. *Antimicrob. Agents Chemother.* **32:**1537–1540.
33. **Frydman, A. M., Y. Le Roux, M. A. Lefebvre, F. Djebbar, J. B. Fourtillan, and J. Gaillot.** 1986. Pharmacokinetics of pefloxacin after repeated intravenous and oral administration (400 mg bid) in young healthy volunteers. *J. Antimicrob. Chemother.* **17**(Suppl. B)**:**65–79.
33a. **Gau, W.** Personal communication.
34. **Golper, T. A., A. I. Hartstein, V. H. Morthland, and J. M. Christensen.** 1987. Effects of antacids and dialysate dwell times on multiple-dose pharmacokinetics of oral ciprofloxacin in patients on continuous ambulatory peritoneal dialysis. *Antimicrob. Agents Chemother.* **31:**1787–1790.
35. **Gonzalez, M. A., A. H. Moranchel, S. Duran, A. Pichardo, J. L. Magana, B. Painter, and G. L. Drusano.** 1985. Multiple-dose ciprofloxacin dose ranging and kinetics. *Clin. Pharmacol. Ther.* **37:**633–637.
36. **Gonzalez, M. A., A. H. Moranchel, S. Duran, A. Pichardo, J. L. Magana, B. Painter, A. Forrest, and G. L. Drusano.** 1985. Multiple-dose pharmacokinetics of ciprofloxacin administered intravenously to normal volunteers. *Antimicrob. Agents Chemother.* **28:**235–239.
37. **Gonzalez, M. A., F. Uribe, S. D. Moisen, A. P. Fuster, A. Selen, P. G. Welling, and B. Painter.** 1984. Multiple-dose pharmacokinetics and safety of ciprofloxacin in normal volunteers. *Antimicrob. Agents Chemother.* **26:**741–744.
38. **Granneman, G. R., P. Carpentier, P. J. Morrison, and A. G. Pernet.** 1991. Pharmacokinetics of temafloxacin in humans after single oral doses. *Antimicrob. Agents Chemother.* **35:**436–441.
39. **Granneman, G. R., K. M. Snyder, and V. S. Shu.** 1986. Difloxacin metabolism and pharmacokinetics in humans after single oral doses. *Antimicrob. Agents Chemother.* **30:**689–693.
40. **Granneman, R.** 1991. The effect of food on the absorption of 600 mg tablet doses of temafloxacin, abstr. 411. *Book Abstr. 17th Int. Congr. Chemother.*
41. **Granneman, R. R. Braeckman, P. Carpentier, and A. G. Pernet.** 1991. Pharmacokinetics of temofloxacin after single intravenous 100, 200, 400, 600 and 800 mg doses, abstr. 383. *Book Abstr. 17th Int. Congr. Chemother.*
42. **Healy, D. P., R. E. Polk, J. Schoenle, and J. Stotka.** 1990. Effect of lomefloxacin on the disposition of caffeine in normal volunteers, abstr. 1008. *Program Abstr. 30th Intersci. Conf. Antimicrob. Agents Chemother.*
43. **Höffken, G., H. Lode, C. Prinzing, K. Borner, and P. Koeppe.** 1985. Pharmacokinetics of ciprofloxacin after oral and parenteral administration. *Antimicrob. Agents Chemother.* **27:**375–379.
44. **Hughes, P. J., D. B. Webb, and A. W. Asscher.** 1984. Pharmacokinetics of norfloxacin (MK 366) in patients with impaired kidney function—some preliminary results. *J. Antimicrob. Chemother.* **13**(Suppl. B)**:**55–57.
45. **Imbimbo, B. P., G. Broccali, M. Cesano, F. Crema, and G. Attardo-Parrinello.** 1991. Inter- and intrasubject variabilities in the pharmacokinetics of rufloxacin after single oral administration to healthy volunteers. *Antimicrob. Agents Chemother.* **35:**390–393.
46. **Joos, B., B. Ledergerber, M. Flepp, J. D. Bettex, R. Luthy, and W. Siegenthaler.** 1985. Comparison of high-pressure liquid chromatography and bioassay for determination of ciprofloxacin in serum and urine. *Antimicrob. Agents Chemother.* **27:**353–356.
47. **Kalager, T., A. Digranes, T. Bergan, and T. Rolstad.** 1986. Ofloxacin: serum and skin blister fluid pharmacokinetics in the fasting and non-fasting state. *J. Antimicrob. Chemother.* **17:**795–800.
48. **Kumasaka, Y., H. Nakahata, K. Imamura, and K. Takebe.** 1981. Fundamental study on AM-715. *Chemotherapy* (Tokyo) **29**(Suppl. 4)**:**56–65.
49. **LeBel, M., F. Vallee, and M. G. Bergeron.** 1986. Tissue penetration of ciprofloxacin after single and multiple doses. *Antimicrob. Agents Chemother.* **29:**501–505.
50. **Lebrec, D., C. Gaudin, and J. P. Benhamou.** 1992. Pharmacokinetics of lomefloxacin in patients with cirrhosis. *Am. J. Med.* **92**(Suppl. 4A)**:**41–44.
51. **Ledergerber, B., J. D. Bettex, B. Joos, M. Flepp, and R. Lüthy.** 1985. Effect of standard breakfast on drug absorption and multiple-dose pharmacokinetics of ciprofloxacin. *Antimicrob. Agents Chemother.* **27:**350–352.
52. **Leroy, A., F. Borsa, G. Humbert, P. Bernadet, and J. P. Fillastre.** 1987. The pharmacokinetics of ofloxacin in healthy adult male volunteers. *Eur. J. Clin. Pharmacol.* **31:**629–630.
53. **Leroy, A., G. Humbert, and J. P. Fillastre.** 1992. Penetration of lomefloxacin into prostatic tissue. *Am. J. Med.* **92**(Suppl. 4A)**:**12–14.
54. **Lettieri, R., W. Frost, G. Krol, K. Lasseter, and E. C. Shamblin.** 1987. *Program Abstr. 27th Intersci. Conf. Antimicrob. Agents Chemother.*, abstr. 1268.
55. **Lockley, M. R., R. Wise, and J. Dent.** 1984. The pharmacokinetics and tissue penetration of ofloxacin. *J. Antimicrob. Chemother.* **14:**647–652.
56. **Lode, H., G. Höffken, P. Olschewski, B. Sievers, A. Kirch, K. Borner, and P. Koeppe.** 1987. Pharmacokinetics of ofloxacin after parenteral and oral administration. *Antimicrob. Agents Chemother.* **31:**1338–1342.
57. **Mahr, G., R. Seelmann, R. Granneman, J. Sylvester, B. Gottschalk, C. Jurgens, P. Muth, U.**

**Stephan, and F. Sorgel.** 1989. The effect of temafloxacin and enoxacin on the pharmacokinetics of theophylline. *Program Abstr. 29th Intersci. Conf. Antimicrob. Agents Chemother.*, abstr. 216.

58. **Mant, T. G. K.** 1992. Multiple-dose pharmacokinetics of lomefloxacin: rationale for once-a-day dosing. *Am. J. Med.* **92**(Suppl. 4A)**:**26–32.
59. **Mattina, R., G. Bonfiglio, C. E. Cocuzza, G. Gulisano, M. Cesana, and B. P. Imbimbo.** 1991. Pharmacokinetics of rufloxacin in healthy volunteers after repeated oral doses. *Chemotherapy* **37:**389–397.
60. **Montay, G., Y. Goueffon, and F. Rogquet.** 1984. Absorption, distribution, metabolic fate, and elimination of pefloxacin mesylate in mice, rats, dogs, monkeys, and humans. *Antimicrob. Agents Chemother.* **25:**463–472.
61. **Montay, G., C. Jacquot, J. Bariety, and R. Cunci.** 1985. Pharmacokinetics of pefloxacin in renal insufficiency. *Eur. J. Clin. Pharmacol.* **29:**345–349.
62. **Morrison, P. J., T. G. K. Mant, G. T. Norman, J. Robinson, and R. L. Kunka.** 1988. Pharmacokinetics and tolerance of lomefloxacin after sequentially increasing oral doses. *Antimicrob. Agents Chemother.* **32:**1503–1507.
63. **Neu, H. C.** 1992. Pharmacokinetics, microbiology, cost: interrelated problems for the 1990s that impact on the use of fluoroquinolone antimicrobial agents. *Am. J. Med.* **92**(Suppl. 4A)**:**2S–7S.
64. **Nix, D. E., R. W. Schultz, R. W. Frost, A. J. Sedman, D. J. Thomas, A. W. Kinkel, and J. J. Schentag.** 1988. The effect of renal impairment and haemodialysis on single dose pharmacokinetics of oral enoxacin. *J. Antimicrob. Chemother.* **21**(Suppl. B)**:**87–95.
65. **On, A., C. H. Nightingale, R. Quintiliani, K. R. Sweeney, H. S. Pasternack, and E. G. Maderazo.** 1992. Lomefloxacin concentrations in bone after a single oral dose. *Am. J. Med.* **92**(Suppl. 4A)**:**15–17.
66. **Ozaki, T., H. Uchida, and T. Irikura.** 1981. Studies on metabolism of AM-715 in humans by high performance liquid chromatography. *Chemotherapy* (Tokyo) **29**(Suppl. 4)**:**128–135.
67. **Pankey, G. A.** 1991. Temafloxacin: an overview. *Am. J. Med.* **91**(Suppl. 6A)**:**166S–172S.
68. **Pecquet, S., A. Andremont, and C. Tancrede.** 1987. Effect of oral ofloxacin on fecal bacterial in human volunteers. *Antimicrob. Agents Chemother.* **31:**124–125.
69. **Percival, A.** 1991. Impact of chemical structure on quinolone potency, spectrum and side effects. *J. Antimicrob. Chemother.* **28**(Suppl. C)**:**1–8.
70. **Perea, E. J., I. Garcia, and A. Pascual.** 1992. Comparative penetration of lomefloxacin and other quinolones into human phagocytes. *Am. J. Med.* **92**(Suppl. 4A)**:**48–51.
71. **Plaisance, K. I., G. L. Drusano, A. Forrest, C. I. Bustamante, and H. C. Standiford.** 1987. Effect of dose size on bioavailability of ciprofloxacin. *Antimicrob. Agents Chemother.* **31:**956–958.
72. **Rohwedder, R. W., and T. Bergan.** 1986. *Proc. Congr. Bacterial Drug Resistance.*
73. **Shalit, I., R. B. Greenwood, M. I. Marks, J. A. Pederson, and D. L. Frederick.** 1986. Pharmacokinetics of single-dose oral ciprofloxacin in patients undergoing chronic ambulatory peritoneal dialysis. *Antimicrob. Agents Chemother.* **30:**152–156.
74. **Singlas, E., A. M. Taburet, I. Landru, H. Albin, and J. P. Ryckelinck.** 1987. Pharmacokinetics of ciprofloxacin tablets in renal failure: influence of haemodialysis. *Eur. J. Clin. Pharmacol.* **31:**589–593.
75. **Somogyi, A. A., F. Bochner, J. A. Keal, P. E. Rolan, and M. Smith.** 1987. Effect of food on enoxacin absorption. *Antimicrob. Agents Chemother.* **31:**638–639.
76. **Sörgel, F.** 1990. Pharmacokinetics of temafloxacin: a review. *9th Int. Symp. Future Trends Chemother.*
77. **Sörgel, F., K. G. Naber, M. Kinzig, G. Mahr, and P. Muth.** 1991. Comparative pharmacokinetics of ciprofloxacin and temafloxacin in humans: a review. *Am. J. Med.* **91**(Suppl. 6A)**:**51S–66S.
78. **Swanson, B. N., V. K. Boppana, P. H. Vlaysses, H. H. Rotmensch, and R. K. Ferguson.** 1983. Norfloxacin disposition after sequentially increasing oral doses. *Antimicrob. Agents Chemother.* **23:**284–288.
79. **Tartaglione, T. A., A. C. Raffalovich, W. J. Poynor, A. Espinel-Ingroff, and T. M. Kerkering.** 1986. Pharmacokinetics and tolerance of ciprofloxacin after sequential increasing oral doses. *Antimicrob. Agents Chemother.* **29:**62–66.
80. **Verho, M., V. Malerczyk, E. Dagrosa, and A. Korn.** 1985. Dose linearity and other pharmacokinetics of ofloxacin: a new, broad-spectrum antimicrobial agent. *Pharmatherapeutica* **4:**376–382.
81. **Webb, D. B., D. E. Roberts, J. B. Williams, and A. W. Asscher.** 1986. Pharmacokinetics of ciprofloxacin in healthy volunteers and patients with impaired kidney function. *J. Antimicrob. Chemother.* **18**(Suppl. D)**:**83–87.
82. **Weidekamm, E., R. Portmann, K. Suter, C. Partos, D. Dell, and P. W. Lucker.** 1987. Single- and multiple-dose pharmacokinetics of fleroxacin, a trifluorinated quinolone, in humans. *Antimicrob. Agents Chemother.* **31:**1909–1914.
83. **Wijnands, W. J. A., T. B. Vree, A. M. Baars, and C. L. A. van Herwaarden.** 1988. Pharmacokinetics of enoxacin and its penetration into bronchial secretions and lung tissue. *J. Antimicrob. Chemother.* **21**(Suppl. B)**:**67–77.
84. **Wijnands, W. J. A., T. B. Vree, and C. L. A. van Herwaarden.** 1986. The influence of quin-

olone derivatives on theophylline clearance. *Br. J. Clin. Pharmacol.* **22:**677–683.

84a. **Wingender, W.** Personal communication.

85. **Wingender, W., D. Beerman, D. Foester, K. H. Graefe, and P. Schacht.** 1984. *4th Mediterranean Congr. Chemother.*, abstr. 621.

86. **Wise, R., D. R. Baldwin, J. M. Andrews, and D. Honeybourne.** 1991. Comparative pharmacokinetic disposition of fluoroquinolones in the lung. *J. Antimicrob. Chemother.* **28**(Suppl. C):65–72.

87. **Wise, R., and I. A. Donovan.** 1987. Tissue penetration and metabolism of ciprofloxacin. *Am. J. Med.* **82**(Suppl. 4A):103–107.

88. **Wise, R., B. Kirkpatrick, J. Ashby, and D. J. Griggs.** 1987. Pharmacokinetics and tissue penetration of Ro 23-6240, a new trifluoroquinolone. *Antimicrob. Agents Chemother.* **31:**161–163.

89. **Wise, R., D. Lister, C. A. M. McNulty, D. Griggs, and J. M. Andrews.** 1986. The comparative pharmacokinetics of five quinolones. *J. Antimicrob. Chemother.* **18**(Suppl. D):71–81.

90. **Wise, R., D. Lister, C. A. M. McNulty, D. Griggs, and J. M. Andrews.** 1986. The comparative pharmacokinetics and tissue penetration of four quinolones including intravenously administered enoxacin. *Infection* **14**(Suppl. 3):S196–S202.

91. **Wise, R., R. M. Lockley, M. Webberly, and J. Dent.** 1984. Pharmacokinetics of intravenously administered ciprofloxacin. *Antimicrob. Agents Chemother.* **26:**208–210.

92. **Wolf, R., R. Eberl, A. Dunky, N. Mertz, T. Chang, J. R. Goulet, and J. Latts.** 1984. The clinical pharmacokinetics and tolerance of enoxacin in healthy volunteers. *J. Antimicrob. Chemother.* **14**(Suppl. C):63–69.

93. **Wolff, M., B. Regnier, C. Daldoss, M. Nkam, and F. Vachon.** 1984. Penetration of pefloxacin into cerebrospinal fluid of patients with meningitis. *Antimicrob. Agents Chemother.* **16:**289–291.

94. **Wolfson, J. S., and D. C. Hooper.** 1985. The fluoroquinolones: structures, mechanisms of action and resistance, and spectra of activity in vitro. *Antimicrob. Agents Chemother.* **28:**581–586.

*Quinolone Antimicrobial Agents, 2nd ed.*
Edited by David C. Hooper and John S. Wolfson


*Chapter 10*

# Pharmacokinetics of Fluoroquinolones in Selected Populations

***Monique Richer and Marc LeBel***

Fluoroquinolones are a burgeoning new class of antibiotics that allow effective oral therapy of serious infections. Tissue penetration is excellent and is a unique feature of these antibiotics. This chapter summarizes peer-reviewed papers on the pharmacokinetics of eight quinolones in special populations. The eight quinolones discussed are ciprofloxacin, enoxacin, fleroxacin, lomefloxacin, norfloxacin, ofloxacin, pefloxacin, and rufloxacin. We have focused this review on fluoroquinolone disposition in patients with renal or hepatic failure, elderly individuals, and patients with cystic fibrosis (CF).

## PHARMACOKINETICS OF FLUOROQUINOLONES IN THE ELDERLY

Most pharmacokinetic studies of a new drug are initially carried out with healthy young volunteers. Later in the development phase, pharmacokinetic studies in elderly subjects may be undertaken. When evaluating such studies, always remember that the elderly are a more heterogeneous group than the young. Aside from the well-documented decrease in renal clearance of certain drugs, other variables including absorption, distribution, and metabolism must be taken into consideration in order to better understand age-related alterations in drug disposition. In fact, age-associated physiologic changes can account for most of the variation seen in the pharmacokinetics of drugs in the elderly population. As an individual ages, the water-to-lipid ratio declines by 10 to 15%, cardiac output can fall by as much as 10%, and the glomerular filtration rate can decline by as much as 40% by the age of 80 (67).

Pharmacokinetic data for selected fluoroquinolones used in the elderly are summarized in Table 1. Several studies included a control group of young subjects. Although some reports do not compare the pharmacokinetics of fluoroquinolones in the elderly with those of a control group, the timing of blood samples and pharmacokinetic analysis allow the inclusion of these reports in this chapter. All data are given in a standardized fashion, and when possible, the same pharmacokinetic calculations were used.

### Absorption

On the basis of a number of reported age-related alterations in the gastrointestinal tract, such as diminished gastric acid secretion, reduced splanchnic blood flow, decreased gastric emptying rate for liquids, and reduced number of functional absorbing cells, one

***Monique Richer and Marc LeBel*** • Laboratoire de Pharmacocinétique Clinique, École de Pharmacie, Université Laval, Québec, Québec G1K 7P4, Canada.

**Table 1.** Pharmacokinetic parameters of quinolones in the elderly[a]

| Drug and reference | Dose[b] | Population studied | Age (yr) | Creatinine clearance (ml/min) | $T_{max}$ (h) | $t_{1/2}$ (h) | $C_{max}$ (μg/ml) | $V_{app}$ (liters/kg) | Clearance (ml/min) | | |
|---|---|---|---|---|---|---|---|---|---|---|---|
| | | | | | | | | | Plasma | Renal | Non-renal |
| Ciprofloxacin | | | | | | | | | | | |
| 2 | 100-mg single dose | 9 elderly patients | 74.0 | | 1.3 | 3.3[c] | 0.8[d] | 2.10[c] | 443.0[c] | 88.0[c] | 355.0[c] |
| | | 6 young patients | <20.0 | | 1.2 | 3.0[c] | 0.4 | 4.55[c] | 1,174.0[c] | 321.0[c] | 853.0[c] |
| 56 | 500-mg single dose | 12 elderly subjects | 75.4 | 41 | 1.1 | 6.8[d] | 3.2[d] | 2.47[d] | 394.0 | 152.0[d] | 236.7[d] |
| | | 12 young subjects | 22.3 | 104 | 1.3 | 3.7 | 2.3 | 3.76 | 908.0 | 908.0 | 512.4 |
| 3 | 250-mg single dose | 10 elderly subjects | 67.0 | 62 | 1.3 | 3.4 | 1.7[d] | 2.60[c] | 560.8[c] | 244.8[d] | 316.0[c] |
| | | 10 young subjects | 24.0 | 106 | 1.3 | 4.4 | 1.2 | 3.65[c] | 750.8[c] | 286.0 | 464.8[c] |
| 39 | 750-mg single dose (acutely ill) | 13 elderly patients | 78.1 | 47 | 1.6 | 5.2 | 5.9 | 3.46 | 415.0 | 100.0 | 383.4 |
| | 750-mg steady state (convalescent) | | | 47 | 1.4 | 4.8 | 8.6 | 3.34 | 336.0 | 172.0 | 259.6 |
| 51 | 200-mg single dose | 14 elderly patients | 74.0 | | 0.5 | 4.2 | 4.2 | | 441.0 | | |
| 43 | 200 mg i.v. q12h or 750 mg p.o. b.i.d. | 6 elderly patients | 78.0 | | 1.9 | 5.7/4.2 | 3.6/7.6 | 1.80 | 274.5[c] | 157.9 | 116.7[c] |
| | 200 mg q12h | 9 elderly patients | 77.1 | | | 5.8 | 3.5 | 2.00 | 289.1[c] | 164.3 | 124.7[c] |
| 74 | 200-mg single dose | 11 elderly patients | 57.0–84.0 | | | 4.3 | 4.2 | 2.09 | 407.0[e] | | |
| | | 12 young volunteers | 19.0–33.0 | | | 3.6 | 3.4[d] | 2.52[d] | 632.0 | 328.0 | 304.0[c] |
| Enoxacin | | | | | | | | | | | |
| 21 | 600-mg single dose | 10 elderly subjects | 74.8 | 63[d] | 1.7 | 6.8 | 6.9 | 1.80[d] | 207.3 | 91.2[d] | 116.1 |
| | | 10 young subjects | 32.6 | 114 | 1.7 | 7.3 | 4.4 | 2.35 | 267.7 | 161.9 | 105.8 |
| 115 | 200-mg single dose | 18 elderly patients | 81.8 | | 1.4 | 6.1 | 1.9 | 1.89[c] | 199.6[c] | | |
| 73 | 400-mg single dose | 19 elderly patients | 70.8 | | 2.3 | 7.3 | 3.6 | 1.56[c] | 177.3[c] | 82.0 | 95.3 |
| Fleroxacin | | | | | | | | | | | |
| 113 | Crossover study (400 mg p.o./100 mg i.v.) | 15 elderly subjects | 60.0–74.0 | | 1.1 | 10.6 | 5.2[d] | 1.1[d] | 106.0[d] | 60.0[d] | 46.0[d] |
| | 400 mg p.o. | 6 young subjects | 18.0–34.0 | | 1.1 | 9.8 | 3.6 | 1.5 | 140.7 | 80.1 | 60.6 |
| 107 | 800-mg single dose | 12 elderly subjects | 75.0 | 61 | 2.7 | 16.0 | 15.6 | 0.9 | 43.0 | 17.0 | |

| | | | | | | | | | | | |
|---|---|---|---|---|---|---|---|---|---|---|---|
| Norfloxacin | | | | | | | | | | | |
| 64 | 400 mg b.i.d. | 8 elderly patients | 81.0 | | 3.2 | 5.0 | 1.5 | | | | |
| 53 | 400 mg b.i.d. | 8 elderly subjects | 83.8 | 41 | | 5.2 | | | | | |
| Ofloxacin | | | | | | | | | | | |
| 111 | 200-mg single dose | 16 elderly subjects | 77.0 | 56 | 2.0 | 13.3 | 3.6 | 1.4 | 82.8 | | |
| 37 | 200-mg single dose | 20 elderly subjects | 75.2 | 44[d] | | 6.1 | 2.9 | 1.7[c] | 189.4 | | |
| | | 8 young subjects | 27.3 | 113 | | 4.6 | 1.9 | 1.7[c] | 262.5 | | |
| 70 | 300-mg single dose | 12 elderly subjects | 85.0 | | 2.1[d] | 6.2[d] | 2.7[e] | | 83.3[e] | | |
| | | 12 young subjects | 24.6 | | 1.5 | 8.5 | 4.70 | | 233.3 | | |
| Pefloxacin | | | | | | | | | | | |
| 23 | 400-mg single dose | 10 elderly subjects | 75.0 | | | 12.6 | 10.7 | 50.5[f] | 48.0[d] | | |
| 33 | 400-mg single dose q12h for 16 doses | 12 young subjects | 24.0 | | 1.3 | 12.0 | 5.4 | 114.2[f] | 123.3 | 7.5 | 115.8 |
| Rufloxacin | | | | | | | | | | | |
| 15 | 400-mg LD, then 400 mg q.d. for 6–9 days | 12 elderly subjects | 71.5 | 62.5 | 4.3 | 28.7 | 6.5 | 77.0[f] | 35.0 | | |
| 66 | 300-mg LD + 150 mg q.d. for 5 days | 11 young subjects | 35.0 | | 4.2 | 29.5 | 2.8 | 111.0[f] | 46.0 | 19.0 | 27.0 |
| | 400-mg LD, then 200 mg q.d. for 5 days | 12 young subjects | 34.8 | | 4.0 | 36.0 | 3.6 | 136.0[f] | 44.0 | 17.0 | 27.0 |

[a]Values are means except where ranges are specified. Abbreviations: $T_{max}$, time to reach maximal concentration in serum; $C_{max}$, maximal concentration in serum; $V_{app}$, apparent volume of distribution; $t_{1/2}$, half-life.

[b]q12h, every 12 h; b.i.d., twice daily; p.o., perorally; i.v., intravenously; LD, loading dose; q.d., once daily.

[c]Calculated from mean data using pharmacokinetic analysis described in reference 56.

[d]$P < 0.05$.

[e]$P < 0.001$.

[f]In liters.

may postulate a priori that absorption may be impaired with age (61). In theory, these changes might lead to a decreased absorption of basic and poorly lipid-soluble drugs in the elderly, since their absorption is enhanced by a higher gastric pH and a decreased gastric emptying time. Conversely, more time would be available for absorption if such drugs were absorbed from a small section of the duodenum.

Clinical conditions such as congestive heart failure, dietary habits, and the edentulousness of elderly patients may also hamper oral absorption of drugs. Moreover, concomitant use of certain drugs, particularly antacids and laxatives, may also modify drug absorption (92).

A priori differences were not observed between young and elderly subjects in the time required to achieve maximal concentration in serum of the fluoroquinolones. However, the elderly showed consistently higher peak concentrations and larger areas under the concentration-time curves (AUC) than did younger subjects for ciprofloxacin, ofloxacin, lomefloxacin, and rufloxacin (2, 3, 15, 16, 56, 66, 70, 74, 90, 113). Increased bioavailability, reduced volume of distribution, reduced clearance, or a combination of these factors may explain these observations. At this point it appears that the absorption of fluoroquinolones is unchanged or possibly increased in elderly populations.

## Distribution

With increasing age, the fraction of total body weight comprising adipose tissue changes and such tissue is redistributed to the trunk, mainly the abdomen. More important, the decrease in total body water and the muscle atrophy observed in old age are responsible for the increased proportion of fat tissue to total body weight.

Smaller apparent volumes of distribution for ciprofloxacin, enoxacin, fleroxacin, lomefloxacin, and rufloxacin have been observed in the elderly compared with young healthy individuals (2, 3, 15, 16, 21, 56, 66, 74, 90, 113). However, one must not exclude the possible contribution of concomitant disease or body habitus in the alteration of volume of distribution in the elderly population. The serum protein binding of fluoroquinolones ranges from 20 to 40% and is too low to be clinically affected by the decrease in albumin levels in serum seen in normal aging.

## Metabolism

Age-associated changes in liver metabolism can be related to a decline in liver mass and a decrease in hepatic blood flow. There is also an age-dependent decline in the activity of hepatic microsomal enzymes responsible for phase I metabolism (67). Fluoroquinolones undergo phase I oxidation reactions through the cytochrome P-450 system. Clinically, nonrenal clearance is the only pharmacokinetic parameter for the fluoroquinolones easily evaluated in the assessment of their metabolism. In single-dose studies performed with elderly patients, the nonrenal clearances of ciprofloxacin (2, 3, 56) and of fleroxacin and its metabolites (107) were reduced, while no difference was seen with enoxacin (21, 73). This suggests some decline in the function of hepatic microsomal enzymes responsible for phase I oxidation.

## Renal Elimination

Elimination of most fluoroquinolones is dependent on glomerular filtration rate. For the fluoroquinolones primarily eliminated unchanged in the urine, the diminished glomerular filtration rate associated with normal aging is the most significant change that could alter drug pharmacokinetics. As a result of aging, renal tubular secretion also undergoes a significant decline. Furthermore, renal atrophy associated with senescence preferentially affects regional cortical flow, resulting in a more pronounced decrease in the cortical perfusion rate compared with that of the medulla.

With the exception of enoxacin, the apparent total clearance of fluoroquinolones from plasma significantly diminishes in the elderly in studies comparing elderly and young healthy volunteers (2, 3, 15, 23, 33, 56, 66, 70, 74). The smaller clearance observed in the elderly population illustrates the decline in glomerular filtration rate observed with aging and translates into significantly longer half-lives for ciprofloxacin and ofloxacin, while a trend toward longer half-lives was observed with fleroxacin and lomefloxacin.

### Conclusion

The concern for drug disposition is triggered by the significant morbidity associated with adverse drug reactions in a population that is more prone to the development of such reactions. This is the case for fluoroquinolones, and in fact, adverse central nervous system reactions seem to occur at an increased rate in the elderly (101). Caution regarding the appropriate use and correct dosage regimen in this group should therefore be exercised. Although significant changes in the pharmacokinetics of fluoroquinolones have been noted in the elderly, most studies do not recommend modification of the dosage regimen solely on the basis of normal aging, except possibly for ofloxacin. In the presence of renal impairment, the lack of compensatory mechanisms through an alternate route of elimination may justify dosage reduction in elderly patients.

## PHARMACOKINETICS OF FLUOROQUINOLONES IN PATIENTS WITH RENAL FAILURE

Fluoroquinolones are primarily eliminated via the kidney by glomerular filtration, but several of these drugs undergo both renal and hepatic elimination. Dosage adjustment in the presence of renal impairment is not required for pefloxacin, since 60% of a pefloxacin dose is recovered mostly as inactive urinary metabolites. In contrast, ofloxacin is largely eliminated unchanged via the renal route, suggesting dosage reduction in renal failure. The other fluoroquinolones lie between these two extremes. This section reviews the available pharmacokinetic studies of fluoroquinolone disposition in subjects with various degrees of renal failure and offers dosing guidelines for patients with renal dysfunction.

### Ciprofloxacin

The absorption of ciprofloxacin is rapid; bioavailability ranges from 60 to 85% in healthy individuals. There is no evidence of decreased absorption (83) or significant alterations in the volume of distribution in the presence of renal dysfunction (112).

In healthy individuals, 50 to 70% of ciprofloxacin is excreted unchanged by the kidneys. Renal excretion far exceeds creatinine clearance, indicating a significant contribution of proximal tubular secretion as an additional elimination pathway (24). In the presence of renal impairment, the contribution of tubular secretion decreases, making creatinine clearance a more precise estimate of renal elimination. Hepatic metabolism accounts for the removal of approximately 20% of the dose, and there is evidence of drug concentrations in the common duct bile, gallbladder bile, and gallbladder wall exceeding concentrations in serum as assessed in patients requiring hepatobiliary surgery (79). A third and more controversial route of excretion is transintestinal excretion across the bowel mucosa into the feces (6). The contribution of this pathway is quite variable but can account for 10 to 40% of ciprofloxacin elimination. Preliminary data have demonstrated evidence of transintestinal excretion of ciprofloxacin, as well as ofloxacin and fleroxacin, in both animals and healthy human subjects (65, 99). Five patients with severe renal failure (creatinine clearance between 8 and 16 ml/min) demonstrated an increase in the amount of metabolites of ciprofloxacin in feces (7.3 to 26.2%) compared with that in healthy volunteers (89). The variable contributions of these three pathways may be altered as a result of the underlying disease process and may explain the differences in half-lives seen in various kinetic studies.

Pharmacokinetic studies assessing the disposition of ciprofloxacin and its metabolites are summarized in Table 2. Results show a decrease in both renal and plasma clearances in the presence of renal impairment (10, 88, 109, 112). Reduced renal function influences the elimination of ciprofloxacin and its three major metabolites, desethyleneciprofloxacin, sulfonylciprofloxacin, and oxociprofloxacin (7). Overall, there is a good correlation between creatinine clearance and renal and plasma clearances. However, elimination half-life does not parallel creatinine clearance owing to an increasing contribution of nonrenal clearance in the face of renal impairment. There is also considerable intersubject variation in drug clearances within groups with similar creatinine clearances. The lack of correlation between half-life and creatinine

**Table 2.** Pharmacokinetic parameters of ciprofloxacin in patients with renal failure[a]

| Reference | Dosage | No. of patients | Clearance (ml/min) | | | $t_{1/2}$ (h) | fe (%) |
|---|---|---|---|---|---|---|---|
| | | | Creatinine | Plasma | Renal | | |
| 88 | 100-mg single dose | 6 | >80 | 538.0 | 300.0 | | |
| | | 6 | 31–80 | 363.0 | 125.0 | | |
| | | 6 | 10–30 | 283.0 | 45.0 | | |
| | | 6 | <10 | 238.0 | 0 | | |
| 10 | 250-mg single dose | 6 | >60[b] | | 232.9 | 4.4 | 37 |
| | | 6 | <20 | | 18.3[c] | 8.7[c] | 5.3[c] |
| | | 5 | Hemodialysis | | | 5.8 | |
| 108 | 500-mg single dose | 5 | Normal | 770.0 | 305.0 | 7.3 | 39.6 |
| | | 5 | 8–20[b] | 440.0 | 60.9 | 10.4 | 16.2 |
| | | 5 | <8 | 378.0 | 21.4 | 7.2 | 8.2 |
| | | 5 | Hemodialysis | 314.0 | 2.8 | 9.3 | 1.0 |
| 112 | 100-mg single dose | 6 | >80 | 624.5 | 464.7 | | |
| | | 6 | 30–80 | 325.3 | 141.8 | | |
| | | 6 | 0–30 | 268.2 | 25.8 | | |
| | | 6 | <10 | 289.8 | 8.2 | | |
| 20 | 100-mg single dose | 11 | ≥60 | 262.1 | | | 63.7 |
| | | 9 | 10–60 | 82.1 | | | 42.2 |
| 24 | 200-mg single dose | 8 | >100[b] | 446.7[b] | 273.3[b] | 4.3 | |
| | | 5 | ≥60–100 | 438.3 | 198.3 | 6.1 | |
| | | 11 | ≥10–60 | 250.0 | 75.0 | 7.7 | |
| | | 8 | <10 | 256.7 | 0 | 8.6 | |
| 34 | 500-mg single dose | 13 | ≥50[b] | 1,002.0 | 245.0 | 4.3 | |
| | 750-mg single dose | | | 1,173.0 | 272.0 | 3.5 | |
| | 500-mg single dose | 14 | <50 | 527.0[c] | 64.0[c] | 7.1[c] | |
| | 750-mg single dose | | | 490.0[c] | 72.0[c] | 6.3[c] | |
| 30 | 750-mg single dose | 8 | 118[b] | 725[b] | 243.3[b] | 5.2 | |
| | | 6 | 62 | 500.0 | 121.7 | 6.4 | |
| | | 10 | 32 | 476.7 | 38.4 | 6.7 | |
| | | 8 | 0 | 423.3 | 0 | 6.9 | |

[a] Values are means except where ranges are specified. Abbreviations: $t_{1/2}$, half-life; fe, percentage of dose excreted unchanged in urine.
[b] Milliliters per minute per 1.73 $m^2$.
[c] $P < 0.01$ compared with the group with the best renal function.

clearance and the wide intersubject variation complicate the implementation of adequate dosing regimens. Most current studies recommend maintaining the 12-h interval and decreasing by one-half or two-thirds the usual dose in patients with creatinine clearances of less than 20 to 30 ml/min (24, 30, 34, 108). According to the North American ciprofloxacin monograph (68), recommended dosages for the oral and intravenous formulations of ciprofloxacin are different. The clinical evidence provided does not justify this discrepancy.

Ciprofloxacin is poorly cleared by hemodialysis. The coefficient of extraction ranges from 18 to 30%, and dialysis clearance ranges from 29 to 47 ml/min (108). Consequently, one can expect approximately 2% of the dose to be removed by hemodialysis (10). In a single-dose study involving eight patients on chronic ambulatory peritoneal dialysis (CAPD), the fraction of the dose eliminated via the peritoneal fluid pathway ranged from 0.4 to 1.6% (93). In a multidose trial, 250 mg of ciprofloxacin was administered orally four times daily for 2 days to 10 patients on CAPD. In contrast with the single-dose study, the mean concentrations in plasma were twice those seen in healthy individuals, and more than half the dialysates contained ciprofloxacin concentrations elevated enough to inhibit the majority of pathogens that are likely to cause peritonitis (29).

Based on an estimated endogenous creatinine clearance of 20 ml/min in individuals on CAPD, the same dosing regimens as the ones used in patients with renal failure could be used. However, because of inconsistent peritoneal dialysate levels, MICs for pathogens should be determined and the dosage should be adjusted accordingly. Alternatively, the intraperitoneal route is being investigated with some success (62, 63). However, the optimal dialysate concentration remains to be determined (25).

## Ofloxacin

More than 90% of the administered dose of ofloxacin is excreted unchanged in the urine 24 h after administration, suggesting that the main route of excretion for this drug is via the kidney.

**Table 3.** Pharmacokinetic parameters of ofloxacin in patients with renal failure[a]

| Reference | Dosage | No. of patients | Clearance (ml/min) | | | $t_{1/2}$ (h) | fe (%) |
|---|---|---|---|---|---|---|---|
| | | | Creatinine | Plasma | Renal | | |
| 44 | 200-mg single dose | 10 | 115.1[b] | 191.9 | 151 | 5.43 | 74.0[c] |
| | | 20 | 28.4 | 57.4[c] | 26.5[c] | 19.37[c] | 36.0[c] |
| 28 | 200-mg single dose | 12 | 119.6 | 241.4[d] | 196.5[d] | 7.9 | 68.4 |
| | | 4 | 45.0 | 109.4 | 60.6 | 15.0 | 37.7 |
| | | 7 | 26.2 | 70.8 | 30.9 | 25.4 | 22.7 |
| | | 5 | 11.5 | 50.6 | 13.7 | 34.8 | 11.8 |
| | | 5 | Hemodialysis | 49.2 | | 37.2 | |
| 109 | 200-mg single dose | 7 | >70 | | 122.4 | 3.2 | 67.7 |
| | | 5 | >50–70 | | 96.4 | 5.1 | 53.0 |
| | | 6 | >30–50 | | 63.4 | 5.3 | 42.7 |
| | | 2 | 30 | | 23.6 | 12.6 | 14.2 |
| 75 | 200 mg t.i.d. for 14 days | 7 | 25–73 | | 17–78 | 6–20 | |

[a]Values are means except where ranges are specified. Abbreviations: $t_{1/2}$, half-life; fe, percentage of dose excreted unchanged in urine; t.i.d., three times daily.
[b]Expressed as glomerular filtration rate.
[c]$P < 0.001$ compared with the group with the best renal function.
[d]In milliliters per minute per 1.73 $m^2$.

Pharmacokinetic studies of ofloxacin in subjects with renal failure are summarized in Table 3. There is a decrease in the clearance of ofloxacin from plasma as reflected by 4- to 10-fold increases in plasma elimination half-life and AUC following small decreases in the clearance of creatinine or the glomerular filtration rate (28, 44, 109). This increase is particularly pronounced when creatinine clearance falls below 20 ml/min. Two metabolites of ofloxacin (desmethylofloxacin and *N*-oxide ofloxacin) have been detected in low concentrations in plasma following the administration of ofloxacin to patients with severe renal failure. Ofloxacin should be adjusted to the degree of renal impairment on the basis of its elimination profile. A dose of 200 mg every 24 h is recommended for subjects with a creatinine clearance exceeding 20 ml/min. The interval should be increased to 36 or 48 h for subjects with a creatinine clearance of less than 20 ml/min (28).

Hemodialysis slightly enhances ofloxacin elimination. The fractional removal of ofloxacin during dialysis is approximately 20% (49). However, this is below the lower limit for the definition of drug dialysability, so an additional postdialysis dose is not required. In patients undergoing dialysis, an initial dose of 200 mg followed by a dose of 100 mg after the first hemodialysis and a daily dose of 100 mg thereafter is recommended (22). In a patient undergoing CAPD, the exchanges remove less than 2% of the total dose of ofloxacin given (14).

## Enoxacin

Fifty percent of enoxacin administered is recovered unchanged in urine in healthy volunteers, and approximately 15% is found in urine as the oxo metabolite.

Limited clinical data show impairment of

**Table 4.** Pharmacokinetic parameters of various quinolones in patients with renal failure[a]

| Drug and reference | Dosage | No. of patients | Clearance (ml/min) | | | | $t_{1/2}$ (h) | fe (%) |
|---|---|---|---|---|---|---|---|---|
| | | | Creatinine | Plasma | Renal | Nonrenal | | |
| Enoxacin | | | | | | | | |
| 77 | 400-mg single dose | —[b] | >60 | 466.0 | 193.0 | 273.0 | 4.9 | |
| | | | 30–60 | 264.0 | 83.0 | 181.0 | 7.5 | |
| | | | 15–30 | 197.0 | 30.0 | 167.0 | 10.5 | |
| | | | <15 | 286.0 | 13.0 | 273.0 | 9.4 | |
| 110 | 400-mg single dose | 4 | 67–146 | 5.0[c] | 2.2 | 3.0 | 4.5 | |
| | | 4 | 34–61 | 4.0 | 1.0 | 2.6 | 8.4 | |
| | | 6 | 18–27 | 1.3 | 0.5 | 0.9 | 13.0 | |
| | | 4 | 9–15 | 1.0 | 0.2[c] | 0.8[c] | 19.8 | |
| | | 5 | 0–10 | 1.7 | | | 19.9 | |
| 12 | 200 mg b.i.d. for 7 days | 5 | 101 | 401.3 | 161.3 | 240.0 | 7.0 | 240.0 |
| | | 10 | 33 | 229.7 | 34.8 | 194.9 | 11.9 | 194.9 |
| Fleroxacin | | | | | | | | |
| 106 | 100-mg single dose | 6 | 101.8[c,d] | 1.4[e] | 0.9[e] | 0.5[e] | 13.0 | 65.2 |
| | | 6 | 55.3 | 0.8 | 0.4 | 0.4 | 17.3 | 44.1 |
| | | 7 | 7.1 | 0.6 | 0.05 | 0.6 | 24.7 | 7.9 |
| | | 7 | 4.3 | 0.6 | 0.02 | 0.5 | 28.6 | 3.0 |
| 96 | 400-mg single dose | 6 | >90 | 81.0 | 43.0 | 38.0 | 14.0 | 53.0 |
| | | 6 | 30–80 | 43.0 | 22.0 | 21.0 | 20.0 | 49.0 |
| | | 6 | 10–29 | 36.0 | 7.0 | 29.0 | 26.0 | 21.0 |
| | | 6 | 2–9 | 30.0 | 3.0 | 27.0 | 30.0 | 10.0 |
| | | 6 | Hemodialysis | | | | 25.0[f] | |

*Continued on following page*

**Table 4.** *Continued*

| Drug and reference | Dosage | No. of patients | Clearance (ml/min) | | | | $t_{1/2}$ (h) | fe (%) |
|---|---|---|---|---|---|---|---|---|
| | | | Creatinine | Plasma | Renal | Nonrenal | | |
| Lomefloxacin | | | | | | | | |
| 9 | 400-mg single dose | 8 | >80[c] | 229.2[c] | 140.4[c] | 88.7[c] | 8.09 | 60.7 |
| | | 8 | >40–80 | 192.7 | 111.2 | 81.5 | 9.11 | 56.0 |
| | | 8 | >10–40 | 77.1 | 28.4 | 48.7 | 20.90 | 29.1 |
| | | 8 | <10 | 33.8 | 0.6 | 33.2 | 44.25 | 1.0 |
| 76 | 400-mg single dose | —[g] | 80–135[c] | 209.0[c] | | | 7.5 | |
| | | | 30–60 | 111.0 | | | 18.2 | |
| | | | 15–30 | 73.0 | | | 20.3 | |
| | | | 5–15 | 43.0 | | | 26.9 | |
| 59 | 400-mg single dose | 6 | 135[c] | 259.0[c] | 199.5[c] | 59.5[c] | 7.8 | 80.6 |
| | | 6 | 47 | 74.6 | 36.3 | 38.3 | 21.3 | 38.3 |
| | | 6 | 21 | 60.6 | 14.8 | 45.8 | 34.3 | 15.7 |
| | | 6 | 7 | 59.6 | 5.1 | 54.5 | 38.1 | 5.5 |
| | | 6 | Hemodialysis | 64.2[f] | | | 29.7[f] | |
| Norfloxacin | | | | | | | | |
| 27 | 400-mg single dose | 5 | >80 | | | | | 17.9 |
| | | 5 | 30–80 | | | | 4.4 | |
| | | 6 | 10–29 | | | | 6.6 | |
| | | 7 | 2–9 | | | | 8.0 | |
| 47 | 400-mg single dose | 5 | >80 | | | | 3.1 | |
| | | 2 | 30–80 | | | | 3.3 | |
| | | 5 | 10–29 | | | | 7.1 | |
| | | 4 | <10 | | | | 8.9 | |
| 26 | 400-mg single dose | 6 | Normal | | | | 4.28 | |
| | | 3 | 15–29 | | | | 6.50 | |
| 1 | 400-mg single dose | 6 | >80 | | 233.8 | | 3.87 | |
| | | 3 | 45–80 | | 138.8 | | 5.85 | |
| | | 6 | 20–44 | | 70.6 | | 7.25 | |
| | | 5 | <20 | | 18.5 | | 8.34 | |
| Pefloxacin | | | | | | | | |
| 45 | 400-mg single dose | 10 | 128.2[d] | 128.3 | 13.4 | 114.9 | 13.0 | 10.7 |
| | | 24 | 17.8 | 90.0[h] | 3.9[i] | 80.0[h] | 16.4 | 5.2[i] |
| 71 | 8-mg/kg single dose | 7 | 10–63 | 109.0[c] | 5.1[c] | 103.9 | 15.2 | |
| | | 8 | <10 | 132.0 | | | 12.1 | |

[a]Values are means except where ranges are specified. Abbreviations: $t_{1/2}$, half-life; fe, percentage of dose excreted unchanged in urine; b.i.d., twice daily.
[b]—, total of 22.
[c]In milliliters per minute per 1.73 $m^2$.
[d]Expressed as glomerular filtration rate.
[e]In milliliters per minute per kilogram.
[f]Interdialysis period.
[g]—, total of 12.
[h]$P < 0.05$ compared with the group with the best renal function.
[i]$P < 0.01$ compared with the group with the best renal function.

the elimination of enoxacin in subjects with severe renal failure (Table 4). The clearance of both enoxacin and its major metabolite oxoenoxacin from plasma decreased and the half-life of enoxacin significantly increased in patients with measured creatinine clearances of less than 15 ml/min (77, 110). Reducing the daily enoxacin dose by half when the estimated creatinine clearance falls below 30 ml/min is therefore recommended (110). Hemodialysis does not remove significant amounts of enoxacin (114).

## Fleroxacin

Urinary recovery of unchanged fleroxacin accounts for 50 to 65% of the dose, while recovery of the *N*-desmethyl and *N*-oxide metabolites accounts for 6.5 to 11% of the dose of the parent compound.

Data concerning the disposition of fleroxacin and its metabolites in patients with renal failure show a correlation of elimination half-life with renal function, suggesting that dosage adjustments may be needed in patients with estimated glomerular filtration rates of less than 30 ml/min/1.73 m$^2$ (96–106). It is therefore recommended that the loading dose remain the same but that subsequent doses be halved. Alternatively, the maintenance dose can remain as for healthy subjects and the dosing interval can be extended to 36 to 48 h, with an additional dose given postdialysis as needed (96, 106).

## Lomefloxacin

No metabolites of lomefloxacin have been identified, and studies of healthy volunteers show that approximately 60 to 80% of a dose is recovered unchanged in urine (9, 59, 76).

In single-dose studies, lomefloxacin elimination half-life increases with increasing renal impairment (Table 4). On the basis of these results and our knowledge of the metabolism of lomefloxacin, dosage need not be adjusted in patients with estimated creatinine clearances exceeding 30 ml/min/1.73 m$^2$ (9, 76). In subjects with severe renal dysfunction, the dosage can be decreased to 200 mg daily. No supplemental dosage seems to be necessary after a hemodialysis session (59).

## Norfloxacin

A review of pharmacokinetic studies of norfloxacin with healthy volunteers reveals a bioavailability of approximately 70% and a urinary recovery of the parent compound of 30% (46). Ten percent of the administered dose is excreted in the urine as metabolites, one or two of which are thought to have some microbial activity. The elimination half-life of norfloxacin ranges from 3.5 to 6.5 h.

Significant increases in norfloxacin half-life and AUC have occurred in patients with creatinine clearances of less than 20 ml/min (Table 4). Half-life in serum has been reported to be twice the normal values for this group of patients (1, 26, 27, 47). At present, no dosage adjustments are recommended when the estimated creatinine clearance exceeds 20 ml/min. However, in the face of severe renal dysfunction, the dose can be halved or the dosing interval can be doubled (27).

## Pefloxacin

Pharmacokinetic studies of pefloxacin with healthy volunteers have demonstrated that this drug is highly metabolized and that 59% of an oral dose is excreted renally as a mixture of parent compound metabolites (33).

The elimination characteristics of patients with renal failure who are receiving pefloxacin are summarized in Table 4. The average extrarenal clearance is significantly less in patients with renal disease, resulting in a significantly higher AUC (45). In addition, patients with renal impairment have a higher renal clearance/glomerular filtration rate ratio that is attributed to the decreased reabsorption capabilities of the diseased kidney. The metabolites *N*-oxide pefloxacin and norfloxacin are more slowly eliminated, resulting in increased metabolite concentrations in plasma (45, 48). However, the rate of clearance from plasma and the volume of distribution of pefloxacin are not altered in the presence of moderate to severe renal impairment (71). This consistency can be attributed to the extensive metabolism of the drug.

While initial recommendations did not support dose modification in the presence of renal disease, subsequent evaluations assessing the possible accumulation of metabolites recommend decreasing the dosage in such situations. Patients with estimated creatinine clearances ranging from 20 to 60 ml/min should receive 55 to 66% of the dose, while those with estimated creatinine clearances of less than 20 ml/min should be given 50% of the usual recommended dose (45). CAPD patients receiving intraperitoneal pefloxacin achieved concentrations in plasma comparable to those obtained 6 h after the administration of an oral or intravenous dose (91). Hemodialysis does not remove pefloxacin to any significant extent (71).

### Conclusion

With their broad antibacterial spectra, the fluoroquinolones offer considerable potential in the treatment of infections in patients with renal diseases. The overall elimination profile favors their use in subjects with impaired renal function. According to single-dose studies performed with patients with various degrees of renal dysfunction, the use of fluoroquinolones in the presence of renal failure appears to be safe as long as the dosage or the dosing interval is adjusted to account for the estimated creatinine clearance. However, when in doubt, MICs for pathogens should be determined and dosages should be adjusted accordingly. Studies assessing parent compound and metabolite accumulations after repeated dosing are needed to further define the safety of the fluoroquinolones in the presence of renal failure.

## PHARMACOKINETICS OF FLUOROQUINOLONES IN PATIENTS WITH HEPATIC FAILURE

Fluoroquinolones can be classified according to their predominant clearance pathways. For example, ofloxacin is eliminated primarily by the kidney, while the clearance of pefloxacin is predominantly hepatic. Renal as well as hepatic mechanisms contribute to the elimination of the other fluoroquinolones. Knowledge of the relative contributions of these pathways can often guide dosing recommendations, since there is an obvious lack of data on the pharmacokinetics of fluoroquinolones in patients with hepatic insufficiency (Table 5).

### Ciprofloxacin

The pharmacokinetics of multidose administration of ciprofloxacin were not altered in seven patients with cirrhosis compared with seven matched healthy controls (32). In addition, hepatic clearance of ciprofloxacin is not altered by changes in hepatic flow or the presence of concomitant renal failure. Mild to moderate cirrhosis does not require dosage adjustments (31).

### Fleroxacin

Altered systemic and renal clearances of fleroxacin and its two major metabolites, *N*-demethylfleroxacin and *N*-oxide fleroxacin, were observed in patients with cirrhosis and ascites compared with both healthy volunteers and cirrhotics without ascites (8). As a result of a significant increase in fleroxacin elimination half-life, a 50% decrease in the fleroxacin dose is recommended for cirrhotic patients with ascites.

### Ofloxacin

Approximately 75% of an oral or intravenous dose of ofloxacin is eliminated unchanged in the urine in 24 h, indicating relatively no first-pass effect (60). According to this pharmacokinetic profile, no dosing changes should be required in the presence of hepatic insufficiency. However, a delayed elimination half-life of ofloxacin was observed in 12 cirrhotic patients with normal serum creatinine. Mean total clearance was 2.3 times lower than clearances in controls as a result of a significant decrease in renal clearance of the drug (94). Since a discrepancy between serum creatinine and creatinine is expected in patients with cirrhosis and can be attributed in part to impairment of the

**Table 5.** Pharmacokinetics of quinolones in patients with hepatic failure[a]

| Drug and reference | Dosage | No. of patients | Clearance (ml/min) | | | $t_{1/2}$ (h) | $V$ (liters/kg) | fe (%) |
|---|---|---|---|---|---|---|---|---|
| | | | Plasma | Renal | Nonrenal | | | |
| Ciprofloxacin (32) | 750 mg p.o. q12h for 5 days | 7 cirrhotics | 764.7 | 213.3 | | 3.5 | 2.8 | 27.6 |
| | | 7 volunteers | 840.3 | 200.0 | | 3.7 | 3.5 | 22.1 |
| Fleroxacin | | | | | | | | |
| 8 | 400 mg p.o. or i.v. | 6 with no ascites | 91.6[b] | 33.3 | 58.3 | 16.6 | 94[c] | 37.2 |
| | | 6 with ascites | 50.0 | 20.0 | 30.0 | 29.6 | 98[c] | 32.1 |
| | | 12 volunteers | 113.3 | 48.3 | 65.0 | 14.1 | 100[c] | 36.2 |
| 42 | 800 mg p.o. daily for 5 days | 9 cholecystectomies | 85.1 | 37.7 | 27.4 | 10.5 | 1.4 | |
| Lomefloxacin (58) | 400-mg single dose | 12 cirrhotics | 150.3[d] | 88.9[d] | 61.6[d] | 9.2 | | 55.7 |
| Ofloxacin (94) | 200-mg single dose | 12 cirrhotics | 96.0[e] | 77.0[e] | 28.0 | 11.6[e] | 1.2[e] | 64.0[f] |
| | | 12 volunteers | 222.0 | 190.0 | 30.0 | 7.0 | 1.8 | 88.0 |
| Pefloxacin | | | | | | | | |
| 17 | 8-mg/kg single dose | 16 cirrhotics | 44.3[d] | 12.6[d] | 38.2[d] | 35.1 | 1.5 | |
| 13 | 400-mg single dose | 10 cirrhotics | 45.2[g] | | | 29.0[g] | 1.1[g] | |
| | | 8 volunteers | 114.2 | | | 12.3 | 1.7 | |

[a]Values are means. Abbreviations: $t_{1/2}$, half-life; $V$, volume of distribution; fe, percentage of dose excreted unchanged in urine; p.o., perorally; q12h, every 12 h; i.v., intravenously.
[b]Data for intravenous administration.
[c]In liters.
[d]In milliliters per minute per 1.73 $m^2$.
[e]$P < 0.001$.
[f]$P < 0.05$.
[g]$P < 0.01$.

tubular handling of ofloxacin (78), ofloxacin may accumulate in cirrhotic patients despite acceptable estimated creatinine clearances. Therefore, individualized dosing adjustments may be required for patients with cirrhosis.

### Pefloxacin

Pefloxacin disposition is altered in patients with cirrhosis. A smaller volume of distribution has been observed and could be attributed to a reduction in the extent of protein binding, decreased blood volume, impaired tissue penetration, or decreased erythrocyte penetration (95). Clearance is also markedly decreased, leading to an increased half-life of the parent compound. Nonrenal clearance of pefloxacin may also be affected in patients with cirrhosis (13, 17). These results may warrant an increase in the dosing interval of pefloxacin in patients with cirrhosis. However, additional studies are needed to evaluate pharmacokinetic parameters after repeated dosing.

### Lomefloxacin

Information regarding lomefloxacin kinetics in liver impairment is limited. In 12 cirrhotic subjects each receiving a single dose of lomefloxacin, no significant relationship between nonrenal clearance and degree of severity of liver disease was observed. Overall, pharmacokinetic parameters in these patients were comparable to those observed in healthy subjects (58).

### Conclusion

Pharmacokinetic evaluations of fluoroquinolone disposition in patients with cirrhosis are few and involve mostly single-dose administration of the fluoroquinolones to small groups of cirrhotics. Judging from available data, the dosing interval of pefloxacin could be increased in patients with liver failure. Limited data concerning other fluoroquinolones do not at this time warrant dosage alterations in patients with liver failure.

## PHARMACOKINETICS OF FLUOROQUINOLONES IN PATIENTS WITH CF

A long-standing debate in the treatment of patients with CF revolves around the purported benefits of antimicrobial therapy directed against *Pseudomonas aeruginosa*, especially in view of the improved survival rate seen in these patients over the past 20 years. Although the advantages of using antibiotics in acute pulmonary exacerbations have been well demonstrated, the aggressiveness of antibiotic therapy is still debated (11, 35, 40, 52, 54, 55, 72, 80, 82, 87, 97).

The Cystic Fibrosis Center in Copenhagen is among the proponents of an aggressive approach requiring elective admission every 3 to 4 months for a 2-week course of intravenous antipseudomonal antibiotic therapy (80, 82). Workers at the center claim an increased 10-year survival rate when this approach is used. This method of treatment is subject to criticism, as it can lead to selection of resistant colonies, which will eventually require modification of the therapeutic regimen.

Workers at the Cystic Fibrosis Clinic at the Hospital for Sick Children in Toronto recently reported their experience over the last 13 years in treating acute exacerbations with antibiotics only (54). Although the report focused on the prevalence of *P. aeruginosa* colonization and its implication for the survival rate, the authors question the justification for aggressive antimicrobial therapy directed against *P. aeruginosa*. Furthermore, those investigators report a 10-year survival rate, which is similar to that reported by the Danish center.

With the advent of potent oral antipseudomonal antibiotics such as fluoroquinolones, the antimicrobial treatment of CF patients may change. This section critically reviews the pharmacokinetics of fluoroquinolones in CF patients. A recent editorial on ciprofloxacin claims that it is the ideal drug for managing CF patients in their late teens who have persistent *P. aeruginosa* infection

(41). In addition, reviews of the pharmacokinetics of drugs in CF patients have focused on the altered drug disposition observed in this population and have added to the expanding volume of knowledge on the pathophysiology of CF (19, 50, 84, 85, 102).

Data are more convincing when they originate from controlled studies and when healthy subjects are matched for weight, age, and gender. Table 6 displays data from seven controlled studies using ciprofloxacin. Five of these studies demonstrated changes in ciprofloxacin disposition in CF patients compared with controls, indicating a faster rate of elimination as evidenced by increased clearance and a shorter half-life (5, 18, 57, 105). None of those investigators studied the fates of ciprofloxacin metabolites in serum, which could have provided insights into the role of drug metabolism in altered drug disposition in this population. Conflicting results among these studies may be explained by the heterogeneity of CF patients and differences in study conditions, such as when the pharmacokinetic profile is determined on a busy ward after the first dose of an acute-phase treatment as opposed to during an infection-free period in the controlled environment of a clinical pharmacokinetic unit.

The pharmacokinetics of pefloxacin, ofloxacin, enoxacin, and fleroxacin obtained in a controlled manner are summarized in Table 7. Altered disposition was generally observed in the CF group. Patients treated with pefloxacin showed a trend toward increasing nonrenal clearance, while the pharmacokinetic profiles of those receiving enoxacin were not different from those of the control group. Conversely, CF patients receiving ofloxacin showed a significantly shorter half-life, decreased volume of distribution, and increased clearance from plasma compared with the control group. In our own evaluation of fleroxacin pharmacokinetics, the formation clearances of *N*-demethyl and *N*-oxide fleroxacin were significantly greater in CF patients than in control subjects (69). Along with the significant increase in renal clearance of fleroxacin and its metabolites, these results support the theories of generalized induction of drug metabolism

**Table 6.** Controlled pharmacokinetic studies of ciprofloxacin in patients with CF

| Reference | Patient group | No. of patients | Single dose[a] | Results[b] |
|---|---|---|---|---|
| 4 | Control | 11 | 500 mg p.o. | No significant difference in pharmacokinetic parameters |
| | CF | 6 | 1,000 mg p.o. | |
| 57 | Control | 12 | 500 mg p.o. | ↓Plasma concn, $\downarrow t_{1/2}$, $\downarrow V_{ss}/F$ |
| | CF | 11 | | |
| 18 | Control | 12 | 750 mg p.o. | ($\uparrow CL_{NR}$) |
| | CF | 12 | 200 mg i.v. | |
| 100 | Control | 8 | 750 mg p.o. | ($\downarrow t_{1/2}$) |
| | CF | 8 | | |
| 86 | Control | 6 | 750 mg p.o. | No significant difference in pharmacokinetic parameters |
| | CF | 6 | | |
| 105 | Control | 8 | 15 mg/kg p.o. | $\uparrow F$, $\uparrow CL$, $\uparrow V_{ss}$ |
| | CF | 5 | 3–4 mg/kg i.v. | |
| 5 | Control | 9 | 3.5 mg/kg i.v. | ↓Plasma concn, $\uparrow CL$, $\uparrow CL_{NR}$ $\uparrow V_{ss}$ |
| | CF | 9 | | |

[a]p.o., perorally; i.v., intravenously.
[b]Results in parenthesis are not statistically significant. Abbreviations: $t_{1/2}$, half-life; $V_{ss}$, apparent volume of distribution; $F$, bioavailability; $CL_{NR}$, nonrenal clearance; CL, total clearance.

**Table 7.** Controlled pharmacokinetic studies of quinolones in patients with CF

| Drug (reference) | Patient group | No. of patients | Dose[a] | Results[b] |
|---|---|---|---|---|
| Pefloxacin (100) | Control | 8 | 400 mg p.o. | (↑$CL_{NR}$) |
| | CF | 8 | 400 mg i.v. | |
| Ofloxacin (38) | Control | 12 | 200 mg p.o. | ↓$t_{1/2}$, ↓$V_{ss}/F$, ↑$CL/F$ |
| | CF | 8 | | |
| Enoxacin (103) | Control | 8 | 300–400 mg p.o. | No significant difference in pharmacokinetic parameters |
| | CF | 6 | | |
| Fleroxacin (69) | Control | 12 | 800 mg p.o. | ↓$V_{ss}/F$, ↑$CL_R$ |
| | CF | 13 | 800 mg p.o.[c] | |

[a]p.o., perorally; i.v., intravenously. All trials used single doses unless otherwise specified.
[b]Results in parenthesis are not statistically significant. $CL_{NR}$, nonrenal clearance; $t_{1/2}$, half-life; $V_{ss}$, apparent volume of distribution; $F$, bioavailability; CL, total clearance; $CL/F$, apparent total clearance; $CL_R$, renal clearance.
[c]Multiple-dose trial.

and a defective process of renal tubular reabsorption of drugs in patients with CF.

Fluoroquinolones are among the drugs showing modified pharmacokinetic behavior in CF patients. In most controlled studies, patients with CF showed lower concentrations in serum and increased total clearance compared with control subjects. Consequently, a higher-than-usual dosage or a shorter administration interval is often required in CF patients to compensate for these pharmacokinetic changes. Unfortunately, controlled pharmacokinetic studies are few and sample sizes are small as a result of the pathophysiology and prevalence of the disease. In addition, several pharmacokinetic studies of fluoroquinolones did not benefit from a control group (36, 81, 98, 104).

There is evidence of altered disposition of the fluoroquinolones in CF patients. The decreased elimination half-life, increased total body and nonrenal clearances, bioavailability, and volume of distribution warrant caution in the dosing of these drugs in both prophylactic and acute-phase treatments of patients with CF. Dosage regimens for ciprofloxacin (750 mg two or three times daily) in the upper portion of the recommended range seem to be the norm rather than the exception. The rationale for this approach is based not only on the pharmacokinetics but also on the clinical efficacy of this drug.

## REFERENCES


1. **Arrigo, G., G. Cavaliere, G. D'Amico, E. Passarella, and G. Broccali.** 1985. Pharmacokinetics of norfloxacin in chronic renal failure. *Int. J. Clin. Pharmacol. Ther. Toxicol.* **23:**491–496.
2. **Ball, A. P., C. Fox, M. E. Ball, I. R. F. Brown, and J. V. Willis.** 1986. Pharmacokinetics of oral ciprofloxacin, 100 mg single dose, in volunteers and elderly patients. *J. Antimicrob. Chemother.* **17:**629–635.
3. **Bayer, A., A. Gajewska, M. Stephens, J. M. Stark, and J. Pathy.** 1987. Pharmacokinetics of ciprofloxacin in the elderly. *Respiration* **51:**292–295.
4. **Bender, S. W., A. Dlahoff, P. M. Shah, R. Strehl, and H. G. Posselt.** 1986. Ciprofloxacin pharmacokinetics in patients with cystic fibrosis. *Infection* **14:**17–21.
5. **Bentur, Y., M. Spino, R. Gold, et al.** 1990. Enhanced ciprofloxacin clearance in cystic fibrosis patients. *Clin. Pharmacol. Ther.* **47:**185.
6. **Bergan, T., A. Dalhoff, and R. Rohwedder.** 1988. Pharmacokinetics of ciprofloxacin. *Infection* **16**(Suppl. 1):S3–S13.
7. **Bergan, T., S. B. Thorsteinsson, R. Rohwedder, and H. Scholl.** 1989. Elimination of ciprofloxacin and three major metabolites and consequences of reduced renal function. *Chemotherapy* **35:**395–405.
8. **Blouin, R. A., B. A. Hamelin, D. A. Smith, T. S. Foster, W. J. John, and H. A. Welker.** 1992. Fleroxacin pharmacokinetics in patients with liver cirrhosis. *Antimicrob. Agents Chemother.* **36:**632–638.

9. **Blum, R. A., R. W. Schultz, and J. J. Schentag.** 1990. Pharmacokinetics of lomefloxacin in renally compromised patients. *Antimicrob. Agents Chemother.* **34:**2364–2368.
10. **Boelaert, J., Y. Valcke, M. Schurgers, et al.** 1985. The pharmacokinetics of ciprofloxacin in patients with impaired renal function. *J. Antimicrob. Chemother.* **16:**87–93.
11. **Bosso, J. A., and P. G. Black.** 1988. Efficacy of ciprofloxacin in patients with cystic fibrosis. *DICP Ann. Pharmacother.* **22:**551–553.
12. **Bury, R. W., G. J. Becker, P. S. Kincaid-Smith, R. F. W. Moulds, and J. A. Withworth.** 1987. Elimination of enoxacin in renal disease. *Clin. Pharmacol. Ther.* **41:**434–438.
13. **Cardey, J., C. Silvain, S. Bouquet, et al.** 1987. Oral pharmacokinetics and ascitic fluid penetration of pefloxacin in cirrhosis. *Eur. J. Pharmacol.* **33:**469–472.
14. **Chan, M. K., P. Y. Chau, and W. W. N. Chan.** 1987. Ofloxacin pharmacokinetics in patients on continuous ambulatory peritoneal dialysis. *Clin. Nephrol.* **28:**277–280.
15. **Cogo, R., R. Rimoldi, R. Mattina, and B. P. Imbimbo.** 1992. Steady-state pharmacokinetics of rufloxacin in elderly patients with lower respiratory tract infections. *Ther. Drug Monit.* **14:**36–41.
16. **Crome, P., and P. J. Morrison.** 1991. Pharmacokinetics of a single dose of lomefloxacin in healthy elderly volunteers. *Drug Invest.* **3:**183– 187.
17. **Danan, G., G. Montay, R. Cunci, and S. Erlinger.** 1985. Pefloxacin kinetics in cirrhosis. *Clin. Pharmacol. Ther.* **38:**439–442.
18. **Davis, R. L., J. R. Koup, J. Williams-Warren, A. Weber, L. Heggen, D. Stempel, and A. L. Smith.** 1987. Pharmacokinetics of ciprofloxacin in cystic fibrosis. *Antimicrob. Agents Chemother.* **31:**915–919.
19. **de Groot, R., and A. L. Smith.** 1987. Antibiotic pharmacokinetics in cystic fibrosis: differences and clinical significance. *Clin. Pharmacokinet.* **13:**28–53.
20. **Dirksen, M. S. C., and T. B. Vree.** 1986. Pharmacokinetics of intravenously administered ciprofloxacin in intensive care patients with acute renal failure. *Pharm. Weekbl.* **8:**359.
21. **Dobbs, B. R., L. R. Gazely, A. J. Campbell, and I. R. Edwards.** 1987. The effect of age on the pharmacokinetics of enoxacin. *J. Clin. Pharmacol.* **33:**101–104.
22. **Dörfler, A., W. Schultz, F. Burkhardt, and M. Zichner.** 1987. Pharmacokinetics of ofloxacin in patients on haemodialysis treatment. *Drugs* **34**(Suppl. 1):62–70.
23. **Dow, J., and A. M. Frydman.** 1988. Single- and multiple-dose pharmacokinetics of pefloxacin in ly patients. *Rev. Infect. Dis.* **10**(Suppl. 1):S107.
24. **Drusano, G. L., M. Weir, A. Forrest, K. Plaisance, T. Emm, and H. C. Standiford.** 1987. Pharmacokinetics of intravenously administered ciprofloxacin in patients with various degrees of renal function. *Antimicrob. Agents Chemother.* **31:**860–864.
25. **Dryden, M. S., A. J. Wing, and I. Phillips.** 1991. Low dose intraperitoneal ciprofloxacin for the treatment of peritonitis in patients receiving continuous ambulatory peritoneal dialysis (CAPD). *J. Antimicrob. Chemother.* **28:**131–139.
26. **Eandi, M., I. Viano, F. Di Nola, L. Leone, and E. Genazzani.** 1983. Pharmacokinetics of norfloxacin in healthy volunteers and patients with renal and hepatic damage. *Eur. J. Clin. Microbiol. Infect. Dis.* **2:**253–259.
27. **Fillastre, J. P., T. Hannedouche, A. Leroy, and G. Humbert.** 1984. Pharmacokinetics of norfloxacin in renal failure. *J. Antimicrob. Chemother.* **14:**439.
28. **Fillastre, J. P., A. Leroy, and G. Humbert.** 1987. Ofloxacin pharmacokinetics in renal failure. *Antimicrob. Agents Chemother.* **31:**156–160.
29. **Fleming, L. W., T. A. Moreland, A. C. Scott, W. K. Stewart, and L. O. White.** 1987. Ciprofloxacin in plasma and peritoneal dialysate after oral therapy in patients on continuous ambulatory peritoneal dialysis. *J. Antimicrob. Chemother.* **19:**493–503.
30. **Forrest, A., M. Weir, K. I. Plaisance, et al.** 1988. Relationships between renal function and disposition of oral ciprofloxacin. *Antimicrob. Agents Chemother.* **32:**1537–1540.
31. **Fraise, A. P., and S. P. Smith.** 1990. Ciprofloxacin in combined renal and hepatic impairment. *J. Antimicrob. Chemother.* **25:**297–303.
32. **Frost, R. W., J. T. Lettieri, G. Krol, E. C. Shamblen, and K. C. Lasseter.** 1989. The effect of cirrhosis on the steady-state pharmacokinetics of oral ciprofloxacin. *Clin. Pharmacol. Ther.* **45:**608–616.
33. **Frydman, A. M., Y. Le Roux, M. A. Lefebvre, F. Djebbar, J. B. Fourtillan, and J. Gaillot.** Pharmacokinetics of pefloxacin after repeated intravenous and oral administration (400 mg bid) in young healthy volunteers. *J. Antimicrob. Chemother.* **17**(Suppl. B):65–79.
34. **Gasser, T. C., S. C. Ebert, P. H. Graversen, and P. O. Madsen.** 1987. Ciprofloxacin pharmacokinetics in patients with normal and impaired renal function. *Antimicrob. Agents Chemother.* **31:**709–712.
35. **Gold, R., S. Carpenter, H. Heurter, M. Corey, and H. Levison.** 1987. Randomized trial of ceftazidime versus placebo in the management of acute respiratory exacerbations in patients with cystic fibrosis. *Pediatrics* **111:**907–913.

36. **Goldfarb, J., G. P. Wormser, M. A. Inchiosa, Jr., et al.** 1986. Single-dose pharmacokinetics of oral ciprofloxacin in patients with cystic fibrosis. *J. Clin. Pharmacol.* **26:**222-226.
37. **Graber, H., E. Ludwig, M. Arr, and P. Lanyi.** 1988. Pharmacokinetics of ofloxacin in young and elderly patients. *Rev. Infect. Dis.* **10**(Suppl. 1):S106.
38. **Grenier, B., R. Thompson, M. Guillot, et al.** 1989. Use of quinolones in cystic fibrosis. *Rev. Infect. Dis.* **11**(Suppl. 5):1245-1252.
39. **Guay, D. R. P., W. M. Auni, P. K. Peterson, S. Obaid, R. Breitenbucher, and G. R. Matzke.** 1987. Pharmacokinetics of ciprofloxacin in acutely ill and convalescent elderly patients. *Am. J. Med.* **82**(Suppl. 4A):124-129.
40. **Guggenbichler, J. P., and J. Schneeberger.** 1987. Antimicrobial chemotherapy in patients with cystic fibrosis. *Infection* **15:**397-402.
41. **Hawkey, P. M.** 1989. Where are we now with ciprofloxacin? *J. Antimicrob. Chemother.* **24:**477-483.
42. **Hayton, W. L., V. Vlahov, N. Bacracheva, et al.** 1990. Pharmacokinetics and biliary concentrations of fleroxacin in cholecystectomized patients. *Antimicrob. Agents Chemother.* **34:**2375-2380.
43. **Hirata, C. A., R. P. Guay, W. M. Awni, D. J. Stein, and P. K. Peterson.** 1989. Steady-state pharmacokinetics of intravenous and oral ciprofloxacin in elderly patients. *Antimicrob. Agents Chemother.* **33:**1927-1931.
44. **Höffler, D., and P. Koeppe.** 1987. Pharmacokinetics of ofloxacin in healthy subjects and patients with impaired renal function. *Drugs* **34**(Suppl. 1):51-55.
45. **Höffler, D., I. Schäfer, P. Koeppe, and F. Sörgel.** 1988. Pharmacokinetics of pefloxacin in normal and impaired renal function. *Drug Res.* **38:**739-743.
46. **Holmes, B., R. N. Brogden, and D. M. Richards.** 1985. Norfloxacin. A review of its antibacterial activity, pharmacokinetic properties and therapeutic use. *Drugs* **30:**482-513.
47. **Hughes, P. J., D. B. Webb, and A. W. Asscher.** 1984. Pharmacokinetics of norfloxacin (MK 366) in patients with impaired kidney function—some preliminary results. *J. Antimicrob. Chemother.* **13**(Suppl. B):55-57.
48. **Jungers, P., D. Ganeval, B. Prieur, and G. Montay.** 1987. Steady-state levels of pefloxacin and its metabolites in patients with severe renal impairment. *Eur. J. Clin. Pharmacol.* **33:**463-467.
49. **Kampf, D., K. Borner, and A. Pustelnik.** 1990. Pharmacokinetics of ofloxacin and adequacy of maintenance dose for patients on hemodialysis. *J. Antimicrob. Chemother.* **26**(Suppl. D):61-68.
50. **Kearns, G. L., and M. D. Reed.** 1989. Clinical pharmacokinetics in infants and children: a reappraisal. *Clin. Pharm.* **17**(Suppl. 1):29-67.
51. **Kees, F., K. G. Naber, G. P. Meyer, and H. Grobecker.** 1989. Pharmacokinetics of ciprofloxacin in elderly patients. *Drug Res.* **39:**523-527.
52. **Kelly, H. W.** 1984. Antibiotic use in cystic fibrosis. *DICP Ann. Pharmacother.* **18:**772-784.
53. **Kelly, K. G., N. B. Deany, J. Lavan, and J. Noel.** 1988. Chronic dose urinary and serum pharmacokinetics of norfloxacin in the elderly. *Br. J. Clin. Pharmacol.* **26:**787-790.
54. **Kerem, E., M. Corey, R. Gold, and H. Levison.** 1990. Pulmonary function and clinical course in patients with cystic fibrosis after pulmonary colonization with *Pseudomonas aeruginosa. J. Pediatr.* **116:**714-719.
55. **Kuhn, R. J., and M. C. Nahata.** 1985. Therapeutic management of cystic fibrosis. *Clin. Pharm.* **4:**555-565.
56. **LeBel, M., G. Barbeau, M. G. Bergeron, D. Roy, and F. Vallée.** 1986. Pharmacokinetics of ciprofloxacin in elderly subjects. *Pharmacotherapy* **6:**87-91.
57. **LeBel, M., M. G. Bergeron, F. Vallée, C. Fiset, G. Chassé, P. Bigonesse, and G. Rivard.** 1986. Pharmacokinetics and pharmacodynamics of ciprofloxacin in cystic fibrosis patients. *Antimicrob. Agents Chemother.* **30:**260-266.
58. **LeBrec, D., C. Gaudin, and J. P. Benhamour.** 1992. Pharmacokinetics of lomefloxacin in patients with cirrhosis. *Am. J. Med.* **92**(Suppl. 4A):41S-44S.
59. **Leroy, A., J. P. Fillastre, and G. Humbert.** 1990. Lomefloxacin pharmacokinetics in subjects with normal and impaired renal function. *Antimicrob. Agents Chemother.* **34:**17-20.
60. **Lode, H., P. Hoffken, B. Olschewski, A. Sievers, A. Kirch, K. Borner, and P. Koeppe.** 1987. Pharmacokinetics of ofloxacin after parenteral and oral administration. *Antimicrob. Agents Chemother.* **31:**1338-1342.
61. **Loi, C. M., and R. E. Vestal.** 1988. Drug metabolism in the elderly. *Pharmacol. Ther.* **36:**131-149.
62. **Ludlam, H. A., I. Barton, and I. Phillips.** 1990. Short course ciprofloxacin therapy for CAPD peritonitis. *J. Antimicrob. Chemother.* **26:**162-164.
63. **Ludlam, H. A., I. Barton, L. White, C. McMullin, A. King, and I. Phillips.** 1990. Intraperitoneal ciprofloxacin for the treatment of peritonitis in patients receiving continuous ambulatory peritoneal dialysis. *J. Antimicrob. Chemother.* **25:**843-851.
64. **MacGowan, A. P., M. A. Greig, E. A. Clarke, L. O. White, and D. S. Reeves.** 1988. The pharmacokinetics of norfloxacin in the aged. *J. Antimicrob. Chemother.* **22:**721-727.

65. **Mahr, G., F. Sörgel, K. G. Naber, et al.** 1991. Principles of gastrointestinal secretion of quinolones in human, abstr. 585. *Program Abstr. 31st Intersci. Conf. Antimicrob. Agents Chemother.*
66. **Mattina, R., G. Bonfiglio, C. E. Cocuzza, G. Gulisano, M. Cesana, and B. P. Imbimbo.** 1991. Pharmacokinetics of rufloxacin in healthy volunteers after repeated oral doses. *Chemotherapy* **37:**389–397.
67. **Mayersohn, M. B.** 1992. Special pharmacokinetic considerations in the elderly, p. 9.1–9.43. *In* W. E. Evans, J. J. Schentag, and W. J. Jusko (ed.), *Applied Pharmacokinetics. Principles of Therapeutic Drug Monitoring.* Applied Therapeutics Inc., Vancouver, Wash.
68. **Miles Canada Inc.** CIPRO® (ciprofloxacin). Etobicoke, 1990.
69. **Mimeault, J., F. Vallée, R. Seelman, F. Sörgel, M. Ruel, and M. LeBel.** 1990. Altered disposition of fleroxacin in patients with cystic fibrosis. *Clin. Pharmacol. Ther.* **47:**618–628.
70. **Molinaro, M., P. Villani, M. B. Regazzi, R. Rondanelli, and G. Doveri.** 1992. Pharmacokinetic of oflòxacin in elderly patients and in healthy young subjects. *Eur. J. Clin. Pharmacol.* **43:**105–107.
71. **Montay, G., C. Jacquot, J. Bariety, and R. Cunci.** 1985. Pharmacokinetics of pefloxacin in renal insufficiency. *Eur. J. Clin. Pharmacol.* **29:**345–349.
72. **Mouton, J. W., and K. F. Kerrebijn.** 1990. Antibacterial therapy in cystic fibrosis. *Med. Clin. N. Am.* **74:**836–851.
73. **Naber, K. G., F. Sörgel, F. Gutzler, and B. Bartosik-Wich.** 1986. In vitro activity, pharmacokinetics, clinical safety and therapeutic efficacy of enoxacin in the treatment of patients with complicated urinary tract infections. *Infection* **14**(Suppl. 3)**:**S203–S208.
74. **Naber, K. G., F. Sörgel, F. Kees, U. Jaehde, and H. Schumacher.** 1989. Brief report: pharmacokinetics of ciprofloxacin in young (healthy volunteers) and elderly patients, and concentrations in prostatic fluid, seminal fluid, and prostatic adenoma tissue following intravenous administration. *Am. J. Med.* **87**(Suppl. 5A)**:**57S–59S.
75. **Nakano, H., A. Nihira, A. Kamiya, and R. Hori.** 1985. Influence of renal impairment on multiple-dose pharmacokinetics of ofloxacin, p. 63–68, abstr. 11. *24th Intersci. Conf. Antimicrob. Agents Chemother.*
76. **Nilsen, O. G., E. Saltvedt, R. A. Walstad, and S. Marstein.** 1992. Single-dose pharmacokinetics of lomefloxacin in patients with normal and impaired renal function. *Am. J. Med.* **92**(Suppl. 4A)**:**38S–40S.
77. **Nix, D. E., R. W. Schultz, R. W. Frost, et al.** 1988. The effect of renal impairment and haemodialysis on single dose pharmacokinetics of oral enoxacin. *J. Antimicrob. Chemother.* **21**(Suppl. B)**:**87–95.
78. **Papadakis, M. A., and A. I. Arieff.** 1987. Unpredictability of clinical evaluation of renal function in cirrhosis. *Am. J. Med.* **82:**945–952.
79. **Parry, M. F., D. A. Smego, and M. A. Digiovanni.** 1988. Hepatobiliary kinetics and excretion of ciprofloxacin. *Antimicrob. Agents Chemother.* **32:**982–985.
80. **Pedersen, S. S., T. Jensen, N. Hoiby, C. Koch, and E. W. Flensborg.** 1987. Management of *Pseudomonas aeruginosa* lung infection in Danish cystic fibrosis patients. *Acta Paediatr. Scand.* **76:**955–961.
81. **Pedersen, S. S., T. Jensen, and E. F. Hvidberg.** 1987. Comparative pharmacokinetics of ciprofloxacin and ofloxacin in cystic fibrosis patients. *J. Antimicrob. Chemother.* **20:**575–583.
82. **Pedersen, S. S., T. Jensen, T. Pressler, N. Hoiby, and K. Rosendal.** 1986. Does centralized treatment of cystic fibrosis increase the risk of *Pseudomonas aeruginosa* infection? *Acta Paediatr. Scand.* **75:**840–845.
83. **Plaisance, K., G. Drusano, A. Forrest, M. Weir, and H. Standiford.** 1987. The effect of renal function on the bioavailability of ciprofloxacin. *Clin. Pharmacol. Ther.* **41:**195.
84. **Prandota, J.** 1987. Drug disposition in cystic fibrosis: progress in understanding pathophysiology and pharmacokinetics. *Pediatr. Infect. Dis. J.* **6:**11–26.
85. **Prandota, J.** 1988. Clinical pharmacology of antibiotics and other drugs in cystic fibrosis. *Drugs* **35:**542–578.
86. **Reed, M. D., R. C. Stern, C. M. Myers, T. S. Yamashita, and J. L. Blumer.** 1988. Lack of unique ciprofloxacin pharmacokinetic characteristics in patients with cystic fibrosis. *J. Clin. Pharmacol.* **28:**691–699.
87. **Regelmann, W. E., G. R. Elliot, W. J. Warwick, and C. C. Clawson.** 1990. Reduction of sputum *Pseudomonas aeruginosa* density by antibiotics improves lung function in cystic fibrosis more than do bronchodilators and chest physiotherapy alone. *Am. Rev. Respir. Dis.* **141:**914–921.
88. **Roberts, D. E., D. B. Webb, and A. W. Ascher.** 1985. Ciprofloxacin pharmacokinetics in subjects with normal and impaired renal function. *J. Pharm. Pharmacol.* **37:**159P.
89. **Rohwedder, R., T. Bergan, S. B. Thorsteinssen, and H. Scholl.** 1990. Transintestinal elimination of ciprofloxacin. *Chemotherapy* **36:**77–84.

90. **Schentag, J. J., and F. Goss.** 1992. Quinolone pharmacokinetics in the elderly. *Am. J. Med.* **92**(Suppl. 4A):33S–37S.
91. **Schmit, J. L., L. Hary, P. Bou, H. Renaud, P. F. Westeel, M. Andrejak, and A. Fournier.** 1991. Pharmacokinetics of single-dose intravenous, oral, and intraperitoneal pefloxacin in patients on chronic dialysis. *Antimicrob. Agents Chemother.* **35:**1492–1494.
92. **Shah, P. M.** 1986. Effect of co-medication on absorption of ciprofloxacin and ofloxacin from gastrointestinal tract. *Quinolones Bull.* **2:**12.
93. **Shalit, I., R. B. Greenwood, M. I. Marks, J. A. Pederson, and D. L. Frederick.** 1986. Pharmacokinetics of single-dose oral ciprofloxacin in patients undergoing chronic ambulatory peritoneal dialysis. *Antimicrob. Agents Chemother.* **30:**152–156.
94. **Silvain, C., S. Bouquet, J. P. Breux, B. Brecq-Giraudon, and M. Beauchamp.** 1989. Oral pharmacokinetics and ascitic fluid penetration of ofloxacin in cirrhosis. *Eur. J. Clin. Pharmacol.* **37:**261–265.
95. **Silvain, C., J. P. Breux, E. Rochard, S. Bouquet, B. Becq-Giraudon, and M. Beauchant.** 1987. Decreased erythrocyte penetration of pefloxacin in cirrhotic patients. *J. Antimicrob. Chemother.* **20:**290–292.
96. **Singlas, E., A. Leroy, E. Sultan, et al.** 1990. Disposition of fleroxacin, a new trifluoroquinolone, and its metabolites. Pharmacokinetics in renal failure and influence of haemodialysis. *Clin. Pharmacokinet.* **19:**67–79.
97. **Smith, A. L., B. Ramsey, G. Redding, and J. Haas.** 1989. Endobronchial infection in cystic fibrosis. *Acta Paediatr. Scand.* **363:**31–36.
98. **Smith, M. J., L. O. White, H. Bowyer, J. Willis, M. E. Hodson, and J. C. Batten.** 1986. Pharmacokinetics and sputum penetration of ciprofloxacin in patients with cystic fibrosis. *Antimicrob. Agents Chemother.* **30:**614–616.
99. **Sörgel, F., K. G. Naber, U. Jaehde, A. Reiter, R. Seelman, and G. Sigl.** 1989. Brief report: gastrointestinal secretion of ciprofloxacin. *Am. J. Med.* **87**(Suppl. 5A):62S–65S.
100. **Sörgel, F., U. Stephan, H. G. Wiesemann, et al.** 1987. High dose treatment with antibiotics in cystic fibrosis—a reappraisal with special reference to the pharmacokinetics of betalactams and new fluoroquinolones in adult CF patients. *Infection* **15:**385–396.
101. **Spino, M.** 1987. The quinolones: an important new group of drugs for the elderly? *Can. Pharm. J.* **120:**242–252.
102. **Spino, M.** 1991. Pharmacokinetics of drugs in cystic fibrosis. *Clin. Rev. Allergy* **9:**169–210.
103. **Spino, M., Y. Bentur, S. Martin, et al.** 1989. Enoxacin disposition in patients with cystic fibrosis (CF) and healthy control subjects. *Eur. J. Clin. Pharmacol.* **169:**A84.
104. **Steen, H. J., E. M. Scott, M. I. Stevenson, A. E. Black, A. O. E. Redmond, and P. S. Collier.** 1989. Clinical and pharmacokinetic aspects of ciprofloxacin in the treatment of acute exacerbation of pseudomonas infection in cystic fibrosis patients. *J. Antimicrob. Chemother.* **24:**787–795.
105. **Strandvik, B., L. Hjelte, A. Lindblad, B. Ljungberg, A. S. Malmborg, and I. Nilsson-Ehle.** 1989. Comparison of efficacy of tolerance of intravenously and orally administered ciprofloxacin in cystic fibrosis patients with acute exacerbations of lung infection. *Scand. J. Infect. Dis.* **60**(Suppl):84–88.
106. **Stuck, A. E., F. Frey, P. Heizmann, R. Brandt, and E. Weidekamm.** 1989. Pharmacokinetics and metabolism of intravenous and oral fleroxacin in subjects with normal and impaired renal function and in patients on continuous ambulatory peritoneal dialysis. *Antimicrob. Agents Chemother.* **33:**373–381.
107. **Taburet, A. M., A. Devillers, P. Thomare, J. P. Fillastre, P. Veyssier, and E. Singlas.** 1990. Disposition of fleroxacin, a new trifluoroquinolone, and its metabolites. Pharmacokinetics in elderly patients. *Clin. Pharmacokinet.* **19:**80–88.
108. **Taburet, A. M., I. Landru, E. Singlas, D. Doucet, and J. P. Ryckelinck.** 1985. Pharmacocinétique de la ciprofloxacine dans l'insuffisance rénale. *J. Pharm. Clin.* **4:**511–520.
109. **Tsugaya, W., H. Washida, N. Hirao, et al.** 1985. Absorption and excretion of ofloxacin in patients with impaired renal function, p. 1769–1770. *In* J. Ishigami (ed.), *Recent Advances in Chemotherapy.* University of Tokyo Press, Tokyo.
110. **Van der Auwera, P., J. C. Stolear, and M. N. Dudley.** 1990. Pharmacokinetics of enoxacin and its oxometabolite following intravenous administration to patients with different degrees of renal impairment. *Antimicrob. Agents Chemother.* **34:**1491–1497.
111. **Veyssier, P., J. B. Fourtillan, J. Modai, et al.** 1986. Pharmacocinétique de l'ofloxacine chez le sujet âgé (65 à 85 ans) à fonction rénale normale après prise orale unique de 200 mg. *Pathol. Biol.* **34:**596–599.
112. **Webb, D. B., D. D. Roberts, J. D. Williams, and A. W. Asscher.** 1986. Pharmacokinetics of ciprofloxacin in healthy volunteers and patients with impaired kidney function. *J. Antimicrob. Chemother.* **18**(Suppl. D):83–87.
113. **Weidekamm, E.** 1987. Pharmacokinetics of fleroxacin in elderly subjects. Department of Clinical Research, Hoffmann-La Roche Inc., Nutley, N.J.
114. **White, L. O., A. P. MacGowan, I. G. Mackay, and D. S. Reeves.** 1988. The pharmacokin-

etics of ofloxacin, desmethylofloxacin N-oxide in hemodialysis patients with end-stage renal failure. *J. Antimicrob. Chemother.* **22**(Suppl. C)**:**65–72.

115. **Wise, R., S. L. Baker, M. Misra, and D. Griggs.** 1987. The pharmacokinetics of enoxacin in elderly patients. *J. Antimicrob. Chemother.* **19:**343–350.

*Quinolone Antimicrobial Agents, 2nd ed.*
Edited by David C. Hooper and John S. Wolfson


*Chapter 11*

# Drug-Drug Interactions with Fluoroquinolone Antimicrobial Agents

*David E. Nix*

Fluoroquinolones have been a welcome addition to our selection of antimicrobial agents. The in vitro potency of these agents against members of the family *Enterobacteriaceae* and *Pseudomonas aeruginosa* is unsurpassed among the orally absorbed antimicrobial agents. Current medical practice is shifting toward shorter hospital stays and more outpatient treatment of infections. Because of the intensive resources required for use of outpatient parenteral antimicrobial agents, oral agents are preferred. There is also a trend toward increased use of oral antimicrobial agents in the hospital setting, since they are less expensive to administer. Moreover, oral antimicrobial agents may be used following a short-course parenteral treatment regimen after the patient shows improvement. Because of the extensive and potentially increasing use of fluoroquinolones, concomitant use of them with other drugs will be frequent. Drug interactions must be anticipated and prevented.

## INTERACTIONS WITH FLUOROQUINOLONE ABSORPTION

Because the oral fluoroquinolones are being used increasingly for moderate to severe infections, reliability of absorption is essential. Most fluoroquinolones appear to be absorbed in the fasting state with an absolute bioavailability of 50 to 100%. The absolute bioavailability of norfloxacin is unknown but is probably about 50%. The systemic absorption of ciprofloxacin was reported as 69%, however; intersubject variability increases with higher (750-mg) oral doses (19, 65). The absolute oral bioavailability of enoxacin was 87% in patients with complicated urinary tract infections (53). Lomefloxacin and ofloxacin are completely absorbed in the fasting state (104).

Food in general has not been shown to reduce the oral bioavailability of fluoroquinolones. The time of maximal concentration is delayed slightly by food, but no change in the total area under the plasma drug concentration-time curve (AUC) is observed (25). Some of the meals have included milk, which did not appear to affect absorption (25, 37, 48). However, the ingestion of milk and yogurt in a fasting state reduced ciprofloxacin absorption by 30 and 36%, respectively (56).

### Antacids

Nalidixic acid forms chelation complexes with various metal ions that associate with the 3-carboxyl and 4-oxo substituents (55). The complex exhibits decreased lipophilicity and may not be absorbed throughout the gastro-

*David E. Nix* • The Clinical Pharmacokinetics Laboratory, Millard Fillmore Hospital, and Center for Clinical Pharmacy Research, State University of New York at Buffalo, Buffalo, New York 14209.

intestinal tract. No formal study has documented the interactions between nalidixic acid and antacids containing metal cations. In 1985, reports of reduced absorption of ciprofloxacin in the presence of antacids first appeared (35). Administration of an aluminum-magnesium antacid (Maalox; 10 30-ml doses) resulted in a decrease in the maximal ciproflaxacin concentration from 1.7 to 0.1 $\mu$g/ml following a single 500-mg ciprofloxacin dose (35). Unfortunately, the timing of antacid doses relative to ciprofloxacin administration was not reported, nor were other details of the study. A second letter to the editor reported that patients who received antacids exhibited lower antibiotic concentrations than those who did not receive antacids (67). The results were apparently collected retrospectively from a clinical study, and the details of antacid doses and time of administration were not provided.

Three studies were performed to determine the characteristics of the interaction between Maalox (aluminum-magnesium hydroxide) and a 750-mg dose of ciprofloxacin (61). Single 30-ml doses of Maalox were administered at various times before and after ciprofloxacin administration. Figure 1 shows the individual and mean relative bioavailabilities of ciprofloxacin following antacid administration at selected intervals before and after ciprofloxacin administration. Relative bioavailabilities were determined on the basis of the AUC from time 0 to infinity for ciprofloxacin administered alone for each subject. Marked reductions in ciprofloxacin absorption were observed following pretreatment with Maalox within 2 h of ciprofloxacin administration. This interaction also exhibited marked interindividual variation, particularly with the 2- and 4-h Maalox pretreatments. Although the aluminum cation has a higher affinity for ciprofloxacin than magnesium cations do, magnesium can reduce ciprofloxacin absorption when it is administered as magnesium citrate solution (12). Ciprofloxacin absorption also decreased by 40% following administration of calcium chloride tablets and by 85% following administration of aluminum hydroxide tablets (26).

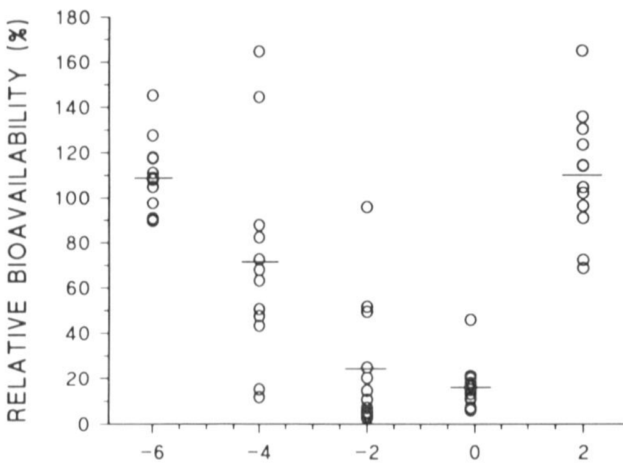


**Figure 1.** Individual (○), and mean (–) ciprofloxacin bioavailabilities when 30 ml of Maalox was administered at various times relative to administration of a single 750-mg dose of ciprofloxacin.

The magnitude of norfloxacin absorption is reduced similarly to that of ciprofloxacin following antacid pretreatments. When Maalox (30 ml) was administered 5 min prior to a 400-mg norfloxacin tablet, norfloxacin bioavailability was reduced by more than 90% (62). When the same dose of Maalox was administered 2 h after the norfloxacin dose, a 20% reduction in bioavailability resulted, which remained statistically significant. Further observations revealed that the reduction in absorption was apparent prior to the dose of Maalox, and this may reflect intraindividual variation in the rate of norfloxacin absorption. Norfloxacin absorption was also reduced 63% by a 5-min pretreatment with calcium carbonate antacid (62). Another study confirmed the reduction in norfloxacin urinary excretion following administration with aluminum and magnesium hydroxides but found no significant interaction with bismuth subsalicylate (14).

Studies with enoxacin used a high dose of antacid, i.e., 30 ml of aluminum-magnesium hydroxide therapeutic concentration (Maalox TC). Following pretreatment with Maalox TC, the mean relative bioavailabilities of enoxacin (400 mg) were 49 and 73% when the antacid was administered 2 and 0.5 h prior to the enoxacin dose, respectively (27). Enoxacin and Maalox TC were not administered concurrently. This interaction is primarily due to decreased enoxacin absorption, since a very intensive Maalox TC regimen caused only a small decrease in nonrenal clearance of intravenous enoxacin and did not affect the total clearance of enoxacin (unpublished data).

Results of studies of antacid interaction with ofloxacin are conflicting. Pretreatment with 10 doses of Maalox over 24 h resulted in a 74% decrease in ofloxacin absorption in one study (36). The timing of Maalox administration was not specified. Administration of a smaller dose of Maalox (15 ml) 2 h prior to administration of ofloxacin led to a 21% reduction in bioavailability, while ofloxacin bioavailability was not affected when the 15-ml Maalox dose was administered 2 h after ofloxacin (23). Administration of aluminum hydroxide (500 mg) with ofloxacin reduced bioavailability by 30% (3). These results suggest that ofloxacin does interact with Maalox but perhaps to a lesser extent than do ciprofloxacin, norfloxacin, and enoxacin. In contrast, concurrent administration of an aluminum phosphate (11 g) colloidal suspension did not affect ofloxacin absorption as assessed by urinary excretion data (54). In this study, aluminum phosphate was employed rather than the hydroxide salt; perhaps aluminum affinity for phosphate is higher than for ofloxacin. However, the same authors reported no reduction in ofloxacin diffusion across a rat intestinal sack in the presence of a soluble aluminum salt [$KAl(SO_4)_2 \cdot 6H_2O$] (54). Reasons for the differences are not entirely clear. When a low dose of calcium carbonate antacid (Titralac, 5 ml) was used, ofloxacin absorption was not affected when the antacid was administered 2 h prior or 2 h after ofloxacin (23). However, concurrent administration of calcium carbonate and ofloxacin led to a 26% reduction in bioavailability (3).

Administration of Maalox 2 or 4 h prior to administration of lomefloxacin produced 20 and 10% reductions in bioavailability, respectively (24). Concurrent administration of lomefloxacin and Maalox reportedly led to a 50% reduction in oral bioavailability, while administration of Maalox 2 h after administration of lomefloxacin reduced bioavailability by only 12%. Administration of lomefloxacin with aluminum hydroxide-magnesium oxide granules led to a 40% reduction in lomefloxacin absorption (83). The existence of quinolone-metal cation chelates was also further substantiated by $^{13}C$ nuclear magnetic resonance spectroscopy. Although these reductions were statistically significant, the bioavailability of lomefloxacin appears to be less affected by antacid than are the bioavailabilities of ciprofloxacin and norfloxacin.

The current treatment of peptic ulcers involves the use of antacids primarily for symptomatic relief, and dose schedules are not fixed. Moreover, antacids are available over the counter and are often used without medical supervision. Avoidance of antacids is most prudent, considering potential problems with patient compliance. However, if antacid and fluoroquinolone treatment are required, ofloxacin and lomefloxacin may be less likely than enoxacin, ciprofloxacin, and norfloxacin to interact. The antacid clearly should not be given within 2 h of a quinolone dose. Moreover, the longest possible spacing between antacid administration and the next fluoroquinolone dose should be utilized.

### Acid Suppressants

Pretreatment with ranitidine for 24 h had no effect on the oral bioavailability of ciprofloxacin or ofloxacin (36). Ranitidine was administered as 3 150-mg tablets (presumably one every 8 h), but the specific timing relative to the fluoroquinolone administrations was not stated. In a subsequent study, administration of 150 mg of ranitidine 2 h prior to administration of ciprofloxacin also had no effect on ciprofloxacin bioavailability (61). Ranitidine also did not affect the bioavailability of lomefloxacin (59). In contrast, intravenous ranitidine administered 2 h prior to administration of enoxacin led to a 40% reduction in enoxacin bioavailability (27). A second study confirmed the interaction and demonstrated that the decrease in absorption was due to an increase in the pH of gastric contents (47). Ranitidine's effect on enoxacin bioavailability was prevented by concurrent administration of ranitidine and pentagastrin such that the gastric pH remained $\leq 3$.

The absorption of temafloxacin did not appear to be affected by concomitant cimetidine administration; however, slight reductions (18 to 19%) in both renal and total clearances were noted (87). Although temafloxacin is no longer available, the inhibition of tubular secretion due to cimetidine may be a potential problem with other quinolones. Cimetidine may also decrease the nonrenal clearance of quinolones such as pefloxacin that undergo significant oxidative metabolism (86).

### Sucralfate

Sucralfate is a poorly absorbed basic aluminum salt of sucrose octasulfate. Each gram of sucralfate (Carafate) contains approximately 20 mg of aluminum cations. Administration of a 1-g sucralfate tablet 2 h prior to administration of norfloxacin or concomitantly with it led to 43 and 98% reductions in norfloxacin's bioavailability, respectively (63). Concomitant administration of ciprofloxacin and sucralfate resulted in a 98% reduction in bioavailability (60). Two hours of pretreatment with sucralfate also reduced ciprofloxacin absorption by 30%.

Interactions of sucralfate and antacids with fluoroquinolones appear to be related to the presence of metal cations in the upper gastrointestinal tract. The number of subjects exhibiting an interaction and the mean extent of interaction decrease as the time between drug administrations is increased. Moreover, sucralfate can be safely administered following the fluoroquinolone as long as sufficient time is allowed for the fluoroquinolone to be absorbed; this is usually about 2 h. Sucralfate is not currently approved by the Food and Drug Administration for twice-daily administration; however, a regimen of 2 g every 12 h may be as effective as the approved regimen of 1 g four times daily (17). It is most prudent to avoid the use of fluoroquinolones and sucralfate in combination; however, if required, the fluoroquinolone should be administered first in the morning and sucralfate can be administered 2 to 6 h later (95). This timing allows at least 6 h before the subsequent fluoroquinolone dose is given.

### Other Metal Cations

Administration of ferrous sulfate (Feosol, 325 mg) with ciprofloxacin resulted in a 64% decrease in ciprofloxacin absorption (66). Likewise, a 70% reduction in ciprofloxacin absorption resulted from ferrous fumarate administered concomitantly as a 200-mg suspension (13). Following administration of FeroGradumet (1,050 mg, two tablets) with ofloxacin, a small (10.9%) but significant reduction in ofloxacin bioavailability was observed (3). FeroGradumet is a sustained-release formulation of ferrous sulfate. It is possible that ofloxacin was absorbed prior to substantial release of iron from the formulation. Oral ferrous sulfate also produced more than a 50% reduction in norfloxacin urinary excretion (14). Considering the many different formulations and release characteristics of iron, results based on one formulation may not be generalizable.

Several multiple-vitamin preparations contain trace metals that could theoretically interact with fluoroquinolones. A multiple-vitamin preparation with zinc (Stress Tabs 600 with zinc) was shown to have a small effect on ciprofloxacin absorption, reducing bioavailability by 24% (66). Zinc sulfate decreased norfloxacin urinary excretion as well (14).

Ciprofloxacin may be useful in the treatment of patients who cannot swallow tablets, such as home health care and nursing home patients. Because there is no liquid formulation of ciprofloxacin, the tablet may be crushed and administered via nasogastric tube. Two studies have demonstrated that ciprofloxacin can be administered in this fashion with enteral feeding despite the fact that enteral feed contains some metal cations (105, 106). The metal cations are probably less available to associate with fluoroquinolones in these complex mixtures. This may also explain why milk ingested alone alters fluoroquinolone absorption (56) but milk ingested with meals does not (25, 36, 48).

## EFFECTS OF FLUOROQUINOLONES ON DRUG METABOLISM

### Theophylline

Enoxacin was the first quinolone reported to increase theophylline concentrations and lead to severe adverse reactions (51, 100). Theophylline was subsequently administered to six patients by continuous infusion until steady state was achieved (101). Then enoxacin treatment (400 to 600 mg twice daily) was initiated. On the third day of concomitant administration, the mean theophylline concentration was increased to 15.1 μg/ml from a baseline of 8.4 μg/ml, corresponding to a 42% reduction in theophylline clearance. The half-life of theophylline was prolonged such that steady state may not have been achieved by day 3. A followup study in patients receiving maintenance theophylline therapy revealed a 63.6% reduction in theophylline clearance after the addition of 400 mg of enoxacin twice daily (102). Several studies have confirmed the interaction between enoxacin and theophylline, with reported decreases in theophylline clearance of 50 to 73.6% (7, 74–76, 85). Empiric reduction in theophylline dose by 50% resulted in no significant change in theophylline concentrations (43). Once enoxacin is discontinued, the resumption of pretreatment theophylline doses should be delayed 24 to 48 h to prevent increases in theophylline concentrations.

The percentages of various quinolones eliminated as oxometabolites correlated with the extent of their theophylline interactions (102). Wijnands et al. proposed that the oxometabolites were responsible for the interaction; however, correlation does not prove causation. Studies in a rat model (21) and studies employing human liver microsomes in vitro (77) show that enoxacin rather than the oxometabolite of enoxacin produces the greatest interaction with xanthines. The extent of interaction depends on the enoxacin dose over the range of 50 to 400 mg (74). All major metabolic pathways are affected as the formations of 3-methylxanthine, 1-methyluric acid, and 1,3,-dimethyluric acid are reduced to similar extents (75).

Adverse reactions in patients treated with enoxacin and theophylline, including nausea and events involving the central nervous system, have been common (51). Seizures in patients taking fluoroquinolones have been reported only rarely, and most of the patients had an underlying neurologic problem or were receiving theophylline or certain nonsteroidal anti-inflammatory agents (42, 79, 80). In a rat model, enoxacin had no direct effect on theophylline-induced seizures (37). The total theophylline dose required to cause seizures was no different among rats receiving no treatment and rats receiving 100 or 400 mg of enoxacin per kg of body weight. Thus, at least some of the reported cases are due to elevated theophylline concentrations. Seizures have also been reported to be more common in patients receiving nonsteroidal anti-inflammatory agents, although the reason for this is not clear (79) (see chapter 27).

Theophylline clearance is inhibited by ciprofloxacin and pefloxacin; however, the magnitude of the clearance reduction is lower than that caused by enoxacin. Ciprofloxacin reduced theophylline clearance by 30.4%, while pefloxacin caused a 29.4% decrease in theophylline clearance (102). Other studies have reported 17 to 30% reductions in theophylline clearance attributable to ciprofloxacin (57, 68, 72, 78, 97, 98). Several cases involving adverse events resulting from this interaction have been reported (8, 20, 38, 70, 91). In patients with respiratory tract infections who were administered a continuous infusion of theophylline, serum theophylline concentrations increased from a mean of 7.8 to 14.6 μg/ml after the addition of ciprofloxacin twice daily (68). This interaction is probably clinically significant in patients with theophylline concentrations that are initially in the upper range of normal.

Norfloxacin, lomefloxacin, and ofloxacin appear to have minimal or no effect on theophylline clearance. In three separate studies, norfloxacin reduced theophylline clearance by 7.4, 11.3, and 14.9%, and a significant difference was detected in the latter study (11, 34, 76). Ofloxacin had no effect on theophylline clearance in two studies (4, 76), but one study detected a significant 12.1% decrease in theophylline clearance (28). Significant interactions between lomefloxacin and theophylline have not been observed (46, 58, 72, 88, 99).

Clinicians should empirically reduce theophylline doses when initiating treatment with enoxacin. Empiric decreases in theophylline dose should be considered when ciprofloxacin or pefloxacin treatment is begun in patients who have theophylline concentrations in the upper therapeutic range or who have difficulty tolerating theophylline. Moreover, serum theophylline concentrations should be monitored frequently when treatment with any of these three quinolones is initiated. In contrast, clinically significant interactions with norfloxacin, ofloxacin, and lomefloxacin are unlikely. Additional monitoring of serum theophylline concentrations should not be needed unless a problem is suspected.

### Caffeine

The same quinolones that reduce theophylline metabolism also reduce the metabolism of caffeine. Caffeine undergoes metabolic transformations that involve the enzyme systems responsible for theophylline metabolism. Enoxacin administration resulted in a 78 to 79% decrease in caffeine clearance (64, 89). Moreover, this interaction appeared to be dose dependent. Caffeine clearance was inhibited approximately 58, 64, and 78% with doses of 100, 200, and 400 mg twice daily, respectively (31). Over a dose range of 250 to 750 mg twice daily, ciprofloxacin caused a 32 to 38% reduction in caffeine clearance (30, 32, 52). However, at lower doses (100 mg of ciprofloxacin twice daily), the reduction in caffeine clearance was only 14.3% (30). Norfloxacin, ofloxacin, and lomefloxacin have not been shown to alter caffeine clearance (31, 33).

The clinical importance of the quinolone-caffeine interaction has not been well evaluated. In volunteers administered a fixed dosage of caffeine and enoxacin, caffeine concentrations were markedly increased, resulting in more adverse events involving the gastrointestinal and central nervous systems (64). Similar but less severe reactions were noted with the coadministration of caffeine and ciprofloxacin (32). In clinical settings, patients control their own caffeine intake and may actually lower their caffeine intake in response to greater central nervous system stimulation from caffeine. Further surveillance of ciprofloxacin and enoxacin use along with measurement of caffeine intake and adverse events is required to determine the significance of this interaction. Patients who are prescribed these quinolones, however, should be advised of a possible interaction with caffeine.

### Warfarin

Warfarin consists of a racemic mixture of the enantiomers *R*- and *S*-warfarin. The *S*-warfarin enantiomer is responsible for most of the pharmacologic activity and is approximately eight times more potent than *R*-warfarin. Enoxacin was shown to reduce the clearance of the *R*-enantiomer by 31.8%; however, the clearance of the *S*-enantiomer was unaffected

(93). No significant difference in the prothrombin time or factor VII concentration was observed. Ciprofloxacin was demonstrated not to prolong prothrombin time in patients stabilized on warfarin (9, 71). Similarly, norfloxacin did not alter warfarin pharmacokinetics or prothrombin times in healthy subjects (73). Despite these negative results from studies, several case reports have been published or received by the Food and Drug Administration (41, 49, 69). It is difficult to ascertain whether the reports reflect an unusual or idiosyncratic interaction or whether some other factor caused a prolongation in prothrombin time. Most reports included a patient who developed an acute infection and was treated with norfloxacin or ciprofloxacin. One patient also developed diarrhea, nausea, and vomiting prior to discovery of a prolonged prothrombin time. It is possible that the infectious process alone alters warfarin pharmacodynamics or that dietary changes related to the illness are responsible for isolated cases. To delineate whether quinolones prolong prothrombin time in patients, a large prospective controlled trial is needed.

## Miscellaneous Drugs

### Rifampin

Rifampin has been used in combination with ciprofloxacin for the treatment of staphylococcal infections. Concomitant administration of these drugs did not appear to affect the pharmacokinetics of either drug; however, the study had methodologic flaws (15). No significant alterations of either enoxacin or rifampin pharmacokinetic parameters were noted during concomitant administration of these agents following an initial 10-day pretreatment with rifampin (56a).

### Cyclosporine

Case reports have implicated fluoroquinolones for causing increases in cyclosporine concentrations (92) and for enhancing the nephrotoxicity of cyclosporine (5, 22). In contrast, to avoid the known interactions of ciprofloxacin with erythromycin and rifampin (39), others have suggested ciprofloxacin as a preferred agent in patients with legionella infections who are receiving cyclosporine. Studies performed in healthy volunteers (90) and in renal and bone marrow transplant recipients (44, 45) have not detected evidence of a pharmacokinetic or pharmacodynamic interaction between ciprofloxacin and cyclosporine.

### Probenecid

Most fluoroquinolones exhibit a renal clearance that exceeds creatinine clearance, suggesting that net tubular secretion occurs. Probenecid inhibits this tubular secretion, leading to reduced total and renal clearances of the fluoroquinolone (18, 82, 84). One study did not detect a significant interaction between fleroxacin and probenecid; however, a 26% increase in plasma AUC was observed, and only five subjects were studied (96). Ciprofloxacin exhibited a significant reduction in renal clearance when administered in combination with probenecid, but there was no significant change in total clearance (18).

### Nonsteroidal anti-inflammatory agents

Convulsions have been reported among several patients receiving both enoxacin and fenbufen, a nonsteroidal anti-inflammatory drug available in Japan. Fluoroquinolones were shown to inhibit the binding of $\gamma$-aminobutyric acid (GABA) to its brain receptors in a concentration-dependent manner (1, 40, 94). The concentrations required to inhibit 50% of the GABA binding were $10^{-5}$ M for norfloxacin and ciprofloxacin, $10^{-4}$ M for fleroxacin and enoxacin, $\geq 10^{-4}$ M for lomefloxacin, and $10^{-3}$ to $\geq 10^{-4}$ M for ofloxacin 1,40). When a constant concentration of fluoroquinolones ($1.0 \times 10^{-5}$ M) was used, the rank order of potency in inhibiting GABA receptor binding was norfloxacin > nalidixic acid > enoxacin > ofloxacin >

ciprofloxacin (94). Other investigators found enoxacin and lomefloxacin to be the most potent epileptogenic quinolones (16). It appears that the ranking of fluoroquinolones is somewhat dependent on the model system utilized. Not only do fluoroquinolones antagonize GABA receptor binding, but decreases in neuron response to GABA were also observed (29, 103). It is possible that the piperazine ring at position 7 on quinolones is responsible, since this structure closely mimics GABA (1). Nalidixic acid lacks a piperazine ring and did not induce seizures in mice. Fenbufen and biphenylacetate, a metabolite of fenbufen, greatly enhanced the effect of quinolones on inhibiting GABA receptor binding (1, 2, 29, 40, 103). The 50% inhibitory concentrations (ICs) of quinolones were reduced up to 100-fold in the presence of fenbufen and up to 1,000-fold in the presence of biphenylacetate. Other nonsteroidal anti-inflammatory agents, such as indomethacin, enhanced the effects of some quinolones on GABA binding (40).

Despite the inhibitory activity of fluoroquinolones on GABA neurons, seizures have been reported only rarely when these agents are used. The $IC_{50}$s for quinolones in the in vitro binding studies are similar to or higher than those achieved in plasma. Moreover, concentrations of quinolones in brain tissue are considerably lower than concentrations in plasma. Since most of the studies were performed using rodent or frog neurons, potential quantitative differences in the effects on human neurons must be considered. Clearly, the concomitant use of fenbufen and quinolones should be avoided. Further research is needed to establish the risk factors for quinolone-induced neurotoxicity so that this toxicity can be avoided.

See chapter 27 for further information on these agents.

## Clindamycin and metronidazole

Currently available quinolones exhibit poor activity against anaerobic bacteria; thus, concomitant use with antianaerobic agents is frequently necessary. Quinolones, including ciprofloxacin, ofloxacin, enoxacin, and fleroxacin, have been administered in combination with clindamycin and metronidazole (10). No significant pharmacokinetic interactions among these agents have been detected. Metronidazole and its metabolites can cause neurotoxicity, especially in patients with renal insufficiency when the metabolites accumulate. Case reports have implicated the combinations ciprofloxacin-metronidazole and pefloxacin-metronidazole as causes of symptoms of neurotoxicity, including seizures, involuntary movements, confusion, disorientation, and slurred speech (50, 80). However, these cases were very complicated, and several other factors may have contributed. Patients receiving a quinolone and metronidazole should be carefully monitored for any central nervous system effects.

## β-Lactams

Combinations of ciprofloxacin and an antipseudomonal penicillin have been advocated as an alternative for treating infections caused by *P. aeruginosa*. In one study, ciprofloxacin did not affect the disposition of azlocillin (6). However, the total clearance, renal clearance, nonrenal clearance, and steady-state volume of distribution of ciprofloxacin were significantly decreased. The total clearance of ciprofloxacin was reduced by 35%. Decreases in ciprofloxacin's renal clearance probably resulted from a competition with azlocillin for renal tubular secretion. The mechanism for decreased nonrenal clearance remains undetermined.

Several penicillins have been implicated in seizures in patients with renal insufficiency. The carbapenem imipenem has also been associated with seizures in a small number of patients. Seizures in a patient receiving the combination of imipenem and ciprofloxacin have been reported (81).

## CONCLUSIONS

All fluoroquinolones appear to interact with antacids containing aluminum-magnesium salts and with sucralfate. Many of the fluoroquinolones have been shown to interact with antacids containing calcium carbonate. Every patient treated with fluoroquinolones should be warned about taking these substances, as most are available over the counter and usage is widespread. Any substance containing significant amounts of a metal cation should be avoided unless the substance has been demonstrated not to interact with fluoroquinolones. Although spacing the administration times of interacting substances and fluoroquinolones may avoid an interaction, several factors must be considered. (i) Most interaction studies were performed with healthy volunteers, and patients with altered gastric emptying may react differently. (ii) Many patients are not compliant in taking medications. Expecting compliance with exact dosing times may be unreasonable. (iii) Patients may become confused or may not remember the specific instructions. If acid suppression is needed, histamine-2 antagonists may be used except with enoxacin.

Fluoroquinolones differ in their effects on theophylline metabolism. Enoxacin causes the largest decrease in theophylline metabolic clearance, while ciprofloxacin causes an intermediate effect. Norfloxacin, lomefloxacin, and ofloxacin exhibit little or no effect on theophylline metabolism. The clinical importance of this interaction varies with the fluoroquinolone employed and the initial theophylline concentration. The theophylline dose should be reduced empirically when enoxacin is started; however, theophylline dose adjustments after ciprofloxacin has been started should be made on a case-by-case basis. If the initial theophylline concentration is greater than 14 $\mu$g/ml, reduction of the theophylline dose should be considered. In any case, theophylline concentrations should be closely monitored when treatment with enoxacin or ciprofloxacin is initiated. Interactions between ofloxacin, norfloxacin, lomefloxacin, and theophylline are probably clinically unimportant or nonexistent.

Patients should be educated regarding the potential of enoxacin and ciprofloxacin to increase caffeine concentrations and pharmacologic effects. If adverse events involving the central nervous system or gastrointestinal system are experienced, caffeine consumption should be evaluated and minimized. The role of caffeine in more-serious adverse events including psychotic reactions and seizures requires further study. In addition, the potential interaction between quinolones and warfarin deserves further study.

Azlocillin, cimetidine, and probenecid appear to compete with quinolones for tubular secretion, thereby reducing renal clearance. With some quinolones, reduction of nonrenal clearance has been reported with azlocillin and cimetidine. In contrast, pharmacokinetic interactions between quinolones and rifampin, metronidazole, and clindamycin have not been seen.

Since fluoroquinolones can cause various central nervous system effects, interactions with other agents that cause neurotoxicity have been suggested. These agents have included caffeine, theophylline, imipenem, and metronidazole. In addition, fenbufen, a nonsteroidal anti-inflammatory agent, appears to enhance the epileptogenic effects of quinolones through inhibition of GABA receptors in the brain. Further study is needed to establish risk factors for quinolone-induced neurotoxicity. At present, seizures are reported rarely in patients without underlying conditions that predispose them to seizures.

The new fluoroquinolones are associated with a large number of potential interactions with other drugs that must be considered when these agents are used. Some of the interactions may compromise therapy by altering the bioavailability of the quinolone. Other drug combinations may lead to a greater probability of toxicity due to pharmacokinetic or pharmacodynamic interactions. Quinolones differ widely in their effects on metabolism of other drugs; therefore, these effects cannot be generalized. Clearly, more epidemiologic research is needed to identify those interactions that are likely to be clinically important so that they can be avoided.

## REFERENCES


1. **Akahane, K., M. Sekiguchi, T. Une, and Y. Osada.** 1989. Structure-epileptogenicity relationship of quinolones with special reference to their interaction with γ-aminobutyric acid receptor sites. *Antimicrob. Agents Chemother.* **33:**1704–1708.
2. **Akaike, N., T. Shiraski, and T. Yakushiji.** 1991. Quinolones and fenbufen interact with $GABA_A$ receptor in dissociated hippocampal cells of rat. *J. Neurophysiol.* **66:**497–504.
3. **Akerele, J. O., and A. O. Ikhamafe.** 1991. Influence of oral co-administered metallic drugs on ofloxacin pharmacokinetics. *J. Antimicrob. Chemother.* **28:**87–94.
4. **Al-Turk, W. A., O. M. Shaheen, S. Othman, R. M. Khalaf, and A. S. Awidi.** 1988. Effect of ofloxacin on the pharmacokinetics of a single intravenous theophylline dose. *Ther. Drug Monit.* **10:**160–163.
5. **Avent, C. K., D. Krinsky, J. K. Kirklin, R. C. Bourge, and W. D. Figg.** 1988. Synergistic nephrotoxicity due to ciprofloxacin and cyclosporine. *Am. J. Med.* **85:**452–453.
6. **Barriere, S. L., D. H. Catlin, P. L. Orlando, A. Noe, and R. W. Frost.** 1990. Alteration in the pharmacokinetic disposition of ciprofloxacin by simultaneous administration of azlocillin. *Antimicrob. Agents Chemother.* **34:**823–826.
7. **Beckmann, J. W. Elsaβer, U. Gendert-Remy, and R. Hertampf.** 1987. Enoxacin—a potent inhibitor of theophylline metabolism. *Eur. J. Clin. Pharmacol.* **33:**227–230.
8. **Bem, J. L., and R. D. Mann.** 1988. Danger of interaction between ciprofloxacin and theophylline. *Br. Med. J.* **296:**1131.
9. **Bianco, T. M., H. I. Bussey, L. E. Farnett, W. D. Linn, M. K. Roush, and Y. W. James-Wong.** 1992. Potential warfarin-ciprofloxacin interaction in patients receiving long-term anticoagulation. *Pharmacotherapy* **12:**435–439.
10. **Boeckh, M., H. Lode, K. M. Deppermann, S. Grineisen, F. Shokry, R. Held, K. Wernicke, P. Koeppe, J. Wagner, C. Krasemann, and K. Borner.** 1990. Pharmacokinetics and serum bactericidal activities of quinolones in combination with clindamycin, metronidazole, and ornidazole. *Antimicrob. Agents Chemother.* **34:**2407–2414.
11. **Bowles, S. K., Z. Popovski, M. J. Rybak, H. B. Beckman, and D. J. Edwards.** 1988. Effect of norfloxacin on theophylline pharmacokinetics at steady state. *Antimicrob. Agents Chemother.* **32:**510–512.
12. **Brouwers, J. R. B. J., H. J. Van der Kam, J. Sijtsma, and J. H. Proost.** 1990. Important reduction of ciprofloxacin absorption by sucralfate and magnesium citrate solution. *Drug Invest.* **2:**197–199.
13. **Brouwers, J. R. B. J., H. J. Van der Kam, J. Sijtsma, and J. H. Proost.** 1990. Decreased ciprofloxacin absorption with concomitant administration of ferrous fumarate. *Pharm. Weekbl.* **12:**182–183.
14. **Campbell, N. R., M. Kara, B. B. Hasinoff, W. M. Haddara, and D. W. McKay.** 1992. Norfloxacin interaction with antacids and minerals. *Br. J. Clin. Pharmacol.* **33:**115–116.
15. **Chandler, M. H., S. M. Toler, R. P. Rapp, R. R. Muder, and J. A. Korvick.** 1990. Multiple-dose pharmacokinetics of concurrent oral ciprofloxacin and rifampin in elderly patients. *Antimicrob. Agents Chemother.* **34:**442–447.
16. **Christ, W., K. Gindler, S. Gruene, W. Hecker, M. Jacobsen, H. Junge, and H. H. Park.** 1989. Interactions of quinolones with opioids and fenbufen, a nonsteroidal anti-inflammatory drug: involvement of dopaminergic neurotransmission. *Rev. Infect. Dis.* **11**(Suppl. 5):S1393–S1394.
17. **Coste, T., J. Rautureau, M. Beaugrand, et al.** 1987. Comparison of two sucralfate dosages presented in tablet form in duodenal ulcer healing. *Am. J. Med.* **83**(Suppl. 3B):86–90.
18. **Davies, B. I., and P. V. Maesen.** 1989. Drug interactions with quinolones. *Rev. Infect. Dis.* **11**(Suppl. 5):S1083–S1090.
19. **Drusano, G. L., H. C. Standiford, K. Plaisance, A. Forrest, J. Leslie, and J. Caldwell.** 1986. Absolute oral bioavailability of ciprofloxacin. *Antimicrob. Agents Chemother.* **30:**444–446.
20. **Duraksi, R. M.** 1988. Ciprofloxacin-induced theophylline toxicity. *South. Med. J.* **81:**1206.
21. **Edwards, D. J., N. M. Waite, and C. K. Svensson.** 1988. Effect of enoxacin and 4-oxo-enoxacin on antipyrine disposition in the rat. *Drug Metab. Dispos.* **16:**653–654.
22. **Elston, R. A., and J. Taylor.** 1988. Possible interaction of ciprofloxacin with cyclosporin A. *J. Antimicrob. Chemother.* **21:**679–680.
23. **Flor, S., D. R. P. Guay, J. A. Opsahl, K. Tack, and G. R. Matzke.** 1990. Effects of magnesium-aluminum hydroxide and calcium carbonate antacids on bioavailability of ofloxacin. *Antimicrob. Agents Chemother.* **34:**2436–2438.
24. **Foster, T., and R. Blouin.** 1989. The effect of antacid timing on lomefloxacin bioavailability, abstr. 1277. *Program Abstr. 29th Intersci. Conf. Antimicrob. Agents Chemother.*

25. **Frost, R. W., J. D. Carlson, A. J. Dietz, Jr., A. Heyd, and J. T. Lettieri.** 1989. Ciprofloxacin pharmacokinetics after a standard high-fat/high calcium breakfast. *J. Clin. Pharmacol.* **29:**953-955.
26. **Frost, R. W., K. C. Lasseter, A. J. Noe, E. C. Shamblen, and J. T. Lettieri.** 1992. Effects of aluminum hydroxide and calcium carbonate antacids on the bioavailability of ciprofloxacin. *Antimicrob. Agents Chemother.* **36:**830-832.
27. **Grasela, T. H., J. J. Schentag, A. J. Sedman, J. H. Wilton, D. J. Thomas, R. W. Schultz, M. E. Lebsack, and A. W. Kinkel.** 1989. Inhibition of enoxacin absorption by antacids or ranitidine. *Antimicrob. Agents Chemother.* **33:**615-617.
28. **Gregoire, S. L., T. H. Grasela, J. P. Freer, K. J. Tack, and J. J. Schentag.** 1987. Inhibition of theophylline clearance by coadministered ofloxacin without alteration of theophylline effects. *Antimicrob. Agents Chemother.* **31:**375-378.
29. **Halliwell, R. F., P. G. Davey, and J. J. Lambert.** 1991. The effects of quinolones and NSAIDs upon GABA-evoked currents recorded from rat dorsal root ganglion neurons. *J. Antimicrob. Chemother.* **27:**209-218.
30. **Harder, S., U. Fuhr, A. H. Staib, and T. Wolff.** 1989. Ciprofloxacin-caffeine: a drug interaction established using *in vivo* and *in vitro* investigations. *Am. J. Med.* **87**(Suppl. 5A):89S-91S.
31. **Harder, S., A. H. Staib, C. Beer, A. Papenburg, W. Stille, and P. M. Shah.** 1988. 4-Quinolones inhibit biotransformation of caffeine. *Eur. J. Clin. Pharmacol.* **35:**651-656.
32. **Healy, D. P., R. E. Polk, L. Kanawati, D. T. Rock, and M. L. Mooney.** 1989. Interaction between oral ciprofloxacin and caffeine in normal volunteers. *Antimicrob. Agents Chemother.* **33:**474-478.
33. **Healy, D. P., J. R. Schoenle, J. Stotka, and R. E. Polk.** 1991. Lack of interaction between lomefloxacin and caffeine in normal volunteers. *Antimicrob. Agents Chemother.* **35:**660-664.
34. **Ho, G., M. G. Tierney, and R. E. Dales.** 1988. Evaluation of the effect of norfloxacin on the pharmacokinetics of theophylline. *Clin. Pharmacol. Ther.* **44:**35-38.
35. **Höffken, G., K. Borner, P. D. Glatzel, P. Koeppe, and H. Lode.** 1985. Reduced enteral absorption of ciprofloxacin in the presence of antacids. *Eur. J. Clin. Microbiol.* **4:**235.
36. **Höffken, G., H. Lode, R. Wiley, T. D. Glatzel, D. Sievers, T. Olschewski, K. Borner, and T. Koeppe.** 1988. Pharmacokinetics and bioavailability of ciprofloxacin and ofloxacin: effect of food and antacid intake. *Rev. Infect. Dis.* **10**(Suppl. 1):S138-S139.
37. **Hoffman, A., and G. Levy.** 1989. Effect of enoxacin on theophylline neurotoxicity. *Life Sci.* **44:**1803-1806.
38. **Holden, R.** 1988. Probable fatal interaction between ciprofloxacin and theophylline. *Br. Med. J.* **297:**1339.
39. **Hooper, T. L., F. K. Gould, C. R. Swinburn, G. Featherstone, N. J. Odom, P. A. Corris, R. Freeman, and C. G. A. McGregor.** 1988. Ciprofloxacin, a preferred treatment for legionella infections in patients receiving cyclosporin A. *J. Antimicrob. Chemother.* **22:**952-953.
40. **Hori, S., J. Shimada, A. Saito, M. Matsuda, and T. Miyahara.** 1989. Comparison of the inhibitory effects of new quinolones on $\gamma$-aminobutyric acid receptor binding in the presence of anti-inflammatory drugs. *Rev. Infect. Dis.* **11**(Suppl. 5):S1397-S1398.
41. **Johlson, H. M., L. A. Tanner, L. Green, and T. H. Grasela.** 1991. Adverse reaction reporting of interaction between warfarin and fluoroquinolones. *Arch. Intern. Med.* **151:**1003-1004.
42. **Karki, S. D., D. W. Bentley, and M. Raghavan.** 1990. Seizure with ciprofloxacin and theophylline combined therapy. *D.I.C.P. Ann. Pharmacother.* **24:**595-596.
43. **Koup, J. R., R. D. Toothaker, E. Posvar, A. J. Sedman, and W. A. Colburn.** 1990. Theophylline dosage adjustment during enoxacin coadministration. *Antimicrob. Agents Chemother.* **34:**803-807.
44. **Krüger, H. U., U. Schuler, B. Proksch, M. Göbel, and G. Ehninger.** 1990. Investigation of potential interaction of ciprofloxacin with cyclosporine in bone marrow transplant recipients. *Antimicrob. Agents Chemother.* **34:**1048-1052.
45. **Lang, J., J. F. DeVillaine, R. Garraffo, and J. L. Touraine.** 1989. Cyclosporine (cyclosporin A) pharmacokinetics in renal transplant patients receiving ciprofloxacin. *Am. J. Med.* **87**(Suppl. 5A):82S-85S.
46. **Lebel, M., F. Vallee, and M. St.-Laurent.** 1990. Influence of lomefloxacin on the pharmacokinetics of theophylline. *Antimicrob. Agents Chemother.* **34:**1254-1256.
47. **Lebsack, M. E., D. Nix, B. Ryerson, R. D. Toothaker, L. Welage, A. Norman, J. J. Schentag, and A. J. Sedman.** 1992. Effect of gastric acidity on enoxacin absorption. *Clin. Pharmacol. Ther.* **52:**252-256.
48. **Ledergerber, B., J. D. Bettex, B. Joos, M. Flepp, and R. Luthy.** 1985. Effect of standard breakfast on drug absorption and multiple-dose pharmacokinetics of ciprofloxacin. *Antimicrob. Agents Chemother.* **27:**350-352.
49. **Linville, D., C. Emory, and L. Graves.** 1991. Ciprofloxacin and warfarin interaction. *Am. J. Med.* **90:**765.

50. **Lucet, J. C., H. Tilly, G. Lerebours, J. J. Gres, and H. Piguet.** 1988. Neurological toxicity related to pefloxacin. *J. Antimicrob. Chemother.* **21:**811–812.
51. **Maesen, F. P. V., J. P. Teengs, C. Baur, and B. I. Davies.** 1984. Quinolones and raised plasma concentration of theophylline. *Lancet* **ii:**530.
52. **Mahr, G., F. Sorgel, M. Noje, B. Gottschalk, R. Granneman, J. Sylvester, and V. Stephan.** 1992. Effects of temafloxacin and ciprofloxacin on the pharmacokinetics of caffeine. *Clin. Pharmacokinet.* **11**(Suppl. 1):90–97.
53. **Marchbanks, C. R., D. J. Mikolich, D. J. Mayer, S. H. Zinner, and M. N. Dudley.** 1990. Pharmacokinetics and bioavailability of intravenous-to-oral enoxacin in elderly patients with complicated urinary tract infection. *Antimicrob. Agents Chemother.* **34:**1966–1972.
54. **Martinez-Cabarga, M., A. Sanchez Navarro, C. I. Colino Gandarillas, and A. Dominguez-Gil.** 1991. Effects of two cations on gastrointestinal absorption of ofloxacin. *Antimicrob. Agents Chemother.* **35:**2102–2105.
55. **Nakano, M., M. Yamamoto, and T. Avita.** 1978. Interactions of aluminum, magnesium, and calcium ions with nalidixic acid. *Chem. Pharm. Bull.* **26:**1505–1510.
56. **Neuvonen, P. J., K. T. Kivisto, and P. Lehto.** 1991. Interference of dairy products with the absorption of ciprofloxacin. *Clin. Pharmacol. Ther.* **50:**498–502.
56a. **Nix, D. E.** Unpublished data.
57. **Nix, D. E., J. M. DeVito, M. A. Whitbread, and J. J. Schentag.** 1987. Effect of multiple dose oral ciprofloxacin on the pharmacokinetics of theophylline and indocyanine green. *J. Antimicrob. Chemother.* **19:**263–269.
58. **Nix, D. E., A. Norman, and J. J. Schentag.** 1989. Effect of lomefloxacin on theophylline pharmacokinetics. *Antimicrob. Agents Chemother.* **33:**1006-1008.
59. **Nix, D. E., and J. J. Schentag.** 1989. Lomefloxacin absorption kinetics when administered with ranitidine and sucralfate, abstr. 1276. *Program Abstr. 29th Intersci. Conf. Antimicrob. Agents Chemother.*
60. **Nix, D. E., W. A. Watson, L. Handy, R. W. Frost, D. L. Rescott, and H. R. Goldstein.** 1989. The effect of sucralfate pretreatment on the pharmacokinetics of ciprofloxacin. *Pharmacotherapy* **9**(Suppl. 6):377–380.
61. **Nix, D. E., W. A. Watson, M. E. Lener, R. W. Frost, G. Krol, H. Goldstein, J. Lettieri, and J. J. Schentag.** 1989. Effects of aluminum and magnesium antacids and ranitidine on the absorption of ciprofloxacin. *Clin. Pharmacol. Ther.* **46:**700–705.
62. **Nix, D. E., J. H. Wilton, B. Ronald, L. Distlerath, V. C. Williams, and A. Norman.** 1990. Inhibition of norfloxacin absorption by antacids. *Antimicrob. Agents Chemother.* **34:**432–435.
63. **Parpia, S. H., D. E. Nix, L. G. Hejmanowski, H. R. Goldstein, J. H. Wilton, and J. J. Schentag.** 1989. Sucralfate reduces the gastrointestinal absorption of norfloxacin. *Antimicrob. Agents Chemother.* **33:**99–102.
64. **Peloquin, C. A., D. E. Nix, A. J. Sedman, J. H. Wilton, R. D. Toothaker, N. J. Harrison, and J. J. Schentag.** 1989. Pharmacokinetics and clinical effects of caffeine alone and in combination with oral enoxacin. *Rev. Infect. Dis.* **2:**S1095.
65. **Plaisance, K. I., G. L. Drusano, A. Forrest, C. I. Bustamante, and H. C. Standiford.** 1987. Effect of dose size on bioavailability of ciprofloxacin. *Antimicrob. Agents Chemother.* **31:**956–958.
66. **Polk, R. E., D. P. Healy, J. Sahai, L. Drwal, and E. Racht.** 1989. Effect of ferrous sulfate and multivitamins with zinc on absorption of ciprofloxacin in normal volunteers. *Antimicrob. Agents Chemother.* **33:**1841–1844.
67. **Preheim, I. C., T. A. Cuevas, J. S. Roccaforte, M. A. Mellencamp, and M. J. Bittner.** 1986. Ciprofloxacin and antacids. *Lancet* **ii:**48.
68. **Raoof, S., C. Wollschlager, and F. A. Khan.** 1987. Ciprofloxacin increases serum levels of theophylline. *Am. J. Med.* **82**(Suppl. 4A):115–118.
69. **Renzi, R., and S. Finkbeiner.** 1991. Ciprofloxacin interaction with sodium warfarin: a potentially dangerous side effect. *Am. J. Emerg. Med.* **9:**551–552.
70. **Richardson, J. P.** 1990. Theophylline toxicity associated with the administration of ciprofloxacin in a nursing home patient. *J. Am. Geriatr. Soc.* **38:**236–238.
71. **Rindone, J. P., C. L. Keuey, W. N. Jones, and H. S. Garewal.** 1991. Hypoprothrombinemic effect of warfarin not influenced by ciprofloxacin. *Clin. Pharm.* **10:**136–138.
72. **Robson, R. A., E. J. Begg, H. C. Atkinson, D. A. Saunders, and C. M. Frampton.** 1990. Comparative effects of ciprofloxacin and lomefloxacin on the oxidative metabolism of theophylline. *Br. J. Clin. Pharmacol.* **29:**491–493.
73. **Rocci, M. L., P. H. Vlasses, L. M. Distlerath, M. H. Gregg, S. C. Wheeler, W. Zing, and T. D. Bjornsson.** 1990. Norfloxacin does not alter warfarin's disposition or anticoagulant effect. *J. Clin. Pharmacol.* **30:**728–732.
74. **Rogge, M. C., W. R. Solomon, A. J. Sedman, P. C. Welling, R. D. Toothaker, and J. G. Wagner.** 1988. The theophylline-enoxacin interaction. I. Effect of enoxacin dose size on theophylline disposition. *Clin. Pharmacol. Ther.* **44:**579–587.
75. **Rogge, M. C., W. R. Solomon, A. J. Sedman, P. C. Welling, R. D. Toothaker, and J. G. Wagner.** 1989. The theophylline-enoxacin interaction.

II. Changes in the disposition of theophylline and its metabolites during intermittent administration of enoxacin. *Clin. Pharmacol. Ther.* **46:**420–428.

76. **Sano, M., K. Kawakatsu, C. Ohkita, I. Yamamoto, M. Takeyama, H. Yamashina, and M. Goto.** 1988. Effects of enoxacin, ofloxacin and norfloxacin on theophylline disposition in humans. *Eur. J. Clin. Pharmacol.* **35:**161–165.
77. **Sarkar, M., R. E. Polk, P. S. Guzelian, C. Hunt, and H. T. Karnes.** 1990. In vitro effect of fluoroquinolones on theophylline metabolism in human liver microsomes. *Antimicrob. Agents Chemother.* **34:**594–599.
78. **Schwartz, J., L. Jauregui, J. Lettieri, and K. Bachmann.** 1988. Impact of ciprofloxacin on theophylline clearance and steady-state concentrations in serum. *Antimicrob. Agents Chemother.* **32:**75–77.
79. **Segev, S., M. Rehavi, and E. Rubinstein.** 1988. Quinolones, theophylline, and diclofenac interactions with the gamma-aminobutyric acid receptor. *Antimicrob. Agents Chemother.* **32:**1624–1626.
80. **Semel, J. D., and N. Allen.** 1989. Combination effects of ciprofloxacin, clindamycin, and metronidazole intravenously in volunteers. *South. Med. J.* **84:**465–468.
81. **Semel, J. D., and N. Allen.** 1991. Seizures in patients simultaneously receiving theophylline and imipenem or ciprofloxacin or metronidazole. *South. Med. J.* **84:**465–468.
82. **Shimada, J., S. Hori, M. Kaji, T. Miyahara, H. Kusajima, S. Kaneko, S. Saito, and H. Uchida.** 1989. Interactions of fleroxacin with dried aluminum hydroxide and probenecid. *Rev. Infect. Dis.* **11**(Suppl. 5)**:**S1097–S1098.
83. **Shimada, J., K. Shiba, T. Oguma, H. Miwa, Y. Yoshimura, T. Nishikawa, Y. Okabayashi, T. Kitagawa, and S. Yamamoto.** 1992. Effect of antacid on absorption of the quinolone lomefloxacin. *Antimicrob. Agents Chemother.* **36:**1219–1224.
84. **Shimada, J., T. Yamaji, Y. Ueda, H. Uchida, H. Kusajima, and T. Irikura.** 1983. Mechanism of renal excretion of AM-715, a new quinolonecarboxylic acid derivative, in rabbits, dogs, and humans. *Antimicrob. Agents Chemother.* **23:**1–7.
85. **Sörgel, F., G. Mahr, R. Granneman, and U. Stephan.** 1992. Effects of two quinolone antibacterials, temafloxacin and enoxacin, on theophylline pharmacokinetics. *Clin. Pharmacokinet.* **22**(Suppl. 1)**:**65–74.
86. **Sörgel, F., G. Mahr, H. U. Koch, U. Stephan, H. G. Wisemann, and U. Malter.** 1988. Effects of cimetidine on the pharmacokinetics of pefloxacin in healthy volunteers. *Rev. Infect. Dis.* **10**(Suppl. 1)**:**S137.
87. **Sörgel, F., R. Selmann, R. Granneman, and C. Locke.** 1992. Effect of cimetidine on the pharmacokinetics of temafloxacin. *Clin. Pharmacokinet.* **22**(Suppl. 1)**:**75–82.
88. **Staibe, A. H., S. Harder, U. Furh, and C. Wack.** 1989. Interaction of quinolones with the theophylline metabolism in man: investigations with lomefloxacin and pipemidic acid. *Int. J. Clin. Pharmacol. Ther. Toxicol.* **26:**289–293.
89. **Stille, W., S. Harder, S. Mieke, C. Beer, P. M. Shah, K. Frech, and A. H. Staib.** 1987. Decrease of caffeine elimination in man during coadministration of 4-quinolones. *J. Antimicrob. Chemother.* **20:**729–734.
90. **Tan, K. K. C., A. K. Trull, and S. Shawket.** 1989. Co-administration of ciprofloxacin and cyclosporine: lack of evidence for a pharmacokinetic interaction. *Br. J. Clin. Pharmacol.* **28:**185–187.
91. **Thomson, A. H., G. D. Thomson, M. Hepburn, and B. Whiting.** 1987. A clinically significant interaction between ciprofloxacin and theophylline. *Eur. J. Clin. Pharmacol.* **33:**435–436.
92. **Thomson, D. J., A. H. Menkis, and F. N. McKenzie.** 1988. Norfloxacin-cyclosporine interaction. *Transplantation* **46:**312–313.
93. **Toon, S., J. J. Hopkins, F. M. Garstan, L. Aarons, A. Sedman, and M. Rowland.** 1987. Enoxacin-warfarin interaction: pharmacokinetic and stereochemical aspects. *Clin. Pharmacol. Ther.* **42:**33–41.
94. **Tsuji, A., H. Sato, E. Okezaki, O. Nagata, and H. Kato.** 1988. Effect of the anti-inflammatory agent fenbufen on the quinolone-induced inhibition of $\gamma$-aminobutyric acid receptor binding to rat brain membranes in-vitro. *Biochem. Pharmacol.* **37:**4408–4411.
95. **VanSlooten, A. D., D. E. Nix, J. H. Wilton, J. H. Love, J. M. Spivey, and H. R. Goldstein.** 1991. Combined use of ciprofloxacin and sucralfate. *D.I.C.P. Ann. Pharmacother.* **25:**578–582.
96. **Weidekamm, E., R. Portmann, K. Suter, C. Partos, D. Dell, and P. W. Lücker.** 1987. Single- and multiple-dose pharmacokinetics of fleroxacin, a trifluorinated quinolone, in humans. *Antimicrob. Agents Chemother.* **31:**1909–1914.
97. **Wijnands, W. J., T. B. Vree, A. M. Baars, and C. L. VanHerwaarden.** 1987. Steady-state kinetics of the quinolone derivatives ofloxacin, enoxacin, ciprofloxacin and pefloxacin during maintenance treatment with theophylline. *Drugs* **34:**159–169.
98. **Wijnands, W. J., T. B. Vree, A. M. Baars, and C. L. VanHerwaarden.** 1987. The influence of the 4-quinolones ciprofloxacin, pefloxacin and ofloxacin on the elimination of theophylline. *Pharm. Weekbl.* **12:**S72–S75.
99. **Wijnands, W. J. A., J. H. Cornel, M. Martea, and T. B. Vree.** 1990. The effect of multiple dose oral lomefloxacin on theophylline metabolism in man. *Chest* **98:**1440–1444.

100. **Wijnands, W. J. A., C. L. A. VanHerwaarden, and T. B. Vree.** 1984. Enoxacin raises plasma concentrations of theophylline. *Lancet* **ii:**108–109.

101. **Wijnands, W. J. A., T. B. Vree, and C. L. VanHerwaarden.** 1985. Enoxacin decreases the clearance of theophylline in man. *Br. J. Clin. Pharmacol.* **20:**583–588.

102. **Wijnands, W. J. A., T. B. Vree, and C. L. VanHerwaarden.** 1986. The influence of quinolone derivatives on theophylline clearance. *Br. J. Clin. Pharmacol.* **22:**677–683.

103. **Yakushiji, T., T. Shiraski, and N. Akaike.** 1992. Noncompetitive inhibition of $GABA_A$ responses by a new class of quinolones and non-steroidal anti-inflammatories in dissociated frog sensory neurons. *Br. J. Pharmacol.* **105:**13–18.

104. **Yuk, J. H., C. H. Nightingale, R. Quintiliani, and K. R. Sweeney.** 1991. Bioavailability and pharmacokinetics of ofloxacin in healthy volunteers. *Antimicrob. Agents Chemother.* **35:**384–486.

105. **Yuk, J. H., C. H. Nightingale, R. Quintiliani, N. S. Yeston, R. Orlando, E. D. Dobkin, J. C. Kambe, K. R. Sweeney, and E. A. Buonpane.** 1990. Absorption of ciprofloxacin administered through a nasogastric or a nasoduodenal tube in volunteers and patients receiving enteral nutrition. *Diagn. Microbiol. Infect. Dis.* **13:**99–102.

106. **Yuk, J. H., C. H. Nightingale, K. R. Sweeney, R. Quintiliani, J. T. Lettieri, and R. W. Frost.** 1989. Relative bioavailability in healthy volunteers of ciprofloxacin administered through a nasogastric tube with and without enteral feeding. *Antimicrob. Agents Chemother.* **33:**1118–1120.

*Quinolone Antimicrobial Agents, 2nd ed.*
Edited by David C. Hooper and John S. Wolfson


*Chapter 12*

# Pharmacodynamics of the Fluoroquinolones

***Jerome J. Schentag, David E. Nix, and Alan Forrest***

Pharmacodynamics refers to drug action versus concentration in serum and should be clearly distinguished from pharmacokinetics, the time course of drug concentrations in serum. Quinolone pharmacokinetics are summarized in chapters 9 and 10. Quinolone pharmacodynamics can be expressed in terms of concentration versus bacterial killing capabilities and concentration (or dose) relationships to toxicities. An example of toxicity versus concentration is the well-known nephrotoxicity of the aminoglycoside antibiotics (44). Since fluoroquinolone toxicity is the subject of chapter 26, this chapter will focus primarily on the main aspect of quinolone pharmacodynamics, i.e., the killing of bacteria versus drug concentration. These bacterial killing rates are usually expressed as change in CFU over time, although time to sterile cultures is also a valid expression of killing rate. Finally, cure of infection is also a relevant pharmacodynamic end point in that clinical cure is a composite parameter, the components of cure being bacterial killing versus concentration and the rates of host repair and resolution of inflammation.

***Jerome J. Schentag, David E. Nix, and Alan Forrest*** • Center for Clinical Pharmacy Research, School of Pharmacy, State University of New York at Buffalo, and The Clinical Pharmacokinetics Laboratory, Millard Fillmore Hospital, Buffalo, New York 14209-1194.

The MIC or MBC and the serum bactericidal titers are pharmacodynamic parameters that express concentration-dependent quinolone actions on bacteria. Bactericidal rates are pharmacodynamic expressions of bacterial killing versus time, although these rates of killing also exhibit marked dependence on quinolone concentration.

## IN VITRO PHARMACODYNAMICS

Most of the information regarding fluoroquinolone pharmacodynamics is gleaned from in vitro studies of antibiotic action on bacteria. When a graded array of known concentrations is exposed to bacteria in broth, the lowest concentration capable of growth inhibition, i.e., the concentration of the lowest dilution in which growth is absent, is the MIC. Subculturing the chamber in which growth was inhibited determines the MBC, which for fluoroquinolones is usually the same as or only 1 dilution higher than the MIC. Many MIC tests have been performed for all of the fluoroquinolones, and the results are usually summarized in the form of large tables like Table 1 or, in more comprehensive fashion, those in chapter 8. We have chosen representative bacteria for Table 1 and have provided MICs derived from many separate studies. Considerable attention was devoted to relative differences in the concentrations that inhibited each bacterium, and Table 1 provides MICs in our best attempts to gauge relative activity profiles for each drug listed. Many investigators and clinicians review MIC data like these and tend to select the drug that produces the lowest MIC. This approach equates MIC with potency. While low MICs do indicate greater potency, the drugs also must be compared on the basis of their achievable concentrations in vivo. Both kinetics and dynamics can be simultaneously considered by integrating these end points to form activity indices during comparative evaluation of the fluoroquinolones. Later in this chapter, we will use the MICs in Table 1 along with each agent's in vivo pharmacokinetics to calculate in vivo activity indices for each of these fluoroquinolones.

Many time kill (bactericidal-rate) studies have been performed for fluoroquinolones (9, 25, 52). Usually, the quinolones kill bacteria more rapidly than $\beta$-lactam antibiotics do (52). In most cases, these bactericidal rates are similar to the killing rates of aminoglycosides (9). The mechanism for the rapid killing action of aminoglycosides and quinolones is largely unknown (13, 26). Perhaps $\beta$-lactams kill relatively slowly because the actively expanding cell walls associated with growing bacteria are necessary for killing. If this is true, then bacterial growth rate would influence killing rate. Evidence in favor of this arises from the slower killing of pseudomonads versus *Escherichia coli,* even when the ratio of concentration to MIC is the same. Rapid bacterial killing may confer clinical advantages on quinolones and aminoglycosides over $\beta$-lactams in the form of shorter duration of therapy (23).

To a certain extent, all antibiotics display concentration-dependent bacterial killing. Killing usually begins just as concentrations of the drug approach the MIC for the organism. For $\beta$-lactams, the rate of killing increases with concentration only until the concentration reaches four to eight times the MIC. Then and thereafter, further increases

**Table 1.** $MIC_{90}$ for selected bacteria versus fluoroquinolones[a]

| Agent | *Escherichia coli* | *Staphylococcus aureus* | *Bacillus fragilis* | *Enterobacter cloacae* | *Pseudomonas aeruginosa* | *Serratia* spp. | *Haemophilus influenzae* | *Streptococcus pneumoniae* |
|---|---|---|---|---|---|---|---|---|
| Norfloxacin | 0.125 | 6.3 | >32 | 0.25 | 2.0 | 4 | 0.06 | 16 |
| Ciprofloxacin | 0.01 | 0.5 | 8.0 | 0.2 | 0.5 | 0.68 | 0.008 | 2.0 |
| Ofloxacin | 0.125 | 0.25 | 8 | 0.50 | 2–8 | 1.0 | 0.06–0.12 | 2.0 |
| Pefloxacin | 0.125 | 0.5 | 32 | 0.50 | 2–8 | | 0.06 | 8.0 |
| Enoxacin | 0.25 | 2.0 | 16 | 0.50 | 2–8 | 2 | 0.06–0.5 | 8.0 |
| Fleroxacin | 0.125 | 0.5 | 8 | 0.50 | 2–8 | 2 | 0.06–0.12 | 8.0 |
| Lomefloxacin | 0.50 | 4.0 | 32 | 2.0 | 12.5 | | 0.12 | 8.0 |
| Sparfloxacin | 0.12 | 0.1 | 2 | | 2 | | 0.1 | 0.5 |
| Tosufloxacin | 0.2 | 0.2 | | | 1.6 | | 0.1 | 0.25 |
| L-Ofloxacin | 0.1 | 0.8 | | | 1.6 | | 0.08 | 1.6 |
| CI-960 | 0.2 | 0.1 | 0.5 | | 0.25 | | 0.08 | 0.20 |
| OPC 17116 | 0.06 | 0.25 | 3.1 | 0.125 | 0.5 | 0.05 | 0.06 | 0.125 |
| WIN 57273 | 0.08 | 0.05 | 0.5 | 0.2 | 4 | 2 | | |

[a]Data are from references 7, 27, and 28.

in concentration do not further increase the rate of bacterial killing (60). In contrast, the quinolone killing rate continually increases as concentrations increase to 30 to 60 times the MIC. Thus, quinolone killing rates are considered concentration dependent above the MIC (51). Not surprisingly, some studies note a plateau in quinolone killing rate at very high multiples of the MIC (11). Since the killing rate with quinolones depends on concentration, in vitro evaluation of the bacterial killing rate should employ a concentration-time profile that mimics the concentration in serum decline observed after a dose is given to humans. In vitro models that mimic changing serum drug concentrations are now fairly common, and studies of these types have been conducted by Dudley and coworkers (17) and others (2, 34, 35). In these models, quinolones kill rapidly at peak serum drug concentrations, and they continue to kill bacteria as long as concentrations exceed the MIC. Most of these workers argue for quinolone-dosing regimens that divide the daily dose in such a way as to produce high peak concentrations in patients (16, 30). A modest postantibiotic effect (PAE), ranging from 2 to 6 h depending on the bacterium, can be demonstrated in vitro as well (10). In these in vitro models, killing rates of fluoroquinolones exceed those of $\beta$-lactams and are similar to those of aminoglycosides. The other observation in these models that is of great relevance is the emergence of an initially small population of resistant organisms ($< 10^3$) that eventually becomes the dominant flora after 24 h of exposure (17, 18). High peak concentrations prolong the time before this emergence, presumably by killing even greater numbers (those with the highest MICs) of the small minority population of highly resistant microbes (4). This argument has been used to support regimens that provide high peak concentrations and high doses for quinolones (32), and it supports the arguments in favor of high peak concentrations for aminoglycosides as well (5).

## ANIMAL MODELS

While in vitro time-killing rate studies can explore bacterial killing in relation to an array of static concentrations, the modeling of quinolone pharmacodynamics in animals and humans necessitates some consideration of changing serum drug concentrations. Thus, the study of antibiotic killing actions on bacteria in animal models needs a strong companion focus on animal pharmacokinetics. The reliable extrapolation of animal data to human treatment requires careful consideration of the pharmacokinetic differences between animals and humans. Pharmacokinetics describes the time course of antibiotic exposure to the bacteria. Exposure time in conjunction with concentration-dependent killing rate determines the time course of bacterial eradication. Host defense mechanisms also play a role in bacterial eradication, but their influence may not be as great as was once thought, since the best animal models now show that effective concentrations in vitro are also effective in vivo. These studies have devoted considerable attention to the pharmacokinetics of exposure as well as to MICs. Dosing matched to pharmacokinetics ensures that in vivo exposure is matched to the in vitro target concentration. Dosing is a special concern when it is realized that virtually all antibiotics have shorter half-lives in commonly used small mammals such as mice and rats. Thus, the animals are exposed to antibiotic peaks and troughs radically different from those that occur in humans or even large animals. As a consequence, the doses for small animals that produce results that match the peaks and troughs in humans must be very frequent (i.e., small doses every 1 to 2 h). Most mouse, rat, and rabbit studies give doses one or two times daily and, as a consequence, test markedly different serum exposure profiles than are observed in humans. Failure to consider these pharmacokinetic differences makes it difficult to compare bacterial killing in animal and human studies, particularly when the antibiotic exhibits killing rates that depend on concentration. For example, animal models nearly always favor drugs with concentration-dependent killing (i.e., aminoglycosides and quinolones) over $\beta$-lactams. This is largely a consequence of high quinolone and aminoglycoside peak concentrations, the considerably shorter half-lives of these drugs, and rapid killing versus concentration. In humans, where half-lives in serum are much longer, doses are less frequent, and peaks are considerably lower, the aminoglycosides are much less effective than the $\beta$-lactams. Thus, the $\beta$-lactams nearly always have the advantage over aminoglycosides in humans. They appear to be more active in humans (21) because the truly active concentrations of the aminoglycosides are never attained in patients out of concern for toxicity (21, 49). Table 2 summarizes some animal studies of quinolones. In animals, quinolones often perform better than aminoglycosides because of greater in vitro activity (50) and often perform better than $\beta$-lactams because of longer half-lives (22, 24, 42). The data in Table 2 largely point to parameters like the ratios of the area under the curve (AUC) to the MIC and the peak concentration to the MIC as indicative of favorable antibacterial actions with these drugs.

A second major difference between animal models and humans is the pharmacodynamic end point. Animal models virtually all use end points reflective of bacterial killing. Examples are colony count reductions versus time or the time required to sterilize the site cultures (Table 2). A few animal models have focused on clinical cure (20), but no recent studies used quinolones. Human trials of antibiotics primarily focus on clinical end points like cure and failure and seem more relevant to the day-to-day practices of clinicians. These end points, however, are exceedingly insensitive for pharmacodynamic analysis. As a consequence, end points like cure and failure largely preclude clinical trials from showing real differences between drugs or between different doses of the same drug. Animal models typically show clear relationships between quinolone concentration and bacterial killing rates (54), and most argue on this basis for high peaks and concentration-dependent killing (Table 2). Animal models can also provide a concentration range for reliable killing, while the strengths of these relationships can deteriorate markedly as investigators search for the same correlates of clinical cure in humans. Later in this chapter, we attempt to correlate the in vitro data and data for animals in order to demonstrate that these pharmacodynamic relationships also apply to humans if the human trials are properly designed to take advantage of sensitive end points like bacterial killing rates and if pharmacokinetic differences between humans are simultaneously considered.

Animal models have been developed to overcome the problems of host defense and different pharmacokinetics. In particular, humanizing factors in models like neutropenic mouse (21, 55), rat (43), or guinea pig (22) make the findings more relevant to the human with compromised or absent neutrophil function. Results with these models are also summarized in Table 2. The use of animals with uranyl nitrate-induced acute renal failure produces pharmacokinetic profiles similar to those of humans (12). With these two "humanizing" adjustments made, mice can and have provided data remarkably similar to those for humans. These animal models become exceedingly useful, because a greater range of doses can be explored in direct comparisons between antibiotics. The studies of Craig and others (12, 21, 30, 55) represent some of the most clinically relevant examples of animal model systems. Table 2 summarizes some important pharmacodynamic relationships for quinolones that arise out of animal model studies. In general, these studies confirm the concentration-related killing rates of quinolones observed in vitro, although many of these models should devote greater attention to dose ranging or to the differences in pharmacokinetics between animals and humans. Parameters like peak concentration/MIC ratio are important predictors

**Table 2.** Important pharmacodynamic relationships as derived from animal model studies[a]

| Animal | Organism | Infection or site | Humanizing factor | End point of response | Quinolone(s) | Peak concn ($\mu$g/ml) | Kinetic-dynamic relationship | Conclusion(s) | Reference |
|---|---|---|---|---|---|---|---|---|---|
| Mouse | *K. pneumoniae* | Pneumonia | Neutropenia | CFU decline; $E_{max}$, P50 | Ciprofloxacin | | AUC/MIC<br>Peak/MIC | Concn-dependent killing | 30 |
| Mouse | *P. aeruginosa* | Thigh | Neutropenia | CFU decline; $E_{max}$, P50 | Ciprofloxacin | | AUC/MIC<br>Peak/MIC | Concn similar to that for humans yields similar kill rates | 30 |
| Rat | *K. pneumoniae* | Pneumonia | Neutropenia | CFU decline vs time | Ciprofloxacin | 0.67 | Peak/MIC<br>Time > MIC<br>No PAE | Intermittent doses slightly better than continuous infusions | 43 |
| Mouse | *P. aeruginosa* | Peritonitis | None | CFU decline vs time | Ciprofloxacin<br>Pefloxacin | 5.6 | Time > MIC<br>No PAE? | Higher doses, less resistance; CI had less resistance than intermittent dosing | 32 |
| Guinea pig | *P. aeruginosa* | Pneumonia | None | CFU decline vs time | Ciprofloxacin<br>Enoxacin<br>Ofloxacin | 2.4<br>3.4<br>10.1 | None noted | Concn-related killing for enoxacin only | 29 |
| Mouse | *S. pneumoniae* | Pneumonia | None | CFU decline and survival | Ofloxacin<br>Ciprofloxacin<br>Temafloxacin | ND | None noted | Dose-related survival | 1 |
| Rabbit | *E. coli* | Endocarditis | None | CFU decline after 1 dose | Ciprofloxacin<br>Pefloxacin | NR | Peak/MIC<br>Long $t_{1/2}$ > short | Dose-dependent ↓ CFU | 42 |
| Rabbit | *P. aeruginosa* | Osteomyelitis | None | Serial site culture | Ciprofloxacin every 8 h | 2.1 | Time > MIC | Cure of *P. aeruginosa* osteomyelitis better than cure of AMG or BL | 40 |
| Rabbit | *E. coli* | Meningitis | None | CFU decline in CSF | Pefloxacin | 29 | Peak/MIC<br>Dose/MIC | Dose- and concn-dependent killing in CSF | 50 |
| Rabbit | *P. aeruginosa* | Meningitis | None | CFU decline in CSF | Ciprofloxacin | 6.7 | Peak/MIC<br>Dose/MIC | Dose- and concn-dependent killing in CSF | 24 |
| Guinea pig | *P. aeruginosa* | Pneumonia | Neutropenia | CFU decline in lung | Ciprofloxacin<br>Pefloxacin | 3.3<br>12 | Peak/MIC | At same peak/MIC, both drugs had same killing rate in vivo | 22 |
| Rabbit | *E. coli* | Endocarditis | None | CFU decline in valve | Pefloxacin | 6.1 | Peak/MIC | At 5 times MBC, killing was same as 20 times MBC | 11 |
| Mouse | *P. aeruginosa* | Granuloma pouch | None | CFU decline at site | Ciprofloxacin | 1.5 | Peak/MIC | At same concn, killing rate depends on MIC | 59 |

[a]Abbreviations: AMG, aminoglycoside antibiotic; BL, $\beta$-lactam antibiotic; CI, continuous infusion; CSF, cerebrospinal fluid; $E_{max}$, maximal effect; ND, not done; NR, not reported; P50, point of 50% effect; $t_{1/2}$, half-life.

of bacterial killing. A PAE is often noted in short-term exposure of animal models, as quantitated by CFU versus time (43). However, there are also some indications that the PAE disappears after multiple dosing begins (32, 33). In contrast to in vitro models (4, 5, 18), animal models (8) have only begun to examine the correlations between exposure concentration, MIC, and the development of bacterial resistance for quinolones. What has been done generally confirms the in vitro dependence of resistance development on peak concentration (32). There has also been some work on resistance in animal models with β-lactams (2). Part of the problem thus far has been the short period (usually $<24$ h) of treatment that is common in these models. Resistance seldom develops in vivo over such short periods. The human treated for 14 days is much more likely to develop resistant bacteria, particularly when foreign bodies are also present.

## HUMANS

A large body of human pharmacokinetic data has been accumulated during studies of the various quinolones (6, 14, 27, 36, 39, 56, 58). Much of this information has been reviewed and summarized in earlier chapters of this book. A pharmacodynamic perspective on these kinetic data comes from attempts to correlate either microbiological or clinical end points with these kinetic indices. This has not yet been done, and the consequence is the current high degree of uncertainty over the proper dosage for these drugs in patients. A similar problem dominates the literature regarding the β-lactams, vancomycin, and the macrolides. For most of these antibiotics, There are often only vague notions of the effective concentration in vivo. For reasons explained elsewhere (37, 38), the effective concentration in vivo is considered to be the concentration in serum for all the fluoroquinolones. We have consistently disagreed with the position that links high ratios of tissue to serum drug concentrations from homogenate studies to antibacterial response (38).

The primary factor in the conduct and interpretation of successful human pharmacodynamic studies is the chosen end point of drug effect (44). The traditional clinical trial end points of cure and failure have some clinical relevance but are too insensitive to detect any but the most dramatic changes in the time course of antibacterial effects. In an attempt to identify more-sensitive end points of effect for pharmacodynamic analysis, we have been exploring the time course of bacterial eradication from the infection site by using serial cultures (19, 31, 41, 47, 48). The site most amenable to serial cultures is the respiratory tract, particularly in nosocomial settings, where intubated patients offer ready access to suctioned endotracheal secretions (19, 31). This site and these methods are readily applicable to pharmacokinetic-pharmacodynamic model development (19). Relevance to these models can be established by correlating the derived pharmacokinetic-pharmacodynamic relationships with both bacterial eradication and clinical cure, and we have recently conducted such an analysis with ciprofloxacin (19). Other fluoroquinolones have not yet been studied, and it is unknown whether our findings with ciprofloxacin apply to other fluoroquinolones, although we have advanced the hypothesis that they should behave similarly (46).

Our clinical trials have been designed to establish a correlation between ciprofloxacin pharmacokinetics, the MIC for the organism, and the speed of bacterial eradication. Other end points have been the traditional ones: clinical cure and microbiological cure. Essentially all of our study patients have been older, critically ill adults with nosocomial pneumonia. This model requires the assessment of daily infection site cultures to precisely determine the day of bacterial eradication. Thus far, ciprofloxacin clearly shows a correlation between pharmacodynamics and both clinical and microbiological outcomes

(19). The most useful parameter descriptive of these relationships is the AUIC, the quotient of the area under the curve and the bacterial MIC (19, 46). The AUIC mathematical relationship has its roots in the bactericidal titer (15, 53, 57) and the concept of area under the bactericidal titer curve (3). Table 3 outlines some of our results in greater detail and summarizes an analysis of the bacterial and clinical outcomes of ciprofloxacin in relation to AUIC and MIC. Perhaps the most striking relationship of this analysis was the threshold AUIC for the onset of effective antibacterial action. This threshold was 125, the value predicted earlier by simulations (46). As shown in Fig. 1, the achieved AUIC for each patient produced bacterial outcomes in direct relationship to the magnitude of AUC divided by MIC. Specifically, a survival-type datum plot of AUICs showed that patients with AUICs below 125 failed, while AUICs between 125 and 250 predicted slow bacterial killing, and bacterial eradication in this case required about 7 days. Regardless of the species, bacterial killing when AUICs exceeded 250 was extremely rapid, as many cultures were already sterile at 24 h after initiating treatment and the bacteria were eradicated in an average of 1.9 days. Overall, the datum plot in Fig. 1 confirms the in vitro concentration-dependent killing of fluoroquinolones in vivo.

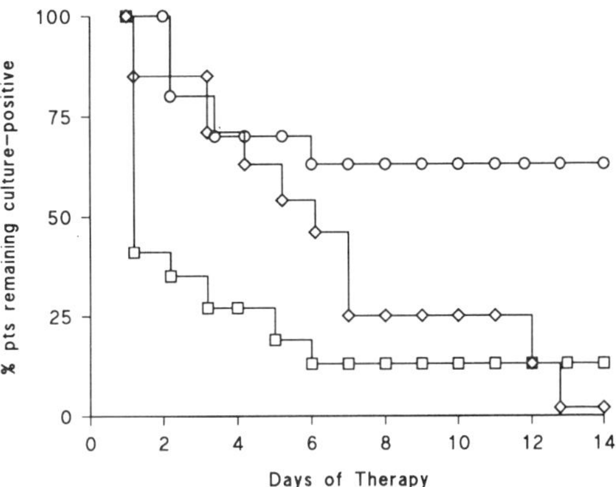


**Figure 1.** Survival plot analysis showing the relationship between the AUIC for intravenous ciprofloxacin in 74 patients (pts) and the percentage of patients remaining with positive cultures at each day of treatment. Three distinct patterns of response were noted: (i) those with an AUIC of <125, with over 60% of patients remaining culture positive after 2 weeks of treatment (○); those with AUICs between 125 and 250, with only 25% remaining culture positive after 7 days of treatment and with most patients having sterile cultures at day 14 (◇); (iii) those with AUICs above 250 (□), with only 40% remaining culture positive on day 2 of treatment and nearly all being negative after 4 days of treatment. This figure is adapted from reference 19.

**Table 3.** Pharmacokinetic and pharmacodynamic relationships to antibacterial outcomes with intravenous ciprofloxacin in patients with nosocomial pneumonia

| Parameter | No. of patients | % Cure | |
|---|---|---|---|
| | | Microbiological | Clinical |
| MIC | | | |
| ≤0.125 | 28 | 82 | 79 |
| 0.125–0.25 | 13 | 75 | 69 |
| 0.5 | 14 | 54 | 79 |
| 1.0 | 9 | 33 | 44 |
| 2.0–4.0 | 2 | 0 | 0 |
| AUIC range | | | |
| 0–125 | 19 | 32 | 42 |
| 125–250 | 16 | 81 | 88 |
| 250–1,000 | 14 | 79 | 71 |
| 1,000–5,541 | 15 | 87 | 80 |
| Dosage | | | |
| 200 mg every 12 h | 36 | 78 | 67 |
| 300 mg every 12 h | 8 | 25 | 38 |
| 400 mg every 8 h | 25 | 70 | 84 |

There are close interrelationships between AUICs and other indices of antimicrobial potency. For example, as AUICs increase, so do ratios of peak concentration to MIC, AUC above MIC, and time above MIC. There are some inherent advantages to integrated parameters of exposure like AUIC over ratios of peak concentration to MIC in that drugs with the same ratios of peak concentration to MIC could have different half-lives and thus produce very different times above MIC or AUC above MIC. However, all of these indices give the same answer if the pharmacokinetics of the drugs being compared are similar. They are highly covariant when the dosing intervals are chosen to provide reasonable coverage above MICs. We prefer AUIC only because it is the same target regardless of the antibiotic being analyzed or used (46). This feature facilitates use of the AUIC in computerized assessment strategies of drug exposure versus outcomes.

Analyses using end points like AUIC show that quinolones display concentration-dependent killing rates in human infections. In order to discriminate among these relationships during the conduct of the usual fixed-dose clinical trials, we measure MIC, measure blood drug levels, determine the AUC, and then calculate the AUIC for each study patient. We then measure day of eradication via serial culturing of the site of infection and correlate day of eradication with AUIC as in Table 3 or Fig. 1. These three procedures must be done for each patient, because there is tremendous variability between patients in the AUC (even if the dose is the same) and the MIC for the organism (even if the organism is the same). This can be illustrated for ciprofloxacin. Table 4 shows the calculated AUCs for ciprofloxacin versus dose, renal function, and weight. As shown, the AUC data for intravenous ciprofloxacin are considerably different for volunteers and patients. This has been shown previously (6, 56, 58). If one considers the impact of a variety of MICs in conjunction with these varied AUCs and employs combinations of AUCs and MICs to calculate the AUIC, then it is readily appreciated why the AUIC varies so widely from patient to patient. The AUIC of ciprofloxacin in the study we performed ranged from 6 to over 5,500 (19). A range of this magnitude occurs in any patient population and explains why clinical studies that do not directly measure the AUIC or any other index of the interaction between pharmacokinetics and pharmacodynamics cannot possibly differentiate between two doses of the same antibiotic or between two different antibiotics.

Another way to illustrate the variance in AUIC is shown in Table 5, in which the ciprofloxacin MICs of Table 1 were used in conjunction with the AUCs from Table 4 to calculate AUICs for ciprofloxacin against common organisms. AUICs were calculated for three popular dosing regimens: 300 mg every 12 h, 400 mg every 12 h, and 400 mg every 8 h. This table considers the MICs for common pathogens in relation to AUCs typical of patients with a creatinine clearance of 50 ml/min. If susceptible bacteria have MICs between 0.5 and 0.008, the AUIC would range from 46 to 7,750 (Table 5) depending on the dose and the specific MIC encountered. This range is quite similar to the 6 to 5,500 range we observed in our patient study (19).

Pharmacodynamic parameters like AUIC can be used to differentiate either between different classes of antibiotics or between different members of the same class of antibi-

**Table 4.** Calculated 24-h AUCs for a variety of intravenous ciprofloxacin regimens[a]

| Dose (mg)[b] | AUC for[c]: | | |
|---|---|---|---|
| | Volunteers ($CL_T$ = 600 ml/min) | 70-kg-dose patients ($CL_T$ = 266 ml/min) | 55-kg-dose patients ($CL_T$ = 266 ml/min) |
| 200 i.v. q12h | 9 | 20 | 24.4 |
| 200 i.v. q8h | 14 | 31 | 37.8 |
| 300 i.v. q12h | 14 | 31 | 37.8 |
| 300 p.o. q12h | 10.5 | 23.2 | 28 |
| 300 i.v. q8h | 21 | 47 | 57 |
| 400 i.v. q12h | 18 | 41 | 50 |
| 400 i.v. q8h | 27 | 62 | 76 |
| 750 p.o. q12h | 29 | 64 | 78 |

[a]Creatinine clearances were 100 ml/min for healthy volunteers and 50 ml/min for patients.
[b]i.v., intravenous; q12h, every 12 h.
[c]$CL_T$, total clearance.

**Table 5.** Susceptibilities of pathogenic organisms to ciprofloxacin and expected activity profiles in patients[a]

| Organism | MIC | Calculated AUIC for i.v. dosage of: | | |
|---|---|---|---|---|
| | | 300 q12h | 400 q12h | 400 q8h |
| *H. influenzae* | 0.008 | 3,875 | 5,125 | 7,750 |
| *E. coli* | 0.01 | 3,100 | 4,100 | 6,200 |
| *K. pneumoniae* | 0.12 | 258 | 342 | 517 |
| *E. cloacae* | 0.2 | 155 | 205 | 310 |
| *Serratia* spp. | 0.68 | 46 | 61 | 92 |
| *P. aeruginosa* | 0.5 | 62 | 82 | 124 |
| *S. aureus* (methicillin resistant) | 0.5 | 62 | 82 | 124 |

[a]Creatinine clearance for patients was 50 ml/min. i.v., intravenous; q12h, every 12 h.

otics (46). The required data include MICs (from Table 1) and AUCs for typical doses, which we extracted from pharmacokinetic studies of each agent. This approach is usually advocated based on normal volunteer data and average MICs for 90% of isolates ($MIC_{90}$) (39). However, we used it here to calculate the lowest MIC (i.e., the breakpoint) that would still achieve a minimally acceptable AUIC of at least 125 for each of the quinolones. Pharmacokinetics reflective of volunteers with healthy renal function (Table 6) or of patients (Table 7) were used. These MIC breakpoints were calculated by assuming a creatine clearance of 100 ml/min (Table 6) or 50 ml/min (Table 7). Overall, pharmacokinetic-pharmacodynamic-derived breakpoints from our calculations were considerably lower than the MIC breakpoints of laboratory susceptibility from the National Committee for Clinical Laboratory Standards, and thus what we have identified here is a lower threshold MIC than would be given for the same quinolones in the package inserts for these drugs. It is useful to point out that these relationships predict a higher degree of clinical response than the usual MIC breakpoint. They define a less tolerant rate of failure in this manner. We are supporting our ciprofloxacin breakpoint with pharmacokinetic-pharmacodynamic data derived from simulations (46) and our clinical trials of quinolones (19) and β-lactams (47).

Pharmacokinetic-pharmacodynamic breakpoint data in Tables 6 and 7 show ciprofloxacin and sparfloxacin to have the highest overall breakpoint MICs and thus the greatest potency when kinetics and MIC are both considered. Ofloxacin is also favorably active, particularly in patients with renal impairment. As evidenced by MICs that allow AUICs of at least 125, the most active agents

**Table 6.** Breakpoint AUICs and MICs for fluoroquinolones in healthy volunteers with 100-ml/min creatinine clearance

| Quinolone | Oral dose (mg/24 h) | AUC (mg·h/liter) | Breakpoint MIC for AUIC of 125 | $MIC_{90}$ | | |
|---|---|---|---|---|---|---|
| | | | | *P. aeruginosa* | *Staphylococcus* sp. | *E. coli* |
| Norfloxacin | 800 | 13.6 | 0.10 | 2.0 | 6.3 | 0.125 |
| Ciprofloxacin | 1,500 | 29.6 | 0.25 | 0.5 | 0.5 | 0.01 |
| Ofloxacin | 800 | 46.6 | 0.30 | 2.0 | 0.25 | 0.125 |
| Enoxacin | 800 | 35.6 | 0.30 | 4.0 | 2.0 | 0.25 |
| Lomefloxacin | 400 | 30 | 0.25 | 12.5 | 4.0 | 0.50 |
| Fleroxacin | 400 | 48 | 0.4 | 2.0 | 0.5 | 0.125 |
| Pefloxacin | 800 | 108 | 0.80 | 1.0 | 0.5 | 0.125 |
| Sparfloxacin | 200 | 18 | 0.12 | 2.0 | 0.1 | 0.12 |

**Table 7.** Breakpoint AUICs and MICs for fluoroquinolones in patients with 50-ml/min creatinine clearance[a]

| Quinolone | Oral dose (mg/24 h) | AUC (mg·h/liter) | Breakpoint MIC for AUIC of 125 | $MIC_{90}$ | | |
|---|---|---|---|---|---|---|
| | | | | *P. aeruginosa* | *Staphylococcus* sp. | *E. coli* |
| Norfloxacin | 800 | 14 | 0.125 | 2.0 | 6.3 | 0.125 |
| Ciprofloxacin | 1,500 | 64 | 0.5 | 0.5 | 0.5 | 0.01 |
| Ofloxacin | 800 | 133 | 1.0 | 2.0 | 0.25 | 0.125 |
| Enoxacin | 800 | 38 | 0.30 | 4.0 | 2.0 | 0.25 |
| Lomefloxacin | 400 | 75 | 0.60 | 12.5 | 4.0 | 0.50 |
| Fleroxacin | 400 | 170 | 1.25 | 2.0 | 0.5 | 0.125 |
| Pefloxacin | 800 | 108 | 0.80 | 1.0 | 0.5 | 0.125 |

[a]Data are from references 14 and 27.

can cover (eradicate) organisms with the highest MICs. Clinical results with any of these quinolones will most certainly depend on the true MIC for the organism in a particular patient and the actual AUC achieved in each individually treated patient. However, this exercise (Tables 6 and 7) makes it quite clear that in vitro potency (low MIC), such as with ciprofloxacin, can offset many of the pharmacokinetic disadvantages that result in a lower serum AUC. Consider ofloxacin (a quinolone that provides a higher AUC but also has a considerably higher MIC for pseudomonads) used against pseudomonads. Ofloxacin does not become more potent against pseudomonads than ciprofloxacin solely because of its higher AUC, because its AUC advantages do not offset its potency disadvantages. While ofloxacin cannot accomplish the same task as ciprofloxacin at its usual dose, a sufficiently higher dose of ofloxacin (e.g., 800 mg twice daily) would raise its AUIC to 125 and produce a regimen equivalent to that of ciprofloxacin.

The calculations of breakpoints in Tables 6 and 7 clearly show that overall antibacterial actions (i.e., pharmacodynamics) are determined for each quinolone only when both the MIC and the pharmacokinetics are considered. Defects in either pharmacokinetics (low AUC) or potency (high MIC) may partially compensate for defects in the other. Of course, one could compensate for either problem by raising the dosage and making any fluoroquinolone more active. This happens naturally in some patient populations. For example, even mild renal insufficiency greatly improves the potency of most quinolones by increasing the AUC, and renal failure helps those quinolones that are renally excreted (ofloxacin, lomefloxacin) more than the two-pathway drugs like ciprofloxacin, norfloxacin, and enoxacin. This is probably the most important message of the AUIC data, given the current marketing-based strategy of giving once-daily doses of quinolones with marginal activities but long half-lives. Whether raising the dosage or shortening the dosing interval on selected patients would increase microbiological cure rates for selected patients remains a subject for further study, as does the question of applicability of these results to other infections beyond nosocomial pneumonia. We have taken the position that actions of all fluoroquinolones can be mathematically described by indices like AUIC even though only ciprofloxacin has been studied to date. This position also must be confirmed by further study. Finally, our data thus far also correlate development of bacterial resistance with low AUC, high MIC, and troughs below the MIC (19, 41). Although this correlation is largely consistent with the results of in vitro animal and human studies, it is hardly proven at this early stage and must be given further study. However, a propensity to resistance development as bacteria are exposed to a low AUIC or troughs below the MIC may become the single greatest reason to counter marketing-driven attempts to lower quinolone dosages or prolong dosing intervals. If a pharmacodynamic perspective can be used to prolong the time that we have useful and microbiologically active fluoroquinolones, then its purpose has been well served indeed.

## REFERENCES


1. **Azoulay-Dupuis, E., J. P. Bedos, E. Vallee, and J. J. Pocidalo.** 1991. Comparative activity of fluorinated quinolones in acute and subacute S. pneumoniae models. *J. Antimicrob. Chemother.* **28**(Suppl. C):45–53.
2. **Bamberger, D. M., L. R. Peterson, D. N. Gerding, J. A. Moody, and C. E. Fasching.** 1986. Ciprofloxacin, azlocillin, ceftizoxime and amikacin alone and in combination against gram negative bacilli in a neutropenic site rabbit model of infection. *J. Antimicrob. Chemother.* **18**:51–63.
3. **Barriere, S. L., E. Ely, J. E. Kapusnik, and J. G. Gambertoglio.** 1985. Analysis of a new method for assessing activity of combinations of antimicrobials: area under the bactericidal activity curve. *J. Antimicrob. Chemother.* **16**:49–59.
4. **Bauernfeind, A., C. Petermuller, and B. Heinrich.** 1986. Dependence of the bactericidal activity and mutant selection of 4-quinolones on their serum concentration levels. *Infection* **14**(Suppl. 1):S26–S30.
5. **Blaser, J., B. B. Stone, M. C. Groner, et al.** 1987. Comparative study with enoxacin and netilmicin in a pharmacodynamic model to determine the importance of ratio of antibiotic peak concentration to MIC for bactericidal activity and emergence of resistance. *Antimicrob. Agents Chemother.* **31**:1054–1060.
6. **Blum, R. A., R. W. Schultz, and J. J. Schentag.** 1990. Pharmacokinetics of lomefloxacin in renally compromised patients. *Antimicrob. Agents Chemother.* **34**:2364–2368.
7. **Canton, E., J. Peman, M. T. Jiminez, M. S. Ramon, and M. Gobernado.** 1992. In vitro activity of sparfloxacin compared with those of five other quinolones. *Antimicrob. Agents Chemother.* **36**:558–565.
8. **Carpenter, T. C., C. J. Hackbarth, H. F. Chambers, and M. A. Sande.** 1986. Efficacy of ciprofloxacin for experimental endocarditis caused by methicillin susceptible or resistant strains of *Staphylococcus aureus*. *Antimicrob. Agents Chemother.* **30**:382–384.
9. **Chalkley, L. J., and H. J. Koornhof.** 1985. Antimicrobial activity of ciprofloxacin against *Pseudomonas aeruginosa*, *Escherichia coli*, and *Staphylococcus aureus* determined by the killing curve method. *Antimicrob. Agents Chemother.* **28**:331–342.
10. **Chin, N. X., and H. C. Neu.** 1987. Post antibiotic suppressive effect of ciprofloxacin against gram positive and gram negative bacteria. *Am. J. Med.* **82**(Suppl. 4A):58–62.
11. **Contrepois, A., C. Daldoss, B. Pangon, J. J. Garaud, M. Kecir, C. Sarrazin, J. M. Vallois, and C. Carbon.** 1984. Pefloxacin in rabbits: protein binding, extravascular diffusion, urinary excretion, and bactericidal effects in experimental endocarditis. *J. Antimicrob. Chemother.* **14**:51–57.
12. **Craig, W. A., J. Redington, and S. C. Ebert.** 1991. Pharmacodynamics of amikacin in vitro and in experimental infections. *J. Antimicrob. Chemother.* **27**(Suppl. C):29–40.
13. **Diver, J. M.** 1989. Quinolone uptake by bacteria and bacterial killing. *Rev. Infect. Dis.* **11**(Suppl. 5):S941–S946.
14. **Drusano, G. L.** 1989. Pharmacokinetics of the quinolone antimicrobial agents, p. 71–105. *In* J. S. Wolfson and D. C. Hooper (ed.), *Quinolone Antimicrobial Agents*. American Society for Microbiology, Washington, D.C.
15. **Drusano, G. L., H. Standiford, P. Ryan, W. McNamee, B. Tatem, and S. Schimpff.** 1986. Correlation of predicted serum bactericidal activities and values measured in volunteers. *Eur. J. Clin. Microbiol.* **5**:88–92.
16. **Dudley, M. N.** 1991. Pharmacodynamics and pharmacokinetics of antibiotics with special reference to the fluoroquinolones. *Am. J. Med.* **91**(Suppl. 6A):45S–50S.
17. **Dudley, M. N., J. Blaser, D. Gilbert, and S. H. Zinner.** 1988. Bactericidal activity of ciprofloxacin against P. aeruginosa and other bacteria in an invitro two compartment capillary model. *Rev. Infect. Dis.* **10**(Suppl.):S34–S35.
18. **Dudley, M. N., and S. H. Zinner.** 1987. Simultaneous pharmacokinetic and pharmacodynamic modeling of the antipseudomonal activity of ciprofloxacin: importance of bacterial subpopulations, abstr. 445. *Program Abstr. 27th Intersci. Conf. Antimicrob. Agents Chemother.*
19. **Forrest, A., D. E. Nix, C. H. Ballow, T. F. Goss, M. C. Birmingham, and J. J. Schentag.** 1993. Pharmacodynamics of intravenous ciprofloxacin in seriously ill patients. *Antimicrob. Agents Chemother.* **37**:1073–1081.
20. **Gengo, F. M., T. W. Mannion, C. H. Nightingale, and J. J. Schentag.** 1984. Integration of pharmacokinetics and pharmacodynamics of methicillin in curative treatment of experimental endocarditis. *J. Antimicrob. Chemother.* **14**:619–631.
21. **Gerber, A. U., H. P. Brugger, C. Feller, T. Stritzko, and B. Stadler.** 1986. Antibiotic therapy of infections due to Pseudomonas aeruginosa in normal and granulocytopenic mice: comparison of murine and human pharmacokinetics. *J. Infect. Dis.* **153**:90–97.
22. **Gordin, F. M., C. J. Hackbarth, K. G. Scott, and M. A. Sande.** 1985. Activities of pefloxacin

and ciprofloxacin in experimentally induced pseudomonas pneumonia in neutropenic guinea pigs. *Antimicrob. Agents Chemother.* **27**:452–454.

23. **Goss, T. F., A. Forrest, D. E. Nix, C. H. Ballow, M. C. Birmingham, T. J. Cumbo, and J. J. Schentag.** Mathematical examination of dual individualization principles. II. The rate of bacterial eradication versus AUIC in lower respiratory tract infection patients treated with cefmenoxime or ciprofloxacin. *Ann. Pharmacother.*, in press.
24. **Hackbarth, C. J., H. F. Chambers, F. Stella, A. M. Shibl, and M. A. Sande.** 1986. Ciprofloxacin in experimental Pseudomonas aeruginosa meningitis in rabbits. *J. Antimicrob. Chemother.* **18**(Suppl. D):65–69.
25. **Hirose, T., E. Okezaki, H. Kato, Y. Ito, M. Inoue, and S. Mitsuhashi.** 1987. In vitro and in vivo activity of NY 198 (lomefloxacin), a new difluorinated quinolone. *Antimicrob. Agents Chemother.* **31**:854–859.
26. **Hooper, D. C., and J. S. Wolfson.** 1989. The mode of action of the quinolone antimicrobial agents: review of recent information. *Rev. Infect. Dis.* **11**(Suppl. 5):S902–S911.
27. **Hooper, D. C., and J. S. Wolfson.** 1991. Fluoroquinolone antimicrobial agents. *N. Engl. J. Med.* **324**:384–394.
28. **Imada, T., S. Miyazaki, M. Nishida, K. Yamaguchi, and S. Goto.** 1992. In vitro and in vivo antibacterial activities of OPC 17116, a new quinolone. *Antimicrob. Agents Chemother.* **36**:573–579.
29. **Kemmerich, B., G. J. Small, and J. E. Pennington.** 1986. Comparative evaluation of ciprofloxacin, enoxacin, and ofloxacin in experimental *Pseudomonas aeruginosa* pneumonia. *Antimicrob. Agents Chemother.* **29**:395–399.
30. **Leggett, J. E., S. Ebert, B. Fantin, and W. A. Craig.** 1991. Comparative dose-effect relations at several dosing intervals for beta-lactam, aminoglycoside and quinolone antibiotics against gram-negative bacilli in murine thigh-infection and pneumonitis models. *Scand. J. Infect. Dis.* **74**(Suppl.):179–184.
31. **Luzier, A., T. F. Goss, T. J. Cumbo, and J. J. Schentag.** 1992. Mathematical examination of dual individualization principles. III. Development of a scoring system for pneumonia staging and quantitation of response to antibiotics: results in cefmenoxime treated patients. *Ann. Pharmacother.* **26**:1358–1364.
32. **Michea-Hamzehpour, M., R. Auckenthaler, P. Regamey, and J. C. Pechere.** 1987. Resistance occurring after fluoroquinolone therapy of experimental *Pseudomonas aeruginosa* peritonitis. *Antimicrob. Agents Chemother.* **31**:1803–1808.
33. **Michea-Hamzehpour, M., J.-C. Pechere, B. Marchou, and R. Auckenthaler.** 1986. Combination therapy: a way to limit emergence of resistance? *Am. J. Med.* **80**(Suppl. 6B):138–142.
34. **Moody, J. A., D. N. Gerding, and L. R. Peterson.** 1987. Evaluation of ciprofloxacin synergism with other agents by multiple in vitro methods. *Am. J. Med.* **82**(Suppl. 4A):44–54.
35. **Muranaka, K., and D. Greenwood.** 1988. The response of Streptococcus faecalis to ciprofloxacin, norfloxacin, and enoxacin. *J. Antimicrob. Chemother.* **21**:545–554.
36. **Neuman, M.** 1988. Clinical pharmacokinetics of the newer antibacterial 4-quinolones. *Clin. Pharmacokinet.* **14**:96–121.
37. **Nix, D. E., D. Goodwin, C. A. Peloquin, D. L. Rotella, and J. J. Schentag.** 1991. Antibiotic tissue penetration and its relevance: models of tissue penetration and their meaning. *Antimicrob. Agents Chemother.* **35**:1947–1952.
38. **Nix, D. E., D. Goodwin, C. A. Peloquin, D. L. Rotella, and J. J. Schentag.** 1991. Antibiotic tissue penetration and its relevance: impact of tissue penetration on infection response. *Antimicrob. Agents Chemother.* **35**:1953–1959.
39. **Nix, D. E., and J. J. Schentag.** 1988. The quinolones: an overview and comparative appraisal of their pharmacokinetics and pharmacodynamics. *J. Clin. Pharmacol.* **28**:169–178.
40. **Norden, C. W., and E. Shinners.** 1985. Ciprofloxacin as therapy for experimental osteomyelitis caused by Pseudomonas aeruginosa. *J. Infect. Dis.* **151**:291–294.
41. **Peloquin, C. A., T. J. Cumbo, D. E. Nix, M. F. Sands, and J. J. Schentag.** 1989. Intravenous ciprofloxacin in patients with nosocomial lower respiratory tract infections: impact of plasma concentrations, organism MIC, and clinical condition on bacterial eradication. *Arch. Intern. Med.* **149**:2269–2273.
42. **Potel, G., N. P. Chau, B. Pangon, B. Fantin, J. M. Vallois, F. Faurisson, and C. Carbon.** 1991. Single daily dosing of antibiotics: importance of in vitro killing rate, serum half life and protein binding. *Antimicrob. Agents Chemother.* **35**:2085–2090.
43. **Roosendaal, I. A., J. Bakker-Woudenberg, M. Vandenberghe-Van Raffe, V. Vandenberg, and M. F. Michel.** 1989. Impact of dosage schedule on the efficacy of ceftazidime, gentamicin and ciprofloxacin in Klebsiella pneumoniae pneumonia and septicemia in leukopenic rats. *Eur. J. Clin. Microbiol. Infect. Dis.* **8**:878–887.
44. **Schentag, J. J.** Correlation of pharmacokinetic parameters to efficacy of antibiotics: relationships between serum concentrations, MIC values, and bacterial eradication in patients with gram negative pneumonia. 1991. *Scand. J. Infect. Dis.* **74**(Suppl.):218–234.
45. **Schentag, J. J., T. J. Cumbo, W. J. Jusko, and M. E. Plaut.** 1978. Gentamicin tissue accumula-

tion and nephrotoxic reactions. *J. Am. Med. Assoc.* **240:**2067–2069.

46. **Schentag, J. J., D. E. Nix, and M. H. Adelman.** 1991. Mathematical examination of dual individualization principles. I. Relationships between AUC above MIC and area under the inhibitory curve for cefmenoxime, ciprofloxacin, and tobramycin. *D.I.C.P. Ann. Pharmacother.* **25:**1050–1057.
47. **Schentag, J. J., I. L. Smith, D. J. Swanson, C. DeAngelis, J. E. Fracasso, A. Vari, and J. W. Vance.** 1984. Role for dual individualization with cefmenoxime. *Am. J. Med.* **77**(Suppl. 6A):43–50.
48. **Schentag, J. J., D. J. Swanson, and I. L. Smith.** 1985. Dual individualization—antibiotic dosage calculation from the integration of in vitro pharmacodynamics and in vivo pharmacokinetics. *J. Antimicrob. Chemother.* **15**(Suppl. A):47–57.
49. **Schentag, J. J., A. J. Vari, N. E. Winslade, D. J. Swanson, I. L. Smith, G. W. Simons, and A. Vigano.** 1985. Treatment with aztreonam or tobramycin in critical care patients with gram negative pneumonia. *Am. J. Med.* **78**(Suppl. A):34–41.
50. **Shibl, A. M., C. H. Hackbarth, and M. A. Sande.** 1986. Evaluation of pefloxacin in experimental *Escherichia coli* meningitis. *Antimicrob. Agents Chemother.* **29:**409–411.
51. **Smith, J. T.** 1986. The mode of action of 4-quinolones and possible mechanisms of resistance. *J. Antimicrob. Chemother.* **18**(Suppl. D):21–29.
52. **Stratton, C. W., J. J. Franke, L. S. Weeks, and F. A. Manion.** 1989. Comparison of the bactericidal activity of ciprofloxacin alone and in combination with selected antipseudomonal $\beta$-lactam agents against clinical isolates of Pseudomonas aeruginosa. *Diagn. Microbiol. Infect. Dis.* **11:**41–52.
53. **Stratton, C. W., M. P. Weinstein, and L. B. Reller.** 1982. Correlation of serum bactericidal activity with antimicrobial agent level and MBC. *J. Infect. Dis.* **145:**160–168.
54. **Vallee, E., E. A. Dupuis, J. J. Pocidalo, and E. Bergogne-Berezin.** 1991. Pharmacokinetics of four fluoroquinolones in an animal model of infected lung. *J. Antimicrob. Chemother.* **28**(Suppl. C):39–44.
55. **Vogelman, B., S. Gudmundsson, J. Turnidge, J. E. Leggett, and W. A. Craig.** 1988. The in vivo post antibiotic effect in a thigh infection in neutropenic mice. *J. Infect. Dis.* **157:**287–298.
56. **Webb, D. B., D. E. Roberts, J. D. Williams, and A. W. Asscher.** 1986. Pharmacokinetics of ciprofloxacin in healthy volunteers and patients with impaired kidney function. *J. Antimicrob. Chemother.* **18**(Suppl. D):83–87.
57. **Wolfson, J. S., and M. N. Swartz.** 1985. Serum bactericidal activity as a monitor of antibiotic therapy. *N. Engl. J. Med.* **312:**968–975.
58. **Yuen, G. J., G. L. Drusano, K. Plaisance, A. Forrest, and E. S. Caplan.** 1989. Ciprofloxacin pharmacokinetics in critically ill trauma patients. *Am. J. Med.* **87**(Suppl. 5A):70S–75S.
59. **Zeiler, H. J., and W. H. Voigt.** 1987. Efficacy of ciprofloxacin in stationary-phase bacteria in vivo. *Am. J. Med.* **82**(Suppl. 4A):87–90.
60. **Zinner, S. H., M. N. Dudley, D. Gilber, and M. Bassignani.** 1988. Effect of dose and schedule on cefoperazone pharmacodynamics in an in vitro model of infection in a neutropenic host. *Am. J. Med.* **85**(Suppl. 1A):56–58.

*Quinolone Antimicrobial Agents, 2nd ed.*
Edited by David C. Hooper and John S. Wolfson


*Chapter 13*

# Treatment of Urinary Tract Infections with Quinolone Antimicrobial Agents

*S. Ragnar Norrby*

When first introduced, quinolones were classified as "urinary antiseptics" and used exclusively for treatment of lower urinary tract infections (UTIs). They were commonly perceived as having no systemic effects, and it was not unusual to allow the use of nonfluorinated quinolones, for example, nalidixic acid, in parallel with other antibiotics in trials of treatment of systemic infections. It is now obvious that older, nonfluorinated quinolones are also bactericidal antibiotics active in systemic infections. In this chapter, fluorinated quinolone antimicrobial agents and their use for the treatment of various types of UTIs are emphasized. Definitions of these types of UTIs, if they are defined at all, tend to vary from one trial to another. Recently, Rubin et al. (52) proposed definitions of acute uncomplicated UTI, acute uncomplicated pyelonephritis, and complicated UTI (Table 1). They also proposed that the definition of significant bacteriuria be changed from the classical $\geq 10^5$ CFU/ml in a midstream urine sample to $\geq 10^3$ CFU/ml in women with uncomplicated cystitis and $\geq 10^4$ CFU/ml in women with uncomplicated pyelonephritis and in men with symptomatic UTI. The definition of bacteriuria was proposed to remain at $\geq 10^5$ in patients with complicated UTI or asymptomatic bacteriuria. These definitions will increase the sensitivity of urine cultures without markedly decreasing the specificity.

*S. Ragnar Norrby* • Department of Infectious Diseases, Lund University Hospital, University of Lund, S-22185 Lund, Sweden.

## IN VITRO ACTIVITIES OF NEWER QUINOLONE AGENTS AGAINST URINARY TRACT PATHOGENS

The in vitro activity of this group of antibiotics is dealt with in detail in chapter 8. For a quinolone to be used in the treatment of a UTI, it must show activity against members of the family *Enterobacteriaceae*, nonfermenting gram-negative aerobes such as *Pseudomonas* spp. and *Acinetobacter* spp., and some gram-positive aerobes, mainly *Staphylococcus saprophyticus*, *Staphylococcus aureus*, coagulase-negative staphylococci, *Enterococcus* spp., and *Streptococcus agalactiae* (group B streptococci). Table 2 summarizes the activities of some of the newer fluoroquinolones against these pathogens. Taking into account the pharmacokinetics of these antibiotics with very high concentrations in urine and the accumulation of the drugs in renal tissues, the differences between the various derivatives should be of clinical importance in only a few cases, when the MICs for 90% of isolates ($MIC_{90}$) exceed 8 mg/liter. This is especially the case when pyelonephritis is treated. High systemic levels of antibiotic are then required, since the patient may have bacteremia.

**Table 1.** Definitions of UTIs[a]

| Term | Definition |
|---|---|
| Acute uncomplicated cystitis . . . . . . . | Dysuria, urgency, frequency, gross hematuria, lower back and/or abdominal discomfort in woman with bacteriuria[b] ($\geq 10^3$ CFU/ml) and pyuria ($\geq$ 10 WBC[c]/mm$^3$) |
| Acute uncomplicated pyelonephritis . | Fever, chills and flank pain in woman with bacteriuria ($\geq 10^4$ CFU/ml) and pyuria ($\geq$ 10 WBC/mm$^3$) |
| Complicated UTI . . . . . . . . . . . . . . . . | Cystitis or pyelonephritis in patient who is catheterized or has anatomical or functional abnormality of the urinary tract and has bacteriuria ($\geq 10^5$ CFU/ml) and pyuria ($\geq$ 10 WBC/mm$^3$). All UTIs with bacteriuria and pyuria in men are complicated. |
| Asymptomatic bacteriuria . . . . . . . . . | Bacteriuria ($\geq 10^5$ CFU/ml in two consecutive urine samples) and pyuria ($\geq$ 10 WBC/mm$^3$) in patient with none of the symptoms listed above. |

[a]Modified from reference 52.
[b]Definition of bacteriuria is based on midstream urine samples. Any bacterial count in a sample obtained by suprapubic aspiration is considered significant. In patients with UTI caused by *S. saprophyticus*, counts should be reduced by 1 $\log_{10}$.
[c]WBC, leukocytes.

**Table 2.** Summary of in vitro activities of newer quinolones against bacterial species causing UTI[a]

| Species | Agents[b] with $MIC_{90}$ ($\mu$g/ml) of: | | |
|---|---|---|---|
| | <1 | 1–8 | >8 |
| *Escherichia coli* | All | | |
| *Klebsiella* spp. | All | | |
| *Enterobacter* spp. | All | | |
| *Citrobacter* spp. | CIP, ENO, FLE, LOM, NOR, TOS | OFL, PEF, SPA | |
| *Proteus mirabilis* | All | | |
| *Proteus vulgaris* | CIP, FLE, LOM, NOR, OFL, PEF, SPA, TOS | ENO | |
| *Providencia stuartii* | | All | |
| *Morganella morganii* | All | | |
| *Pseudomonas aeruginosa* | CIP, SPA | ENO, FLE, LOM, NOR, OFL, PEF, TOS | |
| *Pseudomonas* spp. | | CIP, ENO, FLE, PEF, TOS, TOS | LOM, NOR, OFL |
| *Xanthomonas maltophilia* | | CIP, ENO, FLE, PEF, SPA, TOS | LOM, NOR, OFL |
| *Acinetobacter* spp. | CIP | ENO, FLE, LOM, PEF, SPA, TOS | NOR, OFL |
| *Staphylococcus* spp. | FLE, SPA, TOS | CIP, ENO, LOM, NOR, PEF, OFL | |
| *Enterococcus* spp. | SPA | CIP, FLE, NOR, OFL, TOS | LOM, ENO, PEF |
| *Streptococcus agalactiae* | | CIP, FLE, LOM, NOR, OFL, SPA, TOS | ENO, PEF |

[a]Data are from references 2, 5, 6, 7, 14, 15, 17, 22, 25, 28, 34, 35, 47, 53, 61, and 65.
[b]CIP, ciprofloxacin; ENO, enoxacin; FLE, fleroxacin; LOM, lomefloxacin; NOR, norfloxacin; OFL, ofloxacin; PEF, pefloxacin; SPA, sparfloxacin; TOS, tosufloxacin.

Newer fluoroquinolones such as tosufloxacin and sparfloxacin differ from the older ones (for example, norfloxacin, ofloxacin, and ciprofloxacin), especially in their improved activities against gram-positive pathogens. That advantage is less important when treatment of UTI is considered; gram-positive pathogens are less common in cases of UTI, and only rarely do they disseminate to the blood.

Low pH and high concentrations of $Mg^{2+}$ or $Ca^{2+}$ decrease the in vitro effect of this group of antibiotics (18, 19). Thus, when bacterial strains have been tested in human urine, MICs higher than those in conventional media have been reported (10, 56). The clinical relevance of these in vitro findings has not been studied.

## PHARMACOKINETICS OF FLUOROQUINOLONES WITH SPECIAL REFERENCE TO TREATMENT OF UTI

Details of the pharmacokinetics of new quinolones are dealt with in chapter 9. Pharmacokinetic characteristics that should be considered for an antibiotic intended for use in the treatment of UTIs are concentrations obtained in plasma, urine, renal tissue, and feces. In patients with reduced renal function, the effect of such reductions on the elimination half-life and on the risk of drug accumulation should be taken into account. Concentration in urine is always important for the elimination of bacteriuria. In patients with cystitis, it is the most important pharmacokinetic parameter. Fecal concentrations may influence the degree of suppression of the aerobic fecal flora and hence the risk of early reinfection. High fecal concentrations of quinolones were previously believed to be the result only of poor gastrointestinal absorption. It is now clear that one of the routes of elimination for this group of antibiotics is the transintestinal one. Also, quinolones with a high bioavailability after oral administration, for example, ofloxacin, are excreted to a considerable extent into the feces (38, 67).

Table 3 gives some pharmacokinetic parameter values for ciprofloxacin, enoxacin, fleroxacin, lomefloxacin, norfloxacin, ofloxacin, sparfloxacin, and temafloxacin. Pefloxacin has not been included because of the complicated kinetics of that antibiotic due to extensive liver metabolism. No published kinetic data have been found for tosufloxacin.

Considerable differences exist between the kinetics of the various fluoroquinolones. However, all of them, even sparfloxacin, achieve concentrations in urine that are well above 8 $\mu$g/ml for 24 h or more after a dose. Most of them maintain concentrations in urine above 100 $\mu$g/liter for 12 h or more after a dose. Thus, the concentrations in urine are sufficient to inhibit an absolute majority of pathogens causing cystitis, including *Pseudomonas aeruginosa* and gram-positive organisms. Concentrations in blood vary, and few of the compounds give concentrations in serum above the $MIC_{90}$ for most strains of *P. aeruginosa*. However, with all of them, concentrations in serum well above the $MIC_{90}$s for *Enterobacteriaceae* are achieved.

The half-lives of the compounds vary. Sparfloxacin has a considerably longer half-life than the others. With all of them, high concentrations in urine will be maintained for at least 12 h and in most patients for 24 h or more. Renal impairment results in marked prolongation of the half-life of quinolones that are not metabolized in the liver to a high degree (for example, ofloxacin). With the derivatives that undergo hepatic metabolism (for example, norfloxacin, enoxacin and pefloxacin), renal impairment results in a less-marked effect on the half-life. Because of the very high volume of distribution, hemodialysis does not affect the elimination of any of the fluoroquinolones to a noticeable extent.

The concentrations achieved in renal tissue have consistently been reported to be considerably higher than the concurrent ones in serum or plasma (20, 30, 39, 60). This should

**Table 3.** Summary of pharmacokinetics of orally administered single doses of fluoroquinolones in healthy volunteers

| Quinolone (reference) | Dose (mg) | Pharmacokinetic parameter[a] (mean) | | | |
|---|---|---|---|---|---|
| | | $C_{max}$ (μg/ml) | $T_{max}$ (h) | $t_{1/2}$ (h) | $UR_{0-24}$ (%) |
| Ciprofloxacin (8) | 100 | 0.7 | 0.9 | 3.0 | 12 |
| | 250 | 1.7 | 1.1 | 3.2 | 28 |
| | 500 | 2.3 | 1.5 | 3.2 | 27 |
| | 1,000 | 5.9 | 1.8 | 3.4 | 28 |
| Enoxacin (66) | 200 | 1.2 | 0.8 | 4.2 | 45 |
| | 400 | 2.0 | 1.5 | 4.2 | 47 |
| | 800 | 4.3 | 1.3 | 5.4 | 36 |
| | 1,600 | 8.1 | 2.0 | 6.4 | 42 |
| Fleroxacin (64) | 100 | 2.9 | 0.3 | 8.6 | 67[b] |
| | 200 | 2.3 | 1.1 | 8.9 | 65[b] |
| | 400 | 4.4 | 1.3 | 9.2 | 50[b] |
| | 800 | 7.0 | 1.2 | 10.9 | 50[b] |
| Lomefloxacin (55a) | 100 | 1.0 | 0.8 | 7.1 | 72[c] |
| | 200 | 2.2 | 0.7 | 7.3 | 66[c] |
| | 400 | 2.7 | 1.3 | 7.8 | 69[c] |
| | 600 | 4.3 | 1.6 | 8.0 | 49[c] |
| | 800 | 6.8 | 1.0 | 8.0 | 60[c] |
| Norfloxacin (57) | 200 | 0.8 | 1.1 | 7.3 | 55 |
| | 400 | 1.6 | 1.3 | 7.4 | 52 |
| | 800 | 2.4 | 1.5 | 6.2 | 51 |
| | 1,600 | 3.9 | 1.9 | 6.8 | 27 |
| Ofloxacin (41) | 100 | 1.0–1.3 | 0.5–2.2 | 2.6–6.7 | 70–99 |
| | 200 | 2.6 | 0.8–1.0 | 5.7–7.0 | 74–87 |
| | 400 | 4.0–5.6 | 0.7–1.4 | 5.0–7.4 | 74–81 |
| | 600 | 6.8–6.9 | 1.0–2.8 | 5.9–6.7 | 75–94 |
| Sparfloxacin (42) | 200 | 0.7 | 4 | 20.8 | 10[d] |
| | 400 | 1.2 | 5 | 18.2 | 10[d] |
| | 600 | 1.7 | 5 | 20.3 | 9[d] |
| | 800 | 2.0 | 5 | 20.0 | 9[d] |

[a] $C_{max}$, maximum concentration of drug in serum or plasma; $T_{max}$, time to $C_{max}$; $t_{1/2}$, half-life in serum or plasma in the β phase; $UR_{0-24}$, proportion of dose recovered in urine as unchanged drug during the first 24 h after dose is administered.
[b] Values are for 0 to 60 h.
[c] Values are for 0 to 48 h.
[d] Values are for 0 to 120 h.

be an advantage when pyelonephritis is treated.

## Efficacy in Uncomplicated Cystitis

Uncomplicated cystitis accounts for more than 85% of all patients with UTI who seek medical attention. Table 4 summarizes the largest of the many studies now published on the use of fluoroquinolones in this infection. Studies included have all been comparative, and most of them were double-blind. However, few fulfilled the requirements for study design proposed by Fihn and Stamm (23). Common weaknesses were lack of data from a late follow-up 3 to 6 weeks after treatment and study groups too small to demonstrate equivalences between treatments with a reasonable statistical power. The comparator used in each trial was either trimethoprim-sulfamethoxazole or another quinolone. No studies of reasonable size comparing ciprofloxacin with other antibiotics for UTIs have been found. Several factors caused the rate of elimination of bacteriuria to vary in the different trials. Reasons for these differ-

**Table 4.** Results of clinical trials of fluoroquinolones in patients with uncomplicated cystitis[a]

| Reference | Quinolone | | | Comparator | | | Failure rate (%)[b] | |
|---|---|---|---|---|---|---|---|---|
| | Drug | No. of patients | Dosage (mg)[c] | Drug | No. of patients | Dosage | Quinolone | Comparator |
| 4 | ENO | 33 | 600 SD | ENO | 36 | 300 b.i.d./3 | 24.2 | 11.1 |
| 29a | FLE | 103 | 400 SD | CIP | 127 | 250 b.i.d./7 | 18.4 | 4.7 |
| | FLE | 115 | 200 q.d./7 | | | | 7.0 | |
| 24 | LOM | 134 | 400 q.d./3 | NOR | 139 | 400 b.i.d./7 | 6.4 | 1.8 |
| | LOM | 141 | 400 q.d./7 | | | | 1.2 | |
| 59 | NOR | 248 | 200 b.i.d./7 | T/S | 138 | 960 b.i.d./7 | 2.4 | 1.4 |
| | NOR | 238 | 400 b.i.d./7 | | | | 2.5 | |
| 50 | NOR | 163 | 400 b.i.d./3 | NOR | 162 | 400 b.i.d./7 | 2.5 | 1.9 |
| 58 | NOR | 193 | 400 b.i.d./3 | NOR | 175 | 200 b.i.d./7 | 7.4 | 3.4 |
| 11 | OFL | 97 | 100 b.i.d./3 | T/S | 92 | 960 b.i.d./3 | 8.2 | 12.0 |
| 31 | OFL | 26 | 200 b.i.d./3 | T/S | 55 | 960 b.i.d./7 | 3.7 | 7.3 |
| | OFL | 56 | 200 b.i.d./7 | | | | 8.9 | |
| | OFL | 25 | 300 b.i.d./7 | | | | 0.0 | |
| 46 | OFL | 60 | 100 SD | T/S | 59 | 960 b.i.d./3–7 | 40.0 | 6.8 |
| 49 | PEF | 140 | 800 SD | T/S | 145 | 960 b.i.d./5 | 2.9 | 4.8 |
| 63 | PEF | 75 | 800 SD | NOR | 75 | 400 b.i.d./5 | 12.0 | 13.3 |

[a]Includes trials in which >90% of the patients were women with uncomplicated cystitis. If possible, patients with other types of infections have been excluded. Abbreviations: CIP, ciprofloxacin; ENO, enoxacin; FLE, fleroxacin; LOM, lomefloxacin; NOR, norfloxacin; OFL, ofloxacin; PEF, pefloxacin; T/S, trimethoprim-sulfamethoxazole.
[b]Patients with persistence or reinfection at first posttreatment follow-up 5 to 9 days after last dose.
[c]Number of doses per day/number of days. SD, single dose; q.d., every day; b.i.d., twice daily.

ences could be (i) that the time of assessment relative to the last treatment dose varied; (ii) that the half-lives of the various drugs are different, perhaps leading to residual concentrations in urine in patients who received drugs with long half-lives; and (iii) that the selection of patients seems to have been different; i.e., in some studies, more than 90% of the women had *E. coli* as their pathogen, while in other studies, that species accounted for only 75 to 80% of the isolates. Irrespective of these differences, it seems clear that when quinolones are compared and when treatment times of 3 days or longer are used, no major differences exist between the quinolones in terms of efficacy in this type of UTI. Such differences may exist if single-dose treatment is compared, since the elimination half-life varies. It also seems evident that these antibiotics are highly efficient in the treatment of uncomplicated cystitis. The same was true when follow-up results 3 to 6 weeks after treatment were compared in the few trials that included such controls in a reasonable proportion of patients in the study.

The treatment time in patients with uncomplicated cystitis is a controversial issue (45). With enoxacin and fleroxacin, rates of elimination of bacteriuria were significantly lower when these drugs were given as single doses instead of multiple doses (4, 29a). The same was true for ofloxacin, although the dose given (100 mg) may have been too low (46). In another trial, when enoxacin given as a 400-mg single dose was compared with a 3-g single dose of amoxicillin, considerably better results were obtained with enoxacin (9). Thus, at 6 weeks after treatment, 35 of 40 enoxacin-treated patients had no bacteriuria, while as many as 24 of 40 who received amoxicillin had bacteriuria. In general, it appears that optimal treatment results are obtained with 3 to 7 days of treatment. However, other factors, such as cost of medication, improved compliance, and reduced risks of adverse effects, may justify shorter treatment times.

A special group of patients with uncomplicated UTI are the elderly. These patients often have unidentified complications such as atrophic vaginal mucosa or residual bladder urine. They should therefore not be mixed with younger women with cystitis in any study. In a large study, Jonsson et al. (32) compared 200 mg of norfloxacin given twice daily with 200 mg of pivmecillinam given twice daily for 7 days. At 2 to 8 days post-treatment, 87 of 111 (78.4%) of the patients in the norfloxacin group and only 47 of 91 (51.6%) in the pivmecillinam group had no bacteriuria ($P < 0.0001$; Wilcoxon two-sample test).

The place of fluoroquinolones in the treatment of sporadic uncomplicated cystitis in young women should be questioned. These drugs are highly efficient antibiotics with extremely broad spectra of activity against urinary tract pathogens. Uncomplicated cystitis is in a majority of cases caused by *E. coli* or *S. saprophyticus*, which are susceptible to a wide range of other antibiotics, for example, trimethoprim, trimethoprim-sulfamethoxazole, nitrofurantoin, and ß-lactams, that are well proven against these infections. If properly dosed, these antibiotics have a high degree of safety. For the treatment of women with sporadic uncomplicated cystitis, they should be preferred to the fluoroquinolones in order to avoid emergence of resistance, which may result from their widespread use for treatment of an infection as common as uncomplicated cystitis. Fluoroquinolones should be reserved mainly for treatment of recurrent uncomplicated cystitis, where species other than *E. coli* are more common. Nonfluorinated quinolones such as nalidixic acid, cinoxacin, and pipemidic acid should not be used. These antibiotics have 1/10 or less of the antibacterial activity of the fluorinated quinolones. A single mutation is likely to result in resistance in most of the UTI pathogens. Strains that have undergone such mutations will in most cases still be interpreted as susceptible to fluoroquinolones in a routine susceptibility test. However, the MICs of these compounds will be markedly increased, and a second mutation would result in emergence of clinically relevant resistance to the fluorinated derivatives as well.

## Efficacy in Complicated UTI and Pyelonephritis

Complicated UTI is a broad concept. In the forthcoming guidelines for clinical trials in patients with UTIs, it has been defined as a UTI in a patient with a congenital or acquired malformation that facilitates acquisition of bacteriuria (52). However, also included in the definition is renal parenchymal damage, that is, a factor that in itself does not affect the risk of bacteriuria but that may lead to a more serious course of a UTI. These guidelines also propose that patients with complicated upper or lower UTIs could be pooled with patients with uncomplicated pyelonephritis because of the difficulty in enrolling enough pyelonephritis patients in trials to allow meaningful conclusions to be drawn.

The results of several hundred trials in which fluorinated quinolones have been studied in the treatment of complicated UTIs have been published. Most of these trials are of poor scientific quality. A majority of the studies have been uncontrolled and/or very small (<30 patients per study arm). The larger trials whose results have been published or for which data have been available through new-drug application data are summarized in Table 5. Similar to the situation with trials in patients with uncomplicated cystitis, there is a marked variability in rates of elimination of bacteriuria. This variability seems to be due mainly to differences in patient characteristics. However, it is obvious that the fluoroquinolones were at least as effective as trimethoprin-sulfamethoxazole and considerably more effective than ß-lactam antibiotics.

These types of UTI should be considered main indications for the fluoroquinolones. In comparison to other UTI antibiotics, they offer a better antibacterial spectrum and less-frequent occurrence of resistance.

**Table 5.** Results of clinical trials of fluoroquinolones in patients with complicated UTIs and pyelonephritis[a]

| Reference | Quinolone | | | Comparator | | | Failure rate (%)[b] | |
|---|---|---|---|---|---|---|---|---|
| | Drug | No. of patients | Dosage (mg)[c] | Drug | No. of patients | Dosage | Quinolone | Comparator |
| 26 | CIP | 43 | 250 b.i.d. | | | | 11.6 | |
| | CIP | 37 | 500 b.i.d. | | | | 13.5 | |
| | CIP | 43 | 750 b.i.d. | | | | 14.0 | |
| 48 | CIP | 16 | 100 b.i.d. i.v. | MEZ | 14 | 2,000 b.i.d. | 12.5 | 42.9 |
| 18 | ENO | 28 | 400 b.i.d. | T/S | 28 | 960 b.i.d. | 10.7 | 0.0 |
| 29a | FLE | 284 | 400 q.d. | NOR | 243 | 400 b.i.d. | 9.5 | 15.3 |
| 55a | LOM | 61 | 400 q.d. | NOR | 75 | 400 b.i.d. | 8.2 | 18.7 |
| 55 | NOR | 65 | 400 b.i.d. | CEF | 63 | 1,000 b.i.d. | 1.5 | 33.8 |
| 54 | NOR | 101 | 400 b.i.d. | T/S | 125 | 960 b.i.d. | 3.0 | 9.6 |
| 12 | OFL | 113 | 100 b.i.d. | T/S | 101 | 960 b.i.d. | 5.0 | 10.9 |
| | OFL | 223 | 200 b.i.d. | T/S | 202 | 960 b.i.d. | 18.4 | 21.3 |
| | OFL | 91 | 100 b.i.d. | NOR | 58 | 400 b.i.d. | 22.0 | 34.5 |

[a]Abbreviations: CIP, ciprofloxacin; ENO, enoxacin; FLE, fleroxacin; LOM, lomefloxacin; NOR, norfloxacin; OFL, ofloxacin; MEZ, mezlocillin given intravenously; T/S, trimethoprim-sulfamethoxazole; CEF, cefadroxil.
[b]Patients with persistence or reinfection at first posttreatment follow-up 5 to 12 days after last dose.
[c]Treatment times varied between 7 and 14 days. b.i.d., twice daily; q.d., every day; i.v., intravenously.

### Efficacy in Patients with Renal Transplants

UTI patients with renal transplants form a subgroup that offers special therapeutic problems. An infection in a transplanted kidney may have serious consequences and may even lead to rejection of the transplant. All patients with transplants receive cyclosporin A to prevent rejections. That drug interacts with a multitude of other agents metabolically in the liver and creates an increased risk of nephrotoxic reactions. Well-performed studies have shown no interaction between cyclosporin A on the one hand and pefloxacin, ciprofloxacin, norfloxacin, or ofloxacin on the other hand (36, 37, 51). These reports are contradicted by two case reports of possible nephrotoxic reactions in renal transplant patients receiving ciprofloxacin (3, 21). However, in both of these cases, other factors may have contributed to the reactions reported. Ofloxacin, which undergoes minimal hepatic metabolism, has been studied for the treatment of UTI in renal transplant patients, and the results indicate a high degree of efficacy without signs of interaction with cyclosporin A (43, 52). Fluoroquinolones seem to have advantages over many other antibiotics in this group of patients, and more-extensive studies on their efficacy are warranted.

## PROPHYLAXIS IN PATIENTS UNDERGOING UROLOGICAL SURGERY

The use of fluoroquinolones in surgical prophylaxis was recently reviewed by Mandell (40). One of the areas in which this group should be useful is in urological surgery, where the main threat is infections with gram-negative aerobic bacteria and where anaerobes are less important than in abdominal and gynecological surgery. Kanaiyalal et al. (33) performed a double-blind, placebo-controlled trial in patients undergoing transurethral prostatectomy who had had sterile urine before surgery. The patients received 200 mg of enoxacin or placebo the night before the operation, at 2 to 4 h postoperatively, and then every 12 h for 36 h. After surgery, 3 of 39 (7.7%) of enoxacin-treated patients and 15 of 39 (38.5%) receiving placebo had bacteriuria. The three enoxacin-treated patients with bacteriuria were all detected at the control 2 weeks after surgery, while 11 patients with bacteriuria in the placebo group were found at the control 48 h or 5 days postoperatively. In another, considerably smaller, placebo-controlled trial, pefloxacin or placebo was given intravenously for one preoperative dose and then followed by oral treatment until the catheter was withdrawn (1). Blood for culture was drawn during surgery, and cultures were positive in three patients receiving pefloxacin and eight receiving placebo. Bacteriuria was seen in two pefloxacin-treated patients, while 12 patients in the placebo group had positive urine cultures at removal of the catheters. The overall success rates were 86.1% with pefloxacin and 45.9% with placebo. Several other studies both with intravenous and with oral fluoroquinolones have demonstrated that ciprofloxacin, ofloxacin, and lomefloxacin are more effective than no treatment and have efficacies similar to those of intravenous ß-lactams (13, 16, 19, 27, 29, 40, 44).

## SUMMARY

The fluoroquinolones have well-established high degrees of efficacy in various types of UTIs. In comparison with other antibiotics used for UTIs, such as trimethoprim, trimethoprim-sulfamethoxazole, and various ß-lactams, they are at least as effective and safe, and in most cases, their spectra of activity are also more favorable. The latter factor is a result mainly of the fact that the new quinolones have been used for only a limited time. Reports on resistance to the fluoroquinolones are becoming increasingly frequent. These reports all indicate that resistance is more common in gram-positive pathogens than in gram-negative ones and that in the latter, resistance occurs when the consumption of these antibiotics is very high. To preserve the usefulness of the fluoroquinolones against UTIs and other types of infections, these drugs should not be routinely used for treatment of asymptomatic cystitis in young women unless the infection is a recurrence or the causative bacterial strain is known to be resistant to other antibiotics used against UTIs. By reserving the fluoroquinolones for recurrent uncomplicated cystitis, complicated cystitis, and pyelonephritis (complicated and uncomplicated), the life span of this important group of drugs is likely to be prolonged.

### REFERENCES

1. **Abbou, C., D. Chopin, M. Nguyen, P. Theodon, P. Antiphon, R. Goulois, and D. Bouleau.** 1989. Short term pefloxacin prophylaxis in transurethral resection of the prostate. *Rev. Infect. Dis.* **11**(Suppl. 5):1361.
2. **Aoyama, H., M. Inoue, and S. Mitsuhashi.** 1988. In-vitro and in-vivo antibacterial activity of fleroxacin, a new fluorinated quinolone. *J. Antimicrob. Chemother.* **22**(Suppl. D):99–114.
3. **Avent, C. K., D. Krinsky, J. K. Kirklin, R. C. Borrge, and W. D. Figg.** 1988. Synergistic nephrotoxicity due to ciprofloxacin and cyclosporin. *Am. J. Med.* **85:**452–453.
4. **Backhouse, C. I., and J. A. Matthews.** 1989. Single-dose enoxacin compared with 3-day treatment for urinary tract infections. *Antimicrob. Agents Chemother.* **33:**877–880.
5. **Barry, A. L., and R. N. Jones.** 1987. In vitro activity of ciprofloxacin against Gram-positive cocci. *Am. J. Med.* **82**(Suppl. 4A):27–32.
6. **Barry, A. L., and R. N. Jones.** 1989. In-vitro activity of temafloxacin, tosufloxacin (A-61827) and five other fluoroquinolone agents. *J. Antimicrob. Chemother.* **24:**415–424.
7. **Barry, A. L., C. Thornsberry, and R. N. Jones.** 1986. In vitro evaluation of A-56619 and A-56620, two new quinolones. *Antimicrob. Agents Chemother.* **29:**40–43.
8. **Bergan, T., S. B. Thorsteinsson, R. Solberg, L. Bjornskau, I. M. Kolstad, and S. Johnsen.** 1987. Pharmacokinetics of ciprofloxacin: intravenous and increasing oral doses. *Am. J. Med.* **82**(Suppl. 4A):97–102.
9. **Bischoff, W.** 1986. Vergleichende Untersuchung von Enoxacin mit Amoxicillin be der akuten unkomplizierten Zystitis der Frau. *Infection* **14**(Suppl. 3):209–210.
10. **Blaser, J., M. N. Dudley, D. Gilbert, and S. H. Zinner.** 1986. Influence of media and method on the in vitro susceptibility of *Pseudomonas aeruginosa* and other bacteria to ciprofloxacin and enoxacin. *Antimicrob. Agents Chemother.* **29:**927–929.
11. **Block, J. M., R. A. Walstad, A. Bjertnaes, P. E. Hafstad, M. Holte, I. Ottemo, P. L. Svarva, T.**

**Rolstad, and L. E. Peterson.** 1987. Ofloxacin versus trimethoprim-sulphamethoxazole in acute cystitis. *Drugs* **34**(Suppl. 1):100–106.

12. **Blomer, R., K. Bruch, and R. N. Zahltne.** 1986. Zusammengefasste Ergebnisse der Klinische Phase II- und III-Studien mit Ofloxacin (HOE 280) in Europa. *Infection* **14**(Suppl. 1):102–107.
13. **Charton, M., A. Mombet, and D. Praponich.** 1989. Ideal duration of pefloxacin prophylaxis of urinary tract infection following transurethral resection of the prostate. *Rev. Infect. Dis.* **11**(Suppl. 5):1345.
14. **Chin, N. X., and H. C. Neu.** 1983. In vitro activity of enoxacin, a quinolone carboxylic acid, compared to those of norfloxacin, new ß-lactams, aminoglycosides, and trimethoprim. *Antimicrob. Agents Chemother.* **24**:754–763.
15. **Chin, N. X., A. Novelli, and H. C. Neu.** 1988. In vitro activity of lomefloxacin (SC-47111; NY-198), a difluoroquinolone 3-carboxylic acid, compared with those of other quinolones. *Antimicrob. Agents Chemother.* **32**:652–662.
16. **Christensen, M. M., K. T. Nielsen, J. Knes, and P. O. Madsen.** 1989. Single-dose preoperative prophylaxis in transurethral prostatic surgery. *Am. J. Med.* **87**(Suppl. 5A):258–260.
17. **Clarke, A. M., S. J. V. Zemcov, and M. E. Campbell.** 1985. In-vitro activity of pefloxacin compared with enoxacin, norfloxacin, gentamicin, and new ß-lactams. *J. Antimicrob. Chemother.* **15**:39–44.
18. **Cox, C. E.** 1988. A comparison of enoxacin and co-trimoxazole in the treatment of patients with complicated urinary tract infections. *J. Antimicrob. Chemother.* **21**(Suppl. B):113–118.
19. **Cox, C. E.** 1989. Comparison of intravenous ciprofloxacin and intravenous cefotaxime for antimicrobial prophylaxis in transurethral surgery. *Am. J. Med.* **87**(Suppl. 5A):252–254.
20. **Daschner F. D., M. Westenfelder, and A. Dahlof.** 1986. Penetration of ciprofloxacin into kidney, fat, muscle and skin tissue, p. 81–84. *In* H. C. Neu and D. S. Reeves (ed.), *Current Topics in Infectious Diseases and Clinical Microbiology*, vol. 1. *Ciprofloxacin. Microbiology. Pharmacokinetics-Clinical Experience.* Vieweg & Sohn, Braunschweig/Wiesbaden, Germany.
21. **Elston, R. A., and J. Taylor.** 1988. Possible interaction of ciprofloxacin with cyclosporin. *J. Antimicrob. Chemother.* **21**:679–680.
22. **Fass, R. J.** 1983. In vitro activity of ciprofloxacin (Bay o 9867). *Antimicrob. Agents Chemother.* **24**:568–574.
23. **Fihn, S. D., and W. E. Stamm.** 1985. Interpretation and comparison of treatment studies for uncomplicated urinary tract infections in women. *Rev. Infect. Dis.* **7**:468–478.
24. **Forsgren, A., C. Hansson, R. Neinger, B. Ode, and the South Sweden LOLEX Study Group.** 1991. Lomefloxacin versus norfloxacin in the treatment of uncomplicated urinary tract infections: three-day versus seven-day treatment, p. 505–506. *In* E. Rubinstein (ed.), *Proc. 3rd Int. Symp. New Quinolones. Eur. J. Clin. Microbiol.* (Special Issue).
25. **Fujimaki, K., T. Noumi, I. Saikawa, M. Inoue, and S. Mitsuhashi.** 1988. In vitro and in vivo antibacterial activities of T-3262, a new fluoroquinolone. *Antimicrob. Agents Chemother.* **32**:827–833.
26. **Gasser, T. C., P. H. Graversen, and P. O. Madsen.** 1987. Treatment of complicated urinary tract infections with ciprofloxacin. *Am. J. Med.* **82**(Suppl. 4A):278–279.
27. **Gombert, M. E., L. DuBochet, T. M. Aulicino, L. B. Berkowitz, and R. J. Machia.** 1989. Intravenous ciprofloxacin versus cefotaxime prophylaxis during transurethral surgery. *Am. J. Med.* **87**(Suppl. 5A):250–251.
28. **Hardy, D. J., R. N. Swanson, D. N. Hensey, N. R. Ramer, R. R. Bower, C. W. Hanson, D. T. Chu, and P. B. Fernandes.** 1987. Comparative antibacterial activities of temafloxacin hydrochloride (A-62254) and two reference fluoroquinolones. *Antimicrob. Agents Chemother.* **31**:1768–1774.
29. **Hellsten, S., A. Forsgren, T. Björk, and M. Grabe.** 1989. Use of ciprofloxacin in patients undergoing transurethral prostatic surgery. *Scand. J. Infect. Dis. Suppl.* **60**:104–107.

29a. **Hoffmann-La Roche Inc.** Data on file. Hoffmann-La Roche Inc., Nutley, N.J.

30. **Holmes, B., R. N. Brogden, and D. M. Richards.** 1985. Norfloxacin. A review of its antimicrobial activity, pharmacology and therapeutic use. *Drugs* **30**:482–513.
31. **Hooton, T. M., R. H. Latham, E. S. Wong, C. Johnson, P. L. Roberts, and W. E. Stamm.** 1989. Ofloxacin versus trimethoprim-sulfamethoxazole for treatment of acute cystitis. *Antimicrob. Agents Chemother.* **33**:1308–1312.
32. **Jonsson, M., G. Englund, and K. Nörgård.** 1990. Norfloxacin versus pivmecillinam in the treatment of uncomplicated lower urinary tract infections in hospitalized elderly patients. *Scand. J. Infect. Dis.* **22**:339–344.
33. **Kanaiyalal, D. M., P. H. Abrams, and L. O. White.** 1988. A double-blind comparative trial of short-term orally administered enoxacin in the prevention of urinary infections after elective transurethral prostatectomy: a clinical and pharmacokinetic study. *J. Urol.* **139**:1232–1234.
34. **King, A., and I. Phillips.** 1986. The comparative in vitro activity of pefloxacin. *J. Antimicrob. Chemother.* **17**(Suppl. B):1–10.
35. **Kojima, T., M. Inoue, and S. Mitsuhashi.** 1989. In vitro activity of AT-4140 against clinical bacte-

rial isolates. *Antimicrob. Agents Chemother.* **33**:1980–1988.

36. **Lang, J., J. Finaz de Villaine, R. Garaffo, and J. L. Touraine.** 1989. Cyclosporin A. Pharmacokinetics in renal transplant patients receiving ciprofloxacin. *Am. J. Med.* **87**(Suppl. 5A):82–85.
37. **Lang, J., J. Finaz de Villaine, J. Guemie, J. L. Touraine, and C. Faucon.** 1989. Absence of pharmacokinetic interaction between pefloxacin and cyclosporin A in patients with renal transplants. *Rev. Infect. Dis.* **11**(Suppl. 5):1094.
38. **Leigh, D. A., B. Walsh, K. Harns, P. Hancock, and G. Travers.** 1988. Pharmacokinetics of ofloxacin and the effect on faecal flora of healthy volunteers. *J. Antimicrob. Chemother.* **22**(Suppl. C):115–125.
39. **Malmborg, A. S., and S. Ranniko.** 1988. Enoxacin distribution in renal tissues after multiple oral administration. *J. Antimicrob. Chemother.* **21**(Suppl. B):57–60.
40. **Mandell, L. A.** 1991. Role of quinolones in surgical prophylaxis. *Eur. J. Clin. Microbiol. Infect. Dis.* **10**:368–377.
41. **Monk, J. P., and D. M. Campoli-Richards.** 1987. Ofloxacin. A review of its antibacterial activity, pharmacokinetic properties and therapeutic use. *Drugs* **33**:346–391.
42. **Montay, G., R. Bruno, J. J. Thebault, J. C. Vergniol, D. Chassard, M. Ebmier, and J. Gaillot.** 1990. Dose-dependent pharmacokinetic study of sparfloxacin (SPFX) in healthy young volunteers, abstr. 1248. *Program Abstr. 30th Intersci. Conf. Antimicrob. Agents Chemother.*
43. **Muolo, A., and G. Ancona.** 1988. Comparative evaluation of ofloxacin and trimethoprim-sulfamethoxazole in the treatment of urinary tract infections following renal transplantation. *Rev. Infect. Dis.* **10**(Suppl. 1):165–166.
44. **Murdoch, D. A., D. F. Badenoch, and E. R. Gatchalian.** 1987. Oral ciprofloxacin as prophylaxis in transurethral surgery. *Br. J. Urol.* **60**:153–156.
45. **Norrby, S. R.** 1990. Short-term treatment of uncomplicated urinary tract infections in women. *Rev. Infect. Dis.* **12**:458–467.
46. **Ode, B., M. Walder, and A. Forsgren.** 1987. Failure of single dose of 100 mg ofloxacin in lower urinary tract infections in females. *Scand. J. Infect. Dis.* **19**:677–679.
47. **Paganoni, R., C. Herzog, A. Braunsteiner, and P. Hohl.** 1988. Fleroxacin: in-vitro activity worldwide against 20,807 clinical isolates and comparison to ciprofloxacin and norfloxacin. *J. Antimicrob. Chemother.* **22**(Suppl. D):3–17.
48. **Peters, H. J.** 1986. Comparison of intravenous ciprofloxacin and mezlocillin in treatment of complicated urinary tract infections, p. 124–126. *In* H. C. Neu and D. S. Reeves (ed.), *Current Topics in Infectious Diseases and Clinical Microbiology*, vol. 1. *Ciprofloxacin. Microbiology-Pharmacokinetics-Clinical Experience.* Vieweg & Sohn, Braunschweig/Wiesbaden, Germany.
49. **Petersen, E. E., F. Wingen, K. L. Fairchild, A. Halfhide, A. Hendrischk, M. Links, M. Schad, H. R. Scholz, N. Schürmann, S. Siegmann, and A. J. Yassin.** 1990. Single dose pefloxacin compared with multiple dose co-trimoxazole in cystitis. *J. Antimicrob. Chemother.* **26**(Suppl. B):147–152.
50. **Piipo, T., T. Pitkäjärvi, and S. A. Salo.** 1990. Three-day versus seven-day treatment with norfloxacin in acute cystitis. *Curr. Ther. Res.* **47**:644–653.
51. **Rios, M., E. Renoult, D. Hestin, and M. Kessler.** 1990. Quinolones et ciclosporin chez le transplanté rénal. *Pharmacol. Clin. Ther.* **29**:321–323.
52. **Rubin, R. H., E. D. Shapiro, V. T. Andriole, R. J. Davis, and W. E. Stamm.** 1992. Guidelines for the evaluation of new anti-infective agents for the treatment of urinary tract infections. *Clin. Infect. Dis.* **15**(Suppl.):216–227.
53. **Rylander, M., S. R. Norrby, and R. Svärd.** 1987. Norfloxacin versus co-trimoxazole for treatment of urinary tract infections in adults: microbiological results of a coordinated multicentre study. *Scand. J. Infect. Dis.* **19**:551–557.
54. **Sabbaj, J., V. L. Hoagland, and W. J. Shih.** 1985. Multiclinic comparative study of norfloxacin and trimethoprim-sulfamethoxazole for treatment of urinary tract infections. *Antimicrob. Agents Chemother.* **27**:297–310.
55. **Sandberg, T., G. Englund, K. Lincoln, and L. G. Nilsson.** 1990. Randomized double-blind study of norfloxacin and cefadroxil in the treatment of acute pyelonephritis. *Eur. J. Clin. Microbiol. Infect. Dis.* **9**:317–323.

55a. **Searle.** Data on file. Searle, Chicago.

56. **Shah, P., S. Müller, J. Kipp, and W. Stille.** 1989. In vitro activity of lomefloxacin (NY-198 or SC-47111). *Diagn. Microbiol. Infect. Dis.* **12**:97S–101S.
57. **Swanson, B. N., V. K. Boppana, P. H. Vlasse, H. H. Rotmensch, and R. K. Ferguson.** 1983. Norfloxacin disposition after sequentially increasing doses. *Antimicrob. Agents Chemother.* **23**:284–288.
58. **The Inter-Nordic Urinary Tract Infection Study Group.** 1988. Double-blind comparison of three-day versus seven-day treatment with norfloxacin in symptomatic urinary tract infections. *Scand. J. Infect. Dis.* **20**:619–624.
59. **The Urinary Tract Infection Study Group.** 1987. Coordinated multicenter study of norfloxacin versus trimethoprim-sulfamethoxazole treatment of symptomatic urinary tract infections. *J. Infect. Dis.* **177**:170–177.

60. **Todd, P. A., and D. Faulds.** 1991. Ofloxacin. A reappraisal of its antimicrobial activity, pharmacology and therapeutic use. *Drugs* **42:**825–876.
61. **Van Caekenberghe, D. L., and S. R. Pattyn.** 1984. In vitro activity of ciprofloxacin, compared with those of other new fluorinated piperazinyl-substituted quinolone derivatives. *Antimicrob. Agents Chemother.* **25:**518–521.
62. **Vogt, P., T. Schorn, and U. Frei.** 1988. Ofloxacin in the treatment of urinary tract infection in renal transplant recipients. *Infection* **16:**175–178.
63. **von Balen, F. A. M., F. W. M. M. Touw-Otten, and R. A. de Melker.** 1990. Single dose pefloxacin versus five-days treatment with norfloxacin in uncomplicated cystitis in women. *J. Antimicrob. Chemother.* **26**(Suppl. B):153–160.
64. **Wiedekamm, E., R. Portmann, K. Suter, C. Partos, D. Dell, and P. W. Lücker.** 1987. Single- and multiple-dose pharmacokinetics of fleroxacin, a trifluorinated quinolone, in humans. *Antimicrob. Agents Chemother.* **31:**1909–1914.
65. **Wise, R., J. Andrews, J. Ashby, and R. Matthews.** 1988. In vitro activity of lomefloxacin, a new quinolone antimicrobial agent, in comparison with those of other agents. *Antimicrob. Agents Chemother.* **32:**617–622.
66. **Wolf, R., R. Eberl, A. Dunky, N. Mertz, T. Chang, J. R. Goulet, and J. Latts.** 1984. The clinical pharmacokinetics and tolerance of enoxacin in healthy volunteers. *J. Antimicrob. Chemother.* **14**(Suppl. C):63–69.
67. **Wolfson, J. S., and D. C. Hooper.** 1991. Pharmacokinetics of quinolones: newer aspects. *Eur. J. Clin. Microbiol. Infect. Dis.* **10:**267–274.

*Quinolone Antimicrobial Agents, 2nd ed.*
Edited by David C. Hooper and John S. Wolfson


*Chapter 14*

# Role of Quinolones in Treatment of Chronic Bacterial Prostatitis

*K. G. Naber*

Bacterial prostatitis, whether acute or chronic, is a rare infection but difficult to treat (33); only a few antibiotics are suitable for sufficiently penetrating prostatic fluid (64). Usually, co-trimoxazole and to a smaller extent trimethoprim alone have been used, but with poor results (Table 1). Other antibiotics also did not improve the clinical outcome as shown in patients who were followed up for a sufficient time (Table 2). One exception seems to be the study by Mobley (37), in which patients were treated initially with a 2-week course of erythromycin (500 mg orally four times daily) combined with sodium bicarbonate (10 g with each dose of erythromycin), a lipid-soluble basic macrolide with a $pK_a$ of >8.6. Since erythromycin is not active at acid pH because virtually all of the molecules are charged, Mobley added sodium bicarbonate for urine alkalinization to increase the activity and antibacterial spectrum of the drug (59, 71). Whether the addition of sodium bicarbonate had any influence on the pH of the prostatic fluid was not measured in the study. According to studies by Pfau et al. (56), Anderson and Fair (1), and Blacklock and Beavis (5), the pH of prostatic fluid in patients with chronic bacterial prostatitis is alkaline rather than acidic and is therefore significantly different from the secretions with lower pHs observed in dogs (31) and healthy human males.

The newer quinolones, which exist as zwitterions with $pK_a$ in acid as well as alkaline milieus (Table 3), should theoretically be concentrated in both acid and alkaline prostatic fluids. Because of their unique and favorable pharmacokinetic properties and their broad antibacterial spectra, these antibacterial drugs may be good alternatives in the treatment of chronic bacterial prostatitis.

## CONCENTRATIONS OF QUINOLONES IN PROSTATIC TISSUE AND SECRETIONS AND IN SEMINAL SECRETIONS

In contrast to ß-lactam antibiotics, the newer quinolones show concentrations in prostatic fluid, prostatic tissue, and seminal fluid that are relatively high in comparison with the corresponding concentrations in plasma. Under steady-state conditions in a dog model, Madsen et al. (27), Døorflinger et al. (15) and Gasser et al. (17) demonstrated that the mean ratios of concentrations in prostatic fluid to concentrations in plasma were 0.34 for norfloxacin, 0.67 for ciprofloxacin, 1.12 for fleroxacin, and 1.35 for enoxacin. Investigations in humans are somewhat hindered by the fact that prostatic fluid can usually be obtained in small amounts only by

*K. G. Naber* • Urologic Clinic, Elisabeth Hospital, Straubing, Germany.

**Table 1.** Eradication of pathogens in patients with chronic bacterial prostatitis treated with trimethoprim-sulfamethoxazole or trimethoprim alone[a]

| Duration of treatment (days) | No. of patients | % Bacteriological cure | Duration of follow-up (mo) | Study | | |
|---|---|---|---|---|---|---|
| | | | | Date | Author(s) | Reference |
| 10 | 10 | 0 | 3 | 1979 | Smith et al. | 63 |
| 14 | 9 | 14 | 6 | 1978 | Meares | 32 |
| 14 | 13 | 15 | 6 | 1973 | Meares | 29 |
| 28 | 18 | 33 | 3 | 1974 | Drach | 16 |
| 90 | 19 | 31 | 3 | 1975 | Meares | 30 |
| 90 | 13 | 38 | 6 | 1978 | Meares | 32 |
| 90 | 15 | 40 | 12 | 1976 | McGuire and Lytton | 35 |
| 90 | 8 | 50 | 3 | 1979 | Smith et al. | 63 |
| 90 | 15 | 67 | 12 | 1978 | Paulson and White | 51 |
| 120–140 | 15 | 40 | 12 | 1986 | Pfau | 53 |
| 120–180 | 8[b] | 50 | 12 | 1986 | Pfau | 53 |

[a]Patients were treated with trimethoprim (160 mg)-sulfamethoxazole (800 mg) twice daily. In all patients, infections were localized to the prostate by the technique of Meares and Stamey (34). Data are according to Hanus and Danzinger (22).
[b]Patients were treated with trimethoprim (100 mg) three times daily.

**Table 2.** Eradication of pathogens in patients with chronic bacterial prostatitis treated with various antibiotics[a]

| Antibiotic | Dosage[b] (mg) | Duration of treatment (days) | No. of patients | % Bacteriologic cure | Duration of follow-up (mo) | Study | | |
|---|---|---|---|---|---|---|---|---|
| | | | | | | Date | Author | Reference |
| Minocycline | 100 b.i.d. | 14[c] | 14 | 70 | 12 | 1978 | Paulson and White | 51 |
| Erythromycin | 500 q.i.d. | 14 | 26 | 88 | 6–18 | 1974 | Mobley | 37 |
| Cephalexin | 500 q.i.d. | 28 | 9 | 22 | 1 | 1979 | Oliveri et al. | 50 |
| Carbenicillin | 764 q.i.d. | 28 | 22 | 68 | 1 | | | |
| Cephalexin | 500 q.i.d. | 28 | 5 | 40 | 1 | 1981 | Mobley | 38 |
| Carbenicillin | 764 q.i.d. | 28 | 12 | 67 | 1 | | | |

[a]In all patients, the infection was localized to the prostate by the technique of Meares and Stamey (34). Data are according to Hanus and Danzinger (22).
[b]b.i.d., twice daily; q.i.d., four times daily.
[c]Four patients were withdrawn because of side effects.

**Table 3.** Dissociation constants of newer quinolones[a]

| Quinolone | $pK_{a1}$ | $pK_{a2}$ |
|---|---|---|
| Ciprofloxacin | 6.1 | 8.7 |
| Enoxacin | 6.3 | 8.7 |
| Fleroxacin | 5.5 | 8.1 |
| Lomefloxacin | 5.8 | 9.3 |
| Norfloxacin | 6.3 | 8.4 |
| Ofloxacin | 6.0 | 8.2 |
| Pefloxacin | 6.3 | 7.6 |
| Temafloxacin | 5.6 | 8.8 |
| Sparfloxacin | 6.2 | 8.6 |

[a]$pK_{a1}$, pK for dissociation of $H^+$ of COOH; $pK_{a2}$, pK for protonation of the 4′ N of piperazine. Data are from reference 16a.

prostatic massage. Low-level contamination with urine containing high concentrations of these quinolones can therefore alter the results tremendously.

In studies of drug levels in prostatic fluid (41–47), my coworkers and I made sure that volunteers did not void urine before the prostatic sample was taken. In addition, a renal contrast medium, e.g., ioxitalamic acid or iohexol, excreted almost exclusively by glomerular filtration was administered intravenously at the same time as the drug and served as an internal standard. In many experiments, the ratios of concentrations in prostatic fluid to concentrations in plasma for the contrast medium were markedly below unity. Significant urinary contamination is considered to have occurred if this ratio becomes unexpectedly high (above unity). However, only experiments done up to 4 h after a single dose has been administered can be analyzed in this manner, because then the subject has to void, resulting in urinary contamination of the urethra.

After administration of a single dose, the following median prostatic fluid/plasma drug concentration ratios were found (Table 4): for 800 mg of oral norfloxacin, 0.12 (1 to 4 h); for 200 mg of intravenously administered ciprofloxacin, 0.26 and 0.18 (0.5 to 2 h and 4 h, respectively); for 400 mg of oral fleroxacin, 0.28 (2 to 4 h); for 400 mg of orally administered temafloxacin, 0.36 (4 h); for 400 mg of oral and 428 mg of intravenous enoxacin, 0.39 and 0.47 (2 to 4 h), respectively; and for 400 mg of oral lomefloxacin, 0.48 (4 h).

Data on the penetration of ciprofloxacin (7, 13) and ofloxacin (25, 66) into prostatic fluid of healthy volunteers and patients have been reported, but no effort was made in those studies to assess possible urinary contamination. The high prostatic fluid/plasma ratios reported for some individuals may not reflect true concentrations in prostatic fluid. Therefore, the mean values cannot be compared with our results, in which urinary contamination was excluded.

Concentrations of ciprofloxacin in seminal fluid were measured by Dalhoff and Weidner (13), and concentrations of ofloxacin were measured by Mizoguchi et al. (36) and Schramm (62), with levels usually exceeding corresponding concentrations in plasma severalfold. In my laboratory, we measured the penetration of five newer quinolones into seminal fluid of volunteers (Table 5) (41–43, 45–47). Ciprofloxacin (200 mg intravenously) showed the highest seminal fluid/plasma ratio, and fleroxacin (400 mg orally) showed the highest absolute concentrations. Drug concentrations in fraction 2 of the split ejaculate were usually somewhat higher than those in fraction 1 but were significantly higher ($P < 0.05$) only after intravenous administration (over 60 min) of 428 mg of enoxacin.

Drug concentrations in prostatic tissue are usually measured in patients undergoing transurethral resection of the prostate and thus actually represent concentrations in prostatic adenoma tissue. Levels in prostatic tissue have been studied for most of the newer quinolones.

In general, concentrations in tissue exceeded the corresponding concentrations in plasma, with some differences between the quinolones. The results are not directly com-

**Table 4.** Concentrations of newer quinolones in prostatic fluids of volunteers[a]

| Quinolone | Dose[b] (mg) | Time (h) | No.[c] | Median (range) concn (mg/liter) in: | | Median (range) ratio of prostatic fluid/plasma drug concn |
|---|---|---|---|---|---|---|
| | | | | Plasma | Prostatic fluid | |
| Norfloxacin | 800 p.o. | 1–4 | 8 (2) | 1.40 (0.69–2.71) | 0.14 (0.08–0.43) | 0.12 (0.08–0.19) |
| Ciprofloxacin | 200 i.v. | 0.5–2 | 10 (1) | 0.67 (0.45–1.12) | 0.16 (0.10–0.50) | 0.26 (0.15–0.53) |
| | 200 i.v.[d] | 4 | 8 | 0.44 (0.35–0.59) | 0.08 (0.03–0.19) | 0.18 (0.05–0.33) |
| Fleroxacin | 400 p.o. | 2–4 | 8 | 3.71 (3.30–4.70) | 1.00 (0.84–1.69) | 0.28 (0.22–0.37) |
| Temafloxacin | 400 p.o. | 4 | 4 | 2.23 (1.70–2.65) | 0.78 (0.56–0.92) | 0.36 (0.29–0.40) |
| Enoxacin | 400 p.o. | 2–4 | 10 | 1.09 (0.51–1.91) | 0.39 (0.18–1.33) | 0.39 (0.27–1.22) |
| | 428 i.v. | 2–4 | 9 (1) | 1.26 (1.10–1.71) | 0.57 (0.29–0.96) | 0.47 (0.20–0.56) |
| Lomefloxacin | 400 p.o. | 4 | 5 | 1.81 (1.39–3.00) | 1.38 (0.60–3.06) | 0.48 (0.40–1.53) |

[a]Data are from references 41–47.
[b]p.o., peroral; i.v., intravenous.
[c]A prostatic fluid/plasma value above unity (numbers in parentheses) for ioxitalamic acid was taken as the index for urinary contamination. Results for patients with these values are not included in the table.
[d]Short, steady-state infusion.

**Table 5.** Concentrations of newer quinolones in plasma and seminal fluids of volunteers[a]

| Quinolone | Dose[b] (mg) | Time (h) | No. of volunteers | Concn (mg/liter) in: | | | Ratio | |
|---|---|---|---|---|---|---|---|---|
| | | | | Plasma | SF1 | SF2 | SF1/plasma | SF2/plasma |
| Lomefloxacin | 400 p.o. | 4 | 6 | 1.75 (1.39–3.00) | 1.80 (1.48–2.65) | 2.04 (1.87–2.65) | 1.0 (0.7–1.3) | 1.3 (1.0–1.4) |
| | 400 p.o. | 24 | 6 | 0.19 (0.16–0.24) | 0.17 (0.08–0.51) | 0.20 (0.16–0.32) | 1.1 (0.4–2.2) | 1.1 (0.9–1.3) |
| Temafloxacin | 400 p.o. | 4 | 12 | 2.16 (1.32–3.49) | 2.30 (1.38–4.06) | 2.52 (1.66–5.62) | 1.1 (0.8–1.5) | 1.3 (1.0–2.1) |
| | 400 p.o. | 12 | 6 | 0.93 (0.69–1.17) | 1.39 (0.68–4.96) | 1.31 (0.82–1.77) | 1.4 (0.8–5.3) | 1.3 (1.0–2.0) |
| Fleroxacin | 400 p.o. | 2–4 | 8 | 3.71 (2.98–4.70) | 5.52 (3.05–8.13) | 5.80 (3.95–8.61) | 1.3 (0.8–2.2) | 1.7 (0.9–2.3) |
| | 400 p.o. | 12 | 4 | 1.69 (1.23–1.87) | 2.76 (1.78–2.89) | 2.89 (1.96–3.11) | 1.5 (1.4–1.8) | 1.7 (1.6–1.8) |
| Enoxacin | 400 p.o. | 2–4 | 11 | 1.00 (0.51–1.91) | 2.07 (1.21–4.60) | 2.19 (1.13–3.17) | 2.2 (1.4–3.3) | 2.2 (1.5–3.3) |
| | 428 i.v. | 2–4 | 11 | 1.24 (0.86–1.71) | 2.53 (1.63–3.89) | 3.50 (1.69–5.78) | 2.1 (1.6–2.4) | 2.8 (1.6–3.7) |
| Ciprofloxacin | 200 i.v.[c] | 4 | 8 | 0.44 (0.35–0.58) | 2.53 (1.75–4.11) | 2.53 (1.75–4.14) | 5.8 (4.0–8.6) | 7.1 (3.0–10.6) |
| | 200 i.v. | 12 | 4 | 0.09 (0.06–0.10) | 0.61 (0.54–1.38) | 0.70 (0.44–1.37) | 7.9 (6.7–13.8) | 9.4 (4.9–13.7) |

[a]Data are from references 41–43 and 45–47. Values are medians and ranges. Seminal fluid was collected as a split ejaculate in two fractions. SF1, seminal fluid fraction 1; SF2, seminal fluid fraction 2.
[b]p.o., peroral; i.v., intravenous.
[c]Short, steady-state infusion.

parable, however, because different techniques of tissue preparation and analysis were used. Results obtained in my laboratory (39, 41–45) with five quinolones are presented in Table 6.

In the three studies in which the Stomacher and Ultra Turrax (Typ-Lab-Blender 80 [Kleinfeld, Hannover, Germany] and Typ TP 18-10 [IKA, Staufer, Germany]) preparation techniques were used at the same time, concentrations after the Stomacher technique was used were generally lower. This difference could be explained by the fact that cells in which high concentrations of quinolones are expected were more thoroughly broken down by the Ultra Turrax technique.

For ciprofloxacin and enoxacin, concentrations in prostatic tissue are about twice as high as concentrations in plasma. For norfloxacin, concentrations in prostatic tissue are about 1.5 times higher, and for ofloxacin and fleroxacin, they are about 10% higher. Because of higher concentrations in plasma, ofloxacin and fleroxacin show the highest absolute levels in tissue.

## RESULTS OF CLINICAL STUDIES

Thirty-three studies (2, 3, 6, 8–12, 14, 18–21, 23, 24, 26, 28, 40, 48, 49, 52, 54, 55, 56a, 58, 60, 61, 65, 67, 68, 70) with newer quinolones could be analyzed (Tables 7 through 10). Only studies in which the method of diagnosis of prostatitis was mentioned were considered. Patients with prostatitis who were treated as a subgroup had to be evaluated separately.

In order to present the results of the studies in a comparable way, the bacteriological cure rate per patient, i.e., the number of patients without pathogens at the site of infection as a percentage of the total number of evaluable patients, was calculated for the total time of follow-up. Patients dropping out earlier who had no pathogens at the site of infection were considered unevaluable. Patients dropping out any time during the follow-up who pre-

**Table 6.** Concentrations of newer quinolones in plasma and prostatic tissues of elderly patients undergoing transurethral resections of prostate[a]

| Quinolone | Dose[b] (mg) | Time (h) | No. of values | Median concn (range) | | |
|---|---|---|---|---|---|---|
| | | | | Plasma (mg/liter) | Prostatic tissue (mg/kg) | Median tissue/ plasma ratio (range) |
| Ofloxacin | 400 p.o. | 2.0–4.5 | 7 | 3.99 (2.80–4.86) | 4.08 (2.40–5.58)[c] | 1.12 (0.86–1.32)[c] |
| | 400 p.o. | 14.5–19.5 | 10 | 1.87 (0.41–3.34) | 1.20 (<0.1–1.99)[d] | 0.95 (0.57–1.81)[d] |
| Fleroxacin | 400 p.o. | 1.5–4.0 | 11 | 3.73 (0.44–5.54) | 4.24 (2.98–6.82)[c] | 1.10 (1.00–1.92)[c] |
| Norfloxacin | 800 i.v. | 1.0–2.5 | 13 | 1.56 (0.40–5.07) | 1.68 (0.68–4.30)[c] | 1.52 (0.67–4.20)[c] |
| Ciprofloxacin | 200 i.v. | 1.0–2.5 | 14 | 0.81 (0.64–1.54) | 1.71 (0.89–4.54)[c] | 1.88 (1.30–4.24)[c] |
| | 200 i.v. | 1.0–2.5 | 14 | 0.81 (0.64–1.54) | 1.87 (1.02–5.81)[d] | 2.57 (1.41–5.43)[d] |
| Enoxacin | 400 p.o. | 1.0–4.0 | 7 | 0.95 (0.14–2.07) | 1.65 (0.29–4.29)[c] | 1.91 (1.26–2.25)[c] |
| | | | 12 | 0.96 (0.14–2.07) | 2.25 (0.37–5.02)[d] | 2.56 (0.37–5.02)[d] |

[a]Data are from references 39 and 41–45.
[b]p.o., peroral; i.v., intravenous.
[c]Values were obtained by the Stomacher method.
[d]Values were obtained by the Ultra Turrax method.

sented pathogens at the site of infection were considered failures according to the principle of the least-favorable outcome. Therefore, the number of patients and the bacteriological cure rates may differ from the figures presented in the abstracts by the authors.

The presentations of clinical results also differed among the studies. In some studies, clinical cure and improvement were considered successes, making a comparison difficult. In a considerable number of patients, especially when follow-up periods were short, clinical results did not correlate well with bacteriological results. For all these reasons, only the "objective" bacteriological results were considered in the following analysis. However, even these results are difficult to compare, since in some studies, not only chronic but also acute prostatitis episodes were treated, and the results were not reported separately. In addition, the investigators did not use the same criteria for the diagnosis of chronic bacterial prostatitis. The standard four-specimen technique of Meares and Stamey (34) for localizing the infection to the prostate was not used by all the investigators. French colleagues usually diagnosed prostatitis only according to clinical symptoms and digital rectal examination of the prostate in combination with exacerbation of a urinary tract infection. The causative pathogens were cultured from a clean-catch midstream specimen of urine ($>10^4$ CFU/ml) (18, 20, 21). In two studies (3, 4), the pathogens were cultured from an ejaculate specimen without the standard localization study (34).

There was also a wide range of treatment durations, from 7 to 259 days, and the follow-up periods ranged from evaluation during treatment or immediately at the end of treatment (Japanese studies) to as long as 1 year after completion of therapy (55, 67, 68).

In two studies, no information concerning the follow-up period was available (2, 49). Therefore, the results must be interpreted with great caution, since the issues involved in the treatment of prostatitis are those of relapses and in particular late relapse. Thus, the reported results depend very much on the time of follow-up.

If the only studies considered are those in which patients were included according to the standard localization of the infection (34) and a follow-up of at least 1 month was available, then only a few studies remain for detailed discussion.

Of the studies with norfloxacin (Table 7), only three (8, 52, 61) meet these criteria. Bologna et al. (8) treated 20 patients aged 24 to 62 years. Twelve patients were infected by gram-negative rods (*Escherichia coli*, eight patients; *Klebsiella pneumoniae*, two patients; *Pseudomonas aeruginosa*, two patients), and eight patients were infected by gram-positive cocci (enterococci and *Staphylococcus aureus* in monoinfections and mixed infection). Norfloxacin (400 mg twice daily) was administered for 10 days with serratiopeptidase (20,000 U twice a day for 10 days), a fibrinolytic enzyme, to prevent postinflammatory fibrinolytic damage. The patients were followed up for at least 5 weeks. Three patients (15%) (two infected with *E. coli* and one infected with enterococcus) suffered a relapse, and one patient (5%) suffered a reinfection (*Staphylococcus epidermidis*). Schaeffer and Darras (61) treated 15 men who had chronic bacterial prostatitis (13 infected with *E. coli* and 2 infected with *P. aeruginosa*) refractory to trimethoprim-sulfamethoxazole and/or carbenicillin with 400 mg of norfloxacin twice daily for 28 days. One patient was lost to follow-up at 1 month. Of the 14 patients followed up for at least 6 months, 9 (64%) were cured of the original infection (*E. coli* only), including 6 who remained uninfected for at least 2 years (1 patient), 1 year (2 patients), or 6 months (3 patients). In three patients, urinary tract infections recurred with new pathogens at 6, 560, and 820 days after prostatic fluid cultures had been negative posttherapy.

Bacterial prostatitis with the original pathogen recurred in five patients within 2 months of completion of therapy. The bacteria remained susceptible to norfloxacin but could not be eradicated with 30 to 90 days of additional norfloxacin therapy.

Petrikkos et al. (52) treated 42 patients with norfloxacin at a dose of 400 mg twice daily reduced to 200 mg twice daily after 3 months for a mean duration of 5.8 months. During the median follow-up duration of 8

**Table 7.** Eradication of pathogens (bacteriological cure) in patients with bacterial prostatitis treated with norfloxacin

| Drug[a] | Dose[b] (mg) | Duration of therapy (days) | No. of evaluable patients | % Bacteriological cure | Duration of follow-up[c] (mo) | Type of infection | Study: Date | Study: Author(s) | Study: Reference |
|---|---|---|---|---|---|---|---|---|---|
| NFX | 400 b.i.d. | 28–42 | 25 | 92 | 1 | Chronic | 1986 | Sabbaj et al. | 60 |
| TMS | 160/800 b.i.d. | 15 | 15 | 67 | 1 | Chronic | | | |
| NFX | 400 b.i.d. | 10 | 20[d] | 85 | 1 | Chronic | 1985 | Bologna et al. | |
| NFX | 400 b.i.d. | 10 | 50 | 88 | 0.1 | Not specified | 1985 | Bischoff | 8 |
| RSX | 150 b.i.d. | 14 | 20[d] | 20 | NS | Bacterial-chlamydial | 1986 | Asbach and Mekelos | 2 |
| NFX | 400 b.i.d. | 14 | 15[d] | 75 | NS | Bacterial-chlamydial | | | |
| OFX | 200 b.i.d. | 14 | 20[d] | 75 | NS | Bacterial-chlamydial | | | |
| NFX | 400 b.i.d. | 28 | 14[d] | 64 | 6 | Chronic[e] | 1990 | Schaeffer and Darras | 61 |
| NFX | 400 b.i.d. | 28 | 15[d] | 93 | 0.2 | *E. coli* | 1990 | Rauch and Taylor | 57 |
| CAR | 764 q.i.d. | 28 | 10[d] | 60 | 0.2 | *E. coli* | | | |
| NFX | 4–200 b.i.d. | 174 | 42[d] | 60 | 8 | Chronic | 1991 | Petrikkos et al. | 52 |

[a]NFX, norfloxacin; TMS, trimethoprim-sulfamethoxazole; RSX, rosoxacin; OFX, ofloxacin; CAR, carbenicillin.
[b]b.i.d., twice daily; q.i.d., four times daily.
[c]NS, not stated.
[d]Localization study performed.
[e]Refractory to trimethoprim-sulfamethoxazole with or without carbenicillin.

months, 60% of the patients remained uninfected.

Of the studies with ciprofloxacin (Table 8), six (9, 23, 26, 53, 54, 67, 68) meet the criteria given above. Childs (9) collected data on 42 adult men aged 19 to 85 years who had documented chronic bacterial prostatitis. The most frequently isolated organisms were *E. coli* (17 patients), *P. aeruginosa* (13 patients), *Serratia marcescens* (2 patients), *K. pneumoniae* (2 patients), *Proteus vulgaris* (2 patients), and *Proteus mirabilis* (2 patients). The patients were treated with oral ciprofloxacin at a dosage of 500 mg twice a day for periods ranging from 10 to 259 days. Most patients were treated either for 20 to 29 days (United States) or for 85 days (Europe). Six patients had 10 to 14 days of therapy, and one patient had a 259-day course. In 29 (78%) of 37 evaluable patients, the pathogens remained eradicated during a follow-up period of at least 10 weeks after completion of therapy. One patient required surgery for persisting symptoms.

Weidner et al. (68) evaluated 15 men with chronic bacterial prostatitis (duration of symptoms, more than 1 year) who had previously been treated with trimethoprim and/or trimethoprim-sulfamethoxazole for at least 6 weeks without showing any improvement. The patients were treated with oral ciprofloxacin (500 mg twice daily) for 2 weeks. Eradication for up to 1 year after completion of therapy was achieved in 9 of 15 patients (60%). For six patients (*E. coli* prostatitis) who had acquired infections with chlamydiae or ureaplasmas during follow-up, additional therapy with tetracycline hydrochloride (1,000 mg daily for 1 week) was prescribed.

In a second study, Weidner et al. (67) evaluated 16 men with proved chronic bacterial prostatitis treated with oral ciprofloxacin (500 mg twice a day for 4 weeks). All the men had been pretreated with co-trimoxazole, trimethoprim, or norfloxacin (two cases). Two patients stopped treatment early because of central nervous system side effects. After a median follow-up of 30 months (range, 21 to 36 months), 10 of 16 patients were considered cured. Langenmeyer et al. (26) treated 32 men for 28 days with ciprofloxacin (500 mg twice daily) and had a cure rate of 75% after a 2-month follow-up, and Heidler (23) treated 34 patients for between 21 and 42 days (if not free of symptoms after 21 days) with a lower dose of 250 mg twice daily and had a bacteriological cure rate of 62% after a 6-month follow-up. Pfau (54, 55) cured six of seven patients (84%) with ciprofloxacin (500 mg twice daily) with follow-up periods of at least 12 months.

With ofloxacin (Table 9), four localization studies were performed (2, 11, 56a, 66). In one study (56a) the requirements of segmented culture and sufficient follow-up are present. Fourteen of 21 patients (67%) followed for up to 1 year were cured.

Of the studies with other quinolones (Table 10), the comparative study with enoxacin versus carbenicillin (10), the two studies with temafloxacin (12, 40), and the study with rufloxacin (6) fulfilled the criteria given above. In the other studies, either the infection was not localized or the evaluation was performed at the completion of therapy.

Christensen et al. (10) analyzed the data on patients treated with 400 mg of oral enoxacin twice daily versus 764 mg of oral carbenicillin four times a day for 28 days. Four to 6 weeks after therapy, gram-negative rods were eradicated in 8 (89%) of 9 patients by enoxacin but in only 7 (41%) of 17 patients by carbenicillin. Gram-positive cocci were eradicated in 13 (45%) of 29 patients by enoxacin and in 17 (61%) of 28 patients by carbenicillin. The overall eradication rates of 55 and 53%, respectively, were almost identical.

In the two studies with temafloxacin (12, 40), 76 and 42 men could be evaluated, respectively. Bacteriological cures occurred in 72 and 68% of patients, respectively.

Boerema et al. (6) analyzed an uncontrolled multicenter study with rufloxacin. Twenty-four men with chronic bacterial prostatitis treated orally with 400 mg on the first

**Table 8.** Eradication of pathogens (bacteriological cure) in patients with bacterial prostatitis treated with ciprofloxacin

| Drug[a] | Dose[b] (mg) | Duration of therapy (days) | No. of evaluable patients | % Bacteriological cure | Duration of follow-up[c] (mo) | Type of infection | Study | | |
|---|---|---|---|---|---|---|---|---|---|
| | | | | | | | Date | Author(s) | References |
| CFX | 100 t.i.d. | 12, 17 | 2 | 100 | NS | Chronic | 1985 | Okada | 49 |
| CFX | 250 b.i.d. | 7 | 10 | 60 | 1 | Acute or chronic | 1985 | Zamfirescu and Chysky | 70 |
| CFX | 500 b.i.d. | 84 | 15 | 67 | 3 | *P. aeruginosa* | 1986 | Guibert et al. | 20 |
| CFX | 500 b.i.d. | 28 or 84 | 26 | 77 | 1 | Not specified | 1986 | Guibert et al. | 21 |
| CFX | 500 b.i.d. | 14 | 15[d] | 60 | 12 | Chronic[e] | 1987 | Weidner et al. | 68 |
| CFX | 500 b.i.d. | 28 | 16[d] | 63 | 21–36 | Chronic[e] | 1991 | Weidner et al. | 67 |
| CFX | 500 b.i.d. | 10–259 | 37[d] | 78 | 2.5 | Chronic | 1987 | Childs | 9 |
| CFX | 500 b.i.d. | 28 | 32[d] | 75 | 2 | Chronic | 1987 | Langenmeyer et al. | 26 |
| CFX | 4–600/day | 7–21 | 21[d] | 83 | 0 | Acute or chronic | 1987 | Matsumoto et al. | 28 |
| CFX | 250 b.i.d. | 14 | 40 | 78 | 6 | Not specified | 1989 | Bischoff | 4 |
| TMS | 160/800 b.i.d. | 14 | 40 | 61 | 6 | Not specified | | | |
| CFX | 500 b.i.d. | 60–150 | 7[d] | 86 | 12 | Chronic | 1987, 1991 | Pfau | 54, 55 |
| CFX | 250 b.i.d. | 21–42 | 34[d] | 62 | 6 | Chronic | 1990 | Heidler | 23 |
| CFX | 300 b.i.d. | 14 | 20[d] | 100 | 0 | Chronic | 1991 | Yoshida et al. | 69 |
| CFX | 200 b.i.d. | 14 | 20[d] | 75 | 0 | Chronic | 1991 | Suzuki et al. | 65 |

[a]CFX, ciprofloxacin; TMS, trimethoprim-sulfamethoxazole.
[b]t.i.d., three times a day; b.i.d., twice daily.
[c]NS, not stated.
[d]Localization study performed.
[e]Refractory to trimethoprim with or without sulfamethoxazole.

**Table 9.** Eradication of pathogens (bacteriological cure) in patients with bacterial prostatitis treated with ofloxacin

| Drug[a] | Dose[b] (mg) | Duration of therapy (days) | No. of evaluable patients | % Bacteriological cure | Duration of follow-up[c] (mo) | Type of infection | Study | | |
|---|---|---|---|---|---|---|---|---|---|
| | | | | | | | Date | Author(s) | Reference |
| OFX | 1–200 t.i.d. | 5–21 | 22[d] | 82 | 0 | Acute or chronic | 1984 | Suzuki et al. | 66 |
| OFX | 200 b.i.d. | 40 | 14 | 79 | 3–12 | Not specified | 1986 | Guibert and Acar | 18 |
| OFX | 200 b.i.d. | 60 | 23 | 91 | 7–13 | Acute or chronic | 1988 | Remy et al. | 58 |
| RSX | 150 b.i.d. | 14 | 20[d] | 20 | NS | Bacterial-chlamydial | 1986 | Asbach and Melekos | 2 |
| NXF | 400 b.i.d. | 14 | 15[d] | 75 | NS | Bacterial-chlamydial | | | |
| OFX | 200 b.i.d. | 14 | 20[d] | 75 | NS | Bacterial-chlamydial | | | |
| OFX | 200 b.i.d. | 14 | 21[d] | 67 | 12 | Chronic bacterial | 1989 | Pust et al. | 56a |
| OFX | 300 b.i.d. | 42 | 43[d] | 85 | NS | Not specified | 1991 | Corrado[e] | 11 |
| CAR | 764 t.i.d. | 42 | 42[d] | 53 | NS | Not specified | | | |

[a]OFX, ofloxacin; RSX, rosoxacin; NFX, norfloxacin; CAR, carbenicillin.
[b]t.i.d., three times a day; b.i.d., twice daily.
[c]NS, not stated.
[d]Localization study performed.
[e]Data include results of study (11a).



**Table 10.** Eradication of pathogens (bacteriological cure) in patients with bacterial prostatitis treated with various quinolones

| Drug[a] | Dose[b] (mg) | Duration of therapy (days)[c] | No. of evaluable patients | % Bacteriological cure | Duration of follow-up (mo) | Type of infection | Study | | |
|---|---|---|---|---|---|---|---|---|---|
| | | | | | | | Date | Author(s) | Reference |
| PFX | 400 b.i.d. | NS | 31 | 65 | 3 | Not specified | 1986 | Desplaces et al. | 14 |
| PFX | 400 b.i.d. | 28 | 31 | 74 | 1 | Acute or chronic | 1990 | Guibert et al. | 19 |
| ENX | 200 t.i.d. | 14 | 97[d] | 55 | 0 | Chronic | 1986 | Kumamoto et al. | 24 |
| ENX | 400 b.i.d. | 28 | 38[d] | 55 | 1 | Chronic | 1989 | Christensen et al. | 10 |
| CAR | 764 b.i.d. | 28 | 46[d] | 53 | 1 | Chronic | | | |
| TFX | 400 b.i.d. | 28 | 76[d] | 72 | 1 | Chronic | 1991 | Cox and Childs | 12 |
| TFX | 400 b.i.d. | 28 | 42[d] | 68 | 1 | Chronic | 1991 | Naber et al. | 40 |
| RFX | 4–200 q.i.d. | 28 | 24[d] | 79 | 1 | Chronic | 1990 | Boerema et al. | 6 |
| FLX | 2–300 q.i.d. | 7–26 | 11[d] | 100 | 0 | Chronic | 1991 | Nishitani et al. | 48 |

[a]PFX, pefloxacin; ENX, enoxacin; CAR, carbenicillin; TFX, temafloxacin; RFX, rufloxacin; FLX, fleroxacin.
[b]b.i.d., twice daily; t.i.d., three times a day; q.i.d., four times a day.
[c]NS, not stated.
[d]Localization study performed.

day followed by 200 mg once daily over 4 weeks could be evaluated. Up to 1 month after completion of therapy, 79% of the patients showed bacteriological cure.

## CONCLUSION

Even though it appears that the newer quinolones have been used to quite an extent for the treatment of chronic bacterial prostatitis, the analysis of the published studies has not yet established a definite conclusion concerning the role of quinolones compared with standard treatment. Results can be compared only for studies in which the diagnosis was obtained by localization studies and in which the patients were followed up for a sufficient time after completion of therapy, and only a few studies meet these criteria. Of these studies, only three, i.e., one with norfloxacin (61) and four with ciprofloxacin (23, 54, 55, 67, 68), presented results obtained during a follow-up period of at least 6 months. The results of these studies seem to be comparable.

In general, the therapeutic results are good in chronic prostatitis due to *E. coli* and other members of the family *Enterobacteriaceae* but not in prostatitis due to *P. aeruginosa* and enterococci. For chronic prostatitis caused by *E. coli*, a treatment duration of 1 month seems to be superior to the usual 3-month treatment with co-trimoxazole. There is a need for further studies, especially controlled studies with valid protocols, to elucidate the role of the newer quinolones in the treatment of chronic bacterial prostatitis.

### REFERENCES


1. **Anderson, R. U., and W. R. Fair.** 1976. Physical and chemical determinations of prostatic secretion in benign hyperplasia, prostatitis and adenocarcinoma. *Invest. Urol.* **14:**137–140.
2. **Asbach, H. W., and M. Melekos.** 1986. Zur Behandlung der Urethro-Adnexitis des Mannes mit Gyrasehemmern, p. 857–859. *In* D. Adam, H. Knothe, H. Lode, and W. Stille (ed.), *Ofloxacin, Fortsch. Antimicrob. Antineopl. Chemother. FAC 5-5.* Futuramed, Munich.
3. **Bischoff, W.** 1985. Norfloxacin—Behandlung der akuten Zystitis der Frau und der bakteriellen Prostatitis. *Fortsch. Med.* **103:**225–228.
4. **Bischoff, W., and H. Bischoff.** 1989. Bacterial prostatitis: efficacy of ciprofloxacin versus sulfonamide-trimethoprim therapy, abstr. p. 213. *Austr. Int. Congr. Chemother. 1989.*
5. **Blacklock, N. J., and J. P. Beavis.** 1974. The response of fluid pH in inflammation. *Br. J. Urol.* **46:**537–542.
6. **Boerema, J. B., W. Bischoff, J. Focht, and K. G. Naber.** 1991. An open multicentre study on the efficacy and safety of rufloxacin in patients with chronic bacterial prostatitis. *J. Antimicrob. Chemother.* **28:**587–597.
7. **Boerema, J. B., A. Dalhoff, and F. M. Y. Debruyne.** 1985. Ciprofloxacin distribution in prostatic tissue and fluid following oral administration. *Chemotherapy* **31:**13–18.
8. **Bologna, M., L. Vaggi, D. Flammini, G. Carlucci, and C. M. Forchetti.** 1985. Norfloxacin in prostatitis: correlation between HPLC tissue concentrations and clinical results. *Drugs Exp. Clin. Res.* **11:**95–100.
9. **Childs, S. J.** 1987. Treatment of chronic bacterial prostatitis with ciprofloxacin. *Infect. Surg.*, p. 649–651.
10. **Christensen, M. M., J. M. Knes, and P. O. Madsen.** 1990. Chronic prostatitis: pharmacokinetics of enoxacin and clinical trial results, p. 267.1–267.2. *In* E. Rubinstein and D. Adam (ed.), *Proceedings of the 16th International Congress of Chemotherapy, Recent Advances in Chemotherapy.* Lewin-Epstein Ltd., Jerusalem.
11. **Corrado, M. L.** 1991. Worldwide clinical experience with ofloxacin in urological cases. *Urology* **27**(Suppl.)**:**28–32.

11a. **Cox, G. E.** 1989. Ofloxacin in the management of complicated urinary tract infections, including prostatitis. *Am. J. Med.* **87**(Suppl. 6C)**:**61S–68S.

12. **Cox, C. E., and S. J. Childs.** 1991. Treatment of chronic bacterial prostatitis. *Am. J. Med.* **91**(Suppl. 6A)**:**134S–139S.
13. **Dalhoff, A., and W. Weidner.** 1984. Diffusion of ciprofloxacin into prostatic fluid. *Eur. J. Clin. Microbiol.* **3:**360–366.
14. **Desplaces, N., L. Gutmann, J. Cartlet, J. Guibert, and J. F. Acar.** 1986. The new quinolones and their combinations with other agents for therapy of severe infections. *J. Antimicrob. Chemother.* **17**(Suppl. A)**:**25–39.
15. **Dørflinger, T., E. H. Larsen, T. C. Gasser, and P. O. Madsen.** 1986. The concentration of various quinolone derivatives in the dog prostate, p. 35–39. *In* W. Weidner, H. Brunner, W. Krause, and C. F. Rothauge (ed.), *Therapy of Prostatitis.* W. Zuckschwerdt, Munich.

16. **Drach, G. W.** 1974. Trimethoprim-sulfamethoxazole therapy of chronic bacterial prostatitis. *J. Urol.* **111**:637–639.

16a. **Furet, Y. X., J. Deshusses, and J. C. Pechère.** 1992. Transport of pefloxacin across the bacterial cytoplasmic membrane in quinolone-susceptible *Staphylococcus aureus. Antimicrob. Agents Chemother.* **36**:2506–2511.

17. **Gasser, T. C., P. H. Graversen, and P. O. Madsen.** 1987. Fleroxacin (Ro 23-6240) distribution in canine prostatic tissue and fluids. *Antimicrob. Agents Chemother.* **31**:1010–1013.

18. **Guibert, J., and J. F. Acar.** 1986. Ofloxacin (RU 43280): evaluation clinique dans les infections urinaires et prostatiques. *Pathol. Biol.* **34**:494–497.

19. **Guibert, J., R. Boutelier, and A. Guyot.** 1990. A clinical trial of pefloxacin in prostatitis. *J. Antimicrob. Chemother.* **26**(Suppl. B):161–166.

20. **Guibert, J. M., D. M. Destrée, and J. F. Acar.** 1987. Ciprofloxacin (BAY 09867): clinical evaluation in urinary tract infections due to *Pseudomonas aeruginosa. Chemotherapia* **6**(Suppl.):524–525.

21. **Guibert, J. M., D. Destrée, C. Konopka, and J. Acar.** 1986. Ciprofloxacin in the treatment of urinary tract infection due to enterobacteria. *Eur. J. Clin. Microbiol.* **5**:247–248.

22. **Hanus, P. M., and L. H. Danzinger.** 1984. Treatment of chronic bacterial prostatitis. *Clin. Pharm.* **3**:49–55.

23. **Heidler, H.** 1990. Clinical effects of ciprofloxacin: clinical results in chronic bacterial prostatitis, p. 53–56. *In* H. Lode (ed.), *Ciprofloxacin in Clinical Practice: New Light on Established and Emerging Uses.* Zuckschwerdt, Stuttgart, Germany.

24. **Kumamoto, Y., S. Sakai, H. Tamate, T. Gohro, T. Inoke, S. Tabata, H. Tanda, S. Kato, T. Saka, and I. Hemmi.** 1986. Therapeutic studies on chronic prostatitis—use of AT-2266. *Hinyokika Kiyo* **32**:1213–1223.

25. **Kumon, H., A. Mizuno, M. Kishi, K. Miyata, and H. Ohmori.** 1985. The concentration of ofloxacin in human prostatic tissue and fluid, p. 1767–1768. *In* J. Ishigami (ed.), *Proceedings of the 14th International Congress of Chemotherapy. Recent Advances in Chemotherapy.* University of Tokyo Press, Tokyo.

26. **Langenmeyer, T. N., W. H. Ferwerda, J. A. Hoogkamp-Korstanje, E. J. de Leur, and H. van Oort.** 1987. Treatment of chronic bacterial prostatitis with ciprofloxacin. *Pharm. Weekbl.* **9**(Suppl.):78–81.

27. **Madsen, P. O., A. Baumüller, and U. Hoyme.** 1978. Experimental models for determination of antimicrobials in prostatic tissue, interstitial fluid and secretion. *Scand. J. Infect. Dis.* **1**(Suppl. 4):145–150.

28. **Matsumoto, T., M. Tanaka, J. Kumazawa, H. Nagayoshi, H. Hirano, S. Sato, T. Omoto, T. Amano, T. Soejima, K. Jinnouchi, M. Mikuriya, T. Nakao, K. Nanri, H. Hirata, N. Miyazaki, and A. Nagayama.** 1987. Clinical studies of ciprofloxacin (BAY 09867) in the treatment of prostatitis and acute epididymitis. *Nishinikou J. Urol.* **49**:673–690.

29. **Meares, E. M., Jr.** 1973. Observations on the activity of trimethoprim-sulfamethoxazole in the prostate. *J. Infect. Dis.* **129**(Suppl.):679–685.

30. **Meares, E. M., Jr.** 1975. Long-term therapy of chronic bacterial prostatitis with trimethoprim-sulfamethoxazole. *Can. Med. Assoc. J.* **112**(Suppl.):22–25.

31. **Meares, E. M., Jr.** 1975. Prostatitis. A review. *Urol. Clin. N. Am.* **2**:3–27.

32. **Meares, E. M., Jr.** 1978. Serum antibody titers in treatment with trimethoprim-sulfamethoxazole for chronic prostatitis. *Urology* **11**:141–146.

33. **Meares, E. M., Jr.** 1980. Prostatitis syndromes. New perspectives about old woes. *J. Urol.* **123**:141–147.

34. **Meares, E. M., and T. A. Stamey.** 1968. Bacteriologic localization patterns in bacterial prostatitis and urethritis. *Invest. Urol.* **5**:492–518.

35. **McGuire, E. J., and B. Lytton.** 1976. Bacterial prostatitis. Treatment with trimethoprim-sulfamethoxazole. *Urology* **7**:499–500.

36. **Mizoguchi, H., A. Maeda, T. Thimizu, and J. Ishigama.** 1985. An appraisal of ofloxacin levels in semen, p. 1793–1794. *In* J. Ishigami (ed.), *Proceedings of the 14th International Congress of Chemotherapy. Recent Advances in Chemotherapy.* University of Tokyo Press, Tokyo.

37. **Mobley, D. F.** 1974. Erythomycin plus sodium bicarbonate in chronic bacterial prostatitis. *Urology* **3**:60–62.

38. **Mobley, D. F.** 1981. Bacterial prostatitis: treatment with carbenicillin indanyl sodium. *Invest. Urol.* **19**:31–33.

39. **Naber, K. G., D. Adam, and F. Kees.** 1987. In vitro activity and concentrations in serum, urine, prostatic secretion and adenoma tissue of ofloxacin in urological patients. *Drugs* **34**(Suppl. 1):44–50.

40. **Naber, K. G., J. B. J. Boerema, W. Bischoff, H. Blenk, J. Focht, P. Carpentier, and J. Sylvester.** 1991. An assessment of temafloxacin in the treatment of chronic bacterial prostatitis. *J. Antimicrob. Chemother.* **28**(Suppl. C):87–96.

41. **Naber, K. G., F. Sörgel, F. Kees, U. Jaehde, and H. Schumacher.** 1989. Pharmakokinetik von Ciprofloxacin bei Probanden und älteren Patienten und Konzentrationen im Prostatasekret, Ejakulat und im Prostataadenomgewebe nach intravenöser Gabe, p. 75–87. *In* D. Adam, A. Dalhoff, and B. Wiedemann (ed.), *Fortsch. Antimicrob. Antineopl. Chemother. FAC 8-1.* Futuramed, Munich.

42. **Naber, K. G., F. Sörgel, F. Kees, U. Jaehde, and H. Schumacher.** 1989. Brief report: pharmacoki-

netics of ciprofloxacin in young (healthy) volunteers and elderly patients, and concentrations in prostatic fluid, seminal fluid, and prostatic adenoma tissue following intravenous administration. *Am. J. Med.* **87**(Suppl. 5A):57–59.

43. **Naber, K. G., F. Sörgel, F. Kees, U. Jaehde, H. Schumacher, R. Metz, and H. Grobecker.** 1988. In vitro activity of fleroxacin against isolates causing complicated urinary tract infections and concentrations in seminal and prostatic fluid and in prostatic adenoma tissue. *J. Antimicrob. Chemother.* **21**(Suppl. D.):199–207.
44. **Naber, K. G., F. Sörgel, F. Kees, H. Schumacher, R. Metz, and H. Grobecker.** 1987. Norfloxacin concentration in prostatic adenoma tissue (patients) and in prostatic fluid in patients and volunteers, p. 1956–1958. *In Proceedings of the 15th International Congress of Chemotherapy.* Ecomed, Landsberg, Germany.
45. **Naber, K. G., F. Sörgel, F. Kees, H. Schumacher, G. Sigl, J. Zürcher, and S. Berger.** 1989. Enoxacin-Konzentrationen in der Samenflüssigkeit, im Prostatasekret und im Prostatadenomgewebe nach oraler Gabe oder intravenöser Infusion. *Infection* **17**(Suppl. 1):30–36.
46. **Naber, K. G., F. Sörgel, G. Sigl, H. Schumacher, and R. Metz.** 1990. Lomefloxacin: penetration into prostatic and seminal fluid in volunteers, abstr. 248. *Program Abstr. 3rd. Int. Symp. New Quinolones.*
47. **Naber, K. G., F. Sörgel, G. Sigl, H. Schumacher, and J. Zürcher.** 1991. Penetration of temafloxacin into prostatic and seminal fluid in volunteers. *Eur. J. Clin. Microbiol. Infect. Dis.* **Special Issue:**29–30.
48. **Nishitani, Y., S. Uno, M. Tsugawa, K. Kondo, H. Kumon, and H. Ohmori.** 1991. Fleroxacin in the treatment of bacterial prostatitis, abstr. 1307. *Program Abstr. 17th Int. Congr. Chemother.*
49. **Okada, K.** 1985. Clinical studies on Bay 09867 in the field of urology. *Chemotherapy* (Tokyo) **33**(Suppl. 7):601–611.
50. **Oliveri, R. A., R. M. Sachs, and P. G. Castl.** 1979. Clinical experiences with geocillin in the treatment of bacterial prostatitis. *Curr. Ther. Res.* **25:**415–421.
51. **Paulson, D. F., and R. D. White.** 1978. Trimethoprim-sulfamethoxazole and minocycline hydrochloride in the treatment of culture-proved bacterial prostatitis. *J. Urol.* **120:**184–185.
52. **Petrikkos, G., T. Peppas, H. Giamarellou, K. Poulios, P. Zouboulis, and P. Sfikakis.** 1991. Four year experience with norfloxacin in the treatment of chronic bacterial prostatitis, abstr. 1302. *Program Abstr. 17th Int. Congr. Chemother.*
53. **Pfau, A.** 1986. Prostatitis. A continuing enigma. *Urol. Clin. N. Am.* **13:**695–715.
54. **Pfau, A.** 1987. Therapie der unteren Harnwegsinfectionen beim Mann unter besonderer Berücksichtingung der chronischen bakteriellen Prostatitis. *Akt. Urol.* **18:**31–33.
55. **Pfau, A.** 1991. The treatment of chronic bacterial prostatitis. *Infection* **19**(Suppl. 3):160–164.
56. **Pfau, A., S. Perlberg, and A. Shapiro.** 1978. The pH of the prostatic fluid in health and disease: implications of treatment in chronic bacterial prostatitis. *J. Urol.* **119:**384–387.

56a. **Pust, R. A., H. R. Ackenheil-Koppe, P. Gilbert, and W. Weidner.** 1989. Clinical efficacy of ofloxacin (Tarivid[R]) in patients with chronic bacterial prostatitis: preliminary results. *J. Chemother.* **1**(Suppl. 4):469–471.

57. **Rauch, A. M., and V. I. Taylor.** 1990. Effective treatment of *E. coli* prostatitis with norfloxacin, abstr. 254. *Program Abstr. 3rd Int. Symp. New Quinolones.*
58. **Remy, G., C. Rouger, P. Chavanet, E. Bernard, P. Dellamonica, and H. Portier.** 1988. Use of ofloxacin for prostatitis. *Rev. Infect. Dis.* **10**(Suppl. 1):173–174.
59. **Sabath, L. D., D. A. Gerstein, F. B. Loder, and M. Finland.** 1968. Excretion of erythromycin and its enhanced activity in urine against gram-negative bacilli with alkalinization. *J. Lab. Clin. Med.* **72:**916–923.
60. **Sabbaj, J., V. L. Hoagland, and T. Cook.** 1986. Norfloxacin versus co-trimoxazole in the treatment of recurring urinary tract infections in men. *Scand. J. Infect. Dis.* **48**(Suppl.):48–53.
61. **Schaeffer, A. J., and F. S. Darras.** 1990. The efficacy of norfloxacin in the treatment of chronic bacterial prostatitis refractory to trimethoprim-sulfamethoxazole and/or carbenicillin. *J. Urol.* **144:**690–693.
62. **Schramm, P.** 1986. Ofloxacin concentration in human ejaculate and influence on sperm motility. *Infection* **14**(Suppl. 4):274–275.
63. **Smith, J. W., S. R. Jones, W. P. Reed, A. D. Tice, R. H. Deuprée, and B. Kaijser.** 1979. Recurrent urinary tract infections in men. *Ann. Intern. Med.* **91:**544–548.
64. **Stamey, T. A., E. M. Meares, Jr., and D. G. Winningham.** 1970. Chronic bacterial prostatitis and the diffusion of drugs into prostatic fluid. *J. Urol.* **103:**187–194.
65. **Suzuki, K., and Study Group on Prostatitis.** 1991. Ciprofloxacin in treatment of chronic prostatitis, abstr. 1304. *Program Abstr. 17th Int. Congr. Chemother.*
66. **Suzuki, K., H. Tamai, Y. Naide, K. Ando, and R. Moriguchi.** 1984. Laboratory and clinical study of ofloxacin in the treatment of bacterial prostatitis. *Hinyokika Kiyo* **30:**1505–1518.
67. **Weidner, W., H. G. Schiefer, and E. Brähles.** 1991. Refractory chronic bacterial prostatitis: a reevaluation of ciprofloxacin treatment after a median followup of refractory 30 months. *J. Urol.* **146:**350–352.

68. **Weidner, W., H. G. Schiefer, and A. Dalhoff.** 1987. Treatment of chronic bacterial prostatitis with ciprofloxacin. Results of a one-year follow-up study. *Am. J. Med.* **82**(Suppl. 4A):280–283.
69. **Yoshida, K., Y. Uuchijima, H. Saitoh, T. Negishi, T. Yamada, T. Watanabe, and K. Kawakami.** 1991. *Program Abstr. 17th Int. Congr. Chemother.*, abstr. 1303.
70. **Zamfirescu, C., and V. Chysky.** 1985. Behandlung von refraktären Harnwegsinfektionen und Prostatitis bei nicht hospitalisierten Patienten mit Ciprofloxacin. *Urologe* (B) **25**:330–333.
71. **Zinner, S. H., L. D. Sabath, J. L. Casey, and M. Finland.** 1971. Erythromycin and alkalinization of the urine in the treatment of urinary tract infections due to gram-negative bacilli. *Lancet* **i**:1267–1268.

*Quinolone Antimicrobial Agents, 2nd ed.*
Edited by David C. Hooper and John S. Wolfson


*Chapter 15*

# Use of Quinolones in Sexually Transmitted Diseases

***Rosanna W. Peeling and Allan R. Ronald***

## INTRODUCTION

Bacterial sexually transmitted infections are a global public health problem. The annual incidence of bacterial sexually transmitted diseases (STDs) exceeds 100,000,000 and may be closer to 200,000,000 (36). The prevalence of bacterial STDs is likely substantially higher than we think because of unrecognized asymptomatic or latent infections.

Table 1 lists the bacterial STDs that will be discussed in this chapter and identifies acute presentations and sequelae.

Bacterial STDs, specifically those caused by *Chlamydia trachomatis* and *Neisseria gonorrhoeae*, are responsible for serious morbidity in women, causing problems such as pelvic inflammatory disease (PID), ectopic pregnancy, tubal infertility, and chronic pelvic pain. The incidence of these sequelae is increasing dramatically in some societies, with consequences to reproductive health in women and the well-being of their offspring (168).

Programs to control STDs are different from programs to control other infectious diseases for the following reasons. (i) Individuals and societies stigmatize and often denigrate individuals with these infections. Also, these infections tend to be more common among individuals who are socioeconomically disadvantaged. Consequently, health programs for STDs are given a lower priority than in other health programs in many societies (7). (ii) STDs are transmitted largely by individuals who are asymptomatic and usually unaware of their infections. (iii) A core group of individuals, the "high-frequency transmitters," is responsible for maintaining these infections in society through their frequent changes of sexual partners and their social mixing patterns. Effective treatment removes them from the chain of transmission and may prevent many individuals from being infected (22). (iv) The sequelae of these infections usually occur months to years after the infection and may not be linked by either health care providers or the patient to previous episodes of STDs. (v) Many treatment programs depend on syndrome recognition, with treatment based on the probability of one or more pathogens being present. In as many as 30% of patients, more than one bacterial pathogen is present, so concurrent treatment is required. (vi) Treatment is frequently empiric because laboratory confirmation is not available or is delayed. (vii) An individual with an STD requires, in addition to treatment, education and counseling with regard

***Rosanna W. Peeling*** • National Laboratory for Sexually Transmitted Diseases, Laboratory Centre for Disease Control, Tunney's Pasture, Ottawa, Canada K1A 0L2. ***Allan R. Ronald*** • Division of Infectious Diseases, St. Boniface Hospital, 409 Tache Avenue, Winnipeg, Canada R2H 2A6.

**Table 1.** Clinical manifestations of bacterial STDs

| STD pathogen | Clinical manifestations | | |
|---|---|---|---|
| | Male | Female | Infant |
| *N. gonorrhoeae*[a] | | | |
| Acute illness | Urethritis<br>Conjunctivitis<br>Proctitis<br>Epididymitis | Cervicitis<br>Endometritis<br>Urethritis<br>Conjunctivitis<br>Proctitis<br>Salpingitis<br>Perihepatitis | Conjunctivitis |
| Sequelae | Urethral stricture | Ectopic pregnancy<br>Tubal infertility<br>Pelvic pain syndrome | Blindness |
| *C. trachomatis*[a] | | | |
| Acute illness | Urethritis<br>Conjunctivitis<br>Proctitis<br>Epididymitis<br>Lymphogranuloma venereum[b] | Cervicitis<br>Urethritis<br>Conjunctivitis<br>Proctitis<br>Salpingitis<br>Endometritis<br>Perihepatitis<br>Lymphogranuloma venereum[b] | Conjunctivitis<br>Pneumonia |
| Sequelae | Reiter's syndrome | Reiter's syndrome<br>Pelvic pain syndrome<br>Ectopic pregnancy<br>Tubal infertility | |
| *T. pallidum* | | | |
| Acute illness | Genital ulcers | Genital ulcers | Congenital syphilis |
| Sequelae | Proctitis<br>Secondary and tertiary syphilis | Proctitis<br>Secondary and tertiary syphilis | Late manifestation of congenital syphilis |
| *H. ducreyi* | Genital ulcer disease with bubos | Genital ulcer disease with bubos | None |
| *M. hominis* | None proven | Possible PID<br>Postpartum pyrexia | None proven |
| *U. urealyticum* | Probable urethritis | None proven | Pneumonia |
| Bacterial vaginosis-associated organisms (*G. vaginalis*, *Mobiluncus* spp.) | None | Bacterial vaginosis | None |

[a]Complications of pregnancy are not included.
[b]Limited to unique serovars of *C. trachomatis*.

to risky sexual behavior and contact tracing. Effective treatment is not the only goal of management. (viii) Some bacterial STDs, specifically those caused by *N. gonorrhoeae* and *Haemophilus ducreyi*, have rapidly developed resistance to a wide variety of treatment regimens. Both plasmid-mediated and chromosomally mediated resistance occur. Strategies to prevent the emergence of resistance to newer agents, particularly the quinolones, need to be considered in their initial clinical evaluation and subsequent use. (ix) Conventional STDs, specifically chancroid and perhaps genital herpes, syphilis, and gonococcal and chlamydial infections, are implicated as cofactors in the transmission of human immunodeficiency virus (HIV). As a result, efforts to control and, if possible, markedly reduce the incidence of these infections are mandated by the importance of strategies to slow the sexual spread of HIV infection (113).

### Ideal Drugs for Bacterial STDs

No treatment regimen meets all expectations. However, criteria that can be used to judge the potential therapeutic values of proposed regimens are being established. Many of these regimens arise from unique features of bacterial STDs. At present, the criteria can be summarized as follows. (i) A single dose can be prescribed and administered so that cure is not dependent on patient compliance. (ii) Oral administration, with confidence in bioavailability of the drug in all patients, is possible. (iii) Costs are affordable, so that they are not a deterrent to individual or government purchases. (iv) Wide distribution in the body, particularly on mucosal surfaces, ensures predictable eradication of the pathogen not only at the genital site but also at other sites in which it may reside. This is especially important for patients with gonococcal infections who may have concurrent rectal or pharyngeal infection. (v) Because the overlapping presentations of *N. gonorrhoeae* and *C. trachomatis* make syndrome diagnosis and treatment essential, the drug needs to be effective against both of these pathogens. (vi) Incubating syphilis in patients presenting with urethritis or other genital syndromes can be cured. *Treponema pallidum* has an incubation period of several weeks before serologic evidence or clinical illness is apparent. Drugs such as amoxicillin that are used against gonococcal infections and that cure incubating *T. pallidum* infection have been considered advantageous. (vii) The probability of cure should be sufficiently high that follow-up cultures are not necessary. For gonococcal infection, this essentially means cure rates in excess of 98%. (viii) The regimens should be safe, as they will usually be administered in outpatient settings and are often prescribed by individuals other than physicians. They need to be safe for pregnant and lactating women as well as adolescents and infants. Quinolones are specifically contraindicated during pregnancy and childhood. (ix) The regimen can be used for empiric treatment of contacts, who are usually asymptomatic and uncertain of the necessity of treatment. (x) Resistance does not appear either during treatment or as a result of an epidemiological shift in bacterial populations.

### Duration of Treatment

During the 1960s, studies by Jaffe et al. (62) showed that the major determinant of cure for gonococcal infection was the MIC for *N. gonorrhoeae* and the length of time that the concentration of the therapeutic agent remained above the MIC. A level in serum of at least four times the MIC for about 10 h was required for penicillin to cure gonococcal urethritis. Similar studies for *H. ducreyi* showed that antibacterial levels need to exceed the MIC for 36 to 48 h to cure chancroid (38). Minimum duration of therapy for chlamydial infections has not been determined, but most regimens are prescribed for 7 to 14 days. It is uncertain whether the mechanism of action or the postantibiotic effect of the quinolones will alter these "minimum" requirements for duration of antibacterial activity.

## GUIDELINES FOR THE TREATMENT OF STDS

For the past 40 years, the Centers for Disease Control of the U.S. Public Health Service and, more recently, the Laboratory Centre for Disease Control in Canada and the World Health Organization have published recommendations for therapy of STDs. In the most recent guidelines, published in 1990 in the United States and in 1992 in Canada, clinical management of all STDs is updated and recommended treatment regimens are identified (26a, 75a). For most bacterial STDs, the quinolones are not the drugs of first choice. However, in the past 2 years, a significant number of publications have identified the increasingly important role of these agents for bacterial STDs.

In the United States, new guidelines for approval of therapeutic agents for STDs and other infectious diseases are being established (53). These guidelines will enable both pharmaceutical companies and investigators to design more-appropriate microbiological and clinical treatment trials. The outcome should be therapeutic regimens that meet the expectations of patients and their care providers.

## *C. TRACHOMATIS*

The biphasic life cycle of *C. trachomatis* presents unique challenges for antimicrobial therapy. The infectious extracellular form, the elementary body, is metabolically inert and is therefore not susceptible to antimicrobial agents whose activities require DNA or protein synthesis. The intracellular reticulate body multiplies inside a membrane-bound inclusion in the host cell. An antimicrobial agent must therefore gain access to the multiplying chlamydia through the host cell and must cross the inclusion membrane (117). Its life cycle (48 to 72 h) is considerably longer than that of *N. gonorrhoeae*, hence requiring that drug levels be maintained above the MIC for several days. This finding is supported by data from Kawada that show that 42% of 67 patients with chlamydial urethritis treated for 5 days with ofloxacin remained culture positive compared with only 3% of 95 men treated for 10 days (70). Clad et al. also observed the survival of *C. trachomatis* in cell culture after 12 days of exposure to doxycycline, erythromycin, or ciprofloxacin (27). The clinical significance of this in vitro observation is uncertain.

About one-third of chlamydial infections in women lead to complications (83). Failure to completely eradicate *C. trachomatis* may permit latent or persistent infections, and these may lead to long-term sequelae (84, 139). A regimen of 7 days or longer often leads to incomplete compliance because of symptomatic resolution prior to microbiological cure. The dual goals of curing the infection and preventing sequelae in the upper genital tract are both essential outcomes of treatment.

### Microbiological Studies

Standardized procedures for in vitro antimicrobial susceptibility testing for chlamydia have not been widely accepted (66). Parameters that can give rise to variability in results have been reviewed by Ehret and Judson (39). For example, a large inoculum size that permits the detection of heterotypic resistance to tetracycline may also be important for the determination of resistance to the quinolones (59, 67). Inoculum size, time of antimicrobial addition, and definition of end points (MICs and MBCs) must be standardized. Above all, studies to determine the relevance of these values to immediate and long-term therapeutic outcomes are required (66).

The range of $MIC_{90}$s of the quinolones and other relevant therapeutic agents for *C. trachomatis* isolates compiled from studies in the last few years are shown in Table 2. The newer fluoroquinolones such as ofloxacin, temafloxacin, tosufloxacin, and sparfloxacin are clearly superior to norfloxacin, enoxacin, rosoxacin, and ciprofloxacin (15, 40, 72, 100, 101, 102, 107, 131, 134, 135, 137, 142, 147, 154). Fleroxacin and pefloxacin show only moderate activity against *C. trachomatis*

**Table 2.** In vitro activities of quinolones and other agents against *C. trachomatis*[a]

| Drug | $MIC_{90}$ range ($\mu$g/ml) | Estimated therapeutic ratio |
|---|---|---|
| Quinolones | | |
| Ciprofloxacin | 0.25–2.0 | 1 |
| Enoxacin | 2.0–8.0 | <1 |
| Fleroxacin | 0.5–2.0 | 1–2 |
| Lomefloxacin | 0.5–4.0 | <1 |
| Norfloxacin | 4.0–16.0 | <1 |
| Ofloxacin | 0.5–2.0 | 1–2 |
| Pefloxacin | 2.0–8.0 | 1 |
| Rosoxacin | 5.0–40.0 | <1 |
| Sparfloxacin | 0.01–0.05 | 8–16 |
| Temafloxacin | 0.03–0.25 | 4–8 |
| Tosufloxacin | 0.06–0.25 | 4–8 |
| OPC-17116 | 0.06–0.125 | 4–8 |
| Other agents | | |
| Erythromycin | 0.063–0.25 | 4–8 |
| Doxycycline | 0.015–0.5 | 4–8 |

[a]References: 15, 37, 40, 72, 100–102, 107, 131, 134, 136, 137, 142, 147, 148, 153, 154.

(37, 148). However, both have a long half-life in serum (10 to 12 h) and may be able to sustain activity against *C. trachomatis* with appropriate dosing. The therapeutic ratio for each quinolone, i.e., the ratio of its estimated concentration in serum or tissue to its mean in vitro activity, suggests that ofloxacin, temafloxacin, sparfloxacin, and tosufloxacin achieve adequate concentration-in-tissue–to–MIC ratios (47, 87) (Table 2).

Resistance of *C. trachomatis* to the quinolones has not been reported. However, the mechanism of action of the quinolones has led to some interesting questions regarding their use for the treatment of chlamydial infections. Peeling and Gauthier noted that chlamydial growth in the presence of subinhibitory concentrations of ofloxacin led to the expression of the chlamydial GroEL heat shock protein (HSP60) (112). Immune response to chlamydial HSP60 has been correlated with the development of sequelae such as PID, ectopic pregnancy, and tubal infertility in women with chlamydial infections (20, 21, 166). The induction of the heat shock response is associated with the bacterial SOS DNA repair mechanism. Although HSP60 is produced during the normal chlamydial life cycle, the significance of its overproduction in the presence of quinolones and a possible relationship to the development of long-term sequelae need to be further evaluated.

## Clinical Studies

New treatment regimens for *C. trachomatis* must at least show equivalence to regimens with doxycycline. Recent clinical trials of the newer quinolone agents show an improvement over cure rates achieved with ciprofloxacin and norfloxacin (Table 3) (58, 108, 129, 157). Hooton et al. reported a recurrence of chlamydial infections in 52 and 38% of men treated with 7-day regimens of ciprofloxacin at 750 and 1,000 mg twice daily, respectively (59).

In clinical trials with ofloxacin, 90 to 100% cure rates were achieved with 7 days of twice-daily dosing (41, 73, 96, 125). Single-dose therapy with ciprofloxacin or fleroxacin prescribed for gonococcal infection is not effective for patients coinfected with *C. trachomatis* (8, 77, 156). Once-daily therapy with fleroxacin appears to be effective for chlamydial infections, possibly because of the long half-life of fleroxacin (85). However, frequent adverse reactions are reported (17).

The follow-up periods in these clinical trials vary from 1 to 4 weeks after completion of treatment. Late treatment failures of up to 19% have been documented when follow-up continues for longer than a week (16, 50, 59, 69). Unfortunately, reinfections are more likely and relapse is more difficult to distinguish from reinfection as the follow-up period is lengthened. Future studies should also evaluate long-term reproductive health following treatment of acute or asymptomatic chlamydial infection.

No studies in which the quinolones were used to treat lymphogranuloma venereum have been reported.

**Table 3.** Treatment trials of oral quinolones for genital chlamydial infections

| Drug and dosage[a] | Location of study | Reference(s) | Infection site[b] | Microbiological cure rate (no. of patients cured/ total no. treated [%]) |
|---|---|---|---|---|
| Ciprofloxacin | | | | |
| 1,500 mg, 7 days | Canada | 43 | U | 10/22 (45) |
| 500 mg b.i.d., 5 days | Germany | 12 | U | 22/27 (81) |
| 1,000 mg b.i.d., 14 days | The Netherlands | 156 | C | 24/35 (69) |
| 500 mg b.i.d., 7 days | United Kingdom | 3 | C | 20/26 (77) |
| Fleroxacin | | | | |
| 400 mg, 7 days | Austria | 146 | U, C | 21/22 (95) |
| | Norway | 50 | U, C | 6/10 (60) |
| 600 mg, 7 days | United States | 85, 86 | U, C | 100/104 (97) vs doxycycline[c] (122/129 [95]) |
| 600 mg, 7 days | Denmark | 171 | U, C | 49/58 (86) vs doxycycline[c] (44/50 [89]) |
| 600 mg, 7 days | Finland | 65 | U, C | 45/48 (94) vs doxycycline[c] (33/34 [97]) |
| 800 mg, 7 days | United States | 120 | U | 10/10 (100) |
| 400 mg, 7 days | Canada | 17 | U, C | 5/8 (63) |
| 600 mg, 7 days | Canada | 17 | | 3/4 (75) |
| 800 mg, 7 days | Canada | 17 | | 3/7 (43) |
| Ofloxacin | | | | |
| 200 mg b.i.d., 7 days | United Kingdom | 103 | U | 11/11 (100) |
| | Yugoslavia | | | 17/17 (100) |
| | United Kingdom | 125 | U, C | 49/49 (100) |
| 200 mg, 9 days | | 105 | U, C | 171/180 (95) vs doxycycline[c] (176/180 [98]) |
| 200 mg b.i.d., 28 days | Japan | 106 | C | 30/32 (94) |
| 300 mg b.i.d., 7 days | United States | 16 | U | 15/18 (83) vs doxycycline (10/10 [100]) |
| 300 mg b.i.d., 7 days | United Kingdom | 73 | U, C | 38/38 (100) vs doxycycline[c] (28/28 [100]) |
| 300 mg b.i.d., 7 days | United States | 96 | | 23/24 (96) vs doxycycline[c] (17/18 [100]) |
| 300 mg b.i.d., 7 days | United States | 41 | C | 20/20 (100) vs doxycycline[c] (18/20 [90]) |

[a]b.i.d., twice daily.
[b]U, urethra; C, cervix.
[c]All doxycycline regimens are 100 mg twice daily for 7 days.

## Summary

Ofloxacin and fleroxacin are effective therapeutic agents for *C. trachomatis*. Completion of a 7-day regimen is essential to achieve cure rates equivalent to those achieved with doxycycline.

## GONOCOCCAL INFECTION

The quinolones are proving to be excellent drugs for the treatment of gonococcal infection. Several of the fluoroquinolones are very effective when prescribed as a single oral dose, with cure rates approaching 100%. Many of these studies have included substantial numbers of penicillinase-producing *N. gonorrhoeae* (PPNG) and tetracycline-resistant *N. gonorrhoeae* (TRNG). Studies in both men and women have shown gonococcal eradication not only from genital sites but also from the pharynx and the rectum (122). The ease of administration, safety, and efficacy of the quinolones for the treatment of gonococcal infection may permit treatment strategies that will rapidly reduce the prevalence of gonococcal infection in populations at increased risk.

Despite this very encouraging scenario, the development of resistance of the gonococci in association with the use of rosoxacin in the Philippines and enoxacin in The Netherlands has generated considerable concern (28, 165). Antibacterial resistance to the quinolones among gonococci was first reported for nalidixic acid in 1982 (80), for enoxacin in 1986 (165), and for ciprofloxacin and norfloxacin in 1990 (28, 64, 172–174). The potential for widespread dissemination of resistance remains unknown.

**Table 4.** In vitro activities of quinolones against *N. gonorrhoeae*[a]

| Quinolone | $MIC_{90}$ range ($\mu$g/ml) | Estimated therapeutic ratio |
|---|---|---|
| Ciprofloxacin | 0.002–0.1 | 10–100 |
| Enoxacin | 0.025–0.25 | 5–10 |
| Fleroxacin | 0.002–0.06 | 20–100 |
| Lomefloxacin | 0.008–0.063 | 10–100 |
| Norfloxacin | 0.0015–0.5 | 10–100 |
| Ofloxacin | 0.004–0.1 | 10–100 |
| Pefloxacin | 0.008–0.06 | 10–100 |
| Rosoxacin | 0.001–0.25 | 5–10 |
| Temafloxacin | 0.004–0.125 | >100 |
| Tosufloxacin | 0.002–0.008 | >100 |

[a]References: 1, 63, 72, 75, 82, 90, 93, 118, 124, 132, 142, 143, 153, 154.

## Microbiological Studies

The in vitro efficacy of the fluoroquinolones against *N. gonorrhoeae* is depicted in Table 4. Ciprofloxacin is extremely effective, with ratios of level in serum to $MIC_{90}$ of 100 or more. Although somewhat less active, fleroxacin and ofloxacin also are very effective in vitro. Sparfloxacin and tosufloxacin are even more effective in vitro and presumably will have serum drug concentration-to-$MIC_{90}$ ratios in excess of 100. Although unproven, it is possible that these high ratios of concentration in serum to maximum MIC for gonococci prevent the emergence of resistance due to gonococcal mutants that require multiple-step mutations in order to survive the presence of the fluoroquinolones.

However, resistance to the quinolones has developed (49). Mutants with low-level resistance can be detected among susceptible populations if appropriate conditions are provided. The increase in resistance is usually 2- to 10-fold, and it occurs at a very low frequency of between $10^{-8}$ and $10^{-9}$. Further resistance is difficult to develop in vitro, and organisms with stable resistance to 0.1 $\mu$g of ciprofloxacin per ml have not been induced in the laboratory (48).

Among patients, it is considered unlikely for resistance to appear, as mutants with MICs below 0.1 $\mu$g of ciprofloxacin per ml, selected out during therapy, would presumably be killed following a usual therapeutic dose of ciprofloxacin. However, resistance could be postulated to occur in two scenarios. First, if patients are reinfected while quinolone levels are falling, these very low drug levels may select out strains with small increases in resistance. This would be most likely to occur in individuals who have frequent reinfections or who use the quinolones for prophylaxis against gonococcal infection. Second, the quinolones with lower ratios of concentration in serum to MIC, such as rosoxacin and enoxacin, may more readily select out low-level incremental resistance. This is of particular concern, as experience suggests that both of these agents have been associated with the emergence of resistance. Additional studies should be done in order to determine whether quinolones with therapeutic ratios of less than 10 are appropriate choices for treating gonococcal infection.

A recent study suggests that resistance to the quinolones can be detected by screening during routine disk diffusion susceptibility testing with a 30-$\mu$g nalidixic acid disk (158). Gonococci resistant to any of the quinolones will show no zone around the 30-$\mu$g nalidixic acid disk.

Recent studies have very clearly demonstrated the genetic basis of gonococcal resistance (149). Resistance is chromosomally mediated, and as yet, there is no evidence of plasmid-mediated quinolone resistance. Among isolates from patients, quinolone resistance in the gonococcus may develop from mutations in the *gyrB* gene (150) encoding DNA gyrase or the outer membrane porin proteins. Resistance emerging in this situation appears to be stable, and MICs as high as 0.5 μg of ciprofloxacin per ml have been reported for patient isolates (150). Patients infected with these resistant organisms will fail treatment with ciprofloxacin (159).

The mechanism of gonococcal resistance to the quinolones is currently under investigation. The gonococci can acquire the resistant genotype from a resistant gonococcal strain in a process known as transformation. Corkill et al. showed that in vitro ciprofloxacin resistance could be transferred to other gonococci that share the same porin protein type (30). The transformants showed a 20-fold increase in MICs, from <0.003 to 0.064 μg/ml. However, this increase was 10-fold less than that of the parent strain. Resistance to tetracycline and chloramphenicol was not cotransferred with ciprofloxacin resistance, suggesting that these resistance genes are not linked. The uptake of ciprofloxacin was reduced in resistant strains, and this reduction was enhanced by further exposure to subinhibitory concentrations of ciprofloxacin. This suggests that the mechanism controlling intracellular concentration is inducible rather than constitutive. The protein 1-B is the porin that acts as the diffusion pathway through the outer membrane for the quinolones, and mutations of this protein are a possible mechanism for slowing quinolone diffusion (30).

A great deal more needs to be learned about mechanisms of resistance among gonococci. Will the widespread use of the quinolones result in the rapid appearance of resistance, or is the emergence of resistance an isolated rare phenomenon that will be sporadic and perhaps unimportant? Can the development of resistance be prevented by the use of quinolones with very high therapeutic ratios of levels in serum to $MIC_{90}$? Are there any other ways of thwarting the emergence of resistance among the quinolones other than restricting their use?

## Clinical Studies

In studies conducted around the world, single-dose therapy with ciprofloxacin, fleroxacin, norfloxacin, and ofloxacin achieved microbiological cure rates approaching 100% (Tables 5, 6, and 7). A dose-ranging study with enoxacin showed that two doses of 400 mg each or a single dose of 600 mg is required for predictable cure in all patients (4). Difficulty in eradication of PPNG or TRNG has not been a problem with any of the quinolone regimens (23, 104, 110, 144).

Since one-third or more of individuals with genital gonococcal infection have concomitant chlamydial infection, the efficacy of these single-dose regimens against *C. trachomatis* is a concern. Several studies have documented the failure of these regimens to eradicate chlamydial infection following single-dose therapy (8, 59, 76, 125, 155). As a result, these single-dose regimens must be either extended to a full 7-day course if the quinolones are prescribed or combined with doxycyline or some other regimen that will be effective against *C. trachomatis*. Otherwise, patients will have inadequate therapy for *C. trachomatis*.

It is presumed that the quinolones would be an excellent choice for disseminating gonococcal infection as well as for gonococcal infection localized to joints or other sites of focal infection. Two patients with gonococcal arthritis were cured with a 10-day course of oral ciprofloxacin (121a).

## Summary

The fluoroquinolones are an effective single-dose therapeutic agent for *N. gonorrhoe-*

**Table 5.** Comparative treatment trials of oral quinolones for gonococcal infections, 1988 through 1991

| Drug and dosage[a] | Location of study | Reference | Microbiological cure rate (no. of patients cured/ no. of patients treated [%]) | Comments[b] |
|---|---|---|---|---|
| Ciprofloxacin, 250 mg | Zambia | 23 | 83/83 (100) | 31% PPNG and 25% CMRNG; all men |
| Ceftriaxone, 250 mg i.m. | Zambia | 23 | 81/82 (99) | 37% PPNG and 23% CMRNG; all men |
| Ciprofloxacin, 500 mg | Kenya | 104 | 33/34 (97) | All women |
| Ceftriaxone, 250 mg i.m. | Kenya | 104 | 20/21 (95) | All women |
| Ciprofloxacin, 250 mg | Kenya | 104 | 79/79 (100) | All men 67% PPNG |
| Kanamycin, 2 g i.m. | Kenya | 104 | 56/67 (84) | All men |
| Amoxicillin, 3 g + augmentin, 500/250 mg + probenicid, 1 g | Kenya | 104 | 74/78 (95) | All men |
| Penicillin, 4.8 MU + augmentin + 500/250 mg + probenecid, 1 g | Kenya | 104 | 63/68 (93) | All men |
| Enoxacin, 400 mg | United States | 53 | 74/75 (99) | 6% PPNG |
| Ceftriaxone, 250 mg i.m. | United States | 53 | 72/74 (97) | 7% TRNG |
| | United States | | | |
| Enoxacin, 400 mg | | 4 | 22/23 (96) | 12.5% PPNG; 12/12 men (100%) and 10/11 women (91%) cured |
| Ceftriaxone, 250 mg i.m. | | 4 | 25/25 (100) | 14 men and 11 women treated and cured |
| Enoxacin, 400 mg | United States | 109 | 74/75 (99) | 59/60 men (98%) and 15/15 women (100%) cured |
| Ceftriaxone, 250 mg i.m. | United States | 109 | 72/74 (97) | 58/59 men (98%) and 14/15 women (93%) cured |
| Fleroxacin, 400 mg | Finland | 77 | 48/48 (100) | Men only |
| Penicillin G, $2.4 \times 10^6$ U i.m. + probenecid, 1 g | Finland | 77 | 48/48 (100) | Men only |

*Continued on following page*

**Table 5.** *Continued*

| Drug and dosage[a] | Location of study | Reference | Microbiological cure rate (no. of patients cured/ no. of patients treated [%]) | Comments[b] |
|---|---|---|---|---|
| Norfloxacin, 800 mg | Thailand, Singapore | 110 | 94/94 (100)<br>145/145 (100) | PPNG<br>Non-PPNG } 142 men and 97 women treated and cured |
| Spectinomycin, 2 g i.m. | Thailand, Singapore | 110 | 82/82 (100)<br>159/161 (99) | PPNG<br>Non-PPNG } 145 men and 98 women treated, of whom 144 men and 97 women cured |
| Ofloxacin, 300 mg b.i.d., 7 days | United States | 16 | 30/30 (100) | 10% PPNG, all men |
| Doxycycline, 100 mg b.i.d., 7 days | United States | 16 | 32/34 (94) | |
| Ofloxacin, 400 mg | United States | 13 | 99/100 (99) | 1 PPNG; 47/48 men (98%) and 52/52 (100%) women cured |
| Amoxicillin, 3 g + probenecid, 1 g | United States | 13 | 97/101 (96) | 51/53 men (96%) and 46/48 women (96%) cured |
| Ofloxacin, 400 mg | United States | 79 | 69/70 (99) | 41/42 men (98%) and 28/28 women (100%) cured |
| Amoxicillin, 3 g + probenecid, 1 g | United States | 79 | 76/82 (93) | 51/55 men (93%) and 25/27 women (93%) cured |
| Ofloxacin, 400 mg | United States | 34 | 47/47 (100) | 34–36% PPNG; 27 men, 20 women |
| Ceftriaxone, 250 mg i.m. | United States | 34 | 42/42 (100) | 25 men, 17 women |
| Pefloxacin, 800 mg | The Netherlands | 155 | 35/35 (100) | 9% PPNG, all men |
| Cefotaxime, 1 g i.m. | The Netherlands | 155 | 32/32 (100) | |
| Temafloxacin | United States | 95 | | |
| 200 mg | | | 31/32 (97) | |
| 400 mg | | | 40/40 (100) | |
| Ceftriaxone, 250 mg i.m. | United States | 95 | 40/40 (100) | |

[a]i.m., intramuscular; b.i.d., twice daily.
[b]CMRNG, chromosomally mediated resistant *N. gonorrhoeae*.

**Table 6.** Noncomparative treatment trials of oral quinolones for gonococcal infections, 1988 through 1991

| Drug and dosage[a] | Location of study | Reference | Microbiological cure rate (no. of patients cured/ no. of patients treated [%]) | Comments |
|---|---|---|---|---|
| Ciprofloxacin | Belgium | 8 | | |
| 100 mg | | | 25/25 (100) | 20 men, 5 women |
| 250 mg | | | 22/22 (100) | 17 men, 5 women |
| Ciprofloxacin, 250 mg | United Kingdom | 138 | 59/59 (100) | All women |
| Enoxacin | France | 140 | | |
| 200 mg | | | 65/59 (94) | |
| 400 mg | | | 66/69 (96) | 10% PPNG |
| 400 mg twice | | | 29/29 (100) | 100 men and 100 women were entered |
| 600 mg | | | 29/29 (100) | |
| Ofloxacin | Hong Kong | 55 | | |
| 300 mg | | | 50/50 (100) | |
| 200 mg | | | 49/50 (98) | 44% PPNG, all men |
| Ofloxacin, 400 mg | Malaysia | 121 | 43/43 (100) | |
| Ofloxacin, 400 mg | United Kingdom | 125 | 50/50 (100) | 39 men, 11 women |
| Ofloxacin, 400 mg | United States | 145 | 49/49 (100) | 44% PPNG; 22% TRNG; 36 men, 13 women |
| Ofloxacin | | | | |
| 200 mg b.i.d., 14 days | Japan | 88 | (100) | |
| 200 mg t.i.d., 14 days | | | (92) | |

[a]b.i.d., twice daily; t.i.d., three times daily.

*ae*. It is hoped that widespread resistance will not emerge. Periodic or routine screening for quinolone resistance should be performed with the 30-$\mu$g nalidixic acid disk.

## NSU, CERVICITIS, AND THE GENITAL MYCOPLASMAS

Nonspecific urethritis (NSU) in males is an elusive disease, difficult to diagnose and treat. In most instances, the initial diagnosis is made on the basis of a clinical presentation of dysuria and urethral discharge and a Gram stain in which no gram-negative diplococci are apparent and at least 10 to 15 polymorphonuclear leukocytes per high-power field appear. In about 50% of patients, cultures for *C. trachomatis* are positive. In a minority of patients, usually $<10\%$, herpes simplex virus, *Trichomonas vaginalis*, or urinary tract pathogens such as *Escherichia coli* are the etiologic agents. The etiologic role of *Ureaplasma urealyticum* in NSU remains controversial. Although *Mycoplasma hominis* is isolated from 20% of patients with urethritis, no significant differences in isolation rates in patients and controls are noted. Antimicrobial agents with little or no activity against *M. hominis* are as effective in the treatment of NSU as anti-infective drugs that are active against *M. hominis*. However, some studies suggest that *U. urealyticum* is an etiologic agent for NSU. The most convincing studies are based on quantitative culture of *U. urealyticum*. Although qualitative studies suggest that if sexual activity is controlled, patients with NSU and controls will each have a 50% isolation rate for *U. urealyticum*, placebo-controlled studies show

**Table 7.** Treatment trials of oral quinolones for gonococcal infections of pharynx and rectum, 1988 through 1991

| Drug and dosage[a] | Location of study | Reference | Cure rate (no. of patients cured/no. treated [%]) | |
|---|---|---|---|---|
| | | | Pharynx | Rectum |
| Noncomparative studies | | | | |
| Ciprofloxacin, 250 mg | United Kingdom | 29 | 3/3 (100) | 4/4 (100) |
| Ciprofloxacin, 200 mg | United Kingdom | 138 | 5/5 (100) | 14/14 (100) |
| Enoxacin, 400 mg twice | United Kingdom | 9 | | 15/15 (100) |
| | | | | 18/18 (100) |
| Enoxacin | Canada | 128 | | |
| 200 mg b.i.d., 2 days | | | 6/7 (86) | 13/13 (100) |
| 400 mg b.i.d., 2 days | | | 5/5 (100) | 13/13 (100) |
| Comparative studies | | | | |
| Ofloxacin, 400 mg | United States | 79 | 6/7 (86) | 12/12 (100) |
| Amoxicillin, 3 g + probenecid, 1 g | United States | 79 | 3/5 (60) | 11/12 (92) |
| Ofloxacin, 400 mg | United States | 13 | 7/8 (88) | 13/13 (100) |
| Amoxicillin, 3 g + probenecid, 1 g | United States | 13 | 7/8 (88) | 17/17 (100) |
| Ofloxacin, 400 mg | United States | 34 | 1/1 (100) | 2/2 (100) |
| Ceftriaxone, 250 mg i.m. | United States | 34 | 3/3 (100) | 5/6 (83) |
| Ofloxacin | United States | 31 | | |
| 300 mg b.i.d., 7 days | | | 10/10 (100) | 10/10 (100) |
| 400 mg, 1 dose | | | 8/8 (100) | 20/20 (100) |
| Doxycycline, 100 mg b.i.d., 7 days | United States | 31 | 5/6 (83) | 11/11 (100) |
| Enoxacin, 400 mg | United States | 109 | 0/3 (0) | 1/1 (100) |
| Ceftriaxone, 250 mg i.m. | United States | 109 | 3/3 (100) | 5/5 (100) |
| Enoxacin, 400 mg | United States | 52 | 0/3 (0) | 1/1 (100) |
| Ceftriaxone, 250 mg i.m. | United States | 52 | 2/2 (100) | 5/5 (100) |

[a]b.i.d., twice daily; i.m., intramuscular.

improved outcomes if anti-infective agents that eradicate *U. urealyticum* are prescribed.

The syndromes of NSU and mucopurulent cervicitis from which neither *N. gonorrhoeae* nor *C. trachomatis* is isolated appear to be sexually transmitted. Additional studies are required before we can understand the etiologies, pathogeneses, and epidemiologies of these relatively common illnesses.

As a result of the uncertainty of both of these diagnoses, clinical studies have to be especially carefully designed. In most instances, it is essential to culture for both *N. gonorrhoeae* and *C. trachomatis* before embarking on a treatment regimen for NSU or cervicitis. However, many clinicians investigating these syndromes undertake treatment prior to obtaining positive cultures for either *N. gonorrhoeae* or *C. trachomatis*. As a result, a number of studies have been carried out in which the fluoroquinolones have been prescribed for these diagnoses.

## Microbiological Studies

Most in vitro studies have been directed toward determining MICs for a genital mycoplasma. The results of these studies are shown in Table 8. The fluoroquinolones currently on the market have limited in vitro efficacy against either *M. hominis* or *U. urealyticum*. The MICs are difficult to interpret, but they are in the range in which most pathogens are not effectively treated. Several newer

**Table 8.** In vitro activities of quinolones against *M. hominis* and *U. urealyticum*[a]

| Quinolone | MIC$_{90}$ range (μg/ml) | |
|---|---|---|
| | *M. hominis* | *U. urealyticum* |
| Ciprofloxacin | 0.5–2.0 | 0.5–32.0 |
| Enoxacin | | 4.0–64.0 |
| Lomefloxacin | 4.0–8.0 | 8.0 |
| Norfloxacin | | 8.0–32.0 |
| Ofloxacin | 0.25–2.0 | 0.5–8.0 |
| Rosoxacin | | 0.5–≥62.0 |
| Sparfloxacin | 0.125–1.0 | 0.125–2.0 |
| Temafloxacin | 0.007–0.50 | 1.0–8.0 |

[a]References: 25, 37, 46, 57, 119, 123, 130, 167.

fluoroquinolones such as sparfloxacin and some quinolones that do not yet have generic identification appear to have much lower MICs.

### Clinical Studies

Clinical trials for NSU conducted in the last 3 years are summarized in Table 9. Few studies have identified patients with chlamydial urethritis and/or mucopurulent cervicitis and excluded them prior to patient enrollment (78). A satisfactory clinical response is the resolution of symptoms and signs and fewer than 5 polymorphonuclear leukocytes per high-power field in the urethral smear on a return visit. Batteiger et al. treated seven men who had NSU and positive cultures for *U. urealyticum* (11). Of the three treated with ofloxacin, two had positive cultures at the second return visit, but both of these men had had sexual contact in the interval. Perea et al. reported that *Ureaplasma*-positive NSU patients treated with ciprofloxacin achieved a better clinical response than those treated with ofloxacin (114). They attributed this difference to the superior in vitro efficacy of ciprofloxacin compared with ofloxacin against *Ureaplasma* spp. Moller et al. randomized 200 men to either erythromycin base (500 mg twice daily) or ofloxacin (200 mg twice daily) (97). Of the eight men with positive cultures for *M. hominis*, all five treated with erythromycin and two of the three treated with ofloxacin continued to have positive cultures following treatment. Of the 16 patients with positive cultures for *U. urealyticum*, 1 of 10 treated with erythromycin and 0 of 6 treated with ofloxacin were culture positive on follow-up. Overall, 82% of the erythromycin-treated group and 88% of the ofloxacin-treated group had satisfactory clinical responses. This difference was not significant and was not related to the failure to eradicate *M. hominis* in some patients. Temafloxacin has been reported to be effective in patients with nonchlamydial and nongonococcal urethritis, with clinical responses of 86 to 94% (89, 127).

### Summary

The uncertain etiologies of sexually transmitted NSU and cervicitis make definitive clinical studies difficult. The genital mycoplasmas continue to have a controversial role in the etiology of these syndromes. However, clinical studies suggest that several of the quinolones are effective in the empiric treatment of NSU and perhaps mucopurulent cervicitis. The emergence of tetracycline-resistant ureaplasmas that are also resistant to macrolides, chloramphenicols, and aminoglycosides makes a search for alternative therapeutic agents important (126). Tetracycline-resistant ureaplasmas are a possible cause of persistent nongonococcal urethritis (152). However, at present, the quinolones are not considered the therapeutic agents of first choice for these infections. Additional, more-definitive studies are required to ultimately determine optimal treatment choices.

## CHANCROID AND *H. DUCREYI*

Chancroid is endemic in many developing countries. Impressive evidence links genital ulcerative disease, particularly chancroid, to increased heterosexual transmission of HIV

**Table 9.** Treatment of nongonococcal urethritis and cervicitis: clinical studies

| Drug and dosage[a] | Location(s) of study | Reference | Cure rate (no. of patients cured/no. treated [%])[b] | | | |
|---|---|---|---|---|---|---|
| | | | *C. trachomatis* | *U. urealyticum* | *H. hominis* | Clinical |
| Noncomparative studies | | | | | | |
| Fleroxacin | Canada | 17 | | | | |
| 400 mg, 7 days | | | | | | 5/8 (63) |
| 600 mg, 7 days | | | | | | 3/4 (75) |
| 800 mg, 7 days | | | | | | 3/7 (43) |
| Ofloxacin | Japan | 70 | | | | |
| 200 mg b.i.d., 5 days | | | 39/67 (58) | | | |
| 200 mg b.i.d., 10 days | | | 92/95 (97) | | | |
| Ofloxacin | Israel | 133 | | | | |
| 200 mg b.i.d., 10 days | | | 8/21 (86) | 9/15 (60) | 2/4 (50) | 17/22 (77) |
| 200 mg b.i.d., 20 days | | | 13/14 (82) | 9/12 (75) | 0/3 (0) | 22/24 (92) |
| Comparative studies | | | | | | |
| Ciprofloxacin, 1 g, 7 days | The Netherlands | 161 | 24/32 (85) | 23/32 (72) | | 35/100 (35) |
| Doxycycline | The Netherlands | 161 | | | | |
| 200 mg, 1 day | | | 14/15 (93) | 12/20 (60) | | 38/60 (63) |
| 100 mg b.i.d., 7 days | | | 13/13 (100) | 17/20 (85) | | 20/45 (44) |
| Ciprofloxacin | United States | 59 | | | | |
| 750 mg, 7 days | | | 10/21 (48) | 2/6 (33) | | 20/38 (53) |
| 1,000 mg, 7 days | | | 10/16 (62) | 6/12 (50) | | 21/41 (51) |
| Doxycycline, 100 mg b.i.d., 7 days | United States | 59 | 10/10 (100) | 5/12 (42) | | 20/36 (56) |
| Ofloxacin, 200 mg b.i.d., 7 days | Denmark | 61 | 36/43 (84) | | | 40/43 (93) |
| Erythromycin, 500 mg b.i.d., 7 days | Denmark | 61 | 24/31 (77) | | | 43/51 (84) |
| Ofloxacin, 200 mg b.i.d., 7 days | Sweden and Denmark | 97 | 46/46 (100) | 6/6 (100) | 1/3 (33) | (84) |
| Erythromycin, 500 mg b.i.d., 7 days | Sweden and Denmark | 97 | 34/36 (94) | 9/10 (90) | 0/5 (0) | (77) |

| | | | | | | |
|---|---|---|---|---|---|---|
| Ofloxacin, 300 mg b.i.d., 7 days | United States | 151 | 14/14 (100) | 5/5 (100) | | 16/16 (100) |
| Doxycycline, 100 mg b.i.d., 7 days | United States | 151 | 15/15 (100) | 5/5 (100) | | 17/18 (94) |
| Ofloxacin | Spain | 164 | | | | |
| 200 mg t.i.d., 7 days | | | | | | 35/40 (88) |
| 200 mg b.i.d., 5 days | | | | | | 37/40 (93) |
| Minocycline, 100 mg b.i.d., 7 days | Spain | 164 | | | | 36/40 (90) |
| Ofloxacin, 300 mg b.i.d., 7 days | United States | 96 | 23/24 (96) | 3/4 (75) | | 12/14 (86) |
| Doxycycline, 100 mg b.i.d., 7 days | United States | 96 | 18/18 (100) | 9/11 (82) | | 12/12 (100) |
| Ofloxacin, 400 mg, 7 days | United Kingdom | 73 | 38/38 (100) | | | 36/43 (84) |
| Doxycycline, 100 mg b.i.d., 7 days | United Kingdom | 73 | 28/28 (100) | | | 31/40 (78) |
| Ofloxacin, 200 mg b.i.d., 7 days | Spain | 114 | 11/11 (100) | 13/18 (71) | | 32/43 (74) |
| Ciprofloxacin, 500 mg b.i.d., 7 days | Spain | 114 | 8/13 (62) | 7/12 (58) | | 27/36 (75) |
| Temafloxacin, 400 mg b.i.d., 7 days | United States | 25 | | 18/21F (86)<br>11/11M (100) | | |
| Doxycycline, 100 mg b.i.d., 7 days | United States | 25 | | 10/25F (40)<br>7/8M (88) | | |
| Temafloxacin, 400 mg b.i.d., 7 days | United States | 89 | 25/26 (96) | 49/85 (58) | 48/56 (86) | 72/77 (94) |
| Doxycycline, 100 mg b.i.d., 7 days | United States | 89 | 25/26/ (96) | 38/74 (49) | 71/111 (69) | 80/93 (86) |
| Temafloxacin, 400 mg b.i.d., 7 days | United States | 127 | 6/6 (100) | 12/32 (38) | 29/36 (81) | 18/20 (90) |
| Doxycycline, 100 mg b.i.d., 7 days | United States | 127 | 2/2 (100) | 27/46 (59) | 20/34 (59) | 24/25 (88) |

[a]b.i.d., twice daily; t.i.d., three times daily.
[b]F, women; M, men.

types 1 and 2 (HIV-1 and HIV-2) (113). As a result, strategies to control chancroid with effective regimens are increasingly important.

Penicillin, ampicillin, the tetracyclines, the sulfonamides, and trimethoprim are all now ineffective in many parts of the world because of the emergence of resistance (91). Erythromycin, selected cephalosporins, amoxicillin with clavulanic acid, and the fluoroquinolones are now the agents of choice for treating chancroid (10).

Treatment regimens for chancroid have recently been further complicated by studies that report an increased failure rate in HIV-positive patients (81). A regimen such as ceftriaxone, prescribed as a single injection of 250 mg, cured essentially all patients. It now cures only 60% of ulcers in circumcised HIV-positive patients and less than 20% of ulcers in uncircumcised HIV-positive patients (160).

As a result, both antimicrobial resistance and increasing HIV seroprevalence in many populations in which chancroid is endemic make new treatment regimens a priority.

## MICROBIOLOGICAL STUDIES

The MICs for *H. ducreyi* have been reported for nine of the fluoroquinolones (Table 10). The $MIC_{90}$ for *H. ducreyi* in most instances is comparable to $MIC_{90}$s for other very susceptible gram-negative organisms such as *N. gonorrhoeae* or *Haemophilus influenzae*. The strains are very homogeneous, with essentially all strains susceptible to a narrow range of fluoroquinolone concentration. To date, no resistance to any of the quinolones has been reported. *H. ducreyi* usually develops resistance to antibacterial agents through the acquisition of plasmids containing genes mediating resistance. *H. ducreyi* probably has a limited ability to respond to a drug by effecting mutational changes that develop chromosomal resistance. However, ongoing monitoring of *H. ducreyi* resistance to antimicrobial agents must continue, particularly in patients treated with the fluoroquinolones, to determine whether incremental resistance by mutations of DNA gyrase will occur.

**Table 10.** Activities of quinolones and other agents against *H. ducreyi*[a]

| Quinolone | MIC range (μg/ml) |
|---|---|
| Nalidixic acid | 8.0–32.0 |
| Ciprofloxacin | 0.007–0.016 |
| Enoxacin | 0.12–0.25 |
| Fleroxacin | 0.008–0.25 |
| Lomefloxacin | 0.03 |
| Norfloxacin | 0.12–0.25 |
| Ofloxacin | 0.03–0.06 |
| Pefloxacin | 0.06–0.12 |
| Rosoxacin | 0.004–0.12 |

[a]References: 2, 57, 74, 92, 94, 142.

### Clinical Studies

Four of the quinolones have been investigated in clinical studies with chancroid (10, 58, 92) (Table 11). In all studies, the quinolones cured most patients with chancroid. However, only therapeutic agents with prolonged half-lives will cure chancroid with single-dose therapy.

Rosoxacin was effective in one study, but it is not widely used because of untoward side effects (51). Enoxacin has been used in two studies but requires a long course of treatment because of its shorter half-life and relatively high MIC (98). Ciprofloxacin is effective as single-dose therapy if 1 g is used as the initial dose (10). Lower doses, with 500 mg daily for 3 days, are effective in all patients treated with this regimen (99).

Treatment with fleroxacin is particularly encouraging, as this drug seems to be effective in a single-dose regimen. Either 200 or 400 mg is equally effective (81, 94). Results of this study suggest that the quinolones will be less effective in HIV-positive patients with chancroid. Further studies are needed.

No studies on the efficacy of the fluoroquinolones in the sexual contacts of patients with chancroid have been published. At pre-

**Table 11.** Treatment of infections caused by *H. ducreyi:* clinical trials

| Drug and dosage[a] | Location of study | Reference | Microbiological cure rate (no. of patients cured/ no. treated [%]) |
|---|---|---|---|
| Ciprofloxacin | Thailand | 14 | |
| 500 mg | | | 43/43 (100) |
| 500 mg twice | | | 43/44 (100) |
| Ciprofloxacin | Kenya | 99 | |
| 500 mg | | | 39/41 (95) |
| 500 b.i.d., 3 days | | | 40/40 (100) |
| Enoxacin, 400 mg three times | Kenya | 98 | 65/73 (89) |
| Fleroxacin | | | |
| 200 mg | South Africa | 94 | 14/14 (100) |
| 400 mg | South Africa | 94 | 18/19 (95) |
| 200 mg | Kenya | 81[b] | 23/25 (92) |
| 400 mg | Kenya | 81[b] | 19/23 (83) |
| 400 mg | Kenya | 116 | 39/40 (98) |
| Rosoxacin | Kenya | 51 | |
| 300 mg | | | 17/28 (61) |
| 150 mg b.i.d., 3 days | | | 38/40 (95) |

[a]b.i.d., twice daily.
[b]Microbiologic cure was achieved in 8 (73%) of 11 HIV-1-seropositive patients versus 35 (95%) of 37 HIV-1-seronegative patients ($P = 0.07$).

sent, treatment with a regimen similar to that used for the index case should be prescribed for all sexual contacts of patients with chancroid.

## Summary

The quinolones may quickly become the agents of first choice for patients with chancroid. The effectiveness of single-dose oral regimens, the lack of evidence for emergence of resistance, and the growing significance of programs to control chancroid all support the choice of these agents. The evidence that short courses of therapy will be less effective in patients who are coinfected with HIV requires ongoing investigation to determine which regimens are optimal for these patients.

## PID

PID is usually diagnosed and treated empirically, as microbiological results are not available or are inadequate. It is estimated that about one million women are treated for PID each year in the United States (26). Substantial epidemiological and microbiological evidence argue for the importance of *N. gonorrhoeae* and *C. trachomatis* in 60 to 80% of women with this diagnosis (83). As a result, the empiric therapeutic regimen must provide excellent antibacterial activity against both these pathogens as well as broad-spectrum coverage in selected patients for members of the family *Enterobacteriaceae* and the anaerobes (54). In an area with more than 3% PPNG, all patients should be treated as if all potential gonococci are resistant. Also, at least 20% of patients investigated by laparoscopic examinations have been erroneously diagnosed as having PID. Although laparoscopic diagnosis is now usually required for patients entered into clinical trials, it is not routine practice.

An important therapeutic goal apart from the treatment of clinical symptoms is to preserve fertility by preventing further long-term complications of tubal obstruction and ectopic pregnancy. Most studies have not carried out adequate follow-up in patients, and long-term sequelae and fertility outcomes or prognoses have not been determined. The approach of second-look laparoscopy should be evaluated (18). Brumsted et al. (19) examined the reproductive outcome in a retrospective study of women treated for PID. Of the 27 women who attempted to conceive, 9 (33%) had an intrauterine pregnancy, while 15 (56%) remain involuntarily childless. Three (11%) had tubal damage that resulted in an ectopic pregnancy during an average duration of 4.9 years post-PID.

Since 1985, cefoxitin and doxycycline have been the standard therapies for PID (115). Over 90% of patients appear to respond clinically, and no regimen has been shown to preserve tubal patency more efficiently than any other. The Centers for Disease Control in the 1989 treatment guidelines continued to recommend cefoxitin or cefotetan plus doxycycline (26a). Clindamycin plus gentamicin is a possible alternative regimen. No quinolone regimens are recommended.

## Clinical Studies

Ciprofloxacin has been prospectively studied in five randomized clinical trials (Table 12). In three studies, PID was diagnosed on the basis of clinical criteria (6, 35, 42). In the other two studies, PID was diagnosed by laparoscopy (56, 60). The results were encouraging, with cure rates of 82 to 100% in 81 women treated. In four studies, all 33 women with pretreatment cultures positive for *N. gonorrhoeae* were cured, as were all but 3 of 34 women with pretreatment cultures positive for *C. trachomatis*. Despite these results, the variable clinical efficacy of ciprofloxacin for *C. trachomatis* and the lack of activity against anaerobes in other studies urge caution in the use of this agent for patients with PID (44, 108). The efficacy of other fluoroquinolones in patients with PID is only now being reported. In a small comparative study, orally administered ofloxacin cured 35 of 37 women and was equivalent to cefoxitin and doxycycline (169). All patients with pretreatment cultures positive for *N. gonorrhoeae* had negative posttreatment cultures, and six of seven patients culture positive for *C. trachomatis* were cured. In two other studies, a combination of ofloxacin, amoxicillin, and clavulanic acid achieved cure rates of 97 to 100% (68, 163).

The efficacy of the new quinolone CI-960 (PD 127391) against chlamydial salpingitis was studied by Patton et al. (111) in a monkey model. Although *C. trachomatis* cultures became negative in both primary and chronic infections after treatment, chlamydial DNA could be detected in monkey tissues throughout the study, and inflammation was similar in both treated and untreated animals. Combinations of effective antimicrobial regimens and anti-inflammatory immunomodulating agents should be considered in animal studies and prospective clinical trials.

Combinations of the quinolones with agents active against anaerobes such as metronidazole or clindamycin are currently being investigated. These combinations provide wide-spectrum antibacterial activity against *N. gonorrhoeae, C. trachomatis, Enterobacteriaceae*, and anaerobes. Excellent absorption after oral administration together with limited side effects make this combination very attractive for the treatment of mild to moderately severe PID. Well-designed clinical trials with long-term follow-up to assess reproductive function are necessary.

## Summary

The quinolones, particularly those with increased activity against *C. trachomatis*, are becoming useful agents for the treatment of PID. In combination with therapeutic agents active against anaerobes, the quinolones have the potential to prevent or reduce hospitalization and achieve excellent long-term outcomes.

**Table 12.** PID trials: comparative studies

| Drug and dosage[a] | Location of study | Reference | Diagnosis | Cure rate (no. of patients cured/no. treated [%]) | | |
|---|---|---|---|---|---|---|
| | | | | Clinical | Microbiological | |
| | | | | | Gonococcal | Chlamydial |
| Ciprofloxacin<br>300 mg i.v.<br>750 mg b.i.d. | United States | 6 | Clinical criteria | 10/10 (100) | 7/7 (100) | 11/12 (92) |
| Clindamycin<br>900 mg i.v.<br>450 mg p.o. q.i.d. + gentamicin, 1.5 mg/kg | United States | 6 | | 13/15 (87) | 4/6 (67) | 6/7 (86) |
| Ciprofloxacin<br>300 mg i.v.<br>750 mg p.o. | United States | 35 | Clinical criteria | 31/33 (94) | 22/22 (100) | 6/7 (86) |
| Clindamycin<br>600 mg i.v. + gentamicin, 300 mg p.o. for 2–5 days (14 days for both regimens) | United States | 35 | | 34/35 (97) | 22/22 (100) | 6/6 (100) |
| Ciprofloxacin<br>200 mg i.v.<br>750 mg p.o., 14 days | Finland | 56 | Laparoscopy | 15/16 (94) | 3/3[b] (100) | 6/6 (100) |
| Doxycycline<br>100 mg i.v.<br>150 mg + metronidazole, 500 mg i.v.<br>400 mg t.i.d., 14 days | Finland | 56 | | 14/20 (70) | 2/3[b] (67) | 3/3 (100) |

*Continued on following page*

**Table 12.** *Continued*

| Drug and dosage[a] | Location of study | Reference | Diagnosis | Cure rate (no. of patients cured/ no. treated [%]) | | |
|---|---|---|---|---|---|---|
| | | | | Clinical | Microbiological | |
| | | | | | Gonococcal | Chlamydial |
| Ciprofloxacin 750 mg b.i.d., 10 days | Germany | 60 | Laparoscopy | 18/22 (82) | 1/1 (100) | 8/9 (89) |
| Ofloxacin 200 mg b.i.d., 21 days + amoxicillin-clavulanic acid i.v. p.o. 2–4 times/day | France | 163 | Laparoscopy | 30/30 (100) | 1/1 (100) | 15/15 (100) |
| Ofloxacin, 400 mg b.i.d., 10 days | United States | 169 | Clinical criteria | 35/37 (95) | 21/21 (100) | 6/7 (86) |
| Cefoxitin, 2 g i.m. + probenecid, 1 g p.o. + doxycycline, 100 mg b.i.d., 10 days | United States | 169 | | 34/35 (97) | 16/16 (100) | 10/10 (100) |
| Ofloxacin, 200 mg b.i.d., 3 wk + amoxicillin-clavulanic acid, 1 g b.i.d. | France | 68 | Clinical criteria (84 endometritis, 34 salpingitis) | 58/60 (97) | | 60/60 (100) |
| Doxycycline, 100 mg b.i.d. + amoxicillin-clavulanic acid, 1 g b.i.d. | France | 68 | | 56/58 (97) | | 56/58 (97) |
| Ciprofloxacin + metronidazole | Germany | 42 | Clinical criteria | (92) | | |
| Cefoxitin-doxycycline | Germany | 42 | | (87) | | |
| Ofloxacin | United States | 31 | Not available | | 47/47 (100) | 19/19 (100) |
| Cefoxitin-doxycycline | United States | 31 | | | 23/23 (100) | 13/15 (98) |

[a]i.v., intravenous; b.i.d., twice daily; p.o., peroral; q.i.d., four times a day; t.i.d., three times a day; i.m., intramuscular.
[b]Coinfection with *C. trachomatis*.

## EPIDIDYMITIS

Epididymitis occurs in about 1% of men with urethritis and is equivalent to ascending genital infection in women. The majority of infections occurring prior to age 50 are due to *C. trachomatis* or *N. gonorrhoeae*. In older men, urinary tract pathogens become the predominant etiologic agent. Anaerobic pathogens are uncommon in men with acute epididymitis.

The newer quinolones are potentially excellent therapeutic choices for epididymitis because of their favorable pharmacokinetics and broad-spectrum activities. Few clinical studies have been reported. Costa et al. (32) studied the use of 800 mg of pefloxacin for 21 or 42 days in the treatment of 20 patients with acute epididymitis. A rapid clinical response was evident in all the men. There was no relapse in 18 patients followed up for a year, although small epididymal nodules persisted in 25% of the men. There was no significant difference related to the duration of therapy. Weidner et al. successfully treated nongonococcal epididymitis with ofloxacin (168a).

## SYPHILIS

The quinolones are not effective in animal models of *T. pallidum* infection. Veller-Fornasa et al. (162) reported the failure of a 3-day course of ofloxacin (100 mg/kg of body weight) to suppress *T. pallidum* in experimentally infected rabbits. This lack of efficacy was confirmed by Une et al. (160a). There is no evidence to suggest that the quinolones will have any role in the treatment of *T. pallidum* infection. Presumably, patients coinfected with *T. pallidum* and another pathogen and treated with a quinolone will continue to have unmodified *T. pallidum* infection, and this should be considered in all patients at risk of syphilis.

## BACTERIAL VAGINOSIS

The rationale for the treatment of bacterial vaginosis is increasing as the microbiology of the infection is better understood. Bacterial vaginosis appears to result from a shift of endogenous vaginal flora from hydrogen peroxide-producing lactobacilli to anaerobes and, presumably, *Gardnerella vaginalis*. Therapy with quinolone agents such as ciprofloxacin, norfloxacin, and ofloxacin has not been promising because of their poor in vitro activities against anaerobes (45, 92, 170). A review of MICs for *G. vaginalis* showed that rosoxacin and ciprofloxacin have MICs in the range of 1.0 to 32 μg/ml and that ofloxacin and enoxacin have MICs in the range of 0.25 to 8 μg/ml (92). A clinical trial involving 27 women culture positive for *G. vaginalis* showed that clinical cure was achieved in 70, 70, and 40% of women treated with 7-day courses of ciprofloxacin (500 mg twice daily), ofloxacin (300 mg twice daily), and norfloxacin (400 mg twice daily) (5). A clinical trial of ciprofloxacin (500 mg twice daily) showed that although clinical cure was achieved in 17 of 22 women after 7 days, clue cells persisted in 11 patients, suggesting persistence of infection (24). Covino compared 300 mg of ofloxacin given twice daily for 7 days with 500 mg of oral metronidazole given twice daily for 7 days in a randomized double-blind trial in 27 women (33). Microbiological failure was observed in 57% treated with ofloxacin and in 8% treated with metronidazole ($P = 0.01$).

Among the newer quinolones, temafloxacin has a wide spectrum of activity against anaerobes (141).

## CONCLUSIONS

The quinolones are assuming a significant role in the management of patients with sexually transmitted infections. The efficacy of these drugs for gonococcal infection and chancroid is well established. The risk of emergence of resistance continues to haunt their use, although resistance has not yet occurred to any significant extent. Some of the newer fluoroquinolones promise to provide equivalence to doxycycline for the treatment of *C. trachomatis* infections. Presumably, syndromes such as PID, epididymitis, and NSU, and cervicitis will be well managed by quinolones used either alone or in combination with drugs effective against anaerobes. However, there have been too few large clinical trials to identify the quinolones as the drugs of choice for any of these syndromes. The quinolones are not effective for syphilis or bacterial vaginosis. No studies have yet been reported in which the quinolones have been used for either lymphogranuloma venereum or granuloma inguinale.

The quinolones are restricted by proscription against their use in adolescents and in women who are pregnant or at significant risk of pregnancy.

The role of the quinolones in strategic efforts to control STDs, particularly those caused by *N. gonorrhoeae* and perhaps to a lesser extent those caused by *C. trachomatis*, requires further study.

## ADDENDUM IN PROOF

Temafloxacin has been withdrawn from commercial use.

## REFERENCES


1. **Abeck, D., A. P. Johnson, F. Alexander, H. C. Korting, and R. C. Ballard.** 1988. In vitro activity of eight antimicrobial agents against non-penicillinase-producing gonococci isolated in Munich. *Genitourin. Med.* **64:**233–234.
2. **Abeck, D., A. P. Johnson, Y. Dangor, and R. C. Ballard.** 1988. Antibiotic susceptibilities and plasmid profiles of *Haemophilus ducreyi* isolates from southern Africa. *J. Antimicrob. Chemother.* **22:**437–444.
3. **Ahmed-Jushuf, I. H., O. P. Arya, D. Hobson, B. C. Pratt, C. A. Hart, S. J. How, I. A. Tait, and P. M. Rao.** 1988. Ciprofloxacin treatment of chlamydial infections of urogenital tracts of women. *Genitourin. Med.* **64:**14–17.
4. **Albrecht, L. M., M. J. Rybak, H. H. Schubiner, and L. M. Weiner.** 1989. Single dose enoxacin for the treatment of uncomplicated urogenital gonorrhea. *Sex. Transm. Dis.* **16:**114–117.
5. **Alegente, G., B. Marchi, F. Mugnaini, L. Toscano, and F. De Lalla.** 1989. Treatment of *Gardnerella vaginalis* syndrome with new quinolones: preliminary results. *Rev. Infect. Dis.* **11**(Suppl. 5)**:**S1308.
6. **Apuzzio, J. J., R. Stankiewicz, V. Ganesh, S. Jain, Z. Kaminski, and D. Louria.** 1989. Comparison of parenteral ciprofloxacin with clindamycin-gentamicin in the treatment of pelvic infection. *Am. J. Med.* **87**(5A)**:**148S–151S.
7. **Aral, S. O., and K. K. Holmes.** 1991. Sexually transmitted diseases in the AIDS era. *Sci. Am.* **264:**62–69.
8. **Avonts, D., L. Fransen, J. Vielfont, A. Stevens, K. Hendrick, and P. Piot.** 1988. Treating uncomplicated gonococcal infection with 250 mg or 100 mg ciprofloxacin in a single oral dose. *Genitourin. Med.* **64:**134.
9. **Bakhtiar, M., and P. L. Samarasinghe.** 1988. Enoxacin as one day oral treatment of men with anal or pharyngeal gonorrhoea. *Genitourin. Med.* **64:**364–366.
10. **Ballard, R. C., M. O. Duncan, H. G. Fehler, Y. Dangor, F. L. Exposto, and A. S. Latif.** 1989. Treating chancroid: summary of studies in southern Africa. *Genitourin. Med.* **65:**54–57.
11. **Batteiger, B. E., R. B. Jones, and A. White.** 1989. Efficacy and safety of ofloxacin in the treatment of nongonococcal sexually transmitted disease. *Am. J. Med.* **87**(Suppl. 6C)**:**75S–77S.
12. **Bishoff, W., and H. Bishoff.** 1989. *Chlamydia trachomatis* urethritis: clinical efficacy of ciprofloxacin. *Rev. Infect. Dis.* **11**(Suppl. 5)**:**S1283–S1284.
13. **Black, J. R., J. M. Long, B. E. Zwickl, B. S. Ray, M. S. Verdon, S. Wetherby, E. W. Hook III, and H. H. Handsfield.** 1989. Multicenter randomized study of single-dose ofloxacin versus amoxicillin-probenecid for treatment of uncomplicated gonococcal infection. *Antimicrob. Agents Chemother.* **33:**167–170.
14. **Bodhidatta, L., D. N. Taylor, A. Chitwarakorn, K. Kuvanont, and P. Echeverria.** 1988. Evaluation of 500- and 1,000-mg doses of ciprofloxacin for the treatment of chancroid. *Antimicrob. Agents Chemother.* **32:**723–725.
15. **Borsum, T., L. Dannevig, G. Storvold, and K. Melby.** 1990. *Chlamydia trachomatis*: in vitro susceptibility of genital and ocular isolates to some quinolones, amoxicillin and azithromycin. *Chemotherapy* **36:**407–415.
16. **Boslego, J. W., C. B. Hicks, R. Greenup, R. J. Thomas, H. A. Wiener, J. Ciak, and E. C. Tramont.** 1988. A prospective randomized trial of ofloxacin vs. doxycycline in the treatment of uncomplicated male urethritis. *Sex. Transm. Dis.* **15:**186–191.

17. **Bowie, W. R., V. Willetts, and D. W. Megran.** 1989. Dose-ranging study of fleroxacin for treatment of uncomplicated *Chlamydia trachomatis* genital infections. *Antimicrob. Agents Chemother.* **33:**1774–1777.
18. **Brihmer, C., I. Kallings, C. E. Nord, and J. Brundin.** 1989. Second look laparoscopy: evaluation of two different antibiotic regimens after treatment of acute salpingitis. *Eur. J. Obstet. Gynecol. Reprod. Biol.* **30:**263-274.
19. **Brumsted, J. R., P. M. Clifford, S. T. Nakajima, and M. Gibson.** 1988. Reproductive outcome after medical management of complicated pelvic inflammatory disease. *Fertil. Steril.* **50:**667-669.
20. **Brunham, R. C., I. W. Maclean, B. Binns, and R. Peeling.** 1985. *Chlamydia trachomatis*: its role in tubal infertility. *J. Infect. Dis.* **152:**1275–1282.
21. **Brunham, R. C., R. W. Peeling, I. W. Maclean, M. L. Kosseim, and M. Paraskevas.** 1992. *Chlamydia trachomatis*-associated ectopic pregnancy: serologic and histologic correlates. *J. Infect. Dis.* **165:**1076–1081.
22. **Brunham, R. C., and F. A. Plummer.** 1990. A general model of sexually transmitted disease epidemiology and its implications for control. *Med. Clin. North Am.* **74:**1339–1352.
23. **Bryan, J. P., S. K. Hira, W. Brady, N. Luo, C. Mwale, G. Mpoko, R. Krieg, E. Siwiwaliondo, C. Reichart, C. Waters, and P. L. Perine.** 1990. Oral ciprofloxacin versus ceftriaxone for the treatment of urethritis from resistant *Neisseria gonorrhoeae* in Zambia. *Antimicrob. Agents Chemother.* **34:**819–822.
24. **Carmona, O., S. Hernandez-Gonzalez, and R. Kobelt.** 1987. Ciprofloxacin in the treatment of non-specific vaginitis. *Am. J. Med.* **82**(Suppl. 4A):321–323.
25. **Cassell, G. H., K. B. Waites, L. Duffy, K. Baldus, D. Crabb, and T. Schmid.** 1991. Comparative efficacy of temafloxacin to doxycycline against *Mycoplasma hominis*, abstr. 1257. *Intersci. Conf. Antimicrob. Agents Chemother.*
26. **Cates, W., R. T. Rolfs, and S. Aral.** 1990. Sexually transmitted diseases, pelvic inflammatory disease, and infertility: an epidemiologic update. *Epidemiol. Rev.* **12:**199–220.
26a. **Centers for Disease Control.** 1989. Sexually transmitted diseases treatment guidelines. *Morbid. Mortal. Weekly Rep.* **38**(Suppl. 8):1–43.
27. **Clad, A., P. Plohr, and E. E. Petersen.** 1990. Genital isolates of *Chlamydia trachomatis* survive 12 day antibiotic treatment in vitro due to delayed cell lysis, p. 523–526. *In* W. R. Bowie, H. D. Caldwell, R. P. Jones, P.-A. Mardh, G. L. Ridgway, J. Schachter, W. E. Stamm, and M. E. Ward (ed.), *Chlamydial Infections.* Cambridge University Press, Cambridge.
28. **Clendennen, T. E., III, C. S. Hames, E. S. Kees, F. C. Price, W. J. Rueppel, A. B. Andrada, G. E. Espinosa, G. Kabrerra, and F. S. Wignall.** 1992. In vitro antibiotic susceptibilities of *Neisseria gonorrhoeae* isolates in the Philippines. *Antimicrob. Agents Chemother.* **36:**277–282.
29. **Coker, D. M., I. Ahmed-Jushuf, O. P. Arya, J. S. Chessbrough, and B. C. Pratt.** 1989. Evaluation of single dose ciprofloxacin in the treatment of rectal and pharyngeal gonorrhoea. *J. Antimicrob. Chemother.* **24:**271–272.
30. **Corkill, J. E., A. Percival, and M. Lind.** 1991. Reduced uptake of ciprofloxacin in a resistant strain of *Neisseria gonorrhoeae* and transformation of resistance to other strains. *J. Antimicrob. Chemother.* **28:**601–604.
31. **Corrado, M. L.** 1991. The clinical experience with ofloxacin in the treatment of sexually transmitted diseases. *Am. J. Obstet. Gynecol.* **164:**1396–1399.
32. **Costa, P., J. F. Louis, N. Mottet, H. Navratil, M. Favier, E. Jarroux, and A. Boccanfuso.** 1991. Acute epididymitis and pefloxacin in monoantibiotic therapy. *Eur. J. Clin. Microbiol. Infect. Dis.* **Special Issue:**626–627.
33. **Covino, J. M., J. R. Black, M. Cummings, S. Smith, B. Zwickl, and W. M. McCormack.** 1991. Comparative evaluation of ofloxacin and metronidazole in the treatment of bacterial vaginosis, abstr. P20–224. *Proc. Int. Soc. Sex. Transm. Dis. Res.*
34. **Covino, J. M., M. Cummings, B. Smith, S. Benes, K. Draft, and W. M. McCormack.** 1990. Comparison of ofloxacin and ceftriaxone in the treatment of uncomplicated gonorrhea caused by penicillinase-producing and non-penicillinase-producing strains. *Antimicrob. Agents Chemother.* **34:**148–149.
35. **Crombleholme, W. R., J. Schachter, M. Ohm-Smith, J. Luft, R. Whidden, and R. L. Sweet.** 1989. Efficacy of single-agent therapy for the treatment of acute pelvic inflammatory disease with ciprofloxacin. *Am. J. Med.* **87**(Suppl. 5A):142S–147A.
36. **De Schryver, A., and A. Meheus.** 1990. Epidemiology of sexually transmitted diseases: the global picture. *Bull. W.H.O.* **68:**639–654.
37. **Dubois, J., and V. Fontaine.** 1988. In vitro activity of fleroxacin against urinary tract and genital tract pathogens. *J. Antimicrob. Chemother.* **22**(Suppl. D):31–34.
38. **Dylewski, J., H. Nsanze, L. D'Costa, L. Slaney, and A. R. Ronald.** 1985. Trimethoprim-sulfamethoxazole in the treatment of chancroid: comparison of two single dose treatment regimens with a five day regimen. *J. Antimicrob. Chemother.* **16:**103–110.

39. **Ehret, J. M., and F. N. Judson.** 1988. Susceptibility testing of *Chlamydia trachomatis*: from eggs to monoclonal antibodies. *Antimicrob. Agents Chemother.* **32:**1295–1299.
40. **Endtz, H., J. M. Ossewaarde, P. J. G. M. van de Korput, and H. T. Weiland.** 1989. In vitro activity of eight quinolones against *Chlamydia trachomatis. Rev. Infect. Dis.* **11**(Suppl. 5):S1278.
41. **Faro, S., M. G. Martens, M. Maccato, H. A. Hammill, S. Roberts, and G. Riddle.** 1991. Effectiveness of ofloxacin in the treatment of *Chlamydia trachomatis* and *Neisseria gonorrhoeae* cervical infection. *Am. J. Obstet. Gynecol.* **164:**1380–1383.
42. **Fishbach, F., R. Deckardt, H. Graeff, and W. Busch.** 1991. Comparison of ciprofloxacin/metronidazole versus cefoxitin/doxycycline in the treatment of pelvic inflammatory disease. *Eur. J. Clin. Microbiol. Infect. Dis.* **Special Issue:** 402–403.
43. **Fong, I. W., W. Linton, M. Simbul, R. Thorup, B. McLaughlin, V. Rahm, and P. A. Quinn.** 1987. Treatment of nongonococcal urethritis with ciprofloxacin. *Am. J. Med.* **82**(Suppl. 4A):311–316.
44. **Friesen, T. R., and R. J. Mangi.** 1990. Inappropriate use of oral ciprofloxacin. *JAMA* **264:**1438–1440.
45. **Fuchs, P. C.** 1989. In vitro antimicrobial activity and susceptibility testing of ofloxacin: current status. *Am. J. Med.* **87**(Suppl. 6C):10S–13S.
46. **Garcia-de-Lomas, J., R. M. Ferreruela, M. A. Farga, M. J. Alcaraz, and C. Gimeno.** 1991. In vitro activity of temafloxacin in comparison with other antimicrobial agents against mycoplasmas. *Eur. J. Clin. Microbiol. Infect. Dis.* **Special Issue:**185–186.
47. **Gerding, G. N., and J. A. Hitt.** 1989. Tissue penetration of the new quinolones in humans. *Rev. Infect. Dis.* **11**(Suppl. 5):S1046–S1057.
48. **Gransden, W. R., C. Warren, and I. Phillips.** 1991. 4-Quinolone-resistant *Neisseria gonorrhoeae* in the United Kingdom. *J. Med. Microbiol.* **34:**23–27.
49. **Gransden, W. R., C. A. Warren, I. Phillips, M. Hodges, and D. Barlow.** 1990. Decreased susceptibility of *Neisseria gonorrhoeae* to ciprofloxacin. *Lancet* **335:**51.
50. **Gundersen, T., and F. Zahm.** 1989. Fleroxacin in the treatment of urogenital infections caused by *Chlamydia trachomatis*: a pilot study. *Rev. Infect. Dis.* **11:**S1278.
51. **Haase, D. A., J. O. Ndinya-Achola, R. A. Nash, L. J. D'Costa, D. Hazlett, S. Lubwama, H. Nsanze, and A. R. Ronald.** 1986. Clinical evaluation of rosoxacin for the treatment of chancroid. *Antimicrob. Agents Chemother.* **30:**39–41.
52. **Handsfield, H. H., J. R. Black, and E. W. Hook III.** 1989. Comparative trial of single-dose enoxacin vs. ceftriaxone for treatment of uncomplicated gonorrhea. *Rev. Infect. Dis.* **11**(Suppl. 5):S1315–S1316.
53. **Handsfield, H. H., J. A. McCutchan, L. Corey, and A. R. Ronald.** 1992. Special issues in clinical trials of new anti-infective drugs for the treatment of sexually transmitted diseases. *Clin. Infect. Dis.* **15**(Suppl. 1):596–598.
54. **Hasselquist, M. B., and S. Hillier.** 1991. Susceptibility of upper tract isolates from women with pelvic inflammatory disease to ampicillin, cefpodoxime, metronidazole and doxycycline. *Sex. Transm. Dis.* **18:**146–149.
55. **Heap, B. J.** 1989. Low dose oral ofloxacin to treat gonorrhoea in Hong Kong. *Genitourin. Med.* **65:**198.
56. **Heinonen, P. K., K. Teisala, R. Aine, and A. Miettinen.** 1989. Intravenous and oral ciprofloxacin in the treatment of proven pelvic inflammatory disease. A comparison with doxycycline and metronidazole. *Am. J. Med.* **87**(Suppl. 5A):152S–156S.
57. **Hoban, D., P. DeGagne, and E. Witwicki.** 1989. In vitro activity of lomefloxacin against *Chlamydia trachomatis, Neisseria gonorrhoeae, Haemophilus ducreyi, Mycoplasma hominis*, and *Ureaplasma urealyticum. Diagn. Microbiol. Infect. Dis.* **12**(Suppl. 3):83S–86S.
58. **Hooper, D. C., and J. S. Wolfson.** 1989. Treatment of genitourinary tract infections with fluoroquinolones: clinical efficacy in genital infections and adverse effects. *Antimicrob. Agents Chemother.* **33:**1662–1667.
59. **Hooton, T. M., M. E. Rogers, T. G. Medina, L. E. Kuwamura, C. Ewers, P. L. Roberts, and W. E. Stamm.** 1990. Ciprofloxacin compared with doxycycline for nongonococcal urethritis. Ineffectiveness against *Chlamydia trachomatis* due to relapsing infection. *JAMA* **264:**1418–1421.
60. **Hoyme, U. B., K. Buhler, C. Krasemann, and A. E. Schindler.** 1989. Ciprofloxacin in therapy for uncomplicated salpingitis. *Rev. Infect. Dis.* **11**(Suppl. 5):S1279.
61. **Ibsen, H. H. W., B. R. Moller, L. Halkier-Sorensen, and E. From.** 1989. Treatment of nongonococcal urethritis: comparison of ofloxacin and erythromycin. *Sex. Transm. Dis.* **16:**32–35.
62. **Jaffe, H. W., A. L. Schroeter, G. H. Reynolds, A. A. Zaidi, J. E. Martin, Jr., and J. D. Thayer.** 1979. Pharmacokinetic determinants of penicillin cure of gonococcal urethritis. *Antimicrob. Agents Chemother.* **15:**587–591.
63. **Jephcott, A. E., and K. Gough.** 1988. In vitro activity of enoxacin against gonococcal isolates in comparison with that of five other antibiotics. *J. Antimicrob. Chemother.* **21**(Suppl. B):43–48.
64. **Jephcott, A. E., and A. Turner.** 1990. Ciprofloxacin resistance in gonococci. *Lancet* **335:**165.

65. **Jeskanen, L., and A. Lassus.** 1991. Fleroxacin (Ro 23-6240) versus doxycycline in the treatment of chlamydial urethritis and/or cervicitis. *Eur. J. Clin. Microbiol. Infect. Dis.* **Special Issue:**457–458.

66. **Jones, R. B.** 1990. Treatment of *Chlamydia trachomatis* infections of the urogenital tract, p. 509–518. *In* W. R. Bowie, H. D. Caldwell, R. B. Jones, P.-A. Mardh, G. L. Ridgway, J. Schachter, W. E. Stamm, and M. E. Ward (ed.), *Chlamydia Infections.* Cambridge University Press, Cambridge.

67. **Jones, R. B., B. Van Der Pol, D. H. Martin, and M. K. Shepard.** 1990. Partial characterization of *Chlamydia trachomatis* isolates resistant to multiple antibiotics. *J. Infect. Dis.* **162:**1309–1315.

68. **Judlin, P., C. Scheffler, M. Dailloux, and P. Landes.** 1991. Shorter duration of treatment in chlamydial pelvic infections with ofloxacin-amoxicillin-clavulanate, compared with doxycycline-amoxicillin-clavulanate. *Eur. J. Clin. Microbiol. Infect. Dis.* **Special Issue:**314–315.

69. **Judson, F. N., B. S. Beals, and K. J. Tack.** 1986. Clinical experience with ofloxacin in sexually transmitted disease. *Infection* **14**(Suppl. 4):S309–S310.

70. **Kawada, Y.** 1989. Multicentre study of ofloxacin for nongonococcal urethritis in Asia. *Rev. Infect. Dis.* **11**(Suppl. 5):S1318–S1319.

71. **Kenny, G. E., T. M. Hooton, M. C. Roberts, F. D. Cartwright, and J. Hoyt.** 1989. Susceptibilities of genital mycoplasmas to the newer quinolones as determined by the agar dilution method. *Antimicrob. Agents Chemother.* **33:**103–107.

72. **King, A., L. Bethune, and I. Phillips.** 1991. The in vitro activity of temafloxacin compared with other antimicrobial agents. *J. Antimicrob. Chemother.* **27:**769–779.

73. **Kitchen, V. S., C. Donegan, H. Ward, B. Thomas, J. R. Harris, and D. Taylor-Robinson.** 1990. Comparison of ofloxacin with doxycycline in the treatment of non-gonococcal urethritis and cervical chlamydial infection. *J. Antimicrob. Chemother.* **26**(Suppl. D):99–105.

74. **Knapp, J. S., A. F. Back, A. F. Babat, D. Taylor, and R. J. Rice.** 1991. Antimicrobial susceptibility of *Haemophilus ducreyi* from Thailand and the United States, abstr. 1256. *Program Abstr. 31st Intersci. Conf. Antimicrob. Agents Chemother.*

75. **Korting, H. C., and D. Abeck.** 1989. Activity of enoxacin against *Neisseria gonorrhoeae* in relation to pencillinase production. *Rev. Infect. Dis.* **11**(Suppl. 5):S1307–1308.

75a. **Laboratory Centre for Disease Control, Canada.** 1992. Canadian guidelines for the prevention, diagnosis, management and treatment of sexually transmitted diseases in neonates, children and adults. Department of National Health and Welfare, Ottawa, Canada.

76. **Lassus, A., L. Karppinen, L. Ingervo, L. Jeskanen, S. Reitamo, H. P. Happonen, and R. Karkulahti.** 1989. Ciprofloxacin versus amoxycillin and probenecid in the treatment of uncomplicated gonorrhoea. *Scand. J. Infect. Dis. Suppl.* **60:**58–61.

77. **Lassus, A., O. V. Renkonen, and J. Ellmen.** 1988. Fleroxacin versus standard therapy in gonococcal urethritis. *J. Antimicrob. Chemother.* **22**(Suppl. D.):223–225.

78. **Lee, Y. H., M. T. Chen, and L. S. Chang.** 1991. Ofloxacin in the treatment of urethritis. *Eur. J. Clin. Microbiol. Infect. Dis.* **Special Issue:**310–311.

79. **Lutz, F. B., Jr.** 1989. Single-dose efficacy of ofloxacin in uncomplicated gonorrhea. *Am. J. Med.* **87:**69S–74S.

80. **MacAulay, M. E.** 1982. Acrosoxacin resistance in *Neisseria gonorrhoeae. Lancet* **1:**171–172.

81. **MacDonald, K. S., D. W. Cameron, L. D'Costa, J. O. Ndinya-Achola, F. A. Plummer, and A. R. Ronald.** 1989. Evaluation of fleroxacin (RO 23-6240) as single-oral-dose therapy of culture-proven chancroid in Nairobi, Kenya. *Antimicrob. Agents Chemother.* **33:**612–614.

82. **Magalhaes, M., and V. Magalhaes.** 1989. In vitro activity of lomefloxacin against *Neisseria gonorrhoeae. Rev. Infect. Dis.* **11**(Suppl. 5):S1311.

83. **Mardh, P. A., and C. Lowing.** 1990. Treatment of chlamydial infections. *Scand. J. Infect. Dis. Suppl.* **68:**23–30.

84. **Mardh, P. A., J. Paavonen, and M. Puolakkainen.** 1989. Persistance, relapses and reinfections of chlamydial infections, p. 117–119. *In Chlamydia.* Plenum Medical Book Co., New York.

85. **Martin, D. H., T. F. Mroczknowski, Z. Dalu, A. Iravani, K. Patrick, B. Richelo, P. St. Clair, and D. Pizzuti.** 1991. Double-blind, randomized trial of fleroxacin versus doxycycline for *Chlamydia trachomatis*, abstr. 80. *Program Abstr. 31st Intersci. Conf. Antimicrob. Agents Chemother.*

86. **Martin, D. H., T. F. Mroczkowski, T. Richelo, P. St. Clair, and S. Pizzuti.** 1991. Randomized double-blind study of fleroxacin and doxycycline for the treatment of *Chlamydia trachomatis* genital tract infections. *Eur. J. Clin. Microbiol. Infect. Dis.* **Special Issue:**458–459.

87. **Matsuda, S., K. Oh, and H. Hirayama.** 1991. Penetration of sparfloxacin into the tissues of female genital organs. *Eur. J. Clin. Microbiol. Infect. Dis.* **Special Issue:**576–577.

88. **Matsuda, T., H. Takeuchi, and O. Yoshida.** 1991. Clinical efficacy of ofloxacin against male urethritis. *Eur. J. Clin. Microbiol. Infect. Dis.* **Special Issue:**311–312.

89. **McCarty, J., M. Rodriguez, J. Segreti, G. Cassell, J. Cerasoli, and J. C. Craft.** 1991. Temafloxacin versus doxycycline in the treatment of non-gonococcal urethritis or cervicitis. *Eur. J. Clin. Microbiol. Infect. Dis.* **Special Issue:**202–203.

90. **McEwen, A., and G. Roberts.** 1988. In-vitro activity of ofloxacin against isolates of *Neisseria gonorrhoeae*. *J. Antimicrob. Chemother.* **22**(Suppl. C):21–25.

91. **McNichol, P. J., W. L. Albritton, and A. R. Ronald.** 1984. The plasmids of *Haemophilus ducreyi*. *J. Antimicrob. Chemother.* **14:**561–573.

92. **Megran, D. W.** 1989. Quinolones in the treatment of sexually transmitted diseases. *Clin. Invest. Med.* **12:**50–60.

93. **Melby, K., and A. Faegri.** 1989. The in vitro activity of norfloxacin, ofloxacin and ciprofloxacin and other antibiotics in current use against *Neisseria gonorrhoeae*. *APMIS* **97:**347–350.

94. **Miller, S. D., F. da L. Exposto, Y. Dangor, S. Kaka, H. G. Fehler, and H. J. Koornhof.** 1989. A dose-finding study of fleroxacin in the treatment of chancroid. *Rev. Infect. Dis.* **11**(Suppl. 5):S1310–S1311.

95. **Mogabgab, W., and D. M. Buntin.** 1991. Single-dose therapy of uncomplicated gonococcal urethritis or cervicitis: oral temafloxacin versus intramuscular ceftriaxone. *Eur. J. Clin. Microbiol. Infect. Dis.* **Special Issue:**205–206.

96. **Mogabgab, W. J., B. Holmes, M. Murray, R. Beville, F. B. Lutz, and K. J. Tack.** 1990. Randomized comparison of ofloxacin and doxycycline for chlamydia and ureaplasma urethritis and cervicitis. *Chemotherapy* **36:**70–76.

97. **Moller, B. R., B. Herrmann, H. H. Ibsen, L. Halkier-Sorensen, E. From, and P.-A. Mardh.** 1990. Occurrence of *Ureaplasma urealyticum* and *Mycoplasma hominis* in non-gonococcal urethritis before and after treatment in a double-blind trial of ofloxacin versus erythromycin. *Scand. J. Infect. Dis.* **68**(Suppl.):31–34.

98. **Naamara, W., D. Y. Kunimoto, L. D'Costa, J. O. Ndinya-Achola, H. Nsanze, A. R. Ronald, and F. A. Plummer.** 1988. Treating chancroid with enoxacin. *Genitourin. Med.* **164:**189–192.

99. **Naamara, W., F. A. Plummer, R. Greenblatt, L. J. D'Costa, J. O. Ndinya-Achola, and A. R. Ronald.** 1987. Treatment of chancroid with ciprofloxacin: a prospective, randomized clinical trial. *Am. J. Med.* **82:**S317–S320.

100. **Nagayama, A., S. Kitajima, and T. Nakao.** 1991. In vitro activities of sparfloxacin and other new quinolones against *Chlamydia trachomatis*. *Eur. J. Clin. Microbiol. Infect. Dis.* **Special Issue:**567–568.

101. **Nagayama, A., and T. Nakao.** 1991. In vitro activities of OPC17116 and other new quinolones against *Chlamydia trachomatis*, abstr. 1470. *Program Abstr. 31st Conf. Antimicrob. Agents Chemother.*

102. **Nagayama, A., T. Nakao, and H. Taen.** 1988. In vitro activities of ofloxacin and four other new quinolone-carboxylic acids against *Chlamydia trachomatis*. *Antimicrob. Agents Chemother.* **32:**1735–1737.

103. **Nayagam, A. T., G. L. Ridgway, and J. D. Oriel.** 1988. Efficacy of ofloxacin in the treatment of non-gonococcal urethritis in men and genital infections caused by *Chlamydia trachomatis* in men and women. *J. Antimicrob. Chemother.* **22**(Suppl. C):155–158.

104. **Ndinya-Achola, O., F. A. Odhiambo, P. Wambugu, L. Slaney, M. Bosire, J. Kimata, M. Malisa, F. Plummer, and A. R. Ronald.** 1991. Ciprofloxacin treatment of gonococcal infections in Nairobi, Kenya, abstr. P-20-258. *Proc. 9th Meet. Int. Soc. Sex. Transm. Dis. Res.*

105. **Nedeljkovic, M., S. Vesic, and V. Drenovac.** 1991. Treatment of *Chlamydia trachomatis* genital infections with ofloxacin and doxycycline—a comparative study. *Eur. J. Clin. Microbiol. Infect. Dis.* **Special Issue:**315–316.

106. **Obata, I., M. Hayashi, N. Imagawa, S. Hayashi, T. Yamata, Y. Terashima, K. Saito, and T. Niki.** 1989. Efficacy of ofloxacin against obstetric and gynecologic infections due to *Chlamydia trachomatis*. *Rev. Infect. Dis.* **11:**S1281–1282.

107. **Orfila, J., and F. Haider.** 1991. In vitro susceptibility of *C. trachomatis* (serotype L2) to a new fluoroquinolone, sparfloxacin, compared to other molecules. *Eur. J. Clin. Microbiol. Infect. Dis.* **Special Issue:**568–569.

108. **Oriel, J. D.** 1989. Use of quinolones in chlamydial infections. *Rev. Infect. Dis.* **11**(Suppl. 5):S1273–1276.

109. **Pabst, K. M., N. A. Siegel, S. Smith, J. R. Black, H. H. Handsfield, and E. W. Hook III.** 1989. Multicentre, comparative study of enoxacin and ceftriaxone for treatment of uncomplicated gonorrhea. *Sex. Transm. Dis.* **16:**148–151.

110. **Panikabutra, K., C. T. Lee, B. Ho, and P. Bamberg.** 1988. Single dose oral norfloxacin or intramuscular spectinomycin to treat gonorrhoea (PPNG and non-PPNG infections): analysis of efficacy and patient preference. *Genitourin. Med.* **64:**235–240.

111. **Patton, D. L., Y. T. Cosgrove, C.-C. Kuo, and L. A. Campbell.** 1991. Effects of CI-960 (PD 127391) in a monkey model of *C. trachomatis*

salpingitis, abstr. 1152. *Program Abstr. 31st Intersci. Conf. Antimicrob. Agents Chemother.*

112. **Peeling, R. W., and M. Gauthier.** 1991. Production of heat shock proteins by *Chlamydia trachomatis* in the presence of ofloxacin in cell culture, abstr. P-06-269. *Proc. 9th Meet. Int. Soc. Sex. Transm. Dis. Res.*
113. **Pepin, J., F. A. Plummer, R. C. Brunham, P. Piot, D. W. Cameron, and A. R. Ronald.** 1989. The interaction of HIV infection and other sexually transmitted diseases: an opportunity for intervention. *AIDS* **3**:3–9.
114. **Perea, E. J., J. Aznar, A. Herrera, J. Mazuecos, and A. Rodriguez-Pichardo.** 1989. Clinical efficacy of new quinolones for therapy of nongonococcal urethritis. *Sex. Transm. Dis.* **16**:7–10.
115. **Peterson, H. B., C. K. Walker, J. G. Kahn, A. E. Washington, D. A. Eschenbach, and S. Faro.** 1991. Pelvic inflammatory disease: key treatment issues and options. *J. Am. Med. Assoc.* **266**:2605–2612.
116. **Plourde, P. J., L. J. D'Costa, E. Agoki, J. Ombette, J. O. Ndinya-Achola, L. A. Slaney, A. R. Ronald, and F. A. Plummer.** 1991. A randomized double-blind study of the efficacy of fleroxacin vs. trimethoprim-sulfamethoxazole in male prostitutes with culture-proven chancroid. *J. Infect. Dis.* **165**:949–952.
117. **Pocidalo, J.-J.** 1989. Use of fluoroquinolones for intracellular pathogens. *Rev. Infect. Dis.* **11**:S979–S984.
118. **Ponticas, S., D. L. Shungu, and C. J. Gill.** 1989. Comparative in vitro activity of norfloxacin against resistant *Neisseria gonorrhoeae*. *Eur. J. Clin. Microbiol. Infect. Dis.* **8**:626–628.
119. **Poulin, S., and R. B. Kundsin.** 1991. Susceptibility of *Ureaplasma urealyticum* and *Mycoplasma hominis* to sparfloxacin (CI-978, AT4140). *Eur. J. Clin. Microbiol. Infect. Dis.* **Special Issue**:570–571.
120. **Pust, R. A., H. R. Ackenheil-Koppe, W. Weidner, and H. Meier-Ewert.** 1988. Clinical efficacy and tolerance of fleroxacin in patients with urethritis caused by *Chlamydia trachomatis*. *J. Antimicrob. Chemother.* **22**(Suppl. D):227–230.
121. **Rajakumer, M. K., Y. F. Ngeow, B. S. Khor, and K. F. Lim.** 1988. Ofloxacin, a new quinolone for the treatment of gonorrhoea. *Sex. Transm. Dis.* **15**:25–26.

121a. **Ramirez, C. A., J. L. Bran, C. R. Mejia, and J. F. Garcia.** 1985. Open, prospective study of the clinical efficacy of oral ciprofloxacin. *Antimicrob. Agents Chemother.* **28**:128–132.

122. **Rein, M. F.** 1991. Gonorrhoea. *Curr. Opin. Infect. Dis.* **4**:12–21.
123. **Renaudin, H., and C. Bebear.** 1990. Comparative in vitro activity of azithromycin, clarithromycin, erythromycin and lomefloxacin against *Mycoplasma pneumoniae, Mycoplasma hominis* and *Ureaplasma urealyticum*. *Eur. J. Clin. Microbiol. Infect. Dis.* **9**:838–841.
124. **Rice, R. J., J. S. Knapp, S. A. Morse, and D. M. Buntin.** 1991. In vitro activity of temafloxacin against *Neisseria gonorrhoeae* exhibiting resistance to penicillin and decreased susceptibility to ceftriaxone, abstr. 135. *Program Abstr. 31st Intersci. Conf. Antimicrob. Agents Chemother.*
125. **Richmond, S. J., M. N. Bhattacharyya, H. Maiti, F. H. Chowdhury, R. M. Stirland, and J. A. Tooth.** 1988. The efficacy of ofloxacin against infection caused by *Neisseria gonorrhoeae* and *Chlamydia trachomatis*. *J. Antimicrob. Chemother.* **22**(Suppl. C):149–153.
126. **Robertson, J. A., G. W. Stemke, S. G. Maclellan, and D. E. Taylor.** 1988. Characterization of tetracycline-resistant strains of *Ureaplasma urealyticum*. *J. Antimicrob. Chemother.* **21**:319–332.
127. **Rodriguez, M., and J. C. Craft.** 1991. Temafloxacin versus doxycycline in the treatment of non-gonococcal urethritis or cervicitis. *Eur. J. Clin. Microbiol. Infect. Dis.* **Special Issue**:204–205.
128. **Romanowski, B., J. S. Hardy, M. S. Rafter, and J. Draker.** 1989. Enoxacin in the therapy of anal and pharyngeal gonococcal infections. *Sex. Transm. Dis.* **16**:190–191.
129. **Ronald, A. R., and R. W. Peeling.** 1991. Chlamydial infections and the quinolones. *Eur. J. Clin. Microbiol. Infect. Dis.* **10**:352–354.
130. **Sanghrajka, M., D. Felmingham, and G. L. Ridgway.** 1991. Comparative in vitro activity of the quinolone DR-3355 against *Mycoplasma pneumoniae, Mycoplasma hominis* and *Ureaplasma urealyticum*. *Eur. J. Clin. Microbiol. Infect. Dis.* **Special Issue**:237–238.
131. **Schachter, J., and J. V. Moncada.** 1989. In vitro activity of ofloxacin against *Chlamydia trachomatis*. *Am. J. Med.* **87**(Suppl. 6C):14S–16S.
132. **Schwarez, S. K., J. M. Zenilman, D. Schnell, J. S. Knapp, E. Hook, S. Thompson, F. N. Judson, and K. K. Holmes.** 1990. The gonococcal isolate surveillance project. National Surveillance of Antimicrobial Resistance in *Neisseria gonorrhoeae*. *J. Am. Med. Assoc.* **264**:1413–1417.
133. **Segev, S., M. Dulitsky, Z. Samra, N. Rosen, and E. Rubinstein.** 1991. Comparison of ten- versus twenty-day course of ofloxacin therapy in nongonococcal urethritis. *Eur. J. Clin. Microbiol. Infect. Dis.* **Special Issue**:313–314.
134. **Segreti, J., D. J. Hirsch, A. A. Harris, K. S. Kapell, H. Orbach, and H. A. Kessler.** 1990. In vitro activity of tosufloxacin (A-61827; T-3262) against selected genital pathogens. *Antimicrob. Agents Chemother.* **34**:971–973.

135. **Segreti, J., D. J. Hirsch, K. S. Kapell, and H. A. Kessler.** 1991. In vitro activity of temafloxacin and doxycycline against clinical isolates of *Chlamydia trachomatis. Eur. J. Clin. Microbiol. Infect. Dis.* **Special Issue:**201–202.
136. **Segreti, J., H. A. Kessler, K. Kapell, and G. M. Trenholme.** 1989. In vitro activity of lomefloxacin (SC 47111 or NY-198) against *Chlamydia trachomatis* strains. *Diagn. Microbiol. Infect. Dis.* **12**(Suppl. 3)**:**87S–88S.
137. **Segreti, J., H. A. Kessler, K. S. Kapell, and G. M. Trenholme.** 1989. In vitro activities of temafloxacin (A-62254) and four other antibiotics against *Chlamydia trachomatis. Antimicrob. Agents Chemother.* **33:**118–119.
138. **Shanmugaratnam, K., M. S. Sprott, R. S. Pattman, A. M. Kearns, and P. G. Watson.** 1989. Single dose ciprofloxacin to treat women with gonorrhoea. *Genitourin. Med.* **65:**129.
139. **Shepard, M. K., and R. B. Jones.** 1989. Recovery of *Chlamydia trachomatis* from endometrial and fallopian tube biopsies in women with infertility of tubal origin. *Fertil. Steril.* **52:**232–238.
140. **Siboulet, A., J. M. Bohbot, and A. Catalan.** 1988. Enoxacin in the treatment of sexually transmitted diseases. *J. Antimicrob. Chemother.* **21**(Suppl. B)**:**119–124.
141. **Sinn, L., L. R. Peterson, and D. N. Gerding.** 1991. Efficacy of temafloxacin against anaerobes in an *in vivo* rabbit model, abstr. 1211. *Program Abstr. 31st Intersci. Conf. Antimicrob. Agents Chemother.*
142. **Slaney, L., H. Chubb, A. Ronald, and R. Brunham.** 1990. In vitro activity of azithromycin, erythromycin, ciprofloxacin and norfloxacin against *Neisseria gonorrhoeae, Haemophilus ducreyi*, and *Chlamydia trachomatis. J. Antimicrob. Chemother.* **25**(Suppl. A)**:**1–5.
143. **Slaney, L., P. Odhiambo, J. O. Ndinya-Achola, A. R. Ronald, F. A. Plummer, and J. Ombette.** 1991. Increasing antimicrobial resistance of gonococcal isolates in Nairobi, Kenya, abstr. P-09-269. *Proc. 9th Meet. Int. Soc. Sex. Transm. Dis. Res.*
144. **Smith, B. L., M. Cummings, S. Benes, K. Draft, and W. M. McCormack.** 1989. Evaluation of difloxacin in the treatment of uncomplicated urethral gonorrhea in men. *Antimicrob. Agents Chemother.* **33:**1721–1723.
145. **Smith, B. L., M. C. Cummings, J. M. Covino, S. Benes, K. Draft, and W. M. McCormack.** 1991. Evaluation of ofloxacin in the treatment of uncomplicated gonorrhea. *Sex. Transm. Dis.* **18:**18–20.
146. **Soltz-Szots, J., S. Schneider, and H. Mailer.** 1989. Efficacy of and tolerance to fleroxacin in the treatment of chlamydia urethritis and cervicitis. *Rev. Infect. Dis.* **11:**S1280–S1281.
147. **Stamm, W. E., and K. G. Wong.** 1991. Antimicrobial activity of sparfloxacin (AT-4140, PD 131501, CI-978) against *Chlamydia trachomatis* in cell culture. *Eur. J. Clin. Microbiol. Infect. Dis.* **Special Issue:**566–567.
148. **Steele-Mortimer, O., and H. Meier-Ewert.** 1988. In-vitro activity of fleroxacin against *Chlamydia trachomatis. J. Antimicrob. Chemother.* **22**(Suppl. D)**:**65–70.
149. **Stein, D. C.** 1991. Transformation of *Neisseria gonorrhoeae*: physical requirements of transforming DNA. *Can. J. Microbiol.* **37:**345–349.
150. **Stein, D. C., R. J. Danaher, and T. M. Cook.** 1991. Characterization of a gyrB mutation responsible for low-level nalidixic acid resistance in *Neisseria gonorrhoeae. Antimicrob. Agents Chemother.* **35:**622–626.
151. **Stein, G. E., and L. D. Saravolatz.** 1989. Randomized clinical study of ofloxacin and doxycycline in the treatment of nongonococcal urethritis and cervicitis. *Rev. Infect. Dis.* **11:**S1277.
152. **Stimson, J. B., J. Hale, W. R. Bowie, and K. K. Holmes.** 1981. Tetracycline-resistant *Ureaplasma urealyticum*: a cause of persistent non-gonococcal urethritis. *Ann. Intern. Med.* **94:**192–194.
153. **Talbot, H., and B. Romanowski.** 1989. In vitro activities of lomefloxacin, tetracycline, penicillin, spectinomycin, and ceftriaxone against *Neisseria gonorrhoeae* and *Chlamydia trachomatis. Antimicrob. Agents Chemother.* **33:**2049–2051.
154. **Talbot, H., and B. Romanowski.** 1991. In vitro susceptibility of sparfloxacin (CI-978, AT-4140) against *Neisseria gonorrhoeae* and *Chlamydia trachomatis. Eur. J. Clin. Microbiol. Infect. Dis.* **Special Issue:**569–570.
155. **Tio, T. T., I. R. Sindhunata, J. H. T. Wagenvoort, A. F. Angulo, L. Habbema, M. F. Michel, and E. Stolz.** 1990. Pefloxacin compared with cefotaxime for treating men with uncomplicated gonococcal urethritis. *J. Antimicrob. Chemother.* **22**(Suppl. B)**:**141–146.
156. **Tio, T. T., J. H. T. Wagenvoort, H. L. Moesker, L. Habbema, M. F. Michel, and E. Stolz.** 1991. Evaluation of ciprofloxacin in the treatment of chlamydial cervicitis, abstr. P-20-027. *Proc. 9th Meet. Int. Soc. Sex. Transm. Dis. Res.*
157. **Toomey, K. E., and R. C. Barnes.** 1990. Treatment of *Chlamydia trachomatis* genital infection. *Rev. Infect. Dis.* **12**(Suppl. 6)**:**S645–S655.
158. **Turner, A., A. E. Jephcott, and K. R. Gough.** 1991. Laboratory detection of ciprofloxacin resistant *Neisseria gonorrhoeae. J. Clin. Pathol.* **44:**169–170.
159. **Turner, A., A. E. Jephcott, T. C. Haji, and P. C. Gupta.** 1990. Ciprofloxacin resistant

*Neisseria gonorrhoeae* in the UK. *Genitourin. Med.* **66:**43.

160. **Tyndall, M., M. Malisa, F. A. Plummer, J. Ombetti, J. O. Ndinya-Achola, and A. R. Ronald.** 1993. Ceftriaxone no longer predictably cures chancroid in Kenya. *J. Infect. Dis.* **167:**469–471.

160a. **Une, T., R. Nakajima, T. Otani, K. Katami, Y. Osada, and M. Otani.** 1987. Lack of effectiveness of ofloxacin against experimental syphilis in rabbits. *Arzneim. Forsch.* **37:**1048–1051.

161. **van der Willigen, A. H., A. A. Polak-Vogelzang, L. Habbema, and J. H. Wagenvoort.** 1988. Clinical efficacy of ciprofloxacin versus doxycycline in the treatment of nongonococcal urethritis in males. *Eur. J. Clin. Microbiol. Infect. Dis.* **7:**658–661.

162. **Veller-Fornasa, C., M. Tarantello, R. Cepriani, L. Gurerra, and A. Peserico.** 1987. Effect of ofloxacin on *Treponema pallidum* in incubating experimental syphilis. *Genitourin. Med.* **63:**214.

163. **Verhoest, P., H. Fernandez, J. C. Boulanger, J. Orfila, and E. Papiernik.** 1989. Use of ofloxacin plus amoxicillin-clavulanic acid for the treatment of acute genital tract infections. *Rev. Infect. Dis.* **11**(Suppl. 5):S1307.

164. **Vilata, J. J., J. Garcia-De-Lomas, J. Sanchez, A. Lloret, M. Evole, and J. M. Nogueira.** 1989. A double-blind randomized study comparing two ofloxacin regimens vs. minocycline in the treatment of nongonococcal urethritis. *Rev. Infect. Dis.* **11**(Suppl. 5):S1285–S1286.

165. **Wagenvoort, J. H. T., A. H. van der Willingen, H. J. van Vliet, M. F. Michel, and B. van Klingeren.** 1986. Resistance of *Neisseria gonorrhoeae* to enoxacin. *J. Antimicrob. Chemother.* **18:**429.

166. **Wager, E. A., J. Schachter, P. Bavoil, and R. S. Stephens.** 1990. Differential human serologic response to two 60,000 molecular weight *Chlamydia trachomatis* antigens. *J. Infect. Dis.* **162:**922–927.

167. **Waites, K. B., G. H. Cassell, K. C. Canupp, and P. B. Fernandes.** 1988. In vitro susceptibilities of mycoplasmas and ureaplasmas to new macrolides and aryl-fluoroquinolones. *Antimicrob. Agents Chemother.* **32:**1500–1502.

168. **Wasserheit, J.** 1989. The significance and scope of reproductive tract infections among Third World women. *Int. J. Gynecol. Obstet.* **3**(Suppl.):145–168.

168a. **Weidner, W., H. G. Schiefer, and C. Garbe.** 1987. Acute non-gonococcal epididymitis. Aetiological and therapeutic aspects. *Drugs* **34**(Suppl. 1):111-117.

169. **Wendel, G. D., Jr., S. M. Cox, R. E. Bawdon, S. K. Theriot, M. C. Heard, and B. J. Nobles.** 1991. A randomized trial of ofloxacin versus cefoxitin and doxycycline in the outpatient treatment of acute salpingitis. *Am. J. Obstet. Gynecol.* **164:**1390–1396.

170. **Wolfson, J. S., and D. C. Hooper.** 1989. Treatment of genitourinary tract infections with fluoroquinolones: activity in vitro, plasma pharmacokinetics, and clinical efficacy in urinary tract infections and prostatitis. *Antimicrob. Agents Chemother.* **33:**1655–1661.

171. **Worm, A. M., and M. Stangerup.** 1991. Fleroxacin and doxycycline for genitourinary chlamydial infections, abstr. P20-119. *Proc. 9th Meet. Int. Soc. Sex. Transm. Dis. Res.*

172. **Yeung, K. H., and J. R. Dillon.** 1990. Norfloxacin resistant *Neisseria gonorrhoeae* in North America. *Lancet* **336:**759.

173. **Yeung, K. H., and J. R. Dillon.** 1991. First isolates of norfloxacin-resistant penicillinase-producing *Neisseria gonorrhoeae* (PPNG) in Canada. *Can. Dis. Weekly Rep.* **17:**1–3.

174. **Young, H., A. Moyes, I. B. Tait, A. C. McCartney, and G. Gallacher.** 1990. Non-typable quinolone-resistant gonococci. *Lancet* **335:**604.

*Quinolone Antimicrobial Agents, 2nd ed.*
Edited by David C. Hooper and John S. Wolfson


*Chapter 16*

# Use of the Quinolones for Treatment and Prophylaxis of Bacterial Gastrointestinal Infections

*Herbert L. DuPont*

While fluid-and-electrolyte therapy has received appropriate emphasis as a lifesaving technique in the management of acute diarrhea in areas where severe diarrhea and malnutrition coexist, the value of antimicrobial treatment is less established except in certain forms of organism-specific illness. It is generally agreed that antimicrobial therapy is absolutely indicated for typhoid fever and dysenteric disease caused by *Shigella dysenteriae* type 1 (the Shiga bacillus) and appears to be useful against other forms of shigellosis, campylobacteriosis, and enterotoxigenic *Escherichia coli* (ETEC) diarrhea. The drugs traditionally employed for enteric infection are of questionable value in the management of uncomplicated intestinal salmonellosis. These antimicrobial agents have limitations in treating bacterial diarrhea because of the occurrence of a high frequency of resistance among enteric pathogens (ampicillin, tetracycline) or because of ineffectiveness against both *Campylobacter* and *Shigella* strains (trimethoprim-sulfamethoxazole [TMP-SMX]).

In view of their activities against aerobic enteric gram-negative bacilli and their low frequencies of resistance, the quinolones are logical agents to evaluate for use against intestinal and biliary tract infectious diseases. This review focuses on in vitro susceptibility of enteric bacterial pathogens to the quinolones and reviews efficacy trials of the drugs as they are used in the therapy of enteric infections.

*Herbert L. DuPont* • Medical School/School of Public Health, University of Texas Health Science Center, Houston, Texas 77030.

## IN VITRO SUSCEPTIBILITY OF ENTERIC PATHOGENS TO QUINOLONES

Resistance to ampicillin and tetracycline is currently widespread among enteric bacterial pathogens in most regions of the world (61). TMP-SMX resistance has been documented in enteropathogens in selected areas (7, 8, 61, 71). In vitro studies of antimicrobial susceptibility, performed more than 10 years ago with the first-generation quinolones (nalidixic acid, cinoxacin, and oxolinic acid), demonstrated a high degree of activity against bacterial enteropathogens (11, 28). Several studies have been performed more recently to examine the in vitro activities of the newer, more active quinolones against the broad range of bacterial enteropathogens isolated in diverse areas of the world (12, 21, 26, 35, 38, 53, 60, 64, 72, 74, 80, 81). Table 1 presents the results of in vitro susceptibility testing of a variety of bacterial enteropathogens and selected antimicrobial agents, including several of the newer quinolone preparations

**Table 1.** MICS of various antimicrobial agents against 90% of strains tested

| Bacterial enteropathogen | No. of strains tested | MIC (μg/ml) against 90% of strains tested with[a]: | | | | | | | |
|---|---|---|---|---|---|---|---|---|---|
| | | AMP | DOX | ERY | TMP-SMX | FUR | NOR | ENO | CIP |
| *Salmonella* spp. | 50 | 128 | 64 | 64 | 1 | 1 | ≤0.5 | ≤0.5 | ≤0.5 |
| *Shigella* spp. | 80 | >128 | 16 | 64 | 4 | 2 | ≤0.5 | ≤0.5 | ≤0.5 |
| ETEC | 50 | >128 | 32 | 128 | 8 | 1 | ≤0.5 | ≤0.5 | ≤0.5 |
| *C. jejuni* | 30 | 8 | 8 | ≤0.5 | >128 | ≤0.5 | 1 | 2 | ≤0.5 |

[a]Abbreviations: AMP, ampicillin; DOX, doxycycline; ERY, erythromycin; TMP-SMX, trimethoprim-sulfamethoxazole; FUR, furazolidone; NOR, norfloxacin; ENO, enoxacin; CIP, ciprofloxacin.

(12, 26). The quinolone antimicrobial agents studied (norfloxacin, enoxacin, and ciprofloxacin) showed the lowest MICs (highest susceptibility) when *Campylobacter jejuni*, as well as the other pathogens, was tested. Not shown in the table, the three quinolones employed in these in vitro studies had MICs of <0.5 μg/ml for 90% of 29 strains of miscellaneous bacterial pathogens, including *Aeromonas hydrophila* (6 strains), *Vibrio parahaemolyticus* (9 strains), and *Yersinia enterocolitica* (14 strains). The only other drug tested in our in vitro studies that had such a high degree of in vitro activity against the wide range of strains tested was furazolidone. The quinolones have been shown in other studies to have excellent in vitro activity against *Aeromonas* (72), *Plesiomonas* (64), and *Vibrio* (60) species and *Helicobacter pylori* (4, 5, 34, 58, 73, 79). These drugs show variable to low activities against strains of *Clostridium difficile* (15, 21, 74).

## CLINICAL EVALUATIONS OF QUINOLONES IN ENTERIC INFECTIONS

### Shigellosis

Soon after the first quinolone, nalidixic acid, was introduced, it was successfully employed in the therapy of shigellosis (59). When ampicillin- and TMP-SMX-resistant Shiga dysentery (illness due to *S. dysenteriae* type 1) emerged as a problem in selected areas, nalidixic acid was found to be a useful therapy (7, 8, 71). In a limited trial, oxolinic acid appeared to have some value in the therapy of experimentally induced human shigellosis (27). One study of shigellosis in a small group of hospitalized children dampened enthusiasm for this class of drugs by suggesting that nalidixic acid was of only marginal effectiveness in severe disease (44). Seventeen infants received nalidixic acid, and 19 were treated with ampicillin. Of these, 4 of 17 (24%) receiving nalidixic acid and none of the ampicillin-treated subjects were still experiencing diarrhea after 5 days of therapy.

Several studies carried out more recently with the newer, more active quinolones have established the clinical efficacy of these drugs in patients with shigellosis. Norfloxacin is as effective as nalidixic acid in the treatment of Shiga dysentery (71). Norfloxacin eliminated *Shigella* strains from stools more rapidly than nalidixic acid did in that study. In a clinical trial (29) in which ciprofloxacin was compared with TMP-SMX versus a placebo in the therapy of traveler's diarrhea, 15 adults with shigellosis were included. The average durations of diarrhea after initiation of therapy when the causal agent was a *Shigella* strain were 28 h for the ciprofloxacin group (five patients), 16 h for those receiving TMP-SMX (four patients), and 84 h for those receiving a placebo (six patients). In a study of Peruvian adults with shigellosis, norfloxacin in a single dose was as effective as the standard treatment of 5 days of oral TMP-SMX (41).

### Salmonellosis

Conventional antimicrobial therapy appears to be of limited, if any, benefit in treating intestinal salmonellosis. In fact, antimicrobial agents may encourage the development of resistance and increase the duration of post-convalescent-stage shedding of the infecting strain (3). Recently, Pichler et al. (67) demonstrated that ciprofloxacin effectively reduced the duration of diarrheal illness and the length of time the infecting strain could be isolated from stool specimens of adults with intestinal salmonellosis. A total of 16 patients with salmonellosis received ciprofloxacin, and 21 were given a placebo. The mean duration of diarrhea was 1.9 days for the active-drug group and 3.4 days for the group receiving a placebo ($P < 0.01$). Two additional reports also provided evidence that the newer quinolones could reduce the period of intestinal shedding of *Salmonella* strains in those excreting the organism asymptomatically (22, 48). In a more recent study, ciprofloxacin given orally for 2 weeks failed to eradicate convalescent-stage fecal excretion of *Salmonella* spp. in patients with intestinal salmonellosis (62). While resistance acquisition by the infecting strain did not explain the prolongation in excretion in this study, resistance to the new quinolones may occur during therapy (14). In the treatment of *Salmonella enteritidis* carriers, stool cultures should be performed 1 or 2 weeks after the course of therapy has been completed.

In view of a low MIC of the quinolones for *Salmonella typhi*, representatives from this class of drug have been evaluated in typhoid fever and typhoid carriers. In an open trial, ciprofloxacin was effective in the therapy of 38 patients with blood culture-proven typhoid fever (69). Ciprofloxacin was given in a dose of 500 mg every 12 h for an average of 14 days. There was one treatment failure in a patient developing acute cholecystitis. Defervescence occurred on the average after 4.2 days of therapy. Pefloxacin was shown to favorably influence the course of typhoid fever compared with TMP-SMX therapy in another trial (43). In a third clinical study, norfloxacin compared with a placebo successfully eradicated *S. typhi* carriage in a group of chronic typhoid carriers (41). Chronic typhoid carriers were treated with either 400 mg of norfloxacin or a matching placebo every 12 h for 28 days. Of 12 treated with norfloxacin, 11 had negative stool and bile cultures at the completion of therapy. All 12 placebo-treated subjects had positive cultures at the completion of therapy. The overall bacteriologic cure rate in the Peru study when 11 of the placebo-treated cases received the same norfloxacin therapy was 18 of 23 (78%). The investigators showed an equivalent high rate of organism eradication in those with or without cholelithiasis. Successful eradication of *S. typhi* intestinal carriage has also been reported after oral administration of ciprofloxacin (31, 48).

## Campylobacteriosis

An important advantage of the quinolones compared with other available antimicrobial agents used against diarrhea is their high degree of in vitro activity against *C. jejuni*. Few data are available to establish the values of antimicrobial therapy of any sort in intestinal *Campylobacter* infection. Chronic infection of marmosets was successfully treated with ciprofloxacin (36). A preliminary report for humans suggested that ciprofloxacin could reduce symptoms and the duration of excretion of the causative agent in patients with *Campylobacter* infection (67). Nineteen adults with intestinal campylobacteriosis who received ciprofloxacin experienced on the average 1.1 days of diarrhea after therapy was initiated compared with 2.2 days for 11 placebo-treated subjects ($P < 0.01$). It remains to be determined whether resistance is likely to occur among infecting strains of *C. jejuni* during therapy with the newer quinolones. Emergence of resistance of the infecting *Campylobacter* strain during therapy has been described for nalidixic acid (1) and the newer quinolones (66, 70), and this resistance may limit their value in the therapy of intestinal campylobacteriosis. A single-step mutation in the genes encoding DNA gyrase in *C. jejuni* may be responsible for producing clinically important resistance to the newer quinolones (39).

Gastric infection secondary to *H. pylori* infection has been treated with fluoroquinolones with or without either ranitidine or bismuth subsalicylate (4, 5, 34, 77). In one of the studies, therapy with the quinolone led to more rapid healing and eradication of the organism from posttreatment biopsy samples (4). In the other three studies, resistance to the quinolone occurred, limiting the value of the treatment (5, 34, 77).

### Traveler's Diarrhea and ETEC Diarrhea

Ciprofloxacin was as effective as TMP-SMX and both were significantly more effective than a placebo in treating traveler's diarrhea (26, 29). The average duration of diarrhea was 29 or 20 h after the initiation of therapy with ciprofloxacin or TMP-SMX, respectively, compared with 81 h for those receiving a placebo. The durations of ETEC illness, the most common form of traveler's diarrhea, for the three groups were 33, 26, and 84 h, respectively. In a separate study (82), norfloxacin given for 3 days was effective in eradicating pathogens causing traveler's diarrhea and shortening the duration of diarrhea. In a recent clinical trial, 3 days of ofloxacin given orally was as effective as 5 days of the drug in eradicating the causative enteropathogens and shortening the illness (25).

In other studies, norfloxacin prevented 88% of diarrhea cases that would be expected to occur without prophylaxis in a placebo-controlled trial among U.S. travelers during a 2-week stay in Mexico (50), and ciprofloxacin taken daily gave a protection rate of 94% among Finnish travelers to Morocco (68). In the first study, norfloxacin treatment led to a significant decline in normal flora during prophylaxis. After norfloxacin was discontinued in the study, fecal flora returned to pretreatment levels. No resistant gram-negative aerobic flora was found during weekly quantitative cultures before, during, or after therapy.

### Other Bacterial Causes of Diarrhea

In clinical trials conducted in seven countries, two regimens of norfloxacin, i.e., 400 mg twice daily or 400 mg three times daily for 5 days, were shown to be equivalent to conventional TMP-SMX treatment for acute diarrhea in adults (24). Clinical cure occurred in 89% (lower dose) and 91% (higher dose) of those treated with norfloxacin compared with 78% of those receiving TMP-SMX. Cure rates were greater in all treatment groups when the patient's stool specimen contained numerous leukocytes. This is the second study we have carried out in which antimicrobial agents showed the greatest clinical effect in patients with fecal leukocytes (63). This undoubtedly relates to the fact that patients in whom numerous fecal leukocytes are found microscopically are often infected with an invasive bacterial pathogen (45). In a study of Thai patients with diarrhea, 3 days of norfloxacin was effective in eliminating intestinal carriage of diarrhea due to *Vibrio* sp., *Plesiomonas shigelloides,* and *Aeromonas* sp., yet clinical courses were unaffected by the therapy (55). In another blinded comparative study, ciprofloxacin was more effective than placebo or TMP-SMX in shortening clinical illness in patients with bacterial diarrheas of diverse causes (37).

### Intra-Abdominal and Biliary Tract Infections

The quinolone agents hold promise for use in treating intra-abdominal and biliary tract infections (20, 42–51). The quinolones are active against nearly all of the aerobic bacterial pathogens that commonly produce peritonitis, cholangitis, and biliary sepsis (83). Quinolones can be found in clinically important concentrations in bile and hepatic tissue. The agents appear to be effective in most patients with peritonitis secondary to chronic ambulatory peritoneal dialysis (CAPD), spontaneous bacterial peritonitis, and biliary sepsis (13, 32, 75). In treating intra-abdominal infection related to bowel disease, an antianaerobic drug should be added, since the fluoroquinolones do not have predictable activity against *Bacteroides fragilis* (75). The biliary pharmacokinetics and in vitro activities against aerobic enteric gram-negative organisms of the quinolones make them effective drugs in biliary tract infections (42, 51). Dan et al. (19) found concentrations of norfloxacin in bile ranging from 0.6 to 15.6 μg/ml in patients given a single 400-mg oral dose prior to cholecystectomy. The mean ratio of bile to serum concentrations was 7, and the mean level of drug in gallbladder tissue was 1.8 ± 0.8 μg/g. Grozinger et al. (42) showed high biliary concentrations of ciprofloxacin in the common duct following intravenous or oral administration of drug to cholecystectomy patients with indwelling T-tubes. In another study, ofloxacin given orally for 2 days before cholecystectomy was found in concentrations of 5.3 μg/g of gallbladder tissue, 24.6 μg/ml of gallbladder bile, and 10 μg/ml of common duct bile (51). Ciprofloxacin has been used successfully in preliminary studies to treat biliary tract infection (16, 47, 56).

The quinolones appear to hold promise in the prevention and therapy of bacterial peritonitis in selected patients. In hospitalized cirrhotic patients with reduced total protein levels in ascitic fluid (<1.5 g/dl), norfloxacin at 400 mg every day given orally provided selective intestinal decontamination, resulting in a lower incidence of spontaneous bacterial peritonitis and extrapulmonary infections compared with incidences in a similar group of untreated patients (76). In patients with peritonitis associated with CAPD, ciprofloxacin in a dose of 25 or 50 mg/liter of dialysate for 5 to 7 days was shown to be effective therapy (23, 57). In a related trial, ciprofloxacin at 20 mg/liter added to each dialysate bag for 10 days was as effective as standard intraperitoneal vancomycin and gentamicin (33). Finally, oral ciprofloxacin for 10 days (250 to 500 mg at the time of each dialysate exchange) was as effective as intraperitoneal vancomycin plus netilmicin in CAPD peritonitis (78). Primary resistance to quinolones by coagulase-negative staphylococci was reported in 8% of cases (23), limiting the value of this approach.

## COMMENT

Antibacterial agents play an important role in the therapy and selected prevention of certain forms of enteric infection. There are two major limitations of the drugs commonly used in the treatment of intestinal infections: prevalence or development of antimicrobial resistance and failure to achieve a satisfactory clinical response to therapy, as seen for certain forms of bacterial diarrhea (salmonellosis and campylobacteriosis). The properties of an ideal drug for therapy of bacterial diarrhea include the following: low frequency or absence of resistance among bacterial pathogens; low potential for inducing R-factor (plasmid) resistance; activity against both *Shigella* and *Campylobacter* strains; and achievement of high levels of antibacterial drug in the gut, tissue, and blood. The newly developed drugs with perhaps the greatest potential regarding these attributes are the newer quinolone derivatives as well as bicozamycin, aztreonam, amdinocillin, and furazolidone (26). Of these agents, the quinolones may hold the greatest promise. They show a high degree of activity against enteric pathogens, they are well absorbed after oral administration, and they have large volumes of distribution with long elimination half-lives (see also chapter 9). Norfloxacin given in a dose of 400 mg to healthy volunteers led to levels in feces of between 207 and 2,716 μg/g of stool (17), while a similar study of ciprofloxacin in noninfected volunteers showed that levels in feces ranged between 185 and 2,220 μg/g (10). Ciprofloxacin therapy of traveler's diarrhea produced mean drug levels in feces exceeding 500 μg/g (26). Many of the new quinolones are well absorbed from the gastrointestinal tract, producing levels in serum well above the inhibitory concentrations for most enteric pathogens (8). The quinolones produce profound changes in intestinal aerobic flora during therapy (6, 30, 46, 65). The aerobic enterobacteria are essentially eliminated without producing resistance, and the anaerobic flora is not altered in most cases (see also chapter 8). While *C. difficile* levels have not usually been shown to increase during quinolone therapy, antibiotic-associated colitis has been reported (2, 18). Studies to establish the usefulness of the quinolones in the broad range of bacterial enteric infections are currently under way. Clearly, the most important limitation of the quinolones in the management of diarrhea is the current lack of application to therapy in children. When one considers that diarrhea is numerically a greater problem in children, the hope remains that one or more of the quinolones will be shown to be safe for administration to infants and young children.

The new quinolones will undoubtedly play an important role in the therapy of bacterial enteric infection in adults (52). Currently, they should be considered agents of choice for adults with severe diarrhea that occurs in areas where TMP-SMX-resistant *Shigella* strains and ETEC are known to be prevalent, such as Southeast Asia, Africa, and South America (61). In any area where empiric antimicrobial therapy is indicated for clinical bacillary dysentry in postpubertal children and adults, where either *Shigella* or *Campylobacter* strains may be the responsible agents, a quinolone might ideally be employed. Further study of patients with intestinal and typhoidal salmonelloses is indicated. The quinolones appear to be promising in treating typhoid carriers. Finally, the quinolones should prove to be useful in the treatment of biliary tract infection and possibly, when combined with an agent active against anaerobes, in the therapy of intra-abdominal infections when mixed organisms are suspected. Adverse reactions (detailed in chapter 26) appear to be rare when these drugs are used for short periods for bacterial enteric infection. The most common reactions (occurring in 2 to 3% of treated cases) are gastrointestinal complaints, insomnia, headache, and rash.

*Acknowledgments.* Research activities described in this chapter were supported by the National Institutes of Health (RO1 AI-72534 and RO1 AI-230491) and by grants from Merck Sharp and Dohme Research Laboratories, East Point, Pa.; Miles Pharmaceuticals Inc., West Haven, Conn.; and Ortho Pharmaceutical Corporation, Raritan, N.J.

Betty Morris was responsible for manuscript preparation.

## REFERENCES

1. **Altwegg, M., A. Burnens, J. Zollinger-Iten, and J. L. Penner.** 1987. Problems in identification of *Campylobacter jejuni* associated with acquisition of resistance to nalidixic acid. *J. Clin. Microbiol.* **25:**1807–1808.
2. **Arcieri, G., E. Griffith, G. Grunewaldt, A. Heyd, B. O'Brien, N. Becker, and R. August.** 1987. Ciprofloxacin: an update on clinical experience. *Am. J. Med.* **82**(Suppl. 4A)**:**381–386.
3. **Aserkoff, B., and J. V. Bennett.** 1969. Effect of antibiotic therapy in acute salmonellosis on the fecal excretion of salmonellae. *N. Engl. J. Med.* **281:**636–640.
4. **Bayerdörffer, E., G. Kasper, T. Pirlet, A. Sommer, and R. Ottenjann.** 1987. Ofloxacin in der Therapie Campylobacter-pylori-positive Ulcera duodeni. Eine prospektive kontrollieste randomisierte Studie. *Dtsch. Med. Wochenschr.* **112:**1407–1411.
5. **Bayerdörffer, E., T. Simon, C. Bästlein, R. Ottenjann, and G. Kasper.** 1987. Bismuth/ofloxacin combination for duodenal ulcer. *Lancet* **ii:**1467–1468.
6. **Bergan, T., C. Delin, S. Johansen, I. M. Kolstad, C. E. Nord, and S. B. Thorsteinsson.** 1986. Pharmacokinetics of ciprofloxacin and effect of repeated dosage on salivary and fecal microflora. *Antimicrob. Agents Chemother.* **29:**298–302.
7. **Bhattacharya, D., G. Sen, G. B. Nair, M. K. Bhattacharya, P. Datta, and D. Datta.** 1986. Multiple drug-resistant *Shigella dysenteriae* type 1 and travelers' diarrhea. *J. Infect. Dis.* **154:**729–730.
8. **Bose, R., J. N. Nashipuri, P. K. Sen, P. Datta, S. K. Bhattacharya, D. Datta, D. Sen, and M. K. Bhattacharya.** 1984. Epidemic of dysentery in West Bengal: clinician's enigma. *Lancet* **ii:**1160.

9. **Brogard, J.-M., F. Jehl, H. Monteil, M. Adloff, J.-F. Blickie, and P. Levy.** 1985. Comparison of high-pressure liquid chromatography and microbiological assay for the determination of biliary elimination of ciprofloxacin in humans. *Antimicrob. Agents Chemother.* **28:**311–314.
10. **Brumfitt, W., I. Franklin, D. Grady, J. M. T. Hamilton-Miller, and A. Iliffe.** 1984. Changes in the pharmacokinetics of ciprofloxacin and fecal flora during administration of a 7-day course to human volunteers. *Antimicrob. Agents Chemother.* **26:**757–761.
11. **Byers, P. A., H. L. DuPont, and M. C. Goldschmidt.** 1976. Antimicrobial susceptibilities of shigellae isolated in Houston, Texas, in 1974. *Antimicrob. Agents Chemother.* **9:**288–291.
12. **Carlson, J. R., S. A. Thornton, H. L. DuPont, A. H. West, and J. J. Mathewson.** 1983. Comparative in vitro activities of ten antimicrobial agents against bacterial enteropathogens. *Antimicrob. Agents Chemother.* **24:**509–513.
13. **Chan, M. K., P. Y. Chou, and W. W. Chan.** 1988. Oral treatment of peritonitis in CAPD patients with two dosage regimens of ofloxacin. *J. Antimicrob. Chemother.* **22:**371–375.
14. **Cherubin, C. E., and R. H. K. Eng.** 1991. Quinolones for the treatment of infections due to *Salmonella. Rev. Infect. Dis.* **13:**343–344.
15. **Chow, A. W., N. Cheng, and K. H. Bartlett.** 1985. In vitro susceptibility of *Clostridium difficile* to new β-lactam and quinolone antibiotics. *Antimicrob. Agents Chemother.* **28:**842–844.
16. **Chrysanthopoulos, C. J., A. T. Skoutelis, J. C. Starakis, E. D. Anastassiou, and H. P. Bassaris.** 1987. Use of intravenous ciprofloxacin in respiratory tract infections and biliary sepsis. *Am. J. Med.* **82**(Suppl. 4A):357–359.
17. **Cofsky, R. D., L. DuBouchet, and S. H. Landesman.** 1984. Recovery of norfloxacin in feces after administration of a single oral dose to human volunteers. *Antimicrob. Agents Chemother.* **26:**110–116.
18. **Dan, M., and Z. Samra.** 1989. *Clostridium difficile* colitis associated with ofloxacin therapy. *Am. J. Med.* **87:**479.
19. **Dan, M., F. Serour, A. Gorea, A. Levenbert, M. Krispin, and S. A. Berger.** 1987. Concentration of norfloxacin in human gallbladder tissue and bile after single-dose oral administration. *Antimicrob. Agents Chemother.* **31:**352–353.
20. **Delalla, E., L. Peruzzo, P. Ferraris, B. Biamonti, and S. Savio.** 1988. Chemoprophylaxis in elective biliary tract surgery: oral norfloxacin vs. intravenous piperacillin. *Rev. Infect. Dis.* **10**(Suppl. 1):S215–S216.
21. **Delmee, M., and V. Avesani.** 1986. Comparative in vitro activity of seven quinolones against 100 clinical isolates of *Clostridium difficile. Antimicrob. Agents Chemother.* **29:**374–375.
22. **Dirdl, G., H. Pichler, and D. Wolf.** 1986. Treatment of chronic salmonella carriers with ciprofloxacin. *Eur. J. Clin. Microbiol.* **5:**260–261.
23. **Dryden, M. S., A. J. Wing, and I. Phillips.** 1991. Low-dose intraperitoneal ciprofloxacin for the treatment of peritonitis in patients receiving continuous ambulatory peritoneal dialysis. *Antimicrob. Agents Chemother.* **28:**131–139.
24. **DuPont, H. L., M. L. Corrado, and J. Sabbaj.** 1987. Use of norfloxacin in the treatment of acute diarrheal disease. *Am. J. Med.* **82**(Suppl. 6B):79–83.
25. **DuPont, H. L., C. D. Ericsson, J. J. Mathewson, and M. W. DuPont.** 1992. Five versus three day of ofloxacin therapy for traveler's diarrhea: a placebo-controlled study. *Antimicrob. Agents Chemother.* **36:**87–91.
26. **DuPont, H. L., C. D. Ericsson, A. Robinson, and P. C. Johnson.** 1987. Current problems in antimicrobial therapy for bacterial enteric infection. *Am. J. Med.* **82**(Suppl. 4A):324–328.
27. **DuPont, H. L., and R. B. Hornick.** 1973. Adverse effect of lomotil therapy in shigellosis. *J. Am. Med. Assoc.* **226:**1525–1528.
28. **DuPont, H. L., A. H. West, D. G. Evans, J. Olarte, and D. J. Evans, Jr.** 1978. Antimicrobial susceptibility of enterotoxigenic *Escherichia coli. J. Antimicrob. Chemother.* **4:**100–102.
29. **Ericsson, C. D., P. C. Johnson, H. L. DuPont, D. R. Morgan, J. A. Bitsura, and F. J. Cabada.** 1987. Ciprofloxacin or trimethoprim/sulfamethoxazole as initial therapy for acute traveler's diarrhea. *Ann. Intern. Med.* **106:**216–220.
30. **Erizensberger, R., P. M. Shah, and H. Knothe.** 1985. Impact of oral ciprofloxacin on the faecal flora of healthy volunteers. *Infection* **13:**273–275.
31. **Ferreccio, C., J. G. Morris, Jr., C. Valdivieso, I. Prenzel, V. Sotomayor, G. L. Drusano, and M. M. Levine.** 1988. Efficacy of ciprofloxacin in the treatment of chronic typhoid carriers. *J. Infect. Dis.* **157:**1235–1239.
32. **Fleming, L. W., G. Phillips, W. K. Stewart, and A. C. Scott.** 1990. Oral ciprofloxacin in the treatment of peritonitis in patients on continuous ambulatory peritoneal dialysis. *J. Antimicrob. Chemother.* **25:**441–448.
33. **Friedland, J. S., T. J. Iveson, A. P. Fraise, C. G. Winearls, J. B. Selkon, and D. O. Oliver.** 1990. A comparison between intraperitoneal ciprofloxacin and intraperitoneal vancomycin and gentamicin in the treatment of peritonitis associated with continuous ambulatory peritoneal dialysis (CAPD). *J. Antimicrob. Chemother.* **26**(Suppl. F):77–81.
34. **Glupczynski, Y., M. Labbe, A. Burette, M. Delmee, V. Avesani, and C. Bruck.** 1987. Treatment failure of ofloxacin in *Campylobacter pylori* infection. *Lancet* **i:**1096.

35. **Goodman, L. J., R. M. Fliegelman, G. M. Trenholme, and R. L. Kaplan.** 1984. Comparative in vitro activity of ciprofloxacin against *Campylobacter* spp. and other bacterial enteric pathogens. *Antimicrob. Agents Chemother.* **25:**504–506.
36. **Goodman, L. J., R. L. Kaplan, R. M. Petrak, R. M. Fliegelman, D. Taff, F. Walton, J. L. Penner, and G. M. Trenholme.** 1986. Effects of erythromycin and ciprofloxacin on chronic fecal excretion of *Campylobacter* species in marmosets. *Antimicrob. Agents Chemother.* **29:**185–187.
37. **Goodman, L. J., G. M. Trenholme, R. L. Kaplan, J. Segreti, D. Hines, R. Petrak, J. A. Nelson, K. W. Mayer, W. Landau, G. W. Parkhurst, and S. Levin.** 1990. Empiric antimicrobial therapy of domestically acquired acute diarrhea in urban adults. *Arch. Intern. Med.* **150:**541–546.
38. **Goossens, H., P. De Mol, H. Colgnau, J. Levy, O. Grados, G. Ghysels, H. Innocent, and J. Butzler.** 1985. Comparative in vitro activities of aztreonam, ciprofloxacin, norfloxacin, ofloxacin, HR 810 (a new cephalosporin), RU 28965 (a new macrolide), and other agents against enteropathogens. *Antimicrob. Agents Chemother.* **27:**388–392.
39. **Gootz, T. D., and B. A. Martin.** 1991. Characterization of high-level quinolone resistance in *Campylobacter jejuni. Antimicrob. Agents Chemother.* **35:**840–845.
40. **Gotuzzo, E., R. A. Oberhelman, C. Maguiña, S. J. Berry, A. Yi, M. Guzman, R. Ruiz, R. Leon-Barua, and R. B. Sack.** 1989. Comparison of single-dose treatment with norfloxacin and standard 5-day treatment with trimethoprim-sulfamethoxazole for acute shigellosis in adults. *Antimicrob. Agents Chemother.* **33:**1101–1104.
41. **Gotuzzo, E. J., G. Guerra, L. Benavente, J. C. Palomino, C. Carrillo, J. Lopera, E. Delgado, D. R. Nalin, and J. Sabbaj.** 1988. Use of norfloxacin to treat chronic typhoid carriers. *J. Infect. Dis.* **137:**1221–1225.
42. **Grozinger, K. H., D. Beermann, and S. Elsas.** 1989. Biliary kinetics of ciprofloxacin in humans. *Rev. Infect. Dis.* **11**(Suppl. 5):S1132–S1133.
43. **Hajji, M., N. E. Mdaghri, M. Benbachir, K. M. El Filali, and H. Himmich.** 1988. Prospective randomized comparative trial of pefloxacin versus co-trimoxazole in the treatment of typhoid fever in adults. *Eur. J. Clin. Microbiol. Infect. Dis.* **7:**361–363.
44. **Haltalin, K. C., J. D. Nelson, and H. T. Kusmiesz.** 1973. Comparative efficacy of nalidixic acid and ampicillin for severe shigellosis. *Arch. Dis. Child.* **48:**305–312.
45. **Harris, J. C., H. L. DuPont, and R. B. Hornick.** 1972. Fecal leukocytes in diarrheal illness. *Ann. Intern. Med.* **76:**697–703.
46. **Holt, H. A., D. A. Lewis, L. O. White, S. Y. Bastable, and D. S. Reeves.** 1986. Effect of oral ciprofloxacin on the fecal flora of healthy volunteers. *Eur. J. Clin. Microbiol.* **5:**201–205.
47. **Houwen, R. H. J., C. M. A. Bijleveld, and H. G. de Vries-Hospers.** 1987. Ciprofloxacin for cholangitis after hepatic portoenterostomy. *Lancet* **i:**1367.
48. **Hudson, S. J., H. R. Ingham, and M. H. Snow.** 1985. Treatment of *Salmonella typhi* carrier state with ciprofloxacin. *Lancet* **i:**1047.
49. **Jacobson, M. A., S. M. Hahn, J. L. Gerberding, B. Lee, and M. A. Sande.** 1989. Ciprofloxacin for Salmonella bacteremia in the acquired immunodeficiency syndrome (AIDS). *Ann. Intern. Med.* **110:**1027–1029.
50. **Johnson, P. C., C. D. Ericsson, D. R. Morgan, H. L. DuPont, and F. J. Cabada.** 1986. Lack of emergence of resistant fecal flora during successful prophylaxis of traveler's diarrhea with norfloxacin. *Antimicrob. Agents Chemother.* **30:**671–674.
51. **Kazmierczak, A., A. Pechinot, J. M. Duez, O. Haas, and J. P. Favre.** 1987. Biliary tract excretion of ofloxacin in man. *Drugs* **34**(Suppl. 1):39–43.
52. **Keusch, G. T.** 1988. Antimicrobial therapy for enteric infections and typhoid fever: state of the art. *Rev. Infect. Dis.* **10**(Suppl. 1):S199–S205.
53. **Ling, J., K. M. Kam, A. W. Lam, and G. L. French.** 1988. Susceptibilities of Hong Kong isolates of multiply resistant *Shigella* spp. to 25 antimicrobial agents, including ampicillin plus sulbactam and new 4-quinolones. *Antimicrob. Agents Chemother.* **32:**20–23.
54. **Löffler, A., and H. G. von Westphalen.** 1986. Successful treatment of chronic salmonella excretor with ofloxacin. *Lancet* **i:**1206.
55. **Lolekha, S., S. Patanachareon, B. Thanangkul, and S. Vibulbandhitkit.** 1988. Norfloxacin versus co-trimoxazole in the treatment of acute bacterial diarrhoea: a placebo controlled study. *Scand. J. Infect. Dis.* **56**(Suppl.):35–45.
56. **Lonka, L., and R. S. Pedersen.** 1987. Ciprofloxacin for cholangitis. *Lancet* **ii:**212.
57. **Ludlam, H. A., I. Barton, L. White, C. McMullin, A. King, and I. Phillips.** 1990. Intraperitoneal ciprofloxacin for the treatment of peritonitis in patients receiving continuous ambulatory peritoneal dialysis (CAPD). *J. Antimicrob. Chemother.* **25:**843–851.
58. **McNulty, C. A. M., J. Dent, and R. Wise.** 1985. Susceptibility of clinical isolates of *Campylobacter pyloridis* to 11 antimicrobial agents. *Antimicrob. Agents Chemother.* **28:**837–838.
59. **Moorhead, P. J., and H. E. Parry.** 1965. Treatment of Sonne dysentery. *Br. Med. J.* **2:**913–915.
60. **Morris, J. G., Jr., J. H. Tenny, and G. L. Drusano.** 1985. In vitro susceptibility of pathogenic *Vibrio* species to norfloxacin and six other antimicrobial agents. *Antimicrob. Agents Chemother.* **28:**442–445.

61. **Murray, B. E.** 1986. Resistance of *Shigella, Salmonella,* and other selected enteric pathogens to antimicrobial agents. *Rev. Infect. Dis.* **8:**S172–S181.
62. **Neill, M. A., S. M. Opal, J. Heelan, R. Giusti, J. E. Cassidy, R. White, and K. H. Mayer.** 1991. Failure of ciprofloxacin to eradicate convalescent fecal excretion after acute salmonellosis: experience during an outbreak in health care workers. *Ann. Intern. Med.* **114:**195–199.
63. **Oberhelman, R. A., F. J. de la Cabada, E. V. Garibay, J. M. Bitsura, and H. L. DuPont.** 1987. Efficacy of trimethoprim/sulfamethoxazole in the treatment of acute diarrhea in a Mexican pediatric population. *J. Pediatr.* **110:**960–965.
64. **O'Hare, M. D., D. Felmingham, G. L. Ridgway, and R. N. Grüneberg.** 1985. The comparative *in vitro* activity of twelve 4-quinolone antimicrobials against enteric pathogens. *Drugs Exp. Clin. Res.* **11:**253–257.
65. **Pecquet, S., A. Andremont, and C. Tancrède.** 1987. Effect of oral ofloxacin on fecal bacteria in human volunteers. *Antimicrob. Agents Chemother.* **31:**124–125.
66. **Petruccelli, B. P., G. S. Murphy, J. L. Sanchez, S. Walz, R. DeFraites, J. Gelnett, L. Haberberger, P. Echeverria, and D. N. Taylor.** 1992. Treatment of traveler's diarrhea with ciprofloxacin and loperamide. *J. Infect. Dis.* **165:**557–560.
67. **Pichler, H. E. T., G. Diridl, K. Stickler, and D. Wolf.** 1987. Clinical efficacy of ciprofloxacin compared with placebo in bacterial diarrhea. *Am. J. Med.* **82**(Suppl. 4A)**:**329–335.
68. **Rademaker, C. M., I. M. Hoepelman, M. J. Wolfhagen, H. Beumer, M. Rosenberg-Arska, and J. Verhoef.** 1989. Results of a double-blind placebo-controlled study using ciprofloxacin for prevention of travelers' diarrhea. *Eur. J. Clin. Microbiol. Infect. Dis.* **8:**690–694.
69. **Ramirez, C. A., J. L. Bran, C. R. Mejia, and J. F. Garca.** 1985. Open, prospective study of the clinical efficacy of ciprofloxacin. *Antimicrob. Agents Chemother.* **28:**128–132.
70. **Rautelin, H., O. Renkonen, and T. U. Kosunen.** 1991. Emergence of fluoroquinolone resistance in *Campylobacter jejuni* and *Campylobacter coli* in subjects from Finland. *J. Antimicrob. Chemother.* **35:**2065–2069.
71. **Rogerie, F., D. Ott, J. Vandepitte, L. Verbist, P. Lemmens, and I. Habiyaremye.** 1986. Comparison of norfloxacin and nalidixic acid for treatment of dysentery caused by *Shigella dysenteriae* type 1 in adults. *Antimicrob. Agents Chemother.* **29:**883–886.
72. **San Joaquin, V. H., R. K. Scribner, D. A. Pickett, and D. F. Welch.** 1986. Antimicrobial susceptibility of *Aeromonas* species isolated from patients with diarrhea. *Antimicrob. Agents Chemother.* **30:**794–795.
73. **Shungu, D. L., D. R. Nalin, R. H. Gilman, H. H. Gadebusch, A. T. Cerami, C. Gill, and B. Weissberger.** 1987. Comparative susceptibilities of *Campylobacter pylori* to norfloxacin and other agents. *Antimicrob. Agents Chemother.* **31:**949–950.
74. **Shungu, D. L., E. Weinberg, and H. H. Gadebusch.** 1983. In vitro antimicrobial activity of norfloxacin (MK-0366, AM-715) and other agents against gastrointestinal tract pathogens. *Antimicrob. Agents Chemother.* **23:**86–90.
75. **Smith, J. A.** 1991. Treatment of intra-abdominal infections with quinolones. *Eur. J. Clin. Microbiol. Infect. Dis.* **10:**330–333.
76. **Soriano, G., C. Guarner, M. Teixidó, J. Such, J. Barrios, J. Enríquez, and F. Vilardell.** 1991. Selective intestinal decontamination prevents spontaneous bacterial peritonitis. *Gastroenterology* **100:**477–481.
77. **Stone, J. W., R. Wise, I. A. Donovan, and J. Gearty.** 1988. Failure of ciprofloxacin to eradicate *Campylobacter pylori* from the stomach. *J. Antimicrob. Chemother.* **22:**92–93.
78. **Tapson, J. S., K. E. Orr, J. C. George, E. Stansfield, A. J. Blint, and M. K. Ward.** 1990. A comparison between ciprofloxacin and intraperitoneal vancomycin and netilmicin in CAPD peritonitis. *J. Antimicrob. Chemother.* **26**(Suppl. F)**:**63–71.
79. **Van Caekenberghe, D. L., and J. Breyssens.** 1987. In vitro synergistic activity between bismuth subcitrate and various antimicrobial agents against *Campylobacter pyloridis. Antimicrob. Agents Chemother.* **31:**1429–1430.
80. **Van der Auwera, P. V., and B. Scorneaux.** 1985. In vitro susceptibility of *Campylobacter jejuni* to 27 antimicrobial agents and various combinations of $\beta$-lactams with clavulanic acid or sulbactam. *Antimicrob. Agents Chemother.* **28:**37–40.
81. **Vanhoof, R., J. M. Hubrechts, E. Roebben, H. J. Nyssen, E. Nulens, J. Leger, and N. De Schepper.** 1986. The comparative activity of pefloxacin, enoxacin, ciprofloxacin and 13 other antimicrobial agents against enteropathogenic microorganisms. *Infection* **14:**294–298.
82. **Wiström, J., M. Jertborn, S. A. Hedström, K. Alestig, G. Englund, B. Jellheden, and S. R. Norrby.** 1989. Short-term self-treatment of travellers' diarrhea with norfloxacin: a placebo-controlled study. *J. Antimicrob. Chemother.* **23:**905–913.
83. **Wolfson, J. S., and D. C. Hooper.** 1985. The fluoroquinolones: structures, mechanisms of action and resistance, and spectra of activity in vitro. *Antimicrob. Agents Chemother.* **28:**581–586.

*Quinolone Antimicrobial Agents, 2nd ed.*
Edited by David C. Hooper and John S. Wolfson


*Chapter 17*

# Therapy of Respiratory Tract Infections with Quinolone Antimicrobial Agents

*Brian E. Scully*

In 1993, quinolones are widely prescribed as therapy for both community- and nosocomially acquired respiratory tract infections. Also, because of the increasing incidence of tuberculosis due to multiply resistant strains, there is increasing interest in the quinolones as antituberculosis agents.

This chapter begins with a discussion of the microbiological activity and pharmacology of the quinolones as they pertain to the respiratory tract. This discussion is followed by a review of the clinical data. The discussion is confined to those drugs for which clinical data currently exist: ciprofloxacin, ofloxacin, temafloxacin, lomefloxacin, tosufloxacin, sparfloxacin, rufloxacin, and fleroxacin.

## MICROBIOLOGICAL ACTIVITY AND PHARMACOKINETICS

Table 1 summarizes the activities of the major approved and investigational quinolones against classic respiratory pathogens and the gram-negative bacilli commonly encountered in nosocomial pneumonia. In general, MICs of greater than 2 mg/ml should be considered to indicate resistance, but when differences in MICs among various drugs are interpreted, consideration should also be given to differences in pharmacokinetics and penetration into respiratory tract tissue and sputum, as indicated in Table 2 (see also chapters 8 and 9). Because of the high volume of distribution of quinolones, levels in tissue and within cells often exceed concentrations in serum.

The main strength of the quinolones as a group is against the aerobic gram-negative bacilli. There is excellent activity by most of the compounds against *Haemophilus influenzae, Moraxella catarrhalis, Legionella* species, *Escherichia coli, Klebsiella pneumoniae,* and *Enterobacter* spp. Ciprofloxacin is the most active of the quinolones. It inhibits 90% of these species at concentrations of less than 0.5 μg/ml. For the most part, differences in activity against these organisms are minor and of little consequence. Significant differences, however, are found in activities against *Pseudomonas* species. Ciprofloxacin is again the most active, inhibiting most strains of *Pseudomonas aeruginosa* at 1 μg/ml. Though less active, ofloxacin, enoxacin, sparfloxacin, temafloxacin, and tosufloxacin all have useful activity (MIC for 90% of strains, 2 to 8 μg/ml). Against organisms such as *Pseudomonas cepacia* and *Acinetobacter* spp., activity is only modest.

Less auspicious is the activity of the quinolones against the gram-positive pathogens: *Streptococcus pneumoniae, Streptococcus*

**Brian E. Scully** • Infectious Diseases/Epidemiology Division, College of Physicians and Surgeons of Columbia University, 630 West 168th Street, New York, New York 10032.

**Table 1.** Comparative in vitro activities of quinolones against respiratory pathogens

| Organism | $MIC_{90}$ (μg/ml)[a] | | | | | | | | | |
|---|---|---|---|---|---|---|---|---|---|---|
| | CIP | OFL | ENO | PEF | LOM | TEM | SPA | TOS | FUL | FLX |
| *Streptococcus pneumoniae* | 2.0 | 2.0 | 16 | 8.0 | 8 | 1 | 0.25 | 0.25 | 64 | 8 |
| *Streptococcus pyogenes* | 2.0 | 2.0 | 25 | 16 | 8 | 0.5 | 0.5 | 0.25 | 32 | 8 |
| *Staphylococcus aureus* | 1.0 | 0.5 | 3.1 | 0.5 | 2 | 0.5 | 0.25 | 0.06 | 8 | 0.5 |
| *Haemophilus influenzae* | 0.01 | 0.1 | 0.05 | 0.06 | 0.12 | 0.03 | 0.15 | 0.03 | 0.05 | 0.12 |
| *Moraxella catarrhalis* | 0.05 | 0.05 | 0.02 | 0.25 | <0.12 | 0.03 | 0.03 | 0.03 | 2.0 | 0.25 |
| *Neisseria meningitidis* | 0.01 | 0.03 | <0.1 | 0.03 | 0.12 | 0.15 | 0.015 | 0.03 | | 0.06 |
| *Mycoplasma pneumoniae* | 3.1 | 2.0 | 5.0 | | 8 | 2 | | | | |
| *Legionella* spp. | 0.06 | 0.06 | 0.2 | 1.0 | 0.25 | 0.25 | 0.06 | 0.25 | | 0.25 |
| *Chlamydia pneumoniae* | 2 | 1 | 8 | 2 | | 0.5 | 0.125 | | | |
| *Klebsiella* spp. | 0.25 | 1 | 0.8 | 2.0 | 1.0 | 1.0 | 1.0 | | 1 | 0.5 |
| *Pseudomonas aeruginosa* | 0.8 | 4.0 | 3.1 | 8.0 | 8.0 | 4.0 | 2.0 | 2.0 | <128 | 8.0 |
| *Acinetobacter* spp. | 1.0 | 1.0 | 1.0 | 6.3 | 4.0 | 0.25 | 0.5 | 0.06 | 128 | 0.5 |
| *Escherichia coli* | 0.25 | 1.0 | 1.0 | 2.0 | 0.25 | 0.12 | 0.12 | | 4 | |
| *Enterobacter* spp. | 0.2 | 1.0 | 1.0 | 2.0 | 0.5 | 0.5 | 0.25 | | 8 | |
| *Xanthomonas maltophilia* | 8.0 | 8.0 | <8 | | 8.0 | 16 | | 2 | 16 | 8 |
| *Bacteroides* spp. | 16 | 8.0 | 32 | 32 | 32 | 1.0 | 1.0 | | | |
| Peptostreptococci, peptococci | 2.0 | 2.0 | 8.0 | 8.0 | 16 | 0.5 | 4 | | | |
| *Mycobacterium tuberculosis* | 1 | 0.5 | 4 | 4 | 4 | 2.3 | 0.2 | | | |
| *Mycobacterium avium-M. intracellulare* | 128 | 128 | 128 | 64 | 32 | 16 | 12.5 | | | |

[a]Data were compiled from the following references: for ciprofloxacin (CIP), 14, 28, 30–32, 119, 125, and 131; for ofloxacin (OFL), 31, 32, 69, 71, 86, 91, 125, 142, and 144; for enoxacin (ENO), 5, 13, 28, and 69; for pefloxacin (PEF), 26, 95, 126, and 142; for lomefloxacin (LOM), 15 and 142; for temafloxacin (TEM), 4, 31, 51, 90, and 131; for sparfloxacin (SPA), 19 and 66; for tosfloxacin (TOS), 4 and 142; for rufloxacin (RUF), 82; for fleroxacin (FLX), 128, 129, and 142. $MIC_{90}$, MIC for 90% of strains.

**Table 2.** Concentrations of quinolones in serum and respiratory tissues

| Drug | concn in[a]: | | | |
|---|---|---|---|---|
| | Serum (mg/ml) | Bronchial biopsy sample (mg/g) | Lung (mg/g) | Sputum (mg/ml) |
| Ciprofloxacin | | | | |
| 500 mg b.i.d. | 3.1 | 4.4 | 1.2–1.7 | 1.4 |
| 200 mg i.v. | | | | |
| Ofloxacin | | | | |
| 400 mg p.o. | 8.0 | 2.5 | | 5.0 |
| 600 mg p.o. | 8.7 | | 17.7 | |
| Enoxacin, 600 mg p.o. | 2.0 | | 7.0 | 3–7 |
| Pefloxacin | | | | |
| 400 mg i.v. | 7.3 | | 13.8 | |
| 400 mg p.o. | 10–15 | | | 5–13 |
| Temofloxacin, 600 mg p.o. | 9.6 | 14.9 | | |
| Lomefloxacin, 400 mg p.o. | 2.5 | 5.0 | | 4.3 |
| Sparfloxacin, 300 mg p.o. | 1.5–3 | | | 2–3.5 |
| Fleroxacin, 400 mg p.o. | 4–6 | 150% of concn in serum | 150–300% of concn in serum | 90% of concn in serum |

[a]Compiled from references 2, 8, 15, 36, 49, 55, 70, 90, 93, 107, 132, 138, 139, and 140.

group A, and, increasingly, *Staphylococcus aureus*. Ciprofloxacin and ofloxacin inhibit most strains of *S. pneumoniae* and *Streptococcus pyogenes* at 1 to 2 mg/ml. In the beginning, *S. aureus* was universally susceptible to ciprofloxacin and ofloxacin, but with widespread quinolone use, 20 to 50% or more of strains are now resistant (106, 117, 121, 141). This is particularly the case with methicillin-resistant *S. aureus*. Neither enoxacin nor pefloxacin possesses useful streptococcal activity. Of the experimental agents, tosufloxacin and sparfloxacin have much improved streptococcal activities, inhibiting 90% of strains at less than 0.25 mg/ml.

In general, the established drugs have only weak activities against the obligate anaerobes and peptostreptococci. Many strains are moderately susceptible, however, to some of the newer compounds, e.g., tosufloxacin, sparfloxacin, and temafloxacin.

Of great interest are the activities of many of the fluoroquinolones against mycoplasmas, chlamydiae, and mycobacteria. Ofloxacin appears to be the best of the compounds approved for use in the United States. It inhibits most strains of *Mycoplasma pneumoniae* at 1 to 2 μg/ml (91, 131), *Chlamydia pneumoniae* at 1 μg/ml (30, 31), and *Mycobacterium tuberculosis* at 1 to 2 μg/ml (125, 144). Sparfloxacin inhibits both *C. pneumoniae* and *M. tuberculosis* at 0.2 μg/ml. Most strains of *Mycobacterium avium-Mycobacterium intracellulare* are resistant, and ciprofloxacin and sparfloxacin are the most active of the quinolones against this complex.

Combinations of quinolones with other agents have been extensively studied (87, 89). In vitro combinations of rifampin with quinolones tested against *S. aureus* can show synergy, indifference, or antagonism, but synergy is often demonstrable in actual experiments. Combinations of ß-lactams and quinolones used against *Pseudomonas* spp. are synergistic for 20 to 50% of isolates. Combinations with aminoglycosides, however, are not synergistic.

Many studies have investigated the penetration of the fluoroquinolones into sputum and bronchial or lung tissue. Some representative results are tabulated in Table 2. In general, concentrations in sputum are close to the peak concentrations in serum, but in pulmonary tissue, concentrations are often severalfold higher than those in serum. Very high concentrations have also been found within leukocytes, including alveolar macrophages. Wise et al. (139, 140) and Perea (93), for example, have found the concentrations of ciprofloxacin, ofloxacin, and temafloxacin within alveolar macrophages to be at least 10-fold higher than in extracellular fluid.

## CLINICAL STUDIES

The criteria for assessment of clinical efficacy among many studies varied but usually included the categories of cure, improvement, and failure. In general, successful outcomes (and the clinical responses listed in Tables 3 through 11) were considered by authors of the studies as cure or improvement. Bacteriologic responses indicated eradication of the presumed pathogen from sputum, bronchial secretions, or, in some cases, blood. Durations of therapy were generally 7 to 14 days.

### Ofloxacin

Ofloxacin for the therapy of lower respiratory tract infections has been evaluated in many comparative and open studies. The results are summarized in Table 3.

In the initial studies, bacteriologic data were sparse, but ofloxacin given orally (p.o.) showed efficacy similar to the efficacies of trimethoprim-sulfamethoxazole (86) and doxycycline (50) and superior to that of cefaclor (35). Improved activity against *H. influenzae* and *P. aeruginosa* appeared to account for the good results. Forsberg et al. (33) more recently compared ofloxacin (200 mg given twice daily [b.i.d.]) with erythromycin (500

**Table 3.** Comparative trials of oral ofloxacin given for treatment of lower respiratory tract infections

| Reference | Diagnosis | Treatment[a] | Response (no. of patients cured/no. treated [%]) | |
|---|---|---|---|---|
| | | | Clinical | Bacteriologic |
| 35 | Bronchitis (acute, 37; chronic, 172) | OFL, 200 mg b.i.d. | 82/103 (80) | 90/103 (87) |
| | | CEF, 250 mg t.i.d. | 52/105 (50) | 50/105 (48) |
| 86 | Bronchitis | OFL, 100–400 mg b.i.d. | 26/32 (81) | |
| | | TMP-SMX, 960 mg b.i.d. | 24/28 (86) | |
| | Pneumonia | OFL, 100–400 mg b.i.d. | 18/19 (95) | |
| | | TMP-SMX, 960 mg b.i.d. | 22/24 (92) | |
| 50 | Bronchitis | OFL, 200–400 mg b.i.d. | 47/52 (90) | |
| | | DOX, 100 mg b.i.d. | 33/36 (92) | |
| | Pneumonia | OFL, 200–400 mg b.i.d. | 60/62 (97) | |
| | | DOX, 100 mg b.i.d. | 62/69 (90) | |
| 33 | Pneumonia | OFL, 200 mg b.i.d. | 28/33 (85) | Insufficient data |
| | | ERY, 500 mg b.i.d. | 28/34 (82) | |
| 97 | Chronic bronchitis | OFL, 400 mg q.d. | 41/40 (84) | 18/23 (78) |
| | | AMOX-CLA, 500 mg t.i.d. | 41/46 (89) | 14/19 (75) |
| 104 | Pneumonia | OFL, 400 mg b.i.d., | 69/69 (100) | 69/69 (100) |
| | | i.v. therapy | 61/64 (93) | 61/64 (93) |

[a]For most studies, the duration of therapy was 1 to 14 days. OFL, ofloxacin; CEF, cefaclor; AMOX-CLA, amoxicillin-clavulanate; TMP-SMX, trimethoprim-sulfamethoxazole; DOX, doxycycline; ERY, erythromycin; q.d., once a day.

mg) in the treatment of community-acquired nonlobar pneumonia. The two drugs were equally effective. Interestingly, satisfactory responses were noticed in 9 of 10 patients with *M. pneumoniae* who received ofloxacin. Rademaker et al. (97), using 400 mg of ofloxacin once daily, observed excellent responses to amoxicillin-clavulanate in patients with acute exacerbations of chronic bronchitis: *S. pneumoniae* persisted in three of five patients treated with ofloxacin but in only one of six treated with amoxicillin-clavulanate. Finally, Sanders et al. (104) compared oral ofloxacin with standard parenteral therapies in patients requiring admission for community-acquired pneumonia. All of the 69 patients in the ofloxacin group and 61 of 64 in the control group had favorable responses to therapy. Included in the ofloxacin group were 22 patients harboring *S. pneumoniae*; 3 of these patients were bacteremic.

The results of open trials are summarized in Table 4. Grassi et al. (45) reported the results of a large multicenter Italian trial, and Saito et al. (102) summarized the Japanese experience with oral ofloxacin. Excellent responses were obtained in cases in which *H. influenzae* or enteric gram-negative bacilli were cultured. *P. aeruginosa* commonly and *S. pneumoniae* occasionally persisted in the sputum. Information regarding relapses or superinfections was not given. Maesen et al. (79) treated 113 patients who had exacerbations of chronic bronchitis with several dosage regimens of ofloxacin (400 to 1,200 mg daily). They reported a clinical response rate of 72% at 1 week after completion of therapy. Failures were due to the persistence of *S. pneumoniae* and, less frequently, *Pseudomonas* species. The best results were obtained when ofloxacin was given as a single daily dose of 800 mg, probably because of higher concentrations of ofloxacin in the sputum. Minor increases in ofloxacin MICs for *S. pneumoniae* and *P. aeruginosa* were noted.

**Table 4.** Open trials of oral ofloxacin given for treatment of lower respiratory tract infections

| Reference | Diagnosis (no. of patients)[a] | Treatment[b] | Response (no. of patients cured/no. treated [%]) | |
|---|---|---|---|---|
| | | | Clinical | Bacteriologic |
| 45 | Lower RTI: pneumonia (234), bronchitis (381), pleurisy (18), lung abscess (4), other (30) | 200, 300, or 400 mg b.i.d. | 612/667 (92) | 287/370 (78): *S. aureus*, 40/47 (85); *H. influenzae*, 11/11 (100); *Klebsiella* spp., 18/20 (90); *P. aeruginosa*, 36/69 (52) |
| 102 | Lower RTI | 300–600 mg q.d. | 418/553 (76) | 279/377 (74): *S. aureus*, 16/20 (80); *S. pneumoniae*, 26/34 (76); *E. coli*, 11/11 (100); *Klebsiella* spp., 25/27 (93); *P. aeruginosa*, 32/99 (32); *H. influenzae*, 99/102 (97) |
| | Chronic bronchitis | | 150/182 (82) | |
| | Panbronchiolitis | | 56/80 (70) | |
| | Secondary infection, chronic respiratory disease | | 28/38 (74) | |
| | Pneumonia | | 102/127 (80) | |
| | Lung abscess | | 4/7 (57) | |
| | Pyothorax | | 1/2 (50) | |
| 79 | Bronchitis | 800–1,200 mg q.d. | 82/113 (73) | See text |
| 39 | Lower RTI | | 22/25 (88) | |
| | Bronchitis | 200 mg b.i.d. for 10 days | 14/16 (88) | 13/16 (81) |
| | Pneumonia | 400 mg b.i.d. for 21 days | 7/7 (100) | 7/7 (100) |
| | Lung abscess | 400 mg b.i.d. for 21 days | 1/2 (50) | 1/2 (50) |
| 109 | Lower RTI | 400 mg b.i.d. | 21/21 (100) | 16/21 (76) |
| 12 | Pneumonia | 200 mg p.o. t.i.d. | 112/117 (96) | 117/117 (100) |
| 83 | *Pseudomonas* bronchitis | 800 p.o. b.i.d. for 7 days | 35/40 (88) | 23/40 (58) |

[a]RTI, respiratory tract infection.
[b]q.d., once a day.

The studies by Giamarellou and Tsagarakis (39) and Scully et al. (109) showed good clinical efficacy of ofloxacin in patients bronchitis and pneumonia, but the persistence of *P. aeruginosa* with the development of resistance to ofloxacin was noted in the latter study. More recently, a multicenter trial from France (12) found ofloxacin (200 mg given p.o. three times a day [t.i.d.]) to be very effective in community-acquired pneumonia: 24 of 27 pneumococcal infections were cured, as were 88 of 90 nonpneumococcal infections. A number of *Legionella*, mycoplasma, and chlamydia cases diagnosed serologically were cured.

In an effort to achieve improved results against *P. aeruginosa*, Meek et al. (83) used ofloxacin (800 mg twice daily) to treat acute exacerbations of chronic bronchitis due to *P. aeruginosa*. At this dosage, peak levels in serum would be expected to be between 10 and 20 $\mu$g/ml. Of 40 patients, 35 had initial eradication of the organism and good clinical response, but in 5, the organism recurred in association with sputum purulence 1 week following therapy. In an additional six, a new pathogen was cultured in association with symptoms. Interestingly, resistance did not develop in this study, and hardly any toxicity was noted despite the very high dosage of ofloxacin.

There have been few complete reports of the efficacy of intravenous (i.v.) ofloxacin in treatment of patients with respiratory tract infections. A multicenter French study (76) utilized 200 mg twice daily to treat 273 patients, 40 of whom had infections of the lower respiratory tract. Twenty-two infections were nosocomially acquired, and 29 of the patients were being artificially ventilated. Satisfactory bacteriologic and clinical responses were noted in 33 (75%) of 44 evaluable patients. Kushner et al. (73a) used sequential i.v. and p.o. ofloxacin to treat community-acquired pneumonia. Satisfactory responses were realized in 25 or 26 patients, including 16 of 17 patients harboring *S. pneumoniae*.

## Ciprofloxacin

Ciprofloxacin has been extensively studied as a therapy for infections of the lower respiratory tract. Comparative studies (Table 5) of patients mainly with bronchitis show that oral ciprofloxacin is at least equivalent to trimethoprim-sulfamethoxazole (81), doxycycline (3), ampicillin (143), amoxicillin (145), and amoxicillin-clavulanate (108) and is superior to cephalexin in achieving clinical improvement and sterilization of the sputum. In these studies, the efficacy of ciprofloxacin was about equivalent to the efficacies of the comparison drugs against gram-positive pathogens such as *S. pneumoniae*. It was superior, however, to the efficacies of ampicillin, cephalexin, and cefaclor against the gram-negative bacilli. Dosages of ciprofloxacin were 500 or 750 mg b.i.d.

The results of a number of open studies of oral ciprofloxacin are summarized in Table 6. Good response rates were noted in patients with bronchitis, pneumonia, or bronchiectasis, although bacteriologic data were often lacking. Bacteriologic cure rates were above 90% for patients harboring *H. influenzae*, *M. catarrhalis*, or enteric gram-negative rods. *P. aeruginosa*, as expected, was always a problematic organism. Persistence of the organism or clinical relapse associated with the development of resistance were common phenomena (29, 62). Infections due to *S. pneumoniae* and *S. aureus* were also problematic. Bacteriologic cure rates were as low as 60% in some of the studies, though clinical response rates were better. Pneumococcal bacteremia and meningitis have, in fact, occurred during ciprofloxacin therapy (18).

Ciprofloxacin given i.v. has also been extensively studied in both comparative and open trials (Table 7). Comparison drugs have included imipenem (78) and, more extensively, ceftazidime (47, 66, 77, 84). Most patients have been seriously ill with pneumonia, often nosocomial. Typically, ciprofloxacin was given i.v. in dosages of 100 to 200 mg every 12 h (q12h) for several days

**Table 5.** Comparative trials of oral ciprofloxacin given for treatment of lower respiratory tract infections

| Reference | Diagnosis | Treatment[a] | Response (no. of patients cured/no. treated [%]) | |
|---|---|---|---|---|
| | | | Clinical | Bacteriologic |
| 143 | Bronchitis | CIP, 750 mg b.i.d. | 41/42 (98) | 40/42 (95) |
| | | AMP, 500 mg q.i.d. | 40/45 (89) | 30/40 (75) |
| 40 | Pneumonia or bronchitis | CIP, 500 mg | 21/26 (81) | 15/18 (83) |
| | | AMX, 250 mg t.i.d. | 18/22 (82) | 8/13 (62) |
| 81 | Pneumonia or bronchitis | CIP, 500 mg b.i.d. | 15/15 (100) | 11/15 (73) |
| | | TMP-SMX, 160 mg, 800 mg b.i.d. | 12/15 (80) | 5/12 (42) |
| 3 | Bronchitis | CIP, 250 mg t.i.d. | 53/55 (96) | |
| | | DOX, 100 mg b.i.d. | 55/55 (100) | |
| 30 | Lower respiratory tract infection | CIP, 500 mg b.i.d. | 27/28 (96) | 23/28 (82) |
| | | CEP, 1,000 mg b.i.d. | 22/23 (96) | 14/23 (61) |
| 108 | Bronchitis | CIP, 500 mg b.i.d. | 14/20 (70) | (90) |
| | | AMX-CA, 250 mg t.i.d. | 14/20 (70) | (70) |

[a]Abbreviations: CIP, ciprofloxacin; AMP, ampicillin; AMX, amoxicillin; TMP-SMX, trimethoprim-sulfamethoxazole; DOX, doxycycline; CEP, cephalexin; CLA, clavulanate; q.i.d., four times a day.

and then was given p.o. In general, the experience with the i.v. form has mirrored that with the p.o. form of the drug. Excellent efficacy was noted against members of the family *Enterobacteriaceae* and *H. influenzae,* but *P. aeruginosa* was less often eradicated. Persistence of this organism with the development of resistance, particularly in intubated patients, was common (92). Higher dosages of ciprofloxacin, e.g., 400 mg i.v. q12h, may prove more effective, but data are lacking at this time.

Because of its bactericidal activity and concentration within leukocytes, ciprofloxacin is an attractive drug for the treatment of *Legionella* infections. It has been effective in animal models of infections (52), but published data for humans are few. Unertl et al. (124) successfully treated 8 of 10 critically ill patients with 200 mg of i.v. ciprofloxacin q12h. Several of these patients have previously failed to respond to erythromycin and rifampin. Winter et al. (138) feel that addition of ciprofloxacin to erythromycin-containing regimens has improved the outcome in patients with severe Legionnaire's disease. Hooper et al. (57) had notable successes in two patients who were receiving cyclosporin A. It should be noted, on the other hand, that failures of ciprofloxacin in patients harboring legionellae (with subsequent responses to erythromycin) have also been reported (73).

The clinical efficacy of ciprofloxacin against *M. pneumoniae* and *C. pneumoniae* is unknown. In vitro activity, though borderline, may be useful in view of the high levels of ciprofloxacin achieved in lung and bronchial tissue.

## Enoxacin

Ishigami (59) has summarized the results of the studies of enoxacin in Japan (Table 8). Most patients were treated with 600 mg of enoxacin p.o. daily. Clinical response rates were 80% in patients with pneumonia but only 67% in patients with exacerbations of chronic lung disease. Several other open studies have been published (21, 94, 134). Excellent efficacy rates (95 to 100%) have been noted for infections due to *H. influenzae* or *M. catarrhalis,* but *S. pneumoniae, S. aureus,* and *P. aeruginosa* often persisted.

**Table 6.** Open trials of oral ciprofloxacin given for treatment of lower respiratory tract infections

| Reference | Diagnosis (no. of patients)[a] | Ciprofloxacin therapy[b] | Response (no. of patients cured/no. treated [%]) | |
|---|---|---|---|---|
| | | | Clinical | Bacteriologic |
| 68 | Lower RTI (total) | 200–1,200 mg q.d. (most, 300 mg b.i.d.) | 397/542 (73) | 254/391 (65): *S. aureus*, 26/42 (68); *S. pneumoniae*, 29/42 (69); *E. coli*, 7/9 (78); *Klebsiella* spp., 13/17 (76); *H. influenzae*, 109/125 (87); *P. aeruginosa*, 21/94 (22) |
| | Pneumonia | | 89/110 (81) | |
| | Bronchitis | | 149/214 (70) | |
| | Bronchiectasis | | 94/121 (78) | |
| | Panbronchiolitis | | 36/66 (55) | |
| | Other | | 29/31 (94) | |
| 20 | Bronchitis | Total | 42/75 (56) | 43/75 (57) |
| | | 500 mg p.o. b.i.d. | 10/19 (53) | |
| | | 750 mg p.o. b.i.d. | 21/38 (55) | |
| | | 1,000 mg p.o. b.i.d. | 11/18 (61) | |
| 29 | Lower RTI (total) | 500 or 750 mg b.i.d. | 42/42 (100) | 35/42 (83): *S. pneumoniae*, 7/7 (100); *H. influenzae*, 21/21 (100); *P. aeruginosa*, 7/12 (58); beta-hemolytic streptococci, 0/2 (0); *Enterobacteriaceae*, 6/7 (86) |
| | Bronchitis | | 22/22 (100) | |
| | Pneumonia | | 20/20 (100) | |
| 56 | Bronchitis | 500 mg b.i.d. | 26/27 (96) | 22/27 (81): *S. pneumoniae*, 5/9 (56); *H. influenzae*, 14/14 (100); *Enterobacteriaceae*, 7/8 (88) |
| 103 | Pneumonia<br>Bronchitis | 500 mg p.o. b.i.d. | 28/28 (100) | 26/28 (93) |
| 27 | Pneumonia | 750 mg b.i.d. | 25/25 (100) | 19/19 (100) |

[a]RTI, respiratory tract infection.
[b]q.d., once a day.

**Table 7.** Trials of i.v. ciprofloxacin given for treatment of lower respiratory tract infections

| Reference | Diagnosis | Treatment[a] | Response (no. of patients cured/no. treated [%]) | |
|---|---|---|---|---|
| | | | Clinical | Bacteriologic |
| 17 | Pneumonia | 200 mg q12h i.v. followed by 500 q12h p.o. | 73/78 (94) | Inadequate data |
| 78 | Bronchitis | CIP, 100 q8h–12h p.o.<br>IMI, 500 q6h | 17/18 (94)<br>14/24 (58) | |
| 120 | Pneumonia | CIP, 200 i.v. q12h and then 500 q12h p.o.<br>CEF, 2,000 q8h i.v. | 23/23 (100)<br>15/21 (71) | 23/23 (100)<br>19/21 (90) |
| 47 | Bronchitis<br>Pneumonia | CIP, 200 q12h p.o.<br>CEF, 1–2 g q8h i.v. | 36/37 (97)<br>33/34 (97) | 22/35 (63)<br>27/35 (77) |
| 67 | Pneumonia | CIP, 200 mg q12h i.v., then p.o.<br>CEF, 1–2 g q8h i.v. | 60/66 (91)<br>50/50 (90) | 43/46 (93)<br>38/41 (93) |
| 77 | Pneumonia | CIP, 200 mg q12h i.v.<br>CEF, 2 g q8h | 10/14 (71)<br>12/15 (80) | 14/20 (70)<br>12/15 (80) |

[a]IMI, imipenem; CEF, ceftazidime; CIP, ciprofloxacin.

**Table 8.** Trials of oral enoxacin given for treatment of lower respiratory tract infections

| Reference | Diagnosis | Treatment[a] | Response (no. of patients cured/no. treated [%]) | |
|---|---|---|---|---|
| | | | Clinical | Bacteriologic |
| 59 | Pneumonia<br>Bronchitis<br>Chronic respiratory infection | 600 mg q.d. | 44/51 (86)<br>63/82 (77)<br>194/291 (67) | Not given |
| 134 | Bronchitis or bronchiectasis | 400 or 600 mg b.i.d. | 39/43 (91) | 12/20 (60)<br>23/43 (56)<br>*Pseudomonas* spp., 6/23 (26) |
| 21 | Bronchitis | 400 mg b.i.d.<br>600 mg b.i.d. | 7/11 (54)<br>3/6 (50) | Not given |
| 94 | Bronchitis, pneumonia, and bronchiectasis | 400 mg b.i.d. | 17/20 (85) | 10/12 (83) |

[a]q.d., once a day.

One small study compared enoxacin with amoxicillin in acute exacerbations of chronic bronchitis due to gram-negative bacteria (96). The majority of infections were due to *H. influenzae* and *M. catarrhalis*. Similarly, good efficacies were noted, but several superinfections due to *S. pneumoniae* occurred in the enoxacin-treated group.

Overall, these studies show only a modest efficacy for enoxacin in the respiratory tract. Failures occurred most frequently in patients infected by *S. pneumoniae* and *P. aeruginosa*. Adverse interactions with theophylline were common.

## Pefloxacin

Because of the weak activity of pefloxacin against *S. pneumoniae*, the majority of the studies of this drug have been with patients with nosocomially acquired infections. Both i.v. and p.o. preparations have been used (Table 9). Giamarellou et al. compared pefloxacin (i.v. versus p.o.) with ceftazidime

**Table 9.** Trials of pefloxacin given for treatment of lower respiratory tract infections

| Reference | Diagnosis[a] | Treatment[b] | Response (no. of patients cured/no. treated [%])[c] | |
|---|---|---|---|---|
| | | | Clinical | Bacteriologic |
| 38 | Nosocomial pneumonia | PEF, 400 mg q12h i.v., then p.o.<br>CEF, 2 g q8h | 13/14 (93)<br>15/15 (100) | 11/13 (85)<br>10/15 (68) |
| 37 | Nosocomial pneumonia and bronchitis | PEF, i.v. p.o. 400 mg q12h<br>IMI, 500 mg q6h | 23/35 (66)<br>19/36 (53) | 26/35 (74) (R in 9)<br>18/35 (50) (R in 12) |
| 127 | Bronchitis, pneumonia | PEF, 400 mg q12h p.o.<br>CEF, 2 g q12h | 45/69 (65)<br>51/89 (73) | Not given; persistence of streptococci in PEF group |
| 74 | Pneumonia | PEF, 400 mg q12h i.v. | 13/14 (93) | 12/14 (71) |
| 11 | ICU pneumonia | PEF, 400 mg q12h i.v. | 31/34 (91) | Not given; 10 cases involved *S. aureus* |
| 44 | Bronchitis, pneumonia | PEF, 400 mg q12h p.o. | 91/101 (90) | 70/77 (91) (no *S. pneumoniae*) |

[a]ICU, intensive care unit.
[b]PEF, pefloxacin; CEF, ceftazidime; IMI, imipenem.
[c]R, development of bacterial resistance.

(38) and subsequently with imipenem (37) in serious infections caused by gram-negative organisms. In the former study, *P. aeruginosa* was the predominant pathogen. Ceftazidime and pefloxacin gave very similar bacteriologic and clinical results. In the latter study, in which there were very resistant gram-negative bacteria, especially *Acinetobacter* spp., patients treated with pefloxacin had more rapid clinical responses to therapy, higher bacterial eradication rates, and lower rates of development of resistance than those treated with imipenem. The remaining studies (11, 44, 127) confirm the efficacy of pefloxacin in patients with nosocomial pneumonia. Notable among these, Carrington da Costa (11) observed favorable responses in 9 of 10 patients with nosocomial pneumonia due to *S. aureus*. Dosages of pefloxacin in these studies were 400 mg q8h or q12h.

Pefloxacin given p.o. in dosages of 400 mg b.i.d. or 800 mg once daily is effective against bronchitis caused by gram-negative bacteria (6, 80). High clinical failure rates and the development of resistance in *S. pneumoniae* were noted by Maesen et al. (80). In their study, 8 of 13 patients with *S. pneumoniae* failed therapy, and the geometric mean MICs rose from a mean of 3.8 $\mu$g/ml prior to therapy to 8.3 $\mu$g/ml following therapy with pefloxacin. They also observed the rapid development of resistance in *P. aeruginosa*.

Like the other fluoroquinolones, pefloxacin has excellent activity in vitro against *Legionella* spp. and is effective in animal models of infections (25). Dournon et al. (24) performed an in-depth retrospective analysis of cases of severe Legionnaire's disease treated with pefloxacin in Paris. Twenty patients treated with pefloxacin-containing regimens and 40 patients treated with erythromycin-containing regimens could be monitored. Interpretation of the data was difficult because of concomitant therapy. Six of seven patients treated with pefloxacin alone survived, and there was a tendency for an improved outcome in patients treated with pefloxacin-containing regimens (pefloxacin and erythromycin or rifampin). In this regard, a cell model using human macrophages has shown an additive effect against *Legionella* spp. if pefloxacin is combined with either erythromycin or rifampin (130).

## Lomefloxacin

Lomefloxacin is available as an oral preparation, and because of its long half-life (28 h), it can be given once daily. To date, published studies have focused on its efficacy in patients with exacerbations of chronic bronchitis. The results of two large comparative studies have been published (Table 10). Grassi et al. (43) found lomefloxacin (400 mg daily) to be superior to amoxicillin (500 mg t.i.d.) in patients with exacerbations of chronic bronchitis due to gram-negative pathogens. There were, in fact, no patients with *S. pneumoniae* infections in this study. In the second study, lomefloxacin was found to be superior to cefaclor (250 mg t.i.d.) (42). Seventeen strains each of *S. pneumoniae* and *P. aeruginosa* were treated in the lomefloxacin arm of the study. Thirteen strains of each group (76%) were eradicated, a cure rate similar to those for these organisms obtained with other fluoroquinolones. Earlier phase II studies in Japan have shown similar efficacy and a good safety profile for lomefloxacin in patients with bronchitis (53, 60) when dosages of 200 mg t.i.d. were used. Also, this dose of lomefloxacin was superior to cefaclor (500 mg t.i.d.) in the therapy of bronchitis and pneumonia due to gram-negative pathogens (113).

## Temafloxacin

Because of improved activity against streptococci and anaerobic organism, temafloxacin had promised to be a useful addition to the available fluoroquinolones. Indeed, its efficacy in patients with community-acquired bronchitis is at least equivalent and perhaps superior to that of ciprofloxacin (16). Unfortunately, severe and unforeseen toxicities experienced after Food and Drug Administration approval have resulted in its removal from the market (see chapter 26).

## Other Quinolones

A multitude of other quinolones are under clinical study. Several have improved activities against streptococci, which would make them attractive drugs for use against respiratory infections. Only very limited data as to their efficacies and toxicities are available.

### Sparfloxacin

Sparfloxacin is very much more active than ofloxacin and ciprofloxacin against *S. pneumoniae* and anaerobic bacteria (Table 1). It also retains good activity against the gram-negative bacteria. Its long half-life (18 h) al-

**Table 10.** Comparative study of trials of lomefloxacin given for treatment of lower respiratory tract infections

| Reference | Diagnosis | Treatment[a] | Response (no. of patients cured/no. treated [%]) | |
|---|---|---|---|---|
| | | | Clinical | Bacteriologic |
| 43 | Chronic bronchitis | LOM, 400 mg q.d. | 68/78 (87) | 67/81 (83) |
| | | AMX, 500 mg t.i.d. | 57/79 (72) | 59/80 (74) |
| 42 | Chronic bronchitis | LOM, 400 mg q.d. | 136/170 (80) | 139/170 (82) |
| | | CFC, 250 mg t.i.d. | 99/153 (65) | 96/153 (63) |
| 113 | Bronchitis | LOM, 200 mg t.i.d. | | (78) |
| | Pneumonia | CFC, 500 mg t.i.d. | | (62) |

[a]q.d., once a day; LOM, lomefloxacin; AMX, amoxicillin; CFC, cefaclor.

lows for once-daily dosing. Two preliminary reports by Soejima et al. (113a) and Hara et al. (49a) indicate good efficacy compared with that of ofloxacin when 300 mg of sparfloxacin is given once daily to patients with bronchitis and pneumonia due to *S. pneumoniae, H. influenzae,* or *S. aureus.*

### Tosufloxacin

Tosufloxacin has a spectrum and potency similar to those of sparfloxacin and can also be given once daily. A preliminary report (52a) indicates satisfactory efficacy and tolerance of a once-daily dosage in patients with lower respiratory infections.

### Rufloxacin

Rufloxacin has an extremely long half-life (35 h). A loading dose of 400 mg followed by 200 mg daily has been very effective in patients with bronchitis, with very high eradication rates for *S. pneumoniae* (23, 81a) despite rather weak in vitro activity, with a MIC for 90% of strains of 64 μg/ml (Table 1).

### Fleroxacin

The activity of fleroxacin against *S. pneumoniae* is only borderline, with many strains requiring 4 or 8 μg/ml for inhibition. Lung and bronchial penetrations are excellent, however, and may offset its disadvantages. One preliminary report of a large study from Germany (123) tends to confirm this and showed fleroxacin (400 mg once daily) to be significantly better than 500 mg of amoxicillin t.i.d. in the therapy of bronchitis. Adverse events, e.g., nausea and central nervous system toxicity, were more frequent in those patients given fleroxacin. A second preliminary report found fleroxacin (400 mg once daily) to be equivalent to ofloxacin (200 mg t.i.d.) in the therapy of pneumonia and bronchitis (48).

## CYSTIC FIBROSIS

Chronic infection of the lower respiratory tract by *P. aeruginosa* is a major complication of cystic fibrosis. By a complex interplay of direct toxic and indirect immune-system-mediated damage to the lung, respiratory failure eventually develops. Recent studies have attested to the benefits of anti-*Pseudomonas* therapy, which produces a temporary improvement in the symptoms of pulmonary infection and also seems to slow the progression of lung disease. The antipseudomonal quinolones, by virtue of their good oral absorption, have the potential to reduce the frequency and length of hospitalization for patients with cystic fibrosis. To date, ciprofloxacin and ofloxacin have been studied.

Before the clinical studies are reviewed, brief mention should be made of the pharmacokinetics of the quinolones in patients with cystic fibrosis (see also chapter 10). Ciprofloxacin has been the most extensively studied of the quinolones in this regard. Most of the studies in which controls were used showed an increased rate of elimination of the drug (7, 22, 75, 114). In one study, the serum elimination half-life was about 3.9 h in patients with cystic fibrosis compared with 4 to 9 h in controls (75). There was also a tendency for the maximal concentration in serum to be reduced. Similar results have been found for ofloxacin (46), pefloxacin (114), and fleroxacin (85) but not in the single study of enoxacin (115). The kinetics of the fluoroquinolones are similar to those of the other antimicrobial agents used for patients with cystic fibrosis. Dosage should be in the upper range and perhaps at an increased frequency, e.g., ciprofloxacin at 500 to 750 mg q8h to q12h and ofloxacin at 400 to 600 mg q12h.

### Ciprofloxacin

Table 11 summarizes the results of seven studies in which oral ciprofloxacin use in the treatment of adults with cystic fibrosis was evaluated. The majority of patients received either 500 mg p.o. t.i.d. or 750 mg p.o. b.i.d. for 2 to 3 weeks. Several patients received longer courses of therapy. These studies show that if susceptible organisms are present, ciprofloxacin is effective in treating pulmonary exacerbations, as judged by changes in clinical symptoms and pulmonary function tests. One study compared the efficacies of p.o. and i.v. ciprofloxacin in equivalent dosages (116). There was little to choose between the two, with a tendency for the p.o. forms to be more effective. In the comparative studies with azlocillin-aminoglycoside, improvement was similar in both groups except in the study by Hodson et al. (54), in which improvement appeared to be more sustained in patients treated with ciprofloxacin. The development of resistance in *P. aeruginosa* during therapy was usual but not uncommonly resolved after treatment was stopped. Resistance is more pronounced in patients receiving longer courses of therapy (>3 weeks). Patients retreated with ciprofloxacin did not always respond as well as during the first course. The reasons for some of these failures were unclear, as resistance was not always detected. No serious toxicity was noted in any of these studies.

Two additional comparative studies are noteworthy. Jensen et al. (62) compared the efficacy of a tobramycin–ß-lactam combination with that of oral ciprofloxacin or ofloxacin in 26 patients. At 3-month intervals, patients received two courses of the combination followed by two courses of the quinolones and, finally, two more courses of the combination. Improvement was noted during all courses but was more marked during the combination therapy. This was particularly true for the most severely affected patients. In the other study, Schaad et al. (105) gave ciprofloxacin for 4 weeks in a follow-up to a standard intravenous regimen with 42 patients. After the i.v. therapy, *Pseudomonas* sp. was temporarily eradicated from the sputum of 64% of patients. During ciprofloxacin therapy, clinical improvement was maintained, but relapse of *Pseudomonas* colonization occurred in one-half of the patients. The authors compared this outcome to a previous study in which the same i.v. regimen was followed by a p.o. regimen (amoxicillin-clavulanate or cefaclor) of a drug(s) not active against *P. aeruginosa.* Colonization relapsed quickly in nearly all of the patients, but in this case, it was associated with deterioration of clinical and pulmonary functions almost to baseline.

Experience with young children with cystic fibrosis has been limited because of the fears of quinolone-induced cartilage damage and arthropathy. Reports thus far indicate that these are infrequent but definite complications of therapy (1, 61, 64, 98). Also of concern is interstitial nephritis, which has been reported from one pediatric center (118).

Ciprofloxacin is thus an effective, well-tolerated therapy of pulmonary exacerbations of cystic fibrosis associated with *P. aeruginosa.* There are well-founded concerns about the development of resistance with prolonged and repeated use. Because of this, therapeutic courses should be limited to 10 to 20 days and ciprofloxacin probably should not be used in consecutive exacerbations. In the more severely affected patients who relapse frequently, it may be worthwhile to follow ß-lactam–aminoglycoside therapy with several weeks of oral ciprofloxacin. There are no good data on using ciprofloxacin in combination with either ß-lactams or aminoglycosides, though it may be synergistic with the former compounds against some isolates.

## Ofloxacin

Because of its inferior antipseudomonal activity in vitro, ofloxacin has been studied less extensively than ciprofloxacin in patients with cystic fibrosis. Kurz et al. (72) compared ofloxacin (400 mg p.o. b.i.d.) with ciprofloxacin (500 mg p.o. b.i.d.) for 10 days. Twenty patients each were treated. Results were similar, with two-thirds responding

**Table 11.** Oral ciprofloxacin given for treatment of lower respiratory tract infections in patients with cystic fibrosis

| Reference | Design[a] | No. of patients | Outcome | Resistance |
|---|---|---|---|---|
| 10 | Randomized, CIP (750 mg b.i.d.) vs AZL + TOB | 20 (10 vs 10) | Equivalent clinical and bacterial responses; 8/9 (CIP) vs 7/10 (AZL + TOB) | None |
| | | | Equivalent; 24/26 vs 11/11 | 1 *Pseudomonas cepacia* strain |
| 101 | Open comparative, CIP (750 mg p.o. b.i.d. for 14 days) vs AZL + TOB i.v. | 23 (37 courses) | Equivalent; 24/26 vs 18/20; improvement sustained longer in CIP-treated patients | 20%; not sustained; similar in both groups |
| | Controlled, CIP (500 mg p.o. b.i.d.) vs AZL + TOB i.v. | 40 | | |
| 112 | Randomized comparison, CIP (750 mg p.o. b.i.d. for 14 days) vs CIP (1,000 mg p.o. b.i.d. for 14 days) | 29 (14 vs 15) | Equivalent; 62% substantial improvement | 45% |
| 41 | Open (750 mg p.o. q8h for 21 days) | 30 | All responded | Elevated MICs in all patients for *P. aeruginosa* |
| 110 | Open (750 mg p.o. q8h–12h) | 18 (39 courses) | Overall, 82% improved, 96% to first course | 50% |
| 116 | Open, p.o. 30 mg/kg/day; i.v., 12 mg/kg/day | 20 (25 courses of therapy) | 11/13 vs 11/12 improved | Uncommon |

[a] Abbreviations: CIP, ciprofloxacin; AZL, azlocillin; TOB, tobramycin.

to either therapy. Jensen et al. (63) reported a double-blind crossover study in which ofloxacin (500 mg p.o. b.i.d.) was compared with ciprofloxacin (750 mg p.o. b.i.d.). Similar response rates of 91 and 96%, respectively, were observed. Resistance to both agents occurred during therapy but resolved within 3 months. As part of a large, open study, Scully et al. (109) treated 10 patients. Seven responded clinically, but resistance in *P. aeruginosa* was noted frequently. On the basis of limited data, it appears that ofloxacin will prove to be effective in the therapy of exacerbations of cystic fibrosis lung disease due to susceptible *P. aeruginosa*. The development of resistance occurs as with ciprofloxacin.

## TUBERCULOSIS

In view of the good activity of some quinolones against *M. tuberculosis* and the rising incidence of isoniazid- and rifampin-resistant strains, there has been much interest in the use of quinolones as antituberculous agents. Because of its better absorption and longer half-life, ofloxacin has been used more extensively than ciprofloxacin. In most of the studies, concomitant effective therapy is also given, making it difficult to accurately assess the contribution of ofloxacin to the regimen. Sputum conversion rates have varied between 15 and 90% by the fourth month of therapy (9, 88, 122, 144). Resistance has been well described, particularly in those patients with persistently positive smears and those receiving no other active agents. The optimal dosage is probably 600 to 800 mg given as a single daily dose. Tolerance is good, i.e., much better than with the other second-line agents.

Ichiyama and Tsukamura (58) and Yew et al. (145) have reported several patients with cavitary lung disease due to *Mycobacterium fortuitum* who were successfully treated with ofloxacin (300 to 600 mg daily) as the sole therapy.

## TOXICITY

While overall the new quinolones have been well tolerated in patients with respiratory tract infections, there is concern about toxicity as a result of interactions with theophylline (see also chapter 11). Wijnands et al. (135) have shown that enoxacin reduces the clearance of theophylline, leading to increased theophylline concentrations in serum and the potential for toxicity. Headaches, hallucinations, and even convulsions have occurred in some patients receiving both enoxacin and theophylline. A similar but milder interaction with ciprofloxacin has been noted by some investigators. Raoff et al. (99) noted elevations of serum theophylline into the toxic range for 6 of 33 patients receiving theophylline and ciprofloxacin. Milder elevations were noted in 14 patients. Theophylline toxicity has not been noted in the other clinical studies of ciprofloxacin, however. Wijnands et al. (137) studied healthy volunteers and concluded that ciprofloxacin and pefloxacin as well as enoxacin reduce theophylline clearance and cause elevations of theophylline concentrations in serum.

On the other hand, extensive studies of ofloxacin (34, 137), lomefloxacin (133), and temafloxacin (100) have failed to reveal any adverse interactions with theophylline.

## CONCLUSIONS

It is clear that the fluoroquinolones are an effective therapy for lower respiratory tract infections due to a variety of different pathogens. Clinical and bacteriologic response rates are generally in the 75 to 90% range and are at least equivalent to those obtained with the comparison agents. Ciprofloxacin and ofloxacin are the most thoroughly studied of the fluoroquinolones.

### Ciprofloxacin

Ciprofloxacin given i.v. or p.o. is highly effective against bacterial bronchitis, bronchiectasis, or pneumonia due to *H. influenzae, M. catarrhalis,* and enteric gram-negative rods. In these conditions it has proved to be equivalent and sometimes superior to the oral cephalosporins, amoxicillin-clavulanate, the third-generation cephalosporins, and imipenem. It is less effective than the ß-lactams against pneumococcal infections, and indeed, pneumococcal bacteremia and meningitis have developed during ciprofloxacin therapy. Ciprofloxacin is effective clinically but not bacteriologically in infections due to *P. aeruginosa,* and it can be given p.o., which is an enormous advantage in many situations. Severe infections due to this organism still are probably best treated with two drugs, one of which could be ciprofloxacin in maximal dosage. Data on legionellosis, though limited, are very encouraging. Resistance developing during therapy is a major difficulty with *P. aeruginosa* and *S. aureus.* Resistance may also occur in *S. pneumoniae* strains and is increasingly being described with the enteric gram-negative rods.

What, then, is the place of ciprofloxacin in the therapy of respiratory tract infections? The most obvious place is in the therapy of nosocomial, gram-negative bronchopneumonia. Depending on local antibiograms, it could be included as part of an empiric program or as an oral follow-up to some i.v. regimen once the cultures had returned. Caution is advisable because of the potential for selecting resistant strains in intubated patients and in patients with infections due to *P. aeruginosa.* For community-acquired infections, since *S. pneumoniae* is the predominant pathogen, other agents are generally preferable unless the Gram strain or history strongly suggests a gram-negative pathogen. For *Legionella* infections, ciprofloxacin appears to be an effective alternative to erythromycin and might be considered for initial therapy in certain groups of patients, e.g., transplant recipients taking cyclosporin. In patients with cystic fibrosis, ciprofloxacin is best used sparingly: no more than brief, 2- to 3-week courses for exacerbations. Consecutive ciprofloxacin courses should be avoided to minimize the risks of entrenched resistance developing.

### Ofloxacin

The data on ofloxacin are very similar to those on ciprofloxacin except that ofloxacin appears to be a more effective therapy for infections due to *S. pneumoniae.* This difference, coupled with the drug's lack of interaction with theophylline, makes it the quinolone of choice, if one is to be used, in chronic obstructive pulmonary disease. It also seems to be effective against nosocomial infection by gram-negative organisms and against legionellosis, but for the latter, data are less extensive than for ciprofloxacin. When choosing empiric therapy in the hospital, it should be remembered that ofloxacin is two- to fourfold less active than ciprofloxacin against *P. aeruginosa.* Limited data suggest that ofloxacin will be a useful drug in the therapy of multiply-drug-resistant tuberculosis.

### Pefloxacin

Pefloxacin is available only in Europe. Its main place is in the therapy of infections caused by nosocomial gram-negative organisms. It can be given either i.v. or p.o. It has no place in the therapy of community-acquired infections because of its lack of activity against *S. pneumoniae.*

### Enoxacin

Enoxacin is effective in many situations, but its lack of antistreptococcal and antipseudomonal activities coupled with the severe theophylline interaction makes it a generally unsuitable drug for therapy of infection of the respiratory tract.

### Lomefloxacin

Lomefloxacin has the advantage of once-daily dosage. Data on responses in patients with pneumococcal infections are few, and few critically ill patients have been treated. It also does not interact with theophylline. These properties make it a possible alternative to ofloxacin for patients with community-acquired infections.

## REFERENCES


1. **Alfaham, M., M. Holt, and M. C. Goodchild.** 1987. Arthropathy in a patient with cystic fibrosis taking ciprofloxacin. *Br. Med. J.* **295:**699.
2. **Baldwin, D. R., D. Honeybourne, J. M. Andrews, J. P. Ashby, and R. Wise.** 1990. Concentrations of oral lomefloxacin in serum and bronchial mucosa. *Antimicrob. Agents Chemother.* **34:**1017–1019.
3. **Bantz, P. M., J. Goote, W. Peters-Hartel, J. Stahmann, J. Tunin, R. Kasten, and H. Bruck.** 1987. Low-dose ciprofloxacin in respiratory tract infections. A randomized comparison with doxycycline in general practice. *Am. J. Med.* **82**(Suppl. 4A):208–210.
4. **Barry, A. L., and R. N. Jones.** 1989. The in-vitro activities of temafloxacin, tosufloxacin (A-6182) and five other fluoroquinolone agents. *J. Antimicrob. Chemother.* **23:**527–535.
5. **Bauerfeind, A., and U. Ullmann.** 1984. In-vitro activity of enoxacin, norfloxacin and nalidixic acid. *J. Antimicrob. Chemother.* **14**(Suppl. C):33–37.
6. **Benard, Y., A. Arnaud, D. Benhamou, J. F. Muir, G. Lerebours, P. David, G. Nouvet, and J. C. Guerin.** 1989. A single daily dose (800mg) of pefloxacin as second-line therapy for bronchial infections. *Rev. Infect. Dis.* **11**(Suppl. 5):S1226.
7. **Bentour, Y., M. Spino, R. Gold, A. Tesoro, S. Martin, R. Pop, M. Levy, H. Heurter, and S. M. MacLeod.** 1990. Enhanced ciprofloxacin clearance in cystic fibrosis patients. *Clin. Pharmacol. Therapeut.* **47:**185.
8. **Bergogne-Berezin, E.** 1985. Pharmacologic parameters of quinolones in respiratory tract infections. *Quinolones Bull.* **1:**17–19.
9. **Besozzi, G., F. Colombo, P. V. Montellini, and A. Miradoli.** 1991. Use of ofloxacin in mycobacterial lung infections. *Am. Rev. Respir. Dis.* **143:**119.
10. **Bosso, J. A., P. G. Black, and J. M. Matsen.** 1987. Ciprofloxacin versus tobramycin plus azlocillin in pulmonary exacerbations in adult patients with cystic fibrosis. *Am. J. Med.* **82**(Suppl. 4A):180–184.
11. **Carrington da Costa, R. B., J. Pimentel, A. Rebvelo, J. Goncalves, J. Janeiro, D. Costa, T. Macedo, and C. A. Fontes Ribeiro.** 1989. Therapy with pefloxacin for secondary pneumonia in an intensive care unit. *Rev. Infect. Dis.* **11**(Suppl. 5):S1227.
12. **Chidiac, C., O. Leroy, C. Beuscart, B. Le Chevalier, G. Beaucaire, Y. Mouton, and Group Study.** 1989. Efficacy and safety of oral ofloxacin for treatment of pneumonia. *Rev. Infect. Dis.* **11**(Suppl. 5):S1223–S1224.
13. **Chin, N. X., and H. C. Neu.** 1983. In vitro activity of enoxacin, a quinolone carboxylic acid, compared with those of norfloxacin, new ß-lactams, aminoglycosides, and trimethoprim. *Antimicrob. Agents Chemother.* **24:**754–763.
14. **Chin, N. X., and H. C. Neu.** 1984. Ciprofloxacin, a quinolone carboxylic acid compound active against aerobic and anaerobic bacteria. *Antimicrob. Agents Chemother.* **25:**319–326.
15. **Chin, N. X., H. Novelli, and H. C. Neu.** 1988. In vitro activity of lomefloxacin, a difluoroquinolone 3-carboxylic acid, compared with those of other quinolones. *Antimicrob. Agents Chemother.* **32:**656–662.
16. **Chodosh, S.** 1991. Temafloxacin compared with ciprofloxacin in mild-to-moderate lower respiratory tract infections in ambulatory patients: a multi-center, double-blind randomized study. *Chest* **100:**1497–1502.
17. **Chrysanthopoulos, C. J., A. T. Skoutelis, J. C. Starakis, E. D. Anastassiou, and H. P. Bassaris.** 1987. Use of intravenous ciprofloxacin in respiratory tract infections and biliary sepsis. *Am. J. Med.* **82**(Suppl. 4A):357–359.
18. **Cooper, B., and M. Lawlor.** 1989. Pneumococcal bacteremia during ciprofloxacin therapy for pneumococcal pneumonia. *Am. J. Med.* **87:**475.
19. **Cooper, M. A., J. M. Andrew, J. P. Ashby, R. S. Matthews, and R. Wise.** 1990. The in-vitro activity of sparfloxacin, a new quinolone antimicrobial agent. *J. Antimicrob. Chemother.* **36:**667–676.
20. **Davies, B. I., F. P. V. Maesen, C. Bair, and J. P. Teengs.** 1986. Clinical efficacy of various dosage regimens of ciprofloxacin in chronic bronchitis, p. 248–251. *In* H. C. Neu and H. Weuta (ed.), *Proceedings of the 1st International Ciprofloxacin Workshop.* Excerpta Medica, Amsterdam.
21. **Davies, B. I., F. P. V. Maesen, J. P. Teegs, and C. Baur.** 1986. The quinolones in chronic bronchitis. *Pharm. Weekbl.* **8:**53–59.
22. **Davis, R. L., J. R. Koup, J. Williams-Warren, A. Weber, L. Heggen, D. Stempel, and A. L. Smith.** 1987. Pharmacokinetics of ciprofloxacin in cystic fibrosis. *Antimicrob. Agents Chemother.* **31:**915–919.
23. **Dieksen, M., J. Focht, and J. Boerema.** 1991. Rufloxacin once daily in acute exacerbations of chronic bronchitis. *Infection* **19:**297–300.
24. **Dournon, E., C. A. Mayard, M. Wolff, B. Schlemmer, D. Samuel, J. P. Sollet, and P.**

**Levasseur-Rajagopalan.** 1990. Comparison of the activity of three antibiotic regimens in severe Legionnaire's disease. *J. Antimicrob. Chemother.* **26**(Suppl. B):129–140.

25. **Dournon, E., P. Rajagopalan, J. L. Vildé, and J. J. Pocidalo.** 1986. Efficacy of pefloxacin in comparison with erythromycin in the treatment of experimental guinea pig legionellosis. *J. Antimicrob. Chemother.* **17**(Suppl. B):41–48.
26. **Eliopoulos, G. M., and C. T. Eliopoulos.** 1989. Quinolone antimicrobial agents: activity in-vitro, p. 35–70. *In* J. S. Wolfson and D. C. Hooper (ed.), *Quinolone Antimicrobial Agents.* American Society for Microbiology, Washington, D.C.
27. **Ernst, J. A., E. R. Sy, H. Colon-Lucca, N. Sandhu, T. Rallos, and V. Lorian.** 1986. Ciprofloxacin in the treatment of pneumonia. *Antimicrob. Agents Chemother.* **29:**1088–1089.
28. **Fallon, R., and W. Brown.** 1985. In-vitro sensitivity of legionellas, meningococci and mycoplasmas to ciprofloxacin and enoxacin. *J. Antimicrob. Chemother.* **15:**787–789.
29. **Fass, R. J.** 1987. Efficacy and safety of oral ciprofloxacin in the treatment of serious respiratory infections. *Am. J. Med.* **82**(Suppl. 4A):202–207.
30. **Feist, H., N. Vetter, M. Drlicek, I. Otupal, and H. Weuta.** 1986. Comparative study of ciprofloxacin and cephalexin in the treatment of patients with lower respiratory tract infections, p. 165–267. *In* H. C. Neu and H. Weuta (ed.), *Proceedings of the 1st International Ciprofloxacin Workshop.* Excerpta Medica, Amsterdam.
31. **Fenelon, L. E., G. Mumtaz, and G. L. Ridgway.** 1990. The in-vitro antibiotic susceptibility of *Chlamydia pneumoniae. J. Antimicrob. Chemother.* **26:**763–767.
32. **Fenton, C. H., and M. H. Cynamon.** 1986. Comparative in-vitro activity of ciprofloxacin and other 4-quinolones against *Mycobacterium tuberculosis* and *Mycobacterium intracellulare. Antimicrob. Agents Chemother.* **29:**386–388.
33. **Forsberg, P., R. Maller, and L. Nilsson.** 1989. Comparative study of oral ofloxacin and erythromycin in the treatment of pneumonia. *Rev. Infect. Dis.* **11**(Suppl. 5):S1229–S1230.
34. **Fourtillan, J. B., B. Branier, J. Saint-Salvi, A. Salmon, A. Surjus, D. Tremblay, M. Vincent Du Laurier, and S. Beck.** 1986. Pharmacokinetics of ofloxacin and theophylline alone and in combination. *Infection* **14**(Suppl. 1):67–69.
35. **Fujimori, I., Y. Kobayashi, M. Obana, A. Saito, and M. Tomizawa.** 1984. Comparative clinical study of ofloxacin and cefaclor in bacterial bronchitis. *Kansenshogaku Zasshi* **58:**832–861.
36. **Gerding, D. N., and J. A. Hitt.** 1989. Tissue penetration of the new quinolones in humans. *Rev. Infect. Dis.* **2**(Suppl. 5):S1046–S1057.
37. **Giamarellou, H., K. Mandragos, P. Bechrakis, K. Pigas, D. Bilalis, and P. Sfikakis.** 1990. Pefloxacin versus imipenem in the therapy of nosocomial lung infections of intensive care unit patients. *J. Antimicrob. Chemother.* **26**(Suppl. B):117–128.
38. **Giamarellou, H., G. Perdikaris, N. Galanakis, G. Davoulos, K. Mandragos, and P. Sfikakis.** 1989. Pefloxacin versus ceftazidime in the treatment of a variety of gram-negative bacterial infections. *Antimicrob. Agents Chemother.* **33:**1362–1367.
39. **Giamarellou, H., and J. Tsagarakis.** 1987. Efficacy and tolerance of oral ofloxacin in treating various infections. *Drugs* **34**(Suppl. 1):119–123.
40. **Gleadhill, I. C., W. Ferguson, and R. C. Lowry.** 1986. Efficacy and safety of ciprofloxacin in patients with respiratory infections in comparison with amoxycillin. *J. Antimicrob. Chemother.* **18**(Suppl. D):133–138.
41. **Goldfarb, J., R. C. Stern, M. D. Reed, T. S. Yamashita, C. M. Myers, and J. L. Blumer.** 1987. Ciprofloxacin monotherapy for acute pulmonary exacerbations of cystic fibrosis. *Am. J. Med.* **82**(Suppl. 4A):174–179.
42. **Gottfried, M. H., and W. T. Ellison.** 1992. Safety and efficacy of lomefloxacin versus cefaclor in the treatment of acute exacerbations of chronic bronchitis. *Am. J. Med.* **92**(Suppl. 4A):108S–135S.
43. **Grassi, C., C. Albera, and E. Pozzi.** 1992. Lomefloxacin versus amoxicillin in the treatment of acute exacerbations of chronic bronchitis: an Italian multi-center study. *Am. J. Med.* **92**(Suppl. 4A):103S–107S.
44. **Grassi, C., E. Catena, G. de Iola, F. Ginesu, M. Gori, M. Lucchini, P. Mangiarotti, E. Micillo, M. Onoscuri, and O. Orlandi.** 1990. Pefloxacin in lower respiratory tract infections. *J. Antimicrob. Chemother.* **26**(Suppl. B):103–110.
45. **Grassi, C., G. C. Grassi, and P. Mangiarotti.** 1987. A multi-center study on clinical efficacy of ofloxacin in lower respiratory tract infections. *Drugs* **34**(Suppl. 1):80–82.
46. **Grenier, B., R. Thompson, M. Guillot, G. Lenoir, J. Navarro, P. Foucaud, P. Reinert, F. de la Rocque, F. Noel, and J. B. Fourtillan.** 1989. Use of quinolones in cystic fibrosis. *Rev. Infect. Dis.* **11**(Suppl. 5):S1245–S1252.
47. **Haddow, A., S. Greene, G. Heinz, and D. Wantuck.** 1989. Ciprofloxacin (intravenous/oral) versus ceftazidime in lower respiratory tract infections. *Am. J. Med.* **87**(Suppl. 5A):113–115.
48. **Hara, K., R. Soejiina, A. Saito, K. Takede, H. Tanimoto, and K. Shimada.** 1991. Double-blind, controlled study of fleroxacin versus ofloxacin in respiratory infections, abstr. 1813. *Abstr. 17th Int. Congr. Chemother.*
49. **Hara, K., M. Vaku, H. Voga, S. Kohno, and K. Yamaguchi.** 1990. In-vitro activity of spar-

floxacin against major clinical pathogens and its penetration into sputum, abstr. 1254. *Program Abstr. 30th Intersci. Conf. Antimicrob. Agents Chemother.*

49a. **Hara, K., H. Kobayashi, H. Tanimoto, K. Matsumoto, and K. Oizumi.** 1991. A multicenter double blind comparative study of sparfloxacin and ofloxacin in the treatment of chronic respiratory tract infections (RTI), abstr. 878. *Program Abstr. 31st Intersci. Conf. Antimicrob. Agents Chemother.*

50. **Harazin, H., J. Winner, and H. P. Mittermayer.** 1987. An open randomized comparison of ofloxacin and doxycycline in lower respiratory tract infections. *Drugs* **34**(Suppl. 1)**:**71–73.

51. **Hardy, D. J.** 1991. Activity of temafloxacin and other fluoroquinolones against typical and atypical community-acquired respiratory tract pathogens. *Am. J. Med.* **91**(Suppl. 6A)**:**12S–14S.

52. **Havlichek, D., D. Pohlod, and L. Saravolatz.** 1987. Comparison of ciprofloxacin and rifampicin in experimental *Legionella pneumophila* pneumonia. *J. Antimicrob. Chemother.* **20:**875–881.

52a. **Hayashi, H., N. Nashima, S. Kimura, T. Akaogi, M. Sakom, and H. Haratt.** 1991. *Program Abstr. 17th Int. Congr. Chemother.*, abstr. 1843.

53. **Hiraga, Y., K. Kikuchi, and A. Yamamoto.** 1988. A clinical study of NY-198 in respiratory infections. *Chemotherapy* **36**(Suppl. 2, Part 1)**:** 475–479.

54. **Hodson, M. E., C. M. Roberts, R. J. A. Batland, M. J. Smith, and J. Batten.** 1987. Oral ciprofloxacin compared with conventional intravenous treatment for *Pseudomonas aeruginosa* infection in adults with cystic fibrosis. *Lancet* **i:**235–237.

55. **Honeybourne, D., J. M. Andrews, J. P. Ashby, R. Lodwick, and R. Wise.** 1988. Evaluation of the penetration of ciprofloxacin and amoxycillin into the bronchial mucosa. *Thorax* **43:**715–719.

56. **Hoogkamp-Korstanje, J. A. A., and S. Klein.** 1986. Efficacy of ciprofloxacin in ambulatory patients with respiratory tract infections, p. 257–259. *In* H. C. Neu and H. Weuta (ed.), *Proceedings of the 1st International Ciprofloxacin Workshop.* Excerpta Medica, Amsterdam.

57. **Hooper, T. L., F. K. Gould, C. R. Swinburn, G. Featherstone, N. J. Odom, P. A. Corris, R. Freeman, and C. G. A. McGregor.** 1988. Ciprofloxacin: a preferred treatment for Legionella infections in patients receiving cyclosporin A. *J. Antimicrob. Chemother.* **22:**952–953.

58. **Ichiyama, S., and M. Tsukamura.** 1987. Ofloxacin and the therapy of pulmonary disease due to *Mycobacterium fortuitum. Chest* **92:**1110–1112.

59. **Ishigami, J.** 1985. Clinical efficacy of enoxacin by disease. *Res. Clin. Forums* **7:**107–108.

60. **Ito, A., M. Ri, T. Okubo, and Y. Kaminaga.** 1988. Basic and clinical studies on NY-198. *Chemotherapy* **36**(Suppl. 2, Part 2)**:**572–579.

61. **Jawad, A. S.** 1989. Cystic fibrosis and drug-induced arthropathy. *Br. J. Rheumatol.* **28:**179–180.

62. **Jensen, T., S. S. Pedersen, N. Hoiby, and C. Koch.** 1987. Efficacy of oral fluoroquinolones versus conventional intravenous antipseudomonal chemotherapy in treatment of cystic fibrosis. *Eur. J. Clin. Microbiol.* **6:**618–622.

63. **Jensen, T., S. S. Pedersen, C. H. Nielsen, H. Hoiby, and C. Koch.** 1987. The efficacy and safety of ciprofloxacin and ofloxacin in chronic *Pseudomonas aeruginosa* infection in cystic fibrosis. *J. Antimicrob. Chemother.* **20:**585–594.

64. **Jones, R. N.** 1991. Activity of sparfloxacin (AT-4140), PD 127391 and PD 131628 against *Legionella* spp. *J. Antimicrob. Chemother.* **27:**389–390.

65. **Kesseler, A., A. Lacassie, J. P. Hugot, P. Talon, D. Thomas, and L. Astier.** 1989. Arthropathies following the administration of pefloxacin to an adolescent with mucoviscidosis. *Anal. Pediatr.* **36:**275–278.

66. **Khan, F. A., and R. Basir.** 1989. Sequential intravenous-oral administration of ciprofloxacin vs ceftazidime in serious bacterial respiratory tract infections. *Chest* **96:**528–537.

67. **King, A., K. Shannon, and I. Phillips.** 1985. The in-vitro activities of enoxacin and ofloxacin compared with that of ciprofloxacin. *J. Antimicrob. Chemother.* **15:**551–558.

68. **Kobayashi, H.** 1987. Clinical efficacy of ciprofloxacin in the treatment of patients with respiratory infection in Japan. *Am. J. Med.* **82**(Suppl. 4A)**:**169–173.

69. **Kohno, S., H. Koga, M. Kaku, S. Maesaki, and K. Hara.** 1992. Prospective comparative study of ofloxacin or ethambutol for the treatment of pulmonary tuberculosis. *Chest* **102:**1815–1818.

70. **Kovarik, J. M., A. I. M. Hoepelmann, J. M. Smit, P. A. Sips, M. Rozenberg-Arska, J. M. Glerum, and J. Verhoef.** 1992. Steady-state pharmacokinetics and sputum penetration of lomefloxacin in patients with chronic obstructive pulmonary disease and acute respiratory infections. *Antimicrob. Agents Chemother.* **36:**2458–2461.

71. **Kumada, T., and H. C. Neu.** 1985. In-vitro activity of ofloxacin, a quinolone carboxylic acid, compared to other quinolones and other antimicrobial agents. *J. Antimicrob. Chemother.* **16:**563–574.

72. **Kurz, C. C., W. Marget, K. Harms, and R. M. Bertele.** 1986. Kreuzstudie über die Wirksamkeit von Ofloxacin und Ciprofloxacin bei oraler Anwendung. *Infection* **14**(Suppl. 1)**:**82–86.

73. **Kurz, R. W., W. Graninger, T. P. Egger, H. Pichler, and K. H. Tragl.** 1988. Failure of treatment of Legionella pneumonia with ciprofloxacin. *J. Antimicrob. Chemother.* **22**:389–391.

73a. **Kuschner, R., F. Briones, B. E. Scully, and H. C. Neu.** 1989. Evaluation of IV ofloxacin as therapy of acute lower respiratory tract infections, abstr. 547. *Program Abstr. 29th Intersci. Conf. Antimicrob. Agents Chemother.*

74. **Lauwers, S., A. Vincken, A. Naessens, and D. Pierard.** 1986. Efficacy and safety of pefloxacin in the treatment of severe infections in patients hospitalized in intensive care units. *J. Antimicrob. Chemother.* **17**(Suppl. B):111–116.

75. **LeBel, M., M. G. Bergeron, F. Vallée, C. Fiset, G. Chassé, P. Bigonesse, and G. Rivard.** 1986. Pharmacokinetics and pharmacodynamics of ciprofloxacin in cystic fibrosis patients. *Antimicrob. Agents Chemother.* **30**:260–266.

76. **Leroy O., C. Beuscart, B. Sivery, E. Senneville, Y. Mouton, and Groupe D'Etude.** 1989. Efficacy and tolerance of intravenous ofloxacin: a multi-center French study in 273 patients. *Presse Med.* **18**:2050–2054.

77. **Levine, D. P., P. McNeil, and S. A. Lerner.** 1989. Randomized, double-blind comparative study of intravenous ciprofloxacin versus ceftazidime in the treatment of serious infections. *Am. J. Med.* **87**(Suppl. 5A):160–163.

78. **Lode, H., R. Wiley, G. Höffken, J. Wagner, and K. Borner.** 1987. Prospective, randomized, controlled study of ciprofloxacin versus imipenem-cilastatin in severe clinical infections. *Antimicrob. Agents Chemother.* **31**:1491–1496.

79. **Maesen, F. P. V., B. I. Davies, W. H. Geraedts, and C. Baur.** 1987. The use of quinolones in respiratory tract infections. *Drugs* **34**(Suppl. 1):74–79.

80. **Maesen, F. P. V., B. I. Davies, and J. P. Teengs.** 1985. Pefloxacin in acute exacerbations of chronic bronchitis. *J. Antimicrob. Chemother.* **16**:379–388.

81. **Magnani, C., S. Fregni, G. Valli, R. Consentini, and A. Bisseti.** 1985. Comparative efficacy of ciprofloxacin and co-trimoxazole in respiratory tract infections, p. 260–264. *In* H. C. Neu and H. Weuta (ed.), *Proceedings of the 1st International Ciprofloxacin Workshop.* Excerpta Medica, Amsterdam.

81a. **Mattina, R., M. Cesana, and the Italian Multi-Center LRTI-Rufloxacin Groups.** 1991. *Program Abstr. 17th Int. Congr. Chemother.*, abstr. 1846.

82. **Mattina, R., C. E. Cocuzza, M. Cesana, and G. Bonfiglio.** 1991. In-vitro activity of a new quinolone, rufloxacin, against nosocomial isolates. *Chemotherapy* (Basel) **37**:260–269.

83. **Meek, J. C. E., F. P. V. Maesen, and B. I. Davies.** 1989. A prospective study of ofloxacin in acute exacerbations of chronic respiratory diseases associated with *Pseudomonas aeruginosa. J. Antimicrob. Chemother.* **24**:447–453.

84. **Menon, L., J. A. Ernst, E. R. Sy, D. Flores, A. Pacia, and V. Lorian.** 1989. Brief report: sequential intravenous/oral ciprofloxacin compared with intravenous ceftazidome in the treatment of serious lower respiratory tract infections. *Am. J. Med.* **87**(Suppl. 5A):119–120.

85. **Mimeault, J., F. Vallée, R. Seelman, F. Sorgel, M. Ruel, and M. LeBel.** 1990. Altered disposition of fleroxacin in patients with cystic fibrosis. *Clin. Pharmacol. Chemother.* **47**:618–628.

86. **Monk, J. P., and D. M. Campoli-Richards.** 1987. Ofloxacin: a review of its antibacterial activity, pharmacokinetic properties and clinical use. *Drugs* **33**:346–391.

87. **Moody, J. A., D. M. Gerding, and L. R. Peterson.** 1987. Evaluation of ciprofloxacin's synergism with other agents by multiple in-vitro methods. *Am. J. Med.* **82**(Suppl. 4A):44–54.

88. **Nakae, I., K. Nakatani, S. Inoue, K. Takahasi, N. Ikeda, T. Matsumoto, S. Ozawa, M. Sakatani, N. Kita, and S. Tanaka.** 1991. Therapeutic effect of ofloxacin on intractable pulmonary tuberculosis and ofloxacin resistance of tubercle bacilli isolated from the patients. *Kekkaku* **66**:299–307.

89. **Neu, H. C.** 1991. Synergy and antagonism of combinations with quinolones. *Eur. J. Clin. Microbiol. Infect. Dis.* **10**:255–261.

90. **Nye, K., Y. G. Shi, J. M. Andrews, J. P. Ashby, and R. Wise.** 1989. The in-vitro activity, pharmacokinetics and tissue penetration of temafloxacin. *J. Antimicrob. Chemother.* **24**:415–424.

91. **Osade, Y., and H. Ogawa.** 1983. Anti-mycoplasmal activity of ofloxacin (DL-8280). *Antimicrob. Agents Chemother.* **23**:509–511.

92. **Peloquin, C. A., T. J. Cumbo, D. E. Nix, M. F. Sands, and J. J. Schentag.** 1989. Evaluation of intravenous ciprofloxacin in patients with nosocomial lower respiratory tract infections. *Arch. Int. Med.* **149**:2269–2273.

93. **Perea, E. J.** 1990. Ofloxacin concentrations in tissues involved in respiratory tract infections. *J. Antimicrob. Chemother.* **26**(Suppl. D):55–60.

94. **Philip-Joet, F., J. Nourrit, Y. Frances, and A. Arnaud.** 1988. Enoxacin in the treatment of lower respiratory tract infections. *J. Antimicrob. Chemother.* **21**(Suppl. B):125–129.

95. **Phillips, I., and A. King.** 1986. The comparative in-vitro activity of pefloxacin. *J. Antimicrob. Chemother.* **17**(Suppl. B):1–10.

96. **Prigogine, T., Y. Glupczynski, J. P. Carpiaux, M. Blogie, E. Yourassowsky, and J. S. Schmerber.** 1988. Enoxacin in acute exacerbations of chronic bronchitis: a comparison with amox-

ycillin. *J. Antimicrob. Chemother.* **21**(Suppl. B):131–136.

97. **Rademaker, C. M. A., A. P. Sips, H. M. Beumer, I. M. Hoeplman, B. P. Overbeck, M. J. Mollers, M. Rozenberg-Arska, and J. Verhoef.** 1990. A double-blind comparison of low-dose ofloxacin and amoxicillin/clavulanic acid in acute exacerbations of chronic bronchitis. *J. Antimicrob. Chemother.* **26**(Suppl. D):75–81.
98. **Raeburn, J. A., J. R. Gavan, W. M. McCrae, A. P. Greening, P. S. Collier, M. D. Hodson, and M. C. Goodchild.** 1987. Ciprofloxacin therapy in cystic fibrosis. *J. Antimicrob. Chemother.* **20**:295–296.
99. **Raoff, S., C. Wollschlager, and F. Khan.** 1987. Ciprofloxacin increases serum levels of theophylline. *Am. J. Med.* **82**(Suppl. 4A):115–118.
100. **Riyb, F., E. Santais, E. Callens, J.-P. Chauvin, and J. Hazebroucq.** 1991. Effect of temafloxacin on the pharmacokinetics of temafloxacin. *Am. J. Med.* **91**(Suppl. 6A):76S–80S.
101. **Rubio, T. T.** 1987. Ciprofloxacin comparative data in cystic fibrosis. *Am. J. Med.* **82**(Suppl. 4A):185–188.
102. **Saito, A., M. Katsu, A. Saito, and R. Soejima.** 1987. Ofloxacin in respiratory tract infection: a review of results of clinical trials in Japan. *Drugs* **34**(Suppl. 1):83–89.
103. **Salvati, F., M. Zubiani, A. Antilli, M. Carosi, W. Bianchi, R. Minniti, F. Nunziati, and A. Spano.** 1988. Ciprofloxacin in the oral treatment of severe respiratory tract infections. *Rev. Infect. Dis.* **10**(Suppl. 1):220–221.
104. **Sanders, W. E., P. Alessi, A. T. Madres, R. V. McCloskey, P. Iannuni, and M. J. Bittner.** 1991. Oral ofloxacin for the treatment of acute bacterial pneumonia. Use of a non-traditional protocol to compare experimental therapy with "usual care" in a multicenter clinical trial. *Am. J. Med.* **91**:261–266.
105. **Schaad, U. B., J. Wedgwood-Krucko, K. Guenin, U. Buchlmann, and R. Kraemer.** 1989. Anti-pseudomonal therapy in cystic fibrosis: aztreonam and amikacin vs ceftazidime and amikacin administered intravenously, followed by oral ciprofloxacin. *Eur. J. Clin. Microbiol. Infect. Dis.* **8**:858–865.
106. **Schaefler, S.** 1989. Methicillin-resistant strains of *Staphylococcus aureus* resistant to quinolones. *J. Clin. Microbiol.* **27**:335–336.
107. **Schlenkoff, D., A. Dalhoft, J. Knopf, and W. Opkerkuch.** 1986. Penetration of ciprofloxacin into human lung tissue following intravenous injection. *Infection* **14**:299–300.
108. **Schmidt, E. W., I. Zimmermann, W. Ritzerfeld, E. Voss, and W. T. Ulmer.** 1989. Controlled prospective study of oral amoxycillin/clavulanate vs ciprofloxacin in acute exacerbations of chronic bronchitis. *J. Antimicrob. Chemother.* **24**(Suppl. B):185–193.
109. **Scully, B. E., N. Clynes, and H. C. Neu.** 1991. Oral ofloxacin therapy of infections due to multiply-resistant bacteria. *Diagn. Microbiol. Infect. Dis.* **14**:435–441.
110. **Scully, B. E., M. Nakatomi, C. Ores, S. Davison, and H. C. Neu.** 1987. Ciprofloxacin therapy of cystic fibrosis. *Am. J. Med.* **82**(Suppl. 4A):196–201.
111. **Shah, P. M., R. Strehl, H. G. Posselt, and S. W. Bender.** 1984. Ciprofloxacin bei Mukoviszidose-zystische Fibrose (CF) cine pharmakokinetische Untersuchung. *Fortschr. Antimikrob. Antineoplastischen Chemoter.* **3**:685–690.
112. **Shalit, I., H. R. Stutman, M. I. Marks, S. A. Chartrand, and B. C. Hilman.** 1987. Randomized study of two dosage regimens of ciprofloxacin for treating chronic bronchopulmonary infection in patients with cystic fibrosis. *Am. J. Med.* **82**(Suppl. 4A):189–195.
113. **Shimada, K., Y. Sano, Y. Miyamoto, A. Saito, M. Tomizawa, et al.** 1989. Comparative study on the efficacy of lomefloxacin (NY-198) and cefaclor in respiratory tract infections. *Chemotherapy* **37**:642–645.

113a. **Soejima, R., K. Shimada, F. Matsumoto, F. Miki, and A. Saito.** 1991. A multicenter double blind comparative study of sparfoxacin and ofloxacin in the treatment of bacterial pneumonia, abstr. 877. *Program Abstr. 31st Intersci. Conf. Antimicrob. Agents Chemother.*

114. **Sörgel, F., U. Stephan, H. G. Wiesemann, B. Gottschalk, C. Stehr, M. Rey, H. B. Böwing, H. C. Dominick, and M. Geldmacher von Mallinckrodt.** 1987. High-dose treatment with antibiotics in cystic fibrosis—a reappraisal with special reference to the pharmacokinetics of beta-lactams and new fluoroquinolones in adult CF patients. *Infection* **15**:385–396.
115. **Spino, M., Y. Bentur, S. Martin, H. Heurter, M. Brill-Edwards, J. Tesoro, J. Correia, R. Pop, R. Gold, and S. Macleod.** 1989. Enoxacin disposition in patients with cystic fibrosis and healthy control subjects. *Eur. J. Clin. Pharmacol.* **169**:A84.
116. **Strandvik, B., L. Hjelte, A. Lindblad, B. Ljungberg, A. S. Malmborg, and I. Nilsson-Ehle.** 1989. Comparison of efficacy and tolerance of intravenously- and orally-administered ciprofloxacin in cystic fibrosis patients with acute exacerbations of lung infection. *Scand. J. Infect. Dis.* **60**(Suppl.):84–88.
117. **Strausbaugh, L. J., C. M. Jacobson, D. L. Sewell, and T. T. Ward.** 1989. Emergence of ciprofloxacin (Cip) resistance during an outbreak caused by methicillin-resistant *Staphylococcus au-*

*reus* (MRSA) in a nursing home care unit (NHCU), abstr. 1257. *Program Abstr. 29th Intersci. Conf. Antimicrob. Agents Chemother.*

118. **Stutman, H. R.** 1987. Summary of a workshop on ciprofloxacin use in patients with cystic fibrosis. *Pediatr. Infect. Dis. J.* **6:**932–935.
119. **Sutter, U. L., Y. Y. Kwok, and J. Bulkacz.** 1985. Comparative activity of ciprofloxacin against aerobic bacteria. *Antimicrob. Agents Chemother.* **27:**427–428.
120. **Trenholme, G. M., B. A. Schmitt, J. Spear, L. C. Gvazdinskas, and S. Levin.** 1989. Randomized study of intravenous/oral ciprofloxacin versus ceftazidime in the treatment of hospital and nursing home patients with lower respiratory tract infections. *Am. J. Med.* **87**(Suppl. 5A):116–118.
121. **Trucksis, M., D. C. Hooper, and J. S. Wolfsone.** 1991. Emerging resistance to fluoroquinolones in staphylococci: an alert. *Ann. Intern. Med.* **114:**424–425.
122. **Tsukamura, M., E. Nakamura, S. Yoshii, and H. Amano.** 1985. Therapeutic effect of a new antibacterial substance ofloxacin (DL 8280) on pulmonary tuberculosis. *Am. Rev. Respir. Dis.* **131:**352–356.
123. **Ulmer, W.** 1991. Fleroxacin versus amoxicillin in the therapy of lower respiratory tract infection (LRTI), abstr. 1452. *Abstr. 17th Int. Congr. Chemother.*
124. **Unertl, K. E., F. P. Lenhart, H. Forst, G. Vogler, V. Wilm, W. Ehret, and G. Ruckdeschel.** 1989. Brief report: ciprofloxacin in the treatment of legionellosis in critically-ill patients, including those cases unresponsive to erythomycin. *Am. J. Med.* **87**(Suppl. 5A):128–131.
125. **Van Caekenberg, D.** 1990. Comparative in-vitro activities of 10 fluoroquinolones and fusidic acid against *Mycobacterium spp. J. Antimicrob. Chemother.* **26:**381–386.
126. **Van der Auwera, P., P. Grenier, Y. Glupczynski, and D. Pierard.** 1989. In-vitro activity of lomefloxacin compared with pefloxacin and ofloxacin. *J. Antimicrob. Chemother.* **23:**209–220.
127. **Vanderdonckt, J.** 1990. Comparison of pefloxacin with ceftazidime in severe bronchopulmonary infections. *J. Antimicrob. Chemother.* **26**(Suppl. B):111–116.
128. **Verbist, L.** 1987. Comparative in-vitro activity of RO 23-6240: a new trifluorinated quinolone. *J. Antimicrob. Chemother.* **20:**363–372.
129. **Verschraegen, G., G. Claeps, and A. M. Van den Abeele.** 1988. Comparative in-vitro activity of the new quinolone fleroxacin (RO-236240). *Eur. J. Clin. Microbiol. Infect. Dis.* **7:**63–66.
130. **Vildé, J. L., E. Dournon, and P. Rajagopalan.** 1986. Inhibition of *Legionella pneumophila* multiplication within human macrophages by antimicrobial agents. *Antimicrob. Agents Chemother.* **30:**743–748.
131. **Waites, K. B., G. H. Cassell, K. C. Canupp, and P. B. Fernandes.** 1988. In-vitro susceptibilities of mycoplasmas and ureaplasmas to new macrolides and fluoroquinolones. *Antimicrob. Agents Chemother.* **32:**1500–1502.
132. **Weideblamm, E.** 1991. Pharmacokinetics and tissue penetration of fleroxacin, abstr. 1451. *Abstr. 17th Int. Congr. Chemother.*
133. **Wijnands, W. J. A., J. H. Cornel, M. Martea, and T. B. Vree.** 1990. The effect of multiple-dose oral lomefloxacin on theophylline metabolism in man. *Chest* **98:**1440–1444.
134. **Wijnands, W. J. A., A. J. A. van Griethuysen, T. B. Vree, B. van Klingeren, and C. L. A. van Herwaarden.** 1986. Enoxacin in lower respiratory tract infections. *J. Antimicrob. Chemother.* **18:**719–727.
135. **Wijnands, W. J. A., C. L. H. van Heerwaarden, and T. B. Vree.** 1986. Enoxacin raises plasma theophylline concentrations. *Lancet* **i:**108–109.
136. **Wijnands, W. J. A., T. B. Vree, A. M. Baars, and C. L. H. van Herwaarden.** 1988. Pharmacokinetics of enoxacin and its penetration into bronchial secretions and lung tissue. *J. Antimicrob. Chemother.* **21**(Suppl. B):67–77.
137. **Wijnands, W. J. A., T. B. Vree, and C. L. H. van Heerwaarden.** 1986. The influence of quinolone derivatives on theophylline clearance. *Br. J. Clin. Pharmacol.* **22:**677–683.
138. **Winter, J. H., C. McCartney, J. Bingham, M. Telfer, L. O. White, and R. J. Fallon.** 1988. Ciprofloxacin in the treatment of severe Legionnaire's disease. *Rev. Infect. Dis.* **10**(Suppl. 1):218–219.
139. **Wise, R.** 1992. Comparative penetration of selected fluoroquinolones into respiratory tract fluids and tissues. *Am. J. Med.* **91**(Suppl. 6A):67S–70S.
140. **Wise, R., D. R. Balwin, J. M. Andrews, and D. Honeybourne.** 1991. Comparative pharmacokinetic disposition of fluoroquinolones in the lung. *J. Antimicrob. Chemother.* **28**(Suppl. C):65–72.
141. **Wolff, M., Bure, J. P. Pathe, B. Pangon, B. Regneir, D. Rouger-Barbarier, and F. Vachon.** 1985. Evolution des résistances bactériennes à la péfloxacine dans le service de réanimation de l'hôpital Claude Bernard, p. 213–226. *In* J. J. Pocidalo, F. Vachon, and B. Regnier (ed.), *Les Nouvelles Quinolones.* Editions Arnette, Paris.
142. **Wolfson, J. S., and D. C. Hooper.** 1989. Fluoroquinolone antimicrobial agents. *Clin. Microbiol. Rev.* **2:**378–424.
143. **Wollschlager, C. M., S. Raoff, F. Khan, J. J. Guarneri, V. Labombardi, and Q. Afzal.** 1987.

Controlled comparative study of ciprofloxacin versus ampicillin in the treatment of bacterial respiratory tract infections. *Am. J. Med.* **82**(Suppl. 4A):164–168.

144. **Yew, W. W., S. Y. L. Kwan, W. K. Ma, M. A. Khin, and P. K. Chau.** 1990. In-vitro activity of ofloxacin against *Mycobacterium tuberculosis* and its clinical efficacy in multiply-resistant pulmonary tuberculosis. *J. Antimicrob. Chemother.* **26:**227–236.

145. **Yew, W. W., S. Y. L. Kwan, P. C. Wong, and J. Lee.** 1990. Ofloxacin and imipenem in the treatment of *Mycobacterium fortuitum* and *Mycobacterium chelonae* lung infections. *Tubercle* **71:**131–133.

*Quinolone Antimicrobial Agents, 2nd ed.*
Edited by David C. Hooper and John S. Wolfson


*Chapter 18*

# Treatment of Infections of the Ears, Nose, and Throat and Nasal Carriage

*Jennifer R. Grandis and Victor L. Yu*

The introduction of the quinolones represents an important therapeutic advance in the treatment of certain otolaryngologic infections. The oral route of administration, the low toxicity profile, and the excellent penetration into nares secretions, saliva, and bone are important advantages (1). Unfortunately, objective data from well-controlled studies are scanty; the major weakness in the few studies that have been reported is the failure to adequately document the type of infection being treated.

## TREATMENT OF MALIGNANT EXTERNAL OTITIS

Malignant external otitis is an invasive infection of the external ear canal, mastoid, and base of skull caused almost universally (>98% of cases) by *Pseudomonas aeruginosa* (35). The disease primarily afflicts the elderly patient with diabetes mellitus, although the disease has been reported in children with chronic illness or immunosuppression (36). Prior to the introduction of systemic antipseudomonal antibiotics in the early 1970s, the disease was fatal in the majority of cases despite extensive surgical debridement of infected tissues, primarily because of the multiple cranial neuropathies associated with extensive skull base involvement. With the introduction of aminoglycosides and antipseudomonal penicillins, the mortality rate was reduced to approximately 15 to 30%, but recurrences remained a significant problem (20 to 25%) (35). Prolonged combination parenteral therapy for this disease has been associated with long-term hospitalization as well as vestibular and renal toxicity in addition to the morbidity associated with the disease process itself.

For a number of reasons, quinolone agents, especially ciprofloxacin, have proven to be a major advance in therapy for malignant external otitis. Quinolones have an extensive antimicrobial spectrum, which includes *P. aeruginosa*. They can be administered orally, with high penetration into bone and soft tissue (11, 13, 19, 42, 48), thereby obviating the need for prolonged hospitalization. The dose of ciprofloxacin need not be adjusted in elderly patients with renal failure (15), and the side effects of ototoxicity and nephrotoxicity, which are seen with aminoglycosides and which can be particularly troublesome in elderly diabetics, are only rarely encountered with the quinolones.

Numerous reports have chronicled the successful treatment of patients with malignant external otitis by use of quinolone agents (14,

***Jennifer R. Grandis*** • Department of Otolaryngology, University of Pittsburgh, Pittsburgh, Pennsylvania 15213. ***Victor L. Yu*** • Infectious Disease Section, Veterans Affairs Medical Center, University of Pittsburgh, Pittsburgh, Pennsylvania 15261.

17, 20–23, 34, 38). Ciprofloxacin alone (750 mg twice a day) has been the most popular regimen, with one report of ciprofloxacin plus rifampin (600 mg twice a day) (34) and one of ofloxacin monotherapy (200 mg twice a day). Despite rapid relief of symptoms (pain and otorrhea), prolonged treatment (6 to 12 weeks) is recommended because of the traditionally recalcitrant nature of the infection. A high rate of success (>90%) has been universally reported, with only a few cases of recurrence or persistent disease. In addition to symptomatic relief, the erythrocyte sedimentation rate (ESR) appears to be an accurate objective indicator of disease activity and response to antimicrobial agents. In one study, the ESR fell from a mean pretreatment value of 81 mm/h (range, 41 to 138 mm/h) to a mean of 18 mm/h (range, 3 to 45 mm/h) after the completion of therapy (34). To date, the antibiotic resistance encountered in some *Pseudomonas* infections has not emerged in cases of malignant external otitis.

When reporting and evaluating cases of malignant external otitis, we emphasize that it is important to detail the diagnostic criteria, since there is no single sign or symptom that clearly distinguishes the disease. Rather, it is a constellation of findings, including symptoms (severe and recalcitrant pain, history of otorrhea) in the characteristic host (the elderly diabetic), findings of the physical examination (granulation tissue at the anterior inferior portion of the external auditory canal at the site of the fissures of Santorini), recovery of *P. aeruginosa* from the ear canal, an elevated ESR, and evidence of cartilage or bone destruction on radiographic examination. Some reports of patients with malignant external otitis are difficult to interpret because the diagnostic criteria are not explicitly given. Bone scintigraphy (usually with technetium 99) is almost uniformly positive at presentation (26, 27) and therefore highly sensitive. For one report (38) in which the bone scan was positive in only 65% of the patients, one must speculate whether the patients with negative scans really did have malignant external otitis. On the other hand, bone scanning carries low specificity in diagnosis; in fact, patients with simple external otitis cannot be reliably differentiated from patients with malignant external otitis on the basis of bone scanning (25). In a similar vein, authors of another study reported that fewer than half (41%) of their patients had diabetes mellitus (22). This study is difficult to interpret, since it has been unusual to find this disease in the nondiabetic adult (44).

It is noteworthy that with the advent and widespread availability of ciprofloxacin, patients with malignant external otitis are being diagnosed and treated earlier in the course of the disease, thus changing the clinical spectrum of the disease. These individuals with "Limited-MEO" (malignant external otitis) (21) may present with a lower or even normal ESR and no evidence of bone destruction on computed tomography. One must maintain a high index of suspicion when the typical host presents with otalgia that is out of proportion to physical findings. Furthermore, a history of ear irrigation (usually for cerumen impaction) should be sought because of an association of malignant external otitis with prior aural water exposure (8, 37).

## AURICULAR PERICHONDRITIS

Perichondritis of the auricle caused by *P. aeruginosa* can occur in the burn patient as well as the patient with malignant external otitis. Because of its excellent soft tissue and cartilage penetration and the prolonged duration of therapy, ciprofloxacin seems to be an ideal agent for treating this disease. Oral ciprofloxacin has been successfully used for individuals with auricular perichondritis (24).

## TREATMENT OF CHRONIC EAR DISEASE

In discussing the utility of quinolones in the treatment of chronic ear infections, it is again critical to define the disease process under scrutiny. Specifically, the status of the middle ear and tympanic membrane, presence of cholesteatoma, and prior mastoid surgery are all important parameters in delineating the population being studied. Too often in the few reports of quinolone usage for ear disease other than malignant external otitis, patients with different processes are grouped for evaluation, thus clouding interpretation of the data (10, 29, 46). Furthermore, the assessment of the efficacy of fluoroquinolones for these diseases would benefit from comparison with treatment with another drug or with results for untreated controls, a study design feature that is absent from most reports. *P. aeruginosa* is frequently recovered from the patient with a chronic draining ear, but its pathogenicity is uncertain because of the self-limited nature of otorrhea in many patients without underlying cholesteatoma.

Piccirillo and Parnes administered ciprofloxacin (500 mg twice a day for 2 weeks) to 19 patients with chronic otitis media, an infected mastoid cavity, cholesteatoma, or chronic external otitis (29). The use of topical antimicrobial agents was not controlled; this lack was unfortunate, because in most instances of chronic external otitis with an infected mastoid cavity, topical agents alone are effective. The authors reported a 58% cure rate, but posttreatment cultures were not obtained and follow-up was relatively short compared with the duration of pretreatment drainage. The group with cholesteatoma did not fare as well, which is not surprising, since cholesteatoma is best treated with surgical eradication. For a similar patient population with a combination of chronic ear diseases, Van deHeyning treated 59 patients with a higher dose of ciprofloxacin (750 mg twice a day) with similar rates of clinical and bacteriologic cures (47). Patients with cholesteatoma benefited from surgical intervention in addition to antimicrobial therapy. Although the authors recommended ciprofloxacin for perioperative prophylaxis in otologic surgery, the need for any antibiotic coverage in this setting has never been clearly determined.

The efficacy of topical ciprofloxacin was explored in one study in which 60 patients with chronic otitis media were randomized to receive oral ciprofloxacin alone (250 mg twice a day for 5 to 10 days), topical ciprofloxacin alone (3 drops containing 250 $\mu$g of ciprofloxacin per ml in saline solution twice a day), or oral plus topical ciprofloxacin twice a day (5). The follow-up period was only 14 days; however, topical ciprofloxacin alone appeared to be more efficacious than the oral drug alone or in combination with topical therapy. These results are encouraging and confirm the numerous reports suggesting that topical antimicrobial agents as monotherapy are effective for uncomplicated otorrhea. Furthermore, chronic otorrhea is primarily a disease of children, for whom the use of systemic ciprofloxacin is currently not approved because of the possible deleterious effects on developing joints and cartilage. Topical ciprofloxacin is unlikely to lead to systemic toxicities and may therefore be an ideal candidate for the treatment of chronic otorrhea in the pediatric population unresponsive to traditional therapies.

The only double-blind, randomized trial in this clinical setting compared enoxacin (400 mg twice a day) with amoxicillin (500 mg three times a day) for the treatment of chronic suppurative otitis media in 40 adults (18). The duration of treatment was relatively short (mean, 9.3 days), and data on prior antibiotic therapy were not given. This omission is pertinent, since amoxicillin is most frequently employed as a first-line agent, and prior unsuccessful treatment with amoxicillin may select out patients with more-recalcitrant disease. Enoxacin was more effective than amoxicillin in eradicating the organism as well as in improving bone conduction thresholds on audiogram. Enoxacin has been found in relatively high concentrations in middle ear fluid after a single oral dose of 400 mg (46).

Despite these reports, the use of quinolones in the treatment of chronic otitis remains unestablished. Despite the isolation of *P. aeruginosa* from a large number of chronic draining ears, its pathogenicity in this setting is questionable. The efficacy of systemic therapy for uncomplicated chronic otorrhea has been debated prior to the introduction of the quinolones. The institution of prospective, randomized trials that outline rigorous criteria for entry, specify the disease process being studied, include a comparative antimicrobial agent and/or placebo-treated control group, and evaluate objective end points is sorely needed.

## TREATMENT OF SINUSITIS

It is essential to differentiate between acute and chronic sinusitis when therapies are evaluated. While most cases of acute sinusitis are believed to be the result of bacterial infections, chronic sinusitis is more commonly associated with allergies that result in mucosal edema and obstruction of the osteomeatal complex. A bacteriologic diagnosis in acute sinusitis requires sterile puncture of the maxillary antrum, and while radiography can provide a noninvasive means of diagnosis, therapy is most often instituted empirically on the basis of clinical history and physical examination (12). Aspiration of the maxillary sinus in a number of studies revealed that more than 50% of the isolates are *Streptococcus pneumoniae* and unencapsulated strains of *Haemophilus influenzae*, with anaerobic bacteria, *Staphylococcus aureus, Streptococcus pyogenes, Moraxella catarrhalis*, and gram-negative bacteria being recovered less often (7). Despite the excellent penetration of fluoroquinolones into the tissues of the upper respiratory tract, including the nasal and sinus mucosas, their relatively weak activity against gram-positive cocci argues against their use as a first-line agent in treating sinus infections.

Ofloxacin has been evaluated in two studies including only 18 patients with acute sinusitis (39, 45). In both studies, there was no control group, the duration of treatment was relatively short, three cultures were sterile, and the recovery of *S. aureus* was unusually high (10 of 18 patients). Oral ciprofloxacin has been evaluated for use against chronic sinusitis, but the results were indeterminate (41). *P. aeruginosa* is a rare cause of sinusitis in immunocompetent patients. Moreover, the role of bacteria and hence the utility of antibacterial agents against chronic sinusitis are unclear. Since the fluoroquinolones are not particularly active against the organisms most commonly isolated from patients with acute maxillary sinusitis, there is little rationale for exploring their utility in initial treatment of this disease.

## TREATMENT OF ACUTE PHARYNGOTONSILLITIS

Several reports concerning the efficacies of fluoroquinolones for acute pharyngotonsillitis have been published (6, 16, 40). Amoxicillin (250 mg three times a day) and ofloxacin (200 mg three times a day) were equally effective (40). The other studies did not use comparative control groups but reported good results with either ciprofloxacin (250 mg twice a day) or ofloxacin (600 mg a day). Despite the general success reported in these studies, there is little rationale for employing fluoroquinolones as first-line agents in acute bacterial tonsillitis, given the availability and efficacy of other, less expensive agents.

## NASAL CARRIAGE OF BACTERIA

### *Neisseria meningitidis*

Ciprofloxacin has excellent in vitro activity against *N. meningitidis*, and its concentration in nasal secretions exceeds the MIC for 90% of strains of this organism by 70-fold (30). Concentrations in nasal secretions were as high as 0.40 μg/ml (mean, about 0.14

μg/ml), or approximately 10% of that in serum, while the MIC for 90% of *N. meningitidis* strains was about 0.004 μg/ml.

Short courses of ciprofloxacin (2 to 5 days) at doses of 250 to 500 mg twice a day were effective in eradicating meningococcal carriage in chronic carriers (32, 33). Furthermore, a single oral dose of 750 mg of ciprofloxacin was evaluated in a placebo-controlled, double-blind trial of healthy volunteers (4). One dose proved to be effective in eradicating the organism in 96% of subjects at 7 and 21 days posttherapy. Of note, one of the subjects who was successfully treated carried a minocycline-resistant strain.

Thus, ciprofloxacin may prove to be particularly useful in nasopharyngeal carriers of sulfonamide- or minocycline-resistant organisms.

### *S. aureus*

Ciprofloxacin concentrations in nasal secretions were not sufficient to inhibit either methicillin-sensitive or methicillin-resistant *S. aureus* strains (3). In a study of staphylococcal nasal carriage in hemodialysis patients given 750 mg of ciprofloxacin a day for 6 days, 54% were free of staphylococci 1 day after therapy; however, the number had declined to only 27% 4 weeks later (2).

Not only has prolonged use of ciprofloxacin proven to be relatively ineffective in eradicating carriage by methicillin-resistant *S. aureus*, but emergence of resistance in vitro following such therapy has been commonplace (28, 43).

## SUMMARY

Although infections of the ear, nose, and throat are among the most common outpatient maladies in the world, fluoroquinolones are inappropriate agents for initial therapy of these infections for a number of reasons. These agents possess only intermediate activities against most of the commonly isolated bacterial pathogens and thus may only suppress rather than eradicate the organism. Reports of pneumococcal bacteremia following ciprofloxacin therapy for acute otitis media support this hypothesis (9).

While ciprofloxacin appears to be the drug of choice for infections caused by *P. aeruginosa* (such as malignant external otitis and auricular perichondritis), the utility of fluoroquinolones in the treatment of most ear, nose, and throat infections is not established. The quinolones may be useful as alternative agents for treatment of nasal carriage of *N. meningitidis*. They have proven disappointing for treatment of nasal carriage of *S. aureus*.

## REFERENCES


1. **Barza, M.** 1988. Pharmacokinetics and efficacy of the new quinolones in infections of the eye, ear, nose, and throat. *Rev. Infect. Dis.* **10:**S241–S247.
2. **Chow, J. W., and V. L. Yu.** 1992. Failure of oral ciprofloxacin in suppressing *Staphylococcus aureus* carriage in hemodialysis patients. *J. Antimicrob. Chemother.* **29:**88–89.
3. **Darouiche R., B. Perkins, B. D. Musher, R. Hamill, and S. Tsai.** 1990. Levels of rifampin and ciprofloxacin in nasal secretions: correlation with MIC 90 and eradication of nasopharyngeal carriage of bacteria. *J. Infect. Dis.* **162:**1124–1127.
4. **Dworzack, D. L., C. C. Sanders, E. A. Horowitz, J. Allais, M. Sookpranee, W. E. Sanders, and F. M. Ferraro.** 1988. Evaluation of single-dose ciprofloxacin in the eradication of *Neisseria meningitidis* from nasopharyngeal carriers. *Antimicrob. Agents Chemother.* **32:**1740–1741.
5. **Esposito, S., G. D'Errico, and C. Montanaro.** 1990. Topical and oral treatment of chronic otitis media with ciprofloxacin. A preliminary study. *Otolaryngol. Head Neck Surg.* **116:**557–559.
6. **Esposito, S., G. D'Errico, and C. Montanaro.** 1990. Oral ciprofloxacin for treatment of acute bacterial pharyngotonsillitis. *J. Chemother.* **2:**108–112.
7. **Evans, F. O., Jr., J. B. Sydor, W. E. C. Moore, G. R. Moore, J. L. Manwaring, A. H. Brill, R. T. Jackson, S. Hanna, J. S. Skaar, L. V. Holdeman, G. S. Fitz-Hugh, M. A. Sande, and J. M. Gwaltney, Jr.** 1975. Sinusitis of the maxillary antrum. *N. Engl. J. Med.* **293:**735–739.
8. **Ford, G. R., and R. Courteney-Harris.** 1990. Another hazard of ear syringing: malignant external otitis. *J. Laryngol. Otol.* **104:**709–710.

9. **Frieden, T. R., and R. J. Mangi.** 1990. Inappropriate use of oral ciprofloxacin. *JAMA* **264:**1438–1440.
10. **Giamarellou, H., N. Galanakis, E. Daphnis, J. Stephanou, and P. Sfikakis.** 1988. Treating acute and chronic otitis with ciprofloxacin: a step toward a better prognosis? *Rev. Infect. Dis.* **10**(Suppl. 1)**:**S248.
11. **Gilbert, D., A. D. Tice, P. K. Marsh, P. C. Craven, and L. C. Preheim.** 1987. Oral ciprofloxacin therapy for chronic contiguous osteomyelitis caused by aerobic gram-negative bacilli. *Am. J. Med.* **82:**S254–S258.
12. **Hamory, B. H., M. A. Sande, A. Sydnor, Jr., D. L. Seale, and J. M. Gwaltney, Jr.** 1979. Etiology and antimicrobial therapy of acute maxillary sinusitis. *J. Infect. Dis.* **139:**192–202.
13. **Hessen, M. T., M. J. Ingerman, D. H. Kaufman, P. Weiner, J. Santoro, O. M. Korzenioski, J. Boscia, M. Topiel, L. M. Bush, D. Kaye, and M. E. Levison.** 1987. Clinical efficacy of ciprofloxacin therapy for gram-negative bacillary osteomyelitis. *Am. J. Med.* **83:**S262–S265.
14. **Hickey, S. A., G. R. Ford, A. F. Fitzgerald O'Connor, S. J. Eykyn, and P. H. Sonksen.** 1989. Treating malignant otitis with oral ciprofloxacin. *Br. Med. J.* **299:**550–551.
15. **Hirata, C. A., I. Hirata, D. R. P. Guay, W. M. Awni, D. J. Stein, and P. K. Peterson.** 1989. Steady-state pharmacokinetics of intravenous and oral ciprofloxacin in elderly patients. *Antimicrob. Agents Chemother.* **33:**1927–1931.
16. **Iwasawa, T.** 1984. Fundamental and clinical studies on DL-8280 in the otorhinolaryngologic field. *Chemotherapy* (Tokyo) **32**(Suppl. 1)**:**1001–1012.
17. **Joachims, H. Z., J. Danino, and R. Raz.** 1988. Malignant external otitis: treatment with fluoroquinolones. *Am. J. Otolaryngol.* **9:**102–105.
18. **Krajewski, M. J.** 1988. Effectiveness of enoxacin in the treatment of chronic suppurative otitis media. *Rev. Infect. Dis.* **10**(Suppl. 1)**:**S248.
19. **Leese, A. J., C. Freer, R. A. Salata, J. B. Francis, and W. M. Scheid.** 1987. Oral ciprofloxacin therapy for gram-negative bacillary osteomyelitis caused by aerobic gram-negative bacilli. *Am. J. Med.* **82:**255–262.
20. **Leggett, J. M., and K. Prendergast.** 1988. Malignant external otitis: the use of oral ciprofloxacin. *J. Laryngol. Otol.* **102:**53–54.
21. **Levenson, M. J., S. C. Parisier, J. Dolitsky, and G. Bindra.** 1991. Ciprofloxacin: drug of choice in the treatment of malignant external otitis (MEO). *Laryngoscope* **101:**821–824.
22. **Levy, R., T. Shpitzer, J. Shvero, and S. D. Pitlik.** 1990. Oral ofloxacin as treatment of malignant external otitis: a study of 17 cases. *Laryngoscope* **100:**548–551.
23. **Morrison, G. A. J., and C. M. Bailey.** 1988. Relapsing malignant otitis externa successfully treated with ciprofloxacin. *J. Laryngol. Otol.* **102:**872–876.
24. **Noel, S. B., P. Scallan, M. C. Meadors, T. J. Meek, and G. Pankey.** 1989. Treatment of *Pseudomonas aeruginosa* auricular perichondritis with oral ciprofloxacin. *Dermatol. Surg. Oncol.* **6:**633–637.
25. **Noyek, A. M.** 1979. Bone scanning in otolaryngology. *Laryngoscope* **89**(Suppl. 18)**:**1–29.
26. **Ostfeld, E., A. Aviel, and D. Pelet.** 1981. Malignant external otitis: the diagnostic value of bone scintigraphy. *Laryngoscope* **91:**960–964.
27. **Parisier, S. C., F. E. Lucente, S. Z. Hirschman, P. M. Som, L. M. Arnold, and J. D. Ruffman.** 1982. Nuclear scanning in necrotizing progressive "malignant" external otitis. *Laryngoscope* **92:**1016–1020.
28. **Peterson, L., J. Quick, B. Jensen, S. Homann, and S. Johnson.** 1990. Emergence of ciprofloxacin resistance in nosocomial methicillin-resistant staphylococcus aureus isolation: resistance during ciprofloxacin plus rifampin therapy for methicillin-resistant *S. aureus* colonization. *Arch. Int. Med.* **150:**2151–2155.
29. **Piccirillo, J. F., and S. M. Parnes.** 1989. Ciprofloxacin for the treatment of chronic ear disease. *Laryngoscope* **99:**510–513.
30. **Piercy, E. A., R. Bawdon, and M. P. A. MacKowiak.** 1989. Penetration of ciprofloxacin into saliva and nasal secretion and effect of the drug on the oropharyngeal flora of all subjects. *Antimicrob. Agents Chemother.* **33:**1645–1646.
31. **Pugsley, M. P., D. L. Dworzack, E. Horowitz, T. Cuevas, W. E. Sanders, and C. C. Sanders.** 1987. Efficacy of ciprofloxacin in the treatment of nasopharyngeal carriers of *Neisseria meningitidis*. *J. Infect. Dis.* **156:**211–213.
32. **Pugsley, M. P., D. L. Dworzack, J. Roccaforte, C. C. Sanders, J. Bakken, and W. E. Sanders.** 1988. An open study of the efficacy of a single dose of ciprofloxacin in eliminating the chronic nasopharyngeal carriage of *Neisseria meningitidis*. *J. Infect. Dis.* **157:**852–853.
33. **Renkonen, O. V., A. Sivonen, and R. Visakorpi.** 1987. Effect of ciprofloxacin on carrier rate of *Neisseria meningitidis* in army recruits in Finland. *Antimicrob. Agents Chemother.* **31:**962–963.
34. **Rubin, J., G. Stoehr, V. L. Yu, R. R. Muder, A. Matador, and D. B. Kamerer.** 1989. Efficacy of oral ciprofloxacin plus rifampin for treatment of malignant external otitis. *Arch. Otolaryngol. Head Neck Surg.* **115:**1063–1069.
35. **Rubin, J., and V. L. Yu.** 1988. Malignant external otitis: insights into pathogenesis, clinical manifestations, diagnosis, and therapy. *Am. J. Med.* **85:**391–397.
36. **Rubin, J., V. L. Yu, and S. E. Stool.** 1988. Ma-

lignant external otitis in children. *J. Pediatr.* **113:**965–970.

37. **Rubin, J., V. L. Yu, D. B. Wagener, and M. Wagener.** 1990. Aural irrigation with water: a potential pathogenic mechanism for inducing malignant external otitis? *Ann. Otol. Rhinol. Laryngol.* **99:**117–119.
38. **Sade, J., R. Lang, S. Goshen, and R. Kitzes-Cohen.** 1989. Ciprofloxacin treatment of malignant external otitis. *Am. J. Med.* **87:**5A138S–5A141S.
39. **Sanbe, B., H. Yoshihama, R. Veda, K. Kobayashi, Y. Ito, J. Okada, and M. Inafuku.** 1984. Experimental and clinical studies on DL-8280 in the field of otorhinolarngology. *Chemotherapy* (Tokyo) **32**(Suppl.)**:**1019–1029.
40. **Sasaki, T., T. Unno, T. Tomiyama, O. Yamai, T. Iwasawa, et al.** 1984. Evaluation of clinical effectiveness and safety of DL-8280 in acute lacunar tonsillitis. *Otol. Fukuoka* **30:**484–513.
41. **Scully, B. E., M. F. Parry, H. C. Neu, and W. Mandell.** 1986. Oral ciprofloxacin therapy of infections due to Pseudomonas aeruginosa. *Lancet* **i:**819–822.
42. **Slama, T. G., J. Misinski, and S. Sklar.** 1987. Oral ciprofloxacin therapy for osteomyelitis caused by aerobic gram-negative bacilli. *Am. J. Med.* **82:**S259–S261.
43. **Smith, S. M., R. H. K. Eng, and F. Tomang-Tecson.** 1990. Epidemiology of ciprofloxacin resistance among patients with methicillin-resistant *Staphylococcus aureus. J. Antimicrob. Chemother.* **26:**567–572.
44. **Soliman, A. E.** 1978. A rare case of malignant external otitis externa in a non-diabetic patient. *J. Laryngol. Otol.* **92:**811–812.
45. **Sugita, R., S. Kawamura, Y. Fujimaki, and K. Deguchi.** Clinical experience of DL-8280 in the otorhinolaryngological infections. *Chemotherapy* (Tokyo) **32**(Suppl. 1)**:**1013–1018.
46. **Sundberg, L., and T. Eden.** 1990. Penetration of enoxacin into middle ear fluid effusion. *Acta Otolaryngol.* **109:**438–443.
47. **Van deHeyning, P. H., S. R. Pattyn, H. D. Valcke, D. L. Van Caekenberghe, H. W. Jans, J. B. J. Boerema, and V. Chysky.** 1988. Use of ciprofloxacin in chronic suppurative otitis. *Rev. Infect. Dis.* **10**(Suppl. 1)**:**S250–S251.
48. **Wise, R., and I. A. Donovan.** 1987. Tissue penetration and metabolism of ciprofloxacin. *Am. J. Med.* **82:**S103–S107.

*Quinolone Antimicrobial Agents, 2nd ed.*
Edited by David C. Hooper and John S. Wolfson


*Chapter 19*

# Use of Quinolones for Treatment of Osteomyelitis and Septic Arthritis

*Daniel Lew and Francis Waldvogel*

The continuous interest in the use of fluoroquinolones for the treatment of osteomyelitis and septic arthritis in the past has resulted in more-extensive experience with these drugs. Most of the clinical experience has been acquired with compounds already available on the market, such as ciprofloxacin, ofloxacin (in the United States and Europe), and pefloxacin (in Europe). Additional extensive experience has been gained with experimental models using newer agents or combination therapy. All of these agents have several advantages over other traditional compounds because (i) they penetrate bone at sufficient concentrations to inhibit most members of the family *Enterobacteriaceae*, *Pseudomonas* spp., and a large percentage of *Staphylococcus aureus* strains; (ii) after an initial course of intravenous therapy, they can be administrated orally; and (iii) they are relatively nontoxic.

The purpose of this review is to summarize the knowledge that has been gained in this area since 1989, when a previous review was published (41). Other, often more limited reviews have also been published recently on this same topic (1, 11, 12, 19, 31, 43).

***Daniel Lew and Francis Waldvogel*** • Infectious Diseases Division and Clinique Médicale 2, Department of Medicine, University Hospital, Geneva, Switzerland.

## GENERAL CONSIDERATIONS AND MICROBIOLOGICAL ASPECTS OF OSTEOMYELITIS

The distinctions between acute and chronic osteomyelitis and between osteomyelitis associated with peripheral vascular disease, bacteremia, or contiguous infection become more important when different quinolones are compared with respect to their pharmacokinetics, bone penetration, and antibacterial activity. Thus, some important aspects of these different clinical syndromes will be summarized, since they are pertinent to our present review.

Acute osteomyelitis refers to a disease with symptoms of short duration; there is some bone destruction but usually an absence of new bone formation and/or sclerosis. Bacteremia may be concomitant with or may precede the onset of the osteomyelitis. Acute osteomyelitis is most often diagnosed in children and involves the heavily vascularized growth plates of long bones or, in adults, of vertebrae.

Chronic osteomyelitis refers to a disease with symptoms that have been present for longer than 3 months or for which an initial therapeutic regimen has failed. Chronic osteomyelitis occurs in adults secondary to trauma, particularly to open fracture, contiguous infections such as decubitus ulcers, or surgery, in particular the insertion of prosthe-

**Table 1.** Spectrum of microorganisms responsible for osteomyelitis and arthritis in adults[a]

| Microorganism | Frequency of: | | | |
|---|---|---|---|---|
| | Acute osteomyelitis[b] | Chronic osteomyelitis[c] | Osteomyelitis and diabetes[c] | Infectious arthritis[d] |
| *S. aureus* | +++ | ++ | + | +++ |
| *S. epidermidis* | (+) | ++ | + | − |
| Gram-negative rods | ++ | ++ | + | + |
| Streptococci | (+) | + | + | ++ |
| Anaerobes | (+) | + | + | − |
| *Candida* species | (+) | − | − | |

[a]The problem associated with the use of quinolones in children is discussed in the text. This table was adapted from reference 41. Symbols indicate relative frequencies. The indicated microorganisms are found in different clinical syndromes.
[b]Frequently single culture.
[c]Frequently mixed culture.
[d]Single culture.

tic material. Osteomyelitis of the feet is often associated with peripheral vascular disease, particularly in patients suffering from diabetes.

Both orthopedists and infectious disease specialists agree that in order to choose the optimal antibiotic regimen, it is essential to obtain deep microbiological specimens, ideally a bone biopsy sample, which should be subsequently processed for microbiological and pathological analyses. Superficial swabs or specimens from fistulae have rather low specificities and sensitivities and may lead to erroneous therapy, particularly if the specimens were taken after the introduction of antimicrobial agents.

Clearly, in acute infections, particularly those associated with bacteremia, *S. aureus* and gram-negative rods predominate, but a growing number of reports of nosocomially acquired *Candida* osteomyelitis have also been published (Table 1). In chronic infections, gram-positive microorganisms continue to predominate, i.e., *S. aureus* for open fractures and *Staphylococcus epidermidis* in foreign-body infections, but gram-negative rods (including *Pseudomonas* sp.) and mixed infections are increasingly reported. The microbiology of osteomyelitis associated with peripheral vascular disease is usually complex, involving several microorganisms (including staphylococci, gram-negative rods, anaerobes, and streptococci).

It is believed that in order to be effective, quinolones, like other antibiotics, should achieve bone levels exceeding the MIC for 90% of the responsible microorganisms ($MIC_{90}$) for significant periods. The same comments apply to septic arthritis, for which adequate antibiotic levels above the MIC have to be maintained in the infected joint fluid for prolonged periods. Although this prerequisite is fulfilled for most gram-negative microorganisms, including *Pseudomonas aeruginosa*, it is more difficult to achieve against *Staphylococcus* species and clearly becomes a problem when the agents presently available to treat streptococci and anaerobes are used. Thus, the search for new quinolones with lower MICs for gram-positive bacteria and anaerobes has been pursued. Some gain in MICs has been achieved with recently developed quinolones such as temafloxacin for some anaerobes ($MIC_{90}$ for *Bacteroides fragilis* and anaerobic cocci, $<1$ $\mu$g/ml) and sparfloxacin ($MIC_{90}$ for *Streptococcus pyogenes*, $<0.5$ $\mu$g/ml) (36).

## EXPERIMENTAL OSTEOMYELITIS AND ARTHRITIS

In the past, results from several experimental animal studies indicated that gram-negative infections such as *P. aeruginosa* osteomyelitis had an impressive cure rate of 95%

(2, 30). These excellent results were balanced by the demonstration of important increases in MIC for a significant percentage of the *Pseudomonas* strains isolated during therapy. The data obtained in models of animal infection correlated well with subsequent results observed in humans (15, 18). They underscore the importance of preliminary experiments in animals for deciding on optimal therapeutic regimens and identifying problems leading to therapeutic failures in humans.

More-recent animal studies have attempted to study the role of quinolones in staphylococcal infections, in particular during chronic osteomyelitis and bone infections associated with prosthetic material. Henry et al. (17) studied the treatment of methicillin-resistant *Staphylococcus* osteomyelitis with ciprofloxacin or vancomycin alone or in combination with rifampin for 21 days. Single-drug therapy with vancomycin or ciprofloxacin alone was ineffective, whereas rifampin-containing combinations were successful. Ciprofloxacin-rifampin proved to be the best combination, with no development of resistance to any of these antimicrobial agents. Dworkin et al. (9) also studied the comparative efficacies of ciprofloxacin, pefloxacin, and vancomycin in combination with rifampin in a rat model of methicillin-resistant *S. aureus* chronic osteomyelitis for a duration of 21 to 30 days. In accordance with the results cited above, neither the quinolones nor vancomycin alone was effective in reducing titers of organisms in bone after therapy, while rifampin alone was effective. All combination regimens with rifampin were more effective than rifampin alone, although these differences did not achieve statistical significance. These two studies favor the hypothesis that quinolone-rifampin combinations may offer a nonparenteral option for the treatment of chronic osteomyelitis caused by *S. aureus*.

Various groups have attempted to find successful therapies in a much more difficult experimental situation: the therapy of chronic osteomyelitis associated with foreign implants. In a mixed foreign-body infection with *S. epidermidis* and *Bacteroides thetaiotaomicron*, ciprofloxacin alone for 4 weeks proved ineffective despite the presence of rather high local levels (about 2 μg/ml) of antibiotics (28). This study suggests that ciprofloxacin alone is inadequate in protracted chronic infections because of microorganisms with high MICs for quinolones.

In a series of experiments in our laboratory, we studied the prophylactic activities of various quinolones in a guinea pig animal model of *S. aureus* foreign-body infections (3). Ciprofloxacin and ofloxacin in single doses were poorly effective, owing to the short half-lives of these antibiotics in tissue (respectively, 0 and 25% protection) and an inoculum of $10^3$ CFU; these results could be improved (75% protection) by the administration of a second dose of ofloxacin, allowing antibiotic coverage for the vulnerable period of 24 h after local injection of bacteria. A single dose of fleroxacin, a quinolone with a longer half-life in serum and interstitial fluid, proved to be highly efficient (100% protection) in preventing infection even at high inocula of microorganisms. These results suggest that an antimicrobial agent with prolonged elimination might be more advantageous in the prevention of staphylococcal infection associated with foreign bodies if single-dose regimens are used.

We have also studied the roles of fleroxacin, vancomycin, and rifampin alone and in combination for the short therapy (1 week) of a chronic staphylococcal foreign-body infection in rats (26). The combination fleroxacin-rifampin proved to be the best regimen in decreasing bacterial cell counts as well as in preventing development of resistance to rifampin. More recently, we extended these studies in the same rat model of chronic staphylococcal foreign-body infection by prolonging the antimicrobial therapy for 3 weeks (4). Although fleroxacin-rifampin proved again to be efficient and continued to decrease the number of bacterial cell counts, leading to sterilization of the fluid surrounding the prosthesis, surface-attached bacteria could still be detected. Interestingly, the triple combination vancomycin-fleroxacin-rifampin was highly efficient and sterilized the surface of the implants in most cases.

These experimental animal studies suggest that although presently available quinolones are inefficient in clearing staphylococcal infections associated with chronic bone infection or foreign bodies, combination therapy associating quinolones with rifampin and even additional antimicrobial agents is more successful and may open new therapeutic options in the future, ultimately preventing removal of the prosthetic material.

## CLINICAL STUDIES

Several studies have recently reviewed the literature regarding various antibacterial agents, including quinolones, for the therapy of osteomyelitis. Among the quinolones presently available, ciprofloxacin, ofloxacin, and pefloxacin have been used in large series of patients with bacterial osteomyelitis.

Until now, ciprofloxacin has been the most widely used quinolone for bacterial osteomyelitis, and combined results from almost 400 patients treated in various series are presently available. The usual dosage was 750 mg twice daily (5, 20, 27, 39). The tolerance was excellent (less than 5% of the patients had adverse effects) when this agent was given for prolonged periods (average, more than 2 months). The rates of clinical success after a follow-up of 6 months and of bacteriological eradication approached almost 80% for osteomyelitis due to *S. aureus* and *P. aeruginosa*. The emergence of resistance or persistence of *S. aureus*, however, has been reported in several cases with ciprofloxacin (see chapter 6).

Smaller series of patients (fewer than 50 patients total) have been treated with ofloxacin (24) or pefloxacin. Ofloxacin was given for prolonged periods (average, more than 3 months), with long-term success and bacteriological eradication approaching 70% in published studies.

In France, extensive experience has been acquired with the quinolone pefloxacin used for prolonged periods. French clinicians have treated patients for long periods with regimens that averaged almost 6 months of therapy with excellent tolerance (6, 7), while some of these patients also had surgical debridement. With average follow-up of more than 3 years, the long-term success was 80% and eradication was around 80% for both *S. aureus* and *P. aeruginosa*. A very interesting open therapeutic trial on 32 patients with *Staphylococcus*-infected hip and knee prostheses has been reported recently by Raoult et al. (35). All patients received 900 mg of rifampin plus 600 mg of ofloxacin per day for 6 to 9 months. Fourteen patients underwent prosthesis replacement, and two patients had to stop the antibiotic because of adverse effects. Cure was obtained in 27 cases, with a follow-up ranging from 4 to 48 months. Thus, although this is not a randomized or controlled trial, the results suggest that long-term therapy may cure staphylococcal foreign-body infection in humans as well by using a regimen similar to that of a trial reported with staphylococcal prosthetic infections.

An interesting study has been performed with patients with lower-extremity infections associated with peripheral vascular disease and/or diabetes. Peterson et al. (32) administered ciprofloxacin per os at large doses (750 to 1,000 mg every 12 h) to 29 patients for prolonged periods (90 days); the long-term success rate at the 1-year follow-up was 66%. Bacteriological eradication rates were 57% for *S. aureus* and 83% for *P. aeruginosa*.

Similar results were obtained by Garcia-Rosario and Ramirez-Ronda (10). Their studies suggest that quinolones administered for long periods might be useful for this difficult clinical situation (31). However, caution is warranted because of the poor activities of presently available quinolones against streptococci and anaerobes, the local status (degree of vascularization, neuropathy, and bone involvement), and the importance of optimal timing for surgery in these patients.

Over the last few years, at least three randomized trials have attempted to compare the use of oral ciprofloxacin with that of other antimicrobial agents in the treatment of osteomyelitis.

In a small study (30 adults), Greenberg et al. compared ciprofloxacin (750 mg twice daily) and other antimicrobial therapies adapted to the microorganisms found in lesions, mostly *Enterobacteriaceae* and *Pseudomonas* spp. At 1-year follow-up, 50% of ciprofloxacin-treated patients were cured, whereas 65% treated with other antimicrobial agents were cured (16).

One of the best comparative trials in this area was recently performed by Gentry and Rodriguez (13). Patients were enrolled in a randomized protocol in which they received either oral ciprofloxacin monotherapy or parenteral therapy optimized to culture and sensitivity data. Prior to enrollment, all infections had been surgically debrided and all foreign material had been removed. All 59 patients enrolled had bone biopsies and aerobic and anaerobic cultures. No patient had to stop ciprofloxacin therapy because of the presence of resistant microorganisms (most of the isolated microorganisms were *S. aureus* and various gram-negative rods). Oral ciprofloxacin was as effective and safe as parenteral therapy, with a 2-year success rate of 77%, which was comparable to that of conventional parenteral therapy (79%). In a recent review, Gentry mentioned the persistence of *S. aureus* in three patients in this study who were treated with ciprofloxacin despite in vitro susceptibility to this antimicrobial agent.

In a more recent comparative trial, Gentry and Rodriguez-Gomez (14) compared oral ofloxacin (19 patients treated with 400 mg every 12 h for 8 weeks) and parenteral agents (1 g of cefazolin every 8 h or 2 g of ceftazidime every 12 h for 4 weeks). Hospitalized adult patients with bone biopsy-confirmed osteomyelitis that required antimicrobial therapy were eligible for the study. As in the previous study, most microorganisms (mostly *S. aureus* and gram-negative rods) were susceptible to the antimicrobial agents. Long-term response to therapy was successful for 74% of the subjects who received ofloxacin and 86% of those who received parenteral antibiotics. However, the small number of patients in this study limited its power to detect a statistically significant difference between the two regimens.

One of the major features of the two studies discussed above is that all the patients had biopsy-proven microbiological diagnoses and complete debridement of necrotic bone, soft tissue, and any other foreign material. These features led to the clinical assessment of an optimal antibiotic regimen without the bias of suboptimal surgical therapy. Overall, these clinical studies show excellent results with oral quinolones for the therapy of osteomyelitis, in particular that due to gram-negative microorganisms, with some limitations for therapy of *S. aureus* infections.

## QUINOLONES IN INFECTIOUS ARTHRITIS

In contrast to the situation with osteomyelitis, much less knowledge has been gained about the therapy of infectious arthritis. Bayer et al. have compared the efficacy of ciprofloxacin and ceftriaxone in experimental arthritis in a rabbit model (2). Both agents significantly reduced mean *Escherichia coli* counts in septic joint fluid and also within infected synovial tissue. The ciprofloxacin regimen caused a higher frequency of synovial tissue sterilization (53%) than did ceftriaxone (25%). Several recent case reports (8, 33, 34, 42) illustrate the efficacy of quinolones for the therapy of infectious arthritis, but no study of a large series of patients has been published so far.

## REMAINING ISSUES

### Is There Any Prospect for Optimal Use of Quinolones for Therapy of *S. aureus* Osteomyelitis?

As reviewed above, staphylococci remain one of the most common causative pathogens of osteomyelitis. Because of their antimicrobial activities against staphylococci, quinolones were rapidly considered to be promising therapeutic agents for this indication. Ciprofloxacin is more potent than norfloxacin against staphylococci, with a $MIC_{90}$ of 0.5 mg/liter. Ofloxacin ($MIC_{90}$, 0.2 mg/liter) and pefloxacin ($MIC_{90}$, 0.2 mg/liter) may be more potent than ciprofloxacin against methicillin-resistant *S. aureus* in vitro, and their activities are augmented by higher levels in serum. New fluoroquinolones such as sparfloxacin, with activities greater than or similar to that of ofloxacin against staphylococci ($MIC_{90}$, <0.06 mg/liter for sparfloxacin), might be launched soon. However, the use of quinolones as single agents in *S. aureus* infections has led to a significant percentage of clinical failures, sometimes associated with the development of resistance to these antimicrobial agents. An additional, more worrisome finding has been a generalized epidemiological trend toward development of resistance among staphylococci upon widespread general use of these drugs (23, 25, 40). Thus, in nursing homes in New York, high-level ciprofloxacin resistance in *S. aureus* increased from 0.9 to 5.3%, and in intensive care units in France after widespread use of the drug, high-level resistance to pefloxacin increased from 0% in 1980 to 32% in 1984. Additionally, quinolone resistance is much more common among methicillin-resistant staphylococci, limiting the oral use of these drugs as a replacement for vancomycin. Thus, although a large percentage of staphylococcal strains remain sensitive to quinolones, a strategy should be implemented to limit further the development of resistance and enhance the efficacy of quinolones.

As described above, one of the most promising approaches in this situation is the combination of quinolones with rifampin. Such combinations have been used successfully in small numbers of patients with staphylococcal right-sided endocarditis and chronic osteomyelitis as well as in experimental bone infections. Without large, prospective, randomized clinical trials, however, this approach cannot yet be recommended. One should include in these new strategies the use of optimal doses and the use of new quinolones such as fleroxacin or sparfloxacin with more-prolonged elimination (in order to achieve levels in tissue continuously above the MIC). Finally, new quinolones with higher therapeutic indices, such as sparfloxacin, are promising and will need further animal and human testing (21, 22, 29, 36).

### May Quinolones Be Used for Therapy of Osteomyelitis in Children?

Because of their arthropathic toxicity observed in growing animals, the quinolone antibiotics were not initially recommended for pediatric patients.

So far, unequivocal quinolone-induced skeletal damage has never been documented in humans. Retrospective matched, controlled studies of 268 children treated with nalidixic acid for 9 to 1,689 days did not reveal any drug-associated arthropathy. A recent review of the use of quinolones in pediatrics comprises 540 prepubertal patients treated with one of the fluoroquinolones; results for 68 patients were published in peer-reviewed medical journals. In these children, no quinolone-induced arthropathy was noted, and reversible arthralgia with possible or probable relation to quinolone therapy occurred in approximately 1% (37).

A recent investigation collected clinical, laboratory, radiological, and magnetic resonance imaging data for 18 patients with cystic fibrosis (age range, 14 to 24 years) at the start and the end of a 3-month course of ciprofloxacin (30 mg/kg of body weight/day administered orally in two equal doses) and at follow-up 4 to 6 months later. The results, together with the published data on quinolone use in pediatrics, suggest that ciprofloxacin does not cause arthropathy in children (38).

Further studies on potential quinolone toxicity should, however, be performed with larger numbers of pediatric patients, including infants and young children, and with diseases other than cystic fibrosis. Also, long-term follow-up for many years is needed. In the meantime, the use of quinolone antibiotics must be limited in childhood to carefully monitored trials on safety and efficacy and to specific infections complicated by pathologic or special conditions (for a detailed discussion, see reference 37).

## CONCLUDING REMARKS

Osteomyelitis is difficult to treat, and for optimal therapy, several factors in addition to choosing the optimal antimicrobial agent must be taken into account.

First, the presence of dead bone or a foreign body will lead to failure unless a combined surgical (debridement and removal of sequestra and foreign material) and medical approach is applied.

Second, clinical experience indicates that to obtain cure, the antibiotic must be delivered into bone for prolonged periods (4 to 6 weeks for acute infections and sometimes months for chronic infections).

Upon introduction of the new fluoroquinolones, the ease of oral administration and their potent anti-gram-negative-bacterium activity have led clinicians to try prolonged therapy (weeks to months) for complicated osteomyelitis. This may explain why success rates in some clinical studies are higher than those obtained with experimental infections, where therapy is usually shorter. The presently available quinolones have become the main therapy for gram-negative osteomyelitis and infectious arthritis.

Staphylococcal infections, which remain one of the most frequent causes of osteomyelitis, are still difficult to treat. Although reasonably high success rates have been achieved in several studies with quinolone monotherapy, increasing clinical and experimental evidence suggests that the addition of rifampin would be a promising approach in this area. Randomized and controlled studies are, however, an absolute necessity before it will be possible to recommend this new form of therapy. Finally, newer quinolones with better anti-gram-positive-bacterium and anti-anaerobic activities are being developed and offer exciting new perspectives in this area. Clinical experience, however, is still relatively meager.

*Acknowledgments.* Grant support was from the Swiss National Research Foundation (grant 32-30161.90).

### REFERENCES

1. **Bayer, A. S.** 1989. Clinical utility of new quinolones in treatment of osteomyelitis and lower respiratory tract infections. *Eur. J. Clin. Microbiol. Infect. Dis.* **8:**1102–1110.
2. **Bayer, A. S., D. Norman, and D. Anderson.** 1985. Efficacy of ciprofloxacin in experimental arthritis caused by Escherichia coli in vitro-in vivo correlations. *J. Infect. Dis.* **152:**811–816.
3. **Bouchenaki, N., P. Vaudaux, E. Huggler, F. A. Waldvogel, and D. P. Lew.** 1990. Successful single-dose prophylaxis of *Staphylococcus aureus* foreign body infection in guinea pigs by fleroxacin. *Antimicrob. Agents Chemother.* **34:**21–24.
4. **Chuard, C., P. Rohner, V. Dunand, R. Auckenthaler, and D. P. Lew.** 1992. In-vitro and in-vivo evaluation of the antistaphylococcal activity of S-5556, a new 16-membered macrolide. *J. Antimicrob. Chemother.* **30:**327–337.
5. **Dan, M., Y. Siegman Igra, S. Pitlik, and R. Raz.** 1990. Oral ciprofloxacin treatment of *Pseudomonas aeruginosa* osteomyelitis. *Antimicrob. Agents Chemother.* **34:**849–852.
6. **Dellamonica, P., E. Bernard, H. Etesse, R. Garraffo, and H. B. Drugeon.** 1989. Evaluation of pefloxacin, ofloxacin and ciprofloxacin in the treatment of thirty-nine cases of chronic osteomyelitis. *Eur. J. Clin. Microbiol. Infect. Dis.* **8:**1024–1030.
7. **Desplaces, N., and J. F. Acar.** 1988. New quinolones in the treatment of joint and bone infections. *Rev. Infect. Dis.* **10**(Suppl. 1)**:**S179–S183.
8. **Diaz Tejeiro, R., J. Diez, F. Maduell, N. Esparza, P. Errasti, and A. Purroy.** 1989. Successful treatment with ciprofloxacin of multiresistant

salmonella arthritis in a renal transplant recipient. *Nephrol. Dial. Transplant.* **4:**390–392.

9. **Dworkin, R., G. Modin, S. Kunz, R. Rich, O. Zak, and M. Sande.** 1990. Comparative efficacies of ciprofloxacin, pefloxacin, and vancomycin in combination with rifampin in a rat model of methicillin-resistant *Staphylococcus aureus* chronic osteomyelitis. *Antimicrob. Agents Chemother.* **34:**1014–1016.
10. **Garcia-Rosario, L. N., and C. H. Ramirez-Ronda.** 1990. El uso de ciprofloxacin en pacientes con osteomielitis asociada a insuficiencia vascular. *Bol. Asoc. Med. P.R.* **82:**125–128.
11. **Gentry, L. O.** 1990. Antibiotic therapy for osteomyelitis. *Infect. Dis. Clin. North Am.* **4:**485–499.
12. **Gentry, L. O.** 1991. Oral antimicrobial therapy for osteomyelitis. *Ann. Intern. Med.* **114:**986–987. (Editorial.)
13. **Gentry, L. O., and G. G. Rodriguez.** 1990. Oral ciprofloxacin compared with parenteral antibiotics in the treatment of osteomyelitis. *Antimicrob. Agents Chemother.* **34:**40–43.
14. **Gentry, L. O., and G. Rodriguez-Gomez.** 1991. Ofloxacin versus parenteral therapy for chronic osteomyelitis. *Antimicrob. Agents Chemother.* **35:**538–541.
15. **Gilbert, D. N., A. D. Tice, P. K. Marsh, P. C. Craven, and L. C. Preheim.** 1987. Oral ciprofloxacin therapy for chronic contiguous osteomyelitis caused by aerobic gram-negative bacilli. *Am. J. Med.* **82:**254–258.
16. **Greenberg, R. N., A. D. Tice, P. K. Marsh, P. C. Craven, P. M. Reilly, M. Bollinger, and W. J. Weinandt.** 1987. Randomized trial of ciprofloxacin compared with other antimicrobial therapy in the treatment of osteomyelitis. *Am. J. Med.* **82:**266–269.
17. **Henry, N. K., M. S. Rouse, A. L. Whitesell, M. E. McConnell, and W. R. Wilson.** 1987. Treatment of methicillin-resistant *Staphylococcus aureus* experimental osteomyelitis with ciprofloxacin or vancomycin alone or in combination with rifampin. *Am. J. Med.* **82:**73–75.
18. **Hessen, M. T., M. J. Ingerman, D. H. Kaufman, P. Weiner, J. Santoro, O. M. Korzeniowski, J. Boscia, M. Topiel, L. M. Bush, D. Kaye, and M. E. Levison.** 1987. Clinical efficacy of ciprofloxacin therapy for gram-negative bacillary osteomyelitis. *Am. J. Med.* **82:**262–265.
19. **Hessen, M. T., and M. E. Levison.** 1989. Ciprofloxacin for the treatment of osteomyelitis: a review. *J. Foot Surg.* **28:**100–105.
20. **Hoogkamp-Korstanje, J. A., H. A. van Bottenburg, J. van Bruggen, J. S. Davidson, S. J. Detmar, W. de Graaf, J. Rijnks, J. F. Ypma, and D. F. de Zwart.** 1989. Treatment of chronic osteomyelitis with ciprofloxacin. *J. Antimicrob. Chemother.* **23:**427–432.
21. **Hooper, D. C., and J. S. Wolfson.** 1991. Fluoroquinolone antimicrobial agents. *N. Engl. J. Med.* **324:**384–394.
22. **Jones, R., M. Barrett, M. Erwin, B. Briggs, and D. Johnson.** 1991. In vitro antimicrobial activity of sparfloxacin, compared with numerous other quinolone compounds. *Diagn. Microbiol. Infect. Dis.* **14:**319–330.
23. **Kaatz, G. W., S. M. Seo, and C. A. Ruble.** 1991. Mechanisms of fluoroquinolone resistance in *Staphylococcus aureus. J. Infect. Dis.* **163:**1080–1086.
24. **Ketterl, R., T. Beckurts, B. Stubinger, and B. Claudi.** 1988. Use of ofloxacin in open fractures and in the treatment of post-traumatic osteomyelitis. *J. Antimicrob. Chemother.* **22**(Suppl. C):159–166.
25. **Kotilainen, P., J. Nikoskelainen, and P. Huovinen.** 1990. Emergence of ciprofloxacin-resistant coagulase-negative staphylococcal skin flora in immunocompromised patients receiving ciprofloxacin. *J. Infect. Dis.* **161:**41–44.
26. **Lucet, J. C., M. Herrmann, P. Rohner, R. Auckenthaler, F. A. Waldvogel, and D. P. Lew.** 1990. Treatment of experimental foreign body infection caused by methicillin-resistant *Staphylococcus aureus. Antimicrob. Agents Chemother.* **34:**2312–2317.
27. **Mader, J. T., J. S. Cantrell, and J. Calhoun.** 1990. Oral ciprofloxacin compared with standard parenteral antibiotic therapy for chronic osteomyelitis in adults. *J. Bone Joint Surg.* **72:**104–110.
28. **Mayberry Carson, K. J., B. Tober Meyer, L. R. Gill, D. W. Lambe, Jr., and F. E. Hossler.** 1990. Effect of ciprofloxacin on experimental osteomyelitis in the rabbit tibia, induced with a mixed infection of *Staphylococcus epidermidis* and *Bacteroides thetaiotaomicron. Microbios* **64:**49–66.
29. **Neu, H. C.** 1991. The place of quinolones in bacterial infections. *Adv. Intern. Med.* **36:**1–32.
30. **Norden, C. W., and E. Shinners.** 1985. Ciprofloxacin as therapy for experimental osteomyelitis caused by *Pseudomonas aeruginosa. J. Infect. Dis.* **151:**291–294.
31. **Norrby, S. R.** 1989. Ciprofloxacin in the treatment of acute and chronic osteomyelitis: a review. *Scand. J. Infect. Dis. Suppl.* **60:**74–78.
32. **Peterson, L. R., L. M. Lissack, K. Canter, C. E. Fasching, C. Clabots, and D. N. Gerding.** 1989. Therapy of lower extremity infections with ciprofloxacin in patients with diabetes mellitus, peripheral vascular disease, or both. *Am. J. Med.* **86:**801–808.
33. **Praet, J. P., A. Peretz, H. Goossens, Y. Van Laethem, and J. P. Famaey.** 1989. Salmonella septic arthritis: additional 2 cases with quinolone treatment. *J. Rheumatol.* **16:**1610–1611.
34. **Raffi, F., P. Poirier, and A. E. Reynaud.** 1989. Arthrite septique à *Pasteurella multocida.* Traite-

ment par une fluoroquinolone. *Presse Med.* **18:**1482. (Letter.)

35. **Raoult, D., M. Drancourt, J. N. Argenson, and J. M. Aubaniac.** 1991. Rifampin plus ofloxacin for treatment of staphylococcal-infected hip and knee prosthesis, abstr. 1281. *Program Abstr. 31st Intersci. Conf. Antimicrob. Agents Chemother.*
36. **Rohner, P., M. Peebo, D. P. Lew, R. Auckenthaler, and J. C. Pechère.** 1992. Comparative in-vitro activity of new quinolones against clinical isolates and resistant mutants. *J. Antimicrob. Chemother.* **29:**41–48.
37. **Schaad, U. B.** 1991. Use of quinolones in pediatrics. *Eur. J. Clin. Microbiol. Infect. Dis.* **10:**355–360.
38. **Schaad, U. B., C. Stoupis, J. Wedgwood, H. Tschaeppeler, and P. Vock.** 1991. Clinical, radiologic and magnetic resonance monitoring for skeletal toxicity in pediatric patients with cystic fibrosis receiving a three-month course of ciprofloxacin. *Pediatr. Infect. Dis. J.* **10:**723–729.
39. **Swedish Study Group.** 1988. Therapy of acute and chronic gram-negative osteomyelitis with ciprofloxacin. *J. Antimicrob. Chemother.* **22:**221–228.
40. **Trucksis, M., D. C. Hooper, and J. S. Wolfson.** 1991. Emerging resistance to fluoroquinolones in staphylococci: an alert. *Ann. Intern. Med.* **114:**424–426. (Editorial.)
41. **Waldvogel, F. A.** 1989. Use of quinolones for the treatment of osteomyelitis and septic arthritis. *Rev. Infect. Dis.* **11:**S1259–S1263.
42. **Widmer, A. F., V. E. Colombo, A. Gachter, G. Thiel, and W. Zimmerli.** 1990. Salmonella infection in total hip replacement: tests to predict the outcome of antimicrobial therapy. *Scand. J. Infect. Dis.* **22:**611–618.
43. **Wispelwey, B., and W. M. Scheld.** 1990. Ciprofloxacin in the treatment of *Staphylococcus aureus* osteomyelitis. A review. *Diagn. Microbiol. Infect. Dis.* **13:**169–171.

*Quinolone Antimicrobial Agents, 2nd ed.*
Edited by David C. Hooper and John S. Wolfson


*Chapter 20*

# Treatment of Bacterial Meningitis

*Allan R. Tunkel and W. Michael Scheld*

Bacterial meningitis is an illness that continues to have a high mortality rate despite the availability of effective bactericidal antimicrobial agents. Case fatality rates for meningitis due to the three most common etiologic agents of bacterial meningitis, *Haemophilus influenzae, Neisseria meningitidis,* and *Streptococcus pneumoniae,* were 6.0, 10.3, and 26.3%, respectively, in the United States from 1978 to 1981 (48). Case fatality rates in a subsequent study of five states and Los Angeles County during 1986 (67) were lower (e.g., 19% for *S. pneumoniae*), suggesting that improvements in early detection and antibiotic treatment may have occurred in the 1980s. Bacterial meningitis also remains a significant problem in other parts of the world. In a review of all cases of purulent, nontuberculous meningitis in an isolation-fever hospital in Salvador, Brazil, for the decade 1973 through 1982 (4), the three common meningeal pathogens (see above) accounted for 72% of all cases and 70% of the deaths. The case fatality rate for *H. influenzae*-caused disease was 38%, much higher than that encountered in the United States. The mortality for meningitis due to members of the family *Enterobacteriaceae* was 86% in that study, with more than half of the cases in children less than 24 months of age being caused by *Salmonella* species, a rare cause of bacterial meningitis in the United States. In addition to these unacceptable case fatality rates, recent antimicrobial susceptibility patterns of meningeal pathogens have documented resistance of these organisms to many conventional antimicrobial agents. For example, ß-lactamase-producing strains accounted for approximately 24% of cerebrospinal fluid (CSF) isolates of *H. influenzae* type b overall in the United States in 1981 (48) and for about 32% of CSF isolates in 1986 (67). The etiologic agents of gram-negative bacillary meningitis (e.g., *Escherichia coli, Klebsiella pneumoniae, Pseudomonas aeruginosa*) also have demonstrated increased resistance to standard antibiotics, including expanded-spectrum cephalosporins, particularly in the hospital setting. These data indicate the continued need to investigate the potential effectiveness of alternative antimicrobial agents for the therapy of bacterial meningitis.

The new fluoroquinolones have two important properties that suggest they may be good candidates for the treatment of central nervous system (CNS) infections: excellent in vitro activity against gram-negative men-

***Allan R. Tunkel*** • Department of Internal Medicine (Infectious Diseases), Medical College of Pennsylvania, Philadelphia, Pennsylvania 19129. ***W. Michael Scheld*** • Departments of Internal Medicine (Infectious Diseases) and Neurosurgery, University of Virginia Health Sciences Center, Charlottesville, Virginia 22908.

ingeal pathogens and good penetration into extravascular spaces, including CSF. However, despite these favorable properties, the fluoroquinolones have been used infrequently to treat CNS infections such as bacterial meningitis (22, 28, 41). The following sections review the basic therapeutic principles for the use of antimicrobial agents against bacterial meningitis as well as the in vitro spectra of activity of the fluoroquinolones against meningeal pathogens, their CSF penetration, and clinical results in both experimental animal models and humans to place in perspective the potential usefulness of the fluoroquinolones in the treatment of bacterial meningitis.

## BASIC THERAPEUTIC PRINCIPLES FOR BACTERIAL MENINGITIS

The definition of bacteriologic cure or response in patients with bacterial meningitis is based on bacteriologic eradication from CSF, and several factors determine whether bactericidal activity is achieved (60, 62). The first factor is entry, or penetration, of the antimicrobial agent into CSF, which depends on the status of the blood-brain barrier and other variables. The barrier separates the brain and CSF from the intravascular compartment and acts as a regulatory interface, with functions including active transport, facilitated diffusion of various substances (e.g., hexoses, amino acids), aqueous secretion forming CSF, and most important, maintenance of homeostasis within the CNS. All ß-lactam antibiotics penetrate into CSF poorly (about 0.5 to 2.0% of concurrent peak or steady-state concentrations in serum for penicillin) in the absence of meningeal inflammation (normal blood-brain barrier). In the presence of meningeal inflammation, drug penetration into CSF is generally enhanced. Altered blood-brain barrier permeability is manifested morphologically by separation of intercellular tight junctions and increased numbers of pinocytotic vesicles in cerebral capillary endothelial cells (31). Agents (e.g., methylprednisolone) that decrease subarachnoid space inflammation may reduce the blood-brain barrier permeability of certain antimicrobial agents (e.g., ampicillin or gentamicin) (44). In addition, antibiotic entry into CSF declines as inflammation subsides during the course of therapy for bacterial meningitis; therefore, doses of antimicrobial agents should not be reduced late in therapy. Other factors that enhance penetration of an antimicrobial agent into CSF include low molecular weight (27), low degree of ionization at physiologic pH, high lipid solubility (40), and low degree of protein binding in serum (36, 55). The CSF penetration of selected fluoroquinolone antimicrobial agents in experimental animal models and humans is discussed in detail below.

A second factor contributing to cure of bacterial meningitis relates to the activities of antimicrobial agents in purulent CSF. Once the drug enters the CSF, other factors influence its activity. For example, the pH of CSF decreases in patients with bacterial meningitis because of lactate accumulation and other processes. An acid environment reduces the in vitro activities of the aminoglycosides, possibly explaining, in part, the poor response obtained with these agents in the therapy of gram-negative meningitis (56). Antibiotics can also be metabolized in vivo to less active metabolites. For example, cephalothin is metabolized in vivo to desacetylcephalothin, which is less active in vitro against major meningeal pathogens than the parent compound and contributes to the poor therapeutic results obtained with cephalothin in infections of the CNS (25). In contrast, the metabolite of cefotaxime, desacetylcefotaxime, is as active in vitro as the parent compound (26). In addition, there is an active transport system in the choroid plexus that can remove some antibiotics (generally weak bases) from CSF to blood. This process has been demonstrated for removal of the penicillins and cephalosporins from CSF and can be inhibited by concurrent administration of probenecid, which increases the CSF concentrations of many ß-lactam antibiotics (60).

Antimicrobial activity within purulent CSF may also be influenced by other drugs, including other antimicrobial agents. Studies of experimental animal models of meningitis have demonstrated antagonism of the bactericidal effect in CSF when a bactericidal agent is coadministered with a bacteriostatic antibiotic. Chloramphenicol antagonized the effects of penicillin in an experimental canine model of pneumococcal meningitis (66), a characteristic most apparent when the administration of chloramphenicol preceded that of penicillin. Chloramphenicol therapy also antagonized the action of gentamicin in an experimental rabbit model of *Proteus mirabilis* meningitis (56). This result has been confirmed by clinical experience. In a review of cases of meningitis caused by the *Enterobacteriaceae*, case fatality rates were highest when chloramphenicol was included in the therapeutic regimen (generally an aminoglycoside) (5). However, in other instances, bactericidal efficacy within CSF can be enhanced by the addition of a second drug that also has bactericidal activity, as demonstrated by the addition of gentamicin to either ampicillin or penicillin in experimental models of meningitis caused by *Listeria monocytogenes* (46) or *Streptococcus agalactiae* (43).

The mode of antibiotic administration is a third factor contributing to the response to therapy of bacterial meningitis. The choice of intermittent bolus versus continuous administration by the intravenous route of an antimicrobial agent has been the subject of considerable debate. The two modes of administration were equally efficacious in an experimental animal model of pneumococcal meningitis in which the animals were treated with penicillin G (35), although the test regimens resulted in concentrations of penicillin in CSF above the MBC for the test strain for the entire dosage interval. When intermittent intravenous doses of ampicillin that achieved concentrations in CSF below the MBC for a portion of the treatment period were given, a "postantibiotic effect" characterized by a continued decline or stable pneumococcal concentrations in CSF was observed in vivo. However, there is no demonstrable postantibiotic effect for ß-lactam agents in general against gram-negative aerobic bacilli in vivo or in vitro, suggesting that therapeutic strategies in patients with gram-negative meningitis should be devised to maintain concentrations of this class of drugs in CSF above the MBC for the entire treatment interval.

Finally, there is a need for bactericidal activity in CSF for optimal treatment of bacterial meningitis. Bacterial meningitis is an infection in an area of impaired host resistance in which antibody and complement concentrations are low in CSF, and functional humoral-mediated opsonic or bactericidal activity is usually undetectable early in the disease course (62). Because of this relative and localized host defense deficiency, phagocytosis of major encapsulated pathogens is inefficient, permitting bacteria to attain huge concentrations in purulent CSF. Several experimental studies have demonstrated that rapid bacterial killing is observed only when the CSF concentrations of ß-lactams or aminoglycosides exceed the MBC of the inoculated strain by 10- to 20-fold (38, 45, 47, 56). This concept has also been substantiated by clinical data.

## IN VITRO ACTIVITIES OF FLUOROQUINOLONES AGAINST MENINGEAL PATHOGENS

The in vitro activities of selected fluoroquinolones against meningeal pathogens are shown in Table 1 (14, 24, 28, 65). The fluoroquinolones are extremely active in vitro against the gram-negative bacteria (e.g., *H. influenzae, N. meningitidis,* and *E. coli*). Ciprofloxacin is the most active fluoroquinolone against these organisms currently available in the United States and in addition has the best in vitro activity of the fluoroquino-

**Table 1.** In vitro activities of selected fluoroquinolones against major meningeal pathogens[a]

| Organism | MIC$_{90}$ ($\mu$g/ml) | | | | | | | |
|---|---|---|---|---|---|---|---|---|
| | Norfloxacin | Ciprofloxacin | Ofloxacin | Enoxacin | Pefloxacin | Temafloxacin | Fleroxacin | Lomefloxacin |
| *H. influenzae* | 0.06 | 0.01 | 0.03 | 0.12 | 0.06 | 0.25 | 0.12 | 0.12–0.25 |
| *N. meningitidis* | 0.03 | 0.01 | 0.02 | 0.03 | 0.03 | 0.12 | 0.12 | 0.12 |
| *S. pneumoniae* | 16.0 | 2.0 | 2.0 | 16.0 | 8.0 | 1.0 | 8.0 | 8.0–16.0 |
| *E. coli* | 0.12 | 0.03 | 0.12 | 0.4 | 0.25 | 0.25 | 1.0 | 0.25 |
| *Salmonella* species | 0.06 | 0.02 | 0.06–0.12 | 0.12 | 0.12–0.25 | 0.5 | 0.12 | 0.25 |
| *P. aeruginosa* | 2.0 | 0.5 | 2.0 | 4.0 | 2.0 | 4.0 | 2.0 | 4.0 |
| *S. agalactiae* | 8.0 | 1.0 | 2.0 | 16.0 | 16.0 | 0.5 | 8.0 | 8.0 |
| *S. aureus* | 6.3 | 1.0 | 0.4 | 3.1 | 0.5 | 0.5 | 1.0 | 2.0 |
| Coagulase-negative staphylococci | 3.1 | 0.25 | 0.8 | 6.3 | 0.5 | 2.0 | 1.0 | 1.0 |
| *L. monocytogenes* | 4.0 | 0.5 | 1.0 | 16.0 | 8.0 | 0.25 | 8.0 | |

[a]Data are from references 14, 24, 28, and 65.

lones with activity against *P. aeruginosa*. The fluoroquinolones are also highly active in vitro against pathogens rarely encountered in patients with bacterial meningitis (e.g., *Salmonella* species and other *Enterobacteriaceae*); these pathogens are associated with high mortality rates and are frequently resistant to other antibiotics. Although the MBC is more important than the MIC in determining the optimal response to antimicrobial therapy in patients with bacterial meningitis (see above), the concentrations in CSF achieved with these agents are in general about 4- to >50-fold higher than the MICs for 90% of strains of gram-negative pathogens.

Although gram-negative pathogens are in general highly susceptible to the new fluoroquinolones, gram-positive organisms are considerably less susceptible and are much more variable in their in vitro susceptibility patterns. In addition, while several of the new fluoroquinolones possess in vitro activity against staphylococci, including methicillin-resistant strains, the concentrations in CSF of these agents that are achieved with systemic administration are barely equal to and usually do not exceed the MICs for these isolates. Furthermore, clinical experience with these agents in the therapy of staphylococcal meningitis is virtually nonexistent. For other gram-positive organisms that are important meningeal pathogens (e.g., *S. pneumoniae, S. agalactiae,* and *L. monocytogenes*), susceptibility to the currently available fluoroquinolones is marginal. Because of these in vitro data and other factors (see below), clinical experience with the use of the fluoroquinolones in the treatment of patients with bacterial meningitis has in large part been appropriately restricted to cases involving multidrug-resistant gram-negative bacilli. Certain newer fluoroquinolones (e.g., sparfloxacin, tosufloxacin, etc.) have improved activity against gram-positive pathogens but have not yet been studied extensively in animal models or humans with CNS disease.

## ENTRY OF FLUOROQUINOLONES INTO CSF IN EXPERIMENTAL ANIMAL MODELS OF MENINGITIS

As stated above, the penetration of an antimicrobial agent into CSF is an important factor in determining whether bactericidal activity is achieved in patients with bacterial meningitis. The fluoroquinolones have been evaluated in several experimental animal models to determine their efficiencies of entry into normal or purulent CSF (34, 42). Table 2 compares the CSF penetration of several of the fluoroquinolones with those of conventional antimicrobial agents in the experimental rabbit model of bacterial meningitis.

Early experimental studies that examined the penetration of fluoroquinolones into CSF revealed that concentrations of pefloxacin in CSF were 76% of those in sera of dogs with experimental *Staphylococcus aureus* meningitis (2) (penetration in healthy uninfected dogs was 44.6%). In another experimental canine model (59), a 1-h intravenous injection of either 12.5 or 25 mg of enoxacin per kg of body weight in uninfected animals produced average concentrations in CSF of 2.6 and 6.5 μg/ml, respectively, within 90 to 240 min; these corresponded to percent penetration values into CSF, as calculated by the area under the curve method, of 33% (12.5-mg/kg dose) and 47% (25-mg/kg dose). In animals infected intracisternally with *S. aureus*, an intravenous dose of enoxacin (12.5 mg/kg) given 18 to 20 h later led to a peak concentration in CSF of 6.9 μg/ml (CSF penetration of 67.3%). In both uninfected and infected animals, the concentrations in CSF greatly exceeded the MICs for enoxacin (and other marketed fluoroquinolones) against meningococci and *H. influenzae*.

**Table 2.** Percent penetration of selected antimicrobial agents into CSF of rabbits with experimental meningitis

| Antimicrobial agent | Percent penetration[a] |
|---|---|
| Penicillin G | 2.6–4.9 |
| Ampicillin | 12.1–18.4 |
| Cefotaxime | 2.1–11.1 |
| Ceftriaxone | 2.7–12.0 |
| Ceftazidime | 11.1–32.6 |
| Gentamicin | 18.9–28.7 |
| Amikacin | 19.0–35.3 |
| Vancomycin | 8.4–11.7 |
| Chloramphenicol | 22.3–34.3 |
| Ciprofloxacin | 15.0–27.5 |
| Pefloxacin | 46.0–51.3 |
| Ofloxacin | 20.0 |
| Fleroxacin | 81.9–107 |

[a]Data are from references 13, 42, 52, 53, and 60. Values are calculated as (concentration in CSF/concentration in serum) × 100. These calculations are derived from peak concentrations, mean concentrations, or areas under the curve.

Pefloxacin has also been evaluated in an experimental rabbit model of *E. coli* meningitis (52). In uninfected rabbits, the percent penetration of pefloxacin into CSF after a 3-h infusion of 5, 15, or 30 mg/kg/h ranged from 26.4 to 39.2%. In animals with *E. coli* meningitis, the mean percent penetration of pefloxacin given at various dosages (1 to 30 mg/kg/h for 7 h after an initial bolus) was assessed 16 h after induction of meningitis. The mean percent penetration of pefloxacin into CSF was 51.3% in all rabbits with meningitis compared with percent penetration of 11.1% for cefotaxime (100 mg/kg/h) and 22.3% for chloramphenicol (60 mg/kg/h). In another animal study (23), mean CSF pefloxacin concentrations (8.8 μg/ml) were 44.7% of serum pefloxacin concentrations (19.7 μg/ml) in three healthy dogs after 6 weeks of therapy.

Other fluoroquinolones have been examined with respect to CSF penetration in animal models of bacterial meningitis. In an experimental model of *P. aeruginosa* meningitis (13), the mean percent penetration of ciprofloxacin was 18.4 versus 4.1% in uninfected rabbits. Similar findings have been observed in experimental models of gram-negative bacillary meningitis utilizing ciprofloxacin and ofloxacin (42, 53). Following a single intramuscular injection of ciprofloxacin (50 mg/kg) or ofloxacin (30 mg/kg), mean peak concentrations of ciprofloxacin and ofloxacin in CSF were 2.55 μg/ml (CSF penetration of 27.5%) and 7.67 μg/ml (CSF penetration of 20.0%), respectively. Fleroxacin has been evaluated in the rabbit model of *E. coli* meningitis (7), in which the mean percent penetrations of the drug into animals without meningitis were 46.5 and 71.8% after dosages of 0.5 and 5 mg/kg/h, respectively; in animals with meningitis, the respective percent penetration values were 81.9 and 107%. Taken collectively, these data suggest that as a class, newer fluoroquinolones penetrate into CSF in the presence of bacterial meningitis comparably to other agents (e.g., ß-lactams; Table 2) that have proven useful for the therapy of this disease. Despite favorable penetration ratios, however, the absolute peak concentrations in CSF attained are marginal for the therapy of some forms of meningitis (see below) because of the low concentrations in serum compared with those of ß-lactam agents, which are achieved with normal systemic doses.

**Table 3.** Percent penetration of selected fluoroquinolones into CSF of humans without and with meningitis

| Fluoroquinolone | Percent penetration into patients[a]: Without meningitis | With meningitis |
|---|---|---|
| Pefloxacin | 60 | 52–58 |
| Ciprofloxacin | 5–10 | 6–37 |
| Ofloxacin | 47–87 | 50–73 |
| Temafloxacin | 38 | |
| Sparfloxacin | 25–35 | |

[a]Data are from references 17, 18, 21, 29, 54, 57, 63, 68, and 69. Values are calculated as (concentration in CSF/concentration in serum) × 100. These calculations are derived from peak concentrations, mean concentrations, or areas under the curve.

## ENTRY OF FLUOROQUINOLONES INTO HUMAN CSF

The percent penetration of the fluoroquinolones into human CSF has also been examined (Table 3). Pefloxacin was administered intravenously (7.5 or 15 mg/kg) or orally to 15 patients with meningitis or ventriculitis, 14 of whom were treated with a variety of other antibiotics, from days 3 to 20 of illness (69). Two hours after the end of the third intravenous infusion or 4 h after the third oral ingestion, concentrations of pefloxacin in CSF were measured by high-performance liquid chromatography. The results revealed a wide variability in peak concentrations of pefloxacin in plasma (6.8 to 16.0 μg/ml after a 7.5-mg/kg dose and 14.0 to 18.6 μg/ml after a 15-mg/kg dose) and in CSF (2.4 to 9.0 μg/ml after a 7.5-mg/kg dose and 6.5 to 13.0 μg/ml after a 15-mg/kg dose). The percent penetration was good (Table 3), however, and appeared to persist beyond the point at which the meningitis was cured; concentrations of pefloxacin in CSF exceeded the MICs for most strains (except streptococci), especially when the higher dose was used. In another study (8), pefloxacin was administered as a single 400-mg intravenous dose over 1 h to nine patients with or without meningitis; CSF was sampled frequently through an external ventricular drain. Concentrations in CSF peaked at ~3 μg/ml 4 h later. The ratio of the CSF/serum concentration of pefloxacin was maintained at 0.57 to 0.64 between 6 and 48 h after infusion, which agrees with results of other studies. The apparent duration of transfer of pefloxacin from plasma into ventricular CSF was 1.26 h, with a CSF elimination half-life of 13.4 h (similar to the elimination half-life of pefloxacin from plasma).

The penetration of ciprofloxacin into noninflamed CSF was examined 48 h after oral ingestion of a single 500-mg tablet (18). Concentrations of ciprofloxacin in CSF ranged from 0.06 to 0.14 μg/ml, with a percent penetration into CSF (calculated as the area under the concentration curve of ciprofloxacin in CSF relative to the area under the concentration curve of ciprofloxacin in serum) of about 10%. Higher concentrations of ciprofloxacin in CSF (0.25 and 0.4 μg/ml) were observed in two patients with bacterial meningitis when levels were measured 2 to 3 h after oral ingestion. Similar results were obtained in a 65-year-old female without meningitis who had frequent sampling of CSF through an Ommaya intraventricular reservoir after a single 500-mg ciprofloxacin dose (63), with peak concentrations in serum and CSF of 3.5 and 0.15 μg/ml, respectively. In another study (68), three successive 200-mg doses of intravenous ciprofloxacin at 12-h intervals were administered to 23 patients with bacterial meningitis in addition to standard regimens. CSF sampling between days 2 and 4 of therapy and again between days 10 and 20 at 1 to 8 h after injection revealed mean concentrations in CSF of 0.35 to 0.56 and 0.15 to 0.27 μg/ml, respectively. Penetration, utilizing peak concentrations, ranged from 6.5 to 16.2% during the acute stage and from 4.0 to 9.9% during the late stage of the disease, suggesting that diffusion of the drug into CSF persists (but to a lesser extent) beyond the point at which meningitis is "cured." Additionally, eight adult males hospitalized for reasons other than meningitis received three oral doses of ciprofloxacin at 750 mg every 12 h (20). They underwent lumbar punctures during myelography for lumbar disc disease. The mean ciprofloxacin concentration in CSF was 0.20 μg/ml, with a CSF/serum ratio of 0.082. The penetration of ciprofloxacin (200 mg intravenously for two doses given 12 h apart) into CSF was also studied in 25 patients with noninflamed meninges and in nine patients with inflamed meninges due to a variety of disorders (12). In the patients with noninflamed meninges, the CSF ciprofloxacin concentrations varied from 0.038 to 0.178 μg/ml, with a CSF/plasma ratio of 0.038 to 0.40. In the nine patients with meningitis, the CSF/plasma ratio was markedly increased, ranging from 0.17 to 0.91, with the highest values observed at 7 and 9 h after dosing. However, in this study, the CSF was collected only once from each patient and at variable times, making it impossible to estimate a peak concentration in CSF and compare it with a peak concentration in plasma.

Several studies have investigated the penetration of ofloxacin into human CSF (61). In one report, ofloxacin was administered orally at a dosage of 200 mg twice daily for 2 to 8 days to 17 patients with various neurologic disorders (57). At 1.5 and 12 h after dosing, samples of CSF and serum were obtained. Concentrations of 0.32 to 3.6 and 0.5 to 7.75 μg/ml were demonstrated in CSF and serum, respectively, at 1.5 h, and concentrations of 0.49 to 1.35 and 0.5 to 1.83 μg/ml were demonstrated in CSF and serum, respectively, at 12 h. The authors claimed the percent penetrations to be 47% at 1.5 h and 87% at 12 h, although the original data are difficult to interpret. In a second study, nine patients with proved or presumed bacterial meningitis were treated with amoxicillin plus ofloxacin (200 mg orally twice daily for the first 5 days), and samples of CSF were obtained 2 to 12 h after dosing on days 2 and 5 (54). Concentrations of ofloxacin in CSF were generally 50 to 60% of those in serum. Ofloxacin was also evaluated in 12 patients with or without meningitis (9) to whom a single 300-mg dose of ofloxacin was given orally; blood and CSF samples were analyzed 3 and 6 h later. The mean concentrations in plasma were 3.5 and 1.9 μg/ml at 3 and 6 h after ingestion, respectively, while the mean concentrations in CSF were 1.4 μg/ml at 3 h and 0.7 μg/ml at 6 h after drug administration. In patients with purulent meningitis, mean concentrations in plasma and CSF were 2.5 and 0.7 μg/ml, respectively. In a study of cancer patients without meningitis (3), the CSF penetration of ofloxacin (200-mg single dose) given orally or intravenously was assessed. Peak concentrations of ofloxacin in CSF (0.4 to 1.0 μg/ml) were observed 2 to 4 h after intravenous infusion or oral administration; peak concentrations in serum of 2.0 to 3.5 μg/ml were observed just after infusion, and concentrations of 1.7 to 4.0 μg/ml were documented 1 to 2 h after oral administration. Bactericidal titers against *N. meningitidis*, *H. influenzae*, and *E. coli* in CSF were high, whereas bactericidal titers against *S. aureus*, *L. monocytogenes*, and *S. pneumoniae* were low or nonexistent. In another study of 22 patients with purulent meningitis or ventriculitis treated with conventional antibiotics (29), three successive doses of ofloxacin (200 mg each) were infused at 12-h intervals during the acute stage of the disease. The mean percent penetration into ventricular fluid, expressed as a ratio of areas under the curve for CSF and plasma over 0 to 12 h, was 73%.

Other fluoroquinolones have been examined sparingly for their penetration into human CSF. The mean concentration of temafloxacin in CSF in 30 patients without meningitis following two 600-mg doses given 12 h apart was 1.35 μg/ml, with a CSF/serum ratio of 0.38 (58). The mean CSF/serum ratios of sparfloxacin after a single 200-mg oral dose or 200 mg once daily for 3 days were 0.246 and 0.346, respectively (17).

The fluoroquinolones may also reach potentially therapeutic concentrations in brain tissue. In the only reported study with humans (19), 30 patients received various regimens of pefloxacin prior to removal of a brain tumor. The concentrations of pefloxacin in brain tissue ranged from 3.28 to 4.50 μg/g versus concentrations in plasma of 5.05 to 10.22 μg/ml at the time of removal of brain tissue. In addition, pefloxacin concentrations were higher in tumor tissue than in the surrounding unaffected brain tissue (ratios of tumor/brain concentrations ranged from 1.57 to 3.16), although methods for correction of blood contamination in the samples were not mentioned in this report.

## BACTERICIDAL ACTIVITY OF FLUOROQUINOLONES IN EXPERIMENTAL ANIMAL MODELS OF MENINGITIS

Many of the studies cited above that used fluoroquinolones in experimental models of bacterial meningitis also compared the bactericidal activities of these agents with those of several conventional antibiotics. In an experimental rabbit model of *E. coli* meningitis (52), the rate of bacterial killing in animals treated with pefloxacin was only a mean of $-0.37 \log_{10}$ CFU/ml of CSF per h at dosages of 1 to 15 mg/kg/h, and only 4 of 20 animals had sterile CSF at the end of drug infusion. In contrast, greater bacterial killing ($-0.77 \log_{10}$ CFU/ml of CSF per h) was observed in animals receiving higher doses of pefloxacin (30 mg/kg/h), which is comparable to that obtained with cefotaxime at doses simulating concentrations in serum commonly achieved in humans ($P > 0.1$). Bacterial killing in CSF with pefloxacin therapy at this higher dosage was superior to that obtained with chloramphenicol, with four of four CSF samples sterilized at the end of therapy (versus zero of two CSF samples sterilized with chloramphenicol). No pefloxacin-resistant colonies developed during therapy. However, this result (i.e., rate of eradication of *E. coli* from CSF equivalent to that with cefotaxime) required mean concentrations of pefloxacin in serum of 45.8 μg/ml, levels higher than those achievable in humans receiving standard regimens.

Ciprofloxacin has been evaluated in an experimental model of *P. aeruginosa* meningitis (13). The geometric mean MICs and MBCs against the test strain were 1 and 1 μg/ml for ciprofloxacin, 3.5 and 57 μg/ml for ceftazidime, and 0.8 and 2.6 μg/ml for tobramycin. The rate of bacterial killing in CSF was dose dependent in ciprofloxacin-treated animals ($r = 0.74$; $P < 0.01$); the rate of killing at a ciprofloxacin dosage of 5 mg/kg/h was comparable to that obtained with the combination of ceftazidime and tobramycin. However, these results required mean serum ciprofloxacin concentrations of 6.7 μg/ml, which correspond to concentrations achievable in humans but are higher than those attainable when a dose of 750 mg is administered orally twice daily.

Ciprofloxacin and ofloxacin have also been evaluated in the experimental rabbit model of meningitis (41, 53). The results of therapy were assessed 6 h after the intracisternal inoculation of $10^{8.5}$ CFU of a β-lactamase-producing strain of *H. influenzae*. Although all untreated animals died, bacterial concentrations decreased 2.3 logs in 8 h in untreated animals, whereas bacterial concentrations in CSF decreased 6.9 and 7.2 logs in the ciprofloxacin- and ofloxacin-treated animals, respectively, during this 8-h infusion. These responses were significantly more rapid ($P < 0.01$) than those achieved with ampicillin or chloramphenicol against this ß-lactamase-producing strain of *H. influenzae* and were comparable to the results obtained with ceftriaxone in an experimental model of *E. coli* meningitis. In experimental *P. aeruginosa* meningitis, administration of ciprofloxacin, ofloxacin, or ceftazidime 18 h after intracisternal inoculation of $10^{6.2}$ CFU led to a significant ($P < 0.01$) decrease in CSF concentrations of bacteria compared with those in untreated animals, although the regimens did not differ from one another, producing a decline of only $\sim 2 \log_{10}$ CFU in bacterial concentrations over 8 h, a rate of killing much slower than that achieved against *H. influenzae* with the same duration of therapy at identical dosages. This slower rate of killing is presumably due to the lower concentrations of ciprofloxacin in serum (2.55 $\mu$g/ml) achieved compared with those in other experimental model studies (13).

## FLUOROQUINOLONE THERAPY FOR BACTERIAL MENINGITIS IN HUMANS

The fluoroquinolone antimicrobial agents have been used infrequently to treat bacterial meningitis in humans, and available clinical data are represented by case reports rather than controlled clinical trials comparing the fluoroquinolones with standard therapy. An overview of the clinical efficacy of ciprofloxacin through 1986 in 3,981 patients (1) and an analysis of the new drug application and published clinical experience with ciprofloxacin in 2,018 patients (37) did not include any cases of bacterial meningitis. In another analysis of the results of ciprofloxacin therapy in 8,861 patients treated during clinical trials, among which 3,822 courses satisfied the standards of the Food and Drug Administration (39), only three cases of meningitis (due to *P. aeruginosa, S. aureus,* or *S. pneumoniae*) were identified; no clinical failures were noted, although no other details were reported.

Several isolated case reports have suggested the potential benefits of the fluoroquinolones in the therapy of bacterial meningitis. For example, a 56-year-old male developed *P. aeruginosa* meningitis after a decompression laminectomy (21). Initial therapy with cefotaxime plus gentamicin was ineffective, but the patient made a complete recovery following combination therapy with ciprofloxacin (200 mg every 12 h) and tobramycin (120 mg every 8 h) administered intravenously for 14 days. A 78-year-old woman developed *Morganella morganii* meningitis following an $L_5$-$S_1$ laminectomy; the organism was eradicated by 7 days of intravenous pefloxacin therapy (800 mg every 12 h) (16). A premature infant born at 26 weeks of gestation developed a multidrug-resistant *P. aeruginosa* ventriculitis despite parenteral and ventricular therapy with netilmicin and colistin (15). The administration of ciprofloxacin (4 to 6 mg/kg/day for 28 days, with the last 14 days at the higher dose) and netilmicin (3.5 mg/kg/day administered systemically and 1 mg administered intraventricularly daily for 8 days) eradicated the infection, with no evidence of recurrence at a 3-month follow-up. In addition, oral ciprofloxacin has been successfully utilized to prevent relapses in a patient with chronic pseudomonal meningitis (28). Ciprofloxacin has also been used to successfully treat a neonate with *Salmonella typhimurium* meningitis after the patient experienced relapse due to a chloramphenicol-resistant isolate during chloramphenicol therapy (32).

Data for several larger series in which patients with gram-negative meningitis were treated with fluoroquinolones have been published (Table 4). In one report (22), 11 adult

**Table 4.** Results of clinical trials of fluoroquinolones against bacterial meningitis[a]

| Fluoroquinolone | No. of patients | Organism (no.) | No. of patients | | | Reference |
|---|---|---|---|---|---|---|
| | | | Cured or improved | Relapsed | Failed | |
| Pefloxacin | 11[b] | *S. aureus* (2), *S. epidermidis* (1), *B. cereus* (1), *E. coli* (3), *P. aeruginosa* (2), *A. calcoaceticus* (2) | 8 | 1 | 1 | 22 |
| Pefloxacin | 16[c] | *P. aeruginosa* (5), *A. calcoaceticus* (4), *K. pneumoniae* (3), *E. cloacae* (2), *C. diversus* (1), *Salmonella* group C (1) | 13 | 1 | 1 | 51 |
| Ciprofloxacin | 20 | *E. coli* (6), *P. mirabilis* (3), *K. pneumoniae* (5), *P. aeruginosa* (2), *E. cloacae* (1), *A. calcoaceticus* (3) | 18 | | 2 | 49 |

[a]Data were compiled from references 22, 49, and 51. See text for complete details of these clinical trials, including drug dosages and concomitant use of other antimicrobial agents.
[b]One patient with superinfection.
[c]One patient not accessible.

patients with bacterial meningitis were treated with pefloxacin (400 mg two or three times daily or 800 mg twice daily). Pathogens isolated from CSF in these patients were *S. aureus* (two patients), *S. epidermidis* (one patient), *Bacillus cereus* (one patient), *E. coli* (three patients), *P. aeruginosa* (two patients), and *Acinetobacter calcoaceticus* (two patients). In patients completing therapy, the mean duration of treatment was 19 days (range, 8 to 45 days). Of seven patients treated with pefloxacin alone, six were cured, including one in whom pefloxacin followed previous successful therapy with thienamycin plus amikacin for pseudomonal meningitis. In another case, superinfection due to a pefloxacin-resistant *Klebsiella* strain isolated from blood cultures occurred. In one patient, CSF cultures continued to grow *E. coli* despite 9 days of pefloxacin treatment; cure was then achieved with a combination of cefoxitin and dibekacin. Four patients received a combination of pefloxacin with either vancomycin (two patients), ceftazidime (one patient), or 5-flucytosine (one patient with suspected cryptococcosis). Three patients were apparently cured, and another relapsed at the end of treatment. Overall, 8 of the 11 patients were cured, superinfection occurred in 1, reinfection occurred in 1, and one failed treatment.

In another trial (50), 10 patients with acute meningitis caused by gram-negative bacteria were treated with intravenous pefloxacin (mean daily dose of 19.61 mg/kg) for a mean period of 10 days. All patients had been previously treated ineffectively with a total of 23 courses of other agents (12 of ß-lactams, 7 of aminoglycosides, and 4 of chloramphenicol). Organisms isolated included *P. aeruginosa* (three patients), *A. calcoaceticus* (three patients), *K. pneumoniae* (three patients, including one with a concomitant *S. aureus* isolate), and *Citrobacter diversus* (one patient). Of the 10 patients, 7 were cured, 1 improved, 1 failed to respond, and 1 could not be assessed because of sudden death following an acute myocardial infarction. Of the seven patients who were cured, three died as a result of their underlying diseases. Bacteriologic eradication of gram-negative bacteria was documented in nine of the CSF cultures, but a *Klebsiella* isolate was not eradicated in one patient, and *S. aureus* persisted in another patient. In another report, the same authors compiled data on 16 patients with acute meningitis (10 of whom were reported on in the previous study; see above) caused by gram-negative bacteria and treated with intravenous pefloxacin (800 mg twice daily in adult patients) for a mean period of 11 days (51). The causative organisms were *P. aeruginosa* (five patients), *A. calcoaceticus* (four patients), *K. pneumoniae* (three patients), *Enterobacter cloacae* (two patients), *C. diversus* (one patient) and *Salmonella* group C (one patient). Thirteen patients were cured or clinically improved, 12 were bacteriologically cured, 1 patient failed, 1 patient had reinfection, and 1 patient was not accessible.

In another study from Yugoslavia, ciprofloxacin (200 mg intravenously every 12 h for 10 days) was administered to 20 patients with gram-negative bacillary meningitis, which was most frequently associated with head trauma and neurosurgical procedures (49). In two patients, cefotaxime and penicillin G were also administered. Organisms isolated from CSF included *E. coli, P. mirabilis, K. pneumoniae, P. aeruginosa, E. cloacae,* and *A. calcoaceticus*. Eighteen of 20 patients were apparently cured; in 2 patients, treatment was modified because a positive CSF culture was obtained after 48 h of therapy. These reports demonstrate the potential efficacy of pefloxacin and ciprofloxacin in gram-negative meningitis, although more clinical data are needed to establish their precise roles in this life-threatening infection.

## CHEMOPROPHYLAXIS OF MENINGOCOCCAL CARRIERS

Although not directly pertinent to the treatment of bacterial meningitis, the risk of meningococcal disease among close (e.g., household) contacts of an index case during nonepidemic periods is ~3 in 1,000; this is ~500- to 1,000-fold higher than the background endemic rate (41). These close contacts should receive chemoprophylaxis to eradicate nasopharyngeal carriage. The current antibiotic of choice in this situation is 600 mg of rifampin twice daily for 2 days in adults. However, there are problems with rifampin administration: (i) only 70 to 80% eradication rates of the organism from the nasopharynx are achieved, and this effect is transient; (ii) some adverse reactions occur; (iii) 2 days (four doses) of administration are necessary; and (iv) meningococcal resistance to rifampin has occasionally developed.

Recent reports suggest that ciprofloxacin is highly effective in eliminating *N. meningitidis* from the nasopharynx of a patient carrying the organism (Table 5). Ciprofloxacin was shown to be efficacious among army recruits in Finland: a dose of 250 mg administered twice daily for 2 days eradicated meningococcal carriage from 96% of subjects versus only 13% of those given placebo (33). A single dose of ciprofloxacin (500 or 750 mg for adults) has also been shown in several reports to be effective in eliminating *N. meningitidis* from nasopharyngeal carriers (10, 11, 30), leading some to recommend ciprofloxacin for chemoprophylaxis for meningococcal disease in adults (64). Ciprofloxacin concentrations in nasal secretions have been shown to exceed the MIC for 90% of meningococcal and *H. influenzae* strains (6), suggesting that ciprofloxacin may also be effective in elimination of nasopharyngeal carriage of *H. influenzae*. However, there are no published trials to support this suggestion. Nevertheless, ciprofloxacin is the only oral agent proved effective in eradication of meningococcal carriage after a single dose.

## SUMMARY AND CONCLUSIONS

The fluoroquinolone antimicrobial agents possess several properties that make them potential therapeutic agents for use in patients with bacterial meningitis. Their penetration into CSF is good, with remarkable agreement between values obtained in experimental animal models of meningitis and during therapy in humans. Compared with conventional an-

**Table 5.** Evaluation of ciprofloxacin in eradication of *N. meningitidis* from nasopharyngeal carriers[a]

| Treatment (no. of subjects) | Dose | Carrier reduction | Reference |
|---|---|---|---|
| Ciprofloxacin (56) | 250 mg twice daily for 2 days | 96% at day 8 | 33 |
| Placebo (53) | | 13% | |
| Ciprofloxacin (24) | 750-mg single dose | 96% at day 21 | 10 |
| Placebo | | 9% | |
| Ciprofloxacin (12) | 750-mg single dose | 92% at day 14 | 30 |
| Ciprofloxacin (336) | 500-mg single dose | 97% at day 14 | 11 |
| Ciprofloxacin (104) | | 93% at weeks 6–9 | |

[a]Data were compiled from references 10, 11, 30, and 33.

timicrobial agents utilized for the treatment of bacterial meningitis, the fluoroquinolones enter normal or purulent CSF more rapidly, with percent penetration values into purulent CSF of ~ 50% for enoxacin and pefloxacin and ~ 15 to 30% for ciprofloxacin and ofloxacin. However, despite this efficient penetration, concentrations in CSF are low, primarily because concentrations in serum are low after administration of conventional dosages. The concentrations achievable in CSF are directly correlated with the in vivo potency of each agent (i.e., higher rate of bacterial elimination from CSF as CSF drug concentrations increase), and CSF bactericidal activity correlates with in vitro potency, justifying the selective use of these agents in the therapy of bacterial meningitis due to susceptible gram-negative bacteria but not for meningitis due to gram-positive organisms. The currently available fluoroquinolones should never be used as first-line empiric therapy in patients with meningitis of unknown etiology because of their poor in vitro activity against pneumococci, staphylococci, and *L. monocytogenes*. The limited published literature on the use of fluoroquinolones in humans suggests that the primary area of usefulness of these agents in patients with bacterial meningitis is for therapy of multidrug-resistant gram-negative organisms (e.g., *P. aeruginosa*) or when the response to conventional ß-lactam therapy is slow (e.g., meningitis due to *Salmonella* species). In addition, fluoroquinolones are relatively contraindicated in infants and children, the age groups accounting for the majority of cases of bacterial meningitis. Therefore, the fluoroquinolones have a limited role in the therapy of bacterial meningitis and will not supplant conventional antimicrobial regimens against the major meningeal pathogens. Ciprofloxacin, however, appears promising for use in eradication of the meningococcal carrier state and may replace rifampin for this indication in adults and perhaps even in children. Although no clinical studies are currently available, the fluoroquinolones may also be effective in eliminating nasopharyngeal carriage of *H. influenzae*.

## REFERENCES


1. **Arcieri, G., E. Griffith, G. Gruenwaldt, A. Heyd, B. O'Brien, N. Becker, and R. August.** 1987. Ciprofloxacin: an update on clinical experience. *Am. J. Med.* **46**(Suppl. 4A):381–386.
2. **Armengaud, M., V. T. Tran, and B. DiConstanzo.** 1983. Study of pefloxacin diffusion into serum and CSF in the dog, both with healthy meninges and during experimental meningitis, p. 23–28. *Proc. 13th Int. Congr. Chemother.*
3. **Bitar, N., R. Claes, and P. Van der Auwera.** 1989. Concentrations of ofloxacin in serum and cerebrospinal fluid of patients without meningitis receiving the drug intravenously and orally. *Antimicrob. Agents Chemother.* **33:**1686–1690.
4. **Bryan, J. P., H. R. de Silva, A. Tavares, H. Roche, and W. M. Scheld.** 1990. Etiology and mortality of bacterial meningitis in northeastern Brazil. *Rev. Infect. Dis.* **12:**128–135.
5. **Cherubin, C. E., J. S. Marr, M. F. Sierra, and S. Becker.** 1981. *Listeria* and gram-negative bacillary meningitis in New York City 1972–1979. Frequent causes of meningitis in adults. *Am. J. Med.* **71:**199–209.
6. **Darouiche, R., B. Perkins, D. Musher, R. Hamill, and S. Tsai.** Levels of rifampin and cip-

rofloxacin in nasal secretions: correlation with $MIC_{90}$ and eradication of nasopharyngeal carriage of bacteria. *J. Infect. Dis.* **162:**1124–1127.

7. **Decazes, J. M., J. Mohler, A. Bure, J. M. Vallois, A. Meulemans, and J. Modai.** 1989. Pharmacokinetics of fleroxacin and its metabolites in serum, cerebrospinal fluid, and brain of rabbits with and without experimental *Escherichia coli* meningitis. *Rev. Infect. Dis.* **11:**S1208–S1209.
8. **Dow, J., J. Chazal, A. M. Frydman, P. Janny, R. Woehrle, F. Djebbar, and J. Gaillot.** 1986. Transfer kinetics of pefloxacin into cerebrospinal fluid after one hour iv infusion of 400 mg in man. *J. Antimicrob. Chemother.* **17**(Suppl. B)**:**81–87.
9. **Drancourt, M., H. Gallais, D. Raoult, E. Estrangin, M. W. Mallet, and P. DeMicco.** 1988. Ofloxacin penetration into cerebrospinal fluid. *J. Antimicrob. Chemother.* **22:**263–265.
10. **Dworzack, D. L., C. C. Sanders, E. A. Horowitz, J. M. Allais, M. Sookpranee, W. E. Sanders, Jr., and F. M. Ferraro.** Evaluation of single-dose ciprofloxacin in the eradication of *Neisseria meningitidis* from nasopharyngeal carriers. *Antimicrob. Agents Chemother.* **32:**1740–1741.
11. **Gaunt, P. N., and B. E. Lambert.** 1988. Single dose ciprofloxacin for the eradication of pharyngeal carriage of *Neisseria meningitidis. J. Antimicrob. Chemother.* **21:**489–496.
12. **Gogos, C. A., T. G. Maraziotis, N. Papadakis, D. Beermann, D. K. Siamplis, and H. P. Bassaris.** 1991. Penetration of ciprofloxacin into human cerebrospinal fluid in patients with inflamed and non-inflamed meninges. *Eur. J. Clin. Microbiol. Infect. Dis.* **10:**511–514.
13. **Hackbarth, C. J., H. F. Chambers, F. Stella, A. M. Shibl, and M. A. Sande.** 1986. Ciprofloxacin in experimental *Pseudomonas aeruginosa* meningitis in rabbits. *J. Antimicrob. Chemother.* **18**(Suppl. D)**:**65–69.
14. **Hooper, D. C., and J. S. Wolfson.** 1991. Fluoroquinolone antimicrobial agents. *N. Engl. J. Med.* **324:**384–394.
15. **Isaacs, D., M. P. E. Slack, A. R. Wilkinson, and A. W. Westwood.** 1986. Successful treatment of *Pseudomonas* ventriculitis with ciprofloxacin. *J. Antimicrob. Chemother.* **17:**535–538.
16. **Isaacs, R. D., and R. B. Ellis-Pegler.** 1987. Successful treatment of *Morganella morganii* meningitis with pefloxacin mesylate. *J. Antimicrob. Chemother.* **20:**769–770.
17. **Kawahara, K., M. Kawahara, T. Goto, and Y. Ohi.** 1991. Penetration of sparfloxacin (AT-4140) into human cerebrospinal fluid: a comparative study with five other fluoroquinolones. *Eur. J. Clin. Microbiol. Infect. Dis.* **Special Issue:**580–582.
18. **Kitzes-Cohen, R., A. Miler, A. Gilboa, and D. Harel.** 1988. Penetration of ciprofloxacin into cerebrospinal fluid. *Rev. Infect. Dis.* **10:**S256–S257.
19. **Korinek, A. M., G. Montay, A. Bianchi, M. Guggiari, R. Grob, and P. Viars.** 1988. Penetration of pefloxacin into human brain tissue. *Rev. Infect. Dis.* **10:**S257.
20. **McClain, J. B., J. Rhoads, and G. Krol.** 1988. Cerebrospinal fluid concentrations of ciprofloxacin in subjects with uninflamed meninges. *J. Antimicrob. Chemother.* **21:**808–809.
21. **Millar, M. R., M. A. Bransby-Zachary, D. S. Tompkins, P. M. Hawkey, and R. M. Gibson.** 1986. Ciprofloxacin for *Pseudomonas aeruginosa* meningitis. *Lancet* **i:**1325. (Letter.)
22. **Modai, J.** 1991. Potential role of fluoroquinolones in the treatment of bacterial meningitis. *Eur. J. Clin. Microbiol. Infect. Dis.* **10:**291–295.
23. **Montay, G., Y. Goueffon, and F. Roquet.** 1984. Absorption, distribution, metabolic fate, and elimination of pefloxacin mesylate in mice, rats, dogs, monkeys, and humans. *Antimicrob. Agents Chemother.* **25:**463–472.
24. **Neu, H. C.** 1991. The place of quinolones in bacterial infections. *Adv. Intern. Med.* **36:**1–32.
25. **Nolan, C. M., and C. W. Ulmer, Jr.** 1980. A study of cephalothin and desacetylcephalothin in cerebrospinal fluid in therapy for experimental pneumococcal meningitis. *J. Infect. Dis.* **141:**326–330.
26. **Nolan, C. M., and C. W. Ulmer, Jr.** 1982. Penetration of cefotaxime and moxalactam into cerebrospinal fluid of rabbits with experimentally induced *Escherichia coli* meningitis. *Rev. Infect. Dis.* **4:**S396–S400.
27. **Norrby, S. R.** 1978. A review of the penetration of antibiotics into CSF and its clinical significance. *Scand. J. Infect. Dis. Suppl.* **14:**296–309.
28. **Norrby, S. R.** 1988. 4-Quinolones in the treatment of infections of the central nervous system. *Rev. Infect. Dis.* **10:**S253–S255.
29. **Pioget, J. C., M. Wolff, E. Singlas, M. J. Laisne, B. Clair, B. Regnier, and F. Vachon.** 1989. Diffusion of ofloxacin into cerebrospinal fluid of patients with purulent meningitis or ventriculitis. *Antimicrob. Agents Chemother.* **33:**933–936.
30. **Pugsley, M. P., D. L. Dworzack, J. S. Roccaforte, C. C. Sanders, J. S. Bakken, and W. E. Sanders, Jr.** 1988. An open study of the efficacy of a single dose of ciprofloxacin in eliminating the chronic nasopharyngeal carriage of *Neisseria meningitidis. J. Infect. Dis.* **157:**852–853. (Letter.)
31. **Quagliarello, V. J., W. J. Long, and W. M. Scheld.** 1986. Morphologic alterations of the blood-brain barrier with experimental meningitis in the rat. Temporal sequence and role of encapsulation. *J. Clin. Invest.* **77:**1084–1095.

32. **Ragunathan, P. L., D. V. Potkins, J. G. Watson, A. M. Kearns, and A. Carroll.** 1990. Neonatal meningitis due to *Salmonella typhimurium* treated with ciprofloxacin. *J. Antimicrob. Chemother.* **26:**727–728.
33. **Renkonen, O. V., A. Sivonen, and R. Visakorpi.** 1987. Effect of ciprofloxacin on carrier rate of *Neisseria meningitidis* in army recruits in Finland. *Antimicrob. Agents Chemother.* **31:**962–963.
34. **Sande, M. A., R. A. Brooks-Fournier, and J. L. Geberding.** 1987. Efficacy of ciprofloxacin in animal models of infection: endocarditis, meningitis, and pneumonia. *Am. J. Med.* **82**(Suppl. 4A)**:**63–66.
35. **Sande, M. A., O. M. Korzeniowski, G. M. Alliegro, R. O. Brennan, O. Zak, and W. M. Scheld.** 1981. Intermittent or continuous therapy of experimental meningitis due to *Streptococcus pneumoniae* in rabbits: preliminary observations on the post-antibiotic effect in vivo. *Rev. Infect. Dis.* **3:**98–109.
36. **Sande, M. A., R. J. Sheretz, O. Zak, and L. J. Strausbaugh.** 1978. Cephalosporin antibiotics in therapy of experimental *Streptococcus pneumoniae* and *Haemophilius influenzae* meningitis in rabbits. *J. Infect. Dis.* **137:**S161–S168.
37. **Sanders, W. E., Jr.** 1988. Efficacy, safety, and potential economic benefits of oral ciprofloxacin in the treatment of infections. *Rev. Infect. Dis.* **10:**528–543.
38. **Schaad, U. B., G. H. McCracken, Jr., C. A. Loock, and M. L. Thomas.** 1981. Pharmacokinetics and bacteriological efficacy of moxalactam, cefotaxime, cefoperazone, and Rocephin in experimental bacterial meningitis. *J. Infect. Dis.* **143:**156–163.
39. **Schact, P., G. Arcieri, J. Branolte, H. Bruck, V. Chysky, E. Griffith, G. Gruenwald, R. Hullmann, C. A. Konopka, B. O'Brien, V. Rahm, T. Ryoki, A. Westwood, and H. Weuta.** 1986. Worldwide clinical data on efficacy and safety of ciprofloxacin. *Infection* **16:**S29–S43.
40. **Scheld, W. M.** 1985. Theoretical and practical considerations of antibiotic therapy for bacterial meningitis. *Pediatr. Infect. Dis. J.* **4:**74–83.
41. **Scheld, W. M.** 1989. Quinolone therapy for infections of the central nervous system. *Rev. Infect. Dis.* **11:**S1194–S1202.
42. **Scheld, W. M.** 1991. Evaluation of quinolones in experimental animal models of infections. *Eur. J. Clin. Microbiol. Infect. Dis.* **10:**275–290.
43. **Scheld, W. M., G. M. Alliegro, M. R. Field, and J. P. Brodeur.** 1982. Synergy between ampicillin and gentamicin in experimental meningitis due to group B streptococci. *J. Infect. Dis.* **146:**100.
44. **Scheld, W. M., and J. P. Brodeur.** 1983. Effect of methylprednisolone on entry of ampicillin and gentamicin into cerebrospinal fluid in experimental pneumococcal and *Escherichia coli* meningitis. *Antimicrob. Agents Chemother.* **23:**108–112.
45. **Scheld, W. M., R. S. Brown, Jr., and M. A. Sande.** 1978. Comparison of netilmicin with gentamicin in the therapy of experimental *Escherichia coli* meningitis. *Antimicrob. Agents Chemother.* **13:**899–904.
46. **Scheld, W. M., D. D. Fletcher, F. N. Fink, and M. A. Sande.** 1979. Response to therapy in an experimental rabbit model of meningitis due to *Listeria monocytogenes. J. Infect. Dis.* **140:**287–294.
47. **Scheld, W. M., and M. A. Sande.** 1983. Bactericidal versus bacteriostatic antibiotic therapy of experimental pneumococcal meningitis in rabbits. *J. Clin. Invest.* **71:**411–419.
48. **Schlech, W. F., III, J. I. Ward, J. D. Band, A. Hightower, D. W. Fraser, and C. V. Broome.** 1985. Bacterial meningitis in the United States. The national bacterial meningitis surveillance study. *J. Am. Med. Assoc.* **253:**1749–1754.
49. **Schönwald, S., I. Beus, M. Lisic, V. Car, and B. Gmajnicki.** 1989. Brief report: ciprofloxacin in the treatment of gram-negative bacillary meningitis. *Am. J. Med.* **87**(Suppl. 5A)**:**248S–249S.
50. **Segev, S., A. Barzilai, N. Rosen, G. Joseph, and E. Rubinstein.** 1989. Pefloxacin treatment of meningitis caused by gram-negative bacteria. *Arch. Intern. Med.* **149:**1314–1316.
51. **Segev, S., N. Rosen, G. Joseph, H. Alpern Elran, and E. Rubinstein.** 1990. Pefloxacin efficacy in gram-negative bacillary meningitis. *J. Antimicrob. Chemother.* **26**(Suppl. B)**:**187–192.
52. **Shibl, A. M., C. J. Hackbarth, and M. A. Sande.** 1986. Evaluation of pefloxacin in experimental *Escherichia coli* meningitis. *Antimicrob. Agents Chemother.* **29:**409–411.
53. **Sobieski, M. W., and W. M. Scheld.** 1985. Comparative activity of ciprofloxacin and ofloxacin in experimental *H. influenzae* meningitis, abstr. 216. *Program Abstr. 25th Intersci. Conf. Antimicrob. Agents Chemother.*
54. **Stahl, J. P., J. Croize, M. A. Lefebvre, J. P. Bru, A. Guyot, D. Leduc, J. B. Fourtillan, and M. Micoud.** 1986. Diffusion of ofloxacin into the cerebrospinal fluid in patients with bacterial meningitis. *Infection* **14:**S254–S255.
55. **Strausbaugh, L. J., T. W. Murray, and M. A. Sande.** 1980. Comparative penetration of six antibiotics into the cerebrospinal fluid of rabbits with experimental staphylococcal meningitis. *J. Antimicrob. Chemother.* **6:**363–371.
56. **Strausbaugh, L. J., and M. A. Sande.** 1978. Factors influencing the therapy of experimental *Proteus mirabilis* meningitis in rabbits. *J. Infect. Dis.* **137:**251–260.

57. **Stübner, G., W. Weinrich, and U. Brands.** 1986. Study of the cerebrospinal fluid penetrability of ofloxacin. *Infection* **14:**S250–S253.
58. **Taeger, K., E. Wiethoff, G. Mahr, R. Seelmann, T. Lohr, and F. Sörgel.** 1990. Penetration of temafloxacin into cerebrospinal fluid, abstr. 363. *Proc. 3rd Int. Symp. New Quinolones.*
59. **Tho, T. V., A. Armengaud, and B. Davet.** 1984. Diffusion of enoxacin into the cerebrospinal fluid in dogs with healthy meninges and with experimental meningitis. *J. Antimicrob. Chemother.* **14**(Suppl. C)**:**57–62.
60. **Tunkel, A. R., and W. M. Scheld.** 1989. Applications of therapy in animal models to bacterial infection in human disease. *Infect. Dis. Clin. North Am.* **3:**441–459.
61. **Tunkel, A. R., and W. M. Scheld.** 1991. Ofloxacin. *Infect. Control Hosp. Epidemiol.* **12:**549–557.
62. **Tunkel, A. R., B. Wispelwey, and W. M. Scheld.** 1990. Bacterial meningitis: recent advances in pathophysiology and treatment. *Ann. Intern. Med.* **112:**610–623.
63. **Valainis, G., D. Thomas, and G. Pankey.** 1986. Penetration of ciprofloxacin into cerebrospinal fluid. *Eur. J. Clin. Microbiol.* **5:**206–207.
64. **Visakorpi, R.** 1989. Ciprofloxacin in meningococcal carriers. *Scand. J. Infect. Dis. Suppl.* **60:**108–111.
65. **Walker, R. C., and A. J. Wright.** 1991. The fluoroquinolones. *Mayo Clin. Proc.* **66:**1249–1259.
66. **Wallace, J. F., R. H. Smith, M. Garcia, and R. G. Petersdorf.** 1967. Studies on the pathogenesis of meningitis. VI. Antagonism between penicillin and chloramphenicol in experimental pneumococcal meningitis. *J. Lab. Clin. Med.* **70:**408–418.
67. **Wenger, J. D., A. W. Hightower, R. R. Facklam, S. Gaventa, C. V. Broome, and the Bacterial Meningitis Study Group.** 1990. Bacterial meningitis in the United States, 1986: report of a multistate surveillance study. *J. Infect. Dis.* **162:**1316–1323.
68. **Wolff, M., L. Boutron, E. Singlas, B. Clair, J. M. Decazes, and B. Regnier.** 1987. Penetration of ciprofloxacin into cerebrospinal fluid of patients with bacterial meningitis. *Antimicrob. Agents Chemother.* **31:**899–902.
69. **Wolff, M., B. Regnier, C. Daldoss, M. Nkam, and F. Yachon.** 1984. Penetration of pefloxacin into cerebrospinal fluid of patients with meningitis. *Antimicrob. Agents Chemother.* **26:**289–291.

*Quinolone Antimicrobial Agents, 2nd ed.*
Edited by David C. Hooper and John S. Wolfson


*Chapter 21*

# Treatment of Experimental and Human Bacterial Endocarditis with Quinolone Antimicrobial Agents

*Michael R. Yeaman and Arnold S. Bayer*

The in vivo efficacy of newly developed antimicrobial agents in relevant animal and tissue culture models of infection has been an important transitional link between in vitro activity and human utility. A review of the in vitro activity spectra of the newer quinolones (fluoroquinolones) suggests that these agents might be candidates for the therapy of infective endocarditis, an important human infection. The newer quinolone antibiotics possess in vitro activity spectra encompassing several organisms associated with particularly recalcitrant forms of bacterial endocarditis, including *Staphylococcus aureus* (both methicillin susceptible [MSSA] and methicillin resistant [MRSA]) and *Pseudomonas aeruginosa* (3, 26). These forms of endocarditis have been associated with relatively poor clinical outcomes when treated with standard antimicrobial regimens (42, 50).

Experimental animal models of bacterial endocarditis provide rigorous tests of the efficacy of any antimicrobial regimen. For example, in experimental bacterial endocarditis, the infection is induced in rabbits or rats by the placement of a polyethylene catheter across a heart valve (e.g., aortic or tricuspid) to induce marantic endocarditis followed by the seeding of the sterile vegetation with a large bacterial challenge administered either intravenously or through the catheter. The catheter is generally secured in place for the duration of the study. This procedure, modeled on the methods of Freedman and Valone (27), reliably induces endocarditis in catheterized animals, with infected vegetations containing $>10^7$ to $10^9$ bacteria per g of tissue. Thus, antimicrobial regimens must sterilize vegetations containing high bacterial densities in the presence of an indwelling foreign body (intraventricular catheter). Moreover, many of the organisms in the interstices of the experimental valvular vegetation appear to be in a metabolically inactive phase of growth (stationary [24]), making the efficacy of cell wall-active antibiotics problematic in the treatment of endocarditis.

The newer quinolone antibiotics appear to be particularly promising for the treatment of bacterial endocarditis because these agents possess features in vitro that may overcome the therapeutic problems presented in relevant infection model systems. First, the newer quinolones do not exhibit a pronounced inoculum effect in vitro (an effect seen with many aminoglycosides and ß-lactams [65]), remaining bactericidal at challenge inocula of $\sim 10^6$ to $10^8$ CFU/ml depending on the organism (6, 11, 57). Second, although strain specific, the newer quin-

***Michael R. Yeaman and Arnold S. Bayer*** • UCLA School of Medicine, Los Angeles, California 90024, and Division of Infectious Diseases, Los Angeles County Harbor-UCLA Medical Center, Torrance, California 90509.

olones in some circumstances have bactericidal activity against stationary-phase bacteria in vitro (73). Third, these agents are usually relatively active at acidic pH (5, 6). Last, the quinolones often exhibit concentration-dependent killing kinetics in vivo such that increases in administered doses result in roughly proportional increases in bacterial killing (31).

Since there is little clinical information concerning the efficacies of the newer quinolones in the therapy of human bacterial endocarditis, this chapter concentrates predominantly on a detailed analysis of the results of quinolone treatment protocols in the discriminative animal models outlined above. This chapter emphasizes the lessons learned from these animal models that may be relevant to the treatment of human bacterial endocarditis. Recent reviews addressing the efficacies of quinolone antibiotics in relevant animal models are also available (1, 2, 54, 55, 60).

## TISSUE PENETRATION OF NEWER QUINOLONES IN PATIENTS WITH ENDOCARDITIS

Infected cardiac vegetations represent a nidus of infection in which differential antibiotic penetration due to mechanical (histologic) barriers combines with high densities of bacteria to present special problems in the chemotherapy of endocarditis. There is little information on the clinical efficacy of the newer quinolones in human endocarditis. Data from the experimental endocarditis model, as well as from human pharmacokinetic studies, have, however, suggested that these agents may be useful in the treatment or prophylaxis of human valvular infections caused by selected organisms. Using pefloxacin as a model, Contrepois et al. (22) showed that this agent achieved peak levels of ~20 and 40 μg/g in rabbit aortic valves of healthy animals and of those with *Escherichia coli* endocarditis, respectively, after an intravenous dose of 15 mg/kg of body weight. Moreover, this dosage given repeatedly at 15 mg/kg every 12 h was effective in significantly reducing intravegetation *E. coli* titers in animals with endocarditis compared with untreated controls.

Our laboratory recently examined the ability of pefloxacin to penetrate vegetations of animals with aortic endocarditis due to MRSA; after single intravenous doses of pefloxacin at 20 or 40 mg/kg, mean peak concentrations within aortic vegetations were only ~1.5 and 3 μg/g, respectively (7). In addition, these levels of pefloxacin within vegetations were significantly lower than those achieved after single intravenous doses of vancomycin (15 mg/kg). These latter differences in the abilities of pefloxacin and vancomycin to penetrate MRSA-infected aortic vegetations were roughly mirrored in vivo, as vancomycin caused a more rapid decline in intravegetation MRSA densities than did pefloxacin at both dose regimens. The disparities in the levels of drug achievable in vegetations in our study compared with that of Contrepois et al. may relate either to differences in the route of administration (intravenous infusion [22] versus intravenous bolus [7]) or to methods of preparing vegetations for tissue drug assays. In our study, for example, vegetations after removal from the animals were carefully dried to evaporate extravascular fluid contamination.

As a corollary to the above investigations, Brion et al. (18) studied the penetrability of pefloxacin into abnormal cardiac valves of humans undergoing open heart surgery for prosthetic valve insertion. They showed that a single dose of intravenous pefloxacin at ~10 to 15 mg/kg (800 mg) achieved mean peak levels of ~2 to 9 μg/g in abnormal aortic or mitral valves for 4 to 24 h after infusion; additionally, the mean ratios of valve to plasma pefloxacin concentrations were often >1.0, suggesting complete penetrance from the vascular to the tissue compartment. In addition, the levels of pefloxacin achieved in vegetations were well above the MBCs for 90% of strains of most important valvular pathogens, including the viridans and enterococcal streptococci, MRSA and MSSA, and *P. aeruginosa*. More recently, Carbon reported similar results from investigations of the relationship between antibiotic efficacy and dosage schedule in experimental endocarditis (19). These studies demonstrated that the combination of a rapid bactericidal effect with prolonged in vivo postantibiotic effects of quinolones allowed large intervals between dosing without loss of efficacy. Collectively, these data from human patients and the experimental endocarditis models suggest that in selected circumstances, newer quinolones with long half-lives (such as pefloxacin) may be useful in the prophylaxis or treatment of clinical endocarditis. However, formal chemoprophylactic studies with animals have not been reported to date, and there is little published information on utilizing such agents in humans with confirmed bacterial endocarditis.

## EXPERIMENTAL ENDOCARDITIS

### *P. aeruginosa*

Infective endocarditis due to *P. aeruginosa* remains an important infection among parenteral drug abusers in the United States, particularly in Detroit and Chicago (50, 61). Recent experiences in treating this infection in humans and experimental animals have emphasized the difficulties in achieving cures with aminoglycoside–ß-lactam regimens alone, especially with left-sided valve involvement (12, 50). Such regimens have been limited by primary drug failures, bacteriologic relapses, and the development of antibiotic resistance in vivo (12, 36, 50).

Our laboratory and others have recently reported on the efficacies of newer quinolones in experimental *P. aeruginosa* endocarditis. Ingerman et al. examined the relative efficacies of ciprofloxacin versus ceftazidime or an investigational ß-lactam (BMY-28142), with and without gentamicin, in the rat model of experimental aortic endocarditis due to *P. aeruginosa* (35). In vitro, ciprofloxacin exhibited a significantly faster onset of bactericidal action against the infecting pseudomonal strain than did either ß-lactam (with or without gentamicin added). For example, after 2 h of incubation, ciprofloxacin (1 μg/ml) lowered the initial bacterial inoculum from ~8 to ~4 $\log_{10}$ CFU/ml; in contrast, all ß-lactam regimens lowered the initial pseudomonal inoculum by less than 10-fold. Similarly, when infected aortic valvular vegetations were exposed to drugs ex vivo, ciprofloxacin produced bacterial killing more rapidly or to a greater extent than did ß-lactam regimens (Fig. 1). Of importance, these investigators confirmed that ciprofloxacin (but not the ß-lactams) exerted a persistent suppression of pseudomonal growth in vitro ("postantibiotic effect") for ≥2.5 h after brief exposure (2 h) to the drug (Fig. 2). In vivo, ciprofloxacin therapy produced significantly greater reductions in bacterial density in vegetations and more sterile vegetations than did any of the ß-lactam regimens tested. This therapeutic difference occurred

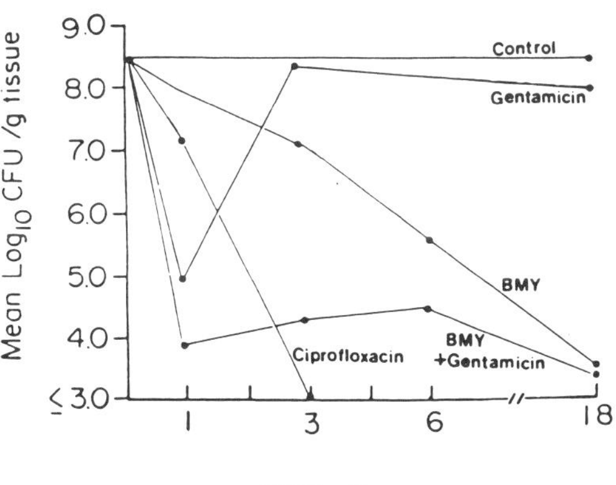


**Figure 1.** Fate of *P. aeruginosa* in vegetations suspended in broth containing 60 μg of BMY-28142 per ml, 6 μg of gentamicin per μl, 2 μg of ciprofloxacin per ml, BMY-28142 plus gentamicin, or broth without drugs. (Reproduced with permission of the University of Chicago Press [35].)

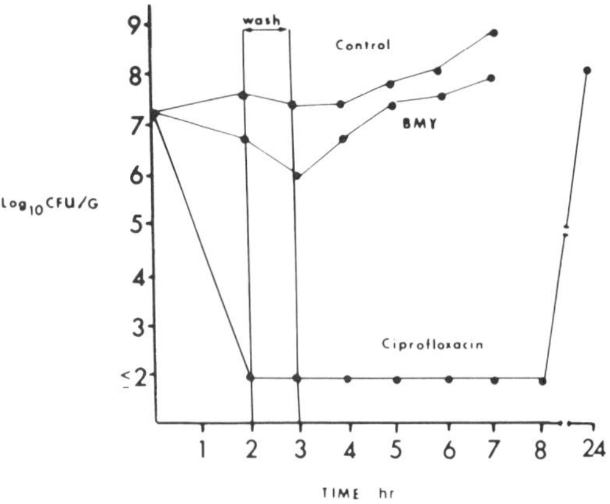


**Figure 2.** Postantibiotic effect of *P. aeruginosa* after 2-h exposure to BMY-28142 (15 μg/ml) or ciprofloxacin (0.5 μg/ml). Drugs were removed by repeated washing. (Reproduced with permission of the University of Chicago Press [35].)

despite the ß-lactam agents being present within infected vegetations at concentrations above the MBC for periods similar to those observed in the ciprofloxacin-treated animals. This study confirmed the importance of pharmacodynamic parameters such as postantibiotic effect and time above MBC at the tissue infection site as dual determinants of ß-lactam therapeutic outcome in experimental infections (28).

Our laboratory studied the efficacy of ciprofloxacin in the rabbit models of experimental tricuspid and aortic valve endocarditis caused by *P. aeruginosa* (6, 9, 10). The comparative drug regimen for the quinolone featured a combination of an aminoglycoside (amikacin or netilmicin) plus an antipseudomonal penicillin (azlocillin) synergistically active against the infecting bacterial strain in vitro. In tricuspid valve endocarditis, ciprofloxacin and a combination of amikacin and azlocillin were equally effective in reducing mortality, preventing pulmonary infarction, and reducing mean pseudomonal densities in vegetations in patients compared with densities untreated controls. Also, both regimens were equivalent in preventing bacteriologic relapse after therapy was discontinued, a substantial problem in the therapy of human pseudomonal endocarditis (9). Moreover, no development of resistance to ciprofloxacin, amikacin, or azlocillin was observed in vivo. The addition of amikacin did not enhance the outcome of ciprofloxacin therapy alone in vivo, despite the frequently additive bactericidal effects of such combinations in vitro (32). In aortic valve endocarditis, ciprofloxacin was significantly more effective than a combination of netilmicin and azlocillin in sterilizing vegetations, reducing pseudomonal densities within vegetations, and preventing bacteriologic relapses after therapy (Table 1).

In contrast, the ciprofloxacin and netilmicin-plus-azlocillin regimens were equally effective in sterilizing renal abscesses. Resistance to azlocillin but not to ciprofloxacin or netilmicin was occasionally seen in vivo among *P. aeruginosa* strains isolated from cardiac vegetations during the second week of treatment. Development of resistance to ß-lactams (e.g., ceftazidime) in the second week of therapy has been previously noted in this model and has been associated with the selection of stably derepressed mutants with constitutive, chromosomally regulated overproduction of ß-lactamase (12). Therefore, the ability of the aminoglycoside and ß-lactam combination to sterilize renal but not endocardial infected tissues in this model suggested differences in the penetration of these agents into renal parenchyma and cardiac vegetations. Strunk et al. (63) have also

**Table 1.** Mortality rates of antibiotic-treated and control rabbits with aortic valve endocarditis due to *P. aeruginosa*[a]

| Treated group | Mortality (no. dead/no. treated [%]) |
|---|---|
| Control[b,c] | 12/19 (63) |
| Netilmicin + azlocillin[c] | 11/23 (47) |
| Ciprofloxacin[b] | 8/23 (34) |

[a]Reproduced with permission of the *Journal of Antimicrobial Chemotherapy* and the British Society of Chemotherapy (6).
[b]$P < 0.05$.
[c]Not significantly different.

confirmed the efficacy of ciprofloxacin in controlling experimental aortic endocarditis due to *P. aeruginosa*. These investigators showed that ciprofloxacin was as effective as the synergistically active combination of tobramycin and azlocillin in reducing intrarenal and intravegetation pseudomonal densities as well as in rendering renal tissue and vegetations sterile. Moreover, none of the surviving bacteria from renal tissue or vegetations were resistant to the pertinent study drug. There was also a suggestion that relapses were less likely to occur after ciprofloxacin therapy than after therapy with the combination of tobramycin and azlocillin, although this difference did not reach statistical significance. The equivalent efficacies of the quinolone and the aminoglycoside–ß-lactam regimens in this latter study are in contrast to the inferior outcome with aminoglycosides and ß-lactams in our study of aortic endocarditis cited above, possibly because of differences in experimental models utilized. In the study by Strunk et al. (63), the catheter was removed approximately 1 h after its placement across the aortic valve and the injection of the pseudomonal inoculum through the catheter; in our study, the catheter remained within the left ventricle for the duration of the study. It seems likely that the persistent presence of the foreign body adversely affected the ability of the aminoglycoside–ß-lactam regimen to eradicate *P. aeruginosa* from vegetations.

Our laboratory has recently reported on the efficacy of pefloxacin, a newer quinolone with a prolonged half-life, in experimental aortic valve *P. aeruginosa* endocarditis (8). Pefloxacin was compared with a combination of high doses of amikacin and ceftazidime that exhibited bactericidal synergy against the infecting pseudomonal strain in vitro. Pefloxacin and the combination regimen both significantly reduced bacterial densities within vegetations compared with densities in untreated controls. As seen in our previous models of aortic pseudomonal endocarditis treated with ß-lactams, bacteria isolated from vegetations after 2 weeks of therapy exhibited ceftazidime resistance related to the constitutive overproduction of ß-lactamase (6, 12). However, as opposed to experiences with ciprofloxacin therapy in this model, intravegetation isolates from pefloxacin recipients showed significant increases (four- to eightfold) in pefloxacin MICs as early as the fourth day of therapy. For these pefloxacin-resistant variants, increases in ciprofloxacin MICS as well as pleiotropic resistance to ticarcillin and chloramphenicol but not to amikacin, ceftazidime, or tetracycline were also exhibited (Table 2). Because of the similarity in the profile of MIC increases for our strain to that induced for *E. coli* with the *cfxB*, *nfxB*, or *norB* gene mutations associated with decreased porin protein OmpF (33, 34), it appeared that altered drug permeability might be the underlying mechanism of resistance in our strain. In collaboration with Chamberland et al. (21), we have recently shown that the major mechanisms of quinolone resistance in our endocarditis variants were the result of at least two distinct alterations of the drug target ("target insensitivity"; altered DNA gyrase). Although a drug permeability defect was also noted, MICs correlated most closely with 50% inhibitory concentrations for inhibition of DNA synthesis.

Over the last decade, a number of ß-lactamase-stable, extended-spectrum cephalosporins have been developed (e.g., cefotaxime and ceftazidime). Recently, increasing numbers of reports have documented the emergence of resistance to these agents by selection of mutants with derepressed ß-lactamase overproduction (36, 46, 56, 58); in addition, several of these multiply ß-lactam-resistant strains exhibited cross-resistance to aminoglycosides (46). This resistance phenomenon has been most commonly seen among bacterial genera within the expanded spectrum of these newer ß-lactams, especially *Enterobacter, Serratia,* and *Pseudomonas* species (56); the quinolones generally retain good in vitro efficacy against these ß-lactam-resistant mutants. We utilized the experimental aortic endocarditis

**Table 2.** Cross- and pleiotropic resistances among selected intravegetation pseudomonal variants isolated during pefloxacin therapy for experimental aortic endocarditis[a]

| Agent | MIC (μg/ml) for: | | | |
|---|---|---|---|---|
| | PA96 (parent) | 22V[b] | $22V_3$[b] | $23V_1$[c] |
| Pefloxacin | 0.19 | 1.56 | 0.78 | 1.56 |
| Ciprofloxacin | 0.19 | 1.56 | 1.56 | 1.56 |
| Ceftazidime | 2 | 2 | 2 | 2 |
| Amikacin | 2 | 2 | 2 | 2 |
| Chloramphenicol | 5 | 1,600 | 800 | 800 |
| Tetracycline | 50 | 50 | 100 | 50 |
| Ticarcillin | 16 | 1,664 | 50 | |

[a]Reproduced with permission of the American Society for Microbiology (8).
[b]Pseudomonal variant isolated on pefloxacin-containing agar (2 μg/ml) after 4 days of pefloxacin therapy.
[c]Pseudomonal variant isolated on pefloxacin-containing agar after 10 days of pefloxacin therapy.

model to evaluate the efficacy of ciprofloxacin against such strains in vivo (10). The infecting strain was a multiply ß-lactam-resistant *P. aeruginosa* variant derepressed for constitutive ß-lactamase overproduction (13). Ciprofloxacin significantly lowered pseudomonal densities within vegetations and rendered significantly more animals abacteremic and with sterile vegetations than did ceftazidime or no therapy. This study suggested that the newer quinolones warrant further evaluation in the treatment of such multiple-drug-resistant, gram-negative bacillary infections due to quinolone-susceptible strains.

### *Enterobacter aerogenes*

*Enterobacter* species rarely cause endocarditis in humans. Such strains, however, are relatively common causes of serious nosocomial infections, especially in patients in intensive care units (17). Boscia et al. (15, 16) performed two studies to evaluate newer oral quinolone agents in *E. aerogenes* aortic endocarditis as a severe test of drug efficacies in this difficult model of bacteremic infection. These investigators first compared oral enoxacin with parenteral cefoperazone in *Enterobacter* endocarditis (15). In vitro, both enoxacin and cefoperazone exerted a rapid and substantial bactericidal effect against the infecting *Enterobacter* strain. However, high-dose enoxacin (100 mg/kg administered every 6 h by the oral syringe method) was significantly better at reducing intravegetation bacterial densities than was lower-dose enoxacin (25 mg/kg given every 6 h) or cefoperazone (60 mg/kg given every 6 h intramuscularly). These findings suggested that the longer half-life of enoxacin (~3 h) versus that of cefoperazone (~1 h) was probably important in the therapeutic differences observed. In a similar study, Boscia et al. (16) compared the efficacies of two oral quinolones, enoxacin and difloxacin, with that of parenterally administered cefoperazone in an experimental aortic endocarditis model caused by *E. aerogenes*. As in their previous study, mentioned above, all three agents were active in vitro against the infecting *Enterobacter* strain, although difloxacin exhibited the most rapid and complete killing of this strain in time-kill experiments. Difloxacin (100 mg/kg given orally every 12 h) was significantly better at reducing intravegetation *Enterobacter* densities than was enoxacin given at the same dose regimen or cefoperazone. As before, the authors ascribed the better efficacy of difloxacin in this model to the greater half-life of this agent (~3.5 h) compared with those of enoxacin (~2.3 h) and cefoperazone (~0.6 h). They also concluded that the relatively inferior outcome of enoxacin therapy in this study compared with that in their prior study was related to differences in the enoxacin dosing intervals utilized in the two studies (every 6 h versus every 12 h).

### *E. coli*

Contrepois et al. (22) reported on the efficacy of 3 days of pefloxacin given at 30 mg/kg/day intramuscularly for experimental *E. coli* aortic valve endocarditis. This regimen significantly lowered intravegetation *E. coli* densities compared with those in untreated controls; unfortunately, these investigators did not include a comparative therapy group for pefloxacin.

### *S. aureus*

Several studies in the animal model of experimental endocarditis have evaluated the efficacies of newer quinolones against both MSSA and MRSA strains. In addition, Pohlod et al. (45) demonstrated that fleroxacin, ciprofloxacin, and difloxacin were active against human endocarditis MRSA and MSSA isolates in vitro, with MICs for 90% of strains of $\leq 1.0$ $\mu$g/ml for these quinolones; other new quinolones were less active. Furthermore, these investigators could not detect selection or emergence of resistance in MRSA or MSSA endocarditis strains exposed to fleroxacin, amifloxacin, or ofloxacin, while resistance in these isolates did develop following exposure to other quinolone drugs.

Sullam et al. (64) compared pefloxacin with cephalothin in MSSA endocarditis and with vancomycin in MRSA endocarditis. Cephalothin and pefloxacin were equally effective in reducing mortality and intravegetation MSSA densities compared with levels in untreated controls. Likewise, both vancomycin and pefloxacin significantly reduced mortality and vegetation MRSA densities versus levels in untreated controls. In a very similar study, Carpenter et al. (20) confirmed that ciprofloxacin was as effective as nafcillin in experimental MSSA aortic endocarditis and as effective as vancomycin in experimental MRSA aortic endocarditis in reducing intravegetation staphylococcal densities. Kaatz et al. (37) also confirmed the equivalent efficacies of intravenously administered ciprofloxacin and vancomycin in reducing intravegetation MRSA densities compared with levels in untreated controls. In addition, this study confirmed a significant reduction in endocarditis-related intrarenal and intrasplenic MRSA infections by both ciprofloxacin and vancomycin (Table 3). Moreover, Kaatz et al. (37, 38) confirmed that the multiple-dose pharmacokinetics of ciprofloxacin in infected animals were markedly different from those that were predicted from single-dose pharmacokinetics in uninfected rabbits. Of particular importance were the higher-than-predicted peak ciprofloxacin levels in the sera of rabbits with endocarditis after multiple drug doses. This difference might have resulted from a decrease in clearance of this agent, but the contribution of endocarditis to renal dysfunction and higher ciprofloxacin levels was not addressed. No development of ciprofloxacin resistance (MIC $>$ 5 $\mu$g/ml) was found among surviving MRSA cells in cardiac vegetations (37).

In subsequent studies, however, resistance to ciprofloxacin during the treatment of experimental endocarditis has been well documented (38, 40). In these studies, *S. aureus* resistance to ciprofloxacin was observed in 12.5% of all animals treated with this drug (38). More recently, the mechanisms by which ciprofloxacin resistance is achieved in *S. aureus* strains recovered from experimental endocarditis were investigated (38, 40). Two such isolates were found to exhibit decreased sensitivity to DNA synthesis inhibition by ciprofloxacin, results similar to our findings with pefloxacin-resistant *P. aeruginosa* strains (suggesting altered DNA gyrase [21]), and a third strain possessed an energy-dependent mechanism that reduced the amount of cell-associated norfloxacin thought to be due to upregulation of the quinolone efflux system. The latter process was

**Table 3.** Counts of MRSA 494 in vegetations and tissues[a]

| Treatment group[b] | Mean ± SD $\log_{10}$ CFU/g[c] | | |
|---|---|---|---|
| | Vegetation | Kidney | Spleen |
| Ciprofloxacin (27) | 3.37 ± 1.58 (14) | 2.01 ± 0.93 (21) | 1.56 ± 0.23 (24) |
| Vancomycin (22) | 3.56 ± 1.67 (12) | 1.91 ± 1.01 (18) | 1.79 ± 0.97 (21) |
| No treatment (controls) (17) | 8.45 ± 0.70 | 5.27 ± 1.55 | 5.15 ± 0.58 |

[a]Reproduced with permission of the American Society for Microbiology (37).
[b]Numbers in parentheses are numbers of rabbits.
[c]Numbers in parentheses are numbers of rabbits rendered culture negative. No significant difference in bacterial counts between the ciprofloxacin and vancomycin treatment groups was observed. Significant differences were noted between the ciprofloxacin-treated animals and the controls and between the vancomycin-treated animals and the controls in all cases ($P < 0.001$).

shown to be independent of alterations in the *gyrA* gene product (A subunit of DNA gyrase) and transferable to a ciprofloxacin-sensitive *E. coli* host by means of a 2.7-kb chromosomal fragment from ciprofloxacin-resistant *S. aureus* cloned on a high-copy-number plasmid. Similar to these findings, resistance to fleroxacin has also recently been reported in experimental MSSA endocarditis (39).

Gilbert et al. studied the comparative efficacies of an orally administered quinolone (enoxacin) versus intravenously administered vancomycin in MRSA aortic endocarditis in rabbits (29). They observed that both agents significantly lowered intravegetation MRSA densities over the 5-day treatment period compared with densities in untreated controls, although the bactericidal effect of enoxacin in vivo was seen earlier than that of vancomycin (3 versus 5 days of treatment). We have recently examined the efficacies of intravenously administered pefloxacin (40 or 80 mg/kg/day) and vancomycin (30 mg/kg/day) in experimental MRSA aortic endocarditis (7). Our results with pefloxacin differ from those of Gilbert et al. (29). As in their study, both the higher-dose pefloxacin regimen and vancomycin significantly lowered intravegetation MRSA densities after 6 days of treatment compared with densities in untreated controls. We, however, observed that the onset of bactericidal activity in vivo was more rapid with vancomycin than with pefloxacin therapy. Significant reductions in intravegetation MRSA densities were seen by the third day of treatment only in vancomycin recipients. We examined various pharmacokinetic and pharmacodynamic parameters that explain in part the superior effect of vancomycin compared with pefloxacin in this model. The in vitro and ex vivo (i.e., intravegetation) postantibiotic effects against the infecting MRSA strain were virtually identical for pefloxacin and vancomycin. Moreover, the trough bactericidal titers in serum were significantly greater in pefloxacin recipients than in animals given vancomycin, reflecting the longer half-life of pefloxacin in serum. Of interest, despite the superior pharmacokinetics of pefloxacin in serum, the penetration of vancomycin in vegetations exceeded that of pefloxacin by 7- to 11-fold. This finding supports the concept of Gengo et al. (28) and suggests that levels of antimicrobial agents achievable in vegetations may correlate better with therapeutic outcome in experimental endocarditis than the levels achievable in serum.

Boscia et al. (14a) reported on the comparative efficacies of oral difloxacin and enoxacin versus parenteral cefazolin in experimental MSSA aortic endocarditis in rabbits. As with their studies in experimental *Enterobacter* endocarditis, difloxacin therapy yielded significantly greater reductions of intravegetation bacterial densities than did enoxacin treatment, presumably reflecting the longer elimination half-life and higher achievable levels for difloxacin in serum. These workers have also reported that enoxacin and vancomycin have equivalent therapeutic efficacies in treating experimental endocarditis in the animal model (29).

### *Staphylococcus epidermidis*

One study of newer quinolones in the treatment of experimental methicillin-resistant *S. epidermidis* endocarditis was performed by Rouse et al. (52). These investigators evaluated ciprofloxacin (alone or with rifampin) in comparison with teicoplanin or vancomycin (alone or in combination with gentamicin, rifampin, or both). Their data showed that ciprofloxacin alone was more effective at reducing intravegetation methicillin-resistant *S. epidermidis* densities than was vancomycin alone or combined with gentamicin. Ciprofloxacin combined with rifampin, and vancomycin combined with gentamicin and rifampin were equally efficacious in the reduction of intravegetation methicillin-resistant *S. epidermidis* densities and were the two most active regimens studied.

### *Coxiella burnetii*

Q fever endocarditis is an important and often devastating form of valvular infection in many countries (e.g., France, Scotland, Australia, New Zealand, etc.). The response of this infection to medical therapy has been poor, and cardiac valve replacement for radical cure has frequently been necessary. Progress toward understanding the fundamental pathogenetic mechanisms of *C. burnetii*-induced endocarditis has been difficult, largely because of the obligate intracellular nature of this bacterial pathogen. There is no experimental animal model of chronic Q fever endocarditis; however, an in vitro tissue culture model of persistent infection of various cell types by *C. burnetii* has been developed (4, 51). This model system has been used extensively to generate new information concerning the efficacies of a variety of the newer quinolones against several *C. burnetii* isolates implicated in distinct clinical syndromes, including endocarditis (49, 67, 68, 70, 71).

Of importance, a correlation has been detected between specific *C. burnetii* clinical disease syndromes (i.e., acute versus chronic Q fever) and isolate antibiotic susceptibility, with isolates from patients with acute Q fever consistently more susceptible to quinolones and other antibiotics than isolates implicated in chronic Q fever (71). Moreover, the process of persistent infection itself appears to result in decreased *C. burnetii* susceptibility to quinolone and other antibiotics, since organisms infecting cells for ≤30 days exhibit significantly lower quinolone MICs than the same isolates infecting cells for ≥400 days. For this reason, new rapid *C. burnetii* antibiotic susceptibility assays such as the shell vial technique, in which organisms typically infect host cells for ≤10 days prior to susceptibility testing (48), provide information pertaining only to acute infection and therefore are difficult to interpret in the context of chronic disease.

The model system of intracellular *C. burnetii* infection has demonstrated several quinolone antibiotics (ciprofloxacin, ofloxacin, pefloxacin, norfloxacin, and difloxacin) to be significantly more effective than tetracyclines (tetracycline, doxycycline) in controlling persistent *C. burnetii* infection in vitro (49, 67, 70, 71). Sparfloxacin has also recently been demonstrated to exert an inhibitory effect on *C. burnetii* within acutely infected host cells in vitro (47). In addition, studies evaluating the efficacies of combinations of quinolones with other antibiotics have revealed evidence of synergy (71), prompting the use of quinolones in combination with rifampin in the treatment of Q fever endocarditis.

Studies suggest that certain quinolone antibiotics are bactericidal versus *C. burnetii*. Such bactericidal action is evidenced by a quinolone-induced reduction in intracellular bacterial counts within host cells that occurs more rapidly than would be expected by host cell elimination of statically inhibited organisms or by dilution of static parasite burden via host cell division (71). Other studies have attempted to differentiate potential bacteriostatic and bactericidal actions of quinolones against *C. burnetii* through the use of cycloheximide treatment to prevent infected host cell division followed by exposure to quinolone antibiotics (48). Quinolones did not lead to the complete elimination of *C. burnetii* from infected, cycloheximide-inhibited host cells in such studies; however, the effects of cycloheximide-induced host cell inhibition on the intracellular metabolic activity of the obligate parasite *C. burnetii* are not well understood. More substantive information is required to address the specific actions of quinolone antibiotics against *C. burnetii*.

Potential mechanisms that may account for differential antibiotic susceptibilities among *C. burnetii* isolates have been examined recently. Although Samuel et al. have correlated plasmid type with clinical syndrome caused by distinct isolates of *C. burnetii* (53), differences in plasmid repertoire have not accounted for the observed differences in quinolone susceptibilities of these isolates. Rather, differential susceptibilities to quinolone antibiotics in *C. burnetii* isolates from acute versus chronic Q fever appear to be the results of differences in drug uptake, with decreased uptake by isolates of the chronic endocarditis group corresponding to their decreased quinolone susceptibilities (69).

## HUMAN ENDOCARDITIS

Daikos et al. (23) have recently reported on experiences with oral quinolone therapy in two patients with infective endocarditis caused by *P. aeruginosa*. One patient was an intravenous-drug addict with mitral valve endocarditis refractory to two mitral valve replacements and three courses of combination parenteral antipseudomonal regimens. Oral ciprofloxacin therapy with daily doses of between 1 and 2 g was continued for 3.5 months (total dose, 150 g). Blood cultures were sterilized during therapy, and fever abated. The patient, however, expired with fulminant endocarditis approximately 1 month after a reduction in the dosage of ciprofloxacin necessitated by drug-induced hepatitis. At autopsy, mitral vegetations contained enormous densities of *P. aeruginosa* ($\sim 10^8$ CFU/g of tissue).

The second patient, who had a permanent cardiac pacemaker, developed mural endocarditis due to *P. aeruginosa*. He failed treatment with parenteral antipseudomonal agents and was treated with 1.5 g of oral ciprofloxacin per day for nearly 2 years, with sterilization of blood cultures and partial abatement of fever. The patient, however, failed a test of cure after 1 year of therapy during a planned discontinuation of the drug. There occurred a rapid return of pseudomonal bacteremia and fever, and progressive biventricular heart failure and anemia developed. At postmortem examination, right ventricular mural endocarditis as well as tricuspid and aortic valvular endocarditis with vegetation bacterial densities of $\sim 10^5$ CFU/g was found. Of interest, selective increases in the MIC of ciprofloxacin (four- to eightfold higher than for the pretreatment strain) were demonstrated for pseudomonal isolates after quinolone therapy in both patients without increases in the MICs of other classes of antibiotics.

The use of quinolones in human staphylococcal endocarditis has been limited to one major study by Dworkin et al. (25). In that investigation, 10 intravenous-drug addict patients with right-sided (tricuspid valve) *S. aureus* endocarditis were treated with a predominantly oral regimen of ciprofloxacin (750 mg twice daily) plus rifampin (600 mg/day) for 3 to 4 weeks following a short course of initial intravenous administration. All 10 patients were cured of their infections. This study was an open, nonrandomized evaluation; however, the excellent results have prompted a multicenter randomized trial comparing ciprofloxacin plus rifampin versus nafcillin plus gentamicin in right-sided *S. aureus* endocarditis. Despite these encouraging results, concern has been expressed about the utility of the quinolones, especially as single agents, in the therapy of staphylococcal infections (66).

The recent report of the failure of ciprofloxacin in controlling right-sided endocarditis illustrates the propensity of *S. aureus* to develop resistance to this drug in vivo when the drug is used as a single-drug regimen in a "high-inoculum" clinical infection such as endocarditis (30). Within 11 days of ciprofloxacin therapy in this patient suspected of ß-lactam allergy, the causative *S. aureus* isolate exhibited an eightfold (2- to 16-$\mu$g/ml) increase in ciprofloxacin MIC and a fourfold (4- to 16-$\mu$g/ml) increase in ciprofloxacin MBC. Of note, high-level ciprofloxacin resistance has now been observed among MRSA strains in a number of medical centers (59) (see chapter 6). Resistance in MSSA isolates, although less than that in MRSA isolates, may be increasing. Similar development of ciprofloxacin resistance in experimental endocarditis *S. aureus* strains supports these observations (37, 38, 40). Findings such as these have given rise to the suggestion that in studies involving ciprofloxacin plus rifampin versus *S. aureus*-induced endocarditis (25), rifampin may be largely responsible for the observed clinical efficacy because of its achievement of concentrations in serum exceeding the MBCs for most *S. aureus* isolates (14, 66). Further investigation involving levels in serum versus those in vegetations relative to the MICs and MBCs of these antibiotics against *S. aureus* endocarditis isolates is needed to define the singular efficacy of ciprofloxacin in such cases.

Chronic Q fever endocarditis, although relatively uncommon, is a life-threatening disease for which an optimal chemotherapeutic regimen has only recently been suggested. As a consequence, chronic *C. burnetii*-induced endocarditis has historically been associated with an alarming mortality rate due to cardiac failure despite cardiac valve resection and prosthetic valve replacement in conjunction with prolonged antibiotic therapy. However, on the basis of recent in vitro findings (68–71), quinolone antibiotics alone and in combination with rifampin or doxycycline may now be considered in the management of chronic Q fever endocarditis in the presence or absence of surgical intervention. Recently, Yerba et al. (72) used ciprofloxacin (orally; 500 mg twice daily) in the treatment of chronic Q fever endocarditis in an elderly patient with previous aortic valve replacement. Within 12 weeks of such therapy, this patient became afebrile, and his phase I complement-fixing-antibody titer dropped from 1:1,024 to 1:128. One year later, the patient was asymptomatic while continuing on ciprofloxacin therapy.

Quinolone antibiotics have also been recently shown to substantially enhance the efficacy of doxycycline in controlling chronic Q fever endocarditis (43). In a study comparing doxycycline alone with doxycycline plus rifampin, doxycycline plus quinolones (ofloxacin or pefloxacin), or doxycycline plus co-trimoxazole, doxycycline used in combination with ofloxacin (200 and 400 mg/day, respectively) or pefloxacin (200 and 400 mg/day, respectively) led to a significant reduction in mortality. However, quinolone therapy did not statistically diminish the prevalence of cardiac valve replacement necessitated by hemodynamic insufficiency, nor did combined doxycycline-quinolone therapy lead to an eradication of *C. burnetii* organisms from cardiac valve tissue despite up to 12 months of antibiotics. Therefore, despite quinolone enhancement of therapeutic efficacy in chronic *C. burnetii* endocarditis, recommended antibiotic therapy duration remains 24 to 36 months, and overall management of the disease may include cardiac valve replacement made necessary by valvular incompetence. Such prolonged antibiotic therapy appears warranted prior to valve replacement surgery in this infection for several important reasons. Autopsy data (44, 62) have suggested that valvular infection seen in chronic Q fever endocarditis generally may involve all four valves histopathologically, despite the dominance of one valve (typically the aortic) in the clinical presentation. Moreover, patients with chronic Q fever endocarditis may have concomitant Q fever hepatitis that may serve as a nidus for subsequent hematogenous seeding of a valve prosthesis.

Pefloxacin in combination with rifampin has recently been used in the treatment of *Brucella melitensis*-induced endocarditis on a Starr-Edwards aortic valve prosthesis (41). This antimicrobial combination failed to prevent periannular abscess formation and valvular deterioration, necessitating subsequent valve replacement as a result of persistent infection and hemodynamic impairment. Fluoroquinolone-resistant *B. melitensis* was subsequently recovered from the infected prosthesis. Following placement of the new valve, continued dual antibiotic chemotherapy did lead to apyrexia and continual patient improvement.

## SUMMARY

The newer quinolones, especially ciprofloxacin, have performed well in the experimental animal models of endocarditis. Most studies have demonstrated that ciprofloxacin is equal to or more effective than synergistically active combinations of aminoglycosides and ß-lactams in the treatment of experimental *P. aeruginosa* endocarditis. Reports documenting the development of increases in the MICs of the newer quinolone agents during the therapy of human and experimental pseudomonal endocarditis are disturbing, however, and further investigation is required to define the relative prevalence of this problem.

The newer quinolones also appear to be highly active in vivo against both MSSA and MRSA strains in experimental endocarditis models. Their efficacy in general appears to be roughly equivalent to that of standard antimicrobial regimens, such as vancomycin for MRSA endocarditis and semisynthetic penicillins or cephalosporins for MSSA endocarditis. Among the quinolones evaluated to date, parenteral ciprofloxacin and pefloxacin appear to be the most active agents in experimental *S. aureus* endocarditis. To date, there is only limited experience with the quinolones in human *S. aureus* endocarditis, although they appear promising in selected cases, particularly when combined with rifampin. Despite these encouraging preliminary results, the development of quinolone resistance in vivo is a growing concern in the therapy of experimental MSSA or MRSA endocarditis, although few of the studies have systematically looked for this phenomenon. Moreover, there is little if any experimental information concerning the utility of the newer quinolone antibiotics in the prophylaxis of MRSA or MSSA endocarditis; such data need to be generated to assess the potential role of these agents in human endocarditis. Information concerning the efficacy of newer quinolones in the prevention of experimental *S. epidermidis* endocarditis remains scanty to date. In vitro studies have motivated the use of newer quinolone antibiotics alone and in combination with other drugs in the treatment of chronic Q fever endocarditis, and results have been promising; extended duration of therapy is required in such cases, however. Further studies are necessary for a more complete evaluation of quinolones for use in controlling difficult endocarditis pathogens such as *C. burnetii* and *Brucella* spp.

### REFERENCES

1. **Andriole, V. T.** 1987. Efficacy of ciprofloxacin in animal models of infection. *Am. J. Med.* **82:**67–70
2. **Andriole, V. T.** 1989. An update on the efficacy of ciprofloxacin in animal models of infection. *Am. J. Med.* **87**(Suppl. 5A)**:**32–34.
3. **Auckenthaler, R. N., M. Michea-Hamzehpour, and J. C. Perchere.** 1986. *In vitro* activity of newer quinolones against aerobic bacteria. 1. *Antimicrob. Chemother.* **17**(Suppl.)**:**29–39.
4. **Baca, O. G., and D. Paretsky.** 1983. Q fever and *Coxiella burnetii*: a model for host parasite interaction. *Microbiol. Rev.* **47:**127–149.
5. **Bauernfeind, A., and C. Petermutier.** 1983. *In vitro* activity of ciprofloxacin, norfloxacin and nalidixic acid. *Eur. J. Clin. Microbiol.* **2:**111–115.

6. **Bayer, A. S., I. K. Blomquist, and K. S. Kim.** 1986. Ciprofloxacin in aortic valve endocarditis due to *Pseudomonas aeruginosa*. *J. Antimicrob. Chemother.* **17:**641–649.
7. **Bayer, A. S., D. P. Greenberg, and J. Yih.** 1988. Correlates of therapeutic efficacy in experimental methicillin-resistant *Staphylococcus aureus* endocarditis. *Chemotherapy* (Basel) **34:**46–55.
8. **Bayer, A. S., L. Hirano, and J. Yih.** 1988. Development of ß-lactam resistance and increased quinolone MICs during therapy of experimental *Pseudomonas aeruginosa* endocarditis. *Antimicrob. Agents Chemother.* **32:**231–235.
9. **Bayer, A. S., K. Lam, D. Norman, K. S. Kim, and J. Morrison.** 1985. *In vivo* efficacy of azlocillin and amikacin versus ciprofloxacin with and without amikacin in experimental right-sided endocarditis due to *Pseudomonas aeruginosa*. *Chemotherapy* (Basel) **32:**364–373.
10. **Bayer, A. S., P. Lindsay, J. Yih, L. Hirano, D. Lee, and I. K. Blomquist.** 1986. Efficacy of ciprofloxacin in experimental aortic valve endocarditis caused by a multiply ß-lactam resistant variant of *Pseudomonas aeruginosa* stably derepressed for ß-lactamase production. *Antimicrob. Agents Chemother.* **30:**528–531.
11. **Bayer, A. S., D. Norman, and D. Anderson.** 1985. Efficacy of ciprofloxacin in experimental arthritis caused by *Escherichia coli: in vitro-in vivo* correlations. *J. Infect. Dis.* **152:**811–816.
12. **Bayer, A. S., D. Norman, and K. S. Kim.** 1985. Efficacy of amikacin and ceftazidime in experimental aortic valve endocarditis due to *Pseudomonas aeruginosa. Antimicrob. Agents Chemother.* **28:**781–785.
13. **Bayer, A. S., J. Peters, T. R. Parr, L. Chan, and R. E. W. Hancock.** 1987. Role of ß-lactamase in in vivo development of ceftazidime resistance in experimental *Pseudomonas aeruginosa* endocarditis. *Antimicrob. Agents Chemother.* **31:**253–258.
14. **Bignardi, G. E.** 1989. Ciprofloxacin resistance and staphylococcal endocarditis. *Lancet* **ii:**1526.
14a. **Boscia, J., W. Kobasa, and D. Kaye.** 1987. *Program Abstr. 27th Intersci. Conf. Antimicrob. Agents Chemother.*, abstr. 934.
15. **Boscia, J. A., W. D. Kobasa, and D. Kaye.** 1985. Enoxacin compared with cefoperazone for the treatment of experimental *Enterobacter aerogenes* endocarditis. *Antimicrob. Agents Chemother.* **27:**708–711.
16. **Boscia, J. A., W. D. Kobasa, and D. Kaye.** 1987. Comparison of difloxacin, enoxacin, and cefoperazone for treatment of experimental *Enterobacter aerogenes* endocarditis. *Antimicrob. Agents Chemother.* **31:**458–460.
17. **Bouza, E., M. Garcia de la Torre, A. Erice, E. Loza, J. M. Diaz-Bnrrega, and L. Buzon.** 1985. *Enterobacter* bacteremia—an analysis of 50 episodes. *Arch. Intern. Med.* **145:**1024–1027.
18. **Brion, N., A. Lessana, F. Mosset, J. J. Lefevre, and G. Montay.** 1986. Penetration of pefloxacin in human heart valves. *J. Antimicrob. Chemother.* **17**(Suppl. B)**:**89–92.
19. **Carbon, C.** 1990. Impact of antibiotic dosage schedule on efficacy in experimental endocarditis. *Scand. J. Infect. Dis.* **74**(Suppl.)**:**163–172.
20. **Carpenter, T. C., C. J. Hackbarth, H. E. Chambers, and M. A. Sande.** 1986. Efficacy of ciprofloxacin for experimental endocarditis caused by methicillin-susceptible or -resistant strains of *Staphylococcus aureus. Antimicrob. Agents Chemother.* **30:**382–384.
21. **Chamberland, S., A. S. Bayer, T. Schollaardt, S. A. Wong, and L. E. Bryan.** 1989. Characterization of mechanisms of quinolone resistance in *Pseudomonas aeruginosa* strains isolated in vitro and in vivo during experimental endocarditis. *Antimicrob. Agents Chemother.* **33:**624–634.
22. **Contrepois, A., C. Daldoss, B. Pangon, J. J. Garaud, M. Kecir, C. Sarrazin, J. M. Valois, and C. Carbon.** 1984. Pefloxacin in rabbits: protein binding, extravascular diffusion, urinary excretion and bactericidal effect in experimental endocarditis. *J. Antimicrob. Chemother.* **14:**51–57.
23. **Daikos, G. L., S. B. Kathpalia, V. T. Lolans, G. C. Jackson, and E. Fosslein.** 1988. Longterm oral ciprofloxacin: experience in the treatment of incurable infective endocarditis. *Am. J. Med.* **84:**786–790.
24. **Durack, D. T., and P. B. Beeson.** 1972. Experimental bacterial endocarditis. II. Survival of bacteria in endocardial vegetations. *Br. J. Exp. Pathol.* **53:**50–53.
25. **Dworkin, R. J., B. L. Lee, M. A. Sande, and H. F. Chambers.** 1989. Treatment of right-sided *Staphylococcus aureus* endocarditis in intravenous drug abusers with ciprofloxacin and rifampin. *Lancet* **ii:**1071–1072.
26. **Eliopoulos, G. M., A. Gardella, and R. C. Moellering, Jr.** 1984. In vitro activity of ciprofloxacin, a new carboxyquinolone antimicrobial agent. *Antimicrob. Agents Chemother.* **25:**331–335.
27. **Freedman, L. R., and J. Valone.** 1979. Experimental infective endocarditis. *Prog. Cardiovasc. Dis.* **22:**169–180.
28. **Gengo, F. M., T. W. Mannion, C. H. Nightingale, and J. J. Schentag.** 1984. Integration of pharmacokinetics and pharmacodynamics of methicillin in curative treatment of experimental endocarditis. *J. Antimicrob. Chemother.* **14:**619–631.
29. **Gilbert, M., J. A. Boscia, W. Kobasa, and D. Kaye.** 1986. Enoxacin compared with vancomycin for the treatment of experimental meth-

icillin-resistant *Staphylococcus aureus* endocarditis. *Antimicrob. Agents Chemother.* **29:**461–463.

30. **Gomez-Jimenez, J., E. Ribera, B. Almirante, O. Del Valle, A. Pahissa, and J. M. Martinez-Vazquez.** 1989. Ciprofloxacin resistance and staphylococcal endocarditis. *Lancet* **ii:**1525–1526.
31. **Hackbarth, C. J., H. F. Chambers, F. Stella, A. M. Shibl, and M. A. Sande.** 1986. Ciprofloxacin in experimental *Pseudomonas aeruginosa* meningitis in rabbits. *J. Antimicrob. Chemother.* **18**(Suppl.):65–69.
32. **Haller, I.** 1985. Comprehensive evaluation of ciprofloxacin-aminoglycoside combinations against *Enterobacteriaceae* and *Pseudomonas aeruginosa* strains. *Antimicrob. Agents Chemother.* **28:**663–666.
33. **Hooper, D. C., J. S. Wolfson, E. Y. Ng, and M. N. Swartz.** 1987. Mechanism of action of and resistance to ciprofloxacin. *Am. J. Med.* **82**(Suppl. 4A):12–20.
34. **Hooper, D. C., J. S. Wolfson, K. S. Souza, C. Tung, L. McHugh, and M. N. Swartz.** 1986. Genetic and biochemical characterization of norfloxacin resistance in *Escherichia coli. Antimicrob. Agents Chemother.* **29:**639–644.
35. **Ingerman, M. J., P. K. Pitsakis, A. E. Rosenberg, and M. E. Levinson.** 1986. The importance of pharmacodynamics in determining the dosing interval in therapy for experimental *Pseudomonas* endocarditis in the rat. *J. Infect. Dis.* **153:**707–714.
36. **Jimenez-Lucho, V. E., L. D. Saravolatz, A. A. Medeiros, and D. Pohlod.** 1986. Failure of therapy in *Pseudomonas* endocarditis—selection of resistant mutants. *J. Infect. Dis.* **154:**64–68.
37. **Kaatz, G. W., S. L. Barriere, D. R. Schaberg, and R. Fekety.** 1987. Ciprofloxacin versus vancomycin in the therapy of experimental methicillin-resistant *Staphylococcus aureus* endocarditis. *Antimicrob. Agents Chemother.* **31:**527–530.
38. **Kaatz, G. W., S. L. Barriere, D. R. Schaberg, and R. Fekety.** 1987. The emergence of resistance to ciprofloxacin during treatment of experimental *Staphylococcus aureus* endocarditis. *J. Antimicrob. Chemother.* **20:**753–758.
39. **Kaatz, G. W., S. M. Seo, S. L. Barriere, L. M. Albrecht, and M. J. Rybak.** 1991. The development of resistance to fleroxacin during therapy of experimental methicillin-susceptible *Staphylococcus aureus* endocarditis. *Antimicrob. Agents Chemother.* **35:**1547–1550.
40. **Kaatz, G. W., S. M. Seo, and C. A. Ruble.** 1990. Mechanisms of fluoroquinolone resistance in *Staphylococcus aureus. J. Infect. Dis.* **163:**1080–1086.
41. **Kamoun, S., A. Hammami, S. Ben Hamed, M. M. Sahnoun, F. Elleuch, and M. Daoud.** 1991. *Brucella* endocarditis on Starr aortic valve prosthesis. *Arch. Mal. Coeur Vaisseaux* **84:**269–271.
42. **Karchmer, A. W.** 1985. Staphylococcal endocarditis—laboratory and clinical basis for antibiotic therapy. *Am. J. Med.* **78**(Suppl. 6B):116–127.
43. **Levy, P. Y., M. Drancourt, J. Etienne, J. C. Auvergnat, J. Beytout, J. M. Sainty, F. Goldstein, and D. Raoult.** 1991. Comparison of different antibiotic regimens for therapy of 32 cases of Q fever endocarditis. *Antimicrob. Agents Chemother.* **35:**533–537.
44. **Palmer, S. R., and S. E. J. Young.** 1982. Q fever endocarditis associated with Q fever in England and Wales, 1975-1981. *Lancet* **iii:**310–321.
45. **Pohlod, D. J., L. D. Saravolatz, and M. M. Somerville.** 1988. *In vitro* susceptibility of staphylococci to fleroxacin in comparison with six other quinolones. *J. Antimicrob. Chemother.* **22**(Suppl. D):35–41.
46. **Preheim, L. C., R. G. Penn, C. C. Sanders, R. V. Goering, and D. K. Giger.** 1982. Emergence of resistance to ß-lactam and aminoglycoside antibiotics during moxalactam therapy of *Pseudomonas aeruginosa* infections. *Antimicrob. Agents Chemother.* **22:**1037–1041.
47. **Raoult, D., P. Bres, M. Drancourt, and G. Vestris.** 1991. In vitro susceptibilities of *Coxiella burnetii, Rickettsia rickettsii,* and *Rickettsia conorii* to the fluoroquinolone sparfloxacin. *Antimicrob. Agents Chemother.* **35:**88–91.
48. **Raoult, D., H. Torres, and M. Drancourt.** 1991. Shell-vial assay: evaluation of a new technique for determining antibiotic susceptibility, tested in 13 isolates of *Coxiella burnetti. Antimicrob. Agents Chemother.* **35:**2070–2077.
49. **Raoult, D., M. R. Yeaman, and O. G. Baca.** 1989. Susceptibility of *Rickettsia* and *Coxiella burnetii* to quinolones. *Rev. Infect. Dis.* **11(**Suppl. 5):986–987.
50. **Reyes, M. P., and A. M. Lerner.** 1983. Current problems in the treatment of infective endocarditis due to *Pseudomonas aeruginosa. Rev. Infect. Dis.* **5:**414–421.
51. **Roman, M. J., P. D. Coriz, and O. G. Baca.** 1986. A proposed model to explain persistent infection of host cells with *Coxiella burnetii. J. Gen. Microbiol.* **132:**1415–1422.
52. **Rouse, M. S., R. M. Wilcox, N. K. Henry, J. M. Steckelberg, and W. R. Wilson.** 1990. Ciprofloxacin therapy of experimental endocarditis caused by methicillin-resistant *Staphylococcus epidermidis. Antimicrob. Agents Chemother.* **34:**273–276.
53. **Samuel, J. E., M. E. Frazier, and L. P. Mallavia.** 1985. Correlation of plasmid type and dis-

ease caused by *Coxiella burnetii*. *Infect. Immun.* **49:**775-779.

54. **Sande, M. A., R. A. Brooks-Fournier, and J. L. Gerberding.** 1987. Efficacy of ciprofloxacin in animal models of infection: endocarditis, meningitis, and pneumonia. *Am. J. Med.* **82:**63-66.
55. **Sande, M. A., R. A. Brooks-Fournier, and J. L. Gerberding.** 1988. Use of animal models in evaluation of the quinolones. *Rev. Infect. Dis.* **10**(Suppl. 1):113-116.
56. **Sanders, C. C., and W. E. Sanders.** 1983. Emergence of resistance during therapy with the new ß-lactam antibiotics: role of inducible ß-lactamases and implications for the future. *Rev. Infect. Dis.* **5:**639-648.
57. **Sanders, C. C., W. E. Sanders, and R. V. Goering.** 1987. Overview of preclinical studies with ciprofloxacin. *Am. J. Med.* **82**(Suppl):196-201.
58. **Sanders, C. C., W. E. Sanders, Jr., R. V. Goering, and V. Werner.** 1984. Selection of multiple antibiotic resistance by quinolones, ß-lactams, and aminoglycosides with special reference to cross-resistance between unrelated drug classes. *Antimicrob. Agents Chemother.* **26:**797-801.
59. **Schaefler, S.** 1989. Methicillin-resistant strains of *Staphylococcus aureus* resistance to quinolones. *J. Clin. Microbiol.* **27:**335-336.
60. **Scheld, W. M.** 1991. Evaluation of quinolones in experimental animal models of infection. *J. Clin. Microbiol. Infect. Dis.* **10:**275-290.
61. **Shekar, R., T. W. Rice, C. H. Zierdt, and C. A. Kallick.** 1985. Outbreak of endocarditis caused by *Pseudomonas aeruginosa* serotype O11 among pentazocine and tripelennamine abusers in Chicago. *J. Infect. Dis.* **151:**203-208.
62. **Spelman, D. W.** 1982. Q fever: a study of 111 consecutive cases. *Med. J. Aust.* **1:**547-553.
63. **Strunk, R. W., J. C. Gratz, R. Maserati, and W. M. Scheld.** 1985. Comparison of ciprofloxacin with azlocillin plus tobramycin in the therapy of experimental *Pseudomonas aeruginosa* endocarditis. *Antimicrob. Agents Chemother.* **28:**428-432.
64. **Sullam, P. M., M. Tauber, C. J. Hackbarth, H. E. Chambers, K. G. Scott, and M. A. Sande.** 1985. Pefloxacin therapy for experimental endocarditis caused by methicillin-susceptible or methicillin-resistant strains of *Staphylococcus aureus*. *Antimicrob. Agents Chemother.* **27:**685-687.
65. **Thrupp, L. D.** 1980. Susceptibility testing of antibiotics in liquid media, p. 73-113. *In* V. Lorian (ed.), *Antibiotics in Laboratory Medicine*. The Williams & Wilkins Co., Baltimore, Md.
66. **Trucksis, M., D. C. Hooper, and J. S. Wolfson.** 1991. Emerging resistance to fluoroquinolones in staphylococci: an alert. *Ann. Intern. Med.* **114:**424-425.
67. **Yeaman, M. R., and O. G. Baca.** 1990. Antibiotic susceptibility of *Coxiella burnetii*, p. 213-223. *In* T. J. Marrie (ed.), *Q Fever*, vol. 1. *The Disease*. CRC Press, Inc., Boca Raton, Fla.
68. **Yeaman, M. R., and O. G. Baca.** 1990. Unexpected antibiotic susceptibility of a chronic isolate of *Coxiella burnetii*. *Ann. N.Y. Acad. Sci.* **590:**297-305.
69. **Yeaman, M. R., and O. G. Baca.** 1991. Mechanisms that may account for differential antibiotic susceptibilities among *Coxiella burnetii* isolates. *Antimicrob. Agents Chemother.* **35:**948-954.
70. **Yeaman, M. R., L. A. Mitscher, and O. G. Baca.** 1987. In vitro susceptibility of *Coxiella burnetii* to antibiotics, including several quinolones. *Antimicrob. Agents Chemother.* **31:**1079-1084.
71. **Yeaman, M. R., M. J. Roman, and O. G. Baca.** 1989. Antibiotic susceptibilities of two *Coxiella burnetii* isolates implicated in distinct clinical syndromes. *Antimicrob. Agents Chemother.* **33:**1052-1057.
72. **Yerba, M., J. Ortigosa, F. Albarran, and M. G. Crespo.** 1990. Ciprofloxacin in a case of Q fever endocarditis. *N. Engl. J. Med.* **323:**614.
73. **Zeiler, H. J.** 1985. Evaluation of the in vitro bactericidal action of ciprofloxacin in cells of *Escherichia coli* in logarithmic and stationary phases of growth. *Antimicrob. Agents. Chemother.* **28:**524-527.

*Quinolone Antimicrobial Agents, 2nd ed.*
Edited by David C. Hooper and John S. Wolfson


*Chapter 22*

# Treatment of Skin and Soft Tissue Infections with Quinolone Antimicrobial Agents

*Layne O. Gentry*

Benign infections of skin and skin structures are not an uncommon cause of visits to physicians' offices. Most of these infections are caused by gram-positive organisms, especially *Staphylococcus aureus* and the beta-hemolytic *Streptococcus* species. With the exception of methicillin-resistant *S. aureus,* which has become an increasing problem as a nosocomial pathogen (5, 29, 55), these organisms are susceptible to a host of oral agents such as penicillin, dicloxacillin, erythromycin, cephalexin, cefaclor, trimethoprim-sulfamethoxazole, clindamycin, and the newer ß-lactamase–ampicillin agents. Because many of these agents have proved to be effective in the treatment of benign infections and because they cost significantly less than the new fluoroquinolones, they remain the agents of choice in many instances.

The more serious infections of skin and skin structures, which frequently occur in postoperative wounds, are often caused by gram-positive and/or gram-negative organisms. Studies from the nationwide survey (Table 1) document the prevalence of gram-positive organisms, gram-negative organisms, and *Candida albicans* in nosocomial wounds (44). These more serious infections are responsible for increased morbidity, prolonged hospital stay, and increased health care costs (26, 28, 45). Infections caused by gram-negative organisms, such as *Pseudomonas aeruginosa*, *Enterobacter* species, and other nosocomial strains, are resistant to most oral antibiotic agents that were available before the introduction of the fluoroquinolones ciprofloxacin and ofloxacin. Thus, the additional expense of parenterally administered broad-spectrum antibiotics was necessary.

Two of the many fluoroquinolones undergoing study worldwide, ciprofloxacin and ofloxacin, are now available for use in treatment of skin infections in the United States. Although briefly available, temafloxacin was removed from the market because of unexpected toxicity. These three agents are active in vitro against gram-positive and gram-negative organisms, including nosocomial strains such as *P. aeruginosa* and members of the family *Enterobacteriaceae*. In addition, the fluoroquinolones provide efficacy combined with convenience and economy.

## CIPROFLOXACIN

There have been numerous studies on the efficacy of ciprofloxacin in the treatment of skin and soft tissue infections. When given orally, ciprofloxacin is usually administered in doses of 500 to 700 mg every 12 h (Table 2)

*Layne O. Gentry* • St. Luke's Episcopal Hospital and Baylor College of Medicine, Houston, Texas 77030.

**Table 1.** Pathogen distribution for nosocomial infections of wounds, National Nosocomial Infections Surveillance System, 1986 through 1989

| Pathogen | n (%)[a] |
|---|---|
| *Staphylococcus aureus* | 3,439 (17) |
| Enterococci | 2,645 (13) |
| Coagulase-negative staphylococci | 2,472 (12) |
| *Escherichia coli* | 1,951 (10) |
| *Pseudomonas aeruginosa* | 1,668 (8) |
| *Enterobacter* sp. | 1,529 (8) |
| *Proteus mirabilis* | 712 (4) |
| *Klebsiella pneumoniae* | 618 (3) |
| Streptococcal species | 539 (3) |
| *Candida albicans* | 481 (2) |
| *Citrobacter* sp. | 321 (2) |
| *Serratia marcescens* | 271 (1) |
| *Candida* sp. | 81 (0) |

[a]A site may have up to four pathogens.

(2, 8, 19, 31, 37, 57, 69). Of this dose, 65% is absorbed by the gastrointestinal tract and 30% is metabolized (see chapter 9). Ciprofloxacin has a high volume of distribution and a moderate degree of biotransformation. In addition, ciprofloxacin has a considerable amount of extrarenal clearance. Its relatively short biologic half-life precludes its accumulation in body tissues at dosing intervals of 12 h.

Ciprofloxacin, like other members of the fluoroquinolone group, has a broad spectrum of activity in vitro against gram-positive and gram-negative microorganisms (Table 3), including methicillin-sensitive staphylococci and most streptococci (1, 34, 35, 59). In vitro activity also extends to some strains of methicillin-resistant staphylococci. Ciprofloxacin is extremely effective against many of the *Enterobacteriaceae,* including strains of *Klebsiella*, *Enterobacter*, and *Serratia* spp. and *P. aeruginosa*. In addition, organisms inhabiting the respiratory and genitourinary tracts are usually extremely susceptible to ciprofloxacin. Unfortunately, ciprofloxacin exhibits poor in vitro activity against most anaerobes.

The efficacy of ciprofloxacin has been evaluated in at least 20 open, noncomparative trials including patients with skin and soft tissue infections (Table 4) (3, 9, 11, 16, 23, 25, 27, 30, 51, 52, 54, 56, 61–66, 70, 71). Oral ciprofloxacin completely or substantially resolved signs and symptoms of infection in 77% of all cases. The rate of adverse gastrointestinal reactions was low (15%), indicating that ciprofloxacin was well tolerated. When data were analyzed from trials in which enrolled patients were initially hospitalized (11, 23, 25, 27, 51, 54, 56, 61–63, 70), ciprofloxacin therapy was successful in 154

**Table 2.** Pharmacokinetic profiles of orally administered quinolones used for treatment of infections of skin and skin structures

| Parameter | Value for indicated agent[a] | | |
|---|---|---|---|
| | Ciprofloxacin | Ofloxacin | Temafloxacin |
| Standard dosage (mg) | 500 q12h | 400 q12h | 400 q12h |
| Availability of i.v. form (United States) | Yes | Yes | Yes |
| Bioavailability (%) | 65 | 95 | 93 |
| Protein binding (%) | 20 | 20 | 26 |
| Half-life (h) | 3.5 | 5.0 | 6.8 |
| Peak level (μg/ml) | | | |
| Serum | 2.3 | 4.0 | 3.3 |
| Tissue | 1.4 | 3.4 | 1.9 |
| Accumulation | No | Yes | Yes |
| Elimination (%) | | | |
| Unabsorbed | 35 | 5 | 7 |
| Unchanged drug | 45 | 80 | 57 |
| Metabolites | 20 | 15 | 6 |

[a]q12h, every 12 h.

**Table 3.** In vitro activities of orally administered quinolones used for treatment of infections of skin and skin structures

| Organism | $MIC_{90}$ (μg/ml) of[a]: | | |
|---|---|---|---|
| | Ciprofloxacin | Ofloxacin | Temafloxacin |
| Gram-positive bacteria | | | |
| *Staphylococcus aureus* | 0.5 | 0.5 | 0.25 |
| Coagulase-negative *Staphylococcus* spp. | 0.25 | 0.5 | 0.25 |
| Group A *Streptococcus* spp. | 0.5 | 1.5 | 0.5 |
| *Streptococcus pneumoniae* | 2.0 | 2.0 | 1.0 |
| *Enterococcus faecalis* | 2.0 | 4.0 | 2.0 |
| Gram-negative and other bacteria | | | |
| *Escherichia coli* | 0.01 | 0.06 | 0.12 |
| *Proteus mirabilis* | 0.13 | 0.25 | 0.5 |
| *Klebsiella pneumoniae* | 0.05 | 0.2 | 1.0 |
| *Enterobacter cloacae* | 0.03 | 0.06 | 0.25 |
| *Serratia marcescens* | 0.06 | 0.25 | 4.0 |
| *Pseudomonas aeruginosa* | 0.5 | 4.0 | 4.0 |
| *Bacteroides fragilis* | R | 8.0 (R) | 4.0 |

[a]$MIC_{90}$, MIC for 90% of strains; R, resistant.

(81%) of 189 cases, and the rate of superinfection was 3%.

Ciprofloxacin has been effective in geriatric patients (71), cancer patients (30), and patients who could not tolerate aminoglycosides (52). Studies have shown that ciprofloxacin may be safely administered for extended periods (56, 66). In addition, ciprofloxacin has been successful against cephalosporin-resistant pathogens (63) and methicillin-resistant *S. aureus* (51, 64). However, resistant strains of *P. aeruginosa* (9, 16, 23, 27, 66, 71) and *S. aureus* (11, 27, 64) have been reported.

Several randomized trials have compared ciprofloxacin with the broad-spectrum cephalosporins cefotaxime (21) and ceftazidime (7, 12, 20) in the treatment of difficult infections of the skin and skin structures in hospitalized patients. In one multicenter trial, the success rate of oral ciprofloxacin (164 of 217 cases [76%]) was similar to that of parenteral cefotaxime (162 of 215 cases [75%]). Oral ciprofloxacin therapy was associated with significantly lower costs and shorter periods of hospitalization than was parenteral cefotaxime therapy.

Three randomized trials comparing ceftazidime (1 to 2 g every 12 h) with sequential parenteral-oral ciprofloxacin (200 mg intravenously every 12 h; 500 to 700 mg orally every 12 h) have been reported (7, 12, 20). Overall, this sequential regimen of ciprofloxacin was effective (i.e., defined as the resolution of or improvement in signs and symptoms of infection) in 46 (79%) of 58 cases, including several cases caused by ceftazidime-resistant organisms (12). Similarly, ceftazidime was successful in 28 (72%) of 39 cases. Patients treated with the ciprofloxacin regimen had significantly more enterococcal superinfections, resulting in an overall superinfection rate of 19% in this group compared with 8% in the ceftazidime-treated group. This difference may possibly be attributed to the fact that oral therapy was continued for 2 days longer than parenteral therapy. Economic advantages, however, were associated with oral therapy.

## OFLOXACIN

Ofloxacin has several advantages over ciprofloxacin. In addition to its wide spectrum

**Table 4.** Noncomparative, open clinical trials of ciprofloxacin for treatment of infections of skin and skin structures[a]

| Reference | Dosage q12h (mg) | Diagnosis[b] | No. of successes[c]/ no. of cases treated (% successful) | No. of infections cured/no. treated (% cured) | | | No. of superinfections (%) |
|---|---|---|---|---|---|---|---|
| | | | | *S. aureus* | *Enterobacter* spp. | *P. aeruginosa* | |
| 31 | 500 | U, A, W, C | 28/33 (85) | 11/17 | 7/7 | 4/8 | 2 (6) |
| 32 | 750 | U, W, C | 15/23 (65) | | | | 0 (0) |
| 33 | 750 | U, A, W | 16/19 (84) | | | | 6 (32) |
| 46 | 750 | U, W | 13/14 (93) | 8/8 | | | 0 (0) |
| 34 | 500 | U, C | 28/30 (93) | 17/19 | 7/7 | 4/6 | |
| 35 | 500 | U, W, C | 21/25 (84) | 3/5 | 10/10 | 11/12 | 0 (0) |
| 37 | 750 | | 18/20 (90) | 12/12 | 9/9 | 7/8 | 1 (5) |
| 38 | 500 | U, W | 15/17 (88) | 3/3 | 3/3 | 7/9 | 1 (6) |
| 40 | 750 | W, C | 4/9 (44) | | | | |
| 41 | 500 | U, W, C | 16/26 (62) | | | | 2 (8) |
| 48 | 750 | W, C | 14/16 (88) | 7/10[d] | | 9/9 | 0 (0) |
| 49 | 500 | W, C | 19/22 (86) | | | 9/16 | |
| 42 | 500 | W | 2/4 (50) | | | 2/4 | |
| 43 | 750 | U, W, C | 8/21 (38) | 8/21[d] | | | |
| 44 | 750 | W | 7/9 (78) | | 6/6 | | 0 (0) |
| 50 | 750 | U, A, W, C | 11/15 (73) | | | 8/15 | 1 (6) |
| 39 | 750 | U | 14/18 (78) | | | 9/11 | 7 (39) |
| 47 | 1,000 | U | 8/16 (50) | | | | |
| 36 | 250[e] | U, C | 10/14 (71) | 5/8 | | | 1 (7) |
| 45 | 750[e] | | 7/7 (100) | 3/3 | 1/1 | 1/1 | 0 (0) |
| Total | | | 274/358 (77) | 77/106 (73) | 43/43 (100) | 71/99 (72) | 21 (8) |

[a]Blanks indicate that no data are available and/or that relevant studies were not done. q12h, every 12 h.
[b]U, infected ulcers; A, abscess; W, wound infection; C, cellulitis.
[c]Success is complete or substantial resolution of signs and symptoms of infection.
[d]Infecting strain was methicillin resistant.
[e]Dose was administered every 8 h.

of antimicrobial activity, ofloxacin has an excellent pharmacokinetic profile (Table 2) (4, 13–15, 32, 33, 39, 41, 68, 69, 72). At the standard dosage (400 mg every 12 h), ofloxacin is readily absorbed by the gastrointestinal tract and undergoes minimal biotransformation. Peak levels of ofloxacin in serum and tissues are higher than those for ciprofloxacin. Its longer biologic half-life allows ofloxacin to accumulate in tissues to a greater degree than does ciprofloxacin.

Although the $MIC_{90}$ for gram-positive cocci is similar for ofloxacin and ciprofloxacin (Table 3), ofloxacin is theoretically superior to ciprofloxacin against gram-positive cocci because of its pharmacokinetic profile (18, 24, 35, 41, 67). Ciprofloxacin is two to four times more active than ofloxacin against most *Enterobacteriaceae* and four to eight times more active against *P. aeruginosa*; however, ofloxacin, unlike ciprofloxacin, is effective against some strains of ß-lactamase-producing *Bacteroides fragilis*.

In an open trial, Fritzen et al. (17) evaluated oral ofloxacin (200 mg every 12 h) in the treatment of surgical infections in 30 hospitalized patients. After 7 days of treatment, the success rate was 100%, with bacteriologic eradication of 17 (74%) of 23 strains of *S. aureus*, all of 3 strains of *Enterobacteriaceae*, and both of 2 strains of *P. aeruginosa*. All enterococci isolated were resistant to ofloxacin. At our center, we compared oral ofloxacin with parenteral cefotaxime in the treatment of serious skin and skin structure infections (22). Cure was defined as the complete resolution of all signs, symptoms, and clinical evidence of infection. Improvement was indicated by marked or moderate reduction in the severity of signs and symptoms of infection. Of the 43 patients treated with ofloxacin, 36 (84%) were cured and 6 (14%) were improved, resulting in a 98% success rate. Of the 50 patients treated with cefotaxime, 29 (58%) were cured and 20 (40%) were improved, resulting in a 98% success rate. Treatment with ofloxacin resulted in a significantly shorter hospital stay.

In a study of 21 patients, Lentino et al. (38) studied the efficacy of ofloxacin given parenterally and then orally in treating serious skin and soft tissue infections, primarily those caused by *S. aureus*. Ofloxacin was successful in 18 cases (86%). The three failures involved the onset of osteomyelitis during therapy for infection of a lower extremity. We recently completed a similar study. For 105 patients, ofloxacin was given sequentially (parenterally-orally) to treat difficult infections, including coagulase-negative staphylococcal surgical wound infections and *P. aeruginosa*-infected ulcers in diabetic patients. The ofloxacin regimen was effective in 91 cases (87%): 28 (93%) of 30 strains of *S. aureus* were eradicated, as were 51 (93%) of 55 strains of *Enterobacteriaceae* and all of 10 strains of *P. aeruginosa*. The rate of superinfection was 7%, and adverse gastrointestinal reactions occurred in 6% of cases.

In studies of the sequential parenteral-oral administration of ciprofloxacin (7, 12, 20), the success rate was 79% and the rate of superinfection was 19%. In larger comparative trials, the rate of superinfection with ciprofloxacin may be significantly higher than that with ofloxacin. This point requires further study but would confirm the theoretical advantages offered by ofloxacin against gram-positive organisms. In addition, the susceptibility of nosocomial pathogens to ciprofloxacin is inversely proportional to consumption of the drug (53).

## TEMAFLOXACIN

Temafloxacin, a new fluoroquinolone, has excellent pharmacokinetic properties. It is rapidly and almost completely absorbed from the gastrointestinal tract. Temafloxacin has an extended biologic half-life compared with those of ciprofloxacin and ofloxacin (Table 2) and broad antimicrobial activity against gram-positive and gram-negative organisms and anaerobic bacteria, including *B. fragilis* (Table 3). In fact, temafloxacin is 2 to 10 times more active than ciprofloxacin and ofloxacin against *B. fragilis* (6, 42, 46).

In a recent comparative study of oral temafloxacin (600 mg twice daily [b.i.d.]) and oral cefadroxil (500 mg b.i.d.) (43), the two drug regimens produced comparable clinical responses and were well tolerated. In 203 patients with mild to moderate soft tissue infections, the clinical success rate (no signs or symptoms of cutaneous infection, or improvement in signs and symptoms) was 98% in the temafloxacin-treated group and 96% in patients receiving cefadroxil. Temafloxacin was significantly more effective in the bacterial eradication of *Staphylococcus epidermidis* than was cefadroxil (100 versus 81%; $P = 0.032$).

In a study by Parish and Jungkind (49), 281 patients with mild to moderate skin infections were treated with either temafloxacin (600 mg b.i.d.) or ciprofloxacin (750 mg b.i.d.). Clinical success (complete resolution of infection, or improvement without complete resolution) was achieved in 136 (96%) of 142 patients treated with temafloxacin and 138 (99%) of 139 patients treated with ciprofloxacin. Both treatment regimens were well tolerated, and bacteriologic eradication rates were similar for patients treated with temafloxacin (95%) and those treated with ciprofloxacin (93%).

## QUINOLONES VERSUS BROAD-SPECTRUM CEPHALOSPORINS

If the experiences with comparative trials of the efficacy of oral quinolones (ciprofloxacin and ofloxacin) and parenteral broad-spectrum cephalosporins (20–22) in treating infections of the skin and skin structures are combined and compared, remarkably similar clinical and bacteriologic results have been obtained with the two therapeutic regimens. A success rate of approximately 90% was achieved in all groups; however, parenteral therapy with cephalosporins was slightly more effective against polymicrobial infections.

The overall rate of bacteriologic eradication was higher for oral quinolones (87%) than for parenteral cephalosporins (79%). Therapy with oral quinolones resulted in more untoward microbiologic events, in that resistance emerged in 5% of all pathogens and superinfections developed in 12% of patients. In the parenteral cephalosporin group, resistance emerged in 2% and superinfection emerged in 3%. As previously noted, these differences may be related to duration of therapy: treatment with oral quinolones required a longer course than did therapy with parenteral cephalosporins.

## RESISTANT ORGANISMS

### *S. aureus*

Methicillin-resistant *S. aureus* remains a serious cause of infection. Often, aggressive parenteral therapy is required to prevent morbidity and mortality in disseminated infections. Ciprofloxacin and ofloxacin are active in vitro against many clinical strains of methicillin-resistant *S. aureus* (40, 53); however, the susceptibility of these organisms to the quinolones may decrease with an increase in antibiotic consumption. Therefore, quinolone therapy is probably not advisable for treating deep-seated methicillin-resistant staphylococcal infections.

### Coagulase-Negative Staphylococci

Frequently, coagulase-negative staphylococci infect surgical wounds and prostheses. More than 65% of these organisms isolated at our institution are resistant to methicillin. Conventional treatment for infection with methicillin-resistant organisms may include a prolonged course of parenteral vancomycin. Because many strains of methicillin-resistant, coagulase-negative staphylococci are susceptible in vitro to the oral quinolones, these agents may be an effective alternative to vancomycin. However, there are reports of ciprofloxacin resistance among coagulase-negative staphylococci isolated from immunocompromised patients (36, 48).

### *Enterococcus faecalis*

Enterococci are a significant cause of nosocomial infections that may arise from endogenous and exogenous contamination of skin and skin structures. These organisms are resistant to cephalosporins. Ciprofloxacin and ofloxacin have exhibited in vitro activity against some strains of enterococci (10, 58, 60).

### *P. aeruginosa*

The quinolones were the first orally administered antibiotics shown to be effective against most strains of *P. aeruginosa*. In fact, ciprofloxacin has been used successfully to treat chronic infected ulcers in patients with diabetes or peripheral vascular disease except in those cases where the organism acquired resistance (51, 66). The rate of quinolone resistance among *P. aeruginosa* as indicated by surveillance data is approximately 6.5% (50). Our review of the published data suggests that the resistance rate among strains of *P. aeruginosa* infecting skin and skin structures is 16% (8 of 50).

### *B. fragilis*

Anaerobes, although frequent pathogens in intra-abdominal and subcutaneous abscesses (47), are not always covered by empirical therapy. Many anaerobes are of limited virulence; however, *B. fragilis* can be a significant pathogen, especially in subcutaneous abscesses and infected ulcers in diabetics. The activities of the quinolones, except for temafloxacin, against anaerobes, including *B. fragilis*, are limited.

## CONCLUSIONS

Two fluoroquinolones, ciprofloxacin and ofloxacin, have been evaluated for the treatment of skin and skin structure infections and are clinically available. The third, temafloxacin, has been withdrawn from the market because of adverse events. All three of these agents have been successfully used for treatment of single or mixed infections caused by susceptible gram-positive and gram-negative organisms. In vitro data and limited published data suggest that ciprofloxacin has an advantage for treating infections caused by *P. aeruginosa*. Ciprofloxacin and ofloxacin have similar in vitro activities, and clinical trials suggest that they are comparable for treating infections caused by all organisms except *P. aeruginosa*. Neither ciprofloxacin nor ofloxacin has activity against *B. fragilis*, and there are no published studies regarding the use of either agent in the treatment of skin and skin structure infections caused by anaerobes. Temafloxacin has an advantage in vitro against gram-positive organisms, especially streptococcal species.

Skin and skin structure infections caused by methicillin-resistant *S. aureus* should not be treated with any quinolone as a single agent until the extent of resistance of these organisms is established worldwide. Clinical trials to assess the efficacy of other fluoroquinolones in the treatment of skin and skin structure infections are under way, but published data are not yet available. Given the potential number of newer fluoroquinolones to be tested, agents that are even more effective may be forthcoming.

## REFERENCES


1. **Barry, A. L., and R. N. Jones.** 1987. In vitro activity of ciprofloxacin against gram-positive cocci. *Am. J. Med.* **82**(Suppl. 4A):27–32.
2. **Bergan, T., S. B. Thorsteinsson, R. Solberg, L. Bjornskau, I. M. Kolstad, and S. Johnsen.** 1987. Pharmacokinetics of ciprofloxacin: intravenous and increasing oral doses. *Am. J. Med.* **82**(Suppl. 4A):97–102.
3. **Berman, S. J., and S. M. Schwartz.** 1987. Clinical evaluation of ciprofloxacin in patients with

moderately severe bacterial infections. *Am. J. Med.* **82**(Suppl. 4A):233–235.

4. **Borner, K., H. Lode, G. Hoffken, P. Koeppe, P. Olschewski, and B. Sievers.** 1988. Comparative pharmacokinetics of ofloxacin and ciprofloxacin. *Rev. Infect. Dis.* **10**(Suppl. 1):91.
5. **Boyce, J. M., and W. A. Causey.** 1982. Increase in occurrence of methicillin-resistant *Staphylococcus aureus* in the United States. *Infect. Control* **3**:377–383.
6. **Chin, N. X., V. M. Figueredo, A. Novelli, and H. C. Neu.** 1988. In-vitro activity of temafloxacin, a new difluoro quinolone antimicrobial agent. *Eur. J. Clin. Microbiol. Infect. Dis.* **7**:58–62.
7. **Dominguez, J., F. Palma, M. E. Vega, et al.** 1989. Brief report: prospective, controlled, randomized non-blind comparison of intravenous/oral ciprofloxacin with intravenous ceftazidime in the treatment of skin or soft-tissue infections. *Am. J. Med.* **87**(Suppl. 5A):136–137.
8. **Drusano, G. L.** 1987. An overview of the pharmacology of intravenously administered ciprofloxacin. *Am. J. Med.* **82**(Suppl. 4A):339–345.
9. **Eron, L. J., L. Harvey, D. L. Hixon, and D. M. Poretz.** 1985. Ciprofloxacin therapy of infections caused by *Pseudomonas aeruginosa* and other resistant bacteria. *Antimicrob. Agents Chemother.* **28**:308–310.
10. **Fabbri, A., G. Manno, A. Tacchella, M. L. Belli, and C. Palmero.** 1986. Susceptibility of enterococci. I. Inhibitory and bactericidal activity of several chemo-antibiotics against *Streptococcus faecalis* and *Streptococcus faecium*. *Chemioterapia* **5**:302–308.
11. **Fass, R. J.** 1986. Treatment of skin and soft tissue infections with oral ciprofloxacin. *J. Antimicrob. Chemother.* **18**(Suppl. D):153–157.
12. **Fass, R. J., J. F. Plouffe, and J. A. Russell.** 1989. Intravenous/oral ciprofloxacin versus ceftazidime in the treatment of serious infections. *Am. J. Med.* **87**(Suppl. 5A):164–168.
13. **Fillastre, J. P., A. Leroy, and G. Humbert.** 1987. Ofloxacin pharmacokinetics in renal failure. *Antimicrob. Agents Chemother.* **31**:156–160.
14. **Flor, S.** 1989. Pharmacokinetics of ofloxacin: an overview. *Am. J. Med.* **87**(Suppl. 6C):24–30.
15. **Flor, S., H. Wentraub, B. Beals, and K. Tack.** 1986. Pharmacokinetics of ofloxacin in humans after single dose and during multiple dose administration, abstr. 483. *Program Abstr. 26th Intersci. Conf. Antimicrob. Agents Chemother.*
16. **Follath, F., M. Bindschedler, M. Wenk, R. Frei, H. Stadler, and H. Reber.** 1986. Use of ciprofloxacin in the treatment of *Pseudomonas aeruginosa* infections. *Eur. J. Clin. Microbiol.* **5**:236–240.
17. **Fritzen, T., E. Marx, and J. Uy.** 1986. Treatment of surgical infections with a modern quinolone: therapy of soft tissue infections and pneumonia with ofloxacin. *Infection* **14**(Suppl. 4):293–296.
18. **Fuchs, P. C.** 1989. In vitro antimicrobial activity and susceptibility testing of ofloxacin. *Am. J. Med.* **87**(Suppl. 6C):10–13.
19. **Gasser, T. C., S. C. Ebert, P. H. Graversen, and P. O. Madsen.** 1987. Pharmacokinetic study of ciprofloxacin in patients with impaired renal function. *Am. J. Med.* **82**(Suppl. 4A):139–141.
20. **Gentry, L. O., and A. Koshdel.** 1989. Intravenous/oral ciprofloxacin versus intravenous ceftazidime in the treatment of serious gram-negative infections of the skin and skin structure. *Am. J. Med.* **87**(Suppl. 5A):132–135.
21. **Gentry, L. O., C. H. Ramirez-Ronda, E. Rodriguez-Noriega, H. Thadepalli, P. L. del Rosal, and C. Ramirez.** 1989. Oral ciprofloxacin vs. parenteral cefotaxime in the treatment of difficult skin and skin structure infections: a multicenter trial. *Arch. Intern. Med.* **149**:2579–2583.
22. **Gentry, L. O., G. Rodriguez-Gomez, B. J. Zeluff, A. Khoshdel, and M. Price.** 1989. A comparative evaluation of oral ofloxacin versus intravenous cefotaxime therapy for serious skin and skin structure infection. *Am. J. Med.* **87**(Suppl. 6C):57–60.
23. **Giamarellou, H., N. Galanakis, C. Dendrinos, J. Stefanou, E. Daphnis, and G. K. Daikos.** 1986. Evaluation of ciprofloxacin in the treatment of *Pseudomonas aeruginosa* infections. *Eur. J. Clin. Microbiol.* **5**:232–235.
24. **Goosens, H., P. de Mol, H. Coignau, J. Levy, O. Grados, G. Ghysels, H. Innocent, and J. Butzler.** 1985. Comparative in vitro activities of aztreonam, ciprofloxacin, norfloxacin, ofloxacin, HR 810 (a new cephalosporin), RU 28965 ( a new macrolide), and other agents against enteropathogens. *Antimicrob. Agents Chemother.* **27**:388–392.
25. **Gorkiewicz-Petkow, A., H. Weuta, S. Jablonska, L. Petkow, S. Bielunska, and M. Gawkonska.** 1988. Bacterial infections of the skin treated with ciprofloxacin. *Infection* **16**(Suppl. 1):55–56.
26. **Green, J. W., and R. P. Wenzel.** 1977. Postoperative wound infection: a controlled study of the increased duration of hospital stay and direct cost of hospitalization. *Ann. Surg.* **185**:264–268.
27. **Greenberg, R. N., D. J. Kennedy, P. M. Reilly, K. L. Luppen, W. J. Weinandt, M. R. Bollinger, F. Aguirre, F. Kodesch, and A. M. K. Saeed.** 1987. Treatment of bone, joint, and soft-tissue infections with oral ciprofloxacin. *Antimicrob. Agents Chemother.* **31**:151–155.
28. **Haley, R. W., D. H. Culver, J. W. White, W. M. Morgan, and T. G. Emori.** 1985. The nationwide nosocomial infection rate: a new need for vital statistics. *Am. J. Epidemiol.* **121**:159–167.
29. **Haley, R. W., A. W. Hightower, R. F. Khabbaz, et al.** 1981. The emergence of methicillin-resistant

*Staphylococcus aureus* infection in United States hospitals: possible role of the house staff-patient transfer circuit. *Ann. Intern. Med.* **97**:297–308.

30. **Haron, E., K. V. I. Rolston, C. Cunningham, F. Holmes, T. Umsawasdi, and G. P. Bodey.** 1989. Oral ciprofloxacin therapy for infections in cancer patients. *J. Antimicrob. Chemother.* **24**:955–962.
31. **Hoffken, G., K. Borner, P. D. Glatzel, P. Koeppe, and H. Lode.** 1985. Reduced enteral absorption of ciprofloxacin in the presence of antacids. *Eur. J. Clin. Microbiol.* **4**:345. [Letter.]
32. **Hoffken, G., P. Olschewski, B. Sievers, et al.** 1986. Absolute bioavailability and interactions in the pharmacology of ofloxacin, abstr. 485. *Program Abstr. 26th Intersci. Conf. Antimicrob. Agents Chemother.*
33. **Kalager, T., A. Digranes, T. Bergan, and T. Rolstad.** 1986. Ofloxacin: serum and skin blister fluid pharmacokinetics in the fasting and non-fasting state. *J. Antimicrob. Chemother.* **17**:795–800.
34. **Kayser, F. H., and J. Novak.** 1987. In vitro activity of ciprofloxacin against gram-positive bacteria. *Am. J. Med.* **82**(Suppl. 4A):33–39.
35. **King, A., and I. Phillips.** 1986. The comparative in-vitro activity of eight newer quinolones and nalidixic acid. *J. Antimicrob. Chemother.* **18**(Suppl. D):1–20.
36. **Kotilainen, P., J. Nikoskelainen, and P. Huovinen.** 1990. Emergence of ciprofloxacin-resistant coagulase-negative staphylococcal skin flora in immunocompromised patients receiving ciprofloxacin. *J. Infect. Dis.* **161**:41–44.
37. **Lebel, M., and M. G. Bergeron.** 1987. Pharmacokinetics in the elderly: studies on ciprofloxacin. *Am. J. Med.* **82**(Suppl. 4A):108–114.
38. **Lentino, J. R., J. B. Augustinsky, T. M. Weber, and C. T. Pachucki.** 1991. Therapy of serious skin and soft tissue infections with ofloxacin administered by intravenous and oral route. *Chemotherapy* **37**:70–76.
39. **Lode, H., G. Hoffken, P. Olschewski, B. Sievers, A. Kirch, K. Borner, and P. Koeppe.** 1987. Pharmacokinetics of ofloxacin after parenteral and oral administration. *Antimicrob. Agents Chemother.* **31**:1338–1342.
40. **Maple, D. A., J. M. T. Hamilton-Miller, and W. Brumfitt.** 1989. World-wide antibiotic resistance in methicillin-resistant *Staphylococcus aureus. Lancet* **i**:537–540.
41. **Monk, J. P., and D. M. Campoli-Richards.** 1987. Ofloxacin: a review of its antibacterial activity, pharmacokinetic properties, and therapeutic use. *Drugs* **33**:346–391.
42. **Nakanishi, N., M. Inoue, K. Inoue, T. Yamaguchi, and S. Mitsuhashi.** 1990. In vitro activity of temafloxacin hydrochloride (TA-167 or A-62254), a new fluorinated 4-quinolone. *Chemotherapy* **36**:345–355.
43. **Nelder, K.** 1991. Double-blind randomized study of oral temafloxacin and cefadroxil in patients with mild to moderately severe bacterial skin infections. *Am. J. Med.* **91**:111–114.
44. **Nichols, R. L.** 1982. Postoperative wound infection. *N. Engl. J. Med.* **307**:1701–1702.
45. **Nichols, R. L.** 1991. Surgical wound infection. *Am. J. Med.* **91**:54S–64S.
46. **Nye, K., Y. G. Shi, J. M. Andrews, J. P. Ashby, and R. Wise.** 1989. The in-vitro activity, pharmacokinetics and tissue penetration of temafloxacin. *J. Antimicrob. Chemother.* **24**:415–424.
47. **Olson, M. M., and M. O. Allen.** 1989. Nosocomial abscess: results of an eight year prospective study of 32,284 operations. *Arch. Surg.* **124**:356–361.
48. **Oppenheim, B. A., J. W. Hartley, W. Lee, and J. P. Burnie.** 1989. Outbreak of coagulase negative staphylococcus highly resistant to ciprofloxacin in a leukaemia unit. *Br. Med. J.* **299**:294–297.
49. **Parish, L., and D. L. Jungkind.** 1991. Systemic antimicrobial therapy in skin and skin structure infections: comparison of temafloxacin and ciprofloxacin. *Am. J. Med.* **91**:115S–119S.
50. **Parry, M. F., K. B. Panzer, and M. E. Yukna.** 1989. Quinolone resistance: susceptibility data from a 300-bed community hospital. *Am. J. Med.* **87**(Suppl. 5A):12–16.
51. **Peterson, L. R., L. M. Lissack, K. Canter, C. E. Fasching, C. Clabots, and D. N. Gerding.** 1989. Therapy of lower extremity infections with ciprofloxacin in patients with diabetes mellitus, peripheral vascular disease, or both. *Am. J. Med.* **86**:801–808.
52. **Pien, F. D., and K. K. Yamane.** 1987. Ciprofloxacin treatment of soft tissue and respiratory infections in a community outpatient practice. *Am. J. Med.* **82**(Suppl. 4A):236–238.
53. **Piercy, P. A. C., D. Barbaro, J. P. Luby, and P. A. Mackowiak.** 1989. Ciprofloxacin for methicillin-resistant *Staphylococcus aureus* infection. *Antimicrob. Agents Chemother.* **33**:128–130.
54. **Powers, T., and D. H. Bingham.** 1990. Clinical and economic effect of ciprofloxacin as an alternative to injectable antimicrobial therapy. *Am. J. Hosp. Pharm.* **47**: 1781–1784.
55. **Preheim, L. C., D. Rimland, and M. J. Bittner.** 1987. Methicillin-resistant *Staphylococcus aureus* in Veterans Administration medical centers. *Infect. Control* **8**:191–194.
56. **Ramirez, C. A., J. L. Bran, C. R. Mejia, and J. F. Garcia.** 1985. Open, prospective study of the clinical efficacy of ciprofloxacin. *Antimicrob. Agents Chemother.* **28**:128–132.
57. **Raoof, S., C. Wollschlager, and F. A. Khan.** 1987. Ciprofloxacin increases serum levels of theophylline. *Am. J. Med.* **82**(Suppl. 4A):115–118.
58. **Sahm, D. F., and G. T. Koburov.** 1989. In vitro activities of quinolones against enterococci resistant

to penicillin-aminoglycoside synergy. *Antimicrob. Agents Chemother.* **33:**71–77.

59. **Sanders, C. C., W. E. Sanders, Jr., and R. V. Goering.** 1987. Overview of preclinical studies with ciprofloxacin. *Am. J. Med.* **82**(Suppl. 4A):2–11.
60. **Sapico, F. L., H. N. Canawati, V. J. Ginunas, et al.** 1989. Enterococci highly resistant to penicillin and ampicillin: an emerging clinical problem? *J. Clin. Microbiol.* **27:**2091–2095.
61. **Scully, B. E., and H. C. Neu.** 1986. Oral ciprofloxacin therapy of infection caused by multiply resistant bacteria other than *Pseudomonas aeruginosa. J. Antimicrob. Chemother.* **18**(Suppl. D):179–185.
62. **Scully, B. E., H. C. Neu, M. F. Parry, and W. Mandell.** 1986. Oral ciprofloxacin therapy of infections due to *Pseudomonas aeruginosa. Lancet* **i:**819–822.
63. **Self, P. L., B. A. Zeluff, D. Sollo, and L. O. Gentry.** 1987. Use of ciprofloxacin in the treatment of serious skin and skin structure infections. *Am. J. Med.* **82**(Suppl. 4A):239–241.
64. **Smith, S. M., R. H. Eng, and F. Tecson-Tumang.** 1989. Ciprofloxacin therapy for methicillin-resistant *Staphylococcus aureus* infections or colonizations. *Antimicrob. Agents Chemother.* **33:**181–184.
65. **Valainis, G. T., G. A. Pankey, H. P. Katner, L. M. Cortez, and J. R. Dalovisio.** 1987. Ciprofloxacin in the treatment of bacterial skin infections. *Am. J. Med.* **82**(Suppl. 4A):230–232.
66. **Valtonen, V., L. Karppinen, and A.-L. Kariniemi.** 1989. A comparative study of ciprofloxacin and conventional therapy in the treatment of patients with chronic lower leg ulcers infected with *Pseudomonas aeruginosa* or other gram-negative rods. *Scand. J. Infect. Dis.* **60**(Suppl.):79–83.
67. **van Caekenberghe, D. L., and S. R. Pattyn.** 1984. In vitro activity of ciprofloxacin compared with those of other new fluorinated piperazinyl-substituted quinolone derivatives. *Antimicrob. Agents Chemother.* **25:**518–521.
68. **Wise, R., D. Griggs, and J. M. Andrews.** 1988. Pharmacokinetics of the quinolones in volunteers: a proposed dosing schedule. *Rev. Infect. Dis.* **10**(Suppl. 1):S83–S89.
69. **Wise, R., D. Lister, C. A. M. McNulty, D. Griggs, and J. M. Andrews.** 1986. The comparative pharmacokinetics of five quinolones. *J. Antimicrob. Chemother.* **18**(Suppl. D):71–81.
70. **Wood, M. J., and M. N. Logan.** 1986. Ciprofloxacin for soft tissue infections. *J. Antimicrob. Chemother.* **18**(Suppl. D):159–164.
71. **Yangco, B. G., V. S. Kenyon, K. D. Halkias, J. A. Bogel, J. F. Toney, and H. Chmel.** 1989. Oral ciprofloxacin treatment of infections in geriatric patients. *Clin. Ther.* **11:**503–510.
72. **Zeiler, H.-J., D. Beermann, W. Wingender, D. Forster, and P. Schacht.** 1988. Bactericidal activity of ciprofloxacin, norfloxacin and ofloxacin in serum and urine after oral administration to healthy volunteers. *Infection* **16**(Suppl. 1):19–23.

*Quinolone Antimicrobial Agents, 2nd ed.*
Edited by David C. Hooper and John S. Wolfson


*Chapter 23*

# Treatment of Eye Infections

*Michael Barza*

The most common site of bacterial infection of the eye is the conjunctiva (conjunctivitis). The major sites of serious bacterial infections of the eye are the cornea (keratitis) and the interior of the eye (endophthalmitis). The fluoroquinolones have promise for the treatment of infections in each of these sites. The drugs are highly potent against gram-negative bacilli, which are causes of conjunctivitis, keratitis, and occasionally endophthalmitis. Applied topically, the drugs are well tolerated and reach appreciable concentrations in the cornea and aqueous humor. Their intraocular penetration after systemic administration is moderate and possibly sufficient to make them useful as adjunctive agents for the treatment of endophthalmitis.

In this chapter, I review the pharmacokinetic and therapeutic studies of the quinolones in experimental animals and humans. Many of the data have been reported in more than one publication. I have tried to cite the more complete or the more readily available reports and to avoid duplication. Adverse ocular effects of the quinolones are discussed in chapter 26.

*Michael Barza* • New England Medical Center, 750 Washington Street, Boston, Massachusetts 02111.

## IN VITRO ACTIVITY AGAINST OCULAR PATHOGENS

The activities of norfloxacin (12, 20, 36, 41) and ofloxacin (36) against ocular pathogens in vitro have been studied. The quinolones are generally as active as any other agent tested against *Staphylococcus aureus*, *Staphylococcus epidermidis*, gram-negative enteric bacilli, *Pseudomonas aeruginosa*, *Neisseria* species, *Haemophilus influenzae*, and *Moraxella* species. The quinolones were only moderately active in vitro against streptococci, including *Streptococcus pneumoniae*; in one study, erythromycin, chloramphenicol, trimethoprim-sulfamethoxazole, and bacitracin were more active than norfloxacin against *S. pneumoniae* (41). Norfloxacin had predictably little activity against obligate anaerobic isolates (12).

## PHARMACOKINETIC STUDIES

In the following sections, the results of pharmacokinetic studies in the rabbit's eye and the human eye are reviewed. For purposes of orientation, a brief description of the major pharmacokinetic issues is given at the beginning of each section.

### Topical Applications in Rabbits

Drops applied to the eye produce high concentrations of drug in the tears; however, the concentrations decrease rapidly because of the "washout" effect of the tears. Penetration of the cornea is modest for most drugs because of the barrier effect of the tight junctions of the corneal epithelium. Corneal penetration is generally better if the drugs are highly lipid soluble or if the corneal epithelium is disrupted. Greater corneal concentrations are produced when highly concentrated solutions (e.g., fortified drops) are applied and when drops are applied at frequent intervals (2). Drug concentrations in the aqueous humor, although commonly measured, are not of great clinical importance in themselves but are a good index of the minimum concentrations in the cornea, which in turn are relevant for the treatment of keratitis. Drugs applied topically rarely produce detectable concentrations in the vitreous humor.

The concentrations of ofloxacin in tears after a single topical application of a 0.3% (3-mg/ml) solution were initially extremely high (2,000 μg/ml) but fell to below 10 μg/ml by 40 min after application. Similar findings were noted for gentamicin and tobramycin (38).

Studies of the penetration of quinolones into the cornea and aqueous humor after topical application are summarized in Table 1. Repeated application of a 2% solution of rosoxacin produced concentrations of 15 to 30 μg/g in the cornea and 5 to 8.7 μg/ml in the aqueous humor but no detectable drug (<0.75 μg/ml) in the vitreous humors of rabbits with healthy eyes. The concentrations in the aqueous humor were highest when the drops were given every 5 min rather than at longer intervals (22). Hourly applications of enoxacin drops (3 mg/ml) produced peak concentrations of 66 μg/g in the cornea and 7 μg/ml in the aqueous humors of the eyes of rabbits from which the corneal epithelia had been removed, whereas levels at these sites in rabbits with healthy eyes were only 12 μg/g and 0.9 μg/ml, respectively (44). In rabbits with *P. aeruginosa* keratitis, application of a single topical dose of enoxacin (5 mg/ml) produced levels of 3.7 μg/ml in the aqueous humor, but no drug was detectable in the vitreous humor (18). The application of ciprofloxacin drops (3 mg/ml) topically every 30 min for six doses produced peak levels of 12.9 μg/ml in the aqueous humors of rabbits with corneal abrasions but only 4.8 μg/ml in rabbits with healthy corneas (33).

Overall, these concentrations in the cornea are in the range of those noted for other agents that are not highly lipid soluble (2). Fortified drops containing higher concentrations of drug, e.g., 6 to 35 mg/ml, would

**Table 1.** Ocular penetration of quinolones after topical application in rabbits[a]

| Drug | Dosage[b] | Concn in eyes: Healthy Cornea (μg/g) | Healthy Aqueous humor (μg/g) | Corneal damage Cornea (μg/g) | Corneal damage Aqueous humor (μg/g) | Reference |
|---|---|---|---|---|---|---|
| Rosoxacin | 200-mg/ml (2%) solution q5–30 min, 6 doses | 15–30 | 5–8.7 | | | 22 |
| Enoxacin | 3-mg/ml (0.3%) solution q1h, 24 doses | 12 | 0.9 | 66 | 7 | 44 |
| Enoxacin | 5-mg/ml (0.5%) solution, 1 dose | | | | 3.7 | 18 |
| Ciprofloxacin | 3-mg/ml (0.3%) solution q30 min, 6 doses | | 4.8 | | 12.9 | 33 |

[a]Peak concentration for each study was selected.
[b]q5–30 min, every 5 to 30 min.

presumably yield higher corneal concentrations. As expected, ocular penetration is much greater in eyes with corneal epithelial damage than in eyes with normal epithelia.

### Systemic and Periocular Administration in Rabbits

Drugs administered systemically penetrate the aqueous and vitreous humors with difficulty because of anatomic barriers (3). Penetration into the aqueous humor is restricted by the blood-aqueous barrier, which exists because the epithelium overlying the capillaries of the ciliary body has tight intercellular junctions. Penetration into the vitreous humor is limited because the endothelial cells of the retinal capillaries and the epithelial cells overlying the choroidal capillaries (the so-called retinal pigment epithelium, or RPE) have tight junctions; together, these constitute the blood-retinal barriers. Drugs administered by periocular, e.g., subconjunctival, injection produce high concentrations in the cornea and aqueous humor but are hindered from entering the vitreous humor by the tight junctions of the RPE. Because of these barriers, drugs that are weakly lipid soluble penetrate the aqueous humor and vitreous humor poorly after systemic administration and penetrate the vitreous humor poorly after periocular injection. The fluoroquinolones are moderately lipid soluble but less so than drugs such as chloramphenicol, rifampin, and metronidazole.

To allow comparison of various studies of drug penetration into the aqueous and vitreous humors after systemic administration, percent penetration values have been calculated; these are the ratio of the peak concentration in the site to the peak concentration in the serum. Because many investigators calculate the penetration ratio from samples obtained simultaneously rather than from the peak concentration measured in each site, the percent penetration values given in this review may differ from those calculated by authors.

Table 2 summarizes data on the concentrations of the quinolones in serum and in aqueous and vitreous humors of the rabbit's eye after systemic administration and periocular (subconjunctival) injection. The data are the peak concentrations reported by the authors, and values for percent penetration are also shown. Only healthy eyes were studied in the reports summarized in Table 2. In all instances, the drug was administered only once; greater intraocular penetration would be expected from repeated administrations.

Several points can be seen from inspection of the data in Table 2. The penetration of the aqueous humor ranged from about 8 to 29%, and that of the vitreous humor ranged from 4 to 27%. The lowest values were obtained by Behrens-Baumann and Martell (6) with ciprofloxacin. The highest values were obtained by Cochereau-Massin et al. (13) with pefloxacin. When penetration was calculated by the latter as the ratio of the area under the curve for the site divided by the area under the curve for serum, a still higher value was obtained for vitreous humor, i.e., 39 to 45%. Cochereau-Massin and coworkers also found a marked difference between albino and pigmented rabbits in the distribution of pefloxacin in pigmented tissues (iris and choroid): accumulation and persistence of the drug in these sites in pigmented animals were about 50-fold greater than in albino animals (13). This suggests binding of the drug to the pigmentary apparatus in the eye, a phenomenon that has been reported for clindamycin and aminoglycosides (4).

A second general point is that penetration of the vitreous humor is similar to that of the aqueous humor after systemic administration of the quinolones. This is in distinction to other classes of drugs, whose penetration into the aqueous humor is usually greater than into the vitreous humor (2) because the tight junctions of the blood-aqueous barrier are leakier than those of the blood-retinal barriers. The quinolones are moderately lipid soluble, so they penetrate the blood-retinal barriers fairly well.

**Table 2.** Ocular penetration after systemic and periocular administration in rabbits[a]

| Drug and route of administration | Dosage and route[b] | Concn, μg/ml (% penetration)[c] | | | Comment | Reference |
|---|---|---|---|---|---|---|
| | | Serum | Aqueous humor | Vitreous humor | | |
| Systemic | | | | | | |
| Ciprofloxacin | 50 mg/kg p.o., 1 dose | 1.5 | 0.32 (21) | 0.33 (21) | | 35 |
| Ciprofloxacin | 12 mg/kg i.v. bolus, 1 dose | 0.7 | 0.06 (8.6) | 0.028 (4) | | 6 |
| Rosoxacin | 5 mg/kg i.v., 1 dose | 5.5 | <0.75 (<14) | <0.75 (<14) | Assay not sensitive | 22 |
| Pefloxacin | 50 mg/kg i.m., 1 dose | 8.9 | 2.6 (29) (ratio of AUCs, 24–33) | 2.4 (27) (ratio of AUCs, 39–45) | Accumulation in pigmented tissues (see text) | 13 |
| Sparfloxacin | 50 mg/kg p.o., 1 dose | 4.0 | 0.74 (18.3) | | | 34 |
| Periocular | | | | | | |
| Ciprofloxacin | 1 mg subconj, 1 dose | | 1.35 | 0.003–0.04 | Small dose | 6 |
| Rosoxacin | 10 mg subconj, 1 dose | 1.66 | 34 | 11 (transient), then 0.33 (20) | Concn of 11 μg/ml in vitreous could be spurious | 22 |

[a]Concentrations were at or near presumed peak except where indicated. All eyes were uninflamed.
[b]p.o., per os; i.v., intravenous, i.m., intramuscular; subconj, subconjunctival.
[c]Percent penetration is concentration in the site as a percentage of the concentration serum. The calculation was not made for subconjunctival injections. AUC, area under the curve (see text).

Corresponding to the moderately good penetration of the vitreous humor, relatively good penetration into the ocular tissues (cornea, iris, choroid, retina, and sclera) after systemic administration was shown for ciprofloxacin (35) and pefloxacin (13). Even the lens showed about 25% penetration with pefloxacin and very long persistence of the drug (13). Accumulation of quinolones in the lens of the eye could be worrisome in terms of toxicity. However, there have been no reports of lens toxicity with pefloxacin (13).

In a small number of rabbits in which one eye was infected experimentally, penetration into the aqueous and vitreous humors was similar in healthy and infected eyes (17). The data are not shown in Table 2 because only four rabbits were studied and several dosing regimens were used.

Subconjunctival injection of 1 mg of ciprofloxacin, a tiny dose, produced a low concentration in the aqueous humor and very low levels in the vitreous humor (Table 2). Subconjunctival injection of 10 mg of rosoxacin produced not only high concentrations in the cornea and aqueous humor but, transiently, concentrations of 11 μg/ml in the vitreous humor. The levels in vitreous are surprisingly high and possibly spurious, because 160 min later they had fallen to 0.33 μg/ml (22). Marked redness and chemosis were produced by the subconjunctival injection of rosoxacin.

Drugs leave the vitreous humor by one of two routes (2). The anterior route involves diffusion through the aqueous humor and egress through the canal of Schlemm. Drugs eliminated by this long and tortuous route, for example, aminoglycosides and vancomycin, have a long vitreal half-life and a high ratio of aqueous/vitreous concentrations after intravitreal injection. The posterior route entails active transport from the vitreous humor by a pump located in the retinal capillaries or the RPE. Drugs eliminated by this route, for example, ß-lactam drugs, have short vitreal half-lives and low ratios of aqueous/vitreous concentrations after intravitreal injection. Probenecid prolongs the vitreal half-life of ß-lactam drugs. Interestingly, the vitreal half-life of pefloxacin after intravitreal injection in rabbits was only 2.2 h (14), and no drug was found in the aqueous humor, suggesting that the drug is actively eliminated by the retinal route. This finding is consistent with the observation that some quinolones are actively secreted by the renal tubule and that secretion is inhibited by probenecid; renal tubular secretion of quinolones may be more pronounced in rabbits than in humans (40).

Ocular tolerance of ciprofloxacin given by intravitreal injection has been reported (43). No retinal or corneal damage was observed in phakic or aphakic eyes of rabbits after an intravitreal dose of up to 100 μg. This dosage would produce a concentration of about 100 μg/ml in the vitreous humor of this species. Larger doses produced dose-dependent acute corneal and retinal toxicities.

### Pharmacokinetic Studies in Humans

Many investigations of the penetration of fluoroquinolones into the ocular humors of humans after systemic administration have been done. Most of the patients from whom aqueous humor was obtained were undergoing cataract extraction. However, vitreous humor was usually obtained from patients undergoing surgery for retinal detachment, vitreal hemorrhage, and diabetic retinopathy. These disorders may have affected the pharmacokinetics of drug penetration. All of the studies were of uninfected eyes, and most were single-dose studies.

A summary of the data for ciprofloxacin, which has been the drug most extensively examined, is shown in Table 3. The percent penetration values for the aqueous humor vary from 6 to 33%, with most being in the range of 10 to 20%. Fewer data are available for concentrations in vitreous humor, but again, most values are in the range of 10 to 20% of the concentration in serum. These percent penetration values and the penetration of the aqueous and vitreous humors are similar to those for rabbits. Penetration increased with repeated dosing (1, 26, 32).

Data for other quinolones are summarized in Table 4. The values for percent penetration of the aqueous humor are remarkably similar for pefloxacin, ofloxacin, and norfloxacin, with all values lying between 15 and 25%. The exception is the only multiple-dose study summarized in Table 4: six doses of pefloxacin were given, and the penetration ratio was 50%. In the only report dealing with vitreous humor, the concentrations of pefloxacin were similar to those in the aqueous humor (17).

## TREATMENT OF EXPERIMENTAL INFECTIONS IN RABBITS

Few studies of the efficacy of the quinolones in the treatment of ocular infections have been done. In rabbits with experimental *Pseudomonas* keratitis, a solution of enoxacin drops (3 mg/ml) applied hourly was as effective as more-concentrated enoxacin drops (10 mg/ml) or as gentamicin drops (3 mg/ml) in reducing bacterial counts in the cornea after 24 h of treatment (44). In rabbits with experimental keratitis caused by an aminoglycoside-resistant strain of *P. aeruginosa*, application of ciprofloxacin drops (3 mg/ml) every 30 min for 12 h reduced bacterial counts in the cornea to undetectable levels compared with counts of $3 \times 10^7$ CFU/g in untreated eyes (33). The strain was unusually susceptible to ciprofloxacin (MIC < 0.125 μg/ml). In a third study, application of enoxacin drops (5 mg/ml) twice daily to the eyes of rabbits with keratitis caused by an aminoglycoside-resistant strain of *P. aeruginosa* also reduced bacterial counts to undetectable levels by the sixth day of treatment (18). In a fourth study, ciprofloxacin (7.5 mg/ml) was significantly more effective than norfloxacin (10 mg/ml) and tobramycin (13.6 mg/ml) for the topical treatment of experimental keratitis caused by an aminoglycoside-resistant strain of *P. aeruginosa* (37).

These studies suggest that the topical application of concentrated solutions of quin-

**Table 3.** Penetration of ciprofloxacin into the human eye

| Dosage and route[a] | Procedure and no. of patients | Concn, $\mu$g/ml (% penetration) | | | Comments | Reference |
|---|---|---|---|---|---|---|
| | | Serum | Aqueous humor | Vitreous humor | | |
| 1 g p.o., 1 dose | Cataract extraction, 22 | 7.36 | 0.56 (7.6) | | | 19 |
| 750 mg p.o., 1 dose | Ocular surgery, 9 | 2.7 | 0.15 (6) | | Many of same data as in reference 26 (below) | 32 |
| 750 mg p.o., 2 doses | | 3.4 | 0.53 (16) | | | |
| 750 mg, 3 doses | | 3.8 | 0.69 (18) | | | |
| 200 mg i.v., 3 doses | Ocular surgery, 3 | 0.7–1.8 | | 0.16–0.29 (17.7) | % penetration calculated from midpoint values of ranges | 26 |
| 400 mg i.v., 1 dose | 4 | 0.9–3.8 | 0.28–0.59 (17.6) | 0.29 (12) | | |
| 400 mg i.v., 2 doses | 2 | 1.6–2.6 | | 0.33–0.55 (21) | | |
| 400 mg i.v., 3 doses | 2 | 1.6–2.5 | | 0.36–0.39 (18) | | |
| 600 mg i.v., 1 dose | 11 | 1.7–6.4 | 0.26–1.1 (17) | 0.13 (3.2) | Vitreous level surprisingly low | |
| 400 mg i.v., 1 dose | Cataract extraction or vitrectomy, 35 | Not stated | 0.24 | 0.4 | | 1 |
| 750 mg p.o., 1 dose | | | 0.16 | | | |
| 750 mg p.o., 2–8 doses | | | 0.80 | | | |
| 200 mg i.v., 1 dose | Cataract extraction, 16 | 1.76 | 0.165 (9.4) | | | 5 |
| 200 mg i.v., 2 doses | Cataract extraction, 25 | 1.4 | 0.21 (15) | | Serum concn inferred from graphs | 42 |
| 1,000 mg p.o., 1 dose | Cataract extraction, 30 | 2.2 | 0.73 (33) | | | 8 |
| 200 mg i.v., 1 dose | Lens implantation, 55 | | 0.136 (14–19) | | Serum concn not stated but % penetration given | 25 |
| 750 mg p.o., 1 dose | Vitreal surgery, 7 | 1.9 | | Mean, 0.17 (9) | Bioassay values 4 h after treatment | 27 |
| 750 mg p.o., 1 dose | 7 | 1.0 | | Mean, 0.2 (20) | Bioassay values 8 h after treatment | |
| 750 mg p.o., 2 doses | 7 | 2.27 | | Mean, 0.35 (15) | Bioassay values 12 h after last dose | |
| 500 mg p.o., 1 dose | Cataract extraction, 8 | 3.1 | 0.52 (17) | | | 45 |
| 1,000 mg p.o., 1 dose | 22 | 6.22 | 0.55 (9) | | | |
| 1,500 mg p.o., 1 dose | 21 | 9.4 | 0.65 (7) | | | |

[a]p.o., per os; i.v., intravenous.

**Table 4.** Penetration of quinolones other than ciprofloxacin into the human eye

| Drug | Dosage[a] | Procedure and no. of patients | Concn, μg/ml (% penetration) | | | Comments | Reference |
|---|---|---|---|---|---|---|---|
| | | | Serum | Aqueous humor | Vitreous humor | | |
| Pefloxacin | 400 mg p.o., 1 dose | Cataract extraction, 14 | 5.0 | 0.89 (18) | | Includes patients studied up to 5 h 30 min after dose | 10 |
| | 400 mg i.v., 1 dose | Cataract extraction, 20 | 6.0 | 1.45 (24) | | Values inferred from graphs | 39 |
| | 400 mg p.o., 6 doses | Cataract extraction, 13 | 15 | 7.5 (50) | | Values inferred from graphs | 29 |
| | 400 mg i.v., 1 dose | Ocular surgery, 27 | 5.2 | 0.8 (15) | 0.5 (10) | 9 patients had vitreal sample | 17 |
| | 800 mg i.v., 1 dose | 31 | 13.0 | 3.3 (25) | 4.0 (31) | 4 patients had vitreal sample | |
| Ofloxacin | 200 mg p.o., 1 dose | Cataract extraction, 30 | 3.0 | 0.6 (20) | | | 9 |
| | 400 mg p.o., 1 dose | Cataract extraction, 20 | 5.2 | 1.14 (22) | | | 29 |
| Norfloxacin | 800 mg p.o., 1 dose | Cataract extraction, 23 | 3.5 | 0.56 (16) | | Serum concn inferred from % penetration values | 11 |
| | 1,600 mg, 1 dose | 9 | 3.3 | 0.8 (24) | | | |

[a]p.o., per os; i.v., intravenous.

olones is effective in the treatment of *P. aeruginosa* keratitis, including infection caused by aminoglycoside-resistant strains. There is no evidence that the quinolones are superior to the aminoglycosides for infection caused by susceptible strains.

Recently, there has been interest in the use of antibiotic-impregnated collagen corneal shields, which act as slow-release devices, to deliver drugs in high concentration to the cornea. In rabbits infected with a tobramycin-resistant strain of *P. aeruginosa*, corneal shields impregnated with ciprofloxacin were more effective than shields impregnated with norfloxacin or tobramycin in reducing corneal counts of bacteria (21).

The bactericidal effect of ciprofloxacin in the vitreous humor was examined in a rabbit model of *P. aeruginosa* endophthalmitis (15). Injection of a high dosage of ciprofloxacin into the vitreous produced a marked bactericidal effect if the drug was given 24 h after infection but little effect if treatment was delayed until 48 h after infection. Similar results were found with imipenem and gentamicin.

## TREATMENT OF OCULAR INFECTIONS IN HUMANS

There have been few studies of the use of quinolones for the treatment of ocular infections in humans. One area of interest concerning these drugs is the treatment of bacterial conjunctivitis. Because this infection is usually self-limited, the main benefit of treatment is a modest reduction in the duration of symptoms. Jacobson et al. (24) compared norfloxacin with tobramycin, both applied topically at a concentration of 0.3% (3 mg/ml), for conjunctivitis. Treatment was given hourly while the patient was awake for the first day and then four times a day for 6 more days. There was no placebo group. Only about half of the infections yielded a bacterial pathogen. The most common isolates were *H. influenzae*, *S. pneumoniae*, alpha-hemolytic streptococci, *S. aureus*, and staphylococcal species. The clinical and bacteriological outcomes were similar in the two groups. No serious side effects of treatment were noted. Leibowitz reported the results of two multicenter studies of ciprofloxacin (3 mg/ml) given topically for bacteriologically proven conjunctivitis (30). In the first study, ciprofloxacin was compared with placebo, with each given for 3 days. Ciprofloxacin was significantly better than placebo in eradicating the infecting organisms ($P < 0.001$). In the second study, ciprofloxacin was compared with tobramycin (3 mg/ml), with each given for 7 days. The drugs were equally effective in eradicating the pathogens. Many treated patients were excluded from the analysis, most often because no bacterial pathogen was isolated. Adverse effects were not reported. The results of these trials suggest that norfloxacin and ciprofloxacin are as effective and safe as tobramycin for ordinary bacterial conjunctivitis.

In one study of patients in a long-term facility (7), an outbreak of purulent conjunctivitis was attributed to infection by methicillin-resistant strains of *S. aureus* (MRSA). Seven of eight patients treated orally with ciprofloxacin and eight of eight treated topically with vancomycin showed clinical resolution of the conjunctivitis. However, the precise role of the MRSA in the conjunctivitis is not clear, and most of the patients received other, potentially effective antibacterial treatments in addition to those noted above. In another study, two patients with keratitis caused by MRSA were successfully treated with topical applications of 3-mg/ml ciprofloxacin. In one patient, an apparent precipitate of the drug appeared on the surface of the cornea but disappeared when the frequency of applications was reduced from hourly to four times a day (23). Because of the widespread emergence of resistance, the quinolones are not favored for the treatment of colonization and infection by MRSA. Therefore, this approach would not be recommended except in selected circumstances.

Keratitis is a far more serious infection than conjunctivitis and may result in the permanent loss of vision. In a multicenter study of patients with culture-proven bacterial keratitis (31), treatment consisted of the frequent topical application of ciprofloxacin drops (3 mg/ml). The most common isolates were *S. epidermidis* and *S. aureus*, but a wide variety of pathogens was encountered. Ninety-two percent of patients were "cured or improved" at the end of treatment. Ciprofloxacin was highly active in vitro against all of the pathogens, and resistance did not emerge during treatment. Adverse effects were mild. The most common adverse effect, occurring in 17% of patients, was the formation of a white precipitate on the cornea. The precipitate sometimes disappeared during continued treatment and led to discontinuation of treatment in only one patient. Comparison groups consisted of patients seen in the same clinics but not enrolled during the study period or seen in the preceding year; they were given the standard treatment regimen of the clinic, usually the combination of "fortified" drops of cefazolin and an aminoglycoside. The results for the control groups were similar to those for the ciprofloxacin-treated patients. These data suggest that the commercially available form of ophthalmic ciprofloxacin, 0.3% (3 mg/ml), may be as effective in the treatment of bacterial keratitis as fortified drops of cefazolin and an aminoglycoside, which must be prepared extemporaneously in the pharmacy. However, a randomized, comparative study to further document this finding would be desirable.

Gonococcal keratoconjunctivitis is a potentially serious ocular infection that may produce corneal damage and, rarely, endophthalmitis. Interestingly, this is one of the bacterial infections of the external eye that is treated primarily by the systemic route. In one study (28), 15 men with gonococcal keratoconjunctivitis were treated with norfloxacin given orally. The first seven patients were treated with 1,200 mg daily for 3 days. Prompted by good results, the authors treated each of the next eight patients with a single dose of 1,200 mg. All patients showed arrest of the disease and eradication of the organisms following treatment. Given the frequency of penicillinase-producing isolates of gonococci, penicillins are probably not a good empiric choice for treating gonococcal ophthalmia. Current options include cefoxitin (1 g intravenously four times daily) or ceftriaxone (1 g intramuscularly once daily) for 5 days or spectinomycin 2 g intramuscularly daily for 3 days. However, on the basis of this small study, a single dose of norfloxacin may be a convenient alternative. Other fluoroquinolones, which produce higher concentrations in serum than norfloxacin, would presumably do as well as norfloxacin.

Good results in the treatment of a variety of external ocular infections were reported by Ooishi et al. (35) with ciprofloxacin given orally. However, the details of the study are scanty.

Although ocular side effects attributable to treatment with quinolones have been mild and infrequent, there is a report of visual scotomata due to bilateral macular bullae in three patients with chronic renal failure who were given flumequine, a quinolone, for urinary tract infection (16). Complete recovery occurred shortly after treatment was discontinued.

## CONCLUSIONS

The spectrum of the new quinolones is reasonably well suited to the treatment of bacterial infections of the eye except for limited activity against streptococci. After repeated topical application to the eyes of rabbits, appreciable concentrations were found in the cornea and aqueous humor, but, predictably, no drug was found in the vitreous humor. The concentrations in the cornea are in the range of those found with penicillins, gentamicin, tetracyclines, or erythromycin (2). As with other antibiotics, penetration of the quinolones is better when the cornea has been damaged. Most of the studies were done with solutions of 3 to 5 mg/ml; higher concentrations would be expected to produce higher ocular levels.

After systemic administration of the quinolones in rabbits and humans, penetration of the aqueous and vitreous humors of healthy eyes following a single dose is generally in the range of 10 to 20%, although some higher values have been reported. Whereas for most other antimicrobial drugs penetration into the aqueous humor is greater than that into the vitreous humor, the quinolones penetrate the two chambers to a similar extent. The vitreal penetration of the quinolones is better than that of ß-lactam drugs, aminoglycosides, and clindamycin given as a single dose (2). Repeated administration of the quinolones produces higher intraocular levels. There is no evidence of a substantial difference in ocular penetration among the congeners. Penetration of the infected eye has been examined only in one small study in rabbits and was found to be similar to the penetration of healthy eyes. In one report of intravitreally injected pefloxacin, the half-life was short and the drug appeared to be eliminated by the retinal route.

Studies of the intraocular penetration of the quinolones after subconjunctival injection in rabbits are limited; in one study, only a very small dosage of drug was used, and in another, a transiently high vitreal concentration was followed by a very low one.

In humans, topical treatment of ordinary bacterial conjunctivitis with norfloxacin or ciprofloxacin was as effective as treatment with tobramycin, even for pneumococcal infection. In rabbits, enoxacin and ciprofloxacin drops were effective for the treatment of pseudomonal keratitis, including infection by aminoglycoside-resistant strains. These data suggest that the quinolones are useful drugs for the topical treatment of infections of the conjunctiva and cornea. Nevertheless, there seems to be no reason to prefer a quinolone over an aminoglycoside for infections caused by aminoglycoside-susceptible organisms. Ciprofloxacin given topically has been reported to be effective for the treatment of conjunctivitis caused by MRSA, but the data are sparse; because of the tendency of these strains to become resistant to quinolones, this approach probably should not generally be recommended. In a nonrandomized study of patients with bacterial keratitis, a commercially available solution of ciprofloxacin was as effective as fortified drops of other antibiotics prepared extemporaneously; however, a randomized study would be desirable. A single dose of norfloxacin (1,200 mg) by mouth cured gonococcal keratoconjunctivitis in a small series of patients, suggesting that the quinolones may be particularly useful for this infection.

The fact that the quinolones penetrate the vitreous humor better than ß-lactams or aminoglycosides after systemic administration raises the possibility that the quinolones may be useful for the treatment of endophthalmitis, especially infections caused by gram-negative bacilli. However, I suggest that the initial empiric treatment of bacterial endophthalmitis should continue to be by direct intravitreal injection of agents such as vancomycin and an aminoglycoside in order to produce immediately high vitreal levels of drugs active against all likely pathogens. The quinolones could be of value as an adjunct to intravitreal injection when vitreal cultures show a susceptible gram-negative organism. When agents with greater activity against gram-positive cocci are available, the consideration of use could be extended to gram-positive coccal infections. Data are too limited to justify speculation about the potential utility of the drugs by periocular administration.

## ADDENDUM

Since this chapter was prepared, several relevant studies on the use of fluoroquinolones for treatment have been reported. In a rabbit model of *P. aeruginosa* keratitis, topical treatments for 12 h with drops of ofloxacin (0.3%) or tobramycin (0.3%) were of similar efficacy in reducing colony counts in the cornea. After 7 days, all treated corneas were sterile, and healing occurred at comparable rates with the two drugs (20a).

In a multicenter, randomized, double-masked study of patients with external ocular infection, ofloxacin (0.3% drops) was similar to tobramycin (0.3% drops) in efficacy and tolerance. There was a more rapid reduction in signs and symptoms with ofloxacin than with tobramycin (20b).

In another multicenter, randomized, double-masked study of patients with external ocular infections, norfloxacin (0.3% drops) was similar to gentamicin (0.3% drops) in efficacy and tolerance (32a).

The intravitreal penetration of ciprofloxacin after a single oral administration of 750 mg in 19 patients about to undergo elective vitreous surgery was reported (17a). Peak concentrations in serum were in the range of 2 to 3 μg/ml. A polynomial regression line showed the peak vitreal concentration, which was reached about 10 h after treatment, to be 0.4 μg/ml. There was no significant difference in penetration in diabetic and nondiabetic patients.

## REFERENCES

1. **Adenis, J. P., F. Dennis, and M. Mounier.** 1987. Ciprofloxacin levels in human eye after oral and intravenous administration, abstr. 1078. *Program Abstr. 27th Intersci. Conf. Antimicrob. Agents Chemother.*
2. **Barza, M.** 1989. Antibacterial agents in the treatment of ocular infections. *Infect. Dis. Clin. North Am.* **3:**533–551.
3. **Barza, M.** 1993. Anatomical barriers for antimicrobial agents. *Eur. J. Clin. Microbiol. Infect. Dis.* **12**(Suppl. 1)**:**S31–S35.
4. **Barza, M., A. Kane, and J. Baum.** 1979. Marked differences between pigmented and albino rabbits in the concentration of clindamycin in iris and choroid-retina. *J. Infect. Dis.* **139:**203–208.
5. **Behrens-Baumann, W., and J. Martell.** 1987. Ciprofloxacin concentrations in human aqueous humor following intravenous administration. *Chemotherapy* (Basel) **33:**328–330.

6. **Behrens-Baumann, W., and J. Martell.** 1988. Ciprofloxacin concentration in the rabbit aqueous humor and vitreous following intravenous and subconjunctival administration. *Infection* **16:**54–57.
7. **Brennen, C., and R. R. Muder.** 1990. Conjunctivitis associated with methicillin-resistant *Staphylococcus aureus* in a long-term-care facility. *Am. J. Med.* **88**(Suppl. 5):14N–17N.
8. **Bron, A., D. Talon, T. Cellier, J. M. Estavoyer, B. Delbosc, and J. Royer.** 1989. La penetration intra-camerulaire de la ciprofloxacin chez l'homme. *Pathol. Biol.* **37:**730–733.
9. **Bron, A., D. Talon, B. Delbosc, J. M. Estavoyer, G. Kaya, and J. Royer.** 1987. La penetration intracamerulaire de l'ofloxacine chez l'homme. *J. Fr. Ophtalmol.* **10:**443–446.
10. **Bron, A., D. Talon, B. Delbosc, J. M. Estavoyer, F. Prost, and M. Montard.** 1986. La penetration intracamerulaire de la pefloxacine chez l'homme. *J. Fr. Ophtalmol.* **9:**317–321.
11. **Bron, A., D. Talon, J. M. Estavoyer, T. Cellier, B. Delbosc, and M. Montard.** 1989. Ocular distribution of the new quinolones. *Rev. Infect. Dis.* **11**(Suppl. 5):S1206–S1207.
12. **Bywater, M. J., H. A. Holt, and D. S. Reeves.** 1988. In vitro activity of norfloxacin in comparison with 11 topical antimicrobial agents against 142 potential ocular pathogens. *Rev. Infect. Dis.* **10**(Suppl. 1):S248–S250.
13. **Cochereau-Massin, I., J. Bauchet, F. Faurisson, J. M. Vallois, P. Lacombe, and J. J. Pocidalo.** 1991. Ocular kinetics of pefloxacin after intramuscular administration in albino and pigmented rabbits. *Antimicrob. Agents Chemother.* **35:**1112–1115.
14. **Cochereau-Massin, I., J. Bauchet, F. Faurisson, J. M. Vallois, and J. J. Pocidalo.** 1989. Ocular kinetics of pefloxacin in rabbits. *Rev. Infect. Dis.* **11**(Suppl. 5):S1063–1064.
15. **Davey, P. G., M. Barza, and M. Stuart.** 1987. Dose response of experimental pseudomonas endophthalmitis to ciprofloxacin, gentamicin, and imipenem: evidence for resistance to "late" treatment of infections. *J. Infect. Dis.* **155:**518–523.
16. **de Ligny, B. H., D. Sirbat, M. Kessler, P. Trechot, and J. Chaniliau.** 1984. Effets secondaires oculaires de la flumequine. *Therapie* **39:**595–600.
17. **Denis, F., M. Mounier, and J. P. Adenis.** 1987. Etude du passage intra-oculaire de la pefloxacine chez l'homme et le lapin. *Pathol. Biol.* **35:**772–776.
17a. **El Baba, F. Z., M. D. Trousdale, W. J. Gauderman, D. G. Wagner, and P. E. Liggett.** 1992. Intravitreal penetration of oral ciprofloxacin in humans. *Ophthalmology* **99:**483–486.
18. **Esposito, S., H. Thadepalli, H. A. Benler, and S. K. Chuah.** 1991. Enoxacin therapy for experimental pseudomonas keratitis. *J. Chemother.* **3:**147–151.
19. **Fern, A. I., G. Sweeney, M. Doig, and G. Lindsay.** 1986. Penetration of ciprofloxacin into aqueous humor. *Trans. Ophthalmol. Soc. UK* **105:**650–652.
20. **Goldstein, E. J. G., D. M. Citron, L. Bendon, A. E. Vagvolgyi, M. D. Trousdale, and M. D. Appleman.** 1987. Potential of topical norfloxacin therapy. *Arch. Ophthalmol.* **105:**991–994.
20a. **Gritz, D. C., P. J. McDonnell, T. Y. Lee, D. Tang-Lui, B. B. Hubbard, and A. Gwon.** 1992. Topical ofloxacin in the treatment of Pseudomonas keratitis in a rabbit model. *Cornea* **11:**143–147.
20b. **Gwon, A.** 1992. Ofloxacin vs tobramycin for the treatment of external ocular infection. Ofloxacin Study Group II. *Arch. Ophthalmol.* **110:**1234–1237.
21. **Hobden, J. A., J. J. Reidy, R. J. O'Callaghan, M. S. Insler, and J. M. Hill.** 1990. Quinolones in collagen shields to treat aminoglycoside-resistant pseudomonal keratitis. *Invest. Ophthalmol. Vis. Sci.* **31:**2241–2243.
22. **Hulem, C. D., S. E. Old, L. D. Zeleznick, and I. H. Leopold.** 1982. Intraocular penetration of rosoxacin in rabbits. *Arch. Ophthalmol.* **100:**646–649.
23. **Insler, M. S., L. A. Fish, J. Silbernagel, J. A. Hobden, R. J. O'Callaghan, and J. M. Hill.** 1991. Successful treatment of methicillin-resistant *Staphylococcus aureus* keratitis with topical ciprofloxacin. *Ophthalmology* **98:**1690–1692.
24. **Jacobson, J. A., N. B. Call, E. M. Kasworm, M. S. Dirks, and R. B. Turner.** 1988. Safety and efficacy of topical norfloxacin versus tobramycin in the treatment of external ocular infections. *Antimicrob. Agents Chemother.* **32:**1820–2824.
25. **Janert, H., B. Schull, and H. P. Geisen.** 1989. Concentrations of ciprofloxacin in aqueous humor following intravenous and oral administration. *Rev. Infect. Dis.* **11**(Suppl. 5):S1077.
26. **Joos, B., F. Gassmann, and R. Luthy.** 1986. Penetration of ciprofloxacin into the human eye, abstr. 475. *Program Abstr. 26th Intersci. Conf. Antimicrob. Agents Chemother.*
27. **Keren, G., A. Alhalel, E. Bartov, R. Kitzes-Cohen, E. Rubinstein, S. Segev, and G. Treister.** 1991. The intravitreal penetration of orally administered ciprofloxacin in humans. *Invest. Ophthalmol. Vis. Sci.* **32:**2388–2392.
28. **Kestelyn, P., J. Bogaerts, A. M. Stevens, P. Piot, and A. Meheus.** 1989. Treatment of adult gonococcal keratoconjunctivitis with oral norfloxacin. *Am. J. Ophthalmol.* **108:**515–523.
29. **Lafaix, C., A. Salvanet, A. Fisch, F. Forestier, G. Montay, and A. Meulemans.** 1987. Diffusion des fluoroquinolones dans l'humeur aqueuse et le cristallin. *Pathol. Biol.* **35:**768–771.
30. **Leibowitz, H. M.** 1991. Antibacterial effectiveness of ciprofloxacin 0.3% ophthalmic solution in

the treatment of bacterial conjunctivitis. *Am. J. Ophthalmol.* **112:**29S–33S.

31. **Leibowitz, H. M.** 1991. Clinical evaluation of ciprofloxacin 0.3% ophthalmic solution for treatment of bacterial keratitis. *Am. J. Ophthalmol.* **112:**34S–47S.
32. **Luthy, R., B. Joos, and F. Gassmann.** 1986. Penetration of ciprofloxacin into the human eye, p. 192–196. *In* H. C. Neu and H. Weuta (ed.), *First International Ciprofloxacin Workshop.* Excerpta Medica, Amsterdam.

32a. **Miller, I., R. Vogel, T. J. Cook, J. Wittreich, and the Worldwide Norfloxacin Ophthalmic Study Group.** 1992. Topically administered norfloxacin compared with topically administered gentamicin for the treatment of external ocular bacterial infections. *Am. J. Ophthalmol.* **113:**638–644.

33. **O'Brien, T. P., M. R. Sawusch, J. D. Dick, and J. D. Gottsch.** 1988. Topical ciprofloxacin treatment of *Pseudomonas* keratitis in rabbits. *Arch. Ophthalmol.* **106:**1444–1446.
34. **Ooishi, M., and M. Miyao.** 1990. Ocular pharmacokinetic studies on AT-4140, abstr. 1258. *Program Abstr. 30th Intersci. Conf. Antimicrob. Agents Chemother.*
35. **Ooishi, M., F., Sakaue, A. Oonomo, and K. Yoneyama.** 1985. Fundamental and clinical studies on BAY o 9867 in ophthalmology. *Chemotherapy* (Tokyo) **33:**1014–1021.
36. **Osato, M. S., H. G. Jensen, M. D. Trousdale, J. A. Bosso, L. R. Borrmann, J. Frank, and P. Akers.** 1989. The comparative in vitro activity of ofloxacin and selected ophthalmic antimicrobial agents against ocular bacterial isolates. *Am. J. Ophthalmol.* **108:**380–386.
37. **Reidy, J. J., J. A. Hobden, J. M. Hill, K. Forman, and R. J. O'Callaghan.** 1991. The efficacy of topical ciprofloxacin and norfloxacin in the treatment of experimental *Pseudomonas* keratitis. *Cornea* **10:**25–28.
38. **Richman, J., H. Zolezio, and D. Tang-Liu.** 1990. Comparison of ofloxacin, gentamicin, and tobramycin concentrations in tears and in vitro MICs for 90% of test organisms. *Antimicrob. Agents Chemother.* **34:**1602–1604.
39. **Salvanet, A., A. Fisch, C. Lafaix, G. Montay, P. Dubayle, F. Forestier, and G. Haroche.** 1986. Pefloxacin concentrations in human aqueous humour and lens. *J. Antimicrob. Chemother.* **18:**199–201.
40. **Shiba, K., A. Saito, J. Shimada, S. Hori, M. Kaji, T. Miyahara, H. Kusajima, S. Kaneko, S. Saito, T. Ooie, and H. Uchida.** 1990. Renal handling of fleroxacin in rabbits, dogs, and humans. *Antimicrob. Agents Chemother.* **34:**58–64.
41. **Shungu, D. L., V. K. Tutlane, E. Weinberg, and H. H. Gadebusch.** 1985. In vitro antibacterial activity of norfloxacin and other agents against ocular pathogens. *Chemotherapy* (Basel) **31:**112–118.
42. **Skoutelis, A. T., S. P. Gartaganis, C. J. Chrysanthopoulos, D. Beermann, C. Papachristou, and H. P. Bassaris.** 1988. Aqueous humor penetration of ciprofloxacin in the human eye. *Arch. Ophthalmol.* **106:**404–405.
43. **Stevens, S. X., B. D. Fouraker, and H. G. Jensen.** 1991. Intraocular safety of ciprofloxacin. *Arch. Ophthalmol.* **109:**1737–1743.
44. **Sugar, A., M. A. Cohen, P. A. Bien, T. J. Griffin, C. L. Heifetz, and S. Mehta.** 1986. Treatment of experimental *Pseudomonas* corneal ulcers with enoxacin, a quinolone antibiotic. *Arch. Ophthalmol.* **104:**1230–1232.
45. **Sweeney, G., A. I. Fern, G. Lindsay, and M. W. Doig.** 1990. Penetration of ciprofloxacin into the aqueous humour of the uninflamed human eye after oral administration. *J. Antimicrob. Chemother.* **26:**99–105.

*Quinolone Antimicrobial Agents, 2nd ed.*
Edited by David C. Hooper and John S. Wolfson


*Chapter 24*

# Use of Quinolone Antimicrobial Agents in Immunocompromised Patients

***Drew J. Winston***

The profile of the fluoroquinolones includes certain antibacterial, pharmacokinetic, and safety features that may be advantageous for the prevention and treatment of infections in immunocompromised patients. These favorable properties have been the basis for an increasing number of laboratory and clinical studies devoted to the use of the fluoroquinolones in immunocompromised patients. This chapter reviews these studies and the current status of the quinolones in relation to the present epidemiology of infections in immunocompromised hosts and the prevention and treatment of these infections with alternative agents.

## PREVENTION OF INFECTIONS IN GRANULOCYTOPENIC PATIENTS

Infections are frequent and almost inevitable complications in severely granulocytopenic patients. Both the level of circulating granulocytes and the duration of granulocytopenia are important. The incidence of infection increases as the granulocyte count falls below 500 cells per $mm^3$ (11). Most serious infections, including nearly all bacteremias, occur when the granulocyte count is less than 100 cells per $mm^3$ (156). Patients who remain granulocytopenic for a prolonged period (>14 days) are also more likely to develop infections. Bacterial organisms causing infections usually arise from the gastrointestinal tract of the patient. These organisms may be part of the endogenous alimentary tract flora of the patient or may be acquired from environmental sources (158).

One approach to the prevention of bacterial infections in granulocytopenic patients is the use of prophylactic oral antimicrobial agents (155). These drugs are designed not only to suppress the endogenous gastrointestinal flora of the patient but also to prevent colonization with potential pathogens from the environment. Initial prophylactic regimens consisted primarily of oral nonabsorbable antibiotics given alone or in conjunction with a protective environment (laminar airflow or a similar isolation) (45, 105, 111, 148, 157, 166, 200). Common regimens were gentamicin, vancomycin, and nystatin; polymyxin, vancomycin, and nystatin; framycetin, colistin, and nystatin; and neomycin, colistin, and nystatin. These oral nonabsorbable antibiotics suppress the microbial flora of the gastrointestinal tract but usually do not completely sterilize it. Several prospective, randomized controlled trials have shown that prophylactic oral nonabsorbable antibiotics decrease the incidence of infection in granu-

***Drew J. Winston*** • University of California Los Angeles Medical Center, Los Angeles, California 90024.

locytopenic patients (105, 157, 166), whereas other studies have not shown this (45, 111, 200). One of the reasons for this disagreement is the variable compliance of patients for oral nonabsorbable antibiotics. These agents cause frequent nausea, vomiting, and diarrhea. They are also expensive and may be associated with the rapid acquisition of organisms after prophylaxis is discontinued (155, 157). Consequently, oral nonabsorbable antibiotics have generally been unpopular with most patients and many physicians.

Another approach to oral chemoprophylaxis is selective decontamination of the gastrointestinal tract. A series of studies by Van der Waaij and colleagues demonstrated that *Escherichia coli, Pseudomonas aeruginosa,* and *Klebsiella pneumoniae* could colonize the alimentary canals of germfree animals when only 100 organisms were given orally (179). In contrast, normal conventional animals required oral inoculation with $10^7$ or more organisms for the gastrointestinal tract to be colonized. This capacity of the normal microbial flora of the alimentary canal to prevent colonization with new organisms was termed "colonization resistance." When these same workers suppressed the aerobic floras of healthy animals with antibiotics while the anaerobic floras persisted, colonization resistance was maintained. An oral inoculation of $10^6$ organisms was still needed to cause colonization. These findings suggested that the normal anaerobic gastrointestinal flora was responsible for preventing colonization with aerobic gram-negative bacilli, perhaps by successfully competing for nutrients in the gut (74). On the basis of these results, drugs such as trimethoprim-sulfamethoxazole and nalidixic acid, which are capable of reducing the aerobic bacterial flora of the gastrointestinal tract without suppressing the anaerobic flora, have been used for selective decontamination.

The results of studies in which either trimethoprim-sulfamethoxazole or nalidixic acid has been used for prophylaxis in granulocytopenic patients have been conflicting. Many controlled trials showed a decrease in infections in patients given prophylactic trimethoprim-sulfamethoxazole or nalidixic acid (37, 68, 75, 76, 160, 182, 185), while others found no benefit (57, 187). Moreover, certain risks are associated with the use of these agents. Trimethoprim-sulfamethoxazole may cause untoward skin rashes and may prolong the period of granulocytopenia by suppressing myelopoiesis (37, 181). Neither trimethoprim-sulfamethoxazole nor nalidixic acid is active against *P. aeruginosa.* Selection of resistant gram-negative bacilli and superinfection with fungi such as *Candida* spp. and *Aspergillus* spp. may also occur during prophylaxis (68, 181, 189). In two separate studies in which trimethoprim-sulfamethoxazole was compared with nalidixic acid, trimethoprim-sulfamethoxazole was found to be superior to nalidixic acid (13, 181). More patients receiving nalidixic acid experienced colonization and infection with gram-negative bacilli. Many of these gram-negative bacilli were resistance to nalidixic acid. These conflicting results and the risk of adverse effects and superinfections have continued to make the prophylactic use of trimethoprim-sulfamethoxazole or nalidixic acid in granulocytopenic patients controversial.

The limitations of oral nonabsorbable antibiotics, trimethoprim-sulfamethoxazole, and nalidixic acid for the prophylaxis of infection have been the impetus for evaluating the fluoroquinolones in granulocytopenic patients. The fluoroquinolones have several favorable properties that may overcome some of the limitations of other agents. The fluoroquinolones have excellent activity against members of the family *Enterobacteriaceae* and inhibit more than 90% of isolates at concentrations of 2 μg/ml or less (84, 197). *P. aeruginosa* isolates are intrinsically resistant to trimethoprim-sulfamethoxazole and nalidixic acid but are susceptible to the fluoroquinolones at concentrations of 2 to 6 μg/ml. Staphylococci are also well inhibited (MIC for 90% of isolates, 1.0 to 6 μg/ml), while streptococci are less susceptible (MIC for 90% of isolates, 2 to 32 μg/ml). On the other hand, the fluoroquinolones have relatively little activity against anaerobic bacteria. In healthy volunteers, high concentrations of the fluoroquinolones (100 to 2,000 μg/g of stool) are achieved in the stool after oral administration and are associated with suppression of the aerobic gram-negative bowel flora with preservation of the anaerobes (19, 30, 53, 84, 93, 129, 139, 140, 146). Similar studies with granulocytopenic patients have shown a reduction of the enteric aerobic gram-negative flora by orally administered fluoroquinolones without a significant change in the anaerobic population (70, 96, 151). Thus, these drugs should maintain colonization resistance. Finally, the fluoroquinolones are not associated with the plasmid-mediated resistance or myelosuppression observed with trimethoprim-sulfamethoxazole (84, 197).

Table 1 compares the effects of the oral fluoroquinolones (norfloxacin, ciprofloxacin, and ofloxacin) with those of a placebo, trimethoprim-sulfamethoxazole, or vancomycin plus polymyxin on the acquisition of gram-negative bacillary organisms during a series of clinical trials of chemoprophylaxis in granulocytopenic patients (12, 39, 96, 102, 194, 196). In each trial, the fluoroquinolone prevented the acquisition of *Enterobacteriaceae* and *P. aeruginosa* and was more effective than the control regimen of a placebo, trimethoprim-sulfamethoxazole, or vancomycin plus polymyxin. Only colonization with non-*P. aeruginosa Pseudomonas* strains or *Acinetobacter* species occurred to a significant degree in the patients receiving the fluoroquinolones, but these organisms rarely caused infection. Some of the non-*P. aeruginosa Pseudomonas* and *Acinetobacter* organisms were resistant to the fluoroquinolones. Otherwise, the acquisition of resistant gram-negative bacilli occurred very infrequently.

The results of different controlled studies in which the efficacies of the fluoroquinolones in the prevention of infection in granulocytopenic patients were evaluated are shown in Table 2. Norfloxacin (six trials) (12, 32, 96, 135, 195, 196), ciprofloxacin (three trials) (39, 119, 130a), ofloxacin (five trials) (72, 79, 102, 113, 194), pefloxacin (two trials) (1, 71), and enoxacin (one trial) (168) have each been evaluated in one or more studies and compared with placebo, trimethoprim-sulfamethoxazole, or oral nonabsorbable antibiotics. Except for one study of ofloxacin prophylaxis in solid-tumor patients (79), the patients in these trials were either receiving conventional chemotherapy for a hematologic malignancy (usually acute leukemia) or having a bone marrow transplant. More than 1,500 patients were enrolled in these studies. Except for a study by Bow et al. comparing norfloxacin with trimethoprim-sulfamethoxazole (12) and a trial by Maschmeyer et al. comparing ciprofloxacin with trimethoprim-sulfamethoxazole plus colistin (119), patients receiving prophylaxis with an oral fluoroquinolone had fewer microbiologically documented infections than did control patients. The overall incidence of microbiologically documented infections was 40% (314 in 774 patients) in the quinolone groups versus 59% (446 in 754 patients) in the control groups. The fluoroquinolones were especially effective in the prevention of gram-negative bacteremia. Twenty-one cases of gram-negative bacteremia occurred in 654 patients (3%) on quinolone prophylaxis compared with 112 cases in 638 control patients (18%). Gram-negative bacteremias reported in patients receiving fluoroquinolones for prophylaxis were usually caused by either *P. aeruginosa* or other *Pseudomonas* species resistant to the quinolones (1, 32, 102, 113). On the other hand, the number of gram-positive bacteremias was similar in the quinolone groups (114 in 590 patients [19%]) and the control groups (145 in 574 patients [25%]). In studies using norfloxacin for prophylaxis, the incidence of gram-positive bacteremia was actually greater in patients receiving norfloxacin (19%) than in patients receiving placebo, trimethoprim-sulfamethoxazole, or oral

**Table 1.** Acquisition of gram-negative bacilli in surveillance cultures of granulocytopenic patients receiving oral antimicrobial prophylaxis

| Organism | No. of patients acquiring gram-negative bacilli[a] | | | |
|---|---|---|---|---|
| | Karp et al. (96) | | Bow et al. (12) | |
| | Placebo ($n$ = 33) | Norfloxacin ($n$ = 35) | Trimethoprim-sulfamethoxazole ($n$ = 28) | Norfloxacin ($n$ = 30) |
| *E. coli* | 8 | 0 | 12 | 5 |
| *Klebsiella-Enterobacter-Serratia* spp. | 14 | 0 | 11 | 3 |
| *Proteus* spp. | 0 | 0 | 2 | 0 |
| *Citrobacter* spp. | 1 | 0 | 4 | 1 |
| *Providencia* spp. | 0 | 0 | 0 | 0 |
| *P. aeruginosa* | 6 | 0 | 9 | 0 |
| Non-*P. aeruginosa Pseudomonas* spp. | 4 | 2 (2) | 3 | 0 |
| *Actinobacter* spp. | 0 | 0 | 1 | 2 |
| Others | 0 | 0 | 0 | 0 |

[a]Numbers in parentheses are numbers of isolates resistant to the fluoroquinolone.

nonabsorbable antibiotics (9%) (Table 2). This increased incidence of gram-positive bacteremia was not observed in the studies using ciprofloxacin, pefloxacin, or enoxacin. The predominant gram-positive organisms causing bacteremia were viridans group streptococci and coagulase-negative staphylococci resistant to the quinolones (1, 12, 39, 96, 102, 168, 194–196). The lack of efficacy of the fluoroquinolones for the prevention of gram-positive infections correlated with a failure of these agents to eradicate colonizing gram-positive organisms (12, 71, 151, 194, 196). Infections with gram-positive bacteria, however, appear to be better tolerated by granulocytopenic patients and generally have a lower mortality rate than gram-negative infections. There was no increased number of fungal infections associated with the prophylactic use of the fluoroquinolones.

Table 3 summarizes the results of controlled trials in which two different oral fluoroquinolones were compared for prophylaxis of infections in granulocytopenic patients. The largest trial was a multicenter study comparing norfloxacin with ciprofloxacin by the Gruppo Italiano Malattie Ematologiche Maligne dell' Adulto Program in Italy (170). This trial found that patients receiving ciprofloxacin had less fever, required fewer antibiotics, and had a lower rate of microbiologically documented infections, particularly of gram-negative bacteremias. Similar results favoring ciprofloxacin or ofloxacin over norfloxacin for prophylaxis of infection were obtained in two other European trials reported by Maschemeyer et al. (120) and D'Antonio et al. (33). These results in Europe are dissimilar to the more favorable results of using routine norfloxacin prophylaxis in granulocytopenic patients at Johns Hopkins, University of California Los Angeles (UCLA), and other oncology centers in the United States (Table 4) (38a, 95, 191). Only four gram-negative infections occurred in 111 consecutive patients (3.6%) receiving routine norfloxacin prophylaxis at Johns Hopkins (95), and only three gram-negative bacteremias developed in 205 consecutive patients (1.5%) receiving routine norfloxacin prophylaxis at UCLA (191). Finally, Arning et al. found no significant difference between ciprofloxacin, ofloxacin, and trimethoprim-sulfamethoxazole plus colistin for prevention of infection (2) (Table 3). There were no gram-negative infections in the quinolone

**Table 1.** *Continued*

| No. of patients acquiring gram-negative bacilli[a] | | | | | | | |
|---|---|---|---|---|---|---|---|
| Winston et al. (196) | | Dekker et al. (39) | | Kern and Kurrle (102) | | Winston et al. (194) | |
| Vancomycin + polymyxin ($n = 30$) | Norfloxacin ($n = 36$) | Trimethoprim-sulfamethoxazole + colistin ($n = 28$) | Ciprofloxacin ($n = 28$) | Trimethoprim-sulfamethoxazole ($n = 58$) | Ofloxacin ($n = 70$) | Vancomycin + polymyxin ($n = 32$) | Ofloxacin ($n = 30$) |
| 0 | 0 | 12 | 0 | 52 | 2 | 0 | 0 |
| 19 | 5 | | | 36 | 7 (2) | 17 | 1 (1) |
| 11 | 1 | 0 | 0 | 0 | 0 | 13 | 0 |
| 1 | 2 | 0 | 0 | 0 | 4 (4) | 4 | 0 |
| 3 | 0 | 0 | 0 | 0 | 0 | 2 | 0 |
| 5 | 1 | 5 | 0 | 8 | 2 (1) | 5 | 0 |
| 10 | 17 (2) | 4 | 4 (4) | 17 | 19 (10) | 0 | 3 (2) |
| 1 | 3 | 6 | 4 (4) | 11 | 18 (16) | 1 | 0 |
| 6 | 3 | 0 | 0 | 7 | 9 | 2 | 0 |

groups compared with one *P. aeruginosa* infection in the trimethoprim-sulfamethoxazole plus colistin group. Both quinolones were better tolerated than trimethoprim-sulfamethoxazole plus colistin, which caused more frequent gastrointestinal intolerance and skin reactions.

Chemoprophylaxis with the fluoroquinolones in granulocytopenic patients was well tolerated (Table 5) (1, 12, 32, 39, 96, 102, 113, 135, 168, 194–196). Compliance was generally better for norfloxacin, ciprofloxacin, or ofloxacin than for trimethoprim-sulfamethoxazole or oral nonabsorbable antibiotics. Gastrointestinal adverse effects were more common in patients given trimethoprim-sulfamethoxazole or oral nonabsorbable antibiotics and occurred less frequently in patients receiving the fluoroquinolones. Skin rashes developed in approximately 10% of the patients on trimethoprim-sulfamethoxazole but, except for four patients given pefloxacin or enoxacin, were uncommon in the patients on the quinolones. Neurological adverse effects were also uncommon and were observed in only three patients who received ofloxacin. Myelosuppression was infrequent in all study groups (three cases with trimethoprim-sulfamethoxazole and none with the quinolones). In the study by Winston et al. of ofloxacin prophylaxis (194), the median duration of severe granulocytopenia (less than 100 cells per $mm^3$) was significantly greater in patients given ofloxacin than in patients receiving vancomycin plus polymyxin (20 versus 12 days). Nevertheless, the other trials of quinolone prophylaxis were not associated with an increased duration of profound granulocytopenia. In vitro, neither ofloxacin nor pefloxacin inhibits myeloid precursor cells except at very high concentrations (137, 141; see also chapter 28). Ciprofloxacin and pefloxacin suppress bone marrow engraftment in mice only at concentrations far beyond the normal therapeutic range (161, 162). Studies of a potential interaction between the fluoroquinolones and cyclosporine in transplant patients have produced conflicting results (55, 92, 110, 130, 147, 169, 171, 175), but most suggest no significant interaction or alteration of cyclosporine blood levels (92, 110, 147, 169, 175; see also chapter 11).

A concern about the use of antimicrobial agents such as the fluoroquinolones for prophylaxis is the emergence of quinolone-

**Table 2.** Controlled trials comparing oral fluoroquinolones with placebo, trimethoprim-sulfamethoxazole, or oral nonabsorbable antibiotics for prophylaxis of infections in granulocytopenic patients

| Drug and reference | Regimen | Dose[a] | Underlying disease | No. of patients | No. (%) of patients with: Microbiologically documented infection | Gram-negative bacteremia | Gram-positive bacteremia | Disseminated fungal infection | Fatal infection |
|---|---|---|---|---|---|---|---|---|---|
| Norfloxacin | | | | | | | | | |
| Karp et al. (96) | Norfloxacin | 400 mg q12h | Acute leukemia and marrow transplant | 35 | 20 (57) | 4 (12) | 4 (12) | 6 (18) | 6 (18) |
| | Placebo | Placebo | | 33 | 26 (79) | 11 (33) | 3 (9) | 5 (15) | 3 (9) |
| Winston et al. (195) | Norfloxacin | 400 mg q8h | Hematologic malignancy | 26 | 10 (38) | 0 (1) | 5 (19) | 2 (8) | |
| | Trimethoprim-sulfamethoxazole | 160mg–800 mg q8h | | 28 | 14 (50) | 1 (4) | 4 (14) | 1 (4) | |
| Bow et al. (12) | Norfloxacin | 400 mg q12h | Acute leukemia | 31 | 10 (32) | 0 (0) | 9 (29) | 0 (0) | |
| | Trimethoprim-sulfamethoxazole | 160 mg–800 mg q12h | | 32 | 8 (25) | 3 (9) | 2 (6) | 2 (6) | |
| Cruciani et al. (32) | Norfloxacin | 20 mg/kg q12h | Hematologic malignancy in children | 21 | 4 (19) | 1 (5) | 3 (14) | 0 (0) | 1 (5) |
| | Trimethoprim-sulfamethoxazole | 15 mg/kg q12h | | 23 | 6 (23) | 3 (13) | 1 (4) | 1 (4) | 1 (4) |
| Orlandi et al. (135) | Norfloxacin | 400 mg q12h | Acute leukemia | 29 | 11 (38) | 6 (21) | 4 (14) | 2 (7) | 2 (7) |
| | Trimethoprim-sulfamethoxazole | 160 mg–800 mg q12h | | 30 | 16 (53) | 7 (23) | 1 (3) | 2 (7) | 3 (10) |
| Winston et al. (196) | Norfloxacin | 400 mg q8h | Hematologic malignancy | 36 | 12 (33) | 0 (0) | 9 (25) | 3 (8) | 3 (8) |
| | Vancomycin-polymyxin | 500 mg–100 mg q8h | | 30 | 16 (53) | 5 (17) | 4 (13) | 6 (20) | 4 (13) |
| Total | | | | | | | | | |
| Norfloxacin | | | | 178 | 67 (38) | 11 (6) | 34 (19) | 13 (7) | |
| Controls | | | | 176 | 86 (49) | 30 (18) | 15 (9) | 17 (10) | |

| | | | | | | | | | |
|---|---|---|---|---|---|---|---|---|---|
| **Ciprofloxacin** | | | | | | | | | |
| Dekker et al. (39) | Ciprofloxacin | 500 mg q12h | Acute leukemia | 28 | 5 (18) | 0 (0) | 3 (11) | 0 (0) | 0 (0) |
| | Trimethoprim-sulfamethoxazole + colistin | 160 mg–800 mg + 200 mg q8h | | 28 | 14 (50) | 5 (18) | 6 (21) | 0 (0) | 1 (4) |
| Maschmeyer et al. (119) | Ciprofloxacin | 500 mg q12h | Acute leukemia | 120 | 66 (55) | | | | 8 (7) |
| | Trimethoprim-sulfamethoxazole + colistin | 160 mg–800 mg + 200 mg q8h | | 116 | 46 (40) | | | | 2 (2) |
| Nazareth et al. (130a) | Ciprofloxacin + colistin | 500 mg + $10^6$ U q12h | Hematologic malignancy and marrow transplant | 64 | 15 (23) | 2 (3) | | | |
| | Neomycin + colistin | 500 mg + $10^6$ U q12h | | 64 | 41 (64) | 17 (26) | | | |
| Total | | | | | | | | | |
| Ciprofloxacin | | | | 212 | 86 (40) | 2/92 (2) | 3/28 (11) | 0/28 (0) | |
| Controls | | | | 208 | 101 (49) | 22/92 (24) | 6/28 (21) | 0/28 (0) | |
| **Ofloxacin** | | | | | | | | | |
| Hartlapp (79) | Ofloxacin | 200 mg q12h | Solid tumors | 42 | 0 (0) | 0 (0) | 0 (0) | 0 (0) | 0 (0) |
| | None | None | | 42 | 7 (17) | 2 (5) | 2 (5) | 0 (0) | 0 (0) |
| Liang et al. (113) | Ofloxacin | 300 mg q12h | Hematologic malignancy | 50 | 6 (12) | 1 (2) | 0 (0) | 2 (4) | 2 (4) |
| | Trimethoprim-sulfamethoxazole | 160 mg–800 mg q12h | | 52 | 13 (25) | 9 (17) | 0 (0) | 1 (2) | 4 (8) |
| Kern and Kurrle (102) | Ofloxacin | 200 mg q12h | Acute leukemia | 70 | 36 (51) | 1 (1) | 13 (19) | 0 (0) | 6 (9) |
| | Trimethoprim-sulfamethoxazole | 160 mg–800 mg q8h | | 58 | 41 (71) | 13 (22) | 12 (21) | 2 (3) | 3 (5) |
| Winston et al. (194) | Ofloxacin | 300 mg q12h | Hematologic malignancy | 30 | 11 (37) | 0 (0) | 6 (20) | 2 (7) | 2 (7) |
| | Vancomycin-polymyxin | 500 mg –100 mg q8h | | 32 | 21 (66) | 5 (16) | 8 (25) | 2 (6) | 3 (9) |
| Gluckman et al. (72) | Ofloxacin + amoxicillin | 200 mg + 1,000 mg q12h | Marrow transplant | 22 | 5 (23) | 1 (5) | 5 (23) | | 0 (0) |
| | Vancomycin + tobramycin + colistin | 150 mg + 150 mg + $10^6$ U q8h | | 22 | 12 (55) | 2 (9) | 10 (45) | | 2 (9) |

*Continued on following page*

**Table 2.** *Continued*

| Drug and reference | Regimen | Dose[a] | Underlying disease | No. of patients | No. (%) of patients with: | | | | |
|---|---|---|---|---|---|---|---|---|---|
| | | | | | Microbiologically documented infection | Gram-negative bacteremia | Gram-positive bacteremia | Disseminated fungal infection | Fatal infection |
| Total | | | | | | | | | |
| Ofloxacin | | | | 214 | 58 (27) | 3 (1) | 24 (11) | 4/192 (2) | |
| Controls | | | | 206 | 97 (47) | 31 (15) | 32 (16) | 5/184 (3) | |
| Pefloxacin | | | | | | | | | |
| Archimbaud et al. (1) | Pefloxacin + vancomycin | 400 mg + 400 mg q12h | Acute leukemia and marrow transplant | 76 | 78 (100) | 3 (4) | 62 (82) | 5 (6) | 4 (5) |
| | Gentamicin + colistin + tobramycin | 50 mg + $10^6$ U + 400 mg q12h | | 74 | 125 (100) | 12 (16) | 83 (100) | 9 (12) | 10 (14) |
| Gluckman et al. (71) | Pefloxacin + penicillin | 400 mg + 400 mg q8h | Marrow transplant | 32 | 5 (16) | 1 (3) | 4 (13) | | 0 (0) |
| | Cephalothin + gentamicin + bacitracin | 1,000 mg + 80 mg + $10^6$ U q8h | | 33 | 8 (24) | 3 (9) | 5 (15) | | 0 (0) |
| Total | | | | | | | | | |
| Pefloxacin | | | | 108 | 83 (77) | 4 (4) | 64 (59) | 5/76 (6) | |
| Controls | | | | 107 | 133 (100) | 15 (14) | 88 (82) | 9/74 (12) | |
| Enoxacin | | | | | | | | | |
| Talbot et al. (168) | Enoxacin | 400 mg q12h | Acute leukemia | 62 | 20 (32) | 1 (2) | 9 (15) | 6 (10) | 2 (3) |
| | Placebo | Placebo | | 57 | 29 (51) | 14 (25) | 10 (18) | 2 (4) | 3 (5) |
| GRAND TOTAL | | | | | | | | | |
| Quinolone | | | | 774 | 314 (40) | 21/654 (3) | 114/590 (19) | 28/536 (5) | |
| Controls | | | | 754 | 446 (59) | 112/638 (18) | 145/574 (25) | 28/519 (5) | |

[a] q12h and q8h, every 12 and 8 h, respectively.

**Table 3.** Controlled trials comparing different oral fluoroquinolones for prophylaxis of infections in granulocytopenic patients

| Reference | Regimen | Dose[a] | Underlying disease | No. of patients | No. (%) of patients with: Microbiologically documented infection | Gram-negative bacteremia | Gram-positive bacteremia | Disseminated fungal infection | Fatal infection |
|---|---|---|---|---|---|---|---|---|---|
| GIMEMA[b] (170) | Norfloxacin | 400 mg q12h | Acute leukemia and marrow transplant | 319 | 76 (24) | 13 (4) | 34 (11) | 2 (1) | 16 (5) |
| | Ciprofloxacin | 500 mg q12h | | 300 | 51 (17) | 7 (2) | 27 (9) | 3 (1) | 16 (5) |
| Maschmeyer et al. (120) | Norfloxacin | 200–400 mg q12h | Acute leukemia | 23 | 9 (39) | 0 (0) | 6 (26) | | |
| | Ciprofloxacin | 500–1,000 mg q12h | | 25 | 5 (20) | 0 (0) | 3 (12) | | |
| D'Antonio et al. (33) | Norfloxacin | 400 mg q12h | Hematologic malignancy | 35 | 15 (43) | 2 (6) | 6 (17) | 1 (3) | |
| | Ofloxacin | 400 mg q12h | | 36 | 6 (17) | 0 (0) | 1 (3) | 0 (0) | |
| Arning et al. (2) | Ciprofloxacin | 500 mg q12h | Acute leukemia | 30 | 7 (23) | 0 (0) | 3 (10) | 3 (10) | |
| | Ofloxacin | 200 mg q12h | | 31 | 7 (23) | 0 (0) | 4 (13) | 3 (10) | |
| | Trimethoprim-sulfamethoxazole + colistin | 160 mg–800 mg + $2 \times 10^6$ U q8h | | 27 | 10 (37) | 1 (4) | 7 (26) | 1 (4) | |

[a]q12h and q8h, every 12 and 8 h, respectively.
[b]GIMEMA, Gruppo Italiano Malattie Ematologiche Maligne dell' Adulto.

**Table 4.** Effects of routine oral fluoroquinolone prophylaxis on colonization and infection during chemotherapy-related granulocytopenia

| Reference | Center | Fluoroquinolone (dose)[a] | Duration of prophylaxis | Gram-negative bacterial colonization | Infection | Gram-negative bacterial fluoroquinolone resistance |
|---|---|---|---|---|---|---|
| Karp et al. (95) | Johns Hopkins | Norfloxacin (400 mg q12h) + i.v. vancomycin (500 mg q12h) | 111 patients in 15 mo | Occasional non-*P. aeruginosa Pseudomonas* spp. (*P. cepacia, Xanthomonas maltophilia, Pseudomonas putida*) | Only 4 gram-negative infections (*P. aeruginosa, Klebsiella oxytoca, K. pneumoniae, Achromobacter* spp.) | None |
| Dekker et al. (38a) | Utrecht | Ciprofloxacin (500 mg q12h) | 194 patients in 4 yr | Occasional non-*P. aeruginosa Pseudomonas* spp. | Only 1 gram-negative infection (*Xanthomonas maltophilia*); 27 gram-positive bacteremias (mostly coagulase-negative staphylococci or viridans group streptococci) but none fatal | None |
| Winston (191) | UCLA | Norfloxacin (400 mg q12h) | 205 patients in 15 mo | Rare non-*P. aeruginosa Pseudomonas* spp. | Only 3 gram-negative bacteremias (*Xanthomonas maltophilia, E. coli, Enterobacter cloacae*); 31 gram-positive bacteremias (mostly coagulase-negative staphylococci or viridans group streptococci) but none fatal | None |

[a]i.v., intravenous; q12h, every 12 h.

**Table 5.** Compliance and adverse effects of oral antimicrobial prophylaxis in granulocytopenic patients

| Reference | Regimen | No. (%) of patients | | No. of patients with adverse effects[a] | | | |
|---|---|---|---|---|---|---|---|
| | | Total | Highly compliant (>90% of doses taken) | GI | Rash | CNS | MYE |
| Karp et al. (96) | Norfloxacin | 35 | 29 (83) | 1 | 0 | 0 | 0 |
| | Placebo | 33 | 29 (88) | 0 | 0 | 0 | 0 |
| Winston et al. (195) | Norfloxacin | 26 | | 0 | 0 | 0 | 0 |
| | Trimethoprim-sulfamethoxazole | 28 | | 0 | 2 | 0 | 0 |
| Bow et al. (12) | Norfloxacin | 31 | 31 (100) | 0 | 0 | 0 | 0 |
| | Trimethoprim-sulfamethoxazole | 32 | 32 (100) | 0 | 0 | 0 | 0 |
| Cruciani et al. (32) | Norfloxacin | 21 | 19 (90) | 2 | 0 | 0 | 0 |
| | Trimethoprim-sulfamethoxazole | 23 | 29 (87) | 3 | 1 | 0 | 0 |
| Orlandi et al. (135) | Norfloxacin | 19 | 19 (100) | 3 | 2 | 0 | 0 |
| | Trimethoprim-sulfamethoxazole | 22 | 22 (100) | 7 | 1 | 0 | 0 |
| Winston et al. (196) | Norfloxacin | 36 | 30 (83) | 1 | 0 | 0 | 0 |
| | Vancomycin-polymyxin | 30 | 16 (53) | 4 | 0 | 0 | 0 |
| Dekker et al. (39) | Ciprofloxacin | 28 | 23 (82) | 6 | 0 | 0 | 0 |
| | Trimethoprim-sulfamethoxazole | 28 | 15 (54) | 12 | 8 | 0 | 0 |
| Liang et al. (113) | Ofloxacin | 50 | 48 (96) | 8 | 2 | 0 | 0 |
| | Trimethoprim-sulfamethoxazole | 52 | 43 (83) | 10 | 8 | 0 | 0 |
| Kern and Kurrle (102) | Ofloxacin | 80 | 75 (94) | 2 | 3 | 1 | 0 |
| | Trimethoprim-sulfamethoxazole | 80 | 61 (76) | 13 | 8 | 0 | 3 |
| Winston et al. (194) | Ofloxacin | 30 | 24 (80) | 1 | 0 | 2[b] | 0 |
| | Vancomycin-polymyxin | 32 | 10 (31) | 9 | 0 | 0 | 0 |
| Archimbaud et al. (1) | Pefloxacin-vancomycin | 76 | 62 (81) | 0 | 13 | 0 | 0 |
| | Gentamicin-vancomycin-colistin | 74 | 64 (87) | 0 | 5 | 0 | 0 |
| Talbot et al. (168) | Enoxacin | 62 | | 6 | 7 | 0 | 0 |
| | Placebo | 57 | | 1 | 2 | 0 | 0 |

[a]GI, gastrointestinal; CNS, central nervous system; MYE, myelosuppression.
[b]One patient each with headaches and vertigo.

resistant organisms. However, colonization or infection with resistant gram-negative organisms has been found infrequently both in controlled studies of prophylaxis in granulocytopenic patients (Table 6) (1, 12, 32, 39, 96, 102, 113, 168, 194, 196) and during routine quinolone prophylaxis (Table 4) (38a, 95, 191). Non-*P. aeruginosa Pseudomonas* organisms and *Acinetobacter* species account for most of the colonization with gram-negative resistant organisms, but they usually do not cause infection. Cases of colonization or infection with quinolone-resistant members of the *Enterobacteriaceae* or *P. aeruginosa* have occurred rarely. In contrast, infections caused by quinolone-resistant gram-positive aerobic bacteria (viridans group streptococci, coagulase-negative staphylococci, corynebacteria, and methicillin-resistant *Staphylococcus aureus*) are common and are associated with the failure of the oral fluoroquinolones to reduce colonization with these organisms (Tables 4 and 6). Indeed, an increased risk for both colonization and bacteremia caused by viridans group streptococci has been associated with quinolone prophylaxis at several oncology centers (25a, 29, 41, 103, 121). Some cases of bacteremia are complicated by shock, adult respiratory distress syndrome, altered mental status, and even mortality (29, 56, 122, 180). These viridans group streptococci are sensitive to vancomycin but sometimes resistant to penicillin and erythromycin in addition to the quinolones (29, 56, 103, 180). The emergence of ciprofloxacin-resistant coagulase-negative staphylococci colonizing the skin flora and causing bacteremia has also been reported in granulocytopenic patients receiving quinolone prophylaxis (108).

The failure of the oral fluoroquinolones to prevent gram-positive infections and the risk of serious infections caused by viridans group streptococci have led to several trials of gram-positive bacterial prophylaxis in granulocytopenic patients receiving oral quinolone prophylaxis (Table 7) (17, 38, 56a, 167a, 190). The agents used for prevention of gram-positive infection were oral roxithromycin or erythromycin, oral or intravenous penicillin, and intravenous vancomycin. Except in the study by Wimperis et al. that used erythromycin plus ciprofloxacin (190), the addition of an agent with gram-positive antibacterial activity to a regimen of quinolone prophylaxis reduced gram-positive bacteremias. However, only streptococcal bacteremias were reduced (15 to 8%). There was no effect on the incidence of staphylococcal bacteremias. Furthermore, some patients developed streptococcal infections resistant to penicillin or erythromycin despite prophylaxis with these agents (17, 190). Vancomycin-resistant infections were not reported but are a concern associated with the routine use of prophylactic intravenous vancomycin. The macrolides may also antagonize the bactericidal activity of the quinolones on gram-negative bacilli in vitro (150), although neither roxithromycin nor erythromycin had any adverse effects on ciprofloxacin's ability to prevent colonization or infection by gram-negative organisms in the trials by Dekker et al. (38) and Wimperis et al. (190) (Table 7).

## TREATMENT OF FEBRILE GRANULOCYTOPENIC PATIENTS

Successful treatment of febrile granulocytopenic patients with suspected or documented infections requires the prompt initiation of appropriate antimicrobial therapy. In most cases, this therapy has consisted of an aminoglycoside plus an antipseudomonal $\beta$-lactam drug (82, 88, 106). Combination therapy is aimed at providing a wide spectrum of antibacterial coverage, obtaining synergistic bactericidal activity (especially against *P. aeruginosa*), and preventing the emergence of resistant organisms. Several recent developments, however, have led to a reevaluation of this traditional approach. Because of the increasing use of nephrotoxic drugs (such as amphotericin B, cyclosporine,

**Table 6.** Colonization and infection with quinolone-resistant organisms during controlled trials of oral fluoroquinolone prophylaxis in granulocytopenic patients

| Reference | Prophylactic fluoroquinolone | No. of patients | Colonization with quinolone-resistant organisms[a] | Infections with quinolone-resistant organisms[a] |
|---|---|---|---|---|
| Karp et al. (96) | Norfloxacin | 35 | *Pseudomonas maltophilia* (3) | None reported, but gram-positive infections occurred on norfloxacin |
| Winston et al. (196) | Norfloxacin | 36 | *Pseudomonas maltophilia* (2) | Viridans group streptococci (3), corynebacteria (2) |
| Bow et al. (12) | Norfloxacin | 31 | None reported | Viridans group streptococci (9), *Streptococcus faecalis* (1), *Micrococcus* spp. (1), *Staphylococcus epidermidis* (4) |
| Cruciani et al. (32) | Norfloxacin | 21 | Gram-negative bacillus (1) | *P. aeruginosa* (1), *Streptococcus mitis* (1), *Streptococcus pneumoniae* (1), *Streptococcus faecalis* (1) |
| Dekker et al. (39) | Ciprofloxacin | 28 | Non-*P. aeruginosa Pseudomonas* species (4), *Acinetobacter* species (4) | None reported, but gram-positive infections occurred on ciprofloxacin |
| Winston et al. (194) | Ofloxacin | 30 | *Pseudomonas maltophilia* (1), *Pseudomonas fluorescens* (1), *P. putida* (1), *Enterobacter aerogenes* (1) | Viridans group streptococci (2), coagulase-negative staphylococci (1), methicillin-resistant *S. aureus* (1), *Pneumocystis carinii* (1) |
| Liang et al. (113) | Ofloxacin | 50 | None reported | *P. aeruginosa* (1) |
| Kern and Kurrle (102) | Ofloxacin | 70 | *Acinetobacter* species (16), non-*P. aeruginosa Pseudomonas* species (10), *Citrobacter* species (4), *P. aeruginosa* (1), *Klebsiella* species (1) | Viridans group streptococci (6), coagulase-negative staphylococci (3), *S. aureus* (3), corynebacteria (2), *P. aeruginosa* (1), *Pseudomonas fluorescens* (1), *Acinetobacter* species (1) |
| Archimbaud et al. (1) | Pefloxacin | 76 | *P. aeruginosa* and non-*P. aeruginosa Pseudomonas* species (4) | *P. aeruginosa* and non-*P. aeruginosa Pseudomonas* species (4), streptococcal and staphylococcal infections occurred on pefloxacin |
| Talbot et al. (168) | Enoxacin | 62 | None reported | None reported, but gram-positive infections occurred on enoxacin |

[a]Numbers in parentheses are numbers of isolates or organisms.

**Table 7.** Controlled trials of gram-positive prophylaxis in granulocytopenic patients receiving oral fluoroquinolone prophylaxis

| Reference | Regimen | Dose[a] | Underlying disease |
|---|---|---|---|
| Dekker et al. (38) | Ciprofloxacin | 500 mg q12h | Acute leukemia and marrow transplant |
| | Ciprofloxacin + roxithromycin | 500 mg q12h + 150 mg q12h | |
| Wimperis et al. (190) | Ciprofloxacin | 250 mg q12h | Marrow transplant |
| | Ciprofloxacin + erythromycin | 250 mg q12h + 250 mg q12h | |
| Szekely et al. (167a) | Ofloxacin | 200 mg q12h | Hematologic malignancy |
| | Ofloxacin + penicillin | 200 mg q12h + 4 × $10^6$ U q12h | |
| EORTC[b] (56a) | Pefloxacin | 400 mg q12h | Hematologic malignancy and marrow transplant |
| | Pefloxacin + penicillin | 400 mg q12h + 500 mg q12h | |
| Broun et al. (17) | Norfloxacin | 400 mg q8h | Marrow transplant |
| | Norfloxacin + penicillin or vancomycin | 400 mg q8h + $10^6$ U q6h or 750 mg q12h | |
| Total | | | |
| Quinolone | | | |
| Quinolone + macrolide, penicillin, or vancomycin | | | |

[a]q12h, q8h, and q6h, every 12, 8, and 6 h, respectively.
[b]EORTC, European Organization for Research and Treatment of Cancer.

and certain chemotherapeutic agents) in granulocytopenic patients, there is a frequent desire to avoid combination therapy with the aminoglycosides (145, 184, 188). The incidence of *P. aeruginosa* infections has declined at many oncology centers, while the proportion of infections caused by gram-positive organisms (coagulase-negative staphylococci, viridans group streptococci, and corynebacteria) has greatly increased (56, 165, 180, 183, 192). Many of these gram-positive pathogens are resistant to the aminoglycosides and β-lactam antibiotics. The availability of newer β-lactam drugs with broader and more potent antibacterial activities has also made it possible to design new approaches to therapy.

The developments described above have been the basis for the recent use of alternative antimicrobial regimens in febrile granulocytopenic patients (88). These include double-β-lactam antibiotic combinations (an expanded-spectrum cephalosporin plus a ureidopenicillin), front loading with an ami-

Table 7. *Continued*

| No. of patients | No. (%) of patients with: | | | | |
|---|---|---|---|---|---|
| | Microbiologically documented infection | Bacteremia | | | |
| | | Gram negative | Gram positive | Streptococcal | Staphylococcal |
| 80 | 23 (29) | 0 (0) | 20 (25) | 16 (20) | 4 (5) |
| 45 | 7 (16) | 0 (0) | 6 (13) | 1 (2) | 5 (11) |
| 16 | 5 (31) | 0 (0) | 5 (31) | 4 (25) | 1 (6) |
| 37 | 23 (62) | 0 (0) | 23 (62) | 13 (35) | 10 (27) |
| 25 | 5 (20) | 2 (8) | 2 (8) | | |
| 25 | 3 (12) | 3 (12) | 0 (0) | | |
| 250 | 58 (23) | 5 (2) | 53 (21) | 27 (11) | 26 (10) |
| 253 | 38 (15) | 2 (1) | 36 (14) | 14 (6) | 22 (9) |
| 21 | 10 (48) | 0 (0) | 10 (48) | 9 (43) | 1 (5) |
| 22 | 3 (14) | 1 (5) | 2 (9) | 1 (5) | 1 (5) |
| 392 | 101 (26) | 7 (2) | 90 (23) | 56/367 (15) | 32/367 (9) |
| 382 | 74 (19) | 6 (2) | 67 (18) | 29/357 (8) | 38/357 (11) |

noglycoside (an expanded-spectrum cephalosporin plus a short course of an aminoglycoside), monotherapy with an expanded-spectrum cephalosporin or imipenem, and vancomycin plus an expanded-spectrum cephalosporin (36, 58, 82, 109, 144, 193). Each of these regimens avoids the nephrotoxicity and ototoxicity associated with the aminoglycosides but has certain limitations. Double-$\beta$-lactam antibiotic combinations are expensive and occasionally may be antagonistic (36). Front loading with an aminoglycoside may not be as effective as the traditional combination of an aminoglycoside plus a $\beta$-lactam antibiotic in patients with prolonged granulocytopenia (58). Monotherapy with ceftazidime does not provide adequate coverage for many gram-positive pathogens and may require the addition of vancomycin for gram-positive superinfections (109, 144, 153). Monotherapy with imipenem is effective as combination therapy but may be associated with an increased number of seizures at high doses (4 g/day) (193). The routine use of vancomycin as part of the initial therapy of all febrile granulocytopenic patients leads to the unnecessary treatment of many patients (153).

Clinical experience in which the fluoroquinolones have been used for the treatment of febrile granulocytopenic patients is still limited. Nevertheless, a number of in vitro and animal studies have provided information suggesting a potential role for these agents in the therapy of infections in granulocytopenic patients. In vitro, the fluoroquinolones, like the aminoglycosides and newer β-lactams, are very active against the common *Enterobacteriaceae* and *P. aeruginosa* strains causing serious infections (84, 197). In addition, the fluoroquinolones are active against many of the methicillin-resistant staphylococci that now cause frequent infections and are resistant to the aminoglycosides and β-lactams. On the other hand, in some centers, ciprofloxacin resistance among methicillin-resistant staphylococci has increased (10a, 108) and the fluoroquinolones are less active than the penicillins, cephalosporins, and vancomycin against viridans group and other streptococci that account for many of the gram-positive infections in granulocytopenic patients. In vitro combinations of the fluoroquinolones with the aminoglycosides or β-lactams for *P. aeruginosa* and the *Enterobacteriaceae* are predominantly indifferent or additive but rarely antagonistic (22, 24, 27, 43, 54, 61, 69, 77, 78, 125, 128, 132, 133, 167). If a synergistic interaction occurs, it is more often seen between a β-lactam agent (azlocillin, mezlocillin, piperacillin, ceftazidime, cefoperazone, or imipenem) and a fluoroquinolone than between an aminoglycoside (gentamicin, tobramycin, or amikacin) and a fluoroquinolone. Similarly, the serum bactericidal activity against *P. aeruginosa, E. coli,* and *K. pneumoniae* in healthy volunteers receiving a fluoroquinolone (ciprofloxacin) plus a β-lactam agent (azlocillin) is more likely to be synergistic than the activity in sera of healthy volunteers receiving a fluoroquinolone (pefloxacin) plus an aminoglycoside (amikacin) (136, 178). Other studies of serum bactericidal activity against the *Enterobacteriaceae* and *P. aeruginosa* found indifference when ofloxacin or pefloxacin was administered in combination with cefotaxime, ceftazidime, piperacillin, or mezlocillin (176, 186). No antagonism occurred. The bactericidal activity of ciprofloxacin plus vancomycin in serum against *S. aureus, Staphylococcus epidermidis,* and corynebacteria is also predominantly indifferent and shows no antagonism (177).

## Studies with Animal Models

Granulocytopenic animal models evaluating the in vivo efficacies of the fluoroquinolones alone or in combination are summarized in Table 8. In most of the studies, animals were treated with dosages of the quinolones and other antimicrobial agents designed to provide levels in serum and tissue similar to those achieved in humans. While only one-half of the studies actually report concentrations in serum and tissues (14–16, 83, 127, 142, 149, 172, 173), an analysis of the results does provide information helpful in the design of clinical trials in humans.

For *P. aeruginosa* bacteremia in granulocytopenic mice or rats, the combinations ciprofloxacin plus gentamicin and ciprofloxacin plus azlocillin were more effective than ciprofloxacin alone in three of four studies (26, 94b, 173). In the fourth study, ciprofloxacin alone was as effective as ciprofloxacin plus azlocillin (147a). For all studies, ciprofloxacin alone was either as effective as or frequently more effective than single-agent therapy with gentamicin, tobramycin, azlocillin, ceftazidime, or imipenem (26, 94b, 147a, 173). In two studies comparing different quinolones as single-agent therapy for *P. aeruginosa* bacteremia in granulocytopenic mice, ciprofloxacin was as effective as or more effective than enoxacin, ofloxacin, pefloxacin, fleroxacin, or lomefloxacin (62, 94b). For *K. pneumoniae* bacteremia in granulocytopenic mice, ciprofloxacin plus ceftazidime was more effective than either agent alone or the combination of ciprofloxacin or ceftazidime plus gentamicin (172).

For *P. aeruginosa* pneumonia in granulocytopenic guinea pigs, ciprofloxacin and pefloxacin each given alone were as effective as ticarcillin plus tobramycin or ceftazidime plus tobramycin and more effective than ceftazidime, ticarcillin, or tobramycin alone (73). Ciprofloxacin alone was more effective than ceftazidime alone for *Klebsiella* pneumonia in granulocytopenic rats (149).

The model of thigh muscle infection in granulocytopenic mice has also been used to evaluate the relative efficacies of the fluoroquinolones and other agents for the treatment of *P. aeruginosa, E. coli,* and *K. pneumoniae* infections (78, 83, 129a, 180a). For *P. aeruginosa,* the combination of ciprofloxacin plus azlocillin was more effective than either drug alone, and ciprofloxacin alone was as effective as cefoperazone plus tobramycin and more effective than tobramycin alone. For *E. coli,* ciprofloxacin plus mezlocillin was more effective than either agent alone, and ciprofloxacin alone was more effective than cefazolin plus gentamicin or gentamicin alone. For *K. pneumoniae* infection, ciprofloxacin alone was more effective than the combination of cefazolin plus gentamicin or gentamicin alone. In a similar model of granulocytopenic chamber site infection in rabbits, ciprofloxacin plus azlocillin was as effective as azlocillin plus amikacin and more effective than ciprofloxacin plus amikacin for *P. aeruginosa,* while ciprofloxacin plus azlocillin was more effective than either mezlocillin plus amikacin or cefotaxime plus amikacin for the *Enterobacteriaceae* (127). The combination of ciprofloxacin plus azlocillin was also as effective as or, in some cases, more effective than azlocillin plus amikacin and more effective than ciprofloxacin alone for streptococcal infections (142).

Different fluoroquinolones have been compared for treatment of bacteremia in mice rendered granulocytopenic by exposure to whole-body irradiation (14–16). Ofloxacin, ciprofloxacin, and pefloxacin were equally effective in treatment of bacteremia caused by the *Enterobacteriaceae,* but the addition of penicillin was required for therapy of streptococcal infections.

In summary, the results from these animal studies suggest a potential synergistic role for the fluoroquinolones in combination with a broad-spectrum ureidopenicillin for the treatment of *P. aeruginosa, Enterobacteriaceae,* and streptococcal infections in granulocytopenic patients.

## Clinical Studies

Table 9 shows the results of controlled, randomized trials in which the effectiveness of the fluoroquinolones in therapy of febrile granulocytopenic patients was compared with that of a standard regimen. Most of these trials used intravenous ciprofloxacin, which was sometimes changed to oral ciprofloxacin after patients improved on intravenous therapy (6, 25, 64, 79a, 89, 94a, 97–99, 115, 124, 143). There were two trials of oral ofloxacin (117, 118). Intravenous pefloxacin has been evaluated mostly in uncontrolled studies involving a small number of granulocytopenic patients (10, 23, 116, 126).

Only one trial used ciprofloxacin in combination with an aminoglycoside and found ciprofloxacin plus netilmicin to be as effective as piperacillin plus netilmicin (25). However, the trial was complicated by superinfections caused by ciprofloxacin-resistant strains of *S. epidermidis* and streptococci. Five trials compared ciprofloxacin plus a penicillin (usually azlocillin) with a combination of an aminoglycoside plus an antipseudomonal $\beta$-lactam drug (azlocillin, piperacillin, or ceftazidime) (64, 79a, 89, 98, 99, 143). The overall response rates of documented infections to ciprofloxacin plus azlocillin or piperacillin (33 to 59%) were similar to the response rates of infections to an aminoglycoside plus a $\beta$-lactam (36 to 52%). There was

**Table 8.** Efficacy of fluoroquinolones in granulocytopenic animal models

| Reference | Animal model[a] | Organism | In vivo antibacterial potency[b] |
|---|---|---|---|
| Jules and Neu (94b) | Bacteremia in granulocytopenic mice challenged i.p. | *Pseudomonas aeruginosa* | Ciprofloxacin + gentamicin > ciprofloxacin > enoxacin > ofloxacin > gentamicin |
| Chin and Neu (26) | Bacteremia in granulocytopenic mice challenged i.p. | *Pseudomonas aeruginosa* | Ciprofloxacin + azlocillin > ciprofloxacin > azlocillin |
| Robson and Cote (147a) | Bacteremia in granulocytopenic rats challenged i.p. | *Pseudomonas aeruginosa* | Ciprofloxacin = ceftazidime = azlocillin = tobramycin = ciprofloxacin + azlocillin |
| Ulrich et al. (173) | Bacteremia in granulocytopenic mice challenged i.p. | *Pseudomonas aeruginosa* | Ciprofloxacin + azlocillin = imipenem + tobramycin > ciprofloxacin = imipenem > azlocillin = tobramycin |
| Fernandez and Swanson (62) | Bacteremia in granulocytopenic mice challenged i.p. | *Pseudomonas aeruginosa* | Ciprofloxacin = pefloxacin = difloxacin = ofloxacin > norfloxacin = enoxacin = fleroxacin = lomefloxacin |
| Trautman et al. (172) | Bacteremia in granulocytopenic mice challenged i.v. | *Klebsiella pneumoniae* | Ciprofloxacin + ceftazidime > ciprofloxacin = ciprofloxacin + gentamicin = ceftazidime + gentamicin > ceftazidime > gentamicin |
| Gordin et al. (73) | Pneumonia in granulocytopenic guinea pigs | *Pseudomonas aeruginosa* | Ciprofloxacin = pefloxacin = ticarcillin + tobramycin = ceftazidime + tobramycin > ceftazidime = ticarcillin = tobramycin |
| Roosendaal et al. (149) | Pneumonia in granulocytopenic rats | *Klebsiella pneumoniae* | Ciprofloxacin > ceftazidime |
| Muszynski et al. (129a) | Thigh muscle infection in granulocytopenic mice | *Pseudomonas aeruginosa* | Ciprofloxacin + azlocillin > ciprofloxacin > azlocillin |
| Haller (78) | Thigh muscle infection in granulocytopenic mice | *Pseudomonas aeruginosa* | Ciprofloxacin + azlocillin > ciprofloxacin > azlocillin |
| | | *Escherichia coli* | Ciprofloxacin + mezlocillin > ciprofloxacin > mezlocillin |

| | | | |
|---|---|---|---|
| Vogelman et al. (180a) | Thigh muscle infection in granulocytopenic mice | *Pseudomonas aeruginosa* | Ciprofloxacin = cefoperazone + tobramycin > tobramycin |
| Hoogeterp et al. (83) | Thigh muscle infection in granulocytopenic mice | *Pseudomonas aeruginosa* | Ciprofloxacin > tobramycin |
| Moody et al. (127) | Granulocytopenic chamber site infection in rabbits | *Pseudomonas aeruginosa* | Ciprofloxacin + azlocillin = azlocillin + amikacin > ceftizoxime + amikacin > ciprofloxacin + amikacin > ciprofloxacin + ceftizoxime |
| | | *Enterobacteriaceae* | Ciprofloxacin + azlocillin > mezlocillin + amikacin > ceftizoxime + amikacin |
| | | Group D streptococci | Ciprofloxacin + azlocillin > azlocillin + amikacin > penicillin + amikacin |
| Peterson et al. (142) | Granulocytopenic chamber site infection in rabbits | *Streptococcus pneumoniae* | Ciprofloxacin + azlocillin = azlocillin > ciprofloxacin |
| | | *Enterococcus faecalis* | Ciprofloxacin + azlocillin = azlocillin + amikacin > azlocillin > ciprofloxacin |
| | | *Streptococcus avium* | Ciprofloxacin + azlocillin > azlocillin + amikacin > azlocillin > ciprofloxacin |
| Brook et al. (15) | Bacteremia in irradiated granulocytopenic mice challenged p.o. | *Klebsiella pneumoniae* | Ofloxacin = pefloxacin = ciprofloxacin |
| Brook and Elliot (14) | Bacteremia in irradiated granulocytopenic mice | *Enterobacteriaceae* | Ofloxacin = ciprofloxacin = pefloxacin |
| Brook and Ledney (16) | Bacteremia in irradiated granulocytopenic mice | *Enterobacteriaceae* and *Streptococcus* sp. | Ofloxacin + penicillin > ofloxacin > penicillin |

[a] i.p., intraperitoneally; i.v., intravenously; p.o., orally.
[b] >, more active than; =, of equal activity.

**Table 9.** Controlled trials of fluoroquinolones for empiric therapy of febrile granulocytopenic patients with documented infections

| Reference | Treatment regimen[a] | Response[b] | Comments |
|---|---|---|---|
| Chan et al. (25) | Ciprofloxacin + netilmicin | 41/76 (54) | Outbreak of infection by ciprofloxacin-resistant strain of *S. epidermidis* during trial; streptococcal superinfection in 3 on ciprofloxacin + netilmicin vs 0 on piperacillin + netilmicin |
| | Piperacillin + netilmicin | 37/71 (52) | |
| Kelsey et al. (98, 99) | Ciprofloxacin + benzylpenicillin | 17/35 (49) | Renal failure in 1 on ciprofloxacin + benzylpenicillin vs 8 on piperacillin + netilmicin |
| | Piperacillin + netilmicin | 14/34 (41) | |
| Flaherty et al. (64) | Ciprofloxacin + azlocillin | 4/12 (33) | Renal failure or ototoxicity in 1 on ciprofloxacin + azlocillin vs 8 on ceftazidime + amikacin |
| | Ceftazidime + amikacin | 14/27 (52) | |
| Philpott-Howard et al. (143) | Ciprofloxacin + azlocillin | 22/38 (58) | |
| | Azlocillin + gentamicin | 16/33 (48) | |
| Hyatt et al. (89) | Ciprofloxacin + azlocillin | 20/37 (54) | |
| | Azlocillin + netilmicin | 13/36 (36) | |
| Herbrecht et al. (79a) | Ciprofloxacin + piperacillin | 13/22 (59) | |
| | Piperacillin + netilmicin | 8/19 (42) | |
| Johnson et al. (94a) | Ciprofloxacin | 15/31 (48) | |
| | Azlocillin + netilmicin | 15/30 (50) | |
| Meunier et al. (124) | Ciprofloxacin | 21/24 (61) | Trial discontinued prematurely owing to poor response of gram-positive bacterial infections to ciprofloxacin |
| | Piperacillin + amikacin | 26/30 (87) | |
| Bayston et al. (6) | Ciprofloxacin | 10/21 (48) | Streptococcal superinfection in 4 on ciprofloxacin vs 0 on ceftazidime |
| | Ceftazidime | 13/25 (52) | |
| Lim et al. (115) | Ciprofloxacin | 23/28 (82) | Gram-positive superinfection in 7 on ciprofloxacin vs 0 on ceftazidime |
| | Ceftazidime | 18/31 (58) | |
| Kelsey et al. (97) | Ciprofloxacin + teicoplanin | 17/23 (74) | *S. epidermidis* infections responded better to ciprofloxacin + teicoplanin (10/12) than to piperacillin + gentamicin (2/8) |
| | Piperacillin + gentamicin | 6/17 (35) | |
| Malik et al. (118) | Ofloxacin (oral) | 14/36 (39) | |
| | Amikacin + carbenicillin, piperacillin, or cloxacillin | 15/36 (42) | |
| Maiche and Teerenhovi (117) | Ofloxacin (oral) + cefotaxime | 13/22 (59) | |
| | Tobramicin + cefotaxime | 13/29 (45) | |
| Total | | | |
| Quinolone regimen | | 230/415 (55) | |
| Control regimen | | 208/418 (49) | |

[a]Drugs given intravenously unless otherwise indicated; some patients changed to oral ciprofloxacin after improvement.
[b]Number of patients improved/number of infections treated (percent improved).

also less risk of nephrotoxicity or ototoxicity in patients treated with ciprofloxacin plus azlocillin or piperacillin. In the four trials of ciprofloxacin monotherapy, gram-positive superinfections were more common in patients receiving ciprofloxacin alone (6, 94a, 115, 124). The poor response of gram-positive infections caused premature discontinuation of the trial by Meunier et al. in which intravenous ciprofloxacin at a low dose of 200 to 300 mg every 12 h was less effective than piperacillin plus amikacin (124). On the other hand, when ciprofloxacin was combined with teicoplanin for empiric therapy, the response rate of gram-positive bacterial infections was much better (10 of 12 infections, or 83%) (97). The two studies of oral ofloxacin alone or in combination with intravenous cefotaxime found oral ofloxacin as effective as the combination of an aminoglycoside plus a $\beta$-lactam, although response rates were low in all patients (117, 118).

In summary, the results from these studies of the fluoroquinolones for empiric therapy of the febrile granulocytopenic patient suggest a need to use the quinolones in combination with an antistreptococcal agent such as a penicillin or vancomycin to reduce the risk for streptococcal superinfections. The use of a potentially synergistic combination such as an antipseudomonal ureidopenicillin (azlocillin or piperacillin) plus a fluoroquinolone might also improve the outcome for infections caused by *P. aeruginosa,* which may develop resistance during treatment with a quinolone alone (9, 18, 66). The coadministration of an aminoglycoside with a fluoroquinolone does not appear to prevent either streptococcal superinfections or the development of quinolone-resistant *P. aeruginosa* and *Enterobacteriaceae* during therapy (4, 25, 65, 66; see also chapter 6).

In an attempt to reduce the costs associated with the admission of febrile granulocytopenic patients to the hospital, oral fluoroquinolones are being evaluated for empiric therapy of patients who are at home or are outpatients (Table 10). Gardembas-Pain

**Table 10.** Ambulatory treatment of febrile granulocytopenic patients with oral fluoroquinolones

| Reference | Treatment regimen[a] | Underlying disease | Response[b] | Comments |
|---|---|---|---|---|
| Gardembas-Pain et al. (67) | Pefloxacin (400 mg q12h) + amoxicillin-clavulanic acid (500 mg–125 mg q8h) | Lymphoma | 59/68 (87) | 9 failures caused by persistent fever requiring hospitalization and i.v. antibiotics; 1 death due to methicillin-resistant *Staphylococcus* bacteremia |
| Rubenstein et al. (152) | Ciprofloxacin (750 mg q8h) + clindamycin (600 mg q8h) | Solid tumors and hematologic malignancy | 28/33 (85) | 5 failures on ciprofloxacin due to bacteremia (2) (*E. cloacae, X. maltophilia*), *Clostridium difficile* colitis (1), and renal failure (2) |
| | i.v. aztreonam + i.v. clindamycin | | 30/30 (100) | |

[a]Drugs given orally unless otherwise indicated. i.v., intravenously; q12h and q8h, every 12 and 8 h, respectively.
[b]Number of patients improved/number of infections treated (percent improved).

et al. instructed a group of lymphoma patients with short-term granulocytopenia (5 days) who were living at home to begin oral pefloxacin and amoxicillin-clavulanic acid at the onset of fever without examination by a physician (67). Fifty-nine of 68 febrile episodes were treated successfully by this approach. Nine patients with persistent fever after 72 h of oral antibiotic therapy required hospitalization for intravenous antibiotics. Rubenstein et al. compared two different regimens for the outpatient treatment of febrile granulocytopenic patients judged to be clinically stable after a physical and laboratory evaluation in an ambulatory treatment center (152). Most patients had solid tumors. Twenty-eight of the 33 patients treated with oral ciprofloxacin and all patients treated with intravenous aztreonam plus clindamycin improved. While these results are impressive, further controlled studies of a large number of febrile patients with moderate or short-term granulocytopenia are needed before empiric outpatient therapy with an oral fluoroquinolone can be recommended as a replacement for standard inpatient treatment with parenteral antibiotics.

## TREATMENT OF BACTERIAL ENTERIC INFECTIONS IN IMMUNOCOMPROMISED PATIENTS

The major bacterial pathogens causing diarrhea (toxigenic *E. coli, Salmonella* spp., *Shigella* spp., *Campylobacter* spp., *Aeromonas* spp., and *Vibrio* spp.) are all inhibited by the fluoroquinolones at concentrations of less than 1 $\mu$g/ml (84, 197; see also chapter 16). Some *Salmonella* strains resistant to ampicillin, chloramphenicol, and trimethoprim-sulfamethoxazole are inhibited by the fluoroquinolones, which are capable of penetrating phagocytic cells and killing salmonellae and other intracellular bacteria (3, 49, 50). In murine models, ciprofloxacin reduces mortality from systemic *Salmonella* infection in mice with no effective immunity as well as in mice with normal immunity (20, 48). For these reasons, ciprofloxacin and norfloxacin have been used for the treatment of *Salmonella* infections complicating malignancy, organ transplant, AIDS, mixed connective disease, and chronic granulomatous disease (21, 31, 44, 59, 80, 81, 91, 104, 107, 138). Of 20 *Salmonella* infections, 18 (90%) responded to ciprofloxacin or norfloxacin (Table 11). Many of these patients had multiple prior clinical episodes of salmonellosis that had not been eradicated with ampicillin or trimethoprim-sulfamethoxazole or were resistant to these conventional agents.

*Shigella* spp. and *Campylobacter* spp. are common causes of diarrhea in homosexual men, including men infected with the human immunodeficiency virus and AIDS. Four (57%) of seven AIDS patients with *Shigella* infection and three (75%) of four AIDS patients with *Campylobacter* infection improved on ciprofloxacin or norfloxacin (35, 60, 81, 131, 154). Six of these patients had the unusual occurrence of *Shigella* or *Campylobacter* bacteremia. A case of *Aeromonas hydrophila* colitis in an AIDS patient has also been treated successfully with oral ciprofloxacin (114).

## TREATMENT OF *LEGIONELLA* INFECTION IN IMMUNOCOMPROMISED PATIENTS

*Legionella* pneumonia is an infrequent but life-threatening infection in immunocompromised patients, especially those with organ transplants (134). Despite treatment with erythromycin and rifampin, many cases are fatal. In addition, some patients tolerate high doses of intravenous erythromycin poorly because of phlebitis, ototoxicity, or alteration of cyclosporine metabolism (94, 134). Alternative agents for treatment are needed. The fluoroquinolones are very active against *Legionella* spp. in vitro and inhibit most isolates at concentrations of less than 1 $\mu$g/ml (84, 197). The uptake and concentra-

**Table 11.** Efficacy of fluoroquinolones for treatment of enteric infection in immunocompromised patients

| Reference | Infection | Underlying disease | Regimen[a] | Response[b] |
|---|---|---|---|---|
| Patton et al. (138) | *Salmonella typhimurium* bacteremia | Acute leukemia | i.v. and oral ciprofloxacin | 1/1 |
| Kiess et al. (104) | *Salmonella tennessee* osteomyelitis | Neuroblastoma | Oral ciprofloxacin | 1/1 |
| Burns and Wallace (21) | *Salmonella typhimurium* urinary infection | Renal transplant | Oral ciprofloxacin | 1/1 |
| Diaz-Tijeiro et al. (44) | *Salmonella typhimurium* arthritis and bacteremia | Renal transplant | i.v. and oral ciprofloxacin | 1/1 |
| Esposito et al. (59) | *Salmonella typhimurium* enteritis | Mixed connective tissue disease | Oral ciprofloxacin | 1/1 |
| Heseltine and Corrado (81) | *Salmonella* bacteremia | Chronic granulomatous disease | Oral norfloxacin | 0/1 |
| Connolly et al. (31) | *Salmonella typhimurium* bacteremia | AIDS | Oral ciprofloxacin | 1/1 |
| Klein et al. (107) | *Salmonella* bacteremia | AIDS | Oral ciprofloxacin | 2/2 |
| Jacobson et al. (91) | *Salmonella* bacteremia | AIDS | Oral ciprofloxacin | 3/4 |
| Heseltine et al. (80) | *Salmonella* enteritis and bacteremia | AIDS | Oral norfloxacin | 7/7 |
| Heseltine and Corrado (81) | *Shigella* enteritis and bacteremia | AIDS | Oral norfloxacin | 0/1 |
| Nelson et al. (131) | *Shigella* enteritis and bacteremia | AIDS | Oral ciprofloxacin | 4/6 |
| Sacks et al. (154) | *Campylobacter cinaedi* bacteremia | AIDS | Oral ciprofloxacin | 1/1 |
| Decker et al. (35) | *Campylobacter cinaedi* bacteremia | AIDS | Oral ciprofloxacin | 1/1 |
| Evans and Riley (60) | *Campylobacter laridis* colitis | AIDS | Oral ciprofloxacin | 0/1 |
| Heseltine and Corrado (81) | *Campylobacter* and *Shigella* enteritis | AIDS | Oral norfloxacin | 1/1 |
| Liao and Chappell (114) | *Aeromonas hydrophila* colitis | AIDS | Oral ciprofloxacin | 1/1 |
| Total | | | | 26/32 (81) |

[a]i.v., intravenously.
[b]Number of patients improved/number of patients treated (percent improved).

**Table 12.** Efficacy of fluoroquinolones for treatment of *Legionella* pneumonia in immunocompromised patients

| Reference | Underlying disease (no. of patients) | Regimen[a] | Response (no. of patients) |
|---|---|---|---|
| Unertl et al. (174) | Lung and liver carcinoma | i.v. ciprofloxacin (200 mg q12h) | Failure |
| | Ovarian carcinoma | i.v. ciprofloxacin (200 mg q12h) | Cure |
| | Kidney and pancreatic transplant | i.v. ciprofloxacin (200 mg q12h) | Cure |
| | Liver transplant | i.v. ciprofloxacin (200 mg q12h) | Failure |
| Hooper et al. (85) | Heart transplant | i.v. ciprofloxacin (200 mg q6h) | Cure |
| | Heart transplant | i.v. ciprofloxacin (200 mg q6h) | Cure |
| Seu et al. (159) | Liver transplant | Oral ciprofloxacin (750 mg q12h) | Cure |
| Meletis et al. (123) | Bone marrow transplant | Oral pefloxacin (400 mg q12h) + erythromycin | Failure |
| | Bone marrow transplant | Oral pefloxacin (400 mg q12h) + erythromycin | Failure |
| Benz-Lemoine et al. (8) | Bone marrow transplant | Pefloxacin + erythromycin | Failure |
| | Bone marrow transplant | Pefloxacin + erythromycin | Failure |
| Douron et al. (46) | Liver or kidney transplant (6) | i.v. ciprofloxacin (400 mg q12h) ± erythromycin ± rifampin | Cure (10) Failure (5) |
| | Hematologic malignancy (3) | | |
| | Solid tumor (3) | | |
| | Vasculitis (1) | | |
| | AIDS (4) | | |
| Total[b] | | | 15/26 (58%) |

[a]i.v., intravenously; q12h and q6h, every 12 and 6 h, respectively.
[b]Number of patients cured/total number of patients treated (percent cured).

tion of quinolones by phagocytic cells are high and correlate with intracellular killing of *Legionella* spp. (42). In animal models of *Legionella* infections in guinea pigs, ciprofloxacin, ofloxacin, pefloxacin, sparfloxacin, and fleroxacin appear to be at least as effective as erythromycin or rifampin (47, 51, 52, 63, 163, 164). Clinical experience in using the fluoroquinolones for treatment of *Legionella* pneumonia in immunocompromised patients is still limited but is summarized in Table 12 (8, 46, 85, 123, 159, 174). Ciprofloxacin or pefloxacin given either alone or in combination with erythromycin was used most often. The majority of patients had either solid-organ or bone marrow transplants. The overall response rate was 58% (15 of 26 cases). The quinolones had no appreciable effect on blood levels of cyclosporine. While further studies are necessary before the fluoroquinolones can be recommended for general use in the treatment of *Legionella* pneumonia, these results suggest a selective role for these agents in patients unable to tolerate erythromycin or rifampin.

## TREATMENT OF *MYCOBACTERIUM AVIUM* COMPLEX INFECTIONS IN AIDS

Serious infections caused by the *M. avium* complex have been increasing and are especially common in patients with AIDS (86, 101). Disseminated disease reportedly affects 20 to 40% of patients with AIDS and is characterized by bacteremia, fevers, chills, night sweats, diarrhea, anorexia, and weight loss.

The therapy of *M. avium* complex infection is limited by the resistance of these organisms to individual standard agents and by the toxicity of combined drug regimens. Among the fluoroquinolones, ciprofloxacin and sparfloxacin are two of the more active anti-*M. avium* agents and are active against isolates from AIDS patients as well (90a, 112, 198, 201). However, only one-fourth to one-half of these isolates are inhibited by ciprofloxacin or sparfloxacin alone. On the other hand, combinations of ciprofloxacin or sparfloxacin plus rifampin and ethambutol and of ciprofloxacin plus imipenem and amikacin are synergistic (198, 199, 201). In the beige mouse model of disseminated *M. avium* complex infection, ciprofloxacin or sparfloxacin as single-agent therapy is less effective than combination therapy with ciprofloxacin, imipenem, and amikacin or sparfloxacin plus ethambutol in reducing mortality and *M. avium* colony counts in blood and tissue (90, 107a, 107b).

Based on the results from the in vitro and animal studies, several trials using ciprofloxacin in combination with other antimycobacterial agents for the treatment of disseminated *M. avium* complex infection in AIDS patients have been performed (Table 13) (7, 28, 40, 87, 91a, 100). The most frequently used combination was ciprofloxacin, ethambutol, rifampin, amikacin, and clofazimine. A reduction in bacteremia and symptoms was achieved in most patients after 2 or more weeks of therapy, but adverse reactions (usually nausea, vomiting, and abdominal pain) were common and frequently led to withdrawal of therapy. Relapse of infection occurred after discontinuation of therapy. In the only controlled study, Jacobson et al. randomized AIDS patients with newly diagnosed disseminated *M. avium* complex infection to receive either placebo or ciprofloxacin, ethambutol, and rifampin for 8 weeks (91a). Patients were then crossed over to the opposite therapy for the next 8 weeks. A decrease in colony counts of *M. avium* in blood cultures and a reduction of clinical symptoms occurred more frequently during treatment, but there was no improved survival. On the other hand, Horsburgh et al. reported that the survival of patients with disseminated *M. avium* complex infection who receive antimycobacterial therapy was prolonged a median of 4 months over survival of a group of matched controls with untreated infection (87).

Other promising drugs for treatment of *M. avium* complex infection are the new macrolides clarithromycin and azithromycin. Both clarithromycin and azithromycin reduce the bacteremia and symptoms associated with *M. avium* complex infection in patients with AIDS (34, 202). De Lalla et al. found similar results in AIDS patients treated with the combination of ciprofloxacin plus clarithromycin and amikacin (Table 13) (40). Whether this combination of a fluoroquinolone and a macrolide would be a more effective and tolerable regimen than other multidrug regimens used for *M. avium* complex infection requires further study. Similarly, additional clinical studies are needed to determine whether the activities of ciprofloxacin, ofloxacin, and the other quinolones against *Mycobacterium tuberculosis* have any benefit in the treatment of tuberculosis in AIDS and other immunocompromised patients (5, 112, 201).

## SUMMARY

The fluoroquinolones are effective agents for the prevention of gram-negative bacillary colonization and infection in granulocytopenic patients. They are better tolerated than oral, nonabsorbable antibiotics or trimethoprim-sulfamethoxazole and have few side effects. Prophylaxis with the quinolones in granulocytopenic patients has not yet been associated with a significant emergence of resistant gram-negative bacilli but may lead to an increase in gram-positive bacterial infections, especially bacteremias caused by viridans group streptococci. Judging from in vitro synergy studies, granulocytopenic animal models, and comparative clinical trials, a combination of a fluoroquinolone plus a

**Table 13.** Efficacy of oral fluoroquinolones for treatment of *M. avium* complex infections in patients with AIDS

| Reference | Regimen[a] | No. of patients treated | Bacteriologic response | Clinical response |
|---|---|---|---|---|
| Chiu et al. (28) | Ciprofloxacin (750 mg q12h)<br>Ethambutol (1,000 mg q24h)<br>Rifampin (600 mg q24h)<br>Amikacin (7.5 mg/kg of body wt q24h) | 17 | Blood culture colony counts decreased after 4 wk of therapy | Systemic symptoms related to infection decreased, but 7 patients stopped therapy because of toxicity |
| Benson et al. (7) | Ciprofloxacin (750 mg q12h)<br>Ethambutol (15 mg/kg q24h)<br>Rifampin (600 mg q24h)<br>Amikacin (7.5 mg/kg q12h)<br>Clofazimine (150 mg q24h) | 5 | Blood culture became negative after 2 mo of therapy | All patients responded by defervescence, improved appetite, and weight gain |
| Kemper et al. (100) | Ciprofloxacin (750 mg q12h)<br>Ethambutol (15 mg/kg q24h)<br>Rifampin (600 mg q24h)<br>Amikacin (7.5 mg/kg q24h)<br>Clofazimine (100 mg q24h) | 41 | Blood culture colony counts decreased after 4 wk of therapy; 13 patients became culture negative | Systemic symptoms related to infection decreased, but drug toxicity occurred in 26 patients; only 19 patients completed therapy |

| | | | | |
|---|---|---|---|---|
| Horsburgh et al. (87) | Ciprofloxacin<br>Ethambutol<br>Rifampin<br>Amikacin<br>Clofazimine | 16 | | 14 patients died, but median survival of treated patients (8 mo) was greater than median survival of untreated matched controls (4 mo) |
| Jacobson et al. (91a) | Ciprofloxacin (750 mg q12h)<br>Ethambutol (25 mg/kg q24h)<br>Rifampin (600 mg q24h) vs crossover to placebo | 13 | Blood culture colony counts decreased on therapy compared with placebo | Karnofsky score greater and fever less on therapy compared with placebo, but drug toxicity occurred in 9 patients |
| De Lalla et al. (40) | Ciprofloxacin (500 mg q8h)<br>Clarithromycin (1,000 mg q12h)<br>Amikacin (7.5 mg/kg q12h) | 12 | Blood cultures became negative after 2–8 wk of therapy | All patients responded by defervescence and weight gain, but drug toxicity occurred in 9 patients |

[a] q24h, q12h, and q8h, every 24, 12, and 8 h, respectively.

ureidopenicillin is at least as effective as an aminoglycoside plus an antipseudomonal $\beta$-lactam for the empiric therapy of febrile granulocytopenic patients and may be more effective than a fluoroquinolone alone by reducing the risk from streptococcal superinfections and the emergence of quinolone-resistant *P. aeruginosa* strains. The fluoroquinolones can be effective alternative drugs for the treatment of enteric bacterial infections and *Legionella* pneumonia in immunocompromised patients, especially those who fail standard therapies as a consequence of drug-related side effects or bacterial resistance. Data establishing the efficacy of the fluoroquinolones for the treatment of mycobacterial diseases in immunocompromised patients are still limited, but results of in vitro and animal model studies as well as initial clinical trials suggest a possible role for these agents as part of combination therapy of *M. avium* complex infections and tuberculosis. The oral administration of the fluoroquinolones also facilitates the outpatient management of immunocompromised patients with specific infections caused by known susceptible organisms but is not yet recommended for empiric therapy of febrile, ambulatory granulocytopenic patients with no defined focus of infection.

## REFERENCES


1. **Archimbaud, E., D. Guyotat, J. Maupas, C. Ploton, A. Nageotte, Y. Devaux, X. Thomas, J. Fleurette, and D. Fiere.** 1991. Pefloxacin and vancomycin vs. gentamicin, colistin sulphate and vancomycin for prevention of infection in granulocytopenic patients: a randomized double-blind study. *Eur. J. Cancer* **27:**174–178.
2. **Arning, M., H. H. Wolf, C. Aul, A. Heyll, R. E. Scharf, and W. Schneider.** 1990. Infection prophylaxis in neutropenic patients with acute leukemia—a randomized, comparative study with ofloxacin, ciprofloxacin, and co-trimoxazole/colistin. *J. Antimicrob. Chemother.* **26**(Suppl. D):137–142.
3. **Asperilla, M. O., R. A. Smego, and L. K. Scott.** 1990. Quinolone antibiotics in the treatment of Salmonella infections. *Rev. Infect. Dis.* **12:**873–889.
4. **Azadian, B. S., J. W. A. Bendig, and D. M. Samson.** 1986. Emergence of ciprofloxacin-resistant *Pseudomonas aeruginosa* after combined therapy with ciprofloxacin and amikacin. *J. Antimicrob. Chemother.* **18:**771.
5. **Barnes, P. F., A. B. Bloch, P. T. Davidson, and D. E. Snider.** 1991. Tuberculosis in patients with human immunodeficiency virus infection. *N. Engl. J. Med.* **324:**1644–1650.
6. **Bayston, K. F., S. Want, and J. Cohen.** 1989. A prospective, randomized comparison of ceftazidime and ciprofloxacin as initial empiric therapy in neutropenic patients with fever. *Am. J. Med.* **87**(Suppl. 5a):269S–273S.
7. **Benson, C. A., H. A. Kessler, J. C. Pottage, and G. M. Trenholme.** 1991. Successful treatment of acquired immunodeficiency syndrome-related *Mycobacterium avium* complex disease with a multiple drug regimen including amikacin. *Arch. Intern. Med.* **151:**582–585.
8. **Benz-Lemoine, E., V. Dewail, O. Castel, F. Guilhot, R. Robert, G. Grollier, F. Rublot-Casenave, C. Gireaud, and J. Tanzer.** 1991. Nocosomial legionnaires' disease in a bone marrow transplant unit. *Bone Marrow Transplant.* **7:**61–63.
9. **Berdig, J. W. A., P. W. Kyle, P. L. F. Giangrande, D. M. Samson, and B. S. Azadian.** 1987. Two neutropenic patients with multiple resistant *Pseudomonas aeruginosa* septicemia treated with ciprofloxacin. *J. R. Soc. Med.* **80:**316–317.
10. **Beun, G. D. M., L. L. Debrus-Palmans, M. S. M. Daniels-Bosman, and G. H. Blijham.** 1988. Therapy with pefloxacin in febrile neutropenic patients. *Rev. Infect. Dis.* **10**(Suppl. 1):S236.

10a. **Blumberg, H. M., D. Rimland, D. J. Carroll, P. Terry, and I. K. Wachsmuth.** 1991. Rapid development of ciprofloxacin resistance in methicillin-susceptible and -resistant *Staphylococcus aureus*. *J. Infect. Dis.* **163:**1279–1285.

11. **Bodey, G. P., M. Buckley, Y. S. Sathe, and E. J. Freireich.** 1966. Quantitative relationship between circulating leukocytes and infection in patients with acute leukemia. *Ann. Intern. Med.* **64:**328–340.
12. **Bow, E. J., E. Rayner, and T. J. Louie.** 1988. Comparison of norfloxacin with cotrimoxazole for infection prophylaxis in acute leukemia. The trade-off for reduced gram-negative sepsis. *Am. J. Med.* **84:**847–854.
13. **Bow, E. J., E. Rayner, B. A. Scott, and T. J. Louie.** 1987. Selective gut decontamination with nalidixic acid or trimethoprim-sulfamethoxazole for infection prophylaxis in neutropenic cancer patients: relationship of efficacy to antimicrobial spectrum and timing of administration. *Antimicrob. Agents Chemother.* **31:**551–557.

14. **Brook, I., and T. B. Elliott.** 1991. Quinolone therapy in the prevention of mortality after irradiation. *Radiat. Res.* **128:**100–103.
15. **Brook, I., T. B. Elliott, and G. D. Ledney.** 1990. Quinolone therapy of *Klebsiella pneumoniae* sepsis following irradiation: comparison of pefloxacin, ciprofloxacin, and ofloxacin. *Radiat. Res.* **122:**215–217.
16. **Brook, I., and G. D. Ledney.** 1991. Ofloxacin and penicillin G combination therapy in prevention of bacterial translocation and animal mortality after irradiation. *Antimicrob. Agents Chemother.* **35:**1685–1687.
17. **Broun, E. R., J. L. Wheat, P. H. Kneebone, K. Sundbald, R. A. Hromas, and G. Tricot.** A randomized trial of the addition of gram positive prophylaxis to standard antimicrobial prophylaxis in patients undergoing autologous bone marrow transplantation. *Bone Marrow Transplant.*, in press.
18. **Brown, A., and G. Smith.** 1989. Treatment of sepsis in patients with neoplastic diseases with intravenous ciprofloxacin. *Am. J. Med.* **87**(Suppl. 5a):266S–268S.
19. **Brumfitt, W., I. Franklin, P. Grady, J. M. T. Hamilton-Miller, and A. Iliffe.** 1984. Changes in the pharmacokinetics of ciprofloxacin and fecal flora during administration of a 7-day course to human volunteers. *Antimicrob. Agents Chemother.* **26:**757–761.
20. **Brunner, H., and H. J. Zeiler.** 1988. Oral ciprofloxacin treatment for *Salmonella typhimurium* infection of normal and immunocompromised mice. *Antimicrob. Agents Chemother.* **32:**57–62.
21. **Burns, B. J., and M. R. Wallace.** 1987. Treatment of *Salmonella typhimurium* infection in a renal transplant patient with ciprofloxacin. *N.Z. Med. J.* **100:**190.
22. **Bustamante, C. I., R. C. Wharton, and J. C. Wade.** In vitro activity of ciprofloxacin in combination with ceftazidime, aztreonam, and azlocillin against multiresistant isolates of *Pseudomonas aeruginosa. Antimicrob. Agents Chemother.* **34:**1814–1815.
23. **Cajozzo, A., R. Carbone, M. Carotenuto, M. Grana, A. La Sala, S. Mancuso, R. Perricone, A. Sgalambro, and F. Dammacco.** 1990. Pefloxacin in the antibacterial treatment of immunodepressed patients. *J. Chemother.* **2:**185–189.
24. **Chalkley, L. J., and H. J. Koornhof.** 1985. Antimicrobial activity of ciprofloxacin against *Pseudomonas aeruginosa, Escherichia coli,* and *Staphylococcus aureus* determined by the killing curve method: antibiotic comparison and synergism interactions. *Antimicrob. Agents Chemother.* **28:**331–342.
25. **Chan, C. C., B. A. Oppenheim, H. Anderson, R. Swindell, and J. H. Scarffe.** 1989. Randomized trial comparing ciprofloxacin plus netilmicin versus piperacillin plus netilmicin for empiric treatment of fever in neutropenic patients. *Antimicrob. Agents Chemother.* **33:**87–91.

25a. **Chenoweth, C., M. Halpern, K. Tibor, and S. Silver.** 1992. *Program Abstr. 32nd Intersci. Conf. Antimicrob. Agents Chemother.*, abstr. 1543.
26. **Chin, N. X., and H. C. Neu.** 1986. Synergy of ciprofloxacin and azlocillin in vitro and in a neutropenic mouse model of infection. *Eur. J. Clin. Microbiol.* **5:**23–28.
27. **Chin, N. X., and H. C. Neu.** 1990. Combination of ofloxacin and other antimicrobial agents. *J. Chemother.* **2:**343–347.
28. **Chiu, J., J. Nussbaum, S. Bozzette, J. G. Tilles, L. S. Young, J. Leedom, P. N. R. Heseltine, J. A. McCutchan, and the California Collaborative Treatment Group.** 1990. Treatment of disseminated *Mycobacterium avium* complex infection in AIDS with amikacin, ethambutol, rifampin, and ciprofloxacin. *Ann. Intern. Med.* **113:**358–361.
29. **Classen, D. C., J. P. Burke, C. D. Ford, S. Evershed, M. R. Alvia, J. K. Wilfahrt, and J. A. Elliott.** 1990. *Streptococcus mitis* sepsis in bone marrow transplant patients receiving oral antimicrobial prophylaxis. *Am. J. Med.* **89:**441–446.
30. **Cofsky, R. D., L. DuBouchet, and S. H. Landesman.** 1984. Recovery of norfloxacin in feces after administration of a single oral dose to human volunteers. *Antimicrob. Agents Chemother.* **26:**110–111.
31. **Connolly, M. J., M. H. Snow, and H. R. Ingham.** 1986. Ciprofloxacin treatment of recurrent *Salmonella typhimurium* septicemia in a patient with acquired immune deficiency syndrome. *J. Antimicrob. Chemother.* **18:**647–648.
32. **Cruciani, M., E. Concia, A. Navarra, L. Perversi, F. Bonetti, M. Arico, and L. Nespoli.** 1989. Prophylactic co-trimoxazole versus norfloxacin in neutropenic children—perspective randomized study. *Infection* **17:**65–69.
33. **D'Antonio, D., A. Iacone, G. Fioritoni, S. Betti, A. Di Girolamo, R. Piccolomini, and G. Torlontano.** 1991. Antibacterial prophylaxis in granulocytopenic patients: a randomized study of ofloxacin versus norfloxacin. *Curr. Ther. Res.* **50:**304–311.
34. **Dautzenberg, B., C. Truffot, S. Legris, M. C. Mehoyas, H. C. Berlie, A. Mercat, S. Chevret, and J. Grosset.** 1991. Activity of clarithromycin against *Mycobacterium avium* infection in patients with the acquired immune deficiency syndrome. *Am. Rev. Respir. Dis.* **144:**564–569.
35. **Decker, C. F., G. J. Martin, W. B. Barham, and S. F. Paparella.** 1992. Bacteremia due to

*Campylobacter cinaedi* in a patient infected with the human immunodeficiency virus. *Clin. Infect. Dis.* **15:**178–179.

36. **Dejace, P., and J. Klastersky.** 1986. Comparative review of combination therapy: two beta-lactams versus beta-lactam plus aminoglycoside. *Am. J. Med.* **80**(Suppl. 6B):29–38.
37. **Dekker, A. W., M. Rozenberg-Arska, J. J. Sixma, and J. Verhoef.** 1981. Prevention of infection by trimethoprim-sulfamethoxazole plus amphotericin B in patients with acute non-lymphocytic leukemia. *Ann. Intern. Med.* **95:**555–559.
38. **Dekker, A. W., M. Rozenberg-Arska, and L. F. Verdonck.** 1990. Prevention of bacteremias caused by alpha-hemolytic streptococci by roxithromycin in patients treated with intensive cytotoxic treatment. *Hematol. Blood Transfusion* **33:**551–554.

38a. **Dekker, A. W., M. Rozenberg-Arska, L. F. Verdonck, and J. Verhoef.** 1990. *Program Abstr. 6th Int. Symp. Infect. Immunocompromised Host,* abstr. 100.

39. **Dekker, A. W., M. Rozenberg-Arska, and J. Verhoef.** 1987. Infection prophylaxis in acute leukemia: a comparison of ciprofloxacin with trimethoprim-sulfamethoxazole and colistin. *Ann. Intern. Med.* **106:**7–12.
40. **De Lalla, F., R. Maserati, P. Scarpellini, P. Marone, R. Nicolin, F. Caccamo, and R. Rigoli.** 1992. Clarithromycin-ciprofloxacin-amikacin for therapy of *Mycobacterium avium–Mycobacterium intracellulare* bacteremia in patients with AIDS. *Antimicrob. Agents Chemother.* **36:**1567–1569.
41. **De Pauw, B. E., J. P. Donelly, T. De Witte, I. R. O. Nováková, and A. Schattenberg.** 1990. Options and limitations of long-term oral ciprofloxacin as antibacterial prophylaxis in allogeneic bone marrow transplant recipients. *Bone Marrow Transplant.* **5:**179–182.
42. **Desnottes, J. F., N. Diallo, C. Loubeyre, and N. Moreau.** 1990. Effect of pefloxacin on microorganism:host cell interaction. *J. Antimicrob. Chemother.* **26**(Suppl. B):17–26.
43. **Desplaces, N., L. Gutmann, J. Carlet, J. Guibert, and J. F. Acar.** 1986. The new quinolones and their combination with other agents for therapy of severe infections. *J. Antimicrob. Chemother.* **17**(Suppl. A):25–39.
44. **Diaz-Tejeiro, R., J. Diez, F. Maduell, N. Esparza, P. Errasti, and A. Purroy.** 1989. Successful treatment with ciprofloxacin of multiresistant Salmonella arthritis in a renal transplant recipient. *Nephrol. Dial. Transplant.* **4:**390-392.
45. **Dietrich, M., W. Gaus, J. Vossen, D. Van der Waaik, and F. Wendt.** 1977. Protective isolation and antimicrobial decontamination in patients with high susceptibility to infection: a prospective cooperative study of gnotobiotic care in leukemia patients. I. Clinical results. *Infection* **5:**107–114.
46. **Douron, E., C. Maynaud, M. Wolff, B. Schlemmer, D. Samuel, J. P. Sollet, and P. Levasseur-Rajagopalan.** 1990. Comparison of the activity of three antibiotic regimens in severe Legionnaires' disease. *J. Antimicrob. Chemother.* **26**(Suppl. B):129–139.
47. **Douron, E., P. Rajagopalan, J. L. Vildé, and J. J. Pocidalo.** 1986. Efficacy of pefloxacin in comparison with erythromycin in the treatment of experimental guinea pig legionellosis. *J. Antimicrob. Chemother.* **17**(Suppl. B):41–48.
48. **Easmon, C. S. F.** 1987. Protective effects of ciprofloxacin in a murine model of Salmonella infection. *Am. J. Med.* **82**(Suppl. 4A):71–72.
49. **Easmon, C. S. F., and J. P. Crane.** 1985. Uptake of ciprofloxacin by human neutrophils. *J. Antimicrob. Chemother.* **16:**67–73.
50. **Easmon, C. S. F., and J. P. Crane.** 1985. Uptake of ciprofloxacin by macrophages. *J. Clin. Pathol.* **38:**442–444.
51. **Edelstein, P. H., M. A. C. Edelstein, and B. Holzknecht.** 1992. In vitro activities of fleroxacin against clinical isolates of *Legionella* spp., its pharmacokinetics in guinea pigs, and use to treat guinea pigs with *L. pneumophila* pneumonia. *Antimicrob. Agents Chemother.* **36:**2387–2391.
52. **Edelstein, P. H., M. A. C. Edelstein, J. Weidenfeld, and M. B. Dorr.** 1990. In vitro activity of sparfloxacin (CI-978; AT-4140) for clinical *Legionella* isolates, pharmacokinetics in guinea pigs, and use to treat guinea pigs with *L. pneumophila* pneumonia. *Antimicrob. Agents Chemother.* **34:**2122–2127.
53. **Edlund, C., A. Lidbeck, L. Kagen, and C. E. Nord.** 1987. Effect of enoxacin on colonic microflora of healthy volunteers. *Eur. J. Clin. Microbiol.* **6:**298–300.
54. **Eliopoulos, G. M., and C. T. Eliopoulos.** 1989. Ciprofloxacin in combination with other antimicrobials. *Am. J. Med.* **87**(Suppl. 5A):17S–22S.
55. **Elston, R. A., and J. Taylor.** 1988. Possible interaction of ciprofloxacin with cyclosporin A. *J. Antimicrob. Chemother.* **21:**679–680.
56. **Elting, L. S., G. P. Bodey, and B. H. Keefe.** 1992. Septicemia and shock syndrome due to viridans streptococci: a case-control study of predisposing factors. *Rev. Infect. Dis.* **14:**1201–1207.

56a. **EORTC International Antimicrobial Therapy Cooperative Group.** 1992. *Program Abstr. 32nd Intersci. Conf. Antimicrob. Agents Chemother.*, abstr. 1692.

57. **EORTC International Antimicrobial Therapy Project Group.** 1984. Trimethoprim-sulfamethoxazole in the prevention of infection in neutropenic patients. *J. Infect. Dis.* **150:**372–379.

58. **EORTC International Antimicrobial Therapy Project Group.** 1987. Ceftazidime combined with a short or long course of amikacin for empirical therapy of gram-negative bacteremia in cancer patients with granulocytopenia. *N. Engl. J. Med.* **317:**1692–1698.

59. **Esposito, S., G. B. Gaeta, D. Galante, and D. Barba.** 1985. Successful treatment with ciprofloxacin of *Salmonella typhimurium* infection in an immunocompromised host. *Infection* **13:**288.

60. **Evans, T. G., and D. Riley.** 1992. *Campylobacter laridis* colitis in a human immunodeficiency virus-positive patient treated with a quinolone. *Clin. Infect. Dis.* **15:**172–173.

61. **Farrag, N. N., J. W. A. Bendig, C. Talboys, and B. S. Azadian.** 1986. In vitro study of the activity of ciprofloxacin combined with amikacin or ceftazidime against *Pseudomonas aeruginosa. J. Antimicrob. Chemother.* **18:**770.

62. **Fernandez, P. B., and R. N. Swanson.** 1988. Correlation of *in vitro* activities of the fluoroquinolones to their *in vivo* efficacies. *Drugs Exp. Clin. Res.* **14:**375–378.

63. **Fitzgeorge, R. B., D. H. Gibson, R. Jepras, and A. Baskerville.** 1985. Studies on ciprofloxacin therapy of experimental Legionnaires' disease. *J. Infect. Dis.* **10:**194–203.

64. **Flaherty, J. P., D. Waitley, B. Edlin, D. George, P. Arnow, P. O'Keefe, and R. A. Weinstein.** 1989. Multicenter, randomized trial of ciprofloxacin plus azlocillin versus ceftazidime plus amikacin for empiric treatment of febrile neutropenic patients. *Am. J. Med.* **87**(Suppl. 5A):278S–282S.

65. **Follath, F., M. Bindschedler, M. Wenk, R. Frei, H. Stalder, and H. Reber.** 1986. Use of ciprofloxacin in the treatment of *Pseudomonas aeruginosa* infections. *Eur. J. Clin. Microbiol.* **5:**236–240.

66. **Frei, R., M. Bindschedler, H. Stalfer, H. Reber, and F. Follath.** 1988. Emergence of resistance to ciprofloxacin during therapy. *Rev. Infect. Dis.* **10**(Suppl. 1):S68.

67. **Gardembas-Pain, M., B. Desablens, L. Sensebe, T. Lamy, C. Ghandour, and M. Boasson.** 1991. Home treatment of febrile neutropenia: an empirical oral antibiotic regimen. *Ann. Oncol.* **2:**485–487.

68. **Gaultier, R. J., G. R. Donowitz, D. L. Kaiser, C. E. Hess, and M. A. Sande.** 1983. Double-blind randomized study of prophylactic trimethoprim-sulfamethoxazole in granulocytopenic patients with hematologic malignancies. *Am. J. Med.* **74:**934–940.

69. **Giamarellou, H., and G. Petrikkos.** 1987. Ciprofloxacin interactions with imipenem and amikacin against multiresistant *Pseudomonas aeruginosa. Antimicrob. Agents Chemother.* **31:**958–961.

70. **Giuliano, M., A. Pantosti, G. Gentile, M. Venditti, W. Arcese, and P. Martino.** 1989. Effects on oral and intestinal microfloras of norfloxacin and pefloxacin for selective decontamination in bone marrow transplant patients. *Antimicrob. Agents Chemother.* **33:**1709–1713.

71. **Gluckman, E., M. Cavazzana, A. Devergie, J. Meletis, G. Arlet, Y. Perol, and M. Boiron.** 1988. Prevention of bacterial infections after bone marrow transplantation using either absorbable broad spectrum antibiotics (pefloxacin and penicillin) or nonabsorbable broad spectrum antibiotics (cephalosporin, gentamicin, and bacitracin). *Pathol. Biol.* **36:**902–906.

72. **Gluckman, E., C. Roudet, I. Hirsch, A. Devergie, H. Bourdeau, C. Arlet, and Y. Perol.** 1991. Prophylaxis of bacterial infections after bone marrow transplantation. *Chemotherapy* (Basel) **37**(Suppl. 1):33–38.

73. **Gordin, F. M., C. J. Hackbarth, K. G. Scott, and M. A. Sande.** 1985. Activities of pefloxacin and ciprofloxacin in experimentally induced *Pseudomonas* pneumonia in neutropenic guinea pigs. *Antimicrob. Agents Chemother.* **27:**452–454.

74. **Guiot, H. F. L.** 1982. Role of competition for substrate in bacterial antagonism in the gut. *Infect. Immun.* **38:**887–892.

75. **Guiot, H. F. L., P. J. Van den Broek, J. W. M. Van der Meer, and R. Van Furth.** 1983. Selective antimicrobial modulation of the intestinal flora of patients with acute nonlymphocytic leukemia: a double-blind, placebo-controlled study. *J. Infect. Dis.* **147:**615–623.

76. **Gurwith, M. J., J. L. Braunton, B. A. Lank, G. K. M. Harding, and A. R. Ronald.** 1979. A prospective controlled investigation of prophylactic trimethoprim-sulfamethoxazole in hospitalized granulocytopenic patients. *Am. J. Med.* **66:**248–256.

77. **Haller, I.** 1985. Comprehensive evaluation of ciprofloxacin-aminoglycoside combinations against *Enterobacteriaceae* and *Pseudomonas aeruginosa* strains. *Antimicrob. Agents Chemother.* **28:**663–666.

78. **Haller, I.** 1986. Comprehensive evaluation of ciprofloxacin in combination with $\beta$-lactam antibiotics against *Enterobacteriaceae* and *Pseudomonas aeruginosa. Drug Res.* **26:**226–229.

79. **Hartlapp, J. H.** 1987. Antimicrobial prophylaxis in immunocompromised patients. *Drugs* **34**(Suppl. 1):131–133.

79a. **Herbrecht, R., K. L. Liu, S. Ortiz, F. Jehl, J. P. Bergerat, P. Dufour, B. Duclos, F. Maloisel, C. Giron, and F. Oberling.** 1990. *Program Abstr. 6th Int. Symp. Infect. Immunocompromised Host,* abstr. 107.

80. **Heseltine, P. N. R., D. M. Causey, M. D. Appleman, M. L. Corrado, and J. M. Leedom.**

1988. Norfloxacin in the eradication of enteric infections in AIDS patients. *Eur. J. Cancer Clin. Oncol.* **24**(Suppl. 1):S25–S28.

81. **Heseltine, P. N. R., and M. L. Corrado.** 1987. Compassionate use of norfloxacin. *Am. J. Med.* **82**(Suppl. 6B):88–92.
82. **Ho, W. G., and D. J. Winston.** 1986. Infection and transfusion therapy in acute leukemia. *Clin. Hematol.* **15:**873–904.
83. **Hoogeterp, J. J., H. Mattie, and P. Terporten.** 1988. The relative efficacies of tobramycin and ciprofloxacin against *Pseudomonas aeruginosa* in vitro and in normal and granulocytopenic mice. *Infection* **16:**58–62.
84. **Hooper, D. C., and J. S. Wolfson.** 1991. Drug therapy: fluoroquinolone antimicrobial agents. *N. Engl. J. Med.* **324:**384–394.
85. **Hooper, T. L., F. K. Gould, C. R. Swinburn, N. J. Odom, P. A. Corris, R. Freeman, and C. G. A. McGregor.** 1982. Ciprofloxacin: a preferred treatment for Legionella infections in patients receiving cyclosporin A. *J. Antimicrob. Chemother.* **22:**952–953.
86. **Horsburgh, C. R.** 1991. *Mycobacterium avium* complex infection in the acquired immunodeficiency syndrome. *N. Engl. J. Med.* **324:**1332–1338.
87. **Horsburgh, C. R., J. A. Havlik, D. A. Ellis, E. Kennedy, S. A. Fann, R. E. Dubois, and S. E. Thompson.** 1991. Survival of patients with acquired immune deficiency syndrome and disseminated *Mycobacterium avium* complex infection with and without antimycobacterial chemotherapy. *Am. Rev. Respir. Dis.* **144:**557–559.
88. **Hughes, W. T., D. Armstrong, G. P. Bodey, R. Feld, G. L. Mandell, J. D. Meyers, P. A. Pizzo, S. C. Schimpff, J. L. Shenep, J. C. Wade, L. S. Young, and M. D. Yow.** 1990. Guidelines for the use of antimicrobial agents in neutropenic patients with unexplained fever. *J. Infect. Dis.* **161:**381–396.
89. **Hyatt, D. S., T. R. F. Rogers, D. M. McCarthy, and D. S. Samson.** 1991. A randomized trial of ciprofloxacin plus azlocillin versus netilmicin plus azlocillin for the empirical treatment of fever in neutropenic patients. *J. Antimicrob. Chemother.* **28:**324–326.
90. **Inderlied, C. B., P. T. Kolonski, M. Wu, and L. S. Young.** 1989. Amikacin, ciprofloxacin, and imipenem treatment for disseminated *Mycobacterium avium* complex infection of beige mice. *Antimicrob. Agents Chemother.* **33:**176–180.

90a. **Inderlied, C. B., F. G. Sandoval, and L. S. Young.** 1990. *Program Abstr. 30th Intersci. Conf. Antimicrob. Agents Chemother.*, abstr. 1241.

91. **Jacobson, M. A., S. M. Hahn, J. L. Gerberding, B. Lee, and M. A. Sande.** 1989. Ciprofloxacin for Salmonella bacteremia in the acquired immunodeficiency syndrome (AIDS). *Ann. Intern. Med.* **110:**1027–1029.

91a. **Jacobson, M. A., D. Yajko, D. Northfeelt, E. Charlebois, D. Gary, C. Brosgart, and K. Hadley.** 1992. *Program Abstr. 32nd Intersci. Conf. Antimicrob. Agents Chemother.*, abstr. 895.

92. **Jadoul, M., Y. Pirson, and C. Van Ypersele de Strihou.** 1989. Norfloxacin and cyclosporine—a safe combination. *Transplantation* **62:**747–748.
93. **Janin, N., H. Meugnier, J. F. Desnottes, R. Woehrle, and J. Fleurette.** 1987. Recovery of pefloxacin in saliva and feces and its action on oral and fecal floras of healthy volunteers. *Antimicrob. Agents Chemother.* **31:**1665–1668.
94. **Jensen, C. W. B., S. M. Flechner, and C. T. Van Buren.** 1987. Exacerbation of cyclosporine toxicity by concomitant administration of erythromycin. *Transplantation* **43:**263–270.

94a. **Johnson, P. R. E., J. A. Liu Yin, and J. A. Tooth.** 1989. *16th Int. Congr. Chemother.*, abstr. 70.

94b. **Jules, K., and H. C. Neu.** 1984. *Program Abstr. 24th Intersci. Conf. Antimicrob. Agents Chemother.*, abstr. 27.

95. **Karp, J. E., J. D. Dick, and W. G. Merz.** 1988. Systemic infection and colonization with and without prophylactic norfloxacin use over time in the granulocytopenic, acute leukemia patient. *Eur. J. Clin. Oncol.* **24**(Suppl. 1):S5–S13.
96. **Karp, J. E., W. G. Menz, C. Hendricksen, B. Laughon, T. Redden, B. Bamberger, J. G. Bartlett, R. Saral, and P. J. Burke.** 1986. Oral norfloxacin for prevention of gram-negative bacterial infections in patients with acute leukemia and granulocytopenia. A randomized double-blind, placebo-controlled trial. *Ann. Intern. Med.* **106:**1–7.
97. **Kelsey, S. M., P. W. Collins, C. Delord, B. Weinhard, and A. C. Newland.** 1990. A randomized study of teicoplanin plus ciprofloxacin versus gentamicin plus piperacillin for the empirical treatment of fever in neutropenic patients. *Br. J. Haematol.* **1990**(Suppl. 2):10–13.
98. **Kelsey, S. M., M. E. Wood, E. Shaw, G. C. Jenkins, and A. C. Newland.** 1990. A comparative study of intravenous ciprofloxacin and benzylpenicillin versus netilmicin and piperacillin for the empirical treatment of fever in neutropenic patients. *J. Antimicrob. Chemother.* **25:**149–157.
99. **Kelsey, S. M., M. E. Wood, E. Shaw, and A. C. Newland.** 1989. Intravenous ciprofloxacin as empirical treatment of febrile neutropenic patients. *Am. J. Med.* **87**(Suppl. 5A):274S–277S.
100. **Kemper, C. A., T. C. Meng, J. Nussbaum, J. Chin, D. F. Feigal, A. E. Bartok, J. M. Leedum, J. G. Tilles, S. C. Deresinski, J. A. McCutchan, and the California Collaborative**

**Treatment Group.** 1992. Treatment of *Mycobacterium avium* complex bacteremia in AIDS with a four-drug oral regimen. Rifampin, ethambutol, clofazimine, and ciprofloxacin. *Ann. Intern. Med.* **116:**466–472.

101. **Kerlikowski, K. M., and M. H. Katz.** 1992. *Mycobacterium avium* complex and *Mycobacterium tuberculosis* in patients infected with the human immunodeficiency virus. *West. J. Med.* **157:**144–148.
102. **Kern, W., and E. Kurrle.** 1991. Ofloxacin versus trimethoprim-sulfamethoxazole for prevention of infection in patients with acute leukemia and granulocytopenia. *Infection* **19:**73–80.
103. **Kern, W., K. Linzmeier, and E. Kurrle.** 1989. Antimicrobial susceptibility of viridans group streptococci isolated from patients with acute leukemia receiving ofloxacin for antibacterial prophylaxis. *Infection* **17:**396–397.
104. **Kiess, W., R. Haas, and W. Marget.** 1984. Chloramphenicol-resistant *Salmonella tennessee* osteomyelitis. *Infection* **12:**359.
105. **Klastersky, J., L. Debusscher, and D. Daneau.** 1974. Use of oral antibiotics in protected environment units: clinical effectiveness and role in the emergence of antibiotic-resistant strains. *Pathol. Biol.* **22:**5–12.
106. **Klastersky, J., S. H. Zinner, T. Calandra, H. Gaya, M. P. Glauser, F. Meunier, M. Rossi, S. C. Schimpff, M. Tattersal, C. Viscoli, and EORTC Antimicrobial Therapy Cooperative Group.** 1988. Empiric antimicrobial therapy for febrile granulocytopenic cancer patients: lessons from four EORTC trials. *Eur. J. Cancer Clin. Oncol.* **24**(Suppl. 1):S35–S45.
107. **Klein, E., M. Trautman, and H. G. Hoffmann.** 1986. Ciprofloxacin bei Salmonellen Infektion und Typhus abdominalis. *Dtsch. Med. Wochenschr.* **111:**1599–1602.

107a. **Kolonski, P. T., M. Wu, C. B. Inderlied, and L. S. Young.** 1990. *Program Abstr. 30th Intersci. Conf. Antimicrob. Agents Chemother.*, abstr. 1247.

107b. **Kolonski, P. T., M. Wu, C. B. Inderlied, and L. S. Young.** 1992. *Program Abstr. 32nd Intersci. Conf. Antimicrob. Agents Chemother.*, abstr. 1666.

108. **Kotilainen, P., J. Nikoskelainen, and P. Huovinen.** 1990. Emergence of ciprofloxacin-resistant coagulase-negative staphylococcal skin flora in immunocompromised patients receiving ciprofloxacin. *J. Infect. Dis.* **161:**41–44.
109. **Kramer, B. S., R. Ramphal, and K. H. Rand.** 1986. Randomized comparison between two ceftazidime-containing regimens and cephalothin-gentamicin-carbenicillin in febrile granulocytopenic cancer patients. *Antimicrob. Agents Chemother.* **30:**64–68.
110. **Krüger, H. U., U. Schuler, B. Proksch, M. Göbel, and G. Ehninger.** 1990. Investigation of potential interaction of ciprofloxacin with cyclosporine in bone marrow transplant recipients. *Antimicrob. Agents Chemother.* **34:**1048–1052.
111. **Levine, A. S., S. E. Siegel, A. D. Schreiber, J. Hauser, H. Preisler, I. M. Goldstein, E. Seidler, R. Simon, S. Perry, J. E. Bennett, and E. S. Henderson.** 1973. Protected environments and prophylactic antibiotics. A prospective controlled study of their utility in the therapy of acute leukemia. *N. Engl. J. Med.* **288:**477–483.
112. **Leysen, D. C., A. Haemers, and S. R. Pattyn.** 1989. Mycobacteria and the new quinolones. *Antimicrob. Agents Chemother.* **33:**1–5.
113. **Liang, R. H. S., R. W. H. Yung, T. K. Chau, P. Y. Chan, W. K. Lam, S. Y. So, and P. Todd.** 1990. Ofloxacin versus co-trimoxazole for prevention of infection in neutropenic patients following cytotoxic chemotherapy. *Antimicrob. Agents Chemother.* **34:**215–218.
114. **Liao, W. C., and M. S. Chappell.** 1989. Treatment with ciprofloxacin of *Aeromonas hydrophila* associated colitis in a male with antibodies to the human immunodeficiency virus. *J. Clin. Gastroenterol.* **11:**552–554.
115. **Lim, S. H., M. P. Smith, A. H. Goldstone, and S. J. Machin.** 1990. A randomized prospective study of ceftazidime and ciprofloxacin with or without teicoplanin as an empiric antibiotic regimen for febrile neutropenic patients. *Br. J. Haematol.* **76**(Suppl. 2):41–44.
116. **Lode, H.** 1989. Pharmacokinetics and clinical results of parenterally administered new quinolones in humans. *Rev. Infect. Dis.* **11**(Suppl. 5):S996–S1004.
117. **Maiche, A. G., and L. Teerenhovi.** 1991. Empiric treatment of serious infections in patients with cancer: randomised comparison of two combinations. *Infection* **19**(Suppl. 6):S326–S329.
118. **Malik, I. A., Z. Abbas, and M. Karim.** 1992. Randomised comparison of oral ofloxacin alone with combination of parenteral antibiotics in neutropenic febrile patients. *Lancet* **339:**1092–1096.
119. **Maschmeyer, G., S. Daenen, B. E. de Pauw, H. G. de Vries-Hospers, A. W. Dekker, J. P. Donnelly, W. Gaus, E. Haralambie, W. Kern, H. Konrad, H. Link, W. Sizoo, D. van der Waaij, M. von Eiff, and F. Wendt.** 1990. Prevention of infection in acute leukemia. *Hematol. Blood Transfusion* **33:**525–530.
120. **Maschmeyer, G., E. Haralambie, W. Gaus, W. Kern, A. W. Dekker, H. G. De Vries-Hospers, W. Sizoo, W. König, F. Gutzler, and S. Daenen.** 1988. Ciprofloxacin and norfloxacin for selective decontamination in patients with severe granulocytopenia. *Infection* **16:**98–104.
121. **McDonnell, R. W., L. J. Istorico, F. Q. Powell, S. Jagannath, and R. W. Bradsher.** 1990.

Streptococcal bacteremia in neutropenic patients treated with ciprofloxacin prophylaxis. *Clin. Res.* **38**:977A.

122. **McWhinney, P. H. M., S. H. Gillespie, C. C. Kibbler, A. V. Hoffbrand, and H. G. Prentice.** 1991. *Streptococcus mitis* and ARDS in neutropenic patients. *Lancet* **337**:429.

123. **Meletis, J., G. Arlet, E. Dournon, S. Pol, A. Devergie, C. Sportes, M. N. Peraldi, C. Mayaud, Y. Perol, and E. Gluckman.** 1987. Legionnaires' disease after bone marrow transplantation. *Bone Marrow Transplant.* **2**:307–313.

124. **Meunier, F., S. H. Zinner, H. Gaya, T. Calandra, C. Viscoli, J. Klastersky, M. Glauser, and EORTC International Antimicrobial Therapy Cooperative Group.** 1991. Prospective randomized evaluation of ciprofloxacin versus piperacillin plus amikacin for empiric antibiotic therapy of febrile granulocytopenic cancer patients with lymphomas and solid tumors. *Antimicrob. Agents Chemother.* **35**:873–878.

125. **Meyer, R. D., and S. Lin.** 1988. In vitro synergy studies with ciprofloxacin and selected beta-lactam agents and aminoglycosides against multidrug-resistant *Pseudomonas aeruginosa. Diagn. Microbiol. Infect. Dis.* **11**:151–157.

126. **Micozzi, A., P. Martino, R. Raccah, C. Eirmenia, G. Gentile, S. Santilli, and B. Monarca.** 1989. Pefloxacin in the treatment of gram-negative infections in patients with hematologic diseases. *Hematologica* **74**:583–585.

127. **Moody, J. A., D. N. Gerding, and L. R. Peterson.** 1987. Evaluation of ciprofloxacin's synergism with other agents by multiple in vitro methods. *Am. J. Med.* **82**(Suppl. 4A):44–54.

128. **Moody, J. A., L. R. Peterson, and D. N. Gerding.** 1985. In vitro activity of ciprofloxacin combined with azlocillin. *Antimicrob. Agents Chemother.* **28**:849–850.

129. **Murray, B. E.** 1989. Quinolones and the gastrointestinal tract. *Eur. J. Clin. Microbiol. Infect. Dis.* **8**:1093–1102.

129a. **Muszynski, M. J., R. K. Scribner, T. D. Lewis, and M. I. Marks.** 1985. *Program Abstr. 25th Intersci. Conf. Antimicrob. Agents Chemother.*, abstr. 1091.

130. **Nasir, M., C. Rotellar, M. Hand, L. Kulczycki, M. R. Alijani, and J. F. Winchester.** 1991. Interaction between ciclosporin and ciprofloxacin. *Nephron* **57**:245–246.

130a. **Nazareth, B., P. Ahmed, A. Bhamra, L. Ghandi, P. Noone, and H. G. Prentice.** 1990. *Program Abstr. 6th Int. Symp. Infect. Immunocompromised Host*, abstr. 192.

131. **Nelson, M. R., D. C. Shanson, D. Hawkins, and B. G. Gazzard.** 1991. Shigella in HIV infection. *AIDS* **5**:1031–1032.

132. **Neu, H. C.** 1989. Synergy of fluoroquinolones with other antimicrobial agents. *Rev. Infect. Dis.* **11**(Suppl. 5):S1025–S1034.

133. **Neu, H. C.** 1991. Synergy and antagonism of combinations with quinolones. *Eur. J. Clin. Microbiol. Infect. Dis.* **10**:255–261.

134. **Nguyen, M. H., J. E. Stout, and V. L. Yu.** 1991. Legionellosis. *Infect. Dis. Clin. N. Am.* **5**:561–584.

135. **Orlandi, E., A. Navarra, M. Cruciani, D. Caldera, E. Morra, C. Castagnola, E. Concia, and C. Bernasconi.** 1990. Norfloxacin versus cotrimoxazole for infection prophylaxis in granulocytopenic patients with acute leukemia. A prospective randomized study. *Hematologica* **75**:296–298.

136. **Orlando, P. L., S. L. Barriere, J. A. Hindler, and R. W. Frost.** 1990. Serum bactericidal activity from intravenous ciprofloxacin and azlocillin given alone and in combination to healthy subjects. *Diagn. Microbiol. Infect. Dis.* **13**:93–97.

137. **Pallivicini, F., A. Antinori, G. Federico, M. Fantoni, and P. Nervo.** 1989. Influence of two quinolones, ofloxacin and pefloxacin, on human myelopoiesis in vitro. *Antimicrob. Agents Chemother.* **33**:122–123.

138. **Patton, W. N., G. M. Smith, M. J. Leyland, and A. M. Geddes.** 1985. Multiply resistant *Salmonella typhimurium* septicemia in an immunocompromised patient successfully treated with ciprofloxacin. *J. Antimicrob. Chemother.* **16**:667–669.

139. **Pecquet, S., A. Andremont, and C. Tancrède.** 1986. Selective antimicrobial modulation of the intestinal tract by norfloxacin in human volunteers and in gnotobiotic mice associated with a human fecal flora. *Antimicrob. Agents Chemother.* **29**:1047–1052.

140. **Pecquet, S., A. Andremont, and C. Tancrède.** 1987. Effect of oral ofloxacin on fecal bacteria in human volunteers. *Antimicrob. Agents Chemother.* **31**:124–125.

141. **Pessina, A., M. G. Neri, A. Muschiato, E. Mineo, and G. Cocuzza.** 1989. Effect of fluoroquinolones on the in-vitro proliferation of myeloid precursor cells. *J. Antimicrob. Chemother.* **24**:203–208.

142. **Peterson, L. R., J. A. Moody, C. E. Fasching, and D. N. Gerding.** 1987. In vivo and in vitro activity of ciprofloxacin plus azlocillin against 12 streptococcal isolates in a neutropenic site model. *Diagn. Microbiol. Infect. Dis.* **7**:127–136.

143. **Philpott-Howard, J. N., K. F. Barker, J. J. Wade, R. S. Kaczmarski, J. C. Smedley, and G. J. Mufti.** 1990. Randomized multicentre study of ciprofloxacin and azlocillin versus gentamicin and azlocillin in the treatment of febrile neutropenic patients. *J. Antimicrob. Chemother.* **26**(Suppl. F):89–99.

144. **Pizzo, P. A., J. W. Hathorn, J. Hiemenz, M. Browne, J. Cummers, D. Cotton, J. Gress, D. Longo, D. Marshall, J. McKnight, M. Rubin, J. Skelton, M. Thaler, and R. Wesley.** 1986. A randomized trial comparing ceftazidime alone with combination antibiotic therapy in cancer patients with fever and neutropenia. *N. Engl. J. Med.* **315:**552–558.
145. **Pizzo, P. A., K. J. Robichaud, F. A. Gill, and F. G. Witebsky.** 1982. Empirical antibiotic and antifungal therapy for cancer patients with prolonged fever and granulocytopenia. *Am. J. Med.* **72:**101–111.
146. **Reeves, D. S.** 1986. The effect of quinolone antibacterials on the gastrointestinal flora compared with that of other antibacterials. *J. Antimicrob. Chemother.* **18**(Suppl. D):89–112.
147. **Robinson, J. A., F. R. Venezio, M. R. Costanzo-Nordin, R. Pifarre, and P. J. O'Keefe.** 1990. Patients receiving quinolones and cyclosporine after heart transplantation. *J. Heart Transplant.* **9:**30–31.
147a. **Robson, H. G., and M. Cote.** 1984. *Program Abstr. 24th Intersci. Conf. Antimicrob. Agents Chemother.*, abstr. 25.
148. **Rodriguez, V., G. P. Bodey, E. J. Freireich, K. B. McCredie, J. U. Gutterman, M. J. Keating, T. L. Smith, and E. A. Gehan.** 1978. Randomized trial of protected environment prophylactic antibiotics in 145 adults with acute leukemia. *Medicine* (Baltimore) **57:**253–266.
149. **Roosendaal, R., I. A. J. M. Bakker-Woudenberg, M. Van Den Berghe-Van Raffe, J. C. Vink-van Den Berg, and M. F. Michel.** 1987. Comparative activities of ciprofloxacin and ceftazidime against *Klebsiella pneumoniae* in vitro and in experimental pneumonia in leukopenic rats. *Antimicrob. Agents Chemother.* **31:**1809–1815.
150. **Rozenberg-Arska, M., A. Dekker, L. Verdonck, and J. Verhoef.** 1989. Prevention of bacteremia caused by alpha-hemolytic streptococci by roxithromycin (RU-28 965) in granulocytopenic patients receiving ciprofloxacin. *Infection* **17:**240–244.
151. **Rozenberg-Arska, M., A. W. Dekker, and J. Verhoef.** 1985. Ciprofloxacin for selective decontamination of the alimentary tract in patients with acute leukemia during remission induction treatment: the effect on fecal flora. *J. Infect. Dis.* **152:**104–107.
152. **Rubenstein, E., K. Rolston, C. Escalante, E. Manzullo, P. Hughes, B. Moreland, and G. P. Bodey.** 1990. Ambulatory treatment of fever in neutropenic patients. *J. Cancer Res. Clin. Oncol.* **116**(Suppl.):1150.
153. **Rubin, M., J. W. Hathorn, D. Marshall, J. Gress, S. M. Steinberg, and P. A. Pizzo.** 1988. Gram-positive infections and the use of vancomycin in 550 episodes of fever and neutropenia. *Ann. Intern. Med.* **108:**30–35.
154. **Sacks, L. V., A. M. Labriola, V. J. Gill, and F. M. Gordin.** 1991. Use of ciprofloxacin for successful eradication of bacteremia due to *Campylobacter cinaedi* in a human immunodeficiency virus-infected person. *Rev. Infect. Dis.* **13:**1066–1068.
155. **Schimpff, S. C.** 1980. Infection prevention during profound granulocytopenia. New approaches to alimentary canal microbial suppression. *Ann. Intern. Med.* **93:**358–361.
156. **Schimpff, S. C.** 1990. Infections in the compromised host—an overview, p. 2258–2265. *In* G. L. Mandell, R. C. Douglas, and J. E. Bennett (ed.), *Principles and Practice of Infectious Diseases,* 3rd ed. Churchill Livingstone, Inc., New York.
157. **Schimpff, S. C., W. H. Greene, V. M. Young, C. L. Fortner, L. Jepsen, N. Cusack, J. B. Block, and P. H. Wiernik.** 1975. Infection prevention in acute nonlymphocytic leukemia: laminar air flow room reverse isolation with oral, nonabsorbable antibiotic prophylaxis. *Ann. Intern. Med.* **82:**351–358.
158. **Schimpff, S. C., V. M. Young, W. H. Greene, G. P. Vermeulen, M. R. Moody, and P. H. Wiernik.** 1982. Origin of infection in acute nonlymphocytic leukemia. Significance of hospital acquisition of potential pathogens. *Ann. Intern. Med.* **79:**707–714.
159. **Seu, P., D. J. Winston, K. M. Olthoff, D. A. Bruckner, and R. W. Busuttil.** 1993. Legionnaires' disease in liver transplant recipients. *Infect. Dis. Clin. Pract.* **2:**109–113.
160. **Sleijfer, D. T., N. H. Mulder, H. G. De Vries-Hospers, V. Fidler, H. O. Nieweg, D. Van der Waaij, and H. K. F. Van Saeve.** 1980. Infection prevention in granulocytopenic patients by selective decontamination of the digestive tract. *Eur. J. Cancer* **16:**859–869.
161. **Somekh, E., B. Lev, E. Schwartz, A. Barzilai, and E. Rubinstein.** 1989. The effect of ciprofloxacin and pefloxacin on bone marrow engraftment in the spleen of mice. *J. Antimicrob. Chemother.* **23:**247–251.
162. **Somekh, E., S. West, A. Barzilai, and E. Rubinstein.** 1989. The lack of long-term suppressive effect of ciprofloxacin on murine bone marrow. *J. Antimicrob. Chemother.* **24:**209–213.
163. **Spito, A., H. Koga, H. Shigeno, K. Watanabe, K. Mori, S. Kohno, Y. Shigeno, Y. Suzuyama, K. Yamaguchi, M. Hirota, and K. Hara.** 1986. The antimicrobial activity of ciprofloxacin against *Legionella* species and the treatment of experimental *Legionella* pneumonia in guinea pigs. *J. Antimicrob. Chemother.* **18:** 251–260.
164. **Spito, A., K. Sawatari, Y. Fukuda, M. Nagasawa, H. Koga, A. Tomonaga, H.**

**Nakazato, K. Fujita, Y. Shigeno, Y. Suzuyama, K. Yamaguchi, K. Izumikawa, and K. Hara.** 1985. Susceptibility of *Legionella pneumophila* to ofloxacin in vitro and in experimental *Legionella* pneumonia in guinea pigs. *Antimicrob. Agents Chemother.* **28:**15–20.

165. **Stamm, W. E., L. E. Tompkins, K. F. Wagner, G. W. Counts, E. D. Thomas, and J. D. Meyers.** 1979. Infection due to *Corynebacterium* species in marrow transplant patients. *Ann. Intern. Med.* **91:**167–173.

166. **Storring, R. A., B. Jameson, T. J. McElwain, E. Wittshaw, A. S. P. Spies, and H. Gaya.** 1977. Oral nonabsorbable antibiotics prevent infection in acute nonlymphoblastic leukemia. *Lancet* **ii:**837–840.

167. **Stratton, C. W., J. J. Franke, L. S. Weeks, and F. A. Manion.** 1989. Comparison of the bactericidal activity of ciprofloxacin alone and in combination with selected antipseudomonal beta-lactam agents against clinical isolates of *Pseudomonas aeruginosa. Diagn. Microbiol. Infect. Dis.* **11:**41–52.

167a. **Szekely, E., T. Magyar, M. Baky, I. Bodrogi, M. Arr, and E. Ludwig.** 1991. *Program Abstr. 17th Int. Congr. Chemother.*, abstr. 988.

168. **Talbot, G. H., P. A. Cassileth, L. Paradiso, R. Correa-Coronas, L. Bond, and the Enoxacin Prophylaxis Study Group.** 1993. Oral enoxacin for infection prevention in adult acute nonlymphocytic leukemia. *Antimicrob. Agents Chemother.* **37:**474–482.

169. **Tan, K. K. C., A. K. Trull, and S. Shawket.** 1989. Co-administration of ciprofloxacin and cyclosporin: lack of evidence for a pharmacokinetic interaction. *Br. J. Clin. Pharmacol.* **28:**185–187.

170. **The GIMEMA Infection Program.** 1991. Prevention of bacterial infection in neutropenic patients with hematologic malignancies. A randomized, multicenter trial comparing norfloxacin with ciprofloxacin. *Ann. Intern. Med.* **115:**7–12.

171. **Thomson, D. J., A. H. Menkis, and F. N. McKenzie.** 1988. Norfloxacin-cyclosporine interaction. *Transplantation* **46:**312–313.

172. **Trautman, M., O. Brüchner, R. Marre, and H. Hahn.** 1988. Comparative efficacy of ciprofloxacin, ceftazidime, and gentamicin given alone or in combination, in a model of experimental septicemia due to *Klebsiella pneumoniae* in neutropenic mice. *Infection* **16:**49–53.

173. **Ulrich, E., M. Trautman, B. Krause, A. Bauernfeind, and H. Hahn.** 1989. Comparative efficacy of ciprofloxacin, azlocillin, imipenem/cilastatin, and tobramycin in a model of experimental septicemia due to *Pseudomonas aeruginosa* in neutropenic mice. *Infection* **17:**311–315.

174. **Unertl, K. E., F. P. Lenhart, H. Forst, G. Vogler, V. Wilm, W. Ehret, and G. Ruckdeschel.** 1989. Brief report: ciprofloxacin in the treatment of legionellosis in critically ill patients including those cases unresponsive to erythromycin. *Am. J. Med.* **87**(Suppl. 5A)**:**128S–131S.

175. **Van Buren, P. H., J. Koestner, A. Adedoyin, T. McCune, R. MacDonell, H. K. Johnson, J. Carroll, W. Nylander, and R. E. Richie.** 1990. Effect of ciprofloxacin on cyclosporine pharmacokinetics. *Transplantation* **50:**888–889.

176. **Van Der Auwera, P., M. Husson, and J. Klastersky.** 1988. Bactericidal activity and killing rate of serum in volunteers receiving pefloxacin alone or in combination with ceftazidime, piperacillin, or mezlocillin against *Pseudomonas aeruginosa. J. Antimicrob. Chemother.* **21:**49–55.

177. **Van Der Auwera, P., and J. Klastersky.** 1986. Bactericidal activity and killing rate of serum in volunteers receiving ciprofloxacin alone or in combination with vancomycin. *Antimicrob. Agents Chemother.* **30:**892–895.

178. **Van Der Auwera, P., J. Klastersky, S. Lieppe, M. Husson, D. Lauzon, and A. P. Lopez.** 1986. Bactericidal activity and killing rate of serum from volunteers receiving pefloxacin alone or in combination with amikacin. *Antimicrob. Agents Chemother.* **29:**230–234.

179. **Van der Waaij, D., J. M. Berghuis, and J. E. C. Lekkerkerk.** 1971. Colonization resistance of the digestive tract in conventional and antibiotic-treated mice. *J. Hyg.* **69:**405–411.

180. **Villablanca, J. G., M. Steiner, J. Kersey, N. K. C. Ramsay, P. Ferrieri, R. Haake, and D. Weisdorf.** 1990. The clinical spectrum of infections with viridans streptococci in bone marrow transplant patients. *Bone Marrow Transplant.* **6:**387–393.

180a. **Vogelman, B., S. Gudmundsson, S. Wolz, and W. Craig.** 1985. *Program Abstr. 25th Intersci. Conf. Antimicrob. Agents Chemother.*, abstr. 1092.

181. **Wade, J. C., C. A. DeJongh, K. A. Newman, J. Crowley, P. H. Wiernik, and S. C. Schimpff.** 1983. Selective antimicrobial modulation as prophylaxis against infection during granulocytopenia: trimethoprim-sulfamethoxazole vs. nalidixic acid. *J. Infect. Dis.* **147:**624–634.

182. **Wade, J. C., S. C. Schimpff, M. T. Hargadon, C. L. Fortner, V. M. Young, and P. H. Wiernik.** 1981. A comparison of trimethoprim-sulfamethoxazole plus nystatin with gentamicin plus nystatin in the prevention of infections in acute leukemia. *N. Engl. J. Med.* **304:**1057–1062.

183. **Wade, J. C., S. C. Schimpff, K. A. Newman, and P. H. Wiernik.** 1982. *Staphylococcus epidermidis:* an increasing cause of infection in patients

with granulocytopenia. *Ann. Intern. Med.* **97**:503-508.

184. **Walsh, T. J., J. Lee, J. Lecciones, M. Rubin, K. Butler, P. Francis, M. Weinberger, E. Roilides, D. Marshall, J. Gress, and P. A. Pizzo.** 1991. Empiric therapy with amphotericin B in febrile granulocytopenic patients. *Rev. Infect. Dis.* **13**:496-503.
185. **Watson, J. G., B. Jameson, H. R. L. Powler, T. J. McElwain, D. N. Lawson, I. Judson, G. R. Morgenstern, H. Lumley, and H. E. M. Kay.** 1982. Co-trimoxazole vs. nonabsorbable antibiotics in acute leukemia. *Lancet* **i**:6-9.
186. **Weber, P., Y. Boussougant, R. Farinotti, and C. Carbon.** 1989. Serum bactericidal activity against *Enterobacteriaceae* producing broad-spectrum beta-lactamases in volunteers administered ofloxacin and cefotaxime, alone or combined. *Eur. J. Clin. Microbiol. Infect. Dis.* **8**:524-526.
187. **Weiser, B., M. Lange, M. S. Fialk, C. Singer, T. H. Szatrowski, and D. Armstrong.** 1981. Prophylactic trimethoprim-sulfamethoxazole during consolidation chemotherapy for acute leukemia: a controlled trial. *Ann. Intern. Med.* **95**:436-438.
188. **Whiting, P. H., I. S. Simpson, and A. W. Thomson.** 1983. Nephrotoxicity of cyclosporine in combination with aminoglycoside and cephalosporin antibiotics. *Transplant. Proc.* **15**:2702-2706.
189. **Wilson, J. M., and D. G. Guiney.** 1982. Failure of oral trimethoprim-sulfamethoxazole prophylaxis in acute leukemia. Isolation of resistant plasmids from strains of Enterobacteriaceae causing bacteremia. *N. Engl. J. Med.* **306**:16-20.
190. **Wimperis, J. Z., T. P. Baglin, R. E. Marcus, and R. E. Warren.** 1991. An assessment of the efficacy of antimicrobial prophylaxis in bone marrow autografts. *Bone Marrow Transplant.* **8**:363-367.
191. **Winston, D. J.** 1993. Prophylaxis and treatment of infection in the bone marrow transplant recipient, p. 293-321. *In* J. S. Remington and M. N. Swartz (ed.), *Current Clinical Topics in Infectious Diseases,* vol. 13. Blackwell Scientific Publications, Inc., Boston.
192. **Winston, D. J., D. V. Dudnick, M. Chapin, W. G. Ho, R. P. Gale, and W. J. Martin.** 1983. Coagulase-negative staphylococcal bacteremia in patients receiving immunosuppressive therapy. *Arch. Intern. Med.* **143**:32-36.
193. **Winston, D. J., W. G. Ho, D. A. Bruckner, and R. E. Champlin.** 1991. Beta-lactam antibiotic therapy in febrile granulocytopenic patients. A randomized trial comparing cefoperazone plus piperacillin, ceftazidime plus piperacillin, and imipenem alone. *Ann. Intern. Med.* **115**:849-859.
194. **Winston, D. J., W. G. Ho, D. A. Bruckner, R. P. Gale, and R. E. Champlin.** 1990. Ofloxacin versus vancomycin/polymyxin for prevention of infections in granulocytopenic patients. *Am. J. Med.* **88**:36-42.
195. **Winston, D. J., W. G. Ho, R. E. Champlin, J. Karp, J. Bartlett, R. S. Finley, J. H. Joshi, G. Talbot, L. Levitt, S. Deresinski, and M. Corrado.** 1987. Norfloxacin for prevention of bacterial infection in granulocytopenic patients. *Am. J. Med.* **82**(Suppl. 6B):40-46.
196. **Winston, D. J., W. G. Ho, S. L. Nakao, R. P. Gale, and R. E. Champlin.** 1986. Norfloxacin versus vancomycin/polymyxin for prevention of infections in granulocytopenic patients. *Am. J. Med.* **80**:884-890.
197. **Wolfson, J. S., and D. C. Hooper.** 1989. Fluoroquinolone antimicrobial agents. *Clin. Microbiol. Rev.* **2**:378-424.
198. **Yajko, D. M., J. Kirihara, C. Sanders, P. Nassos, and W. K. Hadley.** 1988. Antimicrobial synergism against *Mycobacterium avium* complex strains isolated from patients with acquired immune deficiency syndrome. *Antimicrob. Agents Chemother.* **32**:1392-1395.
199. **Yajko, D. M., C. A. Sanders, P. S. Nassos, and K. Hadley.** 1990. In vitro susceptibility of *Mycobacterium avium* complex to the new fluoroquinolone sparfloxacin (CI-978; AT-4140) and comparison with ciprofloxacin. *Antimicrob. Agents Chemother.* **34**:2442-2444.
200. **Yates, J. W., and J. F. Holland.** 1973. A controlled study of isolation and endogenous microbial suppression in acute myelocytic leukemia. Cancer **32**:1490-1498.
201. **Young, L. S., O. G. W. Berlin, and C. B. Inderlied.** 1987. Activity of ciprofloxacin and other fluorinated quinolones against Mycobacteria. *Am. J. Med.* **82**(Suppl. 4A):23-26.
202. **Young, L. S., L. Wiviott, M. Wu, P. Kolonoski, R. Bolan, and C. B. Inderlied.** 1991. Azithromycin for treatment of *Mycobacterium avium-intracellulare* complex infection in patients with AIDS. *Lancet* **338**:1107-1109.

*Quinolone Antimicrobial Agents, 2nd ed.*
Edited by David C. Hooper and John S. Wolfson


*Chapter 25*

# Veterinary Use of Quinolones

***Craig E. Greene and Steven C. Budsberg***

Nalidixic acid, the first antibacterial quinolone developed for clinical use, has been used infrequently for many years in veterinary practice to treat urinary tract infections caused by gram-negative bacilli in dogs and cats. Gastrointestinal, hepatic, and neurologic complications have greatly restricted its use. In the past decade, newer quinolone derivatives such as cinoxacin, oxolinic acid, and flumequine have been used by veterinarians treating gram-negative bacterial infections in mammalian and avian species and farm-raised fish (20, 29, 46). For example, oxolinic acid has been used to treat furunculosis caused by *Aeromonas salmonicida* in freshwater salmon. Flumequine, which is approved for use in several countries, has been effective in treating enteric infections of farm livestock. Since the licensing of the newer fluoroquinolones norfloxacin and ciprofloxacin in 1985, extralabel use has occurred in treatment of canine and feline infections. Enrofloxacin, a fluoroquinolone that was never marketed for human use because it caused adverse psychologic effects, has been licensed exclusively for veterinary purposes since 1987 in Europe and since 1989 in the United States (47). It has received the most widespread experimental study and clinical use in veterinary species. Danofloxacin, another fluoroquinolone, has been directed for veterinary use in the treatment of bacterial respiratory infections of cattle, swine, and chickens (26, 39, 41).

***Craig E. Greene and Steven C. Budsberg*** • Department of Small Animal Medicine, College of Veterinary Medicine, University of Georgia, Athens, Georgia 30602.

## ANTIMICROBIAL ACTIVITY

The newest fluoroquinolones are more active against a variety of gram-negative and some gram-positive veterinary pathogens than are nalidixic acid and the earlier quinolones (9, 33, 59). They also have significant activity against persistent intracellular animal pathogens such as *Brucella, Listeria, Mycoplasma,* and *Chlamydia* spp. As for human bacterial isolates, a MIC of 1 μg/ml or less has been taken as a breakpoint to determine susceptibility or resistance of animal bacterial isolates to quinolones (48, 58). MICs greater than 2 or 4 μg/ml have been regarded as indicating resistance. A drug level of 1.0 μg/ml has also been used as a criterion for attaining adequate concentrations in serum, an indicator of a dosage regimen adequate for therapeutic purposes. Veterinary isolates of clinical importance that are generally highly susceptible to the quinolones (usual mean MICs of 0.008 to 0.06 μg/ml) are *Escherichia coli* and *Salmonella, Klebsiella, Pasteurella, Yersinia, Moraxella,* and *Haem-*

*ophilus* spp. Lower susceptibilities (mean MIC range, 0.125 to 0.5 μg/ml) are seen with *Serratia, Proteus, Campylobacter, Brucella, Bordetella, Vibrio, Staphylococcus, Erysipelothrix, Bacillus,* and *Mycoplasma* spp. (59).

The comparative MICs of ciprofloxacin, enrofloxacin, and norfloxacin for selected veterinary pathogens from cattle, pigs, sheep, goats, and horses have indicated strong activities against gram-negative pathogens such as *Pasteurella multocida, Actinobacillus (Haemophilus) pleuropneumoniae, Actinomyces pyogenes,* and *Haemophilus parasuis;* moderate activities against gram-positive organisms, including *Corynebacterium pseudotuberculosis* and *Erysipelothrix rhusiopathiae;* and low activities against *Streptococcus* spp. and *Rhodococcus equi* (Tables 1 and 2) (33, 59). Norfloxacin has generally been less active than ciprofloxacin and enrofloxacin. Enrofloxacin has been superior in activity against gram-negative veterinary pathogens and comparable for gram-positive organisms compared with oxacillin, penicillin G, and gentamicin (63). Enrofloxacin was also more active than older quinolones, since mean MICs of enrofloxacin were 20 to 30% of those of flumequine (63).

The same generalizations about antimicrobial activity are valid when isolates from particular animals are evaluated. For pathogens from pigs, the new fluoroquinolones have been more active in vitro against a wide variety of mycoplasmas and bacteria commonly associated with porcine respiratory infections than nalidixic acid and the earlier quinolones (33). Of the fluoroquinolones tested, ciprofloxacin has been the most active against the most strains of bacteria, including *Mycoplasma* spp., *Haemophilus* spp., *Bordetella bronchiseptica,* and *P. multocida.* Clinically recommended dosages of enrofloxacin for swine, given by oral (p.o.) or parenteral routes, have produced adequate levels in serum and tissue that exceeded the MICs for these organisms. Enrofloxacin has been highly active against pathogens of calves, including *E. coli, Klebsiella* spp., *Salmonella* spp., and *P. multocida,* and has good activity against *Campylobacter* spp. (60). Ciprofloxacin and norfloxacin also are effective in vitro against bacterial isolates from dogs. The order of susceptibility was *E. coli, Proteus mirabilis, Klebsiella pneumoniae, Staphylococcus intermedius, Pseudomonas aeruginosa,* and the *Bacteroides fragilis* group (71, 73). Many of the new fluoroquinolones show increased bactericidal activity against bacteria such as *A. salmonicida, Vibrio salmonicida,* and *Yersinia ruckeri,* which are pathogenic to fish (42).

## PHARMACOKINETICS

During development of all the 6-fluoroquinolone carboxylic acid compounds, a great deal of pharmacokinetic data has been generated in animal species. However, for practical purposes and to avoid duplication, the major focus of the pharmacokinetic discussion here pertains to agents currently recommended for use in veterinary medicine. In accordance with a previously described classification system, compounds are grouped by their predominant clearance pathways (21). The three compounds most used in veterinary medicine (enrofloxacin, norfloxacin, and ciprofloxacin) are all cleared predominantly by both renal and hepatic mechanisms. Additionally, danofloxacin is currently being developed for use in veterinary medicine and has similar renal and hepatic clearances.

### Enrofloxacin

Enrofloxacin, the first fluoroquinolone approved for veterinary use, is available in p.o. and parenteral formulations. Its structure is similar to that of ciprofloxacin, differing only in the addition of an ethyl group to the piperazinyl ring (Fig. 1). A portion of enrofloxacin is metabolized in vivo by *n*-dealkyation to ciprofloxacin, which is active in the body (24). p.o. administration has been studied in a number of species. Oral absorp-

**Table 1.** Comparative microbial susceptibilities in three fluoroquinolones

| Organism | Origin of isolates | Associated disease(s) | MIC range (no. of strains) | | | Reference(s) |
|---|---|---|---|---|---|---|
| | | | Norfloxacin | Ciprofloxacin | Enrofloxacin | |
| *Mycoplasma* spp. | Many domestic animals | Polyarthritis, conjunctivitis, pneumonia | 0.1–1.0 (40) | 0.025–1.0 (40) | 0.01–1.0 (108) | 33, 56, 59 |
| Gram-negative bacteria | | | | | | |
| *Haemophilus somnus* | Cow | Thromboembolic meningoencephalitis | 0.125 (10) | 0.015 (10) | 0.015 (10) | 56 |
| *Haemophilus parasuis* | Pig | Pneumonia | 0.03–0.06 (19) | 0.001–0.015 (19) | <0.001 (10) | 33, 56 |
| *Actinobacillus pleuropneumoniae* | Pig | Pleuropneumonia | 0.03–0.015 (19) | 0.0014–0.03 (19) | 0.01–0.06 (10) | 33, 56, 64 |
| *Actinomyces pyogenes* | Cow, sheep | Abscesses | 8.0 (10) | 1.0 (10) | 1.0 (10) | 56 |
| *Actinomyces suis* | Pig | Mastitis | 0.03 (7) | <0.001 (7) | 0.001–0.015 (7) | 56 |
| *Bordetella bronchiseptica* | Pig | Rhinitis, pneumonia | 7–16 (9) | 0.5–2 (9) | | 33 |
| *Pasteurella multocida* | Pig | Rhinitis, pneumonia | 0.03–0.25 (93) | 0.007–0.03 (93) | 0.007–0.12 (88) | 33, 56, 59 |
| *Pseudomonas aeruginosa* | Dog | Urinary and nosocomial infections, otitis externa | 0.156–1.25 (41) | ≤0.078–1.2 (41) | 0.25–8.0 (93) | 8, 47, 59, 71, 73 |
| *Escherichia coli* | Dog | Urinary and nosocomial infections | <0.078–0.625 (178) | 0.078–0.16 (178) | 0.01–2.0 (330) | 8, 47, 59, 71, 73 |
| *Proteus mirabilis* | Dog | Urinary and nosocomial infections | <0.078–0.313 (55) | ≤0.078–0.16 (55) | 0.03–0.5 (91) | 47, 59, 71, 73 |
| *Klebsiella pneumoniae* | Dog | Urinary and nosocomial infections | <0.078–0.625 (48) | ≤0.078–0.031 (48) | 0.03–0.5 (144) | 8, 47, 59, 71, 73 |
| Gram-positive bacteria | | | | | | |
| *Staphylococcus intermedius* | Canine | Pyoderma and nosocomial infections | 0.156–1.25 (135) | ≤0.078–0.16 (135) | 0.01–1.0 (147) | 59, 71, 73 |
| *Corynebacterium pseudotuberculosis* | Sheep, goat | Lymphadenopathy, abscesses | 0.3–8.0 (10) | 0.06–1.0 (10) | 0.125–0.5 (10) | 56 |
| *Rhodococcus equi* | Horse | Abscesses, pneumonia | 2.0–4.0 (10) | 0.5–1.0 (10) | 0.5–1.0 (10) | 56 |
| *Streptococcus equi* | Horse | Abscesses, strangles, navel, ill | 8.0 (10) | 1.0 (10) | 1.0 (10) | 56 |
| *Streptococcus suis* | Pig | Meningitis, sepsis | 8.0 (10) | 1.0 (10) | 0.5–1.0 (10) | 56 |
| *Streptococcus zooepidemicus* | Horse | Suppurative and genitourinary infections, septicemia | 8.0 (10) | 1.0 (10) | 1.0 (10) | 56 |
| Anaerobic bacteria | | | | | | |
| *Bacteroides fragilis* group (*B. fragilis*, *B. thetaiotaomicron*) | Canine | Suppurative infections, abscesses | >100 (25) | 12.5–25 (25) | 0.8–12.5 (27) | 47, 59, 71, 73 |

**Table 2.** Microbial susceptibility to enrofloxacin

| Type of bacterium | Origin of isolates (domestic animals) | Associated disease(s) | MIC range (no. of strains) | Reference(s) |
|---|---|---|---|---|
| Gram negative | | | | |
| *Moraxella bovis* | Cow | Infectious keratoconjunctivitis | 0.03–0.05 (5) | 59 |
| *Salmonella* spp. | Many | Enteritis, septicemia, arthritis, pneumonia, abortion | 0.003–1.0 (339) | 8, 59 |
| *Serratia marcescens* | Many | Nosocomial infection | 0.01–1.0 (20) | 59 |
| *Yersinia* spp. | Many | Enteritis, mesenteric adenitis | 0.01–0.04 (5) | 59 |
| *Campylobacter* spp. | Many | Enteritis | 0.03–0.25 (31) | 59 |
| *Brucella canis* | Dog | Infertility, abortion | 0.1–0.25 (5) | 59 |
| *Treponema hyodysenteriae* | Swine | Dysentery | 4.0 (5) | 59 |
| *Enterobacter* spp. | Dog | Urinary and noscomial infections | 0.06–1.0 (10) | 47 |
| *Bordetella bronchiseptica* | Dog | Tracheobronchitis, pneumonia | 0.001–0.12 (34) | 47, 59 |
| Gram positive | | | | |
| *Staphylococcus* spp. | Dog | Pyoderma, nosocomial infection | 0.031–0.5 (47) | 8, 47 |
| *Listeria monocytogenes* | Cattle | Meningoencephalitis | 1.0–2.0 (5) | 59 |
| *Corynebacterium pyogenes* | Sheep | Abscesses, septicemia | 0.06–4.0 (29) | |
| | Cattle | | | 59 |
| *Bacillus cereus* | Cattle | Abortion | 0.06–0.5 (48) | 59 |
| *Streptococcus* spp. | Many | Suppurative infections, mastitis, septicemia | 0.06–8.0 (139) | 8, 47, 59 |
| Anaerobic | | | | |
| *Clostridium perfringens* | Many | Enterotoxemia | 0.2–2.0 (34) | 47, 59 |

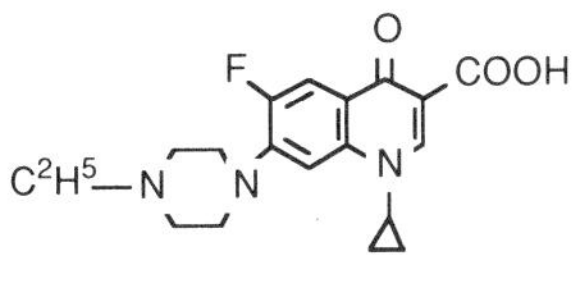

**Figure 1.** Chemical structure of enrofloxacin.

tion is rapid in most species, with peak concentrations in serum following bolus administration occurring at 0.5, 0.9 to 2.5, 1.4, 2.3, 2.3, 2.5, 2.6, 5.4, and 6 to 8 h in the horse, dog, turkey, pig, rabbit, chicken, cat, calf, and trout, respectively (4, 11, 12, 70, 72). Peak concentrations in serum following a 5-mg/kg bolus were 1.63, 1.36 to 1.66, 1.10, 0.45, 2.5, 1.9, and 0.55 $\mu$g/ml in the horse, dog, turkey, rabbit, chicken, cat, and calf, respectively. Table 3 contains additional comparative pharmacokinetic data on the p.o. administration of 5 mg of enrofloxacin per kg of body weight (4). The pharmacokinetics of intramuscularly (i.m.) and intravenously (i.v.) administered enrofloxacin have been studied in rabbits (16). The elimination half-lives ($t_{1/2}$s) for a 5-mg/kg dose were 2.2 $\pm$ 0.3 and 1.8 $\pm$ 0.3 h for i.v. and i.m. administration, respectively. The bioavailability was 92% following i.m. administration. Lower concentrations in serum have been reported when enrofloxacin was administered with milk replacer in calves (58). This decrease is speculated to be due to minerals in the milk replacer that could chelate the enrofloxacin (58, 70). In fingerling trout, enrofloxacin is widely distributed, with an average area-derived volume of distribution ($V_{area}$) of 2.9 liters/kg. This is similar to data for dogs (2.8 liters/kg), turkeys (3.1 liters/kg), and chickens (3.61 liters/kg) (11). Concentrations in serum and tissue fluid for enrofloxacin have been studied in dogs receiving 2.75, 5.5, and 11.0 mg/kg p.o. (72). Peak concentrations in serum increased with each dosage level and from the first to the seventh dose given.

## Norfloxacin

The pharmacokinetics of norfloxacin have been determined in the dog for single i.v. doses and single and multiple p.o. dosages (13). Dosages of 5, 10, and 20 mg/kg p.o. had peak concentrations in serum between 1 to 1.5 h of 0.811 $\pm$ 0.662, 0.525 $\pm$ 0.215, and 1.3 $\pm$ 0.423 $\mu$g/ml, respectively. The ratio of the area under the curve (AUC)/dose (dose-normalized AUC) decreased linearly as the dose increased. The authors of the study attributed this decrease to a dose-dependent

**Table 3.** Comparative pharmacokinetic parameters for enrofloxacin in five species following a single p.o. bolus administration of 5 mg/kg[a]

| Parameter[b] | Value for: | | | | |
|---|---|---|---|---|---|
| | Chicken ($n$ = 10) | Turkey ($n$ = 10) | Calf (10–6 wk old) | Dog ($n$ = 4) | Horse ($n$ = 3) |
| Compartmental model | | | | | |
| Apparent $k_a$ ($h^{-1}$) | 1.91 | 1.74 | 0.438 | 5.385 | 4.74 |
| Apparent $t_{1/2a}$ (h) | 0.36 | 0.40 | 1.58 | 0.13 | 0.15 |
| Apparent $k_e$ ($h^{-1}$) | 0.045 | 0.177 | 0.045 | 0.142 | 0.123 |
| Apparent $t_{1/2e}$ (h) | 15.6 | 3.9 | 15.4 | 4.9 | 5.6 |
| Noncompartmental model | | | | | |
| $t_{max(obs)}$ (h) | 2.5 | 1.4 | 5.4 | 0.90 | 0.51 |
| $C_{max(obs)}$ ($\mu$g/ml) | 1.49 | 1.10 | 0.55 | 1.66 | 1.63 |
| *F (%)* | 101 | 61 | 8 | 91 | 60 |

[a]Data are cited from reference 4 with permission.

[b]$k_a$, apparent first-order absorption rate constant; $t_{1/2a}$, apparent absorption $t_{1/2}$; $k_e$, apparent overall rate of elimination; $t_{1/2e}$, apparent elimination $t_{1/2}$; $t_{max(obs)}$, observed time to maximum serum drug concentration; $C_{max(obs)}$, observed maximum serum drug concentration; *F*, percent of oral dose absorbed.

decrease in absorption for the gastrointestinal tract. Serum pharmacokinetics following single i.v. bolus administration of 5 mg/kg were best described by a two-compartmental open model with first-order elimination (Table 4). The elimination $t_{1/2}$ was 3.56 h (harmonic mean). $V_{area}$ was 1.77 ± 0.69 liters/kg, indicating excellent distribution into the tissues. (In a crossover portion of the study, the bioavailability of oral norfloxacin was 35.0% ± 46.1%, with a mean residence time after p.o. administration of 5.71 ± 2.24 h.)

Despite the moderate bioavailability, concentrations in urine were sustained following p.o. administration over a 12-h period, with urine concentrations of 47.4 ± 20.6, 46.9 ± 28.3, and 80.0 ± 37.7 μg/ml for the 5-, 10-, and 20-mg/kg doses, respectively. In the multiple-dose test, drug accumulation was minimal.

Concentrations of norfloxacin in serum and tissue cage fluid (TCF) have been studied in dogs receiving the drug at 10 and 22 mg/kg p.o. (71).

Norfloxacin was rapidly absorbed, with maximal concentrations in serum observed at 1.5 h. Peak concentrations in serum for an 11-mg/kg dose were 1.0 ± 0.3 and 1.4 ± 0.5 μg/ml for the first and seventh doses, respectively. At 22 mg/kg, the peak concentrations in serum for the first and seventh doses were identical, i.e., 2.8 μg/ml. Tissue cages had slow penetration of norfloxacin, with maximal concentrations reached at 5 h. Peak concentrations were 0.3 ± 0.2 and 0.7 ± 0.3 when the first and seventh doses were 11 mg/kg and 1.2 ± 0.5 and 1.6 ± 0.2 when these doses were 22 mg/kg (Fig. 2). Norfloxacin was eliminated from the TCF slower than from serum. Elimination $t_{1/2}$ for the 11-mg/kg dose was 6.3 h for serum and 7.7 h for TCF, while the 22-mg/kg dose gave a $t_{1/2}$ of 6.7 h for serum and 8.7 h for TCF. The percentages of TCF penetration ($AUC_{TCF}/AUC_{serum}$) were 71% for the 11-mg/kg dose and 90% for the 22-mg/kg dose, indicating the ability of norfloxacin to diffuse into interstitial fluid.

The pharmacokinetics of i.v. and oral norfloxacin and its metabolites have been studied in broiler chickens (1). Peak concentration in plasma for 8 mg/kg given p.o. was 2.89 ± 0.20 μg/ml, occurring at 0.22 ± 0.02 h. Bioavailability of p.o. doses was 57.0 ± 2.4%. Considerable concentrations in tissue were found when the drug was given p.o. for 4 successive days. The concentration in fat, kidneys, and liver was 0.05 μg/ml after the dosing period.

**Table 4.** Pharmacokinetic values of norfloxacin[a]

| Variable[b] | Value (mean ± SD) |
|---|---|
| $C_1$ (μg/ml) | 4.86 ± 4.08 |
| $C_2$ (ng/ml) | 2.490 ± 1.08 |
| 1 ($h^{-1}$) | 1.48 ± 0.712 |
| 2 ($h^{-1}$) | 0.194 ± 0.0347 |
| $AUC_x$ (h·μg/ml) | 16.9 ± 6.38 |
| $AUMC_x$ ($h^2$·μg/ml) | 70.4 ± 25.2 |
| $V_{area}$ (liters/kg) | 1.77 ± 0.688 |
| $V_{ss}$ (liters/kg) | 0.332 ± 0.115 |
| MRT (h) | 4.32 ± 0.98 |
| $t_{1/2,1}$ (h) | 0.467 (0.282 to 1.24)[c] |
| $t_{1/2,2}$ (h) | 3.56 (2.63 to 4.20)[c] |

[a]Dose was 5 mg/kg given i.v. Predictive equations were used. Data are cited from reference 71 with permission.
[b]$C_1$, $C_2$, respective $y$ intercepts of the first and second terms of the equation; 1, 2, respective slopes of the first and second terms of the equation; $AUMC_x$, area under the moment curve; $V_{area}$, area-derived volume of distribution; $V_{ss}$, steady-state $V$; MRT, mean residence time; $t_{1/2,1}$, $t_{1/2,2}$, $t_{1/2}$ derived from the first and second terms in the equation, respectively.
[c]Harmonic mean (range).

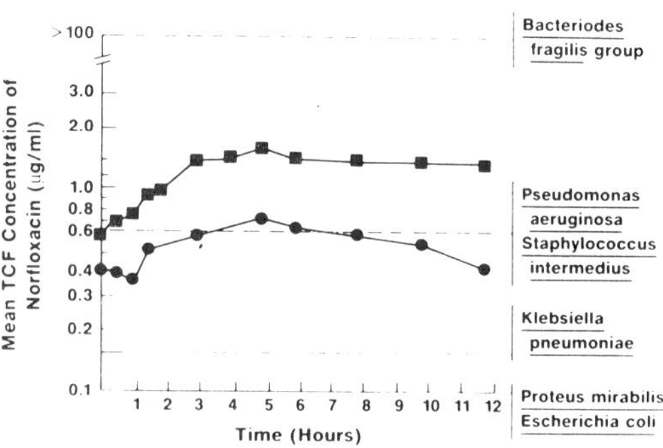


**Figure 2.** Mean concentration of norfloxacin in TCF versus time in four dogs administered 11 mg/kg (●) or, 22 mg/kg (■) p.o. compared with MIC for 90% of 171 clinical isolates from dogs.

## Ciprofloxacin

Concentrations of ciprofloxacin in serum and TCF have been evaluated in the dog in a model identical to that described for norfloxacin and enrofloxacin at 11 and 22 mg/kg, respectively (73). Table 5 summarizes these pharmacokinetic data. Following multiple doses, tissue penetration exceeds 95%. As with the other quinolones tested in this model, ciprofloxacin is rapidly absorbed; however, time to maximum concentration ($t_{max}$) for the TCF was 4 to 8 h, depending on dosage and number of doses. Elimination $t_{1/2}$s were much longer in tissue than in serum. p.o.- and i.v.-dose pharmacokinetics have been studied in calves and pigs (50). Following i.v. bolus administration, rapid distribution with large $V$ was noted. The calculated $V_{area}$ was significantly larger in the piglet, and while the distribution rate ($k_{12}$) was identical, back diffusion out of the peripheral compartment ($k_{21}$) was two to three times faster in the calf. Elimination $t_{1/2}$s for the two species were similar at 2.5 h. p.o. administration to calves showed a $t_{max}$ of 3 h with a maximum concentration in serum of 0.27 $\mu$g/ml and an elimination $t_{1/2}$ of 8.0 h. Bioavailability was calculated at 53.0% for the calf. Urinary recoveries following i.v. administration to calves and pigs were 45.6 and 47.9%, respectively.

The pharmacokinetics of ciprofloxacin have been evaluated in a number of fish species (49). The fish were medicated at 15 mg/kg i.m. and i.v. Similar elimination $t_{1/2}$s of approximately 14 h were noted following i.v. bolus infusion; however, striking differences were noted in $V$ and distribution rates ($k_{12}$, $k_{21}$) between species. i.m. injection showed rapid absorption ($t_{max}$ of less than 1 h) and elimination $t_{1/2}$ of between 20 and 23 h. Bioavailabilities for carp and trout were 61 and 87%, respectively, after i.m. injection. Plasma protein binding levels were 23.1, 21.6, and 20.2 for trout, carp, and catfish, respectively.

In red-tailed hawks, as in other species, there was rapid absorption of ciprofloxacin, with a $t_{max}$ of 0.81 h and good tissue distribution (35). The maximum concentration in serum was 2.96 $\mu$g/ml following a dosage of 50

**Table 5.** Pharmacokinetic values of ciprofloxacin for the dog[a]

| Pharmacokinetic parameter[b] | Value for: | | | |
|---|---|---|---|---|
| | Low dose (11 mg/kg) | | High dose (22 mg/kg) | |
| | Single | Multiple | Single | Multiple |
| Serum | | | | |
| $C_{max}$ ($\mu$g/ml) | 0.93 | 1.18 | 2.33 | 5.68 |
| $T_{max}$ (h) | 1.18 | 1.70 | 1.85 | 1.38 |
| $AUC_{0-12}$ ($\mu$g·h/ml) | 5.95 | 9.58 | 14.80 | 31.95 |
| $t_{1/2}$ (h) | 4.65 | 7.48 | 3.95 | 4.48 |
| TCF | | | | |
| $C_{max}$ ($\mu$g/ml) | 0.43 | 0.83 | 0.95 | 2.90 |
| $T_{max}$ (h) | 7.95 | 4.88 | 8.23 | 4.57 |
| $AUC_{0-12}$ ($\mu$g·h/ml) | 3.87 | 8.98 | 8.07 | 30.50 |
| $t_{1/2}$ (h) | 20.08 | 10.80 | 17.78 | 9.72 |
| $AUC_{TCF}/AUC_{serum}$ (%)[c] | 60.49 | 96.49 | 50.62 | 95.03 |
| Peak concn in TCF/concn in serum (5)[c] | 43.25 | 71.25 | 39.25 | 56.25 |

[a]Reported values represent the means for four dogs for each of the eight combinations of the three factors (dose frequency, size of dose, and site). Data are cited from reference 73 with permission.

[b]$C_{max}$, peak concentration; $t_{max}$, time to peak concentration; $AUC_{0-12}$, AUC from 0 to 12 h after drug administration. MS errors and standard errors of the means were, respectively, 1.16 and 0.54 for $C_{max}$, 1.51 and 0.61 for $t_{max}$, 14.46 and 1.90 for $AUC_{1-12}$, and 26.39 and 2.57 for $t_{1/2}$. The standard errors are calculated as (MS error/4)$^{1/2}$.

[c]Values are means for four dogs for each of the four combinations of two factors (dose frequency, dose size).

mg/kg. The elimination $t_{1/2}$ was 2.98 h, which is shorter than that reported for other species.

### Danofloxacin

Danofloxacin, or 1-cyclopropyl-6-fluoro-1,-4-dihydro-7-[(1*S*,4*S*)-5-methyl-2,5-diazabicyclo[2.2.1] hept-2-yl]-4-oxo-3-quinolinecarboxylic acid, differs from enrofloxacin by changes in the piperazinyl ring at the $R_7$ position. Danofloxacin pharmacokinetic values have been calculated for i.v., i.m., and subcutaneous (s.c.) administration in cattle (26). At 5 mg/kg, the calculated elimination $t_{1/2}$s, peak concentrations in serum, and AUCs for i.v., i.m., and s.c. administrations were 2.9, 2.9, and 4.3 h; 1.63, 0.82, and 0.63 μg/ml; and 6.0, 4.7, and 4.3 μg·h/ml, respectively. Bioavailabilities following i.m. and s.c. administrations were 78 and 72%, respectively. Similarly, in swine, danofloxacin was rapidly absorbed after i.v., i.m., and p.o. administrations of 5 mg/kg. Calculated elimination $t_{1/2}$s, peak concentrations in serum, and AUCs for i.v., i.m., and p.o. administrations were 8.0, 6.8, and 9.8 h; 1.05, 0.80, and 0.42 μg/ml; and 7.9, 6.0, and 7.0 μg·h/ml, respectively. Bioavailabilities for i.m. and p.o. drugs were 76 and 89%, respectively.

## CLINICAL USAGE

Laboratory animals such as rodents, rabbits, and nonhuman primates have been used to conduct many of the preclinical, pharmacodynamic, and toxicologic studies of quinolones. Similarly, many experimental models of infection in laboratory species have been used to evaluate the efficacies of these drugs (36, 48, 51, 52, 57). Although important for comparative and toxicological purposes, use of quinolones in these experimental subjects is not particularly relevant to routine veterinary clinical practice. Therefore, the following discussion focuses on the available information on quinolone usage in domestic animals. In veterinary practice, quinolones have been recommended primarily for therapy of gram-negative bacterial infections of the gastrointestinal respiratory and genitourinary systems and for therapy of secondary spread of such infections.

### Cattle

Enrofloxacin is available for use in cattle in some countries as an injectable solution for parenteral use and as a bolus or a liquid for p.o. administration. Because fermentation in the rumen of mature cattle precludes the p.o. use of quinolones in these animals, parenteral inoculation must be used. In suckling calves, quinolones are often given in milk replacer. The formulation for use in calves is a 5 or 10% parenteral solution, which is usually administered s.c. in divided dosages at a daily rate of 5 ml/100 or 200 kg of body weight (2.5 to 5 mg/kg/day). A viscous 2.5% p.o. solution is available and can be administered at a daily rate of 5 ml/50 kg.

Shipping fever is an acute respiratory infection of recently transported feedlot cattle that results from stress and compromised host defenses. Viruses, *Mycoplasma* spp., and bacteria such as *Pasteurella* spp. are most commonly isolated from sick animals. In spontaneous outbreaks of shipping fever, parenteral enrofloxacin at 5 mg/kg for 3 days has been found to be superior to standard oxytetracycline therapy (10 mg/kg) in improving clinical and blood gas abnormalities (40). Lower dosages of enrofloxacin (2.5 mg/kg) were as effective as oxytetracycline therapy, and all animals in these treatment groups that had not recovered improved when enrofloxacin was given at the higher dosage.

Respiratory disease, also common in congregated young calves that are still receiving milk substitutes, involves organisms similar to those involved in shipping fever. Parenteral tetracycline treatment and p.o. therapy with penicillins in milk substitutes have been routinely used for this condition. Enrofloxacin (2.5 mg/kg) given p.o. in milk substitutes for 8 days was more effective than placebo in producing clinical and bacteriologic cures in naturally infected calves (69). Isolation of *Pasteurella* spp. from nasal and tracheal washings and succeeding recurrence of respiratory disease were lower in treated animals.

In other studies of acute bronchopneumonia in calves treated with progressively graded therapeutic doses of enrofloxacin, doses of 2.5 mg/kg or more were more effective than gentamicin or no treatment (7, 8).

Pathogenic strains of *E. coli* produce diarrhea and septicemic disease in young calves. In experimental infection with *E. coli,* which was lethal if untreated, enrofloxacin (2.5 mg/kg) given p.o. or parenterally daily for 3 days was effective compared with no treatment or treatment with gentamicin, ampicillin, or folic acid antagonists (8). Similar results were obtained in studies of natural infections (7). Enrofloxacin treatment resulted in a reduction of diarrhea, a reduction in numbers of deaths, and recovery.

In colostrum-deprived calves artificially infected with *Salmonella typhimurium,* enrofloxacin given at 5 mg/kg for 3 days was effective in reducing clinical symptomatology (7, 23). Bacteriologic cure was achieved after 6 days of therapy. In older calves that were experimentally infected, dosages of 2.5 mg/kg or greater reduced clinical symptomatology and fecal carriage (10). In naturally infected herds where veal calves have been treated with 5 mg/kg for 5 days, the bacteriologic cure rate has been high but not absolute (7). However, in other herds given 5 or 10 mg/kg for 10 days, the elimination of fecal shedding of *Salmonella* spp. has been more complete (65).

## Pigs

Quinolones are administered to swine by the p.o. and i.m. routes. Enrofloxacin is available in some countries as an injectable for parenteral use and as a food additive. Pending Food and Drug Administration approval it may be similarly marketed in the United States. For swine, the drug has low palatability in drinking water. The 0.5% p.o. solution is given as a gavage to piglets at a rate of 1 ml/3 kg or as a 5% parenteral solution at a dose rate of 1 ml/20 kg (2.5 mg/kg). For piglet scours, a dose of 1.25 mg/kg in feed is effective, although 2.5 mg/kg is better. If the dose is given parenterally, 1 mg/kg is effective in reducing clinical symptomatology. In swine, quinolones have been recommended for treating respiratory diseases such as mycoplasmal (enzootic) pneumonia and polyarthritis; enteric infections such as diarrhea of suckling, weaning, or fattening pigs (coli diarrhea); septicemia caused by pathogenic *E. coli* (edema disease) or *Salmonella* spp.; and mastitis-metritis-agalactia (MMA).

According to MIC data for swine pathogens, enrofloxacin seems to be effective against *E. coli* and *Haemophilus, Mycoplasma, Pasteurella,* and *Salmonella* spp.

Treatment for piglet diarrhea and MMA lasts 2 to 3 days but may be longer and at a higher dose rate if salmonellosis is present. A minimum dose of 2.5 mg/kg daily is recommended for treating most established infections; however, doses as low as 1.25 mg/kg in feed have been effective for prophylaxis following exposure to pathogenic enteric bacteria (3). It is often difficult to achieve sufficient levels of antimicrobial agents given in medicated feed to pigs suffering from respiratory diseases, because these pigs have reduced food intake. Therefore, parenteral therapy is used in those instances. The duration of therapy varies with the type and site of infection and is generally shorter for diarrheic infections and MMA and longer for respiratory infections (7). Treatment of infections in swine by using quinolones usually requires a minimum duration of 8 to 10 days (27, 63).

For respiratory diseases, good antibacterial activities of quinolones against mycoplasmas give these drugs the potential for treating respiratory pathogens of swine, although other antimicrobial agents have similar my-

antimicrobial agents have similar mycoplasmacidal efficacies. Low dose rates of enrofloxacin (1.25 mg/kg) have been 100% effective for prophylaxis against experimental mycoplasma pneumonia, but 2.5 mg/kg has been superior for therapy of existing disease (7). A 6-chloro analog of norfloxacin administered at 400 ppm in food for 21 days markedly reduced the pneumonic lesions in pigs inoculated experimentally with 14 *Mycoplasma hyopneumoniae,* even though organisms persisted at low concentrations in these lesions (32). Concentrations of 200 ppm of the drug were not effective.

In controlled studies of swine infected with *A. pleuropneumoniae,* 60% of the pigs died 18 to 56 h after experimental inoculation. Enrofloxacin, administered i.m. for 3 days at 2.5 or 5 mg/kg beginning 8 h postinfection or at 5 mg/kg starting 12 h postinfection, facilitated recovery in all treated animals (7, 66). Clinical improvement began 12 h after therapy was instituted. In experimental studies of *A. pleuropneumoniae* infection, enrofloxacin given to pigs in the diet at a concentration of 150 ppm was effective in reducing the severity of clinical signs, pulmonary lesions, and isolation of the organism compared with levels in unmedicated control animals.

In pigs artificially infected with *Salmonella derby,* the organism was cleared from tissues and secretions after 10 days of therapy with enrofloxacin in the food at 200 ppm (45). In sows with MMA, parenteral dosing at 2.5 mg/kg was very effective in treating infection (7, 55).

## Dogs and Cats

Quinolones have found the widest use on an individual basis in companion animal practice. Because of the damage to developing cartilage these drugs can cause, their use is restricted to animals that have reached their full stature. Although pharmacologic and toxicologic studies with dogs and cats have been extensive, minimal data on treatment of experimentally infected animals or controlled clinical trials are available. Despite this major limitation, in vitro susceptibility data and limited clinical field studies indicate the benefit of their use (6, 25, 56). Clinical studies have shown benefits from treatment of dermatologic, connective tissue, respiratory, digestive, and genitourinary infections caused by gram-negative organisms. Resolution of lesions has also been reported in treatment of opportunistic mycobacterial infections of cats (67).

To avoid routine use and subsequent development of resistant strains, enrofloxacin should be limited to the treatment of infections caused by otherwise resistant gram-negative organisms or *Pseudomonas* spp. Those types of infections that most warrant the use of quinolones include chronic osteomyelitis, prostatitis, pyelonephritis, and bronchitis or pneumonia in addition to sepsis, bacterial endocarditis, wound infections, or enteritis caused by *Campylobacter* or *Salmonella* spp.

Extralabel use of norfloxacin and ciprofloxacin marketed for humans occurs in treatment of household pets, although enrofloxacin is the only quinolone licensed for use in dogs and cats. Enrofloxacin is available as p.o. and parenteral formulations. In the United States, it is marketed as 5.7-, 22.7-, and 68.0-mg tablets and as a p.o. solution of 22.7 mg/ml. The recommended dose for urinary infections is 2.5 mg/kg given twice daily. Higher doses are indicated for treatment of systemic infections and for those in whom tissue distribution is limited. A dosage of 11 mg/kg given twice daily was effective in maintaining continuous concentrations in serum and tissue fluid that exceeded the MIC for 90% of *P. aeruginosa* isolates (72). The duration of treatment is determined by the type, degree, and course of infection, and treatment is spread over 5 to 10 days. The dose rate in all the trials ranged between 4.5 and 6.7 mg/kg/day with treatment for 5 to 10 days. Use must be restricted to mature dogs and cats.

In a dose titration study in an artificial wound infection with *E. coli* and *Klebsiella*

related antibacterial activity (6). In natural urinary infections in dogs, clinical and bacteriologic improvement resulted, although long-term follow-up was not done (25). Treatment of prostate infections with quinolones may be beneficial, since experimental studies show therapeutic concentrations in the healthy canine gland, although treatment of infected animals has not been extensively studied.

### Horses

Although the fluoroquinolones have good potential for treatment of resistant gram-negative infections of horses, their use has been limited because of potential toxicity. Because cartilaginous and skeletal damage has occurred following treatment of young horses (8), quinolones are not recommended for use in these animals.

### Poultry

The quinolones have high efficacy against gram-negative bacteria and mycoplasmas (*Haemophilus paragallinarum, Salmonella* spp., *Pasteurella* spp., *E. coli, Mycoplasma* spp., and *Erysipelothrix*), the chief pathogens of poultry. In poultry, antibacterial substances are generally given by drinking water, and enrofloxacin is available in some countries as a 10% solution for this purpose. Good palatability and tolerability of quinolones when administered in the drinking water makes them suitable drugs for this purpose (5). As a result of clinical studies, a concentration of 25 to 50 ppm (25 to 50 mg of active ingredient per liter) of enrofloxacin in the drinking water is recommended for chickens and turkeys for therapeutic and prophylactic use. At this concentration, a p.o. intake of 8 to 10 mg/kg/day, considered a therapeutic minimum, is achieved. Quinolones are also available in an injectable form for medication of individual turkey poults. Quinolones are generally given for 3 to 5 days in the treatment of most infections, while those caused by *Salmonella* spp. involve longer treatment periods.

The efficacy of enrofloxacin against poultry pathogens such as *Mycoplasma* spp., *E. coli, H. paragallinarum, Salmonella* spp., *P. multocida,* and *E. rhusiopathiae* has been evaluated in experimental infections (5). When organisms are of low resistance (*Haemophilus* or *Mycoplasma* spp.) or when risk of infection is low, control has been definite. For salmonellosis or *E. coli* infections, elimination of the carrier state has been impossible, and the dose and duration of treatment must be greater than for other infections.

For *Mycoplasma gallisepticum,* infected chicks and turkey pullets have been treated with 12.5 or 25 ppm of the drug in drinking water for 3 to 5 days. Enrofloxacin at either concentration has been more effective than tiamulin or tylosin given for a similar period. Enrofloxacin at 50 ppm has eliminated *M. gallisepticum* from pulmonary tissues. For chicks, similar studies that compared 50 ppm of danofloxacin in drinking water for 3 days with tylosin or no treatment showed a reduction of *M. gallisepticum* in tissues and occurrence of air sac lesions (39).

Similarly, dose rates of enrofloxacin of 25 to 50 ppm for 5 days have been effective in treating artificial infections with *E. coli* alone or in conjunction with infectious bronchitis virus, *M. gallisepticum,* or *S. typhimurium* (5, 8).

Studies involving turkeys with coryza (*Haemophilus gallinarum* infection) showed good clinical and microbiologic control with 50 ppm of enrofloxacin in the drinking water for 3 days. Similarly, in other studies of *P. multocida* infection, disease and mortality rates were lowered by a minimum dose of 25 ppm for 5 days (8, 43).

In salmonellosis, latent and clinical manifestations of disease have been prevented by 50 to 200 ppm of enrofloxacin in the drinking water of chickens and turkeys; however, bacteriologic cures have been uncertain, and reshedding of organisms has often occurred 1 week after medication was discontinued (5). Arizonosis was induced by inoculation of *Salmonella arizonae* into turkey poults (8). Treatment with a single i.m. injection of enrofloxacin over a dose range of 0.25 to 4.0 mg per poult was beneficial compared with no treatment, which resulted in a mortality rate of 45%. Survival paralleled the dosage given, with no mortality noted at the highest dosage level. In *Salmonella pullorum* infections, 25 to 100 ppm for 6 days resolved illness and shedding in 80% of the cases compared with a comparatively poor response to flumequine and furazolidone (5).

## TOXICITY

The target tissues for the fluoroquinolones are juvenile cartilage, digestive tract, central nervous system, urinary tract, and eye. It must be pointed out that other than the capability for cartilage damage, the side effects of the fluoroquinolones in domestic animals are extremely few.

### Juvenile Arthropathies

Administration of any of the quinolone agents to immature animals will induce lesions in the cartilage of the major diarthrodial joints (14, 18, 30, 31, 37, 38, 44). Gross lesions have been generally described as fluid-filled vesicles that project above the contour of the articular surface, with histological lesions occurring in the intermediate zone (14, 30, 31, 38). In dogs given difloxacin daily, gross and microscopic lesions were found after only 2 days (14). Macroscopically, lesions were fluid-filled vesicles or cartilaginous flaps, while microscopically, the earliest lesions were fissures in the cartilage filled with clumps of collagen fibrils and clumps of granular extracellular material. Chondrocytes with shrunken cytoplasms and nuclei were seen adjacent to the fissures along with histologically normal chondrocytes. Ultrastructural changes, seen as early as 24 h, include chondrocyte mitochondrial swelling and enlargement of cytoplasmic vacuoles (15). Extracellular matrix changes were limited to cartilage from dogs of the 48-h group. Thus, the ultrastructural changes in chondrocytes preceded changes in the matrix (15). Histochemically, collagen fibrils were unmasked and proteoglycan was lost from the matrix of the lesions (14). Burkhardt et al. inferred that the different responses of the chondrocytes were due to intrinsic differences in the chondrocytes rather than differences in their microenvironments. Also, there were characteristic sites of lesions on weight-bearing surfaces. This finding combined with earlier data suggested the importance of weight bearing in the pathogenesis of the lesions caused by difloxacin and other quinolones (14, 37). Similar pathologic changes have been found in dogs given oxolinic and pipemidic acids (68). A dose-related incidence of lesions was found in a 500-mg/kg dosage comparison; prevalence and severity of articular cartilage lesions were greater with pipemidic acid than with oxolinic acid (30).

However, animal species have different sensitivities to a given agent, and arthropathy findings reported for one quinolone compound are not necessarily transferable to another (14, 17, 37, 44). The younger the animal, the worse the lesions and the shorter the interval between drug administration and development of the lesion (18). The dog seems to be the most sensitive species tested. Articular cartilage lesions have been documented in 3- to 4-month-old puppies given dosages of 5, 15, or 25 mg of enrofloxacin per kg/day, 20 mg of norfloxacin per kg/day, or 30 mg of ciprofloxacin per kg/day (2, 18). Limited data from the manufacturer also describe cartilaginous abnormalities in cats given 25 mg of a quinolone per kg/day but not in those given 15 mg/kg/day (2). Toxicity problems associated with cartilage and bone development have also occurred with enrofloxacin use in young horses (8).

Many toxicity tests have entailed use of dosage regimens far exceeding those recommended for the given species (e.g., 300 mg/kg/day). Also, many of the studies were done in rats, and comparatively much larger dosages are necessary to create equivalent lesions in the dog (18). Thus, interpretation of these experimental models must be done carefully when data are extrapolated to the clinical situation.

## Other Systems

### Digestive system

Excessive dosages (15 to 50 times the recommended amounts) of quinolones cause vomiting and anorexia. In a more practical situation, the following disturbances have been noted. Vomiting has been occasionally noted in dogs given norfloxacin at a dosage of 20 to 22 mg/kg, but the vomiting abated when the dosage was lowered to 16.5 mg/kg (13, 71). Dogs have vomited following i.v. bolus injections (13). African grey parrots given water medicated with enrofloxacin at concentrations of 1.5 to 3.0 mg/ml have shown anorexia, polydipsia, and weight loss (24).

### Central nervous system

Norfloxacin given in an i.v. bolus caused one dog to have seizures. It was speculated that the high transient initial concentration of norfloxacin in the central nervous system stimulated the centers responsible for vomiting or precipitation of seizures (13). For this reason, it is recommended that if quinolones are given i.v., infusion should be constant. Electroencephalogram changes have been observed in cats and dogs only after i.v. injection at dosages of ≥25 mg/kg (18). One clinical report indicated an increase in the frequency and intensity of seizures in phenobarbital-treated epileptic dogs given enrofloxacin (70).

### Urinary system

Crystalluria is the major renal abnormality noted in animals (17, 18, 61, 70). Renal tolerance of the quinolones is linked to the pH-dependent solubilities of each compound, and doses that induce a distinct crystalluria do not necessarily cause renal damage. However, nephropathologic changes do not seem to occur without crystalluria (18). As noted above, dosages used in most of these studies were far greater than therapeutic dosage regimens.

### Ocular system

Pefloxacin and rosoxacin given at extremely high dosages over a period of months cause lenticular opacities in the dog. The clinical relevance of these findings is unclear (18).

# PUBLIC HEALTH CONSIDERATIONS

## Zoonotic Potential

From a human health standpoint, the greatest risk of acquiring antimicrobial-resistant bacteria from animals resides in ingestion of foodstuffs from animal sources and in direct animal contact with treated animals or antimicrobial agents on the farm or in processing plants by animal handlers. A second source of contact with quinolone-resistant bacteria could arise from contact with household pets that have developed resistant strains as a result of prior treatment. Although many possibilities exist, the greatest sources of human contact with bacterial strains from pets have been saliva from bites or licking of wounds and fecal contamination from animals with diarrhea. Large-scale use of quinolones in veterinary medicine may lead to an increase in infection with antimicrobial-resistant bacteria in people who are otherwise not exposed to these drugs.

## Emerging Resistance

Indirect evidence indicates that quinolone-resistant bacteria are emerging in treated animal populations and that these bacteria may pose a threat to human health. The greatest proof comes from studies of poultry. *Campylobacter jejuni,* which has been recognized as a common cause of human diarrhea, arises from animal sources (28). Contact with uncooked poultry or diarrheic kittens has been shown to be the most common risk factor in affected people in the United States (19). According to in vitro data, *Campylobacter* spp. are more resistant to quinolones than *Salmonella* or *Shigella* spp.; therefore, any increased resistance of *Campylobacter* spp. makes quinolone efficacy questionable. In The Netherlands, *Campylobacter* strains have been examined for antimicrobial susceptibility to ciprofloxacin between the years 1982 and 1989 with the knowledge that veterinary use of quinolones began in 1987 with the licensing of enrofloxacin (22). In the years 1982 to 1983, none of the isolates from humans or poultry were resistant; however, from 1987 to 1988, resistance levels were 8 and 8.4%, respectively, and in 1989, they were 11 and 14%, respectively. Since poultry are of major significance in human campylobacteriosis, the extensive use of quinolones as feed additives may have led to a transfer of resistant bacterial populations to people. Similar increased levels of resistance to nalidixic acid, norfloxacin, ciprofloxacin, and enrofloxacin have been noted in strains of salmonellae isolated from poultry since the use of quinolones as feed additives began (53, 54, 74, 75).

## REFERENCES


1. **Anadón, A., M. R. Martinez-Larrânaga, C. Velez, M. J. Dìaz, and P. Bringas.** 1992. Pharmacokinetics of norfloxacin and its N-desethyl- and oxometabolites in broiler chickens. *Am. J. Vet. Res.* **53:**2084–2089.
2. **Anonymous.** 1991. Quinolones. *Compend. Vet. Pract.* **1:**105–106.
3. **Awas-Masalmeh, M., and H. Willinger.** 1987. Untersuchunger uber die Wirkung von Baytril gegen E. coli-Infektionen von Saug und Absatzterkein. *Wien. Tierarzt. Monatschr.* **7:**105–108.
4. **Babish, J., J. Wilder, and J. Davidson.** The comparative pharmacokinetics of a new quinolone, enrofloxacin in dogs, horses, calves, chickens and turkeys. *J. Vet. Pharmacol. Ther.*, in press.
5. **Bauditz, R.** 1987. Results of clinical studies with Baytril in poultry. *Vet. Med. Rev.* **2:**130–136.
6. **Bauditz, R.** 1987. Results of clinical studies with Baytril in dogs and cats. *Vet. Med. Rev.* **2:**137–140.
7. **Bauditz, R.** 1987. Results of clinical studies with Baytril in calves and pigs. *Vet. Med. Rev.* **2:**122–129.
8. **Berg, J.** 1988. Clinical indications for enrofloxacin in domestic animals and poultry, p. 25–34. *Proc. West. Vet. Conf.*
9. **Berg, J., G. Ling, J. Davidson, J. Newman, D. Copeland, H. McCurdy, and R. Stewart.** 1987. Susceptibility of bacterial isolates to a new quinolone antimicrobial, BAY VP 2674, p. 151. *Proc. XXII World Vet. Congr.*
10. **Berg, J., K. Vogelweid, and D. Wendell.** 1986. Efficiacy of a new quinolone compound (BAY Vp 2674) in treatment of experimentally induced salmonellosis in cattle, abstr. A-39, p. 7. *Abstr. Annu. Meet. Am. Soc. Microbiol. 1986.*
11. **Bowser, P. R., G. A. Wooster, J. St. Leger, and J. G. Babish.** 1992. Pharmacokinetics of enrofloxacin in fingerling rainbow trout (Oncorhynehus mykiss). *J. Vet. Pharmacol. Ther.* **15:**62–71.
12. **Broome, R. L., D. L. Brooks, J. G. Babish, D. D. Copeland, and G. M. Conzelman.** 1991. Pharmacokinetic properties of enrofloxacin in rabbits. *Am. J. Vet. Res.* **52:**1835–1841.
13. **Brown, S. A., J. Cooper, J. J. Gauze, D. S. Greco, D. W. Weise, and J. M. Buck.** 1990. Pharmacokinetics of norfloxacin in dogs after single intravenous and single and multiple oral administrations of the drug. *Am. J. Vet. Res.* **51:**1065–1070.
14. **Burkhardt, J. E., M. A. Hill, W. W. Carlton, and J. W. Kesterson.** 1990. Histologic and histochemical changes in articular cartilages of immature beagle dogs dosed with difloxacin, a fluoroquinolone. *Vet. Pathol.* **27:**162–170.
15. **Burkhardt, J. E., M. A. Hill, J. J. Turek, and W. W. Carlton.** Ultrastructural changes in articular cartilages of immature beagle dogs dosed with difloxacin, a fluoroquinolone. *Vet. Pathol.* **29:**230–238.
16. **Cabanes, A., M. Arbaix, J. M. Garcia Anton, and F. Reig.** 1992. Pharmacokinetics of enrofloxacin after intravenous and intramuscular injection in rabbits. *Am. J. Vet. Res.* **53:**2090–2093.
17. **Corrado, M. L., W. E. Struble, C. Peter, V. Hoagland, and J. Sabbaj.** 1987. Norfloxacin: review of safety studies. *Am. J. Med.* **82**(Suppl. 6B):22–26.
18. **Crist, W., T. Lehnert, and B. Ulbrich.** 1988. Specific toxicologic aspects of the quinolones. *Rev. Infect. Dis.* **10**(Suppl. 1)**:**141–146.
19. **Deming, M. S., R. V. Tauxe, B. A. Blake, et al.** 1987. Campylobacter enteritis at a university: transmission from eating chicken and from cats. *Am. J. Epidemiol.* **126:**526–533.

20. **Dorrestein, G. M., H. Van Gogh, M. N. Buitelarr, and J. F. M. Nouws.** 1983. Clinical pharmacology and pharmacokinetics of flumequine after intravenous intramuscular and oral administration in pigeons (Columba livia). *J. Vet. Pharmacol. Ther.* **6:**281-292.
21. **Drusano, G. L.** 1989. Pharmacokinetics of the quinolone antimicrobial agents, p. 71-105. *In* J. S. Wolfson and D. C. Hooper (ed.), *Quinolone Antimicrobial Agents.* American Society for Microbiology, Washington, D.C.
22. **Endtz, H. P., R. P. Mouton, T. van der Reyden, G. J. Ruijs, M. Biever, and B. van Klingeren.** 1990. Fluoroquinolone resistance in Campylobacter spp isolated from human stools and poultry products. *Lancet* **335:**787.
23. **Espinasse, J., B. Dellac, A. Silmi, C. Prommelet, and M. Viso.** 1986. Essay d'une nouvelle quinolone BAY Vp 2674 (Baytril) dans la Salmonellose experimentale des veau a Salmonella typhimurium, p. 1324-1325. *Proc. 14th World Congr. Dis. Cattle.*
24. **Flammer, K., D. P. Aucoin, D. A. Whitt, and S. A. S. Prus.** 1990. Plasma concentrations of enrofloxacin in African grey parrots treated with medicated water. *Avian Dis.* **3:**1017-1022.
25. **Ford, R. B.** 1988. Enrofloxacin: a new antimicrobial strategy in small animal practice, p. 17-24. *Proc. West. Vet. Conf.*
26. **Giles, C. J., R. A. Magonigle, and W. T. R. Grimshaw.** 1991. Clinical pharmacokinetics of parenterally administered danofloxacin in cattle. *J. Vet. Pharmacol. Ther.* **14:**400-410.
27. **Glawischnig, E., H. Frank, and E. Weber.** 1989. On the efficacy of Bayril in some infectious diseases of pigs caused by different microorganisms. *Wein. Tierarzt. Monatschr.* **76:**91-96.
28. **Goodman, L. J., R. L. Kaplan, R. M. Petrak, R. M. Fliegelman, D. Taff, F. Walton, J. L. Penner, and G. M. Trenholme.** 1986. Effects of erythromycin and ciprofloxacin on chronic fecal excretion of Campylobacter species in marmosets. *Antimicrob. Agents Chemother.* **29:**185-187.
29. **Goren, E., W. A. De Jong, and P. Doornebal.** 1982. Pharmacokinetical aspects of flumequine and therapeutic efficacy in Escherichia coli infection in poultry. *Avian Pathol.* **1:**463-474.
30. **Gough, A., N. J. Barsoum, L. Mitchell, E. J. McGuire, and F. A. de la Iglesia.** 1979. Juvenile canine drug-induced arthropathy: clinicopathological studies on articular lesions caused by oxolinic and pipemidic acids. *Toxicol. Appl. Pharmacol.* **51:**177-187.
31. **Gough, A. W., N. J. Barsoum, R. C. Renlund, J. M. Sturgess, and F. A. de la Iglesia.** 1985. Fine structural changes during reparative phase of canine drug-induced arthropathy. *Vet. Pathol.* **22:**82-84.
32. **Hannan, P. C. T., and R. F. W. Goodwin.** 1990. Treatment of experimental enzootic pneumonia of the pig by norfloxacin or its 6-chloro analogue. *Res. Vet. Sci.* **49:**203-210.
33. **Hannan, P. C. T., P. J. O'Hanlon, and N. H. Rogers.** 1989. In vitro evaluation of various quinolone antibacterial agents against veterinary mycoplasmas and porcine respiratory bacterial pathogens. *Res. Vet. Sci.* **46:**202-211.
34. **Howard, L. C., D. C. Van Sickle, K. Deshmukh, W. J. Griffing, and N. V. Owen.** 1979. Cinoxacin induced arthropathy in juvenile beagle dogs. *Toxicol. Appl. Pharmacol.* **48:**145-154.
35. **Isaza, R., S. C. Budsberg, S. F. Sundlof, and B. Baker.** Pharmacokinetics of ciprofloxacin in red tailed hawks. *J. Zoo Wild Med.*, in press.
36. **Jehl, F., L. Bresler, C. Koechlin, M. Merle-Melet, J. P. Didelot, and J. Hazebrouca.** 1992. Pharmacokinetics and biliary elimination of temafloxacin in pigs. *J. Antimicrob. Chemother.* **30:**189-196.
37. **Kato, M., and T. Onedera.** 1988. Effect of ofloxacin on the uptake of [$^3$H]thymidine by articular cartilage in the rat. *Toxicol. Lett.* **44:**131-142.
38. **Kato, M., and T. Onodera.** 1988. Morphological investigation of cavity formation in articular cartilage induced by ofloxacin in rats. *Fundam. Appl. Toxicol.* **11:**110-119.
39. **Kempf, I., F. Gesbert, M. Guittet, and G. Bennejean.** 1992. Efficacy of danofloxacin in the therapy of experimental mycoplasmosis in chicks. *Res. Vet. Sci.* **53:**257-259.
40. **Lekeux, P., and T. Art.** 1988. Effect of enrofloxacin therapy on shipping fever pneumonia in feedlot cattle. *Vet. Rec.* **123:**205-207.
41. **Mann, D. D., and G. M. Frame.** 1992. Pharmacokinetic study of danofloxacin in cattle and swine. *Am. J. Vet. Res.* **53:**1022-1026.
42. **Martinsen, B., H. Oppegaard, R. Wiehstrøn, and E. Myhr.** 1992. Temperature-dependent in vitro antimicrobial activity of four 4-quinolones and oxytetracycline against bacteria pathogenic to fish. *Antimicrob. Agents Chemother.* **36:**1738-1743.
43. **McMillan, R., J. Davidson, D. Copeland, G. Counzelman, and J. Baggot.** 1986. The pharmacological basis and therapeutic application of a new antimicrobial agent in turkeys, p. 12-13. *West. Poultry Dis. Conf.*
44. **McQueen, C., and J. Williams.** 1987. Effects of quinolone antibiotics in tests for genotoxicity. *Am. J. Med.* **82**(Suppl. 4A):94-96.
45. **Merkdt, M., B. Patel, and G. Amtsberg.** 1986. Efficacy of the quinolone derivative BAY Vp 2674 (Baytril) in latent Salmonella infection in pigs, p. 163. *Proc. 9th Congr. Int. Pig Vet. Soc.*
46. **Michel, C.** 1981. Utilisation des antibiotiques en pisciculture. *Bull. Fr. Piscicult.* **53:**125-127.
47. **Mobay Corp.** 1990. Baytril, brand of enrofloxacin. Product information. Mobay Corp., Shawnee, Kans.

48. **Norden, C. W., and E. Shinners.** 1985. Ciprofloxacin as therapy for experimental osteomyelitis caused by Pseudomonas aeruginosa. *J. Infect. Dis.* **151:**291-294.
49. **Nouws, J. F. M., J. L. Grondel, A. R. Schutte, and J. Laurensen.** 1988. Pharmacokinetics of ciprofloxacin in carp, African catfish and rainbow trout. *Vet. Q.* **10:**211-216.
50. **Nouws, J. F. M., D. J. Mevius, T. B. Vree, A. M. Baars, and J. Laurense.** 1988. Pharmacokinetics, renal clearance and metabolism of ciprofloxacin following intravenous and oral administration to calves and pigs. *Vet. Q.* **10:**156-163.
51. **O'Brien, T. P., M. R. Sawusch, J. D. Kick, and J. D. Gettsch.** 1988. Topical ciprofloxacin treatment of Pseudomonas keratitis in rabbits. *Arch. Ophthalmol.* **106:**1444-1446.
52. **Peterson, L. R.** 1986. Animal models: the in-vivo evaluation of ciprofloxacin. *J. Antimicrob. Chemother.* **18**(Suppl. D):55-64.
53. **Piddock, L. J. V., K. Whale, and R. Wise.** 1990. Quinolone resistance in salmonella: clinical experience. *Lancet* **335:**1459.
54. **Piddock, L. J. V., C. Wray, I. McClaren, and R. Wise.** 1991. Quinolone resistance in Salmonella spp: veterinary pointers. *Lancet* **336:**125.
55. **Plonait, H., A. Wilms-Schultze Kump, and G. Schonig.** 1986. Prophylaxis of the MMA syndrome by antibacterial medication and restricted feeding, p. 16-19. *Proc. 9th Int. Vet. Symp.*
56. **Prescott, J. F., and K. M. Yielding.** 1990. In vitro susceptibility of selected veterinary bacterial pathogens to ciprofloxacin, enrofloxacin and norfloxacin. *Can. J. Vet. Res.* **54:**194-199.
57. **Sande, M. A., R. A. Brooks-Fournier, and J. L. Gerberding.** 1988. Use of animal models in evaluation of the quinolones. *Rev. Infect. Dis.* **10**(Suppl. 1):S113-S116.
58. **Scheer, M.** 1987. Concentrations of active ingredient in the serum and in tissues after oral and parenteral administration of baytril. *Vet. Med. Rev.* **2:**104-118.
59. **Scheer, M.** 1987. Studies on the antibacterial activity of baytril. *Vet. Med. Rev.* **2:**290-299.
60. **Scheer, M., and R. Bauditz.** 1987. Baytril (BAY Vp 2674). Antibacterial activity as well as serum and tissue levels in calves, p. 1322-1325. *14th World Congr. Dis. Cattle.*
61. **Schluter, G.** 1987. Ciprofloxacin: review of potential toxicologic effects. *Am. J. Med.* **82**(Suppl. 4A):91-93.
62. **Schluter, G.** 1989. Ciprofloxacin: toxicologic evaluation of additional safety data. *Am. J. Med.* **87**(Suppl. 5A):37s-39s.
63. **Schroder, J.** 1989. Enrofloxacin: a new antimicrobial agent. *J. Afr. Vet. Assoc.* **60:**122-124.
64. **Smith, I. M., A. Mackie, and J. Lida.** 1991. Effect of giving enrofloxacin in the diet to pigs experimentally infected with *Actinobacillus pleuropneumoniae. Vet. Rec.* **129:**25-29.
65. **Spiecker, R. F.** 1986. Untersuchungen zur Wirksamkeit des chinoloncarbonsaure Derivats. BAY Vp 2674 (Baytril) bei der Behandlung der latenten Salmonellen-Infektion des Rindes. Ph.D. dissertation. University of Hannover, Hannover, Germany.
66. **Stephano, A., F. Vazquez-Rojas, and C. Diaz.** 1987. Enrofloxacin treatment against experimental infection with Haemophilus pleuropneumoniae in weaned pigs, p. 305. *Abstr. 23rd World Vet. Congr.*
67. **Studdert, V. P., and K. L. Hughes.** 1992. Treatment of opportunistic mycobacterial infections with enrofloxacin in cats. *J. Am. Vet. Med. Assoc.* **201:**1388-1390.
68. **Tatsumi, H., H. Senda, S. Yatera, Y. Takemoto, M. Yamoyoshi, and K. Ohnishi.** 1978. Toxicological studies on pipemidic acid. V. Effect on diarthrodial joints of experimental animals. *J. Toxicol. Sci.* **3:**357-367.
69. **Tornquist, M., and A. Franklin.** 1987. A field trial using a new antibacterial substance (Baytril) against respiratory diseases in calves, p. 621-626. *Proc. 14th World Congr. Dis. Cattle.*
70. **Vancutsem, P. M., J. G. Babish, and W. S. Schwark.** 1990. The fluoroquinolone antimicrobials: structure, antimicrobial activity, pharmacokinetics, clinical uses in domestic animals and toxicity. *Cornell Vet.* **80:**173-186.
71. **Walker, R. D., G. E. Stein, S. C. Budsberg, E. J. Rosser, and K. H. MacDonald.** 1989. Serum and tissue fluid norfloxacin concentrations after oral administration of the drug to healthy dogs. *Am. J. Vet. Res.* **50:**154-157.
72. **Walker, R. D., G. E. Stein, J. G. Hauptman, and K. H. MacDonald.** 1992. Pharmacokinetic evaluation of enrofloxacin administered orally to healthy dogs. *Am. J. Vet. Res.* **53:**2315-2319.
73. **Walker, R. D., G. E. Stein, J. G. Hauptman, K. H. MacDonald, S. C. Budsberg, and E. J. Rosser.** 1990. Serum and tissue cage fluid concentrations of ciprofloxacin after oral administration of the drug to healthy dogs. *Am. J. Vet. Res.* **51:**896-900.
74. **Wallis, A. S.** 1991. Use of enrofloxacin in laying birds. *Vet. Rec.* **128:**554-555.
75. **Wray, C., I. McLaren, R. Wise, and L. J. V. Piddock.** 1989. Nalidixic acid-resistant salmonellae. *Vet. Rec.* **124:**489.

*Quinolone Antimicrobial Agents, 2nd ed.*
Edited by David C. Hooper and John S. Wolfson


*Chapter 26*

# Adverse Effects

*David C. Hooper and John S. Wolfson**

It is difficult to assess accurately drug-related adverse experiences in humans. In order to establish rigorously in an individual patient a cause-and-effect relationship between the drug administered and the adverse experience reported or observed, the putative toxic effect should improve with cessation of therapy and return reproducibly on rechallenge with drug but not placebo. Obviously, for ethical reasons and because some toxic effects may not be reversible, it is seldom possible (or desirable to attempt) to fulfill these criteria in humans.

The best estimates of the frequency and types of drug-related adverse experiences come from placebo-controlled, double-blind, randomized trials, which in the population studied allow determination of the statistical likelihood that an observed effect is drug related. Such studies could be performed with healthy volunteers, but the results might not extrapolate reliably to other groups of patients with infections for which the drug is to be tested for efficacy or used clinically. In addition, the use of placebo controls in studies of treatment of infections is limited to those infections that are nonfatal, resolve spontaneously, and have little residual morbidity. Crossover designs of drug trials may overcome some of these problems.

Because of the limitations cited above, information on adverse experiences in clinically relevant populations comes most commonly from open studies or studies comparing fluoroquinolones with other antimicrobial agents. Assessments of adverse experiences are particularly difficult in open studies because the frequency of reporting varies with the method of ascertainment and with the patient population studied. In all studies, the investigators must make clinical judgments as to whether the symptom or sign reported is possibly, probably, or definitely drug related. Even in comparative studies, which should preferably be double blinded to eliminate possible bias in these clinical judgments, the information gained is relative and must be assessed in the context of the general clinical experience with the tolerability of the comparison agent.

## CLINICAL ADVERSE EFFECTS

### Frequencies of Adverse Experiences in Comparative Clinical Studies

Safety profiles of an increasing number of fluoroquinolones are now accumulating, although most clinical experience has been with norfloxacin, ciprofloxacin, ofloxacin,

*David C. Hooper and John S. Wolfson* • Infectious Disease Unit, Medical Services, Massachusetts General Hospital, Boston, Massachusetts 02114-2696.
*Deceased.

and pefloxacin. Although general patterns exist, safety profiles of the newer agents may differ, as was the case with some of the older quinolone analogs (80, 130).

In the English literature are now a large number of double-blind studies comparing fluoroquinolones and other antimicrobial agents or placebo (Table 1). Some double-blind comparative studies from Japan have also been reviewed (Table 1) (136). The incidence of adverse experiences thought to be either possibly, probably, or definitely drug related ranged from 2 to 82%. Such a broad range reflects differences in patient populations, drug doses, durations of therapy, and methods of ascertaining adverse effects (147). The breadth of this range also reemphasizes the importance of comparison with control agents rather than reliance on the apparent adverse effect rate itself. In most double-blind studies, no differences between fluoroquinolone and nonquinolone agents

**Table 1.** Adverse effects of fluoroquinolones compared with other agents or placebo in prospective, randomized, double-blind studies

| Fluoroquinolone | No. of patients with adverse effects/total no. treated (%) | Comparison drug | No. of patients with adverse effects from comparison drug/total no. treated (%) | Reference |
|---|---|---|---|---|
| Ciprofloxacin | 3/31 (10)[a] | TMP-SMX | 10/31 (29) | 82 |
| Ciprofloxacin | 2/47 (4) | TMP-SMX | 0/46 (0) | 141 |
| Ciprofloxacin | 1/22 (5) | TMP-SMX | 6/23 (26) | 4 |
| Ciprofloxacin | 18/103 (17)[a] | TMP-SMX | 32/100 (32) | 78 |
| Ciprofloxacin | 3/51 (6) | TMP-SMX | 8/52 (16) | 84 |
| Ciprofloxacin | 1/60 (2) | TMP-SMX | 1/59 (2) | 61 |
| | | Placebo | 0/62 (0) | |
| Ciprofloxacin | 2/49 (4) | Ampicillin | 3/51 (6) | 175 |
| Ciprofloxacin | 7/42 (17)[a] | Ampicillin | 16/45 (35) | 230 |
| Ciprofloxacin | 18/22 (82) | Ampicillin | 17/22 (77) | 43 |
| Ciprofloxacin | 9/60 (15) | Ampicillin | 7/61 (11) | 26 |
| Ciprofloxacin | 3/29 (10) | Ampicillin | 3/28 (11) | 41 |
| Ciprofloxacin | 10/28 (36) | Cefotaxime | 11/28 (36) | 167 |
| Ciprofloxacin | 8/38 (24) | Cefotaxime | 5/35 (17) | 189 |
| Ciprofloxacin | 40/282 (14) | Cefotaxime | 34/288 (12) | 71 |
| Ciprofloxacin | 14/87 (16) | Doxycycline | 19/83 (23) | 68 |
| Ciprofloxacin | 40/110 (36)[a] | Doxycycline | 10/52 (19) | 92 |
| Ciprofloxacin | 5/44 (11) | Placebo | 2/41 (5) | 160 |
| Ciprofloxacin | 3/61 (5) | Placebo | 3/59 (5) | 171 |
| Enoxacin | 5/18 (28) | Placebo | 2/6 (33) | 216 |
| Enoxacin | 45/62 (73) | Placebo | 36/63 (63) | 211 |
| Fleroxacin | 4/41 (10) | TMP-SMX | 2/41 (5) | 162 |
| Fleroxacin | 42/102 (41)[a] | Amoxicillin | 14/92 (15) | 43 |
| Fleroxacin | 61/313 (19)[a] | Amoxicillin | 27/310 (9) | 218 |
| Fleroxacin | 97/321 (31) | Ciprofloxacin | 84/324 (26) | 102 |
| Fleroxacin | 78/94 (82)[a] | Norfloxacin | 26/95 (27) | 161 |
| Fleroxacin | 75/287 (26)[a] | Norfloxacin | 41/292 (14) | 163 |
| Fleroxacin | 42/65 (65)[a] | Placebo | 25/64 (39) | 203 |
| | 36/61 (59)[a] | | | |
| Fleroxacin | 10/160 (6) | Placebo | 12/170 (7) | 36 |
| | 11/172 (6) | | | |

*Continued on next page*

Table 1. *Continued*

| Fluoroquinolone | No. of patients with adverse effects/total no. treated (%) | Comparison drug | No. of patients with adverse effects from comparison drug/total no. treated (%) | Reference |
|---|---|---|---|---|
| Lomefloxacin | 13/235 (6) | Norfloxacin | 18/223 (8) | 143 |
| Lomefloxacin | 22/84 (26) | Norfloxacin | 20/80 (25) | 144 |
| Norfloxacin | 221/658 (34)[a] | TMP-SMX | 105/216 (49) | 219 |
| Norfloxacin | 9/43 (21) | TMP-SMX | 9/45 (20) | 217 |
| Norfloxacin | 5/81 (6) | TMP-SMX | 7/85 (8) | 231 |
| Norfloxacin | 23/148 (16) | TMP-SMX | 15/148 (10) | 118 |
| | | Placebo | 24/150 (16) | |
| Norfloxacin | 21/97 (22)[a] | Cefadroxil | 37/96 (39) | 180 |
| Norfloxacin | 8/83 (10) | Loracarbef | 4/78 (5) | 96 |
| Norfloxacin | 5/8 (62)[a] | Placebo + norfloxacin | 0/7 (0) | 191 |
| Norfloxacin | 3/63 (5) | Placebo | 6/64 (10) | 227 |
| Norfloxacin | 1/12 (8) | Placebo | 0/12 (0) | 76 |
| Norfloxacin | 3/15 (20) | Placebo | 3/15 (20) | 145 |
| Ofloxacin | 0/41 (0) | Pivampicillin | 1/43 (2) | 59 |
| Ofloxacin | 2/49 (4) | Amoxicillin-clavulanate | 5/46 (11) | 165 |
| Ofloxacin | 20/49 (21)[a] | Erythromycin | 37/96 (39) | 97 |
| Ofloxacin | 9/23 (39) | Ciprofloxacin | 13/24 (54) | 106 |
| Ofloxacin | 2/30 (7) | Ciprofloxacin | 2/31 (6) | 115 |
| Pefloxacin | 21/155 (14) | TMP-SMX | 25/161 (16) | 157 |
| Pefloxacin | 39/98 (40)[a] | Norfloxacin | 23/101 (23) | 221 |
| Temafloxacin | 100/478 (20) | TMP-SMX | 49/196 (25) | 100 |
| Temafloxacin | 40/204 (20) | TMP-SMX | 46/196 (24) | 101 |
| Temafloxacin | 30/123 (24) | Amoxicillin | 19/115 (16) | 39 |
| Temafloxacin | 63/183 (34)[a] | Cefadroxil | 47/191 (25) | 142 |
| Temafloxacin | 33/243 (14) | Ciprofloxacin | 43/249 (17) | 153 |
| Temafloxacin | 81/188 (43)[a] | Ciprofloxacin | 59/188 (31) | 42 |
| Temafloxacin | 12/140 (8) | Ciprofloxacin | 8/138 (6) | 113 |
| Temafloxacin | 7/138 (5) | Norfloxacin | 9/141 (6) | 50 |
| Temafloxacin | 820/2,602 (32) | Fluoroquinolone | 360/1,169 (36) | 147 |
| | | Nonquinolone | 253/862 (29) | |

[a] $P < 0.05$ compared with nonquinolone agent.

were found, although the small numbers of patients in some studies limited the power of the study to detect differences. Likewise, in most comparisons between different fluoroquinolones, no differences in adverse effect rates could be detected (50, 106, 115, 143, 144, 147, 153).

Fluoroquinolones had significantly fewer adverse effects than nonquinolone agents in six studies: ciprofloxacin compared with trimethoprim-sulfamethoxazole (TMP-SMX) (78, 82) and ampicillin (230), norfloxacin compared with TMP-SMX (219) and cefadroxil (180), and ofloxacin compared with erythromycin (97). In contrast, adverse effects were more frequent in the fluoroquinolone group in seven studies: ciprofloxacin compared with doxycycline (92), norfloxacin compared with placebo (191), temafloxacin compared with cefadroxil (142) and ciprofloxacin (42), and fleroxacin compared with amoxicillin (43, 218) and placebo (203). In the only double-blind studies detecting differences between two fluoroquinolones, norfloxacin had fewer adverse effects than pefloxacin (221) and fleroxacin (161, 163). Strikingly, in five of the eight studies with fleroxacin, this fluoroquinolone had significantly more adverse effects than the comparison agent (Table 1).

Comparative data on the adverse effects of intravenously administered fluoroquinolones are few. There have been no double-blind studies, but in a summary of the randomized comparative trials of ciprofloxacin and ceftazidime that included over 1,000 patients in each group, overall adverse effects excluding local reactions at the site of infusion were similar in the two groups. Central nervous system reactions were, however, significantly more frequent with ciprofloxacin (2.2%) than with ceftazidime (0.7%) (14). The tolerability of oral ciprofloxacin appeared to be greater than that of the intravenous formulation in one small nonrandomized study of patients with cystic fibrosis (205).

### Effects of dose and duration of therapy on adverse effects

Reviews of blinded and unblinded clinical trials have identified trends suggesting that the frequency of adverse effects with oral fluoroquinolones increases with the dose and duration of therapy (89, 90, 147, 202). Similar correlations were found for intravenous ciprofloxacin when durations of therapy were compared and when the highest-dosage group (>12.4 mg/kg/day) was compared with a group given lower doses (4.4 to 12.4 mg/kg/day) (14). Dose effects can be most clearly interpreted in studies with randomized, blind comparisons of different doses or durations of treatment. For norfloxacin, a 400-mg dose twice daily had significantly more adverse effects than a 200-mg dose twice daily (219), and at the higher dose, patients receiving 3 days of therapy had fewer adverse effects than those given 7 days of therapy (99). Prolongation of norfloxacin treatment from 12 to 24 weeks also resulted in substantial increases in adverse effects (191). In two relatively small studies, no differences could be detected between the tolerability of a single dose of norfloxacin (179) or ciprofloxacin (26) and each drug given for 3 days (six doses) or for 5 days (10 doses) of therapy. The adverse effects of fleroxacin were also dose related in some studies (33, 161, 202) but not in others (36, 102, 203). Overall, fewer patients receiving single doses of fleroxacin had adverse effects (7.5%) than those receiving multiple doses (26%) (70). In one study (143), photosensitivity reactions to lomefloxacin, some severe and causing discontinuation of therapy, occurred significantly more often in patients treated for 7 days than in those treated for 3 days, although results with once- and twice-daily lomefloxacin did not differ in another small study (110). In phase I studies of temafloxacin, patients receiving 800 to 1,000 mg/day had more adverse effects than those receiving ≤600 mg/day (147), although no particular type of adverse event predominated in the higher-dose group.

In most studies that identified increases in adverse effects related to dose, the particular type of adverse reaction affected was not defined. In a reported accidental overdose with intravenous ofloxacin (3 g), the patient developed predominantly dizziness and nausea (112). For fleroxacin, gastrointestinal, central nervous system (most often insomnia), and photosensitivity reactions all appeared to increase with increasing dose (202), and photosensitivity reactions to lomefloxacin were dose related (143).

### Characteristics of adverse effects

Reviews of adverse effects reported by the manufacturers provide the largest body of information on the tolerability profiles of fluoroquinolones (70, 87, 88, 147, 174, 195, 196, 209, 228) (Table 2). These values are likely an upper estimate of drug-related adverse effects, because experiences thought possibly, probably, and definitely drug related were generally included. In addition, methods of ascertainment of adverse effects differed and do not allow direct comparisons among fluoroquinolones. An additional group of 140 granulocytopenic cancer patients given norfloxacin as prophylaxis had a very high rate

**Table 2.** Clinical adverse effects of oral fluoroquinolones as reported to manufacturers[a]

| Category[b] | No. of patients (%) | | | | | | | | | |
|---|---|---|---|---|---|---|---|---|---|---|
| | Norfloxacin | Cipro-floxacin | Ofloxacin | Pefloxacin | Lome-floxacin | Enoxacin | Tema-floxacin | Fleroxacin | Tosu-floxacin | Sparfloxacin |
| Total no. studied | 2,206 | 9,473 | 15,641 | 1,437 | 2,869 | 2,407 | 2,602 | 4,234 | 3,010 | 2,754 |
| Total no. with AE | 202 (9.1) | 881 (9.3) | 704 (4.5) | 140 (9.7) | | 149 (6.2) | 820 (31.5) | 887 (21) | 109 (3.6) | 133 (4.8) |
| Total requiring cessation of therapy | (<1.0) | 146 (1.5) | 231 (1.5) | 43 (3.0) | | 132 (2.6)[c] | 107 (4.1) | 93 (2)[d] | | |
| Types of AE | | | | | | | | | | |
| GI | 85 (3.9)[e] | 461 (4.8) | 464 (3.0) | | 146 (5.1) | 91 (3.8) | 349 (13.4) | 467 (11) | 70 (2.3) | 54 (2.0) |
| Nausea or vomiting | 44 (2.0) | 196 (2.0) | 160 (1.0)[f] | 68 (4.7) | 106 (3.7) | | | 385 (10) | 44 (1.5) | 37 (1.3) |
| Abdominal discomfort | 26 (1.2) | 75 (0.8) | 171 (1.1)[f] | 20 (1.4) | | | | | | |
| Diarrhea | 9 (1.2) | 113 (1.1) | 73 (0.5) | 6 (0.4) | 40 (1.4) | | | 40 (0.9) | 13 (0.4) | 11 (0.4) |
| Other | 6 (0.3) | 57 (0.6) | 60 (0.4) | 14 (1.0) | | | | 30 (0.7) | 13 (0.4) | 6 (0.2) |
| CNS | 103 (4.4) | 138 (1.4) | 152 (1.0) | 18 (1.2) | 158 (5.5) | 29 (1.2) | 190 (7.4) | 374 (9) | 13 (0.4) | 17 (0.6) |
| Headache | 34 (1.4) | 27 (0.3) | 29 (0.2) | | 92 (3.2) | | | 105 (2) | 4 (0.1) | 6 (0.2) |
| Dizziness | 29 (1.2) | 38 (0.4) | 28 (0.2) | | 66 (2.3) | | | 96 (2) | 4 (0.1) | 5 (0.2) |
| Sleep disorder | 13 (0.6) | 16 (0.2) | 48 (0.3) | | | | | 157 (4) | 3 (0.1) | 2 (0.07) |
| Mood change | 13 (0.6) | 28 (0.3) | 18 (0.1) | | | | | | | |
| Seizures | 4 (0.2) | 2 (0.02) | | | | | | | 1 (0.03) | 1 (0.03) |
| Other | 10 (0.4) | 27 (0.3) | 29 (0.2) | | | | | | 1 (0.03) | 3 (0.1) |
| Skin or allergic | 11 (0.5)[c] | 101 (1.0) | 71 (0.4) | 19 (1.3) | | 14 (0.6) | 62 (2.4) | 111 (3) | 23 (0.8) | 44 (1.6) |
| Rash | 11 (0.5) | 54 (0.6) | 48 (0.3) | | | | | | 12 (0.4) | 25 (0.9) |
| Pruritis | | 29 (0.3) | 14 (0.1) | | | | | | 6 (0.2) | 5 (0.2) |
| Photosensitivity | | 4 (0.04) | | 12 (0.8) | 69 (2.4) | | | 24 (0.6) | | |
| Other | | 14 (0.1) | | | | | | | 5 (0.2) | 14 (0.5) |

[a]Data are from references 225 (norfloxacin), 20 and 183 (ciprofloxacin), 29 and 114 (ofloxacin), 75 (pefloxacin), 174 (lomefloxacin), 65 (enoxacin), 147 and 229 (temafloxacin), 70 (fleroxacin), and 195 (tosufloxacin and sparfloxacin). Data for tosufloxacin and sparfloxacin are data from Japanese open studies only.

[b]Abbreviations: AE, adverse effect; GI, gastrointestinal, CNS, central nervous system.

[c]Data (from reference 79) are based on denominators of 1,181 patients for enoxacin and 5,088 patients for pefloxacin.

[d]Adverse effects listed as severe; discontinuation of therapy not specified.

[e]Granulocytopenic patients are not included, leaving a total of 2,206 patients assessed for gastrointestinal or skin symptoms.

[f]Eighty-seven patients were listed as having nausea, vomiting, or abdominal discomfort; 43 of these were assigned to "nausea or vomiting," and 44 were assigned to "abdominal discomfort."

of total adverse experiences (63%), but in only two patients (1.4%) were the effects thought to be related to norfloxacin; many of the adverse effects were likely related to antitumor chemotherapy (225).

Most adverse reactions reported were mild to moderate in severity. Adverse effects of sufficient severity to prompt cessation of therapy ranged in frequency from <1.0% of patients given norfloxacin to 4.1% of patients given temafloxacin. In the double-blind comparative trials with temafloxacin and nonquinolone agents, significantly more patients discontinued temafloxacin than discontinued the nonquinolone agents (229).

Although the numbers of patients entered into clinical trials and monitored by the manufacturers during drug development (often several thousand) are usually sufficient to define a profile encompassing the common and relatively uncommon adverse effects of new drugs, they are insufficiently reliable to detect toxicities that are rare but serious or that may appear only after substantial delay. Detection of the latter group of toxicities may be possible during postmarketing surveillance of much larger numbers of patients. This reporting mechanism is voluntary and thus may be sporadic, with a greater likelihood of more-severe reactions being reported (104, 107). The system of postmarketing surveillance in the United States was able to detect rare serious adverse effects that unexpectedly occurred shortly after approval of temafloxacin for general clinical use (see section on hematologic reactions below).

## Gastrointestinal reactions

In general, gastrointestinal symptoms were the most frequent symptoms reported, occurring in 3.0 to 13.4% of patients overall. These symptoms have included nausea, vomiting, abdominal discomfort, and anorexia, which in many instances likely resulted from gastric irritation. In some cases, however, nausea and vomiting may have resulted from toxicity to the central nervous system or from theophylline accumulation in patients receiving theophylline and fluoroquinolones (enoxacin and ciprofloxacin) that impair its excretion (see chapter 11).

Diarrhea developing during fluoroquinolone therapy has been infrequent. The development of antibiotic-associated colitis as identified by the presence of pseudomembranes on the colonic mucosa or *Clostridium difficile* cytotoxin in the stool has been associated with fluoroquinolone therapy (20, 24, 37, 40, 53, 60, 79, 85, 104, 120, 127, 149) but appears to be rare when it is considered that fluoroquinolones have been administered to over 40 million patients (74). The minimal effect of many fluoroquinolones on anaerobic bowel flora has been postulated to reduce the likelihood of overgrowth of *C. difficile* (85, 117), and the possible use of fluoroquinolones for treatment of *C. difficile*-associated colitis as been suggested (117, 125).

## Central nervous system reactions

Some early quinolone analogs exhibited notable central nervous system toxicities, with dizziness occurring in as many as half of the patients treated with oxolinic acid (190) or rosoxacin (80). Amfenolic acid, a derivative of nalidixic acid containing a methylbenzene substituent at the 7 position of the naphthyridine ring, was also originally developed as a central nervous system stimulant (1, 108, 133).

For the newer fluoroquinolones, symptoms referable to the nervous system have been reported in 0.9 to 7.4% of patients in clinical trials and usually followed gastrointestinal reactions in frequency of adverse effects. In postmarketing surveillance in Germany, central nervous system adverse effects were the most commonly reported group of reactions for ofloxacin (104, 107), a result in contrast to those of clinical trials with ofloxacin and ciprofloxacin and postmarketing surveillance of ciprofloxacin (170), in which gastrointestinal reactions were most frequent.

Symptoms of mild headache or dizziness have predominated, followed by sleep disturbance (usually insomnia) or mood alteration (agitation, anxiety, or depression). Headache was more frequent with temafloxacin than with cefadroxil in one double-blind study (142). Hallucinations, delirium, and acute psychoses have been uncommon with the newer agents (6, 45, 104, 107, 121, 132, 170, 183, 233). Benign intracranial hypertension has been seen in children given nalidixic acid (32, 139) or ciprofloxacin (226). In two patients, myasthenia gravis appeared to worsen following use of ciprofloxacin, although the contribution of infection (for which ciprofloxacin was used) to the findings of myasthenia is difficult to exclude with certainty (137, 140). Two patients developed confusion and tremors with dysmetria or cog wheel rigidity while receiving pefloxacin and metronidazole concurrently; in both, the neurologic findings resolved when pefloxacin was stopped (121). One patient with vertebral osteomyelitis and prior treatment of Hodgkin's disease with vincristine many years earlier developed peripheral neuropathy following 5 months of therapy with pefloxacin; improvement occurred when pefloxacin was stopped, but neuropathic symptoms recurred when ofloxacin was substituted (11).

Seizures have been reported in small numbers of patients receiving nalidixic acid (103, 177), norfloxacin (7, 225), ciprofloxacin (12, 13, 64, 150, 168, 183, 200), ofloxacin (104, 209), enoxacin (54, 198), and temafloxacin (147). In some patients, underlying conditions have been sufficient to account for seizures, although fluoroquinolone therapy may have lowered the seizure threshold. Concurrent therapy with theophylline and ciprofloxacin or enoxacin and the resultant theophylline accumulation also may have accounted for some (12, 20, 54, 168) but not all (16, 150, 198) cases of seizures (see chapter 11). Interactions between fluoroquinolones and nonsteroidal anti-inflammatory agents (NSAIDs) may also predispose to the development of seizures, possibly by augmentation of the ability of fluoroquinolones to antagonize binding of the inhibitory neurotransmitter $\gamma$-aminobutyric acid (GABA) to its receptors in the central nervous system. This apparent interaction was recognized clinically as seizures occurring in Japanese patients given enoxacin and the NSAID fenbufen (138). Although animal models suggest that an interaction may occur with other quinolones in high doses and with other NSAIDs (185), the extent to which other NSAIDs contribute to the neurologic adverse effects of other fluoroquinolones in humans remains unclear. The interactions with GABA receptors and the possible mechanisms of central nervous system toxicities of fluoroquinolones are discussed in more detail in chapter 27. In mice, high doses of fleroxacin and flumequine but not other quinolones given alone induce seizures (45), and in rats, intraventricular injections of ciprofloxacin, enoxacin, and to a lesser extent pefloxacin also induce seizures (45). Direct effects of temafloxacin and ciprofloxacin on cerebral glucose and oxygen metabolism were not seen in healthy volunteers studies by positron emission tomography (25). Ciprofloxacin was, however, found to reduce cerebral blood flow by about 20%, but the clinical implications of this finding are unknown.

## Skin and hypersensitivity reactions

Dermatologic reactions to fluoroquinolones have been infrequent, occurring in 0.4 to 2.2% of patients. Unspecified rashes have been most frequent, followed by pruritis. Skin reactions have been reversible on cessation of drug administration.

Photosensitivity reactions have been reported in patients receiving a number of quinolones, including nalidixic acid (17, 28, 31, 34, 234), pefloxacin (58, 79), norfloxacin (192), ofloxacin (79, 106, 107), enoxacin (109), ciprofloxacin (20, 67, 77, 183), lomefloxacin (174), and fleroxacin (33, 202). Among these quinolones, the highest frequency of these reactions seems to occur with pefloxacin (75, 104, 146), lomefloxacin (102, 174), and fleroxacin (202). Apparent photoonycholysis has occurred in one patient taking pefloxacin and in one taking ofloxacin (22).

The mechanisms of quinolone photosensitivity reactions are incompletely understood, but the differences in apparent frequency among compounds suggest that the ability to induce a common mechanism or the types of mechanisms may differ. All quinolones absorb light in the UV spectrum (131). For nalidixic acid, skin reactions occur after exposure to light of both UV (320 to 400 nm) and visible (>400 nm) wavelengths (34), have often included subepidermal bulla formation, and have been thought to be an idiosyncratic hypersensitivity phenomenon (31, 34). Dose-response effects have been seen with some quinolones, however, suggesting that the reactions may not be entirely idiosyncratic. In 3 of 20 patients given 800 mg of enoxacin per day, the minimal dose of type A UV (UVA) (320 to 420 nm) but not UVB (270 to 320 nm) needed to produce erythema (MED) was reduced by 45%, whereas at lower doses of enoxacin, no effect on erythema response after UVA or UVB was seen (158). For ciprofloxacin at usual clinical doses, a similar reduction in MED was seen for wavelengths 335 and 365 nm but not 305 nm (66). Also, as noted above, increasing doses or durations of therapy were associated with a higher frequency of photosensitivity reactions for both lomefloxacin (143) and fleroxacin (33, 202). The presence of a fluorine substituent at the 8 position of the quinolone ring (found in lomefloxacin and fleroxacin) appears to enhance UVA-induced chemical alterations of some quinolones associated with loss of antibacterial activity and increased cytotoxicity in vitro (128). These effects of UVA were substantially reduced in a quinolone analog with a methoxy group at the 8 position (128). Notably, for enoxacin and lomefloxacin, these effects were seen at lower doses of UVA than were required for norfloxacin, ofloxacin, and ciprofloxacin (128). The order of potency of quinolones in inducing erythema in mice exposed to UVA was lomefloxacin > enoxacin = nalidixic acid > ofloxacin > ciprofloxacin (224). Thus, there appears to be a correlation with UVA-induced photoinstability and the potential for photosensitivity or phototoxicity among several quinolones. A similar correlation exists for the potential for phototoxic reactions of these quinolones and the generation of toxic oxygen products after exposure of quinolones to UVA (222, 223). Although understanding of the phototoxic mechanisms of quinolones is incomplete, current findings suggest that the likelihood of phototoxic reactions to quinolones may be reduced by the use of sunscreens that block in the UVA range. This possibility remains to be tested in humans.

Drug fever (29, 183), urticaria (183), angioedema (170, 183), vasculitis (44, 93, 152, 207), serum sickness-like syndromes (199), and anaphylactoid reactions (56, 107, 206, 220) have been uncommon. Anaphylactoid reactions to ciprofloxacin have been noted in patients infected with human immunodeficiency virus (27, 156, 232). Individual patients with lobular panniculitis (176) and eosinophilic meningitis (15) associated with ciprofloxacin treatment have also been described. Allergic interstitial nephritis is discussed below under renal reactions.

Administration of the intravenous formulation of ciprofloxacin has been associated with local skin reactions at the site of infusion in 83 of 1,869 patients (4.4%) (14, 188). Local reactions were more common with ciprofloxacin than with ceftazidime in randomized, unblinded trials (14). A similar trend was seen with intravenous fleroxacin compared with ceftazidime (63). For ciprofloxacin, phlebitis was reported in 2% of patients. Local reactions have been more common during infusions in the small veins of the dorsum of the hand (214). Rapid intravenous infusions of fluoroquinolones have also been associated with acute changes in blood pressure (46, 201).

## Arthropathy

Rheumatologic adverse experiences during quinolone treatment are uncommon. Arthralgias and myalgias have been reported in small numbers of patients receiving nalidixic acid (19), norfloxacin (18, 225), ciprofloxacin (3, 20, 105), ofloxacin (29, 136, 186), and pefloxacin (79, 116), and reversible joint swelling and tendonitis have recurred in two patients rechallenged with norfloxacin (18, 57, 111). In one small, single-blind, randomized trial, arthralgias and myalgias were significantly more frequent in patients taking norfloxacin than in those taking nitrofurantoin (148). Achilles tendonitis, in three cases complicated by rupture, has also been seen in seven patients given pefloxacin or ofloxacin (172), and Achilles tendonitis was reported in 5 of 22 dialysis patients given pefloxacin (178).

In animals, quinolones have been shown to produce cartilage erosions and noninflammatory effusions in weight-bearing joints, and inhibition of cartilaginous embryonic limb bud growth has also been reported (46, 47, 49, 98, 136, 185, 213). Repair of cartilage erosions and cavity formation may follow drug withdrawal, with reactive proliferation of chondrocytes (55). In a few animals, nalidixic acid has also produced some disorganization of the epiphyseal plates (98). Arthropathy is dose related and varies among species and among quinolones (46, 181). Juvenile animals appear more susceptible, but arthropathy has developed with less frequency in adult dogs given pefloxacin for prolonged periods and can develop to a lesser degree in immobilized joints (47). The concentrations of norfloxacin and nalidixic acid measured in articular cartilage were similar to or higher than concentrations in serum, and similar concentrations in cartilage were found at the minimal arthropathic doses of both drugs (124). The mechanism of these effects in animals is unknown.

The extent to which arthropathy will pose a limitation to fluoroquinolone therapy in children remains unclear. A retrospective case-control study of a small number of pediatric patients suggested no difference in the occurrence of arthralgia in those patients receiving nalidixic acid (from 9 to 600 days) and those not receiving drug (182). No abnormalities of skeletal growth were seen in the nalidixic acid group. Over 200 children treated with nalidixic acid had no clinical or radiographic evidence of arthropathy (2). Arthropathy also was not seen in 21 leukemic children given norfloxacin as prophylaxis (51). One of 30 pediatric patients with cystic fibrosis is reported to have developed arthropathy while receiving a high dose of ciprofloxacin (1,500 mg/day for a 35-kg patient); all joint symptoms subsided within 2 weeks after cessation of therapy (166). The same report mentioned that 10% of older patients with cystic fibrosis may develop arthropathy, a percentage much higher than was reported from studies of adults. Others, however, have seen little joint toxicity in small numbers of cystic fibrosis patients younger than 17 years who were given ciprofloxacin (187). In contrast, in a review of patients with cystic fibrosis who were given pefloxacin, 14% developed arthralgia and joint swelling (155); arthropathy occurred in 45% of those between the ages of 15 and 20 years. For patients receiving ofloxacin, no arthropathy was identified in a similar retrospective analysis.

Recently, magnetic resonance imaging has been used to evaluate quinolone-induced arthropathy. In animals, small intra-articular effusions were predictive of ciprofloxacin-induced arthropathy (181). In 18 patients (13 of them prepubertal) with cystic fibrosis who were monitored during a 3-month course of ciprofloxacin, no changes were detected by magnetic resonance imaging. Autopsy of two patients who died of the complications of cystic fibrosis and had received repeated courses of ciprofloxacin revealed no cartilage degenerative changes like those seen in animals with arthopathy.

Possible dental effects (green teeth) have been reported in infants given ciprofloxacin as neonates (122).

In sum, concerns about the potential for cartilage damage and the development of arthropathia deformans that may occur in quinolone-treated animals have led to recommendations that the fluoroquinolones not be used in patients whose skeletal growth is incomplete or in pregnant women, particularly in cases for which alternative therapies exist. Accumulating experience, however, suggests that in some pediatric patients (particularly those with cystic fibrosis), the compassionate use of ciprofloxacin may be justified by an anticipated relatively low risk of arthropathy or cartilage damage (126, 181). It is noteworthy, however, that quinolones may differ in the extent to which they produce arthropathy in animals and humans (as suggested by the experience with pefloxacin [155]) and that experience with other quinolones in children is much smaller. In addition, subtle effects on cartilage may not be detectable for years. Thus, the relative benefit of choosing quinolones over other therapies must be carefully weighed in each individual pediatric patient for whom it is considered.

## LABORATORY TEST ABNORMALITIES

Abnormalities of laboratory tests occurring during fluoroquinolone therapy have been noted in 4.5 to 11.6% of patients (Table 3). As with reporting of clinical adverse experiences, these values are likely upper-limit estimates because of the inclusion of abnormalities possibly, probably, and definitely drug related. Some information was available only from Japanese open studies (195). Published summaries of laboratory abnormalities for patients given temafloxacin in clinical trials were not available, but information derived from postmarketing surveillance is discussed under hematologic reactions.

### Hematologic Reactions

Hematologic abnormalities were found in 0.4 to 5.3% of patients and have included leukopenia, eosinophilia, anemia, and thrombocytosis. Leukopenia was frequently mild and generally did not require cessation of therapy. Even in the rare cases in which neutropenia was severe, it was reversible after therapy was stopped (154). Mild anemia has been seen in 0.4 to 0.6% of patients given ofloxacin or pefloxacin (79, 136), and thrombocytosis has been seen in 0.06 to 0.6% of patients given ciprofloxacin, pefloxacin, or ofloxacin (20, 79). The mechanism of these abnormalities is not known, but eosinophilia and leukopenia may represent idiosyncratic hypersensitivity reactions. Changes in coagulation tests and platelet function were not found in volunteers given ciprofloxacin for 7 days (235).

In May 1992, several months after the approval of temafloxacin for clinical use in the United States, the U.S. Food and Drug Administration (FDA) through its postmarketing surveillance mechanism received reports of hemolytic anemia in patients given temafloxacin. Hemolytic anemia had not been seen in the data from clinical trials that constituted the New Drug Application to the FDA. Subsequent investigations by the FDA and the manufacturer identified patients receiving temafloxacin who developed hemolysis, renal failure, and thrombocytopenia with or without disseminated intravascular coagulation, most often after 5 to 7 days of therapy. One patient underwent renal biopsy: acute tubular necrosis with hemoglobin plugging without vasculitis was found. Several patients required dialysis for renal failure. Review of the experience with earlier fluoroquinolones in surveillance in the several months after marketing in the United States did not reveal a similar pattern of adverse effects. The estimated reporting incidence of this pattern of adverse effects, which mimics the hemolytic-uremic syndrome, was around 1/5,000 prescriptions (reported at an open meeting of the FDA Anti-Infective Drugs Advisory Committee on 10 July 1992), an incidence too low to be detected reliably in the usual numbers of patients that are studied for new drug applica-

**Table 3.** Laboratory test abnormalities during fluoroquinolone therapy[a]

| Category[b] | No. of patients (%) | | | | | | | | |
|---|---|---|---|---|---|---|---|---|---|
| | Norfloxacin | Ciprofloxacin | Ofloxacin | Pefloxacin | Lomefloxacin | Enoxacin | Fleroxacin | Tosufloxacin | Sparfloxacin |
| Total no. studied | 2,346 | 9,473 | 15,641 | 1,181 | 3,399 | 2,516 | 1,182 | 3,010 | 2,754 |
| Total no. with AE | 273 (11.6) | 504 (5.3) | 1,189 (7.6) | 53 (4.5) | | | | | |
| Types of AE | | | | | | | | | |
| Hematologic | 98 (5.3)[c] | 90 (1.0) | 78 (0.5) | 30 (2.5) | 24 (0.7) | | | | |
| Leukopenia | 60 (3.3) | 14 (0.1)[d] | 78 (0.5) | 3 (0.2) | | 5 (0.2) | | 2 (0.06) | 11 (0.4) |
| Eosinophilia | 38 (2.1) | 61 (0.6) | 92 (0.6) | 3 (0.2) | | 18 (0.7) | 4 (0.3) | 24 (0.8) | 33 (1.2) |
| Hepatic | 49 (2.7)[c] | 176 (1.8) | 313 (2.0) | 21 (1.8) | 20 (0.6) | | | | |
| Elevated serum transaminases | 49 (2.7) | 141 (1.4)[e] | 375 (2.4)[e] | 21 (1.8)[e] | 14 (0.4) | 23 (0.9) | 7 (0.6) | 69 (2.3) | 88 (3.2) |
| Renal | 25 (1.4)[c] | 42 (0.4) | 125 (0.8) | 2 (0.2) | 7 (0.2) | | | | |
| Elevated serum creatinine | 15 (0.8) | 24 (0.2) | 205 (1.3) | 2 (0.2) | | 13 (0.5) | 8 (0.7) | 12 (0.4) | 3 (0.1) |
| Proteinuria | 10 (0.5) | 6 (0.6) | | | | | | 6 (0.2) | 3 (0.1) |

[a]Data are from references 225 (norfloxacin), 183 (ciprofloxacin), 79 (ofloxacin and pefloxacin), 174 (lomefloxacin), and 195 (enoxacin, fleroxacin, tosufloxacin, and sparfloxacin). Data for tosufloxacin and sparfloxacin are from Japanese open studies only.

[b]AE, adverse effect.

[c]Denominator is 1,841 patients.

[d]From reference 13. Denominator is 2,829 patients.

[e]Elevations in transaminases and alkaline phosphatase were combined.

tions to the FDA. As a result of these findings, temafloxacin was voluntarily withdrawn by the manufacturer from the market worldwide.

As yet, the mechanisms that underlie these unexpected and infrequent adverse effects have not been defined. The structure of temafloxacin differs from that of earlier developed fluoroquinolones in having a difluorophenyl substituent at the 1 position (see chapter 2). The relationship of this substituent to these adverse effects is, however, unknown, and tosufloxacin, which contains the same substituent and has been marketed in Japan, has not yet been reported to produce a hemolytic-uremic-like syndrome. Hemolytic anemia, occasionally associated with renal failure, coagulation abnormalities, or both, has been reported to the FDA Spontaneous Reporting System for other marketed fluoroquinolones. The reporting incidence, however, has been far lower than that for temafloxacin.

### Hepatic Reactions

Abnormalities of liver function have been seen in 0.6 to 3.2% of patients given fluoroquinolones. Elevations of serum transaminases have predominated and have been mild, seldom requiring cessation of treatment. Elevations of serum alkaline phosphatase have also been found, but the frequency of this abnormality is not well defined in the English literature. In one patient who developed hepatitis while receiving norfloxacin for a urinary tract infection, extensive investigation for other causes of hepatitis was negative, and liver biopsy revealed moderate steatosis, small foci of centrilobular necrosis with scattered eosinophilic bodies, and ceroid-laden macrophages (119). No fibrosis, inflammatory infiltrates, or bile duct abnormalities were seen. Serum transaminase levels returned to normal several weeks after cessation of therapy. Hepatic failure secondary to fluoroquinolone therapy has not been reported.

### Renal Reactions

Mild worsening of renal function during fluoroquinolone therapy has been reported in 0.1 to 1.3% of patients. Crystalluria has been seen rarely in patients given norfloxacin (184, 208, 225) and ciprofloxacin (13, 38, 183, 189, 215), has been associated with high doses and an alkaline urine (which is associated with reduced drug solubility) (208, 215), and was not associated with elevations in serum creatinine in humans. Crystalluria was not seen in clinical trials with ofloxacin (209), temafloxacin (147), and lomefloxacin (174). Analysis of urine crystals induced in animals revealed a complex of ciprofloxacin (or its metabolites), magnesium, and protein (185). In animals, high doses of ciprofloxacin produce crystal deposition in tubules, with a slight to moderate inflammatory response and elevations in serum creatinine levels (46).

Acute interstitial nephritis is rare but predominates as the cause of important renal dysfunction in case reports that have included patients given ciprofloxacin (5, 69, 81, 83, 91, 151, 169, 173, 197) and norfloxacin (30). In a number of cases, allergic manifestations (skin rash, fever, and eosinophiluria) have been present (5, 81, 151, 169, 173), suggesting that the renal injury is allergic. Crystalluria has not been noted in these cases, and in some patients, urine pH was documented to be in the acid range, at which crystalluria is unlikely. In renal biopsies or at autopsy in one fatal case (81), edema and lymphocytic infiltrates have been seen in the interstitium with normal glomeruli (5, 30, 81, 151, 173, 197); eosinophils have also been found in the interstitium in some cases (81, 151, 173). In one patient with high concentrations of ciprofloxacin in plasma and a urine pH of 7, acute tubular necrosis developed (72), although crystal deposition was not documented. Recurrent hematuria with erythrocyte casts without renal failure was associated with each of three courses of ciprofloxacin in one patient (20). Renal failure and hematuria have also been identified in postmarketing surveillance in a small number of patients given ofloxacin (107).

Rarely, hyperuricemia has been encountered during fluoroquinolone therapy (62).

## OTHER POTENTIAL ADVERSE EFFECTS BASED ON MICROBIOLOGIC OR ANIMAL STUDIES

### Ocular and Otic Effects

Toxicities of quinolones affecting the eye have been encountered in some animals and rarely in humans. Subcapsular cataracts have developed in rats and cats treated with pefloxacin and in dogs treated with rosoxacin for prolonged periods (21, 46, 47, 185). Alterations in retinal electrophysiology and histology have been seen in cats given nalidixic acid but were not seen when the animals were given norfloxacin (49) or ciprofloxacin (185) systemically. However, cataracts have not been seen in other animals given ciprofloxacin and have not been reported in humans receiving fluoroquinolones (20, 185). Flumequine has produced bulla formation in the maculas of three patients with renal failure (94), but retinal toxicity has not been reported with other fluoroquinolones in humans (129). Injection of ciprofloxacin directly into the vitreous humors of rabbits produced dose-dependent retinal toxicity, and injection into the aqueous humors produced dose-dependent corneal toxicity (204), but local drug concentrations were substantially higher than those achievable with systemic administration (see chapter 23). No fundoscopic or pathologic abnormalities were detected in the eyes of rabbits treated with ofloxacin for 28 days (55).

Repeated application of ciprofloxacin to the round window membranes of guinea pig ears produced either slight reductions in hearing at high frequency (16 to 32 kHz) (48) or no effect (123), results in contrast to a substantial reduction in hearing for controls in whom neomycin was applied to the round window.

### Teratogenicity and Safety in Pregnancy

Norfloxacin failed to produce malformations in the offspring of pregnant mice, rats, or rabbits, but in high doses resulting in serum drug levels threefold higher than are achievable in humans, it produced fetal loss in monkeys (49, 52). No teratogenic effect was seen in monkeys given even higher doses of norfloxacin, and fetal loss was thought to result from suppression of placental progesterone. Ciprofloxacin also produced no evidence of teratogenicity in rats, mice, and rabbits, but weight loss from gastrointestinal toxicity has been associated with an increased incidence of abortion in rabbits (data on file; Miles Inc., Pharmaceutical Division, West Haven, Conn.) (38). Ofloxacin produced similar fetal loss in rabbits (210). Pefloxacin, enoxacin, and fleroxacin also produced no teratogenic effects in rats (46). In macaques, temafloxacin in high doses produced fetal wastage but no fetal malformations (212). Dose-related skeletal abnormalities have been reported in rat fetuses exposed to ofloxacin in utero, but other studies with rats and studies with rabbits found no teratogenic effects (55, 136, 210).

Use of fluoroquinolones in pregnant humans has been infrequent. Postmarketing surveillance identified 39 patients who received ofloxacin during pregnancy (107). In 33 cases (15 exposed before day 17 of pregnancy, 9 exposed after day 17, and 9 with an unspecified time of exposure), babies were born healthy. Six disorders, including one miscarriage and four congenital malformations (malformation of the pinna with partial deafness, proencephalia, enterothorax, and congenital blindness), were reported, although the relation to ofloxacin treatment was not clearly established. The safety of fluoroquinolones in pregnant humans has not been adequately established, and the use of these compounds remains contraindicated during pregnancy.

## Mutagenicity

In bacteria, quinolones interact with DNA gyrase and DNA in a manner that results in the induction of the RecA SOS DNA repair system (see chapter 3); this repair is error prone and may thereby increase the frequency of bacterial mutations (159). The Rec assay of mutagenicity in *Bacillus subtilis* has been slightly positive with norfloxacin (49) and ofloxacin (136); other bacterial tests of mutagenicity (*Salmonella typhimurium* reverse mutation test [Ames assay] with norfloxacin [49] and ciprofloxacin [38] and *Escherichia coli* DNA repair test with ciprofloxacin [38]) have been negative, however.

In eukaryotic cells, the homolog of DNA gyrase, topoisomerase II, is several orders of magnitude more resistant to the action of most fluoroquinolones than is the bacterial enzyme (95) (see chapter 7), suggesting that the ability to produce mutagenic effects by interaction with topoisomerase II and DNA is substantially lower for these compounds in eukaryotic cells. Some quinolone congeners, however, have a substantially enhanced potency against eukaryotic topoisomerase II (see chapter 7), and some of these congeners have been shown to be direct mutagens in mammalian cell culture systems (86).

For norfloxacin, ciprofloxacin, and ofloxacin, most tests of mutagenicity in eukaryotic systems have produced negative results. Included have been tests of cytotoxicity, sister chromatid exchange, chromosomal aberration, V-79 mammalian cell mutagenicity (norfloxacin [49]), and error rates of DNA synthesis in vitro (95); the mouse micronucleus and dominant lethal tests have also been negative (ciprofloxacin [38, 135], ofloxacin [135, 193, 194]). One eukaryotic test of mutagenicity, the in vitro rat hepatocyte primary culture-DNA repair test, has given positive results with norfloxacin, ciprofloxacin, ofloxacin, and pefloxacin but not nalidixic acid (134). The same test conducted in vivo, however, was negative with ciprofloxacin (134); results for the other fluoroquinolones in the in vivo test were not given. Modest unscheduled DNA synthesis in lymphocytes and DNA strand breaks in Raji cells as measured by the alkaline elution technique have been reported with ciprofloxacin at concentrations of $\geq 10\ \mu g/ml$ (35). Thus, the evidence as to the mutagenicity of the newer fluoroquinolones is conflicting, although the preponderance of the current data suggests that the potential for significant mutagenicity of the current antibacterial quinolones in humans is low. Chapter 28 contains a more detailed discussion of the various effects of fluoroquinolones on eukaryotic cells.

## Carcinogenicity

Long-term studies of the carcinogenicity of norfloxacin in rats and mice are negative (21, 47, 49). Information on the carcinogenic potentials of the other newer fluoroquinolones has not yet been reported.

## Effects on Leukocyte Functions

Effects on leukocyte functions are discussed in chapter 28.

## Effects on Reproductive Functions

Long-term toxicity studies using high doses of norfloxacin, pefloxacin, enoxacin, and fleroxacin given for at least several months have identified testicular atrophy, azoospermia, and, in some cases, reduction in prostate weight in rats and dogs (46, 47). Similar studies with ciprofloxacin and ofloxacin have revealed no histologic or functional abnormalities of the reproductive tracts of male rats (46, 55, 129). The mechanisms of these effects are unknown, and they have not been described in humans.

## FINANCIAL TOXICITIES

In the United States, norfloxacin, ciprofloxacin, ofloxacin, lomefloxacin, and enoxacin have been approved for clinical use. The average wholesale cost of 1 day's treatment ranges from $4.26 for norfloxacin (400 mg twice daily) to $10.14 for ciprofloxacin (750 mg twice daily) (Table 4) (8–10). The costs to the patient will likely be higher and may vary. Compared with other generic antimicrobial agents given orally for the treatment of urinary tract infections (e.g., ampicillin, $0.66; TMP-SMX, $0.29), these quinolones are substantially more expensive. When the most suitable alternative agents are parenteral, however, oral quinolone therapy is more cost-effective. Many parenteral agents are more expensive than quinolones (e.g., cefotaxime, $56.64; imipenem-cilastatin, $89.60), and the use of oral agents also avoids the costs of intravenous administration sets and nursing time. Intravenous quinolones are also substantially more expensive than oral quinolones (Table 4). Additional savings may be gained if oral therapy allows avoidance of hospitalization, earlier discharge from the hospital, or avoidance of intravenous therapy at home (23, 164).

## CONCLUSIONS

### Contraindications to Use of Fluoroquinolones

The newer fluoroquinolones are contraindicated (Table 5) in patients with a history of allergic reactions to the older analogs (nalidixic acid, cinoxacin, pipemidic acid, oxolinic acid) or to any of the newer agents. The fluoroquinolones should also be avoided in children with incomplete skeletal growth, in pregnant patients, and in nursing mothers. Breast milk concentrations of ciprofloxacin, pefloxacin, and ofloxacin have been documented to be similar to concentrations in serum (73), and in animals, norfloxacin is also excreted into breast milk (data on file; Merck Sharpe & Dohme, Rahway, N.J.). As discussed above (section on arthropathy), the contraindication for quinolone use in pediatric patients is not absolute. Use of ciprofloxacin in selected pediatric patients, such as those with cystic fibrosis, may be considered when there are important limitations to the use of nonquinolone therapies and when careful monitoring for joint toxicities is possible.

**Table 4.** Costs of fluoroquinolones and selected other antimicrobial agents[a]

| Drug and route of administration | Daily dose | Daily cost[b] |
|---|---|---|
| Norfloxacin, p.o. | 400 mg b.i.d. | $4.68 |
| Ciprofloxacin, p.o. | 250–750 mg b.i.d. | $5.06–10.14 |
| Ofloxacin, p.o. | 200–400 mg b.i.d. | $5.36–6.72 |
| Lomefloxacin, p.o. | 400 mg q.d. | $5.66 |
| Ampicillin, p.o. | 500 mg q.i.d. | $0.66 |
| TMP-SMX, p.o. | 160 mg–800 mg b.i.d. | $0.29 |
| Amoxicillin-clavulanate, p.o. | 250–500 mg t.i.d. | $5.19–7.17 |
| Ciprofloxacin, i.v. | 200–400 mg b.i.d. | $28.82–57.62 |
| Ofloxacin, i.v. | 400 mg b.i.d. | $52.82 |
| Gentamicin, i.v. | 80 mg q8h | $1.98 |
| Cefotaxime, i.v. | 2 g q8h | $56.64 |
| Imipenem-cilastatin, i.v. | 500 mg q6h | $89.60 |

[a]Abbreviations: p.o., peroral; i.v., intravenous; b.i.d., twice a day; q.d., daily; q.i.d., four times a day; t.i.d., three times a day; q8h, q6h, every 8 or 6 h, respectively.
[b]Average wholesale price, February 1993.

**Table 5.** Contraindications and cautions for clinical use of fluoroquinolones

Contraindicated for:
- Patients with previous allergy to old or new quinolone agents
- Pregnant patients
- Lactating mothers
- Children with incomplete skeletal growth

Patients requiring special monitoring and caution
- Those with history of seizures or conditions predisposing to seizures
- Those receiving nonsteroidal anti-inflammatory agents
- Those receiving theophylline preparations[a]

[a]For patients receiving enoxacin or ciprofloxacin (see chapter 11).

## Patients for Whom Special Caution Should Be Exercised

Particular attention should be given to monitoring for central nervous system toxicities in patients with histories of a seizure disorder or structural lesions of the central nervous system that might predispose to seizures or in patients concurrently receiving NSAIDs (Table 5). In addition, serum theophylline levels should be monitored in patients receiving concurrent theophylline preparations and enoxacin, ciprofloxacin, or pefloxacin.

Patients who are receiving higher-than-recommended doses of fluoroquinolones and whose urine has a persistently neutral or alkaline pH because of infection with urea-splitting organisms or because of underlying renal tubular defects should be monitored for the development of crystalluria or rises in serum creatinine.

## Overall Tolerability

Although this chapter has emphasized and detailed the adverse effects of the newer fluoroquinolone agents, the frequencies of toxicities encountered with these agents have overall been quite acceptable compared with those of other antimicrobial agents in clinical use, as is emphasized by the data in Table 1. As more extensive use occurs, additional information about rare or late-developing toxicities with some fluoroquinolones may become available, as it did with temafloxacin. Use of fluoroquinolones in doses higher than those used in most studies reviewed in the foregoing chapters on clinical uses is likely to be associated with more adverse effects. With careful dosing, however, studies indicate that quinolone intolerance is unlikely to present major limitations to the realization of the clinical potential of these agents as measured by their substantial efficacy in a broad range of infections.

## REFERENCES

1. **Aceto, M. D., L. S. Harris, G. Y. Lesher, J. Pearl, and T. G. Brown, Jr.** 1967. Pharmacologic studies with 7-benzyl-1-ethyl-1,4-dihydro-4-oxo-1,8-naphthyridine-3-carboxylic acid. *J. Pharmacol. Exp. Ther.* **158:**286–293.
2. **Adam, D.** 1989. Use of quinolones in pediatrics. *Rev. Infect. Dis.* **11**(Suppl. 5)**:**1113–1116.
3. **Alfaham, M., M. E. Holt, and M. C. Goodchild.** 1987. Arthropathy in a patient with cystic fibrosis taking ciprofloxacin. *Br. Med. J.* **295:**699.
4. **Allais, J. M., L. C. Preheim, T. A. Cuevas, J. S. Roccaforte, M. A. Mellencamp, and M. J. Bittner.** 1988. Randomized, double-blind comparison of ciprofloxacin and trimethoprim-sulfamethoxazole for complicated urinary tract infections. *Antimicrob. Agents Chemother.* 32:1327–1330.
5. **Allon, M., E. J. Lopez, and K.-W. Min.** 1990. Acute renal failure due to ciprofloxacin. *Arch. Intern. Med.* **150:**2187–2189.
6. **Altes, J., J. Gasco, J. de Antonio, A. Salas, and C. Villalonga.** 1989. Ciprofloxacin and delirium. *Ann. Intern. Med.* **110:**170–171.
7. **Anastasio, G. E., D. Menscer, and J. M. Little.** 1988. Norfloxacin and seizures. *Ann. Intern. Med.* **109:**169–170.
8. **Anonymous.** 1987. Norfloxacin (Noroxin). *Med. Lett. Drugs Ther.* **29:**25–27.
9. **Anonymous.** 1988. Ciprofloxacin. *Med. Lett. Drugs Ther.* **30:**11–13.
10. **Anonymous.** 1992. Two new fluoroquinolones. *Med. Lett. Drugs Ther.* **34:**58–60.
11. **Aoun, M., C. Jacquy, L. Debusscher, D. Bron, M. Lehert, P. Noel, and P. van der Auwera.** 1992. Peripheral neuropathy associated with fluoroquinolones. *Lancet* **340:**127.
12. **Arcieri, G., R. August, N. Becker, C. Doyle, E. Griffith, G. Gruenwaldt, A. Heyd, and B. O'Brien.** 1986. Clinical experience with ciproflox-

acin in the USA. *Eur. J. Clin. Microbiol.* **5:**220–225.

13. **Arcieri, G., E. Griffith, G. Gruenwaldt, A. Heyd, B. O'Brien, N. Becker, and R. August.** 1987. Ciprofloxacin: an update on clinical experience. *Am. J. Med.* **82**(Suppl. 4A)**:**381–394.
14. **Arcieri, G. M., N. Becker, B. Esposito, E. Griffith, A. Heyd, C. Neumann, B. O'Brien, and P. Schacht.** 1989. Safety of intravenous ciprofloxacin. A review. *Am. J. Med.* **87**(Suppl. 5A)**:**92S–97S.
15. **Asperilla, M. O., and R. A. Smego.** 1989. Eosinophilic meningitis associated with ciprofloxacin. *Am. J. Med.* **87:**589–590.
16. **Bader, M. B.** 1992. Role of ciprofloxacin in fatal cases. *Chest* **101:**883–884.
17. **Baes, H.** 1968. Photosensitivity caused by nalidixic acid. *Dermatologica* **136:**61–64.
18. **Bailey, R. R., J. A. Kirk, and B. A. Peddie.** 1983. Norfloxacin-induced rheumatic disease. *N.Z. Med. J.* **96:**590.
19. **Bailey, R. R., R. Natale, and A. L. Linton.** 1972. Nalidixic acid arthralgia. *Can. Med. Assoc. J.* **107:**604–605.
20. **Ball, P.** 1986. Ciprofloxacin: an overview of adverse experiences. *J. Antimicrob. Chemother.* **18**(Suppl. D)**:**187–193.
21. **Ball, P.** 1989. Adverse reactions and interactions of fluoroquinolones. *Clin. Invest. Med.* **12:**28–34.
22. **Baran, R., and P. Brun.** 1986. Photoonycholysis induced by the fluoroquinolones pefloxacine and ofloxacine. *Dermatologica* **173:**185–188.
23. **Barriere, S. L.** 1987. Economic impact of oral ciprofloxacin. A pharmacist's perspective. *Am. J. Med.* **82**(Suppl. 4A)**:**387–390.
24. **Bates, C. J., M. H. Wilcox, R. C. Spencer, and D. M. Harris.** 1990. Ciprofloxacin and *Clostridium difficile* infection. *Lancet* **336:**1193.
25. **Bednarczyk, E. M., J. A. Green, A. D. Nelson, G. A. Leisure, D. Little, L. P. Addler, M. S. Berridge, E. A. Panacek, and F. D. Miraldi.** 1991. Comparison of the effect of temafloxacin, ciprofloxacin, or placebo on cerebral blood flow, glucose, and oxygen metabolism in healthy subjects by means of positron emission tomography. *Clin. Pharmacol. Ther.* **50:**165–171.
26. **Bennish, M. L., M. A. Salam, W. A. Khan, and A. M. Khan.** 1992. Treatment of shigellosis. III. Comparison of one- or two-dose ciprofloxacin with standard 5-day therapy. A randomized, blinded trial. *Ann. Intern. Med.* **117:**727–734.
27. **Berger, T. G., and N. Franklin.** 1992. Anaphylactoid reaction to ciprofloxacin in a patient infected with the human immunodeficiency virus. *J. Am. Acad. Dermatol.* **26:**256–257.
28. **Birkett, D. A., M. Barretts, and C. J. Stevenson.** 1969. Phototoxic bullous eruptions due to nalidixic acid. *Br. J. Dermatol.* **81:**342–344.
29. **Blomer, R., K. Bruch, H. Krauss, and W. Wacheck.** 1986. Safety of ofloxacin—adverse drug reactions reported during phase-II studies in Europe and in Japan. *Infection* **14**(Suppl. 4)**:**S332–S334.
30. **Boelaert, J., P. P. de Jaegere, R. Daneels, M. Schurgers, B. Gordts, and H. W. van Lauduyt.** 1986. Case report of renal failure during norfloxacin therapy. *Clin. Nephrol.* **25:**272. (Letter.)
31. **Boisvert, A., and G. Barbeau.** 1981. Nalidixic acid-induced photodermatitis after minimal sun exposure. *Drug Intell. Clin. Pharm.* **15:**126–127.
32. **Boréus, L. O., and B. Sundström.** 1967. Intracranial hypertension in a child during treatment with nalidixic acid. *Br. Med. J.* **2:**744–745.
33. **Bowie, W. R., V. Willetts, and P. J. Jewesson.** 1989. Adverse reactions in a dose-ranging study with a new long-acting fluoroquinolone, fleroxacin. *Antimicrob. Agents Chemother.* **33:**1778–1782.
34. **Brauner, G. J.** 1975. Bullous photoreaction to nalidixic acid. *Am. J. Med.* **58:**576–580.
35. **Bredberg, A., M. Brant, K. Riesbeck, Y. Azou, and A. Forsgren.** 1989. 4-Quinolone antibiotics: positive genotoxic screening tests despite an apparent lack of mutation induction. *Mutat. Res.* **211:**171–180.
36. **Butler, T., S. Loleka, C. Rasidi, A. Kadio, P. L. Del Rosal, H. Iskandar, E. Rubinstein, and G. Pastore.** 1993. Treatment of acute bacterial diarrhea: a multicenter international trial comparing placebo with fleroxacin given as a single dose or once daily for 3 days. *Am. J. Med.* **94**(Suppl. 3A)**:**187S–194S.
37. **Cain, D. B., and M. E. O'Connor.** 1990. Pseudomembranous colitis associated with ciprofloxacin. *Lancet* **336:**946.
38. **Campoli-Richards, D. M., J. P. Monk, A. Price, P. Benfield, P. A. Todd, and A. Ward.** 1988. Ciprofloxacin. A review of its antibacterial activity, pharmacokinetic properties and therapeutic use. *Drugs* **35:**373–447.
39. **Carbon, C., P. Léophonte, P. Petitpretz, J. P. Chauvin, and J. Hazebroucq.** 1992. Efficacy and safety of temafloxacin versus those of amoxicillin in hospitalized adults with community-acquired pneumonia. *Antimicrob. Agents Chemother.* **36:**833–839.
40. **Chew, S. L., R. Daelemans, and R. L. Lins.** 1990. Ciprofloxacin and pseudomembranous colitis. *Lancet* **336:**1509.
41. **Chmel, H., G. Emmanuel, T. Lie, L. Anderson, and J. Ireland.** 1990. A prospective, double-blind randomized study comparing the efficacy and safety of low-dose ciprofloxacin with ampicillin in the treatment of bronchitis. *Diagn. Microbiol. Infect. Dis.* **13:**149–151.
42. **Chodosh, S.** 1991. Temafloxacin compared with ciprofloxacin in mild to moderate lower respiratory tract infections in ambulatory patients. A multicen-

ter, double-blind, randomized study. *Chest* **100:**1497–1502.
43. **Chodosh, S.** 1993. Efficacy of fleroxacin versus amoxicillin in acute exacerbations of chronic bronchitis. *Am. J. Med.* **94**(Suppl. 3A)**:**131S–135S.
44. **Choe, U., B. M. Rothschild, and L. Laitman.** 1989. Ciprofloxacin-induced vasculitis. *N. Engl. J. Med.* **320:**257–258.
45. **Christ, W.** 1990. Central nervous system toxicity of quinolones: human and animal findings. *J. Antimicrob. Chemother.* **26**(Suppl. B)**:**219–225.
46. **Christ, W., and T. Lehnert.** 1990. Toxicity of the quinolones, p. 165–187. *In* C. Siporin, C. L. Heifetz, and J. M. Domagala (ed.), *The New Generation of Quinolones.* Marcel Dekker, Inc., New York.
47. **Christ, W., T. Lehnert, and B. Ulbrich.** 1988. Specific toxicologic aspects of the quinolones. *Rev. Infect. Dis.* **10**(Suppl. 1)**:**S141–S146.
48. **Claes, J., P. J. Govaerts, P. H. Van de Heyning, and S. Peeters.** 1991. Lack of ciprofloxacin ototoxicity after repeated ototopical application. *Antimicrob. Agents Chemother.* **35:**1014–1016.
49. **Corrado, M. L., W. E. Struble, C. Peter, V. Hoagland, and J. Sabbaj.** 1987. Norfloxacin: review of safety studies. *Am. J. Med.* **82**(Suppl. 6B)**:**22–26.
50. **Cox, C. E.** 1991. Oral temafloxacin compared to norfloxacin for the treatment of complicated urinary tract infections. *Am. J. Med.* **91**(Suppl. 6A)**:**129S–133S.
51. **Cruciani, M., G. Di Perri, E. Concia, D. Bassetti, A. Navarra, and L. Nespoli.** 1989. Use of quinolones in childhood. *J. Pediatr.* **115:**1022–1023.
52. **Cukierski, M. A., S. Prahalada, A. G. Zacchei, C. P. Peter, J. D. Todgers, D. L. Hess, et al.** 1989. Embryotoxicity studies of norfloxacin in cynomolgus monkeys. I. Teratology studies and norfloxacin plasma concentration in pregnant and nonpregnant monkeys. *Teratology* **39:**39–52.
53. **Dan, M., and Z. Samra.** 1989. *Clostridium difficile* colitis associated with ofloxacin therapy. *Am. J. Med.* **87:**479.
54. **Davies, B. I., F. P. V. Maesen, and J. P. Teengs.** 1984. Serum and sputum concentrations of enoxacin after single oral dosing in a clinical and bacteriological study. *J. Antimicrob. Chemother.* **14**(Suppl. C)**:**83–89.
55. **Davis, G. J., and B. E. McKenzie.** 1989. Toxicologic evaluation of ofloxacin. *Am. J. Med.* **87**(Suppl. 6C)**:**43S–46S.
56. **Davis, H., E. McGoodwin, and T. G. Reed.** 1989. Anaphylactoid reactions reported after treatment with ciprofloxacin. *Ann. Intern. Med.* **111:**1041–1043.
57. **Deaney, N. B., R. Vogel, M. J. Vandenburg, and W. J. C. Currie.** 1984. Norfloxacin in acute urinary tract infections. *Practitioner* **228:**111-117.
58. **Desplaces, N., L. Gutmann, J. Carlet, J. Guibert, and J. F. Acar.** 1986. The new quinolones and their combinations with other agents for therapy of severe infections. *J. Antimicrob. Chemother.* **17**(Suppl. A)**:**25–39.
59. **Egede, F., and I. Kristensen.** 1988. A clinical comparative trial of ofloxacin and pivampicillin in acute exacerbations of chronic bronchitis. *J. Antimicrob. Chemother.* **22**(Suppl. C)**:**139–142.
60. **Ehrenpreis, E. D., M. W. Lievens, and R. M. Craig.** 1990. *Clostridium difficile*-associated diarrhea after norfloxacin. *J. Clin. Gastroenterol.* **12:**188–189.
61. **Ericsson, C. D., P. C. Johnson, H. L. DuPont, D. R. Morgan, J. A. M. Bitsura, and F. J. de la Cabada.** 1987. Ciprofloxacin or trimethoprim-sulfamethoxazole as initial therapy for travelers' diarrhea. *Ann. Intern. Med.* **106:**216–220.
62. **Eron, L. J., L. Harvey, D. L. Hixon, and D. M. Poretz.** 1985. Ciprofloxacin therapy of infections caused by *Pseudomonas aeruginosa* and other resistant bacteria. *Antimicrob. Agents Chemother.* **27:**308–310.
63. **Farkas, S. A.** 1993. Intravenous fleroxacin versus ceftazidime in the treatment of acute nonpneumococcal lower respiratory tract infections. *Am. J. Med.* **94**(Suppl. 3A)**:**142S–149S.
64. **Fass, R. J.** 1987. Efficacy and safety of oral ciprofloxacin in the treatment of serious respiratory infections. *Am. J. Med.* **82**(Suppl. 4A)**:**202–207.
65. **Fass, R. J.** 1987. Adverse reactions associated with quinolones. *Quinolones Bull.* **3:**5–6.
66. **Ferguson, J., and B. E. Johnson.** 1990. Ciprofloxacin-induced photosensitivity: in vitro and in vivo studies. *Br. J. Dermatol.* **123:**9–20.
67. **Ferguson, J., J. McIntosh, and E. M. Walker.** 1988. Ciprofloxacin-induced photosensitivity: in vitro and in vivo studies. *J. Invest. Dermatol.* **91:**385.
68. **Fong, I. W., W. Linton, M. Simbul, R. Thorup, B. McLaughlin, V. Rahm, and P. A. Quinn.** 1987. Treatment of nongonococcal urethritis with ciprofloxacin. *Am. J. Med.* **82**(Suppl. 4A)**:**311–316.
69. **Garlando, F., M. G. Täuber, B. Joos, O. Oelz, and R. Lüthy.** Ciprofloxacin-induced hematuria. *Infection* **13:**177–178.
70. **Geddes, A. M.** 1993. Safety of fleroxacin in clinical trials. *Am. J. Med.* **94**(Suppl. 3A)**:**201S–203S.
71. **Gentry, L. O., C. H. Ramirez-Ronda, E. Rodriguez-Noriega, H. Thadepalli, P. L. del Rosal, and C. Ramirez.** 1989. Oral ciprofloxacin vs parenteral cefotaxime in the treatment of difficult skin and skin structure infections. A multicenter trial. *Arch. Intern. Med.* **149:**2579–2583.
72. **Gerritsen, W. R., A. Peters, F. C. Henry, and J. R. B. J. Brouwers.** 1987. Ciprofloxacin-induced nephrotoxicity. *Nephrol. Dial. Transplant.* **2:**382–383.

73. **Giamarellou, H., E. Kolokythas, G. Petrikkos, J. Gazis, D. Aravantinos, and P. Sfikakis.** 1989. Pharmacokinetics of three newer quinolones in pregnant and lactating women. *Am. J. Med.* **87**(Suppl. 5A)**:**49S–51S.

74. **Golledge, C. L., C. F. Carson, G. L. O'Neill, R. A. Bowman, and T. V. Riley.** 1992. Ciprofloxacin and *Clostridium difficile*-associated diarrhoea. *J. Antimicrob. Chemother.* **30:**141–147.

75. **Gonzalez, J. P., and J. M. Henwood.** 1989. Pefloxacin. A review of its antibacterial activity, pharmacokinetic properties and therapeutic use. *Drugs* **37:**628–668.

76. **Gotuzzo, E., J. G. Guerra, L. Benavente, J. C. Palomino, C. Carrillo, J. Lopera, F. Delgado, D. R. Nalin, and J. Sabbaj.** 1988. Use of norfloxacin to treat chronic typhoid carriers. *J. Infect. Dis.* **157:**1221–1225.

77. **Granowitz, E. V.** 1989. Photosensitivity rash in a patient being treated with ciprofloxacin. *J. Infect. Dis.* **160:**910.

78. **Grubbs, N. C., H. J. Schultz, N. K. Henry, D. M. Ilstrup, S. M. Muller, and W. R. Wilson.** 1992. Ciprofloxacin versus trimethoprim-sulfamethoxazole: treatment of community-acquired urinary tract infections in a prospective, controlled, double-blind comparison. *Mayo Clin. Proc.* **67:**1163–1168.

79. **Halkin, H.** 1988. Adverse effects of the fluoroquinolones. *Rev. Infect. Dis.* **10**(Suppl. 1)**:**S258–S261.

80. **Handsfield, H. H., F. N. Judson, and K. K. Holmes.** 1981. Treatment of uncomplicated gonorrhea with rosoxacin. *Antimicrob. Agents Chemother.* **20:**625–629.

81. **Helmink, R., and H. Benediktsson.** 1990. Ciprofloxacin-induced allergic interstitial nephritis. *Nephron* **55:**432–433.

82. **Henry, N. K., H. J. Schultz, N. C. Grubbs, S. M. Muller, D. M. Ilstrup, and W. R. Wilson.** 1986. Comparison of ciprofloxacin and co-trimoxazole in the treatment of uncomplicated urinary tract infection in women. *J. Antimicrob. Chemother.* **18**(Suppl. D)**:**103–106.

83. **Hessen, M. T., M. J. Ingerman, D. H. Daufman, P. Weiner, J. Santoro, O. M. Korzeniowski, J. Boscis, M. Topiel, L. M. Bush, D. Kaye, and M. E. Levison.** 1987. Clinical efficacy of ciprofloxacin therapy for gram-negative bacillary osteomyelitis. *Am. J. Med.* **82**(Suppl. 4A)**:**262–265.

84. **Hibberd, P. L., N. E. Tolkoff-Rubin, M. Doran, A. Delvecchio, A. B. Cosimi, F. L. Delmonico, H. Auchincloss, Jr., and R. H. Rubin.** 1992. Trimethoprim-sulfamethoxazole compared with ciprofloxacin for the prevention of urinary tract infection in renal transplant recipients, document 15. *Online J. Curr. Clin. Trials 1992.*

85. **Hillman, R. J., G. Gopal Rao, J. R. W. Harris, and D. Taylor-Robinson.** 1990. Ciprofloxacin as a cause of *Clostridium difficile*-associated diarrhoea in an HIV antibody-positive patient. *J. Infect.* **21:**205–207.

86. **Holden, H. E., J. F. Barrett, C. M. Huntington, P. A. Muehlbauer, and M. G. Wahrenburg.** 1989. Genetic profile of a nalidixic acid analog: a model for the mechanism of sister chromatid exchange induction. *Environ. Mol. Mutagen.* **13:**238–252.

87. **Holmes, B., R. N. Brogden, and D. M. Richards.** 1985. Norfloxacin. A review of its antibacterial activity, pharmacokinetic properties and therapeutic use. *Drugs* **30:**482–513.

88. **Hooper, D. C., and J. S. Wolfson.** 1985. The fluoroquinolones: pharmacology, clinical uses, and toxicities in humans. *Antimicrob. Agents Chemother.* **28:**716–721.

89. **Hooper, D. C., and J. S. Wolfson.** 1989. Adverse effects of quinolone antimicrobial agents, p. 249–271. *In* J. S. Wolfson and D. C. Hooper (ed.), *Quinolone Antimicrobial Agents.* American Society for Microbiology, Washington, D.C.

90. **Hooper, D. C., and J. S. Wolfson.** 1989. Treatment of genitourinary infections with fluoroquinolones: clinical efficacy in genital infections and adverse effects. *Antimicrob. Agents Chemother.* **33:**1662–1667.

91. **Hootkins, R., A. Z. Fenves, and M. K. Stephens.** 1989. Acute renal failure secondary to oral ciprofloxacin therapy: a presentation of three cases and a review of the literature. *Clin. Nephrol.* **32:**75–78.

92. **Hooton, T. M., E. Rogers, T. G. Medina, L. E. Kuwamura, C. Ewers, P. L. Roberts, and W. E. Stamm.** 1990. Ciprofloxacin compared with doxycycline for nongonococcal urethritis. Ineffectiveness against *Chlamydia trachomatis* due to relapsing infection. *J. Am. Med. Assoc.* **264:**1418–1421.

93. **Huminer, D., J. D. Cohen, R. Majadla, and S. Dux.** 1989. Hypersensitivity vasculitis due to ofloxacin. *Br. Med. J.* **299:**303.

94. **Hurault de Ligny, B., D. Sirbat, M. Kessler, P. Trechot, and J. Chanliau.** 1984. Effets secondaires oculaires de la fluméquine. Trois observations d'atteintes maculaires. *Therapie* **39:**595–600.

95. **Hussy, P., G. Maass, B. Tummler, F. Grosse, and V. Schomburg.** 1986. Effect of 4-quinolones and novobiocin on calf thymus DNA polymerase $\alpha$ primase complex, topoisomerases I and II, and growth of mammalian lymphoblasts. *Antimicrob. Agents Chemother.* **29:**2073–2078.

96. **Hyslop, D. L., and W. Bischoff.** 1992. Loracarbef (LY 163892) versus cefaclor and norfloxacin in the treatment of uncomplicated pyelonephritis. *Am. J. Med.* **92**(Suppl. 6A)**:**86S–94S.

97. **Ibsen, H. H. W., B. R. Moller, L. Hankier-Sorensen, and E. From.** 1989. Treatment of non-gonococcal urethritis: comparison of ofloxacin and erythromycin. *Sex. Transm. Dis.* **16:**32–35.
98. **Ingham, B., D. W. Brentnall, E. A. Dale, and J. A. McFadzean.** 1977. Arthropathy induced by antibacterial fused N-alkyl-4-pyridone-3-carboxylic acids. *Toxicol. Lett.* **1:**21–26.
99. **Inter-Nordic Urinary Tract Infection Study Group.** 1988. Double-blind comparison of 3-day versus 7-day treatment with norfloxacin in symptomatic urinary tract infections. *Scand. J. Infect. Dis.* **20:**619–624.
100. **Iravani, A.** 1991. Treatment of uncomplicated urinary tract infections with temafloxacin. *Am. J. Med.* **91**(Suppl. 6A)**:**124S–128S.
101. **Iravani, A.** 1991. Comparative, double-blind, prospective, multicenter trial of temafloxacin versus trimethoprim-sulfamethoxazole in uncomplicated urinary tract infections in women. *Antimicrob. Agents Chemother.* **35:**1777-1781.
102. **Iravani, A.** 1993. Multicenter study of single-dose and multiple-dose fleroxacin versus ciprofloxacin in the treatment of uncomplicated urinary tract infections. *Am. J. Med.* **94**(Suppl. 3A)**:**89S–96S.
103. **Islam, M. A., and T. Sreedharan.** 1965. Convulsions, hyperglycaemia and glycosuria from overdose of nalidixic acid. *J. Am. Med. Assoc.* **192:**1000–1001.
104. **Janknegt, R.** 1989. Fluoroquinolones. Adverse reactions during clinical trials and postmarketing surveillance. *Pharm. Weekbl. (Sci.)* **11:**124–127.
105. **Jawad, A. S. M.** 1989. Cystic fibrosis and drug-induced arthropathy. *Br. J. Rheumatol.* **28:**179–180.
106. **Jensen, T., S. S. Pedersen, C. H. Nielsen, N. Hoiby, and C. Koch.** 1987. The efficacy and safety of ciprofloxacin and ofloxacin in chronic *Pseudomonas aeruginosa* infection in cystic fibrosis. *J. Antimicrob. Chemother.* **20:**585–594.
107. **Jüngst, G., and R. Mohr.** 1988. Overview of postmarketing experience with ofloxacin in Germany. *J. Antimicrob. Chemother.* **22**(Suppl. C)**:**167–175.
108. **Juorio, A. V.** 1982. The effects of amfonelic acid and some other central stimulants on mouse striatal tyramine, dopamine and homovanillic acid. *Br. J. Pharmacol.* **77:**511–515.
109. **Kawabe, Y., N. Mizuno, and S. Sakakibara.** 1989. Photoallergic reactions caused by enoxacin. *Photodermatology* **6:**58–60.
110. **Kemper, P., and D. Köhler.** 1992. A double-blind study of two dosage regimens of lomefloxacin in bacteriologically proven exacerbations of chronic bronchitis of gram-negative etiology. *Am. J. Med.* **92**(Suppl. 4A)**:**98S–102S.
111. **Kirby, C. P.** 1984. Treatment of simple urinary tract infections in general practice with a 3-day course of norfloxacin. *J. Antimicrob. Chemother.* **13**(Suppl. B)**:**107–112.
112. **Kohler, R. B., N. Arkins, and K. J. Tack.** 1991. Accidental overdose of intravenous ofloxacin with benign outcome. *Antimicrob. Agents Chemother.* **35:**1239–1240.
113. **Kosmidis, J.** 1991. A double-blind study of once-daily temafloxacin in the treatment of bacterial lower respiratory tract infections. *J. Antimicrob. Chemother.* **28**(Suppl. C)**:**73–79.
114. **Koverech, A., M. Picari, F. Granata, R. Fostini, D. Toniolo, and G. Recchia.** 1986. Safety profile of ofloxacin: the Italian data base. *Infection* **14**(Suppl. 4)**:**S335–S337.
115. **Kromann-Andersen, B., P. Sommer, C. Pers, V. Larsen, and F. Rasmussen.** 1986. Clinical evaluation of ofloxacin versus ciprofloxacin in complicated urinary tract infections. *Infection* **14**(Suppl. 4)**:**S305–S306.
116. **Le Loët, X., C. Fessard, C. Noblet, L. A. Saït, and N. Moore.** 1991. Severe polyarthropathy in an adolescent treated with pefloxacin. *J. Rheumatol.* **18:**1941–1942.
117. **Lettau, L. A.** 1988. Oral fluoroquinolone therapy in *Clostridium difficile* colitis. *J. Am. Med. Assoc.* **260:**2216–2217.
118. **Loleka, S., S. Patanachareon, B. Thanangkul, and B. Vibulbandhitkit.** 1988. Norfloxacin versus co-trimoxazole in the treatment of acute bacterial diarrhoea: a placebo controlled study. *Scand. J. Infect. Dis. Suppl.* **56:**35–45.
119. **López-Navidad, A., P. Domingo, J. Cadafalch, and J. Farrerons.** 1990. Norfloxacin-induced hepatotoxicity. *J. Hepatol.* **11:**277–278.
120. **Low, N., and A. Harries.** 1990. Ciprofloxacin and pseudomembranous colitis. *Lancet* **336:**1509.
121. **Lucet, J.-C., H. Tilly, G. Lerebours, H.-J. Gres, and H. Piguet.** 1988. Neurologic toxicity related to pefloxacin. *J. Antimicrob. Chemother.* **21:**811–812.
122. **Lumgiganon, P., K. Pengsaa, and T. Sookpranee.** 1991. Ciprofloxacin in neonates and its possible adverse effect on teeth. *Pediatr. Infect. Dis. J.* **10:**619–620.
123. **Lutz, H., T. Lenarz, and R. Götz.** 1990. Ototoxicity of gyrase antagonist ciprofloxacin? *Adv. Otorhinolaryngol.* **45:**175–180.
124. **Machida, M., H. Kusajima, H. Aijima, A. Maeda, R. Ishida, and H. Uchida.** 1990. Toxicokinetic study of norfloxacin-induced arthropathy in juvenile animals. *Toxicol. Appl. Pharmacol.* **105:**403–412.
125. **Maggiolo, F., W. Bianchi, and H. Ohnmeiss.** 1989. A new approach to the treatment of pseudomembranous colitis? *J. Infect. Dis.* **160:**170–171.
126. **Maggiolo, F., S. Caprioli, and F. Suter.** 1990. Risk/benefit analysis of quinolone use in children:

the effect on diarthrodial joints. *J. Antimicrob. Chemother.* **26:**469–471.

127. **Manzione, N. C.** 1992. A note of caution on empiric use of ciprofloxacin for diarrhea. *Arch. Intern. Med.* **152:**213–214.
128. **Matsumoto, M., K. Kojima, H. Nagano, S. Matsubara, and T. Yokota.** 1992. Photostability and biological activity of fluoroquinolones substituted at the 8 position after UV irradiation. *Antimicrob. Agents Chemother.* **36:**1715–1719.
129. **Mayer, D. G.** 1987. Overview of toxicological studies. *Drugs* **34**(Suppl. 1)**:**150–153.
130. **Mayrer, A. R., and V. T. Andriole.** 1982. Urinary tract antiseptics. *Med. Clin. N. Am.* **66:**199–208.
131. **McCaffrey, C., A. Bertasso, J. Pace, and N. H. Georgopapadakou.** 1992. Quinolone accumulation in *Escherichia coli, Pseudomonas aeruginosa,* and *Staphylococcus aureus. Antimicrob. Agents Chemother.* **36:**1601–1605.
132. **McCue, J. D., and J. R. Zandt.** 1991. Acute psychoses associated with the use of ciprofloxacin and trimethoprim-sulfamethoxazole. *Am. J. Med.* **90:**528–529.
133. **McMillen, B. A., and P. A. Short.** 1978. Amfonelic acid, a non-amphetamine stimulant, has marked effects on brain dopamine metabolism but not noradrenaline metabolism: associated with differences in neuronal storage systems. *J. Pharm. Pharmacol.* **30:**464–466.
134. **McQueen, C. A., and G. M. Williams.** 1987. Effects of quinolone antibiotics in tests of genotoxicity. *Am. J. Med.* **82**(Suppl. 4A)**:**94–96.
135. **Mitelman, F., A.-M. Kolnig, B. Strömbeck, R. Norrby, G. Kromann-Andersen, P. Sommer, and J. Wadstein.** 1988. No cytogenetic effects of quinolone treatment in humans. *Antimicrob. Agents Chemother.* **32:**936–937.
136. **Monk, J. P., and D. M. Campoli-Richards.** 1987. Ofloxacin. A review of its antibacterial activity, pharmacokinetic properties and therapeutic use. *Drugs* **33:**346–391.
137. **Moore, B., M. Safani, and J. Keesey.** 1988. Possible exacerbation of myasthenia gravis by ciprofloxacin. *Lancet* **i:**882.
138. **Morikawa, K., O. Nagata, S. Kubo, H. Kato, and K. Yamamoto.** 1987. *Program Abstr. 27th Intersci. Conf. Antimicrob. Agents Chemother.*, abstr. 255.
139. **Mukherjee, A., P. Dutta, M. Lahiri, S. Sinha, A. K. Mitra, and S. K. Bhattacharya.** 1990. Benign intracranial hypertension after nalidixic acid overdose in infants. *Lancet* **335:**1602.
140. **Mumford, C. J., and L. Ginsberg.** 1990. Ciprofloxacin and myasthenia gravis. *Br. Med. J.* **301:**818.
141. **Naamara, W., F. A. Plummer, R. M. Greenblatt, J. D'Costa, J. O. Ndinya-Achola, and A. R. Ronald.** 1987. Treatment of chancroid with ciprofloxacin: a prospective, randomized clinical trial. *Am. J. Med.* **82**(Suppl. 4A)**:**317–320.
142. **Neldner, K. H.** 1991. Double-blind randomized study of oral temafloxacin and cefadroxil in patients with mild to moderately severe bacterial skin infections. *Am. J. Med.* **91**(Suppl. 6A)**:**111S–114S.
143. **Neringer, R., A. Forsgren, C. Hansson, B. Ode, and The South Swedish Lolex Study Group.** 1992. Lomefloxacin versus norfloxacin in the treatment of uncomplicated urinary tract infections: three-day versus seven-day treatment. *Scand. J. Infect. Dis.* **24:**773–780.
144. **Nicolle, L. E., J. DuBois, A. Y. Martel, G. K. M. Harding, S. D. Shafran, and J. M. Conly.** 1993. Treatment of acute uncomplicated urinary tract infections with 3 days of lomefloxacin compared with treatment with 3 days of norfloxacin. *Antimicrob. Agents Chemother.* **37:**574–579.
145. **Nicolle, L. E., G. K. M. Harding, M. Thompson, J. Kennedy, B. Urias, and A. R. Ronald.** 1989. Prospective, randomized, placebo-controlled trial of norfloxacin for the prophylaxis of recurrent urinary tract infection in women. *Antimicrob. Agents Chemother.* **33:**1032–1035.
146. **Norrby, S. R.** 1991. Side-effects of quinolones: comparisons between quinolones and other antibiotics. *Eur. J. Clin. Microbiol. Infect. Dis.* **10:**378–383.
147. **Norrby, S. R., and A. G. Pernet.** 1991. Assessment of adverse events during drug development: experience with temafloxacin. *J. Antimicrob. Chemother.* **20**(Suppl. C)**:**111–119.
148. **Nuñez, U., and Z. Solís.** 1990. Macrocrystalline nitrofurantoin versus norfloxacin as treatment and prophylaxis in uncomplicated recurrent urinary tract infection. *Curr. Ther. Res.* **48:**234–245.
149. **O'Keefe, B. J., and G. S. Tillotson.** 1990. Ciprofloxacin and pseudomembranous colitis. *Lancet* **336:**1509.
150. **O'Mahony, M. S., and M. X. FitzGerald.** 1991. Cystic fibrosis and seizures. *Lancet* **338:**259.
151. **Ortiz, A., J. J. Plaza, and J. Egido.** 1992. Ciprofloxacin-associated tubulointerstitial nephritis with linear tubular basement membrane deposits. *Nephron* **60:**248.
152. **Pace, J. L., and P. Gatt.** 1989. Fatal vasculitis associated with ofloxacin. *Br. Med. J.* **299:**658–659.
153. **Parish, L. C., and D. L. Jungkind.** 1991. Systemic antimicrobial therapy in skin and skin structure infections: comparison of temafloxacin and ciprofloxacin. *Am. J. Med.* **91**(Suppl. 6A)**:**115S–119S.
154. **Patoia, L., R. Guerciolini, F. Menichetti, G. Bucaneve, and A. Del Favero.** 1987. Norfloxacin and neutropenia. *Ann. Intern. Med.* **107:**788–789. (Letter.)

155. **Pertuiset, E., G. Lenoir, M. Jehanne, F. Douchain, M. Guillot, and C. J. Menkès.** 1989. Tolérance articulaire de la péfloxacine et de l'ofloxacine chez les enfents et adolescents atteints de mucoviscidose. *Rev. Rhum.* **56:**735–740.
156. **Peters, B., and A. J. Pinching.** 1989. Fatal anaphylaxis associated with AIDS related complex. *Br. Med. J.* **298:**605.
157. **Petersen, E. E., F. Wingen, K. L. Fairchild, A. Halfhide, A. Hendrischk, M. Links, M. Schad, H. R. Scholz, N. Schürmann, S. Siegmann, and A. J. Yassin.** 1990. Single dose pefloxacin compared with multiple dose co-trimoxazole in cystitis. *J. Antimicrob. Chemother.* **26**(Suppl. B):147–152.
158. **Petri, H., and H. Tronnier.** 1986. Efficacy of enoxacin in the treatment of bacterial infections of the skin with regards to photosensitization. *Infection* **14**(Suppl. 3):S213–S216.
159. **Phillips, I.** Bacterial mutagenicity and the 4-quinolones. *J. Antimicrob. Chemother.* **20:**771–782.
160. **Pichler, H., G. Diridle, K. Stickler, and D. Wolf.** 1987. Clinical efficacy of ciprofloxacin compared with placebo in bacterial diarrhea. *Am. J. Med.* **82**(Suppl. 4A):329–332.
161. **Pittman, W., J. O. Moon, L. C. Hamrick, C. E. Cox, J. Clark, S. Childs, D. Pizzuti, J. Fredericks, and P. St. Clair.** 1993. Randomized double-blind trial of high- and low-dose fleroxacin versus norfloxacin for complicated urinary tract infection. *Am. J. Med.* **94**(Suppl. 3A):101S–104S.
162. **Plourde, P. J., L. J. D'Costa, E. Agoki, J. Ombette, J. O. Ndinya-Achola, L. A. Slaney, A. R. Ronald, and F. A. Plummer.** 1992. A randomized, double-blind study of the efficacy of fleroxacin versus trimethoprim-sulfamethoxazole in men with culture proven chancroid. *J. Infect. Dis.* **165:**949–952.
163. **Plummer, K.** 1993. Fleroxacin versus norfloxacin in the treatment of urinary tract infections: a multicenter, double-blind, prospective, randomized, comparative study. *Am. J. Med.* **94**(Suppl. 3A):108S–113S.
164. **Quintiliani, R., B. W. Cooper, L. L. Briceland, and C. H. Nightingale.** 1987. Economic impact of streamlining antibiotic administration. *Am. J. Med.* **82**(Suppl. 4A):391–394.
165. **Rademaker, C. M. A., A. P. Sips, H. M. Beumer, I. M. Hoepelman, B. P. Overbeek, M. J. Möllers, M. Rozenberg-Arska, and J. Verhoef.** 1990. A double-blind comparison of low-dose ofloxacin and amoxycillin/clavulanic acid in acute exacerbations of chronic bronchitis. *J. Antimicrob. Chemother.* **26**(Suppl. D):75–81.
166. **Raeburn, J. A., J. R. W. Govan, W. M. McCrae, A. P. Greening, P. S. Collier, M. E. Hodson, and M. C. Goodchild.** 1987. Ciprofloxacin therapy in cystic fibrosis. *J. Antimicrob. Chemother.* **20:**295–296.
167. **Ramirez-Ronda, C. H., S. Saavedra, and C. R. Rivera-Vázquez.** 1987. Comparative, double-blind study of oral ciprofloxacin and intravenous cefotaxime in skin and skin structure infections. *Am. J. Med.* **82**(Suppl. 4A):220–223.
168. **Raoof, S., C. Wollschlager, and F. Khan.** 1987. Treatment of respiratory tract infections with ciprofloxacin. *J. Antimicrob. Chemother.* **18**(Suppl. D):139–145.
169. **Rastogi, S., J. L. D. Atkinson, and J. T. McCarthy.** 1990. Allergic nephropathy associated with ciprofloxacin. *Mayo Clin. Proc.* **65:**987–989.
170. **Reiter, C., M. Pfeiffer, and R. N. Hullman.** 1989. Brief report: safety of ciprofloxacin based on phase IV ("Anwendungsbeobachtung") in the Federal Republic of Germany. *Am. J. Med.* **87**(Suppl. 5A):103S–106S.
171. **Renkonen, O.-V., A. Sivonen, and R. Visakorpi.** 1987. Effect of ciprofloxacin on carrier rate of *Neisseria meningitidis* in army recruits in Finland. *Antimicrob. Agents Chemother.* **31:**962–963.
172. **Ribard, P., F. Audisio, M.-F. Kahn, M. de Bandt, C. Jorgensen, G. Hayem, O. Meyer, and E. Palazzo.** 1992. Seven Achilles tendinitis including 3 complicated by rupture during fluoroquinolone therapy. *J. Rheumatol.* **19:**1479–1481.
173. **Rippelmeyer, D. J., and A. Synhavsky.** 1988. Ciprofloxacin and allergic interstitial nephritis. *Ann. Intern. Med.* **109:**170.
174. **Rizk, E.** 1992. The U.S. clinical experience with lomefloxacin, a new once-daily fluoroquinolone. *Am. J. Med.* **92**(Suppl. 4A):130S–135S.
175. **Roddy, R. E., H. H. Handsfield, and E. W. Hook.** 1986. Comparative trial of single-dose ciprofloxacin and ampicillin plus probenecid for treatment of gonococcal urethritis in men. *Antimicrob. Agents Chemother.* **30:**267–269.
176. **Rodríguez, E., J. A. Martínez, M. Torres, A. Nubiola, and J. Buges.** 1990. Lobular panniculitis associated with ciprofloxacin. *Br. Med. J.* **300:**1468.
177. **Ronald, A. R., M. Turck, and R. G. Petersdorf.** 1966. A critical evaluation of nalidixic acid in urinary tract infections. *N. Engl. J. Med.* **275:**1081–1089.
178. **Rose, T. F., R. Ellis-Pegler, J. Collins, and M. Small.** 1990. Oral pefloxacin mesylate in the treatment of continuous ambulatory peritoneal dialysis associated peritonitis: an open non-comparative study. *J. Antimicrob. Chemother.* **25:**853–859.
179. **Saginur, R., L. E. Nicolle, and Canadian Infectious Diseases Society Clinical Trials Study Group.** 1992. Single-dose compared with 3-day norfloxacin treatment of uncomplicated urinary tract infection in women. *Arch. Intern. Med.* **152:**1233–1237.
180. **Sandberg, T., G. Englund, K. Lincoln, and L.-G. Nilsson.** 1990. Randomised double-blind study

of norfloxacin and cefadroxil in the treatment of acute pyelonephritis. *Eur. J. Clin. Microbiol. Infect. Dis.* **9:**317–323.

181. **Schaad, U. B., and J. Wedgwood.** 1992. Lack of quinolone-induced arthropathy in children. *J. Antimicrob. Chemother.* **30:**414–416.
182. **Schaad, U. B., and J. Wedgwood-Krucko.** 1987. Nalidixic acid in children: retrospective matched controlled study for cartilage toxicity. *Infection* **15:**165–168.
183. **Schacht, P., G. Arcieri, and R. Hullmann.** 1989. Safety of oral ciprofloxacin. An update based on clinical trial results. *Am. J. Med.* **87**(Suppl. 5A)**:**98S–102S.
184. **Schaeffer, A. J.** 1987. Multiclinic study of norfloxacin for treatment of complicated or uncomplicated urinary tract infections. *Am. J. Med.* **82**(Suppl. 6B)**:**53–64.
185. **Schlüter, G.** 1987. Ciprofloxacin: review of potential toxicologic effects. *Am. J. Med.* **82**(Suppl. 4A)**:**91–93.
186. **Scully, B. E., N. Clynes, and H. C. Neu.** 1991. Oral ofloxacin therapy of infections due to multiply-resistant bacteria. *Diagn. Microbiol. Infect. Dis.* **14:**435–441.
187. **Scully, B. E., M. Nakatomi, C. Ores, S. Davidson, and H. C. Neu.** 1987. Ciprofloxacin therapy in cystic fibrosis. *Am. J. Med.* **82**(Suppl. 4A)**:**196–201.
188. **Scully, B. E., and H. C. Neu.** 1987. Treatment of serious infections with intravenous ciprofloxacin. *Am. J. Med.* **82**(Suppl. 4A)**:**369–375.
189. **Self, P. L., B. A. Zeluff, D. Sollo, and L. O. Gentry.** 1987. Use of ciprofloxacin in the treatment of serious skin and skin structure infections. *Am. J. Med.* **82**(Suppl. 4A)**:**239–241.
190. **Shapera, R. M., and J. M. Matsen.** 1977. Oxolinic acid therapy for urinary tract infections in children. *Am. J. Dis. Child.* **131:**34–37.
191. **Sheehan, G. J., G. K. Harding, D. A. Haase, M. J. Thompson, B. Urias, J. K. Kennedy, D. J. Hoban, and A. R. Ronald.** 1988. Double-blind, randomized comparison of 24 weeks of norfloxacin and 12 weeks of norfloxacin followed by 12 weeks of placebo in the therapy of complicated urinary tract infection. *Antimicrob. Agents Chemother.* **32:**1292–1293.
192. **Shelley, E. D., and W. B. Shelley.** 1988. The subcorneal pustular drug eruption: an example induced by norfloxacin. *Cutis* **42:**24–27.
193. **Shimada, H., Y. Ebine, Y. Kurosawa, and T. Arauchi.** 1984. Mutagenicity studies of DL-8280, a new antibacterial drug. *Chemotherapy* (Tokyo) **32**(Suppl. 1)**:**1162–1170.
194. **Shimada, H., Y. Ebine, T. Sato, Y. Kurosawa, and T. Arauchi.** 1985. Dominant lethal study in male mice treated with ofloxacin, a new antimicrobial drug. *Mutat. Res.* **144:**51–55.
195. **Shimada, J., and S. Hori.** 1992. Adverse effects of fluoroquinolones. *Prog. Drug Res.* (Basel) **38:**133–143.
196. **Simon, J., and A. Guyot.** 1990. Pefloxacin: safety in man. *J. Antimicrob. Chemother.* **26**(Suppl. B)**:**215–218.
197. **Simpson, J., A. R. Watson, A. Mellersch, C. S. Nelson, and K. Dodd.** 1991. Typhoid fever, ciprofloxacin, and renal failure. *Arch. Dis. Child.* **66:**1083–1084.
198. **Simpson, K. J., and M. J. Brodie.** 1985. Convulsions related to enoxacin. Lancet **ii:**161. (Letter.)
199. **Slama, T. G.** 1990. Serum sickness-like illness associated with ciprofloxacin. *Antimicrob. Agents Chemother.* **34:**904–905.
200. **Slavich, I. L., R. F. Gleffe, and E. J. Haas.** 1989. Grand mal epileptic seizures during ciprofloxacin therapy. *J. Am. Med. Assoc.* **261:**558–559.
201. **Smith, C. R.** 1987. The adverse effects of fluoroquinolones. *J. Antimicrob. Chemother.* **19:**709–712.
202. **Stahlmann, R.** 1990. Safety profile of the quinolones. *J. Antimicrob. Chemother.* **26**(Suppl. D)**:**31–44.
203. **Steffen, R., R. Jori, H. L. DuPont, J. J. Mathewson, and D. Stürchler.** 1993. Efficacy and toxicity of fleroxacin in the treatment of travelers' diarrhea. *Am. J. Med.* **94**(Suppl. 3A)**:**182S–186S.
204. **Stevens, S. X., B. D. Fouraker, and H. G. Jensen.** 1991. Intraocular safety of ciprofloxacin. *Arch. Ophthalmol.* **109:**1737–1743.
205. **Strandvik, B., L. Hjelte, A. Lindblad, B. Ljungberg, A.-S. Malmborg, and I. Nilsson-Ehle.** 1989. Comparison of efficacy and tolerance of intravenously and orally administered ciprofloxacin in cystic fibrosis patients with acute exacerbations of lung infection. *Scand. J. Infect. Dis.* **60:**84–88.
206. **Stricker, B. H. C., G. Slagboom, R. Damaeseneer, V. Slootmaekers, I. Thijs, and S. Olsson.** Anaphylactic reactions to cinoxacin. *Br. Med. J.* **297:**1434–1435.
207. **Stubbings, J., R. Sheehan-Dare, and S. Walton.** 1992. Cutaneous vasculitis due to ciprofloxacin. *Br. Med. J.* **305:**29.
208. **Swanson, B. N., V. K. Boppana, P. H. Vlasses, H. H. Rotmensch, and R. K. Ferguson.** 1983. Norfloxacin disposition after sequentially increasing oral doses. *Antimicrob. Agents Chemother.* **23:**284–288.
209. **Tack, K. J., and J. A. Smith.** 1989. The safety profile of ofloxacin. *Am. J. Med.* **87**(Suppl. 6C)**:**78S–81S.
210. **Takayama, S., T. Watanabe, Y. Akiyama, K. Ohura, S. Harada, K. Matsuhashi, K. Mochida, and N. Yamashita.** 1986. Reproductive toxicity of ofloxacin. *Arzneim. Forsch. Drug Res.* **36:**1244–1248.

211. **Talbot, G. H., P. A. Cassileth, L. Paradiso, R. Correa-Coronas, L. Bond, and the Enoxacin Prophylaxis Study Group.** 1993. Oral enoxacin for infection prevention in adults with acute nonlymphocytic leukemia. *Antimicrob. Agents Chemother.* **37:**474–482.

212. **Tarantal, A. F., S. B. Lehrer, B. L. Lasley, and A. G. Hendrickx.** 1990. Developmental toxicity of temafloxacin hydrochloride in the long-tailed macaque (*Macaca fascicularis*). *Teratology* **42:**233–242.

213. **Tatsumi, H., H. Senda, S. Yatera, Y. Takemoto, M. Yamayoshi, and K. Ohnishi.** 1978. Toxicological studies on pipemidic acid. V. Effect on diarthrodial joints of experimental animals. *J. Toxicol. Sci.* **3:**357–367.

214. **Thorsteinsson, S. B., T. Bergan, G. Johannesson, H. S. Thorsteinsson, and R. Rohwedder.** 1987. Tolerance of ciprofloxacin at injection site, systemic safety and effect on electroencephalogram. *Chemotherapy* (Basel) **33:**448–451.

215. **Thorsteinsson, S. B., T. Bergan, S. Oddsdottir, R. Rohwedder, and R. Holm.** 1986. Crystalluria and ciprofloxacin, influence of urinary pH and hydration. *Chemotherapy* **32:**408–417.

216. **Tsuei, S. E., A. S. Darrach, and I. Brick.** 1984. Pharmacokinetics and tolerance of enoxacin in healthy volunteers administered at a dosage of 400 mg twice daily for 14 days. *J. Antimicrob. Chemother.* **14**(Suppl. C)**:**71–74.

217. **Tungsanga, K., A. Chongthaleong, N. Udomsantisuk, O.-A. Petcharabutr, V. Sitprija, and E. C. K. Wong.** 1988. Norfloxacin versus co-trimoxazole for the treatment of upper urinary tract infections: a double-blind study. *Scand. J. Infect. Dis. Suppl.* **56:**28–34.

218. **Ulmer, W.** 1993. Fleroxacin versus amoxicillin in the treatment of acute exacerbations of chronic bronchitis. *Am. J. Med.* **94**(Suppl. 3A)**:**136S–141S.

219. **Urinary Tract Infection Study Group.** 1987. Coordinated multicenter study of norfloxacin versus trimethoprim-sulfamethoxazole treatment of symptomatic urinary tract infections. *J. Infect. Dis.* **155:**170–177.

220. **Valdivieso, R., J. Pola, E. Losada, J. Subiza, A. Armentia, and C. Zapata.** 1988. Severe anaphylactoid reaction to nalidixic acid. *Allergy* **43:**71–73.

221. **van Balen, F. A. M., F. W. M. M. Touw-Otten, and R. A. de Melker.** 1990. Single-dose pefloxacin versus five-days treatment with norfloxacin in uncomplicated cystitis in women. *J. Antimicrob. Chemother.* **26**(Suppl. B)**:**153–160.

222. **Wagai, N., and K. Tawara.** 1992. Possible direct role of reactive oxygen species in the cause of mouse cutaneous phototoxicity induced by 5 quinolones. *Arch. Toxicol.* **66:**392–397.

223. **Wagai, N., and K. Tawara.** 1992. Possible reasons for differences in phototoxic potential of 5 quinolone antibacterial agents: generation of toxic oxygen. *Free Rad. Res. Commun.* **17:**387–398.

224. **Wagai, N., F. Yamaguchi, M. Sekiguchi, and K. Tawara.** 1990. Phototoxic potential of quinolone antibacterial agents in Balb/c mice. *Toxicol. Lett.* **54:**299–308.

225. **Wang, C., J. Sabbaj, M. Corrado, and V. Hoagland.** 1986. World-wide clinical experience with norfloxacin: efficacy and safety. *Scand. J. Infect. Dis.* **48**(Suppl)**:**81–89.

226. **Winrow, A. P., and G. Supramaniam.** 1990. Benign intracranial hypertension after ciprofloxacin administration. *Arch. Dis. Child.* **65:**1165–1166.

227. **Wiström, J., S. R. Norrby, L. G. Burman, R. Lundholm, B. Jellheden, and G. Englund.** 1987. Norfloxacin versus placebo for prophylaxis against travelers' diarrhea. *J. Antimicrob. Chemother.* **20:**563–574.

228. **Wolfson, J. S., and D. C. Hooper.** 1988. Norfloxacin: a new targeted fluoroquinolone antimicrobial agent. *Ann. Intern. Med.* **108:**238–251.

229. **Wolfson, J. S., and D. C. Hooper.** 1991. Overview of fluoroquinolone safety. *Am. J. Med.* **91**(Suppl. 6A)**:**153S–161S.

230. **Wollschlager, C. M., S. Raoof, F. A. Khan, J. J. Guarneri, V. LaBombardi, and Q. Afzal.** 1987. Controlled, comparative study of ciprofloxacin versus ampicillin in treatment of bacterial respiratory tract infections. *Am. J. Med.* **82**(Suppl. 4A)**:**164–168.

231. **Wong, W. T., M. K. Chan, M. K. Li, W. S. Wong, P. D. Yin, and I. K. P. Cheng.** 1988. Treatment of urinary tract infections in Hong Kong: a comparative trial of norfloxacin and co-trimoxazole. *Scand. J. Infect. Dis. Suppl.* **56:**22–27.

232. **Wurtz, R. M., D. Abrams, S. Becker, M. A. Jacobson, M. M. Mass, and S. H. Marks.** 1989. Anaphylactoid drug reactions to ciprofloxacin and rifampicin in HIV-infected patients. *Lancet* **i:**955–956.

233. **Zaudig, M., and M. von Bose.** 1987. Ofloxacin-associated psychosis. *Br. J. Psychiatry* **151:**563–564.

234. **Zelickson, A. S.** 1964. Phototoxic reaction with nalidixic acid. *J. Am. Med. Assoc.* **190:**556.

235. **Ziemen, M., P. M. Shah, and K. Breddin.** 1988. Haemostasis during treatment with ciprofloxacin. *Infection* **16**(Suppl. 1)**:**S65–S68.

*Quinolone Antimicrobial Agents, 2nd ed.*
Edited by David C. Hooper and John S. Wolfson


*Chapter 27*

# Effects of Quinolones on the Central Nervous System

*Seiji Hori and Jingoro Shimada*

Recently, many fluoroquinolones have been developed and used for the treatment of infectious diseases. As the number of fluoroquinolones used in clinical practice has increased, the number of reports on the adverse effects of these agents has also increased. The most common adverse reactions are gastrointestinal reactions (Table 1). Reactions in the central nervous system (CNS) are the next most frequent. Since nalidixic acid, the first quinolone introduced into clinical use, was reported to have various adverse reactions (Table 2) in the CNS (20), neurotoxicities have been considered intrinsic to quinolones. Newer fluoroquinolones have also been reported to have adverse reactions, including convulsions, in the CNS. It is thus important to know the mechanism of the convulsions induced by fluoroquinolones. In this chapter, we discuss the mechanism of adverse reactions in the CNS and particularly the mechanism of the convulsions induced by fluoroquinolones.

## CONVULSIONS INDUCED BY FLUOROQUINOLONES

Symptoms probably related to toxicity in the CNS have been reported in 0.2 to 1.9% of the patients who were given fluoroquinolones in Japan. Predominant symptoms were headache, dizziness, and sleep disturbance (Table 3). Most of these reactions were not severe, but convulsions have been reported with the older quinolone nalidixic acid (9, 15) and with the newer fluoroquinolones norfloxacin (2, 30), enoxacin (29), ofloxacin (18), and ciprofloxacin (4, 5, 8, 19, 25, 26). In 1986, it was reported that concurrent administration of enoxacin and fenbufen, a nonsteroidal anti-inflammatory drug (NSAID), might be responsible for the onset of the convulsions induced in patients who had taken these agents (16). Since then, investigators have been interested in the neurochemical mechanism of the convulsions induced by fluoroquinolones with or without NSAIDs.

## CONVULSIONS AND γ-AMINOBUTYRIC ACID

γ-Aminobutyric acid (GABA) is known to be an inhibitory transmitter in the mammalian CNS. It is synthesized by decarboxylation of glutamate and is released into the synaptic cleft. GABA binds to its receptor site, which is located on the postsynaptic membrane; increases the influx of $Cl^-$ ion; and then leads to postsynaptic membrane hyperpolarization. The inhibition of GABA-mediated inhibitory

*Seiji Hori and Jingoro Shimada* • Division of Clinical Pharmacology, Institute of Medical Science, St. Marianna University School of Medicine, 2-16-1 Sugao, Miyamae-ku, Kawasaki 216, Japan.

**Table 1.** Clinical adverse effects of fluoroquinolones

| Fluoroquinolone | Total no. of patients | No. showing adverse effect[a] | | | | |
|---|---|---|---|---|---|---|
| | | GI | CNS | Skin, allergy | Other | Total |
| Norfloxacin | 14,730 | 182 | 32 | 35 | 24 | 233 |
| Ofloxacin | 2,856 | 80 | 16 | 21 | 10 | 99 |
| Ciprofloxacin | 2,575 | 54 | 11 | 10 | 18 | 77 |
| Enoxacin | 2,516 | 96 | 25 | 17 | 12 | 117 |
| Tosufloxacin | 3,010 | 70 | 13 | 23 | 3 | 109 |
| Lomefloxacin | 2,546 | 44 | 22 | 8 | 12 | 78 |
| Fleroxacin | 1,182 | 22 | 22 | 6 | 3 | 53 |
| Sparfloxacin | 2,754 | 54 | 17 | 44 | 18 | 133 |

[a]GI, gastrointestinal. Data are from Japanese open studies.

**Table 2.** Adverse effects of nalidixic acid on CNS

| | |
|---|---|
| Headache | Excitement |
| Giddiness | Confusion |
| Drowsiness | Hallucinations |
| Syncope | Weakness |
| Sensory change | Myalgia |
| Visual disturbance | Peripheral neuritis |
| Overbrightness of lights, blurred vision, difficulty in focusing, decreased visual acuity, double vision, alteration in color perception | Convulsions<br>Psychosis<br>Other |

**Table 3.** Adverse effects of fluoroquinolones on CNS

| Fluoroquinolone | Total no. of patients | No. showing[a]: | | | | |
|---|---|---|---|---|---|---|
| | | Headache | Dizziness | Sleep disorder | Seizures, tremor | Other |
| Norfloxacin | 14,730 | 6 | 21 | 4 | 0 | 1 |
| Ofloxacin | 2,856 | 4 | 6 | 4 | 0 | 2 |
| Enoxacin | 2,516 | 8 | 8 | 9 | 0 | 0 |
| Ciprofloxacin | 2,575 | 3 | 8 | 0 | 0 | 0 |
| Tosufloxacin | 3,010 | 4 | 4 | 3 | 1 | 1 |
| Lomefloxacin | 2,546 | 1 | 8 | 3 | 0 | 10 |
| Fleroxacin | 1,182 | 3 | 9 | 7 | 1 | 2 |
| Sparfloxacin | 2,754 | 6 | 5 | 2 | 1 | 3 |

[a]Data are from Japanese open studies.

transmission should increase excitability in the CNS and then lead to convulsions (22). For example, decreasing the amount of GABA in synaptosomes (nerve terminal-rich fraction) and administering GABA receptor-blocking agent have been reported to induce convulsions (1, 10, 21).

As to the convulsions induced by antimicrobial agents, penicillins (7, 24) and cephalosporins (6, 17, 31, 32) have been reported to induce convulsions. They have been reported to inhibit GABA receptor binding, and it has been suggested that this inhibition of GABA receptor binding might be related to the onset of the convulsions induced by penicillins and cephalosporins (3, 11, 23).

## INHIBITORY ACTIVITY OF FLUOROQUINOLONES AGAINST GABA RECEPTOR BINDING IN VITRO

Convulsions associated with the fluoroquinolones have been reported, and concurrent administration of a fluoroquinolone and an NSAID might enhance the convulsant activity of a fluoroquinolone. The neurochemical mechanism of the convulsions induced by fluoroquinolones with or without NSAIDs was studied.

Fluoroquinolones inhibited GABA receptor binding in a concentration-dependent manner (Fig. 1). Nalidixic acid at concentrations up to $10^{-3}$ M did not inhibit GABA receptor binding (data not shown). The concentrations that inhibited 50% of the binding ($IC_{50}$s) are shown in Table 4 (28).

The structure-activity relationships of the inhibitory activities of derivatives of ofloxacin with GABA receptor binding were evaluated. As shown in Table 5 and Fig. 2, the derivatives that had free piperazinyl groups in their chemical structures had stronger inhibitory activities than those with their piperazinyl groups replaced (27).

Fluoroquinolones have been considered to induce convulsions through the inhibition of GABA receptor binding when they accumulated in the CNS.

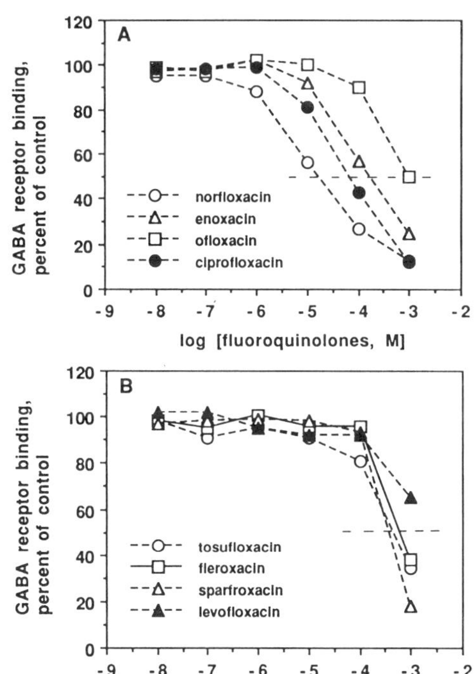


**Figure 1.** Effects of fluoroquinolones on GABA receptor binding.

**Table 4.** $IC_{50}$s of fluoroquinolones

| Fluoroquinolone | $IC_{50}$ (M)[a] |
|---|---|
| Norfloxacin | $1.4 \times 10^{-5}$ |
| Enoxacin | $1.4 \times 10^{-4}$ |
| Ofloxacin | $1.0 \times 10^{-3}$ |
| Ciprofloxacin | $7.6 \times 10^{-5}$ |
| Tosufloxacin | $5.7 \times 10^{-4}$ |
| Fleroxacin | $7.6 \times 10^{-4}$ |
| Sparfloxacin | $9.1 \times 10^{-4}$ |
| Levofloxacin | $>10^{-3}$ |

[a]Each value represents the mean of two or three separate experiments.

## DRUG INTERACTIONS BETWEEN FLUOROQUINOLONES AND NSAIDS

Concurrent administration of enoxacin and fenbufen seemed to enhance the convulsant activity of enoxacin (16). The effect of fluoroquinolones on GABA receptor binding was studied in the presence of various NSAIDs.

In the presence of NSAIDs, the inhibitory activities of norfloxacin, enoxacin, ofloxacin, and ciprofloxacin on GABA receptor binding were remarkably enhanced (Fig. 3). Among NSAIDs, 4-biphenylacetic acid, an active metabolite of fenbufen, enhanced the inhibitory activity of fluoroquinolones. On the other hand, acetylsalicylic acid at $10^{-4}$ M did not change the inhibitory activities of fluoroquinolones (13). The inhibitory activities of newly developed fluoroquinolones such as tosufloxacin (12), sparfloxacin (14), and fleroxacin (13) were little enhanced in the presence of NSAIDs. The $IC_{50}$s of various fluoroquinolones in the presence of NSAIDs are listed in Table 6. These in vitro

**Table 5.** Chemical structures of fluoroquinolones and their $IC_{50}$s

| Compound | R | $IC_{50}$(M) |
|---|---|---|
| 1 | H | $>10^{-3}$ |
| 2 | HN N- | $4.8\times10^{-5}$ |
| 3 | $CH_3$-N N- | $1.0\times10^{-3}$ |
| 4 | $C_2H_5$-N N- | $>10^{-3}$ |
| 5 | $CH_3CO$-N N- | $>10^{-3}$ |
| 6 | N- | $>10^{-3}$ |

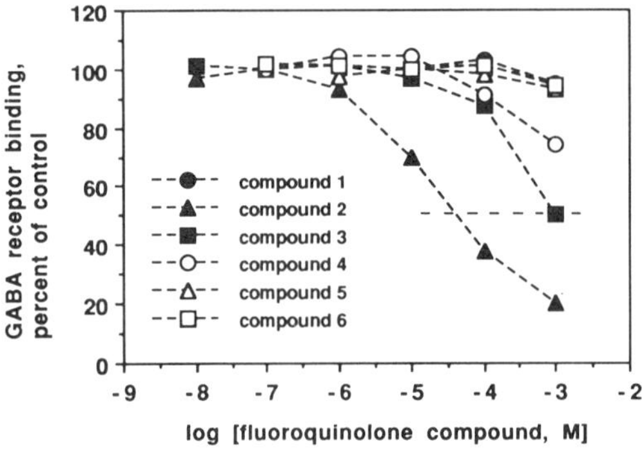


**Figure 2.** Effects of fluoroquinolone compounds on GABA receptor binding.

neurochemical results suggest that the concurrent administration of fluoroquinolones and NSAIDs might induce convulsions with lower concentrations of fluoroquinolones through enhancement of the inhibitory activities of fluoroquinolones.

## CONCLUSION

Today, many fluoroquinolones are used for the treatment of infectious diseases, and the consumption of fluoroquinolones is increasing. Fluoroquinolones might have potent convulsant activities, and the concurrent administration of fluoroquinolones and NSAIDs (except acetylsalicylic acid) might enhance the convulsant activities of fluoroquinolones. It would therefore be better to avoid the concurrent administration of fluoro-

**Table 6.** $IC_{50}$s of fluoroquinolones in the presence of NSAIDs

| Fluoroquinolone | No NSAID | Aspirin | Fenbufen | Indomethacin | Flurbiprofen | 4-Biphenyl-acetate[b] |
|---|---|---|---|---|---|---|
| Norfloxacin | $1.4 \times 10^{-5}$ | $1.4 \times 10^{-5}$ | $1.2 \times 10^{-7}$ | $1.9 \times 10^{-7}$ | $1.4 \times 10^{-8}$ | $<10^{-8}$ |
| Enoxacin | $1.4 \times 10^{-4}$ | $8.3 \times 10^{-5}$ | $1.3 \times 10^{-6}$ | $5.3 \times 10^{-7}$ | $3.3 \times 10^{-8}$ | $1.1 \times 10^{-8}$ |
| Ofloxacin | $1.0 \times 10^{-3}$ | $7.6 \times 10^{-4}$ | $3.6 \times 10^{-5}$ | $1.2 \times 10^{-4}$ | $3.0 \times 10^{-6}$ | $8.3 \times 10^{-7}$ |
| Ciprofloxacin | $7.6 \times 10^{-5}$ | $1.0 \times 10^{-4}$ | $1.3 \times 10^{-6}$ | $1.0 \times 10^{-4}$ | $1.0 \times 10^{-6}$ | $3.0 \times 10^{-8}$ |
| Tosufloxacin | $5.7 \times 10^{-4}$ | $>10^{-3}$ | $>10^{-3}$ | $>10^{-3}$ | NT | $1.2 \times 10^{-4}$ |
| Fleroxacin | $7.6 \times 10^{-4}$ | $7.6 \times 10^{-4}$ | $5.8 \times 10^{-4}$ | $5.8 \times 10^{-4}$ | $2.5 \times 10^{-4}$ | $1.0 \times 10^{-4}$ |
| Sparfloxacin | $9.1 \times 10^{-4}$ | $1.0 \times 10^{-3}$ | $4.0 \times 10^{-4}$ | $2.8 \times 10^{-4}$ | $1.6 \times 10^{-4}$ | $5.2 \times 10^{-5}$ |
| Levofloxacin | $>10^{-3}$ | NT | NT | NT | NT | $3.5 \times 10^{-5}$ |

[a]Each value represents the mean of two or three separate experiments. The concentration of each NSAID was $10^{-4}$ M. NT, not tested.
[b]An active metabolite of fenbufen.

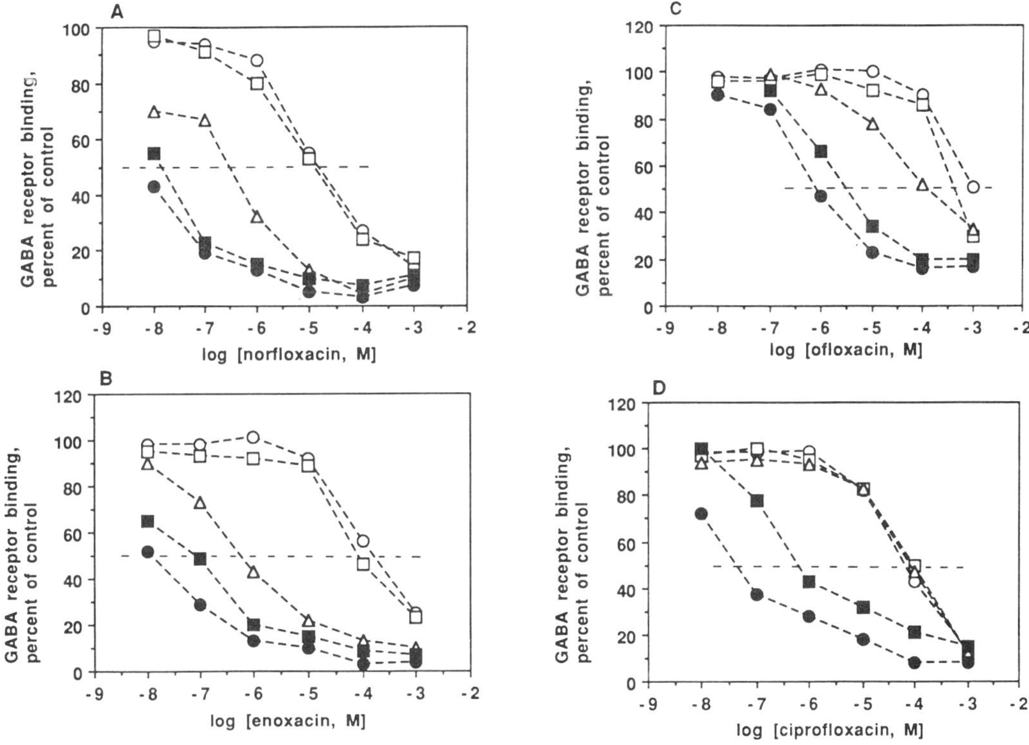


**Figure 3.** Effects of norfloxacin (A), enoxacin (B), ofloxacin (C), and ciprofloxacin (D) on GABA receptor binding in the presence of NSAIDs (all at $10^{-4}$ M). Symbols: ○, no NSAID; □, acetylsalicylic acid; △, indomethacin; ■, flurbiprofen; ●, biphenylacetate.

quinolones and NSAIDs. Some fluoroquinolones are known to be eliminated by the kidney, and the half-lives of these fluoroquinolones have been reported to be prolonged in patients with compromised renal functions. In such patients, the fluoroquinolones may accumulate. Therefore, patients with impaired renal functions should be carefully observed when they are given fluoroquinolones.

## REFERENCES

1. **Abe, M.** 1978. Relationship between γ-aminobutyric acid metabolism and antivitamin $B_6$-induced convulsions. *J. Nutr. Sci. Vitaminol.* **24:**419–427.
2. **Anastasio, G. D., D. Menscer, and J. M. Little.** 1988. Norfloxacin and seizures. *Ann. Intern. Med.* **109:**169–170.
3. **Antoniadis, A., W. E. Muller, and U. Wollert.** 1980. Inhibition of GABA and benzodiazepine receptor binding by penicillins. *Neurosci. Lett.* **18:**309–312.
4. **Arcieri, G., E. Griffith, G. Gruenwaldt, A. Heyd, S. O'Brien, N. Becker, and R. August.** 1987. Ciprofloxacin: an update on clinical experience. *Am. J. Med.* **82**(Suppl. 4A):381–394.
5. **Arcieri, G. M., B. S. Becker, B. Esposito, E. Griffith, A. Heyd, C. Neumann, B. O'Brien, and P. Schacht.** 1989. Safety of intravenous ciprofloxacin. A review. *Am. J. Med.* **87**(Suppl. 5A):92S–97S.
6. **Bechtel, T. P., R. L. Slaughter, and T. D. Moore.** 1980. Seizures associated with high cerebrospinal fluid concentrations of cefazolin. *Am. J. Pharm.* **37:**271–273.
7. **Curtis, D. R., C. J. A. Game, G. A. Johnston, R. M. MuCulloch, and R. M. MacClachlan.** 1972. Convulsive action of penicillin. *Brain Res.* **43:**242–245.

8. **Fass, R. J.** 1987. Efficacy and safety of oral ciprofloxacin in the treatment of serious respiratory infections. *Am. J. Med.* **82**(Suppl. 4A):202–207.
9. **Fraser, A. G., and A. D. B. Harrower.** 1977. Convulsions and hyperglycemia associated with nalidixic acid. *Br. Med. J.* **2:**1518.
10. **Hori, S.** 1982. Study on hyperbaric oxygen induced convulsions with particular reference to γ-aminobutyric acid in synaptosomes. *J. Biochem.* **91:**443–448.
11. **Hori, S., S. Kurioka, M. Matsuda, and J. Shimada.** 1985. Inhibitory effect of cephalosporins on γ-aminobutyric acid receptor binding in rat synaptic membranes. *Antimicrob. Agents Chemother.* **27:**605–651.
12. **Hori, S., A. Saito, J. Shimada, M. Ohmori, K. Shiba, T. Hojo, M. Kaji, S. Okuda, M. Yoshida, and T. Miyahara.** 1988. Effect of T-3262 and its structural derivatives on GABA receptor binding. *Chemotherapy* **36**(Suppl. 9):116–120. (In Japanese.)
13. **Hori, S., J. Shimada, A. Saito, M. Matsuda, and T. Miyahara.** 1989. Comparison of the inhibitory effects of new quinolones on γ-aminobutyric acid receptor binding in the presence of antiinflammatory drugs. *Rev. Infect. Dis.* **11**(Suppl. 5):S1397–S1398.
14. **Hori, S., J. Shimada, K. Shiba, M. Yoshida, A. Saito, and O. Sakai.** 1991. A study on convulsive effects of sparfloxacin with or without nonsteroidal anti-inflammatory drugs. *Chemotherapy* **39**(Suppl. 4):161–166. (In Japanese.)
15. **Islam, M. A., and T. Sreedharan.** 1965. Convulsions, hyperglycemia and glucosuria from overdose of nalidixic acid. *JAMA* **192:**1100–1101.
16. **Japanese Ministry of Welfare.** 1986. Report of clinical adverse reaction. *Nihon-Izishinpou* **3263:**101–102.
17. **Kamei, C., A. Sunami, and K. Tasaka.** 1983. Epileptogenic activity of cephalosporins in rats and their structure-activity relationship. *Epilepsia* **24:**421–439.
18. **Kamota, T., N. Kataoka, M. Shigeta, and C. Nakahara.** 1989. Convulsion associated with ofloxacin in a patient with acute interstitial nephritis. *Jpn. J. Paediatr.* **93:**1188–1194.
19. **Kljucar, S., M. Heimesaat, E. von Pritzbuer, J. Timm, H. Scholl, and D. Beermann.** 1989. Efficacy and safety of higher-dose intravenous ciprofloxacin in severe hospital-acquired infections. *Am. J. Med.* **87**(Suppl. 5A):52S–56S.
20. **Kucers, A., and N. M. Bennett.** 1987. Nalidixic acid, p. 1203–1218. *In The Use of Antibiotics*, 4th ed. Lippincott, Philadelphia.
21. **Meldrum, B.** 1979. Convulsant drugs, anticonvulsants and GABA-mediated neural inhibition, p. 390–405. *In* P. Krogsgaard-Larsen, J. Scheel-Kruger, and H. Kofod (ed.), *GABA-Neurotransmitter.* Munksgaard, Copenhagen.
22. **Meldrum, B. S.** 1975. Epilepsy and γ-aminobutyric acid-mediated inhibition. *Int. Rev. Neurobiol.* **17:**1–36.
23. **Olsen, R. W., M. K. Ticku, P. C. Van Ness, and D. Gleenlee.** 1978. Effect of drugs on γ-aminobutyric acid receptors, uptake, release and synthesis in vitro. *Brain Res.* **139:**277–294.
24. **Raicle, M. E., H. Kutt, S. Louis, and F. McDowell.** 1971. Neurotoxicity of intravenously administered penicillin G. *Arch. Neurol.* **25:**232–239.
25. **Reiter, C., M. Pfeiffer, and R. N. Hullman.** 1989. Brief report: safety of ciprofloxacin based on phase IV studies ("Anwendungsbeobachtung") in the Federal Republic of Germany. *Am. J. Med.* **87**(Suppl. 5A):103S–106S.
26. **Schacht, P., and R. Hullmann.** 1989. Safety of oral ciprofloxacin. An update based on clinical trial results. *Am. J. Med.* **87**(Suppl. 5A):98S–102S.
27. **Shimada, J., and S. Hori.** 1991. Effect of quinolones on GABA receptor binding, p. 196–207. *In* S. Mitsuhashi (ed.), *New Quinolones.* Japan Scientific Societies Press, Tokyo. (In Japanese.)
28. **Shimada, J., and S. Hori.** 1992. Adverse effects of fluoroquinolones. *Prog. Drug Res.* **38:**133–143.
29. **Simpson, K. J., and M. J. Brodie.** 1985. Convulsions related to enoxacin. *Lancet* **ii:**161.
30. **Wolfson, J. S., and D. C. Hooper.** 1986. Norfloxacin: a new targeted fluoroquinolone antimicrobial agent. *Ann. Intern. Med.* **108:**238–251.
31. **Yoshioka, H., H. Nambu, M. Fukita, and H. Uehara.** 1975. Convulsion following intrathecal cephaloridine. *Infection* **3:**123–124.
32. **Yost, R. L., J. D. Lee, and J. P. O'Leary.** 1977. Convulsions associated with sodium cefazolin: a case report. *Am. Surg.* **43:**417–420.

*Quinolone Antimicrobial Agents, 2nd ed.*
Edited by David C. Hooper and John S. Wolfson


*Chapter 28*

# Effects of the Quinolones on the Immune System

***Ethan Rubinstein and Itamar Shalit***

Many antimicrobial agents have been reported to modify human and animal immune responses measured in various assays in vitro and in vivo (23). Interest in the immunomodulatory effects of the quinolones has been raised by several factors: their inhibition of the eukaryotic topoisomerases I and II and the DNA polymerases; the beneficial effect of the quinolones in the treatment of cystic fibrosis patients, which exceeds the expected antibacterial activity against *Pseudomonas aeruginosa*; and the beneficial effect of quinolones in prophylaxis and treatment of bacterial infections in immunocompromised hosts, including AIDS patients, bone marrow transplant recipients, and leukemic patients (42).

A key observation was made by Forsgren and associates, who have repeatedly demonstrated increased [$^3$H]thymidine uptake by stimulated lymphocytes exposed to clinically attainable concentrations of various quinolones (14, 17). These observations varied considerably according to the quinolone chosen (9, 19) and the incubation conditions and concentrations of quinolones used. Dose-related effects could also be demonstrated for various other functions, such as cell proliferation, phagocytosis, regulation of prostaglandin metabolism, and production of other cytokines (4, 31, 41).

***Ethan Rubinstein*** • Infectious Disease Unit, Sheba Medical Center, Tel-Hashomer, Israel. ***Itamar Shalit*** • Tel-Aviv Sourasky Medical Center, Tel-Aviv University, Tel-Aviv, Israel.

## PHAGOCYTOSIS

Most authors agree that quinolones do not exert a direct effect on polymorphonuclear phagocytes. The chemiluminescence response, myeloperoxidase content, superoxide production, and hexose monophosphate shunt index in human polymorphonuclear cells (PMNs) were unaffected in vitro by various quinolones at concentrations of 0.1 to 10 μg/ml (4, 13, 15, 35). Similarly, clinically relevant concentrations of quinolones did not have a direct effect on chemotaxis of PMNs towards several chemoattractants, nor did they adversely affect phagocytosis and intracellular killing of ingested bacteria by human granulocytes (4, 15, 27, 35). In contrast, phagocytosis of bacteria preexposed to subinhibitory concentrations of quinolones was significantly increased. It is apparent that exposure of quinolone-susceptible gram-negative and gram-positive bacteria to low concentrations of these antimicrobial agents results in morphological and structural changes of bacterial surfaces that lead to enhanced ingestion by phagocytic cells (15, 35). This phenomenon has been demonstrated in opsonized as well as nonopsonized bacteria (35).

Another factor influencing phagocytic efficacy is the intracellular activities of quinolones in PMNs. Several investigators have demonstrated that compounds such as ciprofloxacin, norfloxacin, enoxacin, ofloxacin, pefloxacin, and fleroxacin readily penetrate into PMNs and exhibit intracellular bactericidal activities. This uptake is rapid, does not depend on temperature or cell viability, and is followed by rapid efflux when the extracellular concentration of the antimicrobial agent decreases. The mechanism of uptake is unclear but most likely involves diffusion (49). The bactericidal activities of the intracellular quinolones against a variety of ingested microorganisms, including *Staphyloccocus aureus*, *Serratia marcescens*, and classical intracellular pathogens such as *Legionella pneumophila*, *Salmonella typhimurium*, and *Mycobacterium fortuitum*, have been demonstrated (11, 12, 28, 48, 50, 51), even at acidic intracellular pH.

Thus, despite lack of a direct effect on phagocytes, quinolones enhance overall phagocytic activity by their direct effects on bacteria and their persistent bactericidal activities inside the phagocytic cell.

## LYMPHOCYTE PROLIFERATION

[$^3$H]thymidine uptake by stimulated lymphocytes is widely accepted for assessment of lymphocyte proliferation in vitro. The effects of various quinolones on thymidine uptake were studied by several groups, with some discrepancies in results. Forsgren et al. (14, 16, 18) have reported in several studies an increase in [$^3$H]thymidine uptake by human lymphocytes stimulated by phytohemagglutinin (PHA) and exposed to various quinolones at concentrations of 1.25 to 25 $\mu$g/ml (47). In contrast, other investigators (9, 19, 20) have found either no change in nucleoside uptake in lymphocytes exposed to ciprofloxacin or an inhibitory effect in cells exposed to ofloxacin, pefloxacin, norfloxacin, and difloxacin at the same concentration range. Some of these discrepancies may be explained by different incubation periods and different stimulators used by the various researchers. It is generally agreed, however, that the various quinolones at concentrations exceeding 50 $\mu$g/ml result in inhibition of thymidine uptake by stimulated lymphocytes. In addition, Forsgren et al. (18) and Gollapudi et al. (19) have shown that lymphocyte growth and cell cycle progression from the resting phase to the DNA synthesis phase are inhibited by quinolones at concentrations exceeding 20 $\mu$g/ml.

These data suggest that the enhanced thymidine uptake reported by Forsgren et al. (18) was not indicative of true DNA synthesis or cell growth. The possibility that enhanced thymidine uptake is indicative of genotoxic effects of certain quinolones on eukaryotic cells was studied by Bredberg et al. (5). Although some degree of DNA strand breakage and unscheduled DNA synthesis was noted, these effects occurred only at high concentrations of quinolones ($>10$ $\mu$g of ciprofloxacin per ml, $>80$ $\mu$g of ofloxacin per ml, and $>160$ $\mu$g of norfloxacin per ml). No induced mutations were noted with any of the quinolones tested.

It can be concluded, therefore, that at therapeutic concentrations, quinolones have either no effect or a minor inhibitory effect on lymphocyte proliferation in vitro and no genotoxic effects, whereas higher concentrations ($>20$ $\mu$g/ml) are inhibitory to lymphocyte growth in vitro.

Few investigators have studied the lymphocyte proliferative response in animals or in humans treated with quinolones. Pulverer and Peters (35) found no change in [$^3$H]thymidine uptake in splenic lymphocytes obtained from mice treated with ofloxacin (1 to 10 mg/kg of body weight per day) compared with untreated control animals. Similarly, no effect was described by Gollapudi et al. (19) in mice treated with ciprofloxacin (40 mg/kg twice daily for 5 days). Biglino et al. (3) assessed transformation of peripheral blood lymphocytes obtained from patients treated with oral ofloxacin (300 mg twice daily) for urinary tract or lower respiratory tract infections. Lymphocytes obtained before treatment, 1 h after the first dose, and 5 days after onset of treatment were stimulated by various mitogens. Proliferation was enhanced at 1 h and 5 days of therapy compared with the pretreatment baseline in cells stimulated with PHA or pokeweed mitogen but not in those stimulated with concanavalin A or tetanus toxoid.

These results should be interpreted with some reservations, since no comparisons with healthy subjects receiving ofloxacin or with infected patients treated with other antimicrobial agents were made.

## IMMUNOGLOBIN PRODUCTION

Very few studies have evaluated the influence of new quinolones on immunoglobulin production. Ofloxacin at clinically achievable concentrations seems to have no significant effect on production of immunoglobulin G (IgG) and IgM in vitro or in mice treated with 1 to 10 mg/kg/day (13, 35). Ciprofloxacin was reported to inhibit immunoglobulin production in vitro at concentrations of 5 μg/ml (18), whereas animal studies demonstrated IgG and IgM secretion in mice treated with ciprofloxacin for 7 days (5 mg/kg/day) (34). The small number of studies with differing designs and results precludes any definitive conclusion regarding the effect of quinolones on immunoglobulin production in clinical settings.

## IL-1

Two distinct forms of interleukin-1 (IL-1) have been identified and designated IL-1$\alpha$ and IL-1$\beta$. Extracellular IL-1 is predominantly IL-1$\beta$, and intracellular IL-1 is predominantly IL-1$\alpha$. IL-1 activity in the supernatant culture fluids of quinolone-treated mononuclear cells decreased in a dose-dependent manner after exposure of the cells to pefloxacin, ofloxacin, and ciprofloxacin (4). These effects were apparent for drug concentrations of $>100$ μg/ml. Concentrations in the therapeutic range ($<10$ μg/ml), however, were reported to yield an increase in IL-1 activity or to have no effect. Interestingly, cell-associated IL-1 was not affected, whereas extracellular IL-1 concentrations decreased in cells exposed to high concentrations of various quinolones. Extracellular IL-1 was thought to account for the altered proliferative responses of the exposed monocytes (39).

Ciprofloxacin (100 μg/ml) reduced IL-1$\beta$ but not IL-1$\alpha$ released into the medium by lipopolysaccharide-stimulated monocytes (2). Similarly, mouse macrophages increased the production of IL-1 when they were exposed to low concentrations (1 to 2.5 μg/ml) of pefloxacin, ofloxacin, and ciprofloxacin (21, 33, 47).

Taken together, these observations indicate that quinolones increase the production of extracellular IL-1. The biological importance of this observation is not readily apparent, but the data suggest an effect on modulation of the mononuclear-lymphoid cell proliferation response to various stimuli.

## IL-2

Administration of IL-2 enhanced the survival of mice following infection with *Toxoplasma gondii* (45) and lethal challenge with *Escherichia coli* and *P. aeruginosa* (8), possibly because of macrophage activation. Although IL-2 has not been shown to activate macrophages directly, it is capable of inducing murine lymphocytes to produce gamma interferon (IFN-$\gamma$) (24), which in turn activates macrophages and neutrophils (46). Enoxacin and ciprofloxacin at concentrations of 5 to 80 μg/ml caused a dose-dependent increase in IL-2 production in normal PHA-stimulated human lymphocytes (37). The peak level of IL-2 in the presence of 80 μg/ml of enoxacin or ciprofloxacin was 50 to 60 times higher than that of controls (47).

Pefloxacin and ofloxacin at the same concentrations caused 23- and 10-fold-higher IL-2 levels, respectively, than the controls. At a concentration of 5 μg/ml, however, nalidixic acid, pefloxacin, ofloxacin, enoxacin, ciprofloxacin, and amifloxacin exhibited peak activity that was only 1- to 1.5-fold that of the controls (37). IL-2 mRNA was also elevated 16- to 32-fold in PHA-stimulated human lymphocytes exposed to ciprofloxacin at a concentration of 80 μg/ml, while in unstimulated lymphocytes, no IL-2 mRNA was detectable (17). This observation of increased IL-2 production by PHA-stimulated mononuclear cells in the presence of therapeutic levels of quinolones in serum was confirmed by Roche et al. (40) and Zehavi-Willner and Shalit (53). The latter authors also found that without stimulation of the cells with PHA, ciprofloxacin did not augment IL-2 secretion. Biglino et al. (3) demonstrated no change in IL-2 secretion from baseline in tetanus toxoid-stimulated lymphocytes obtained from patients treated with ofloxacin for a variety of minor infections.

In summary, all quinolones augment IL-2 secretion by stimulated lymphocytes in in vitro assays in a dose-dependent manner. This effect, however, could not be demonstrated in the single reported clinical study.

## IFN

Most of the studies evaluating quinolone effects on IFNs dealt with IFN-γ. This cytokine has a central role in the immune network (29). IFN-γ is produced during an immune response mainly by antigen-specific T cells and by IL-2-recruited natural killer cells. Among its important functions, IFN-γ activates macrophages, T cells, and natural killer cells, which themselves produce additional IFN-γ. This cytokine also regulates the humoral response by inducing immunoglobulin synthesis and secretion.

De Simone et al. (9) incubated harvested human lymphocytes in the presence of concanavalin A and several quinolones for 2 days; IFN-γ production was measured by radioimmunoassay. Their results showed that low concentrations of ofloxacin, norfloxacin, and pipemidic acid (3 μg/ml) and nalidixic acid and piromidic acid (10 μg/ml) had no significant effect on IFN-γ production compared with that of controls, whereas with higher concentrations (30 μg of norfloxacin per ml, 100 μg of nalidixic acid per ml, and 100 μg of piromidic acid per ml), a 50% drop in IFN-γ synthesis occurred. High concentrations (30 μg/ml) of ofloxacin and pipemidic acid did not seem to affect IFN-γ synthesis. Riesbeck and Forsgren (38) measured IFN-γ production by lipopolysaccharide-stimulated monocytes exposed to ciprofloxacin. Like ofloxacin, ciprofloxacin at concentrations of 5 and 20 μg/ml did not alter IFN-γ synthesis. At a concentration of 80 μg of ciprofloxacin per ml, a statistically significant decrease in IFN-γ synthesis occurred. Our group (22) has used a bioassay of the antiviral activity of IFN-γ on vesicular stomatitis virus-induced cytopathic effect in HeLa cells to study IFN-γ production in the supernatant fluids of monocytic cultures with and without granulocyte-macrophage colony-stimulating factor (CSF). Ciprofloxacin produced a dose-dependent increase in IFN-γ in PHA-stimulated cells from no increase at a concentration of 1.6 μg/ml to a sevenfold increase at a concentration of 120 μg/ml. It was of interest, however, that a low concentration of ciprofloxacin in the presence of a low concentration of IFN-γ inhibited hematopoietic cell growth (22). Zehavi-Willner and Shalit (53) have also demonstrated an increase in IFN-γ production by PHA-stimulated lymphocytes exposed to 50 to 100 μg of ciprofloxacin per ml. Interestingly, ofloxacin at the same concentrations had no effect (50 μg/ml) or an inhibitory effect (100 μg/ml) on IFN-γ production (53).

Biglino et al. (3) studied the effect of ofloxacin on IFN-γ and IFN-α in patients treated with ofloxacin for a variety of nonserious infections. Mononuclear cells from these patients were stimulated with PHA and tetanus toxoid. IFN-$\gamma$ was measured by a bioassay of inhibition of vesicular stomatitis virus-induced cytopathic effect on a human amniotic cell line, and levels of IFN-$\alpha$ were determined by using monoclonal anti-IFN antibodies. Similarly to the previously mentioned in vitro experiments, production of IFN-$\gamma$ did not differ significantly from baseline following 1 h or 5 days of ofloxacin therapy. IFN-$\alpha$ showed a small but significant decrease with ofloxacin treatment under the same conditions. In cells stimulated with tetanus toxoid, a slight decrease in IFN-$\alpha$ production was noted 1 h after ofloxacin administration.

Because these studies used different experimental conditions and stimuli, their results cannot be easily compared. At clinically attainable concentrations of quinolones, the effects of IFN-$\gamma$ production alone may be insufficient to produce important immunological changes. Such effects in conjunction with those of other cytokines might, however, cause alterations in immune functions or hematopoiesis.

## TNF

Tumor necrosis factor (TNF) has recently become a focus of interest because of its relation to the outcome of several infections (52) as well as its role in induction and regulation of numerous immune and inflammatory processes. At concentrations above 25 $\mu$g/ml (for ofloxacin, 100 $\mu$g/ml), ciprofloxacin, ofloxacin, and pefloxacin decreased extracellular TNF production (1). Cell-associated TNF concentrations were 10% of extracellular levels. Our group (22) could not demonstrate TNF production in mononuclear cells exposed to quinolones in the concentration range 1.6 to 100 $\mu$g/ml. Therapeutic concentrations of quinolones, however, suppressed human hematopoietic stem cells in the presence of low doses of TNF (1 $\mu$g/ml). These findings suggest that quinolones on their own are unlikely to produce any effect that is solely dependent on TNF. An interplay of TNF, quinolones, and possibly other cytokines may, however, be associated with limited immune alterations.

The interplay among cytokine activities does not allow assessment of an effect of quinolones on isolated cytokines. It seems that in most instances in the immunocompetent patient, the net effect of quinolone-cytokine interactions is probably clinically unimportant. It remains possible, however, that in certain as-yet-unstudied circumstances (e.g., in the immunocompromised patient), quinolone-induced immune alterations are important.

## BONE MARROW AND CSF

Bone marrow cells are among the most rapidly dividing eukaryotic cells and therefore are considered most susceptible to agents interfering with DNA synthesis. It was therefore natural to study the quinolones, which may interfere with eukaryotic DNA synthesis in this system. The effects of quinolones on bone marrow function are particularly important because of the potential of these drugs for inhibition of eukaryotic DNA synthesis and because the quinolones are often administered to leukemic patients and bone marrow transplant recipients, both as therapy for infectious episodes and for long-term gastrointestinal decontamination. Pessina et al. (32) measured the ability of murine marrow cells to form granulocyte-macrophage colonies (GM-CFU) in a soft-agar layer system. Significant inhibition of GM-CFU occurred at concentrations above 50 $\mu$g of rufloxacin per ml and 100 $\mu$g of ofloxacin per ml. Therapeutic concentrations of quinolones ($<10$ $\mu$g/ml) did not affect cell proliferation in vitro. Pallavicini et al. (30) extended these observations to include human bone marrow myeloid precursors. Their results, showing inhibition of GM-CFU at high concentrations of quinolones and no effect at therapeutic concentrations, were confirmed by Broide et al. (7) and Hahn et al. (22). Somekh et al. (43) further extended these observations by measuring the effect on bone marrow engraftment of treatment of recipient and donor mice with quinolones. Ciprofloxacin at high doses (100 mg/kg/24 h) suppressed marrow engraftment, while lower doses of ciprofloxacin (25 and 50 mg/kg/24 h) and pefloxacin had no effect. The suppressive effect of ciprofloxacin on murine bone marrow was also shown to be short-lived (44), subsiding less than 3 days after the discontinuation of treatment of recipients. Kletter et al. (25) could even demonstrate enhanced repopulation of hematopoietic organs and survival after the engraftment procedure in sublethally irradiated mice treated with ciprofloxacin. Their results suggest that there is enhanced production of CSF in mice treated with quinolones (25). This suggestion is supported by the demonstration that ciprofloxacin (at therapeutic concentrations) in concert with pokeweed mitogen stimulated murine splenic cells to enhance the production of CSF, an effect that could be antagonized by the use of specific anti-CSF antibodies (25). In an additional study, Broide et al. (7) found no suppressive effect on bone marrow in patients receiving short-term therapy (2 days) with ciprofloxacin. In addition to the direct effect of quinolones on hematopoietic progenitor cells, which is probably mediated through the inhibition of the eukaryotic topoisomerase, quinolones may also affect CSFs, which mediate bone marrow proliferation and maturation. Hahn et al. (22) found that TNF, which alone has little effect on bone marrow proliferation, had in the presence of ciprofloxacin a synergistic suppressive effect.

In summary, quinolones in low doses do not adversely affect the bone marrow of animals and humans. A possible salutary effect may be the result of enhanced secretion of various CSFs by stimulated cells exposed to quinolones at therapeutic concentrations.

Quinolones inhibit eukaryotic topoisomerases. For quinolones currently in clinical use, however, this inhibition occurs only at high, therapeutically irrelevant concentrations (100 $\mu$g/ml). As a possible result of this inhibition, certain immunological functions (e.g., cytokine production and hematopoiesis) may be antagonized. Immunological functions found to be enhanced at low quinolone concentrations ($<10$ $\mu$g/ml) suggest another mechanism, a common feature of which may be increased mRNA expression. Further studies evaluating the effects of low quinolone concentrations on eukaryotic cell function are needed to define the molecular mechanisms involved. In the clinical setting, the importance of these immunomodulating effects induced by quinolones may be of little importance in the immunocompetent host, but the potential for benefit in the immunocompromised patient merits further study.

## REFERENCES


1. **Bailly, S., M. Fay, Y. Roche, and M. A. Gougerot-Pocidalo.** 1990. Effect of quinolones on tumor necrosis factor production by human monocytes. *Int. J. Immunopharmacol.* **12:**31–36.
2. **Bailly, S., Y. Mahe, B. Ferrua, M. Fay, T. Tursz, H. Wakasugi, and M. A. Gougerot-Pocidalo.** 1990. Quinolone induced differential modification of IL-1$\alpha$ and IL-1$\beta$ production by LPS stimulated human monocytes. *Cell. Immunol.* **128:**277–288.
3. **Biglino, A., B. Forno, A. M. Pollono, M. Busso, F. Arpeinelli, M. Benedetti, and A. Pugliese.** 1990. Effect of ofloxacin on cell mediated immune response and lymphokine production. *J. Antimicrob. Chemother.* **25:**797–802.
4. **Boogaerts, M. A., S. Malbrain, W. Scheer, and R. L. Verwilghen.** 1986. Effects of quinolones on granulocyte function in-vitro. *Infection* **14**(Suppl. 2):S258–S262.
5. **Bredberg, A., M. Brant, K. Riesbeck, Y. Azou, and A. Forsgren.** 1989. 4-Quinolone antibiotics: positive genotoxic screening tests despite an apparent lack of mutation induction. *Mutat. Res.* **211:**171–180.
6. **Broide, E., D. Douer, N. Shaked, A. Yellin, Y. Lieberman, N. Rosen, S. Segev, and E. Rubinstein.** 1992. The effect of short term therapy with ciprofloxacin, ceftriaxone and placebo on human peripheral WBC and marrow derived granulocyte macrophage progenitor cells (CFU-GM). *Eur. J. Hematol.* **48:**276–277.

7. **Broide, E., E. Rubinstein, N. Shaked, A. Yellin, Y. Lieberman, N. Rosen, S. Segev, and D. Douer.** In-vitro suppression of normal human bone marrow derived myeloid progenitor cells by antibiotic agents. Submitted for publication.
8. **Chong, K.-T.** 1987. Prophylactic administration of interleukin-2 protects mice from lethal challenge with gram-negative bacteria. *Infect. Immun.* **55:**668–673.
9. **De Simone, C., L. Bandinelli, M. Ferrazzi, S. DeSantis, L. Pugnaloni, and F. Sorice.** 1986. Influence of ofloxacin, norfloxacin, nalidixic acid, piromidic acid and pipemidic acid on human gamma-interferon production and blastogenesis. *J. Antimicrob. Chemother.* **17:**811–814.
10. **Dinarello, C., and J. W. Mier.** 1987. Lymphokines. *N. Engl. J. Med.* **17:**940–945.
11. **Easmon, C. S. F., and J. P. Crane.** 1987. Uptake of ciprofloxacin by human neutrophilis. *J. Antimicrob. Chemother.* **20:**614–615.
12. **Easmon, C. S. F., and L. Verity.** 1987. Effect of Ro 23-6240 on sensitive and resistant intracellular mycobacteria. *Eur. J. Clin. Microbiol.* **6:**165–166.
13. **Fantoni, M., E. Tamburrini, F. Pallavicini, A. Antinori, and P. Nervo.** 1988. Influence of ofloxacin and pefloxacin on human lymphocyte immunoglobulin secretion and on polymorphic leucocyte superoxide anion production. *J. Antimicrob. Chemother.* **22:**193–196.
14. **Forsgren, A., A. K. Bergh, M. Brandt, and G. Hanson.** 1986. Quinolones affect thymidine incorporation in DNA of human lymphocytes. *Antimicrob. Agents Chemother.* **299:**506–508.
15. **Forsgren, A., and P. I. Bergqvist.** 1985. Effect of ciprofloxacin on phagocytosis. *Eur. J. Clin. Microbiol.* **4:**575–578.
16. **Forsgren, A., A. Bredberg, A. B. Pardee, S. F. Schlossman, and T. F. Tedder.** 1987. Effects of ciprofloxacin on eucaryotic pyrimidine nucleotide biosynthesis and cell growth. *Antimicrob. Agents Chemother.* **31:**774–779.
17. **Forsgren, A., A. Bredberg, and K. Riesbeck.** 1989. New quinolones: in vitro effects as a potential source of clinical toxicity. *Rev. Infect. Dis.* **11**(Suppl. 5)**:**S1382–S1389.
18. **Forsgren, A., S. F. Schlossman, and T. F. Tedder.** 1987. 4-Quinolone drugs affect cell cycle progression and function of human lymphocytes in vitro. *Antimicrob. Agents Chemother.* **31:**768–773.
19. **Gollapudi, S. V. S., R. H. Prabhala, and H. Thadepalli.** 1986. Effect of ciprofloxacin on mitogen-stimulated lymphocyte proliferation. *Antimicrob. Agents Chemother.* **29:**337–338.
20. **Gollapudi, S. V. S., B. Vaywegulu, S. Gupta, M. J. Fuk, and A. Thadepalli.** 1986. Aryl fluoroquinolone derivatives A-56619 (difloxacin) and A-56620 inhibit mitogen-induced human mononuclear cell proliferation. *Antimicrob. Agents Chemother.* **30:**390–394.
21. **Guenounou, M., E. Ronco, E. Kodari, F. Vacheron, and V. Momrikof.** 1987. Modulation of quinolones of the in-vitro proliferative response of splenic cells of the mouse and IL-1 production. *Pathol. Biol.* **35:**785–789.
22. **Hahn, T., Y. Barak, E. Leibovich, L. Malach, O. Dagan, and E. Rubinstein.** 1991. Ciprofloxacin inhibits human hematopoietic cell growth synergism with tumor necrosis factor and interferon. *Exp. Hematol.* **19:**157–160.
23. **Hauser, W. E., and J. S. Remington.** 1982. Effect of antibiotics on the immune response. *Am. J. Med.* **72:**711–716.
24. **Kawase, I., C. G. Brooks, K. Kuribagashi, S. Olabuenaga, S. Newman, S. Gillis, and C. S. Henney.** 1982. Interleukin-2 induces gamma interferon production. Participation of macrophages and NK cells. *J. Immunol.* **131:**288–293.
25. **Kletter, Y., I. Riklis, I. Shalit, and I. Fabian.** Enhanced repopulation of murine hematopoietic organs in sublethally irradiated mice following treatment with ciprofloxacin. *Blood*, in press.
26. **Knoller, J., J. Brom, W. Schonfeld, and W. Konig.** 1989. Influence of ciprofloxacin on leukotriene generation from various cells in-vitro. *J. Antimicrob. Chemother.* **25:**605–612.
27. **Lombard, J. Y., J. Descotes, and J. C. Evreux.** 1987. Polymorphonuclear leucocyte chemotaxis little affected by three quinolones in-vitro. *J. Antimicrob. Chemother.* **20:**614–615.
28. **Milatovic, D.** 1987. Intraphagocytic activity of ciprofloxacin and CI934. *Eur. J. Clin. Microbiol.* **5:**659–660.
29. **O'Garra, A.** 1989. Peptide regulatory factors: interleukins and the immune system. II. *Lancet* **i:**1003–1005.
30. **Pallavicini, F., A. Antinori, G. Frederico, M. Funtoni, and P. Neruo.** 1989. Influence of two quinolones, ofloxacin and pefloxacin, on human myelopoiesis in vitro. *Antimicrob. Agents Chemother.* **33:**122–123.
31. **Pascual, A., L. Martinez-Martinez, and E. J. Perea.** 1989. Effects of ciprofloxacin and ofloxacin on human polymorphonuclear leucocyte activity against staphylococci. *Chemotherapy* (Basel) **35:**17–22.
32. **Pessina, A., M. G. Neri, E. Muschiato, E. Mineo, and G. Cocuzza.** 1989. Effect of fluoroquinolones on the in-vitro proliferation of myeloid precursor cells. *J. Antimicrob. Chemother.* **24:**203–208.
33. **Petit, J. C., G. I. Daguet, G. Richard, and B. Burghoffer.** 1987. Influence of ciprofloxacin and piperacillin on IL-1 production of murine macrophages. *J. Antimicrob. Chemother.* **20:**615–617.
34. **Pulverer, G. 1986**. Effects of ciprofloxacin on the humoral and cellular immune response in Balb/c mice. *Zentralbl. Bakteriol. Mikrobiol. Hyg. Abt. A* **262:**396–402.

35. **Pulverer, G., and G. Peters.** 1986. Investigations on ofloxacin: antibacterial activity and influence on the immune system. *Infection* **14**(Suppl. 4):245-247.
36. **Queensbury, P., and L. Levitt.** 1979. Hematopoietic stem cells. *N. Engl. J. Med.* **301:**755-761.
37. **Riesbeck, K., J. Anderson, M. Gulberg, and A. Forsgren.** 1990. New 4-quinolones induce hyperproduction of interleukin-2. *Proc. Natl. Acad. Sci. USA* **86:**2809-2813.
38. **Riesbeck, K., and A. Forsgren.** 1990. Selective enhancement of synthesis of interleukin-2 in lymphocytes in the presence of ciprofloxacin. *Eur. J. Clin. Microbiol. Infect. Dis.* **9:**409-413.
39. **Roche, Y., M. Fay, and M. A. Gougerot-Pocidalo.** 1987. Effect of quinolones on IL-1 production in vitro by human monocytes. *Immunopathology* **13:**99-109.
40. **Roche, Y., M. Fay, and M. A. Gougerot-Pocidalo.** 1988. Enhancement of IL-2 production by quinolone-treated human mononuclear leucocytes. *Int. J. Immunopharmacol.* **10:**161-167.
41. **Roche, Y., M. A. Gougerot-Pocidalo, M. Fay, D. Etienne, N. Forest, and J. J. Pocidalo.** 1987. Comparative effects of quinolones on human mononuclear leucocyte functions. *J. Antimicrob. Chemother.* **19:**781-790.
42. **Shalit, I.** 1991. Immunological aspects of new quinolones. *Eur. J. Clin. Microbiol. Infect. Dis.* **17:**262-266.
43. **Somekh, E., B. Lev, E. Schwartz, A. Barzilai, and E. Rubinstein.** 1989. The effect of ciprofloxacin and pefloxacin on bone marrow engraftment in the spleen of mice. *J. Antimicrob. Chemother.* **23:**247-251.
44. **Somekh, E., S. West, A. Barzilai, and E. Rubinstein.** 1989. The lack of long term suppressive effect of ciprofloxacin on murine bone marrow. *J. Antimicrob. Chemother.* **24:**209-213.
45. **Starma, S. D., J. M. Hoffin, and J. S. Remington.** 1985. In-vivo recombinant IL-2 enhances survival against a lethal challenge with *Toxoplasma gondii*. *J. Immunol.* **135:**4160-4162.
46. **Steinbeck, M. J., and J. A. Roth.** 1989. Neutrophil activation by recombinant cytokines. *Rev. Infect. Dis.* **11:**549-568.
47. **Stünkel, K. G., G. Hewlett, and H.-J. Zeiler.** 1991. Ciprofloxacin enhances T-cell function by modulating interleukin activities. *Clin. Exp. Immunol.* **86:**525-531.
48. **Traub, W. H.** 1984. Intraphagocytic bactericidal activity of bacterial DNA gyrase inhibitors against *Serratia marcescens*. *Chemotherapy* (Basel) **30:**379-386.
49. **Tulkens, P. M.** 1991. Intracellular distribution and activity of antibiotics. *Eur. J. Clin. Microbiol. Infect. Dis.* **10:**100-106.
50. **Van Rensburg, C. E. J., G. Joone, and R. Anderson.** 1989. An in-vitro investigation of the intraphagocytic bioactivity of difloxacin, ciprofloxacin, pefloxacin and fleroxacin. *Chemotherapy* (Basel) **35:**273-277.
51. **Vilde, J. L., E. Dournon, and P. Rajagopalan.** 1986. Inhibition of *Legionella pneumophila* multiplication within human macrophages by antimicrobial agents. *Antimicrob. Agents Chemother.* **30:**743-748.
52. **Waage, A., A. Halstensen, and T. Espevilk.** 1987. Association between TNF in serum and fatal outcome in patients with meningococcal disease. *Lancet* **i:**355-357.
53. **Zehavi-Willner, T., and I. Shalit.** 1989. Enhancement of interleukin-2 production in human lymphocytes by two new quinolone derivatives. *Lymphokine Res.* **8:**35-46.

*Quinolone Antimicrobial Agents, 2nd ed.*
Edited by David C. Hooper and John S. Wolfson


*Chapter 29*

# Quinolone Antimicrobial Agents: Overview and Conclusions

***Robert C. Moellering, Jr.***

It has been over 30 years since the discovery of nalidixic acid, the first of the "quinolone" antimicrobial agents. Now, after the first generation of the quinolone era, it seems reasonable to take stock of the current status of these agents and look forward to the surprises and advances that the next generation of these drugs might bring. The first edition of this book was published 4 years ago and provided an outstanding summary of the state of the art at that time. Since then, a number of important events have taken place, and a great deal of clinical experience has been gained with these agents. This experience is reflected in the increased number of chapters and citations in the second edition of *Quinolone Antimicrobial Agents*. In addition to changes dealing specifically with the antimicrobial agents, the world has lost two individuals who made important contributions to this field. The first is George Lesher, who discovered the first quinolone, nalidixic acid, in the late 1950s. The "In Memoriam: George Y. Lesher" in this volume contains a brief summary of his contributions to quinolone chemistry and to pharmaceutical chemistry in general. The second loss occurred with the untimely death of one of the coeditors of the first edition of this book, John Wolfson, on 11 October 1991. In his brief career, Dr. Wolfson added significantly to our knowledge of the mechanism of action and resistance to the quinolones. A tribute to him is found in the "In Memoriam: John Stone Wolfson."

Clear-cut evidence of the advances that have been made in the past 4 years can be easily found in an examination of a number of subjects covered in chapters that were not included in the first edition of this book. Among these are new chapters on structure-activity relationships, quinolone-DNA interaction, quinolones and eukaryotic topoisomerases, effects of quinolones on the immune system, effects of quinolones on the central nervous system, and drug-drug interactions with the fluoroquinolone antimicrobial agents. The growing clinical importance of resistance to the quinolones is reflected in chapter 6, "Quinolone Resistance in Clinical Practice: Occurrence and Importance." Clinical topics not previously included in separate chapters include the role of quinolones in the treatment of chronic bacterial prostatitis; treatment of infections of the ears, nose, and throat and nasal carriage; treatment of bacterial meningitis; and veterinary use of quinolones. Many of the general comments that I made in the concluding chapter to the first edition of this book remain true. The newer fluoroquinolones continue to represent significant

***Robert C. Moellering, Jr.*** • Department of Medicine, New England Deaconess Hospital and Harvard Medical School, Boston, Massachusetts 02215.

advances compared with older compounds such as nalidixic acid, oxolinic acid, cinoxacin, pipemidic acid, and others. The broader spectra of activity of the newer compounds are clearly a major advantage, and the fact that single-step mutations to high-level resistance to these agents occur with much less frequency than they did with the older agents has prevented the development of wholesale resistance to these agents. Such resistance would undoubtedly have occurred if the newer compounds possessed the ability to select for single-step mutations leading to high-level resistance with frequencies in the range of $10^{-6}$ to $10^{-8}$, as was true for the older compounds. Nonetheless, emergence of resistance is proving to be a significant problem even with the newer agents. The mechanisms and clinical importance of this resistance are detailed in chapters 5 and 6. The development of resistance in gram-positive organisms has been particularly troublesome in some settings. Thus, in certain hospitals in the United States, the majority of methicillin-resistant staphylococci (especially methicillin-resistant *Staphylococcus aureus*) are now resistant to all of the currently available fluoroquinolones. Increasing resistance among non-methicillin-resistant strains is also being seen in some centers, as is resistance in *Streptococcus pneumoniae*. Enterococci also threaten to become rapidly resistant, eliminating even the marginal activity possessed by the currently available fluoroquinolones against these problematic nosocomial pathogens. Resistance to the fluoroquinolones has emerged in *Pseudomonas aeruginosa* somewhat more slowly than among the gram-positive organisms, but such resistance has major clinical consequences, since if it becomes more widespread, it will eliminate the most effective oral agents currently available for the treatment of urinary tract infections and skin and soft tissue infections due to this organism. Emergence of resistance among enteric pathogens (especially *Campylobacter jejuni*) is also very disturbing and will likely destroy one of the most attractive features of the fluoroquinolones for the treatment of bacterial diarrheas; namely, that when originally introduced, they included all known bacterial causes of diarrhea in their effective spectra of activity. Despite the rather gloomy news concerning the development of resistance to the fluoroquinolones associated with their widespread clinical use, one bright spot remains: as noted in chapter 5, there are still no confirmed reports of plasmid-mediated resistance to these agents. Although such resistance is possible, it fortunately has not yet surfaced as a clinically important problem.

Significant advances in the development of new fluoroquinolones have occurred during the past 4 years, aided largely by burgeoning knowledge of structure-activity relationships for this class of antimicrobial agents, as detailed in chapter 2. More than 10,000 quinolone analogs have now been described. These have enabled the pharmaceutical chemists to define a number of structure-activity relationships and to utilize these relationships (although knowledge is not perfect in this area) to synthesize compounds that fill in some of the gaps remaining in the spectra of activity and pharmacokinetics of the presently available fluoroquinolones. Thus, it is possible to produce compounds with markedly enhanced activities against gram-positive organisms and anaerobes in particular. A number of the newer drugs even have activity against ciprofloxacin-resistant strains. If they successfully complete their clinical trials, some of these compounds, such as sparfloxacin, WIN-57273, BAYy3118, and others outlined in Table q in chapter 2, should represent significant advances. However, a major note of caution must be sounded. It is clear that we are "approaching the point of diminishing returns, and successful structural novelty is desperately needed in the quinolone field." Thus, while the newer congeners may at least temporarily stave off the advance of quinolone-resistant organisms, it is unlikely that they will provide anything close to a final answer for this important problem.

From a pharmacokinetic point of view, the fluoroquinolones continue to exhibit very favorable characteristics, as detailed in chapters 9 through 12. They are exceedingly well absorbed when given by the oral route, and a number of them can be given both orally and parenterally. Their long half-lives in serum make them ideal for once-a-day or twice-a-day dosing regimens, and their pharmacokinetics are predictable enough to allow their safe utilization in patients with impaired hepatic and renal functions. Certain drug-drug interactions do occur: the clinician must be aware of the effects of metal ion-containing antacids on absorption when fluoroquinolones are given orally. Fortunately, food has little influence on the bioavailability of presently available compounds. Interference with theophylline metabolism is a particular problem with enoxacin and is seen with certain other compounds, as detailed in chapter 11, which also contains appropriate warnings that foods containing methylxanthines, such as coffee and tea, may enhance the central nervous system side effects of certain of the fluoroquinolones. For the most part, however, major drug-drug interactions (outside of those involving the antacids containing aluminum-magnesium salts or calcium carbonate) are relatively infrequent and not usually of major clinical significance.

In my overview of the first edition, I noted that "the new quinolones are generally exceedingly well tolerated, and in comparative trials to date, the overall rate of side effects seen with these agents has been equivalent to or lower than that seen with older drugs such as trimethoprim-sulfamethoxazole." It was also noted, however, that most of the data on toxicity obtained up to that point had been derived from clinical trials in which relatively low doses had been employed, and there was a possibility that with more-widespread use and dosage escalations, the incidence of dose-related toxic effects such as gastrointestinal intolerance, phototoxicity, and central nervous system irritability or seizures would increase. For the most part, those statements remain true, with one remarkable exception. Temafloxacin has been taken off the market because of an unexpected incidence of severe hemolytic anemia, thrombocytopenia, and renal failure (with or without hypoglycemia) that became obvious in postmarketing surveillance in the United States following clinical approval by the U.S. Food and Drug Administration. Although similar side effects probably occur with much lower frequencies for at least some of the other fluoroquinolones currently available, they occurred with sufficient frequency in patients receiving temafloxacin that the manufacturer of this drug voluntarily stopped marketing it. Thus, while the overall toxicity profiles of these agents remain very favorable, the possibility that agents currently available or under development could cause unexpected side effects remains real. For instance, a higher incidence of phototoxicity than expected has been seen in patients receiving lomefloxacin and will likely require some alteration in the data included in the package insert (at least in the United States) (1). This, too, emerged during postmarketing surveillance of the drug. Because of concerns related to the production of arthropathy in weight-bearing joints of experimental animals, the fluoroquinolones are still not approved for use in children. However, there is increasing experience with the use of ciprofloxacin and other quinolones in children with cystic fibrosis, and cautious trials are being undertaken with short courses of these drugs for diarrhea caused by multiresistant enteropathogens in children in certain developing countries. To date, no serious adverse effects have been discovered in children receiving these drugs. Nonetheless, careful surveillance is indicated before it can be finally proven that they are safe for use in children and adolescents. Reports on the mutagenicity of these drugs continue (5), which is not at all surprising because of their ability to interfere with DNA synthesis. Despite this, there is no need at present to change the statement I made 4 years ago that "despite the fact that there are conflicting data on mutagenicity in bacteria, the available evidence from studies with eukaryotic cells, animal studies, and clinical trials suggests that the potential for mutagenicity in humans is low" (9). The statement that "thus far there has likewise been no evidence of teratogenicity, but there are insufficient data available to permit the use of these drugs in pregnant women" also remains true.

During the past 4 years, the body of published data on clinical use of the fluoroquinolones has increased dramatically. Chapters 13 through 24 provide an extensive review of the useful and potentially useful clinical applications of these agents that were clearly defined in the earlier edition. In addition to the indications such as urinary tract infections, bacterial infections of the gastrointestinal tract, selected sexually transmitted diseases, and infections of the respiratory tract, bones, joints, skin, and soft tissues, we have accumulated further data on their potential uses for upper respiratory tract infections, eye infections, the immunocompromised host, and other settings.

As defined in chapter 13, the fluoroquinolones are firmly established as important agents for the treatment of complicated and uncomplicated urinary tract infections. They fare at least as well as if not better than the older, established agents such as trimethoprim, trimethoprim-sulfamethoxazole, penicillins, and cephalosporins. The fact that they achieve high and prolonged effective concentrations in urine and surrounding tissues in the urinary tract is in part responsible for their effectiveness, as is the fact that they are rapidly bactericidal against many common uropathogens (with the possible exception of *Enterococcus* spp.). In addition, they clearly work well in short-course (single-dose or 3-day) regimens for acute cystitis and uncomplicated urinary tract infections. Although they are highly effective for the treatment of uncomplicated cystitis, I agree with the recommendations made in chapter 13 that in order to prevent widespread emergence of resistance, it makes sense to reserve the fluoroquinolones for complicated urinary tract infections and cases of acute cystitis that are recurrent or caused by resistant microorganisms.

The treatment of bacterial prostatitis is made difficult because many antimicrobial agents do not penetrate well into prostatic tissue, and those that do (such as erythromycin) often have a spectrum of activity that does not include the major gram-negative pathogens responsible for this condition. The fluoroquinolones, on the other hand, not only penetrate well into prostatic tissue and are found in high concentrations in prostatic secretions but also have a spectrum of activity that includes virtually all of the major bacterial pathogens responsible for acute and chronic prostatitis. Thus, they theoretically are ideally suited for the treatment of such infections. Although studies available 4 years ago had suggested that the fluoroquinolones are effective in patients with acute prostatitis, I noted then that "we are in need of much more clinical information before the role of these compounds in the management of prostatitis can be optimally assessed." Chapter 14 of this edition provides a good overview of the current situation. The author defines the methodologic problems in measuring fluoroquinolone levels in prostatic tissue and secretions and provides a summary of the currently available clinical data. Chronic bacterial prostatitis is a particularly difficult entity to evaluate because in many cases the bacterial etiology is not clearly defined. However, on the basis of a small subsample of studies in which adequate bacteriology is available, it appears that therapeutic results with the fluoroquinolones are quite good in cases of chronic prostatitis due to *Escherichia coli* and other members of the family *Enterobacteriaceae* and that in these settings, a treatment duration of 1 month is sufficient. This is important information, since many clinicians routinely treat such patients for a much longer period. The results for the therapy of chronic prostatitis due to enterococci and *P. aeruginosa*, on the other hand, are less promising, and the ultimate role of the fluoroquinolones in these infections remains to be defined.

The fluoroquinolones exhibit outstanding in vitro activity against a number of important sexually transmitted pathogens, including the gonococcus, *Chlamydia trachomatis*, and *Haemophilus ducreyi*. Despite this, they fall short of being ideal agents for treating sexually transmitted diseases because they are not effective against incubating syphilis, they cannot safely be given to adolescents and pregnant women, and, although they work in single-dose therapy for gonorrhea, they do not work in single-dose therapy for genital chlamydial infections. Indeed, a number of these agents have been relatively ineffective in the last setting, even in prolonged dosing regimens, and the most effective drugs studied to date, ofloxacin and fleroxacin, must be given for 7 to 10 days in order to have efficacies equivalent to that of doxycycline for genital chlamydial infections. Although these agents may have utility in treating pelvic inflammatory disease and epididymitis, their ultimate role in these settings remains to be determined. They are not effective against bacterial vaginosis. Thus, their greatest utility appears to be in the treatment of gonorrhea, for which they are effective in single-dose therapy, and as alternative agents against chancroid, for which the data suggest that at least some of the agents with longer half-lives, such as fleroxacin, may be effective in single-dose regimens as well.

From a purely theoretical point of view, the fluoroquinolones should be outstanding agents for the treatment of bacterial diarrhea, and in fact they are. They achieve high concentrations in the gut lumen when given by the oral route, the currently available compounds do not significantly alter anaerobic fecal flora, and they have a spectrum of activity that includes virtually all known causes of bacterial diarrhea in humans. As resistance to trimethoprim-sulfamethoxazole becomes more prevalent in *Shigella* spp., *E. coli*, and other enteropathogens in many parts of the world, the fluoroquinolones are staking out an even more important role in this arena. Recent studies suggest that adjunctive therapy may enhance the effectiveness of the fluoroquinolones in the treatment of diarrhea. For example, the addition of loperamide to a fluoroquinolone (in this case ciprofloxacin) may further enhance the therapeutic efficacy of fluoroquinolone therapy for dysentery caused by *Shigella* spp. (8). It is particularly disturbing, therefore, to see the recent reports of resistance to fluoroquinolones in *C. jejuni*. If this trend continues (as seems highly likely), it will significantly limit the utility of these drugs against bacterial diarrhea, especially in those countries in the northern hemisphere where *C. jejuni* is a major cause of bacterial diarrhea. This fact should not be lost on those physicians who now routinely prescribe fluoroquinolones for "diarrhea of unknown origin." The use of fluoroquinolones to treat *Salmonella* gastroenteritis remains somewhat controversial. Although there are now data suggesting that these drugs are clinically effective for *Salmonella* gastroenteritis, the question of whether they prolong the carrier state remains to be answered definitively. Interestingly, several of these agents, including ciprofloxacin, norfloxacin, and pefloxacin, have been quite effective for the treatment of typhoid fever and, when given in sufficiently long courses of treatment, appear to effectively eradicate gastrointestinal carriage of *Salmonella typhi*. Their role, if any, in treating gastric infection due to *Helicobacter pylori* remains to be determined, but the data suggest a high rate of mutation to resistance among these organisms when they are exposed to the currently available fluoroquinolones alone.

As noted in chapter 17, the use of fluoroquinolones in the treatment of respiratory tract infections continues to engender controversy. These agents penetrate well into pulmonary tissues and secretions and include many important respiratory pathogens in their spectra of activity. However, the effectiveness of the currently available agents against gram-positive respiratory pathogens, particularly *S. pneumoniae*, is less than optimal. Of all of the currently available compounds, ofloxacin appears to have the highest degree of efficacy against infections due to *S. pneumoniae*, but as noted earlier, none of the compounds is ideal. The demise of temafloxacin was unfortunate from many points of view, but perhaps none more so than the fact that it had been studied very well in respiratory tract infections and had demonstrated efficacy for community-acquired pneumonia. Indeed, the major clinical trial of this drug stands as an example of excellence for all future clinical trials of antimicrobial agents in lower respiratory tract infections (3). In general, the fluoroquinolones have outstanding activity against *Haemophilus influenzae, Moraxella (Branhamella) catarrhalis, Mycoplasma pneumoniae, Chlamydia pneumoniae*, and *Legionella* spp. Definitive proof of their clinical effectiveness in mycoplasmal infections is limited primarily by the difficulties in identifying this pathogen in most studies. The limited data available thus far suggest that pefloxacin, ciprofloxacin, and ofloxacin are likely to be effective in treating infections due to *Legionella pneumophila*, although an occasional failure has been reported. Thus, unfortunately, we still do not have enough data to define the ultimate role of the fluoroquinolones in treating legionellosis. Ciprofloxacin has been effective in patients with cystic fibrosis, but its prolonged use here is clearly limited by the development of resistance in *P. aeruginosa* and other gram-negative pathogens that are responsible for infections in patients with cystic fibrosis. Although these agents have considerable efficacy against mycobacteria in vitro, further data are necessary to define their ultimate role in the treatment of tuberculosis and infections due to other mycobacteria. From the data thus far available, however, it is clear that they cannot be used alone in the treatment of any infections due to these organisms.

The lack of outstanding activity against streptococci (especially *S. pneumoniae*) has limited the utility of the presently available fluoroquinolones for the treatment of infections of the ears, nose, and throat, as is well detailed in chapter 18. These drugs should not be used to treat acute pharyngitis or sinusitis unless one is absolutely certain that the pathogen is highly susceptible (which rarely occurs in the clinical setting). This being said, there are several settings in which the fluoroquinolones have shown some utility. The most important is in the treatment of malignant otitis externa. The authors of chapter 18 correctly point out, however, that this condition may be overdiagnosed, and some of the reported "cures" of this condition in the literature were probably of patients who did not have true malignant otitis externa. Nonetheless, the effectiveness of ciprofloxacin in treating this condition (especially if the drug is combined with appropriate surgical debridement) is impressive. While the fluoroquinolones have failed miserably in eradicating *S. aureus* in nasal carriers, these agents (especially ciprofloxacin) are quite effective for meningococcal carriers, and they may be useful as alternatives to rifampin in this setting.

The efficacy of the fluoroquinolones for the treatment of osteomyelitis and septic arthritis and for the therapy of skin and soft tissue infections is detailed in chapters 19 and 22. In both settings, the new fluoroquinolones have selectively demonstrated outstanding efficacy. For example, the facts that the new agents can be given orally and have outstanding activities against a variety of gram-negative organisms make them nearly ideal agents for the treatment of acute and, especially, chronic gram-negative bacillary osteomyelitis. The continued emergence of resistance to the fluoroquinolones in *S. aureus* and especially the striking progress of fluoroquinolone resistance among methicillin-resistant staphylococci makes the use of these agents for the treatment of infections of bones and joints and of infections of skin and soft tissues due to staphylococci, which are the leading cause of infections in these areas, somewhat problematic. The possible addition of rifampin may limit the emergence of resistance during therapy of staphylococcal infections but will do nothing for those organisms that are primarily fluoroquinolone resistant. In this regard, it is a bit disappointing that there still is no definitive proof of the value of adding rifampin to fluoroquinolones for the therapy of staphylococcal infections. Although comparative trials have shown that several of the fluoroquinolones are effective in the therapy of skin and soft tissue infections, it is hard to consider them drugs of first choice, given the alternatives available and the problems with resistant gram-positive organisms alluded to above. Nonetheless, the facts that these agents can be given orally and have high potency against susceptible organisms make them worthy of consideration in carefully selected cases. One potentially valuable use of the fluoroquinolones that was not covered in detail in these chapters is in the outpatient treatment of diabetic foot infections. Coupled with appropriate surgical management, these agents are likely to be quite useful for these infections, and clinical data already attest to their effectiveness in this area (2). The necessity of adding an agent such as metronidazole or clindamycin, with activity against anaerobes, remains to be determined.

The role of the fluoroquinolones in the treatment of bacterial meningitis and endocarditis is a limited one at best. Chapters 20 and 21 provide extensive data on the use of the fluoroquinolones in animal models of meningitis and endocarditis. On the basis of these studies and the limited data from human trials, it appears that the fluoroquinolones may be useful in selected cases of gram-negative meningitis (especially those caused by *P. aeruginosa* and *S. typhi*) and in some cases of endocarditis due to *P. aeruginosa*. The use of an oral regimen consisting of ciprofloxacin plus rifampin for the treatment of right-sided endocarditis in addicts infected with *S. aureus* represents an interesting potential application. However, until a multicenter comparative trial is completed, one cannot routinely recommend this regimen. Of concern is the previously mentioned prevalence of resistance to *S. aureus* and the fact that drug addicts are notoriously unreliable when it comes to taking prolonged (even 2-week) courses of oral medication. The possible role of fluoroquinolones in the treatment of Q fever endocarditis remains to be elucidated.

The penetration of the fluoroquinolones into the vitreous humor of the eye is better than that of most antimicrobial agents used in the treatment of eye infections. Thus, there is a potential for using these agents in the treatment of selected cases of endophthalmitis, as noted in chapter 23. Unfortunately, there are insufficient clinical data available at present to suggest that systemic fluoroquinolone therapy should replace standard direct intravitreal injection of agents such as vancomycin or aminoglycosides for initial therapy of bacterial endophthalmitis. Topical preparations of the fluoroquinolones show considerable promise in the treatment of external ocular infections but have not been proven superior to other topical agents in this setting.

Current information concerning the use of fluoroquinolones in the treatment of bacterial infections of immunocompromised patients is provided in chapter 24. While the use of antimicrobial agents to prevent infections in granulocytopenic patients remains controversial, data currently available clearly show the effectiveness of fluoroquinolones in preventing infections due to gram-negative bacteria in this setting. Often, however, this advantage is offset by an increase in infections due to gram-positive organisms, many of which (e.g., *Staphylococcus epidermidis*) can be argued to be "less virulent" than the gram-negative infections they replace. Although major emergence of resistance among gram-negative bacterial pathogens in this setting has yet to be documented, it remains a major concern.

When used alone, parenteral fluoroquinolones may be less effective than combination therapy in the treatment of febrile neutropenic patients (6). Combining fluoroquinolones with a ureidopenicillin seems to obviate this disadvantage. As noted previously, the fluoroquinolones may be useful for the treatment of legionella infections in immunocompromised patients and, in combination with other agents, will likely play a role in the treatment of infections due to the *Mycobacterium avium* complex in these patients.

Chapter 25 discusses veterinary use of the quinolones. It points out that there is extensive extralabel use of fluoroquinolones approved for human use in a number of veterinary applications, especially for treating feline and canine infections. It should be of interest to physicians that there are fluoroquinolones such as enrofloxacin and danofloxacin that have been developed solely for veterinary use. Enrofloxacin shares many structural similarities (including the N-1 cyclopropyl moiety) with ciprofloxacin and is metabolized to ciprofloxacin in animals. Given these facts, there is reason to worry that its widespread use for veterinary applications is likely to select out organisms resistant to the fluoroquinolones approved for human use. Given the extensive data now available on the propensity of other antimicrobial agents to select for resistant pathogens in animals (which can subsequently be spread to humans) (7), one hopes that veterinarians and farmers will be circumspect in their application of these agents. Of even greater concern is the use of enrofloxacin and agents such as nalidixic acid, norfloxacin, and ciprofloxacin as feed additives, as documented in chapter 25.

It is clear from reading this book that there has been considerable progress in the development of new fluoroquinolones and in the clinical evaluation of those already approved for human (and animal) use during the past 4 years. It seems, however, that the "golden age" of discovery in this area may have passed unless new and unexpected breakthroughs in our understanding of structure-activity relationships are realized. Novel approaches, such as the development of "quinalactams," in which quinolones are chemically linked with ß-lactams (4), are of interest, but thus far the potential clinical value of these compounds, if any, remains to be determined. Nonetheless, this is an area that clearly warrants further investigation and for which more information will be forthcoming. The greatest threat to the fluoroquinolones is still bacterial resistance. Although resistance to these compounds has developed relatively slowly, especially considering the extensive use they have enjoyed during the past 4 years, we are in danger of losing certain organisms from the effective spectra of these drugs. In many parts of the world, the majority of methicillin-resistant staphylococci are already resistant to fluoroquinolones, and some of these strains are resistant to even the newest agents under development. The development of resistance among enterococci, *P. aeruginosa, C. jejuni,* and *Helicobacter pylori* is also of concern, although for obvious reasons, the clinical importance of resistance among the aforementioned agents differs greatly from one to the other.

I ended my summary of the first edition of this book with the following paragraph: "In summary, the new quinolones represent a major advance in the chemotherapy of infectious diseases. Unfortunately, these compounds also have a great potential for overuse and misuse, which, in turn, may result in the emergence of resistance among a number of the organisms currently susceptible to the quinolones. Therefore, the future viability of the quinolones will in large part depend on the ability of the medical community to use them wisely." Nothing that has occurred in the past 4 years alters the truth in that paragraph. As exciting as the new fluoroquinolones are, they are far from invulnerable.

## REFERENCES

1. **Anonymous.** 1993. Searle *Maxaquin* "Dear Prescriber" letter on phototoxicity letter should be sent,

FDA Advisory Committee urges; group is split on "black box" warning. *F-D-C Rep.* **55**:16–17.

2. **Beam, T. R., Jr., I. Gutierrez, S. Powell, R. Hewitt, M. Hocko, and M. Brackett.** 1989. Prospective study of the efficacy and safety of oral and intravenous ciprofloxacin in the treatment of diabetic foot infections. *Rev. Infect. Dis.* **11**(Suppl. 5): S1163.
3. **Carbon, C., P. Leophonte, P. Petitpretz, J. P. Chauvin, and J. Hazebroucq.** 1992. Efficacy and safety of temofloxacin versus those of amoxacillin in hospitalized adults with community-acquired pneumonia. *Antimicrob. Agents Chemother.* **36**:833–839.
4. **Georgopapadakou, N. H., and A. Bertasso.** 1993. Mechanisms of action of cephalosporin 3′-quinolone esters, carbamates, and tertiary amines in *Escherichia coli. Antimicrob. Agents Chemother.* **37**:559–565.
5. **Mamber, S. W., B. Kolek, K. W. Brookshire, D. P. Bonner, and J. Fung-Tomc.** 1993. Activity of quinolones in the Ames *Salmonella* TA102 mutagenicity test and other bacterial genotoxicity assays. *Antimicrob. Agents Chemother.* **37**:213–217.
6. **Meunier, F., S. H. Zinner, H. Gaya, T. Calandara, C. Viscoli, J. Klastersky, M. Glauser, and the European Organization for Research on Treatment of Cancer International Antimicrobial Therapy Cooperative Group.** 1991. Prospective randomized evaluation of ciprofloxacin versus piperacillin plus amikacin for empiric antibiotic therapy of febrile granulocytopenic cancer patients with lymphomas and solid tumors. *Antimicrob. Agents Chemother.* **35**:873–878.
7. **Moellering, R. C., Jr.** 1990. Interaction between antimicrobial consumption and selection of resistant bacterial strains. *Scand. J. Infect. Dis.* **70** (Suppl.):18–24.
8. **Murphy, G. S., L. Bodhidatta, P. Echeverria, S. Tansuphaswadikul, C. W. Hoge, S. Imlarp, and K. Tamura.** 1993. Ciprofloxacin and loperamide in the treatment of bacillary dysentery. *Ann. Intern. Med.* **118**:582–586.
9. **Phillips, I.** 1987. Bacterial mutagenicity and the 4-quinolones. *J. Antimicrob. Chemother.* **20**:771–773.

# Index